RETAVASE™
Reteplase recombinant

FROM THE LIBRARY OF
PATRICK J. HOGAN
2121 ADDISON
HOUSTON, TEXAS 77030

ACUTE CORONARY SYNDROMES

Compliments of

Centocor

RP-99043

ACUTE CORONARY SYNDROMES

SECOND EDITION
REVISED AND EXPANDED

edited by

ERIC J. TOPOL

The Cleveland Clinic Foundation
Cleveland, Ohio

MARCEL DEKKER, INC. NEW YORK • BASEL

ISBN: 0-8247-0416-9

This book is printed on acid-free paper.

Headquarters
Marcel Dekker, Inc.
270 Madison Avenue, New York, NY 10016
tel: 212-696-9000; fax: 212-685-4540

Eastern Hemisphere Distribution
Marcel Dekker AG
Hutgasse 4, Postfach 812, CH-4001 Basel, Switzerland
tel: 41-61-261-8482; fax: 41-61-261-8896

World Wide Web
http://www.dekker.com

The publisher offers discounts on this book when ordered in bulk quantities. For more information, write to Special Sales/Professional Marketing at the headquarters address above.

Current printing (last digit):
10 9 8 7 6 5 4 3 2 1

PRINTED IN THE UNITED STATES OF AMERICA

Preface to the Second Edition

It is remarkable how the field has evolved in the short timeframe since the first edition of this book was published in 1998—in fact, so much progress that we accelerated the schedule of this edition. The advances include a much better understanding of the pathophysiology, especially the underpinning of inflammation and embolization, and new therapeutics including intravenous antiplatelet agents (tirofiban and eptifibatide), oral antiplatelet agents (clopidogrel), and anticoagulants (low-molecular-weight heparins).

The extent of newness in choices of therapeutic strategies has led to another term for ACS instead of acute coronary syndromes, taken from the neurologists: "acute confusional state." That is, we are still left with uncertainty as to which of the new agents to use in individual patients, whether the invasive or conservative strategy of angiography and revascularization is preferable, and many other aspects of patient management. Even the term acute coronary syndromes is used quite liberally and at times inappropriately, as it was intended to refer to the whole gamut of clinical scenarios between unstable angina, non-ST-elevation myocardial infarction (formerly non-Q MI), and classic ST-segment elevation MI.

In the second edition of this monograph, there has been a significant expansion of the coverage, with new chapters dealing with inflammation, embolization, combined fibrin and platelet-lysis for MI, the invasive and conservative management strategies, new oral antiplatelet agents, bedside platelet function testing, aspirin resistance, and cost-effectiveness. The intent is to provide a state-of-the-art, comprehensive approach to the pathophysiology, new diagnostic modalities, therapeutic options, and public health implications for the diverse array of acute coronary syndromes.

Much of the groundwork for this edition has been laid by intensive basic and clinical investigation that has rapidly transformed our knowledge base. Recognition of aspirin resistance was almost unheard of until a few years ago, even though this therapeutic was introduced in 1897! Improvements over heparin with the low-molecular-weight heparins took from 1916 until just the past couple of years. It is quite likely that our whole approach to myocardial reperfusion will be revamped with the promise of combined red and white clot lysis.

Many of the leading investigators of the field have contributed to this project and I remain deeply indebted for their willingness to lend their insights and expertise to this new edition. In the 28 chapters, 45 authors from around the world have come together to refine the only dedicated book that exists in the field. As the Editor, I am deeply thankful to all the authors for their timely submission of high-quality manuscripts that assured the fine makeup of this monograph, and to the production team at Marcel Dekker, Inc., for their supportive effort. In particular, I would like to acknowledge the Managing Editor, Ms. Donna Wasiewicz-Bressan at the Cleveland Clinic Foundation. We hope that this book will serve as a useful resource for all clinicians, including cardiologists, internists, nurses, and paraprofessional staff, who are engaged in caring for patients with acute coronary syndromes. If the book promotes better understanding and care of these patients, we have again achieved our primary objective.

Eric J. Topol

Contents

Contributors

John H. Alexander, M.D. Assistant Professor, Division of Cardiology, Department of Medicine, Duke University Medical Center, Durham, North Carolina

Eric R. Bates, M.D. Professor of Medicine and Director, Cardiac Catheterization Laboratory, Division of Cardiology, Department of Internal Medicine, University of Michigan, Ann Arbor, Michigan

Kevin J. Beatt, Ph.D., F.R.C.P., F.E.B.C., F.A.C.C. Imperial College Medical School and Cardiac Catheter Laboratory, Department of Cardiology, Hammersmith Hospital, London, England

Richard C. Becker, M.D. Professor of Medicine; Director, Coronary Care Unit; Director, Cardiovascular Thrombosis Research Center; and Director, Anticoagulation Services, Department of Cardiology, University of Massachusettts Medical School, Worcester, Massachusetts

Peter B. Berger, M.D. Division of Cardiovascular Diseases, Mayo Clinic, Rochester, Minnesota

Deepak L. Bhatt, M.D. Department of Cardiology, The Cleveland Clinic Foundation, Cleveland, Ohio

Andra L. Blomkalns, M.D. Chief Resident, Department of Emergency Medicine, University of Cincinnati College of Medicine, Cincinnati, Ohio

Sorin J. Brener, M.D. Interventional Cardiologist, Department of Cardiology, The Cleveland Clinic Foundation, and Assistant Professor, Department of Medicine, Ohio State University, Cleveland, Ohio

Robert H. Christenson, Ph.D. Professor, Department of Pathology and Department of Medical and Research Technology, University of Maryland School of Medicine, and Director, Rapid Response and Clinical Chemistry Laboratories, Department of Clinical Pathology, University of Maryland Medical Center, Baltimore, Maryland

Eric L. Eisenstein, D.B.A. Assistant Research Professor, Duke Clinical Research Institute and Duke University Medical Center, Durham, North Carolina

Erling Falk, M.D., D.Sci. Department of Cardiology, Skejby University Hospital and Aarhus University, Aarhus, Denmark

Ole Frøbert, M.D., Ph.D Department of Cardiology, Skejby University Hospital and Aarhus University, Aarhus, Denmark

Peter Ganz, M.D. Cardiovascular Division, Department of Medicine, Brigham and Women's Hospital and Harvard Medical School, Boston, Massachusetts

John P. Gassler, M.D. Fellow, Department of Cardiology, The Cleveland Clinic Foundation, Cleveland, Ohio

W. Brian Gibler, M.D. Richard C. Levy Professor of Emergency Medicine and Chairman, Department of Emergency Medicine, University of Cincinnati College of Medicine, and Director, Center for Emergency Care, University of Cincinnati Hospital, Cincinnati, Ohio

Christopher B. Granger, M.D. Assistant Professor, Department of Medicine, and Director, Cardiac Care Unit, Duke University Medical Center, Durham, North Carolina

James G. Jollis, M.D. Associate Professor, Division of Cardiology, Department of Medicine, Duke University Medical Center and Duke Clinical Research Institute, Durham, North Carolina

Claus S. Jørgensen, M.D., Ph.D. Institute of Experimental Clinical Researach, Skejby University Hospital and Aarhus University, Aarhus, Denmark

David E. Kandzari, M.D. Fellow, Division of Cardiology, Department of Medicine, Duke University Medical Center and Duke Clinical Research Institute, Durham, North Carolina

Samir R. Kapadia, M.D.* Department of Cardiology, The Cleveland Clinic Foundation, Cleveland, Ohio

Philippe L. L'Allier, M.D.† Department of Cardiology, The Cleveland Clinic Foundation, Cleveland, Ohio

Richard T. Lee, M.D. Cardiovascular Division, Department of Medicine, Brigham and Women's Hospital and Harvard Medical School, Boston, Massachusetts

Jeffrey Lefkovits, M.B.B.S Department of Cardiology, The Royal Melbourne Hospital, Melbourne, Australia

Peter Libby, M.D. Chief, Cardiovascular Medicine, Brigham and Women's Hospital and Harvard Medical School, Boston, Massachusetts

A. Michael Lincoff, M.D. Director, Experimental Interventional Laboratory, Department of Cardiology, The Cleveland Clinic Foundation, Cleveland, Ohio

Daniel B. Mark, M.D., M.P.H. Professor of Medicine; Co-Director, Cardiac Care Unit; and Director, Outcomes Research and Assessment Group, Duke Clinical Research Institute and Duke University Medical Center, Durham, North Carolina

David J. Moliterno, M.D. Associate Professor of Medicine, Department of Cardiology, The Cleveland Clinic Foundation, Cleveland, Ohio

Debabrata Mukherjee, M.D. Department of Cardiology, The Cleveland Clinic Foundation, Cleveland, Ohio

K.-L. Neuhaus, Prof. Dr. Med Chief, Medizinische Klinik II, Klinikum Kassel, Kassel, Germany

---

Current affiliations
*Assistant Professor, Department of Medicine, University of Washington, Seattle, Washington.
†Assistant Professor, McGill University and Montreal Heart Institute, Montreal, Quebec, Canada.

L. Kristin Newby, M.D. Assistant Professor, Division of Cardiology, Department of Medicine, Duke University Medical Center and Duke Clinical Research Institute, Durham, North Carolina

Steven E. Nissen, M.D. Vice Chairman, Department of Cardiology, The Cleveland Clinic Foundation, Cleveland, Ohio

E. Magnus Ohman, M.D. Associate Professor, Division of Cardiology, Department of Medicine, Duke University Medical Center, and Coordinator, Interventional Trials (Cardiology), Duke Clinical Research Institute, Durham, North Carolina

Vasant Patel, M.D. Department of Cardiology, The Cleveland Clinic Foundation, Cleveland, Ohio

A. Thomas Pezzella, M.D. Associate Professor, Division of Cardiothoracic Surgery, Department of Surgery, University of Massachusetts Medical School, Worcester, Massachusetts

Louise Pilote, M.D., M.P.H., Ph.D. Assistant Professor of Medicine, Divisions of Internal Medicine and Clinical Epidemiology, McGill University Health Centre, Montreal, Quebec, Canada

Mark Robbins, M.D. Department of Cardiology, The Cleveland Clinic Foundation, Cleveland, Ohio

Frederick J. Schoen, M.D., Ph.D. Department of Pathology, Brigham Women's Hospital and Harvard Medical School, Boston, Massachusetts

Mitchell J. Silver, D.O. Staff, Departments of Cardiology and Vascular Medicine, The Cleveland Clinic Foundation, Cleveland, Ohio

Steven R. Steinhubl, M.D. Director, Cardiovascular Research, and Director, Cardiac Catheterization Laboratory, Department of Cardiology, Wilford Hall Medical Center, San Antonio, Texas

Eric J. Topol, M.D. Chairman and Professor, Department of Cardiology, and Director, Joseph J. Jacobs Center for Thrombosis and Vascular Biology, The Cleveland Clinic Foundation, Cleveland, Ohio

E. Murat Tuzcu, M.D. Interventional Cardiologist, Department of Cardiology, The Cleveland Clinic Foundation, Cleveland, Ohio

Steven Vanderschueren, M.D., Ph.D. Center for Molecular and Vascular Biology and Department of General Internal Medicine, Gasthuisberg University Hospital and University of Leuven, Leuven, Belgium

Frans Van de Werf, M.D., Ph.D. Professor of Medicine and Chairman, Department of Cardiology, Gasthuisberg University Hospital and University of Leuven, Leuven, Belgium

Robert A. Vogel, M.D. Herbert Berger Professor of Medicine; Head, Division of Cardiology; Co-Director, Center for Vascular Biology and Hypertension; and Associate Chairman of Medicine for Clinical Affairs, University of Maryland School of Medicine, Baltimore, Maryland

A. Vogt, Prof. Dr. Med. Medizinische Klinik II, Klinikum Kassel, Kassel, Germany

1

Inflammation in Acute Coronary Syndromes

Mark Robbins and Eric J. Topol
The Cleveland Clinic Foundation
Cleveland, Ohio

INTRODUCTION

The late Russell Ross's assertion that atherosclerosis is an inflammatory disease is now strongly supported by clinical, basic, and pathological research calling for an evolution in thought concerning the evaluation and treatment of acute coronary syndromes (ACS) (1–5). The initial insult is endothelial injury and subsequent dysfunction via the deleterious effects of the known cardiac risk factors such as oxidized LDL, infection, hyperglycemia, hypertension, hyperhomocystenemia, or smoking. Irrespective of the cause of endothelial damage, the resultant activation and proliferation of inflammatory cells, smooth muscle cells, generation of cytokines, growth factors, and many other substances lead to the progression of atherosclerosis. The presence and degree of inflammation and procoagulant state, defined by elevated CRP, fibrinogen, interleukin (IL)-1, IL-6, TNF-α, adhesion molecules, plasminogen activator inhibitor (PAI-1), tissue factor, and composition of the atherosclerotic plaque have been strongly associated with an increased risk of future cardiac events (6–9). Thus, the perpetuation of the inflammatory response likely plays a pivotal role in the pathobiology and vulnerability of the atherosclerotic plaque.

PATHOBIOLOGY OF INFLAMMATION, ATHEROSCLEROSIS, AND ACS

Endothelial Function

The endothelium lies in a critical location between the remaining vascular wall and the circulating blood thereby functioning as the pivotal barrier that protects the arterial wall from injury. This critical monolayer of cells is pluripotential, carrying out the following functions; 1) provision of a non-thrombotic surface; 2) maintenance of vascular tone through the production and release of nitric oxide (NO), prostacyclin, and endothelin; 3) regulation of growth factors and cytokines; 4) provision of a nonadherent surface for leukocytes and platelets; and 5) the modification of lipoproteins as they transverse its permeable barrier (5). Injury to this monolayer plays a key role in the initiation and progression of the atherosclerotic lesion by increasing adhesive cell surface glycoproteins such as vascular cell adhesion molecule-1 (VCAM-1) and intracellular adhesion molecule (ICAM), adherence, migration, and activation of leukocytes, and smooth muscle cells, production of cytokines, chemokines, and growth factors, as well as the reversal from an antithrombotic to a prothrombotic state (4,10–12).

Adhesion Molecules

Cell-cell interactions are a vital component in the pathogenesis of inflammation. Collectively known as cell adhesion molecules, three distinct families exist—the selectins, the integrins, and the immunoglobulin superfamily each with its own specific role in the inflammatory process. The process entails tethering and rolling of leukocytes on the activated endothelium, leukocyte activation, and ultimately firm adhesion and transendothelial migration along a chemotactic gradient generated by mediators of inflammation (13,14).

Selectins are expressed on the cell surface of leukocytes (L-selectin), platelets (P-selectin), and endothelial cells (E-selectin). Upon activation from inflammatory cytokines, mainly TNF-α and IL-1, cell surface expression of each selectin is enhanced (15–17). This process is vital in the early phase of inflammation mediating leukocyte recruitment and transient endothelial cell to leukocyte interactions (tethering and rolling phase). The subsequent steps of firm adhesion and migration of leukocytes is predominantly mediated through the interaction of integrins [leukocyte function associated antigen-1 (LAF-1), macrophage antigen-1 (MAC-1), very late activation antigen-4 (VLA-4) and GPIIb/IIIa receptor], the immunoglobulin superfamily [vascular cell adhesion molecule-1 (VCAM-1), intercellular adhesion molecule-1 (ICAM-1) and intercellular adhesion molecule-2 (ICAM-2)] and potent stimulation by inflammatory cytokines including IL-1, IL-4, IL-8, TNF-α, INF-γ, and chemokines such as chemotactic protein-1 (13,14). In addition to the cell adhesion molecules on endothelial cells, leukocytes, and platelets, ICAM-1 and VCAM-1 are expressed on smooth muscle cells (18). The interaction between leukocytes and smooth muscle cells contributes to smooth muscle cell migration and proliferation, cellular composition of the atherosclerotic plaque, and an increased expression of monocyte tissue factor mRNA, all of which are likely to be vital in influencing plaque stability (18,19). An additional component that ties inflammation and the prothrombotic state involves the adhesion of activated platelets to the endothelium through the P-selectin-GPIIb/IIIa receptor interactions with subsequent platelet aggregation and thrombus formation (20).

Growing evidence supports that the presence of increased cell adhesion molecules in serum or vascular tissue may reflect ongoing active vascular remodeling due to persistent inflammation. Elevated serum levels of the soluble form of the VCAM-1 receptor (sVCAM-1) has been associated with the extent of atherosclerosis in patients with peripheral vascular disease (21). In patients with coronary artery disease, elevated levels of the soluble ICAM-1 (sICAM-1) has been found to be inversely proportional to HDL levels and associated with the presence of other coronary risk factors, unstable angina, myocardial infarction, and importantly to increased risk of future myocardial infarction in apparently healthy men (22,23). Interestingly, immunohistochemical evaluation of coronary athrectomy tissue has shown P-selectin but not E-selectin, or ICAM-1 was expressed significantly greater in the setting of unstable angina versus stable angina (24). This reflects an augmented response between an endothelial cell adhesion molecule and the activated platelet linking thrombus formation and unstable coronary syndromes.

Treatment strategies available based on the inhibition of cell to cell interactions have shown promise in the treatment of chronic inflammatory diseases, and recently coronary artery disease (13,25). This should not be surprising given the marked similarities that exist between the pathophysiology of inflammatory diseases, such as rheumatoid arthritis, and atherosclerosis (Table 1). ASA and other NSAIDS affect the expression and function of cell adhesion molecules, and have been shown to inhibit many phases of the adhesion cascade (18). Direct antagonism via monoclonal antibodies and selectin-blocking agents against ICAM-1 and L-selectin has been shown to reduce neutrophil accumulation and myocardial injury in experimental animal studies (26,27). New approaches using antisense oligonucleotides to inhibit mRNA translation for cell adhesion molecule expression, and inhibition of gene expression by synthetic DNA molecules and triplex-forming oligonucleotides have shown conceptual promise in animal studies (13).

Table 1 Similarities Between Atherosclerosis and Rheumatoid Arthritis

	Atherosclerosis	Rheumatoid arthritis
Macrophage activation		
TNF-α	↑	↑
Metalloproteinases	↑	↑
Interleukin-6	UA ↑	↑
Mast cell activation	↑	↑
T-cell activation		
CD+DR+	UA ↑	↑
CD4+CD28−/INF+	UA ↑	↑
TH1/TH2 balance	TH1 ↑	TH1 ↑
B-cell activation	0 or ↑	0 or ↑
CRP	↑	↑↑
Adhesion molecules	↑	↑
Endothelin	↑	↑
Neoangiogenesis	↑	↑

Source: Modified from Ref. 153.

CELLULAR AND HUMORAL MEDIATED RESPONSE

Monocytes and Macrophages

Monocytes, the circulating precursors of tissue macrophages, are essential in the progression of atherosclerosis and are found in all stages of atherosclerotic lesions (4,28). Their recruitment and infiltration through the endothelium into the intima are tightly coupled to the humoral activity of the T-lymphocyte. The colocalization of CD4+ T-cells and macrophages and the abundant expression of HLA II molecules in atherosclerotic lesions is strong evidence for the role of cell-mediated immunity in the development and progression of atherosclerosis. Population size of CD14dimCD16a+ peripheral blood monocytes has been shown to correlate with degree of hypercholesterolemia and is dramatically reduced with lipid lowering therapy (29). This phenotypic expression, in contrast to other phenotypes of monocytes, is shown to express high levels of inflammatory cytokines such as TNF-α whereas the anti-inflammatory IL-10 is low or absent. In addition, these cells are further characterized by an upregulation of cell surface adhesion molecules, suggesting an increased capacity for cell to cell interactions (30).

The degree of macrophage infiltration has been shown to distinguish between unstable and stable coronary lesions. The preferential localization of macrophages in high-flow shoulder regions of the atherosclerotic plaque correlates with areas at highest risk for plaque instability. In contrast to controls, infiltrates of CD68-positive macrophages and CD3- and CD8-positive T-cells were statistically associated with the severity and frequency of superficial plaque inflammation and rupture (31–33). This plaque instability, in part, stems from metalloproteinase (MMP-1and MMP-2) production and release by activated macrophages within the inflamed atherosclerotic plaque (34).

T-Lymphocyte

Antigen-presenting macrophages induced T-cell activation and results in inflammatory amplification through T-cell release of TNF-α, and INF-γ, further activating macrophages, platelets, and smooth muscle cells (35). Levels of the main specific immune markers CD4+ and CD3+/DR+ T-cells, IL-2, and IgM have all been reported to be higher in unstable than in stable angina patients (36). In addition, a higher percentage of IL-2 receptor positive T-lymphocytes in culprit lesions of patients with acute coronary syndromes indicate recent activation and amplification of the immune response within plaques. These findings support the concept that a burst of inflammatory products could initiate or accelerate the onset of an acute coronary event (37).

Mast Cell

Mast cells have been recently identified to inhabit the vulnerable shoulder regions of the atherosclerotic plaque and to be associated with plaque erosion and rupture (38,39). The population size of mast cell in athrectomy tissue correlates with the clinical severity of coronary syndromes. Their presence in the adventitia of ruptured plaques has led to the postulate that histamine release may provoke coronary spasm and contributes to the onset of myocardial infarction (40,41). Mast cells have a primary role in the perpetuation of the inflammatory response in atherosclerosis, characterized by the production of TNF-α and neutral proteases (tryptase and chymase) (42,43). TNF-α stimulates macrophages and smooth muscle cells to produce two prometalloproteinases-prostomelysin and procollagenase. Subsequent activation of prometalloproteinases by mast cell produced tryptase and chymase leads to fibrous cap degradation and plaque destabilization (44).

Neutrophil

As previously discussed, macrophages and T lymphocytes are the predominant cellular components of local inflammation within the atherosclerotic plaque. Neutrophils, although found sparsely in atherosclerotic plaques, play an integral part in the acute inflammatory response to tissue injury and have been implicated as a major factor in tissue damage in response to ischemia and reperfusion (45). TNF-α, IL-8, IL-6, platelet-activating factor, and leukotrienes enhance neutrophil recruitment to ischemic and reperfused myocardium by augmenting cell adhesion molecule expression. The extent of accumulation has also been correlated to the degree of tissue injury (46,47). A systemic activation of neutrophils has been reported in patients with angiographically documented coronary artery disease as compared with normal controls and a subset of trauma patients providing further proof for a chronic systemic inflammatory state in patients with atherosclerosis (48).

Platelet

Traditionally, platelets have not been classified as inflammatory cells, but recent discoveries have led investigators to believe that platelets are critical constituents that tie in both inflammation and thrombosis. The presence of serologic markers of platelet activation is well established in the setting of an ACS (49–51). Inflammatory cytokines induce the translocation of the cell adhesion molecule P-selectin to the surface of the platelet membrane, facilitating interactions among platelets, endothelial cells, and monocytes. Monocyte expression of tissue factor is induced by P-selectin and may be an initiator of thrombosis in areas of vascular injury (52).

An initial step to answer the question of whether platelet activation is a result of or results in the development of an ACS was recently reported by Furman et al. (53). In a flow cytometric analysis patients with stable coronary artery disease were shown to not only have increased levels of circulating activated platelets with enhanced P-selectin expression, but also to have an increased propensity to form monocyte-platelet aggregates (Fig. 1) (53). Additional evidence to implicate platelets as inflammory mediators is the recent finding of their expression of CD40L. This transmembrane protein found on constituents of both cellular and humoral components of the inflammatory system is structurally related to TNF-α. CD40L is rapidly expressed by activated platelets and induces the expression of chemokines and cell adhesion molecules by endothelial cells thus provoking cell attraction, activation, and migration into the arterial wall (54).

MARKERS AND MEDIATORS OF INFLAMMATION

C-Reactive Protein (CRP)

Although many markers of inflammation have been associated with adverse cardiovascular outcome, CRP has been evaluated in every clinical phase of coronary disease. It therefore provides a superlative avenue to thoroughly

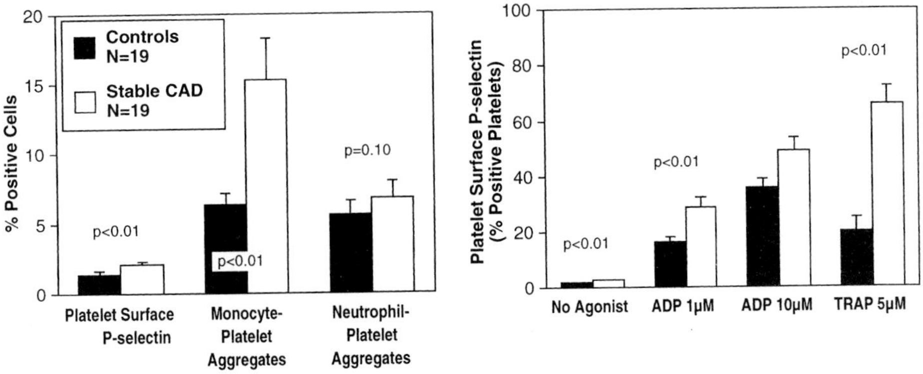

Figure 1 Augmented platelet activity and response to agonist in patients with stable coronary artery disease versus normal controls. (From Ref. 53.)

discuss the prognostic significance of inflammatory markers in cardiovascular disease. CRP is an acute-phase reactant whose concentration in blood rises dramatically in response to nonspecific inflammatory stimuli. It has been convincingly linked to cardiovascular disease, initially in sera of patients after acute myocardial infarction and recently in the wall of human coronary arteries possibly linking its presence directly with the development of atherosclerosis (55–57). Whether the association reflects a casual or direct interaction, elevated levels of CRP are associated with a worse prognosis in the full spectra of atherosclerotic disease.

In the setting of a Q-wave myocardial infarction, Anzai et al. (58) reported that elevated levels of CRP were associated with cardiac rupture, left ventricular aneurysm formation, and 1-year cardiac death. Even though CRP was found to be an independent predictor of these events, there remained a confounding correlation to extent of cardiac enzyme elevation in those patients without revascularization procedures (58). Therefore, CRP levels in this study may reflected infarct size and subsequent risk for adverse outcome.

Tommasi et al. (8) reported on the prognostic value of CRP levels inpatients with a first acute myocardial infarction, uncomplicated in-hospital course, absence of residual ischemia, and normal left ventricular function. Only increased CRP levels were independently associated to the incidence of patients who developed cardiac events (cardiac death, new-onset angina, and recurrent myocardial infarction) (Fig. 2) (8). Importantly, there was no correlation between CRP levels and extent of rise of cardiac enzymes.

Although numerous studies have shown that an elevated CRP in the setting of unstable angina and non-Q-wave myocardial infarction is associ-

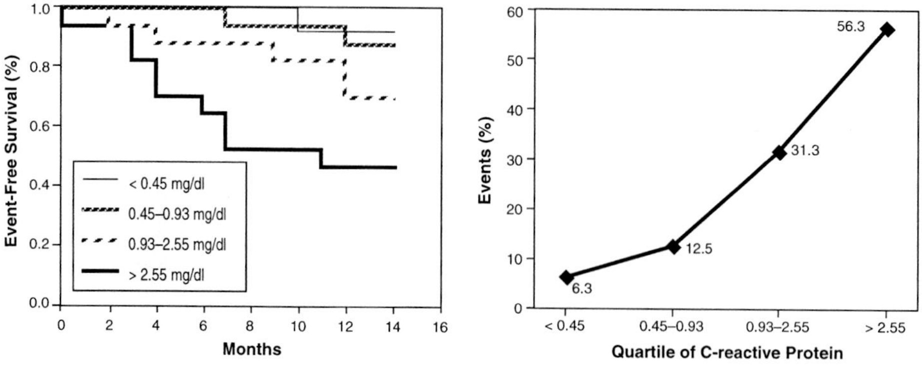

Figure 2 (Left) The event-free survival with respect to level of CRP in patients after an uncomplicated myocardial infarction. (Right) The distribution of events per quartile of CRP elevation. (From Ref. 8.)

ated with worse prognosis (6,7,59–61), Biassicci et al. (62) reported on the prognostic significance of CRP elevation in patients with unstable angina without myocardial injury. They excluded those patients with elevated levels of cardiac enzymes at entry to avoid the interplay of myocardial necrosis on CRP and future events. They reported that an elevated discharge CRP was strongly associated with recurrent coronary instability and myocardial infarction (Fig. 3) and, interestingly, 42% of patients had persistent elevation of CRP 3 months after hospital discharge. Adjunctive evidence that elevated CRP levels possess predictive power exceeding there association with myonecrosis is their independent and additive prognostic value to markers of myocardial injury, such as troponin T and I (63,64).

In the Thrombolysis in Myocardial Infarction (TIMI) IIA trial, a dose-ranging trial for enoxaparin in UA and NQMI, elevated CRP correlated with increased 14-day mortality (Fig. 4). Most importantly, these findings existed even in patients with a negative rapid troponin T assay, thereby dissociating myonecrosis from CRP's prognostic power (64). Milazzo et al. (65) reported that in patients undergoing CABG a preoperative elevation of CRP has prognostic significance (Fig. 5). CRP levels <3 mg/L and ≥ 3 mg/L were associated with new ischemic events in 4% vs. 25% of patients, respectively.

In the setting of percutaneous coronary revascularization, a hyperresponsive reaction of the inflammatory system, defined by elevation of CRP, IL-6, and serum amyloid A after angioplasty, was recently presumed to portend a worse prognosis (66). Gaspardone et al. (67) confirmed this by showing a persistent elevation in CRP 72 hours after coronary artery stenting (excluding patients with periprocedural myocardial infarction) pinpointed all

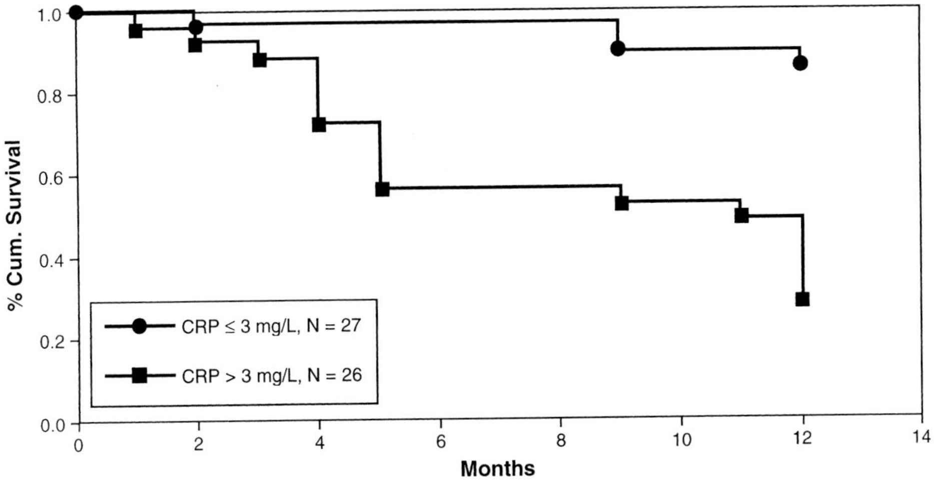

Figure 3 Cumulative event-free survival in patients with unstable angina, negative cardiac enzymes, and elevated discharge CRP. (From Ref. 62.)

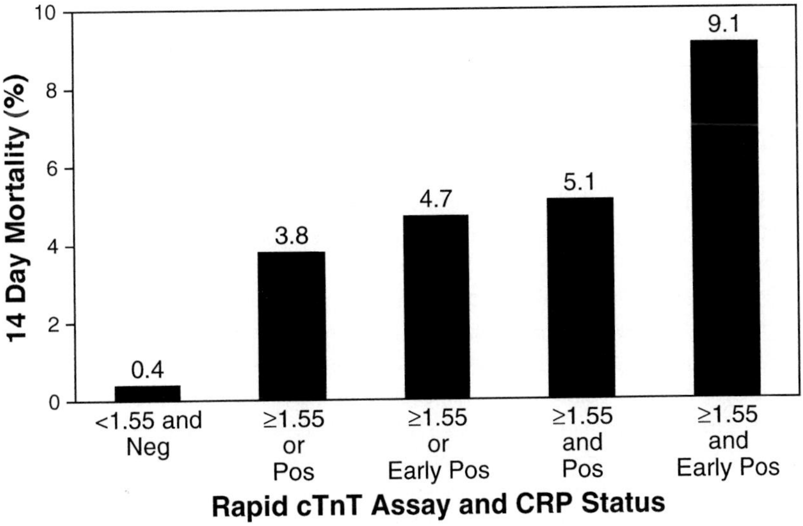

Figure 4 Independent and additive predictive value of CRP and cTNT (early positive defined by being positive in <10 minutes) on 14-day mortality. (From Ref. 64.)

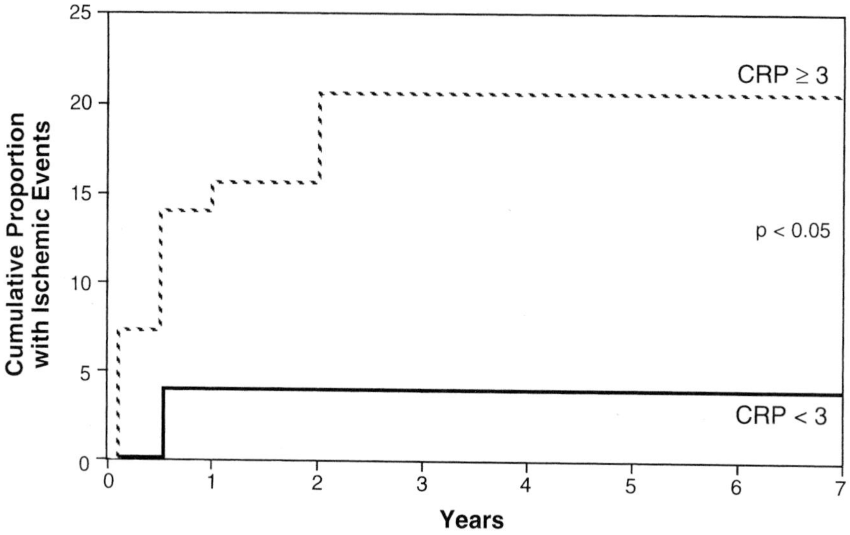

Figure 5 Cumulative proportion of ischemic events in patients with elevated CRP prior to coronary artery bypass grafting. (From Ref. 65.)

patients who later suffered an adverse outcome. In contrast, no cardiac events occurred in those with normal levels at 1 year follow-up (Fig. 6).

Ex vivo studies have recently introduced the concept that detecting heat release by inflammatory cells within an atherosclerotic plaque may predict future instability and rupture (68). Stefanadis et al. (69), using a thermography catheter, demonstrated heterogeneity in heat production of 20%, 40%, and 67% in atherosclerotic plaques of patients with stable angina, unstable angina, and acute myocardial infarction, respectively. Most importantly there was a significant correlation between thermal heterogeneity and baseline CRP (Fig. 7) (69).

More conclusive evidence that chronic, indolent inflammation plays a principal role in the development and progression of atherosclerosis has come from the long-term follow-up of patients with no known atherosclerotic disease but increased levels of CRP. Among 14,916 apparently healthy men participating in the Physician's Health Study an elevated level of high-sensitivity CRP (HsCRP), which detects CRP levels as low as 0.175mg/L, added to the predictive value of elevated lipids in predicting first myocardial infarction (Fig. 8) (70). Similarly, in the Women's Health Study, those who developed cardiovascular events had higher baseline CRP levels than control subjects, with the highest levels at baseline being associated with a five- and

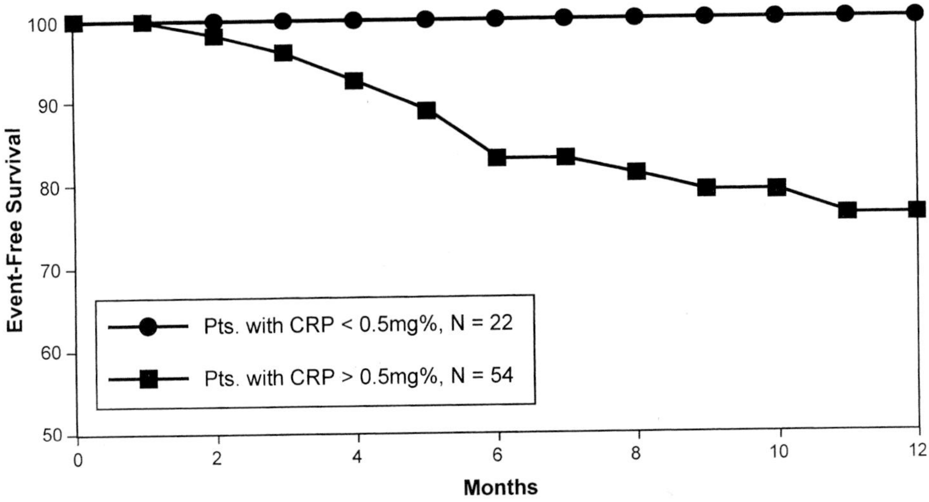

Figure 6 Event-free survival with respect to persistent elevation of CRP >72 hours after coronary stenting. (From Ref. 67.)

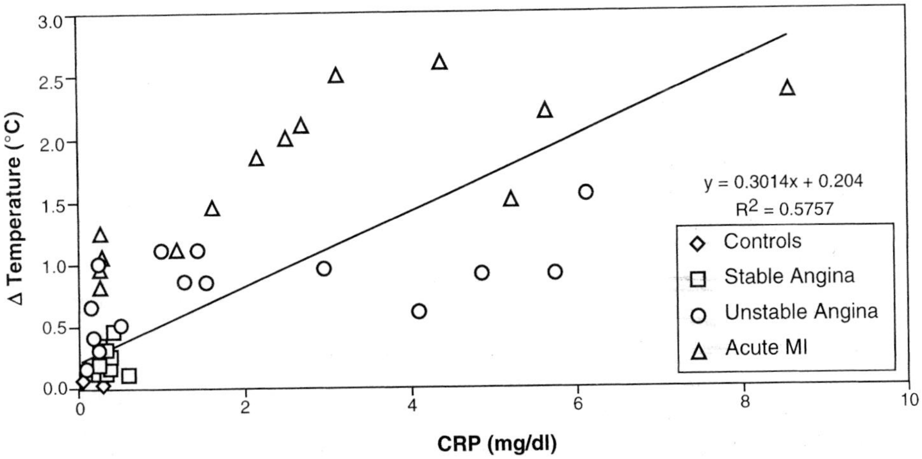

Figure 7 The correlation between thermal heterogeneity and level of CRP in control, stable angina, unstable angina, and acute myocardial infarction patients. (From Ref. 69.)

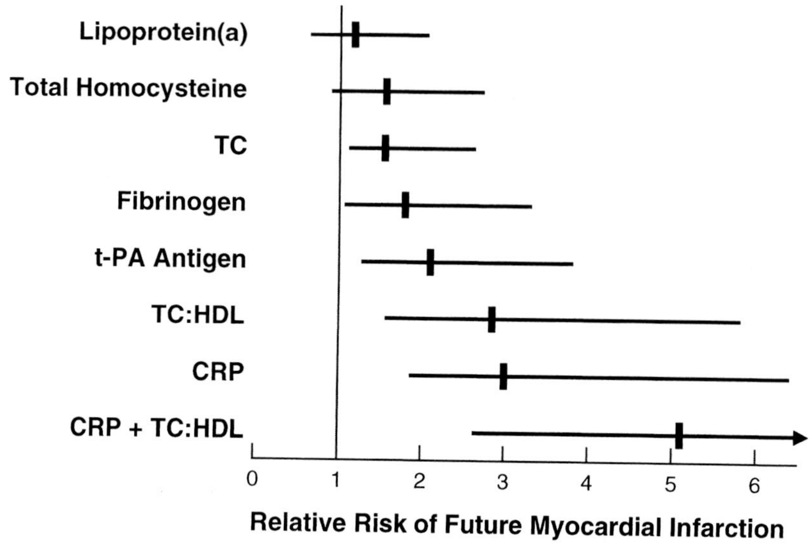

Figure 8 Predictive value for lipoprotein(a), total homocysteine, total cholesterol, fibrinogen, t-PA antigen, ratio of total cholesterol to HDL, CRP, and CRP plus total cholesterol HDL ratio. (From Ridker PM et al., Ann Intern Med 1999;130:933–937.)

seven-fold increase in any vascular event and combined stroke or myocardial infarction, respectively (71).

Additional evidence that CRP levels are strong predictors of future cardiac events in apparently healthy men was recently published from the Monitoring Trends and Determinants in Cardiovascular Disease Study (MONICA). Patients in the highest quintile of CRP level had a 2.6-fold increased risk of suffering a fatal or nonfatal myocardial infarction or sudden cardiac death (72). These findings strongly support the pivotal role that inflammation plays in the destabilization of atherosclerosis.

The question remains what if any direct role CRP plays in the development of atherosclerosis. A possible explanation supporting CRP as an indirect cardiovascular risk factor is that it reflects inflammation related to coronary vessel pathogens, extent of atherosclerosis, myocardial necrosis, myocardial ischemia, and activity of circulating proinflammatory cytokines (73). Direct evidence for CRP's role in the pathogenesis of atherosclerosis is that its presence in the arterial wall predicts severity of atherosclerosis and that it is able to bind to damaged membranes and lipids, activate complement, and stimulate production of tissue factor from activated macrophages (74–77). Irrespective of its pathologic role, there is overwhelming evidence that CRP, a sensitive marker of inflammation, is a powerful predictor of future cardiac events in patients with Q-wave MI, non-Q MI, unstable angina, stable angina, in patients who have undergone CABG and percutaneous coronary stenting, and recently in apparently healthy men and women. Recently the FDA has approved the use of a high-sensitivity CRP assay (Behring) as a prognostic test in the evaluation of patients with or expected atherosclerosis. This test has been most studied in those patients without clinically apparent atherosclerosis as a predictor of future cardiovascular events based on tertile of elevation.

Tumor Necrosis Factor-α (TNF-α) and Other Mediators

TNF-α is a pleiotropic proinflammatory cytokine with a wide range of effects that extend across a spectrum of pathologic conditions. Present in atherosclerotic lesions (78), TNF-α appears to one of the most important influences on the progression of atherosclerosis. Its upregulation is known to mediate and amplify a multitude of interactions resulting in progressive inflammation, plaque destabilization, and prothrombotic tendencies (79–87) (Table 2). Treatment with a chimeric mAb to TNF-α has been shown to suppress inflammation and improve patient well-being in rheumatoid arthritis. Administration of anti-TNF-α Ab was recently shown to rapidly downregulate a spectrum of cytokines (IL-6), cytokine inhibitors (TNF receptors

Table 2 Proinflammatory and Thrombotic Properties of TNF-α

Inflammatory properties
Regulation of macrophage colony-stimulating factor
Regulation of cell adhesion molecules
Modulation of smooth muscle cell phenotype
Induction of IL-1 mRNA
Inhibition of endothelial cell apoptosis
Plaque destabilization
Induces smooth muscle cell interstitial collagenases
Neutral effect on tissue inhibitors of metalloproteinases
Thrombotic properties
Augments transcription and expression of tissue factor
Decreases in activity of thrombomodulin-C and tissue-type plasminogen activator
Increases production of plasminogen activator inhibitor
Increases release of Von Willebrand factor

p75 and p55), and acute-phase proteins (amyloid A, haptoglobin, and fibrinogen) (88). This potent suppression of markers and mediators of inflammation may have tremendous potential in preventing progression of atherosclerosis.

IL-6 and IL-1Ra (IL-1 receptor antagonist) not only have been shown to be elevated in the setting of ACS, but also are associated with increased risk of in-hospital events (89). IL-6, produced by a variety of inflammatory cell types, has been shown to remain elevated up to 4 weeks after a myocardial infarction. Its properties increase fibrinogen and PAI-1, promote adhesion of neutrophils and myocytes during myocardial reperfusion, and produce a negative inotropic effect on the myocardium (90–94). Pannitteri et al. (95) reported that levels of IL-8 not only are elevated in the setting of acute myocardial infarction but that they precede the levels of IL-6 and parallel the kinetics of CPK. IL-8 is a powerful trigger for firm adhesion of monocytes to vascular endothelium, may play a potential atherogenic role by inhibiting local inhibitors of metalloproteinases in atherosclerotic plaques, and stimulates smooth muscle cell migration (96,97). IL-4 and IL-13 have been shown to enhance the ability of activated human monocytes to oxidize LDL, thus potentiating its toxics effects (98). OxLDL induces IFN-γ production by T-helper-1-like cells, which are known to inhibit local collagen synthesis by SMC, stimulate expression of tissue factor and CD40, and selectively induce MCP-1 (98–100). Many other cytokines have been implicated in immunity, inflammation, thrombosis, and angiogenesis (101).

The above discussion underscores the vast trafficking, redundancy, and interplay of the cytokine system. Each mediator, though, must work through specific receptors and ultimately regulate gene expression of proteins vital to the potentiation and regulation of the inflammatory cascade. Nuclear factor κ-B (NF-κB), Peroxisome proliferator-activated receptor activators (PPARs), CD40 receptor and its ligand, and inducible cyclooxygenase enzyme (Cox-2) are avidly being investigated as we attempt to discover the final common pathway of inflammation and its role in atherosclerosis.

NF-κB

NF-κB is a transcription factor located in the cytoplasm of many cells as an inactive complex associated with a specific class of inhibitory proteins, called IκB. This complex binds and prevents nuclear translocation and DNA binding of NF-κB (102). In response to inflammatory stimuli IκB is eventually degraded and NF-κB is released and transported to the nucleus. In the nuclei, NF-κB can initiate or regulate early response gene transcription by binding to promotor or enhancer regions (103). NF-κB is known to regulate or be regulated by genes involved in every aspect of the proinflammatory cascade (104,105). TNF-α and IL-1 are two important inducers, contributing to a positive feedback loop for NF-κB activation. As a consequence, there is a continuous upregulation of cytokines and perpetuation of inflammation (103). NF-κB has been implicated in a variety of inflammatory diseases, such as allograft rejection, rheumatoid arthritis (RA), asthma, and inflammatory bowel disease (104). In RA, NF-κB is overly expressed in synovial tissue, associated with surface expression of cell adhesion molecules, production of cytokines, and upregulation of the inducible isoform of cyclo-oxygenase (Cox-2). These processes are parallel to those found in atherosclerotic lesions (104).

NF-κB activity is enhanced by known cardiac risk factors such as very low-density lipoprotein, OxLDL, hyperglycemia, and elevated levels of angiotensin II. On the contrary, its activity is inhibited by HMG-CoA reductase inhibitors, antioxidants, and gallates (phenolic coumpounds found abundantly in red wine) (106–111). Recently, Ritchie (112) reported data showing that NF-κB is activated in patients with unstable angina without evidence of myonecrosis and is therefore potentially linked in plaque disruption. Immunosuppression with glucocordicoids, gold, cyclosporin, FK506, and, importantly, aspirin and salicylates is known to inhibit NF-κB. Kopp et al. (113) demonstrated that aspirin inhibits NF-κB activity by preventing the degredation of IκB, while Weber et al. (114) established aspirin's ability to inhibit TNF-α-stimulated NF-κB activity.

CD40 and CD40L

CD40 is a phosphorylated 49-kDa glycoprotein expressed on B-lymphocytes, fibroblasts, monocytes, platelets, epithelial cells, and endothelial cells (115). CD40L, also named CD154 or gp39, belongs to the TNF family of cytokines. The presence of CD40 and CD40L has been found in human atheroma, and their association is implicated with expression of cell adhesion molecules, cytokines, matrix metalloproteinases, and tissue factor (54,115). Anti-CD40L has been shown to regulate autoimmune diseases such as lupus nephritis, skin and cardiac allograft rejection, and multiple sclerosis in experimental models (116–118). Mach et al. (119) reported a reduction in aortic atherosclerotic lesion size, fewer T-lymphocytes and macrophages, and a decreased presence of cell adhesion molecules in atheroma in cholesterol-fed mice lacking the LDL receptor when treated with anti-CD40L antibody (119). Aukrust et al. (120) recently reported elevated levels of CD40-CD40L in patients with angina pectoris. Patients with unstable angina had significantly higher levels than those with stable angina, allowing the authors to conclude that presence of CD40-CD40L may have a pathologic role in plaque destabilization and the development of ACS (120) (Fig. 9).

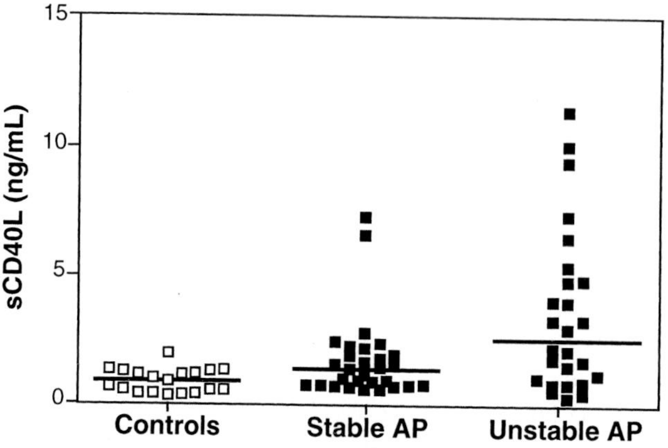

Figure 9 Levels of soluble CD40L in normal controls, stable angina, and unstable angina patients. (From Ref. 120.)

PPAR

Peroxisomal proliferator-activated receptors (PPARs), including PPAR-α, PPAR-γ, and PPAR-δ, are a group of nuclear transcription factors playing a key role in adipogenesis and lipid metabolism (121). Recently, modulation of the development and progression of atherosclerosis has been substantiated by research that appears to link PPAR activity with the regulation of inflammation and plaque stability by their interactions with macrophages, endothelial cells, smooth muscles cells, and metalloproteinases. Ricote et al. (122) found PPAR-γ to be upregulated in activated macrophages and to inhibit gelatinase B, nitric oxide synthase, and scavenger receptors. OxLDL has been shown to induce PPAR-γ expression in macrophages, resulting in monocyte differentiation and enhanced uptake in OxLDL (123,124). Max et al. (125) recently reported elevated levels of PPAR-γ expression on monocytes in human atherosclerotic lesions as compared to normal controls. Furthermore, PPAR-γ stimulation leads to a concentration-dependent decrement in monocyte-derived metalloproteinase activity. Finally, PPAR-α and -γ have been implicated in the induction of macrophage apoptosis through inhibition of NF-κB antiapoptotic pathways (126). Endothelial cells also appear to be under the influence of PPARs by the regulation of leukocyte/endothelial cell interactions. Jackson et al. (127) demonstrated an inhibitory effect of stimulated PPAR on endothelial cell expression of VCAM-1. In addition, stimulated PPAR-α has been shown to inhibit TNF-α-mediated endothelial cell VCAM-1 expression, COX-2 expression, IL-1 induced production of IL-6, and thrombin-induced endothelial-1 production (128–130).

Key stimulatory PPAR ligands are naturally occurring prostaglandins, as well as synthetic antidiabetic and antilipidemic drugs. Gemfibrozil, a finofibrate and stimulator of PPAR-α, has recently been shown to dramatically reduce IL-1-induced production of IL-6, expression of COX-2 in human smooth muscle cells, and cardiovascular events in patients with low HDL levels. Importantly, this reduction in cardiovascular events was independent of LDL levels (130,131). Troglitazone, an insulin sensitizer and PPAR-γ ligand, demonstrates a range of anti-inflammatory and potential plaque-stabilizing activities such as PPAR-γ-induced inhibition of macrophage metalloproteinases (125).

Currently, the complex activities of PPARs and their ligands are not completely understood, although ligands with positive effects on lipid lowering (finofibrates) and glycemic control (troglitazone) would suggest that these transcriptional factors are clinically beneficial and mainly antiatherogenic.

Cyclo-oxygenase-2 (COX-2)

There are two distinct isoforms of cyclo-oxygenase (COX-1 and COX-2). These enzymes are necessary in the conversion of arachidonic acid to prostaglandin G2 and H2, which are potent agonists to the inflammatory cascade (132,133). The ability of ASA and other NSAIDs to inhibit inflammation through their regulation of COX-1 was first described by Vane in 1971 (132). It was not until 1991 that an inducible form of the COX enzyme was discovered, COX-2 (134). Although a weak COX-2 inhibitor, aspirin and most available NSAIDs by virtue of their preferential COX-1 inhibitory effects, provide minimal anti-inflammatory action at doses not associated with significant side effects. COX-2 receptors are scantly expressed in the gastrointestinal tract or platelets and therefore likely provide augmented inflammatory control with few adverse effects (135). COX-2 is felt to be the principal isoform that participates in inflammation and has been recently found to be widely expressed in atherosclerotic tissue (136,137). Macrophage COX-2 mRNA expression has been shown to be induced by inflammatory cytokines such as INF-γ, TNF-α, and lipopolysaccharide, while other cytokines with antiinflammatory properties, such as IL-10, have been shown to inhibit its induction (138,139).

Speir et al. (140) recently demonstrated a reduction in reactive oxygen species generation in CMV infected smooth muscle cells when pretreated with NSAIDs. This reduction was thought mainly to be due to inhibition of the COX-2 enzyme (140). Although most investigations have described COX-2 as a proinflammatory mediator, recent reports by Cockerill et al. (141) and Bishop-Bailey et al. (142) have provided evidence for its anti-

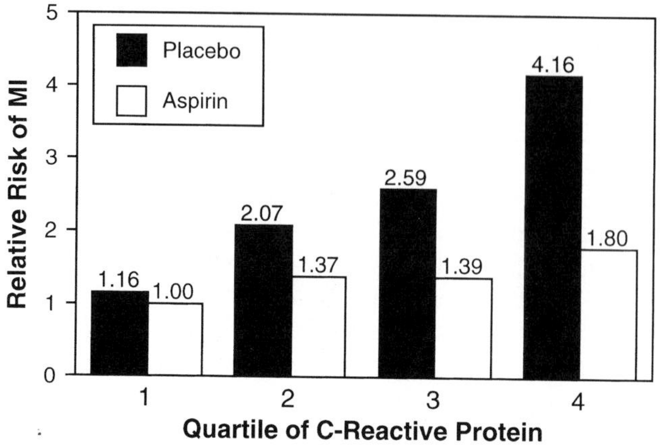

Figure 10 Relative benefit of ASA with respect to quartile of CRP. Data are shown allocated to ASA (open bars) and placebo (solid bars). (From Ref. 144.)

inflammatory potential. They demonstrated that HDL enhanced the expression of COX-2-dependent prostaglandin-I2, which is known to inhibit platelet and leukocyte activity. In addition, inhibition of IL-1-β resulted in upregulation of COX-2 and downregulation of the cell adhesion molecule ICAM-1. Although questions still remain, anti-inflammatory treatment such as aspirin, with its unquestionable beneficial effects, and a recent retrospective analysis of NSAIDs inpatients after myocardial infarction that demonstrated a reduction in cardiac mortality and adverse events (Fig. 10) (143), suggest the potential for augmented clinical benefit with more potent and selective cyclooxygenase inhibition.

THE FUTURE OF INFLAMMATION CONTROL IN ACS

Aspirin, initially thought of mainly as an antiplatelet drug in the battle with atherosclerotic heart disease, is becoming more recognized for its anti-inflammatory properties. In addition to aspirin's COX-1 and weak COX-2 activity, the inhibition of NF-κB activity is achieved by inhibiting both the degradation of IκB and effects of TNF-α. Clinical evidence to support aspirin's anti-inflammatory role has been reported by Ridker et al. (144). Aspirin reduced first MI in the Physicians Health Study, and this effect was directly related to the baseline CRP level (144) (Fig. 11). In addition, the recent negative results of the oral IIb/IIIa receptor inhibitor may be explained in part by the lack of aspirin's anti-inflammatory properties in the group receiving sole oral IIb/IIIa treatment.

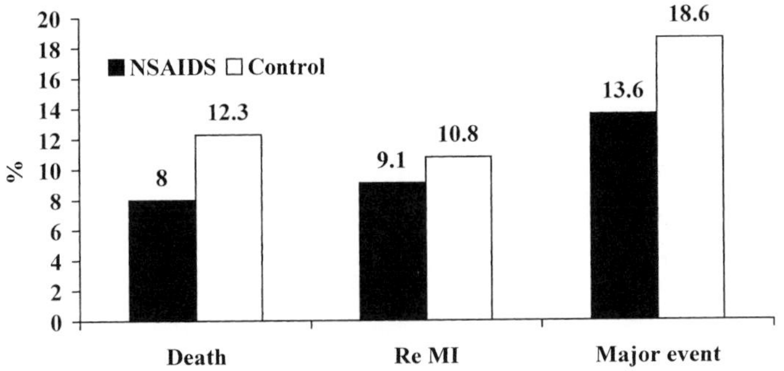

Figure 11 Cardiovascular events allocated to background of NSAID (solid bars) and control (open bars).

A paradigm shift in thought may be evolving in favor of the anti-inflammatory properties of aspirin being more salient than its relatively weak antiplatelet effects in the reduction of ischemic cardiac events. HMG-CoA reductase inhibitors have been shown to dramatically reduce cardiovascular mortality and morbidity although the reduction in events is not linear with the reduction of LDL cholesterol below 125 mg/dL (145). In an analysis of the Cholesterol and Recurrent Events (CARE) trial, Ridker et al. (146) reported a significant 22% drop in CRP over a 5-year period in those treated with pravastatin versus placebo. Interestingly, CRP rose even in the placebo-treated arm which realized a reduction in LDL cholesterol (Fig. 12). Evi-

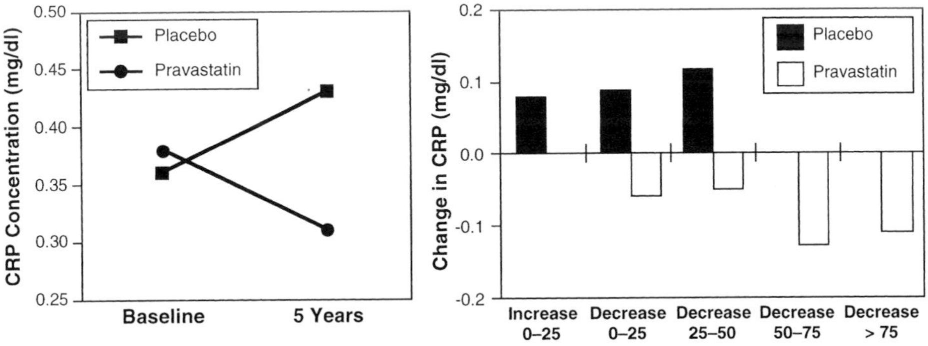

Figure 12 (Left) CRP at baseline and 5 years for patients treated with pravastatin or placebo. (Right) The change in CRP according to LDL level. Data are shown allocated to pravastatin (open bars) and placebo (solid bars). (From Ridker PM et al., Circulation 1999;100:320–335.)

dence continues to mount suggesting an anti-inflammatory role for HMG-CoA reductase inhibitors as these agents has been shown to alter regulation of DNA transcription, regulate natural-killer-cell cytotoxicity, inhibit platelet-derived growth factor-induced DNA synthesis, and decrease macrophage production of metalloproteinases (146–149). ACE inhibitors have recently been demonstrated to possess potent anti-inflammatory properties that may explain their regulating effects on atherosclerotic driven endpoints. ACE inhibitors have been shown to exhibit antiproliferative and antimigratory effects on SMC and leukocytes, restore endothelial function, modulate platelet effects, and promote endogenous fibrinolysis (150). The Heart Outcomes Prevention Evaluation (HOPE) study, a study of patients with vascular disease and no known heart failure, reported a dramatic and significant decrease in cardiovascular death, MI, and stroke in patients treated with ramipril versus placebo (Fig. 13) (151). Finofibrates and insulin sensitizers such as troglitazone are stimulators of PPAR receptors and are currently receiving attention for their anti-inflammatory and antiatherogenic potential. Unfortunately, not all methods of inflammatory control have realized a positive clinical outcome. Prevention of reperfusion injury in patients presenting with ACS by inhibiting leukocyte adhesion was recently reported from the HALT MI study. There was no significant reduction in infarct size and unfortunately a significant increase in infection rates in those randomized to high dose of the CD11/CD18 inhibitor (152). This trial underscores the careful balance needed between adequate anti-inflammatory control and clinically significant immunosuppression.

Even though CRP and HsCRP have been shown to predict risk of future adverse cardiovascular events in virtually all patient subgroups, treat-

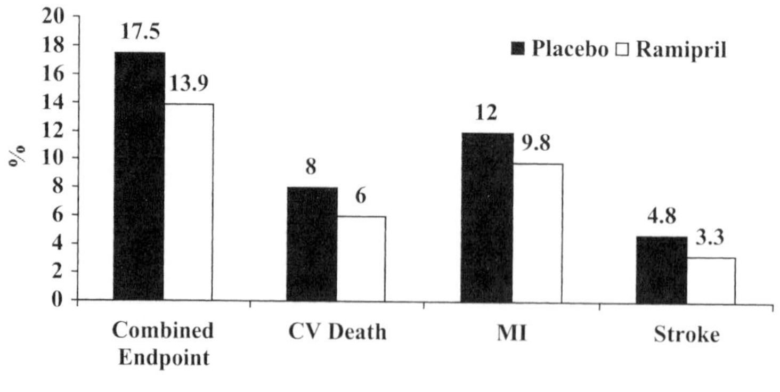

Figure 13 Cardiovascular endpoints allocated by patients receiving ramipril (open bars) or placebo (solid bars).

ment options are limited to drugs not specifically heralded for their anti-inflammatory properties. Novel downstream approaches with the use of TNF-α, CD40L, NF-κB, and COX-2 inhibitors are under in vitro and animal investigations to determine their potential role in the battle against atherosclerosis. Treatment of atherosclerosis as an inflammatory disease should first focus on those pathogens known to initiate and propagate this disease, such as hypercholesterolemia, hypertension, diabetes, hyperhomocysteinemia, smoking, and possible infection. The second approach should be to uncover the etiology of the nearly 50% of patients who present with an ACS without known cardiac risk factors. Finally, further investigation is needed to determine the clinical efficacy of adjunctive anti-inflammatory therapy on the background of pathogen directed treatment.

REFERENCES

1. Alexander RW. Inflammation and coronary artery disease. N Engl J Med 1994;331:468–469.
2. Ross R, Glomset JA. The pathogenesis of atherosclerosis (first of two parts). N Engl J Med 1976;295:369–377.
3. Ross R. The pathogenesis of atherosclerosis—an update. N Engl J Med 1986; 314:488–500.
4. Ross R. The pathogenesis of atherosclerosis: a perspective for the 1990s. Nature 1993;362:801–809.
5. Ross R. Atherosclerosis—an inflammatory disease. N Engl J Med 1999;340: 115–126.
6. Toss H, Lindahl B, Siegbahn A, Wallentin L. Prognostic influence of increased fibrinogen and C-reactive protein levels in unstable coronary artery disease. FRISC Study Group. Fragmin during instability in coronary artery disease. Circulation 1997;96:4204–4210.
7. Liuzzo G, Biasucci LM, Gallimore JR, Grillo RL, Rebuzzi AG, Pepys MB, Maseri A. The prognostic value of C-reactive protein and serum amyloid a protein in severe unstable angina. N Engl J Med 1994;331:417–424.
8. Tommasi S, Carluccio E, Bentivoglio M, Buccolieri M, Mariotti M, Politano M, Corea L. C-reactive protein as a marker for cardiac ischemic events in the year after a first, uncomplicated myocardial infarction. Am J Cardiol 1999; 83:1595–1599.
9. Biasucci LM, Liuzzo G, Caligiuri G, Quaranta G, Andreotti F, Sperti G, van de Greef W, Rebuzzi AG, Kluft C, Maseri A. Temporal relation between ischemic episodes and activation of the coagulation system in unstable angina. Circulation 1996;93:2121–2127.
10. Bhagat K. Endothelial function and myocardial infarction. Cardiovasc Res 1998;39:312–317.
11. Kinlay S, Selwyn AP, Libby P, Ganz P. Inflammation, the endothelium, and the acute coronary syndromes. J Cardiovasc Pharmacol 1998;32:S62–S66.

12. Noll G, Luscher TF. The endothelium in acute coronary syndromes. Eur Heart J 1998;19(suppl C):C30–C38.
13. Gonzalez-Amaro R, Diaz-Gonzalez F, Sanchez-Madrid F. Adhesion molecules in inflammatory diseases. Drugs 1998;56:977–988.
14. Petruzzelli L, Takami M, Humes HD. Structure and function of cell adhesion molecules. Am J Med 1999;106:467–476.
15. Frenette PS, Wagner DD. Adhesion molecules—part I. N Engl J Med 1996; 334:1526–1529.
16. Frenette PS, Wagner DD. Adhesion molecules—part II: blood vessels and blood cells. N Engl J Med 1996;335:43–45.
17. Springer TA. Adhesion receptors of the immune system. Nature 1990;346: 425–434.
18. Braun M, Pietsch P, Schror K, Baumann G, Felix SB. Cellular adhesion molecules on vascular smooth muscle cells. Cardiovasc Res 1999;41:395–401.
19. Marx N NF-J, Fischer A, Heimerl S, Dickfeld T. Induction of monocyte procoagulant activity by adhesion on vascular smooth muscle cells and ICAM-1 transfected CHO-cells. Circulation 1997;96(suppl):I-112.
20. Phillips DR, Charo IF, Parise LV, Fitzgerald LA. The platelet membrane glycoprotein IIb-IIIa complex. Blood 1988;71:831–843.
21. De caterina R BG, Lazzerini G, Dell'Omo G, Petrucci R, Morale M, Carmassi F, Pedrinelli R. Soluble vascular cell adhesion molecule-1 as a biohumoral correlate of athersclerosis. Aterioscler Thromb Vasc Biol 1997;17:2646–2654.
22. Ridker PM, Hennekens CH, Roitman-Johnson B, Stampfer MJ, Allen J. Plasma concentration of soluble intercellular adhesion molecule 1 and risks of future myocardial infarction in apparently healthy men. Lancet 1998;351: 88–92.
23. Rohde LE, Hennekens CH, Ridker PM. Cross-sectional study of soluble intercellular adhesion molecule-1 and cardiovascular risk factors in apparently healthy men. Arterioscler Thromb Vasc Biol 1999;19:1595–1599.
24. Tenaglia AN, Buda AJ, Wilkins RG, Barron MK, Jeffords PR, Vo K, Jordan MO, Kusnick BA, Lefer DJ. Levels of expression of P-selectin, E-selectin, and intercellular adhesion molecule-1 in coronary atherectomy specimens from patients with stable and unstable angina pectoris. Am J Cardiol 1997; 79:742–747.
25. Davis LS, Kavanaugh AF, Nichols LA, Lipsky PE. Induction of persistent T cell hyporesponsiveness in vivo by monoclonal antibody to ICAM-1 in patients with rheumatoid arthritis. J Immunol 1995;154:3525–3537.
26. Buerke M, Weyrich AS, Zheng Z, Gaeta FC, Forrest MJ, Lefer AM. Sialyl $Lewis_x$-containing oligosaccharide attenuates myocardial reperfusion injury in cats. J Clin Invest 1994;93:1140–1148.
27. Silver MJ, Sutton JM, Hook S, Lee P, Malycky JL, Phillips ML, Ellis SG, Topol EJ, Nicolini FA. Adjunctive selectin blockade successfully reduces infarct size beyond thrombolysis in the electrolytic canine coronary artery model. Circulation 1995;92:492–499.
28. Gown AM, Tsukada T, Ross R. Human atherosclerosis. II. Immunocytochem-

ical analysis of the cellular composition of human atherosclerotic lesions. Am J Pathol 1986;125:191–207.
29. Schmitz G, Herr AS, Rothe G. T-lymphocytes and monocytes in atherogenesis. Herz 1998;23:168–177.
30. Frankenberger M, Sternsdorf T, Pechumer H, Pforte A, Ziegler-Heitbrock HW. Differential cytokine expression in human blood monocyte subpopulations: a polymerase chain reaction analysis. Blood 1996;87:373–377.
31. Boyle JJ. Association of coronary plaque rupture and atherosclerotic inflammation. J Pathol 1997;181:93–99.
32. Moreno PR, Falk E, Palacios IF, Newell JB, Fuster V, Fallon JT. Macrophage infiltration in acute coronary syndromes. Implications for plaque rupture. Circulation 1994;90:775–778.
33. Dirksen MT, van der Wal AC, van den Berg FM, van der Loos CM, Becker AE. Distribution of inflammatory cells in atherosclerotic plaques relates to the direction of flow. Circulation 1998;98:2000–2003.
34. Shah PK, Falk E, Badimon JJ, Fernandez-Ortiz A, Mailhac A, Villareal-Levy G, Fallon JT, Regnstrom J, Fuster V. Human monocyte-derived macrophages induce collagen breakdown in fibrous caps of atherosclerotic plaques. Potential role of matrix-degrading metalloproteinases and implications for plaque rupture. Circulation 1995;92:1565–1569.
35. Hansson GK, Jonasson L, Seifert PS, Stemme S. Immune mechanisms in atherosclerosis. Arteriosclerosis 1989;9:567–578.
36. Caligiuri G, Liuzzo G, Biasucci LM, Maseri A. Immune system activation follows inflammation in unstable angina: pathogenetic implications. J Am Coll Cardiol 1998;32:1295–1304.
37. Van der Wal AC, Piek JJ, de Boer OJ, Koch KT, Teeling P, van der Loos CM, Becker AE. Recent activation of the plaque immune response in coronary lesions underlying acute coronary syndromes. Heart 1998;80:14–18.
38. Kaartinen M, Penttila A, Kovanen PT. Accumulation of activated mast cells in the shoulder region of human coronary atheroma, the predilection site of atheromatous rupture. Circulation 1994;90:1669–1678.
39. Kovanen PT, Kaartinen M, Paavonen T. Infiltrates of activated mast cells at the site of coronary atheromatous erosion or rupture in myocardial infarction. Circulation 1995;92:1084–1088.
40. Kaartinen M, van der Wal AC, van der Loos CM, Piek JJ, Koch KT, Becker AE, Kovanen PT. Mast cell infiltration in acute coronary syndromes: implications for plaque rupture. J Am Coll Cardiol 1998;32:606–612.
41. Laine P, Kaartinen M, Penttila A, Panula P, Paavonen T, Kovanen PT. Association between myocardial infarction and the mast cells in the adventitia of the infarct-related coronary artery. Circulation 1999;99:361–369.
42. Irani AA, Schechter NM, Craig SS, DeBlois G, Schwartz LB. Two types of human mast cells that have distinct neutral protease compositions. Proc Natl Acad Sci USA 1986;83:4464–4468.
43. Kaartinen M, Penttila A, Kovanen PT. Mast cells in rupture-prone areas of human coronary atheromas produce and store TNF-alpha. Circulation 1996; 94:2787–2792.

44. Hibbs MS, Hoidal JR, Kang AH. Expression of a metalloproteinase that degrades native type V collagen and denatured collagens by cultured human alveolar macrophages. J Clin Invest 1987;80:1644–1650.
45. Takeshita S, Isshiki T, Ochiai M, Ishikawa T, Nishiyama Y, Fusano T, Toyoizumi H, Kondo K, Ono Y, Sato T. Systemic inflammatory responses in acute coronary syndrome: increased activity observed in polymorphonuclear leukocytes but not T lymphocytes. Atherosclerosis 1997;135:187–192.
46. Dreyer WJ, Smith CW, Michael LH, Rossen RD, Hughes BJ, Entman ML, Anderson DC. Canine neutrophil activation by cardiac lymph obtained during reperfusion of ischemic myocardium. Circ Res 1989;65:1751–1762.
47. Smith EFd, Egan JW, Bugelski PJ, Hillegass LM, Hill DE, Griswold DE. Temporal relation between neutrophil accumulation and myocardial reperfusion injury. Am J Physiol 1988;255:H1060–H1068.
48. Kassirer M, Zeltser D, Prochorov V, Schoenman G, Frimerman A, Keren G, Shapira I, Miller H, Roth A, Arber N, Eldor A, Berliner S. Increased expression of the CD11b/CD18 antigen on the surface of peripheral white blood cells in patients with ischemic heart disease: further evidence for smoldering inflammation in patients with atherosclerosis. Am Heart J 1999;138:555–559.
49. Fuster V, Badimon L, Badimon JJ, Chesebro JH. The pathogenesis of coronary artery disease and the acute coronary syndromes (1). N Engl J Med 1992;326:242–250.
50. Fuster V, Badimon L, Badimon JJ, Chesebro JH. The pathogenesis of coronary artery disease and the acute coronary syndromes (2). N Engl J Med 1992;326:310–318.
51. Fitzgerald DJ, Roy L, Catella F, FitzGerald GA. Platelet activation in unstable coronary disease. N Engl J Med 1986;315:983–989.
52. Celi A, Pellegrini G, Lorenzet R, De Blasi A, Ready N, Furie BC, Furie B. P-selectin induces the expression of tissue factor on monocytes. Proc Natl Acad Sci USA 1994;91:8767–8771.
53. Furman MI, Benoit SE, Barnard MR, Valeri CR, Borbone ML, Becker RC, Hechtman HB, Michelson AD. Increased platelet reactivity and circulating monocyte-platelet aggregates in patients with stable coronary artery disease. J Am Coll Cardiol 1998;31:352–358.
54. Henn V, Slupsky JR, Grafe M, Anagnostopoulos I, Forster R, Muller-Berghaus G, Kroczek RA. CD40 ligand on activated platelets triggers an inflammatory reaction of endothelial cells. Nature 1998;391:591–594.
55. Zimmermann-Gorska I, Kujawa H, Drygas J. Studies of acute phase reactants in myocardial infarction. Pol Med J 1972;11:779–785.
56. Jain VC. An evaluation of C-reactive protein test in acute myocardial infarction. Indian Heart J 1968;20:16–21.
57. Zhang YX, Cliff WJ, Schoefl GI, Higgins G. Coronary C-reactive protein distribution: its relation to development of atherosclerosis. Atherosclerosis 1999;145:375–379.
58. Anzai T, Yoshikawa T, Shiraki H, Asakura Y, Akaishi M, Mitamura H, Ogawa S. C-reactive protein as a predictor of infarct expansion and cardiac rupture

after a first Q-wave acute myocardial infarction. Circulation 1997;96:778–784.

59. Haverkate F, Thompson SG, Pyke SD, Gallimore JR, Pepys MB. Production of C-reactive protein and risk of coronary events in stable and unstable angina. European Concerted Action on Thrombosis and Disabilities Angina Pectoris Study Group. Lancet 1997;349:462–466.
60. Verheggen PW, de Maat MP, Cats VM, Haverkate F, Zwinderman AH, Kluft C, Bruschke AV. Inflammatory status as a main determinant of outcome in patients with unstable angina, independent of coagulation activation and endothelial cell function. Eur Heart J 1999;20:567–574.
61. Biasucci LM, Vitelli A, Liuzzo G, Altamura S, Caligiuri G, Monaco C, Rebuzzi AG, Ciliberto G, Maseri A. Elevated levels of interleukin-6 in unstable angina. Circulation 1996;94:874–877.
62. Biasucci LM, Liuzzo G, Grillo RL, Caligiuri G, Rebuzzi AG, Buffon A, Summaria F, Ginnetti F, Fadda G, Maseri A. Elevated levels of C-reactive protein at discharge in patients with unstable angina predict recurrent instability. Circulation 1999;99:855–860.
63. Rebuzzi AG, Quaranta G, Liuzzo G, Caligiuri G, Lanza GA, Gallimore JR, Grillo RL, Cianflone D, Biasucci LM, Maseri A. Incremental prognostic value of serum levels of troponin T and C-reactive protein on admission in patients with unstable angina pectoris. Am J Cardiol 1998;82:715–719.
64. Morrow DA, Rifai N, Antman EM, Weiner DL, McCabe CH, Cannon CP, Braunwald E. C-reactive protein is a potent predictor of mortality independently of and in combination with troponin T in acute coronary syndromes: a TIMI 11A substudy. Thrombolysis in Myocardial Infarction. J Am Coll Cardiol 1998;31:1460–1465.
65. Milazzo D, Biasucci LM, Luciani N, Martinelli L, Canosa C, Schiavello R, Maseri A, Possati G. Elevated levels of C-reactive protein before coronary artery bypass grafting predict recurrence of ischemic events. Am J Cardiol 1999;84:459–461, A9.
66. Liuzzo G, Buffon A, Biasucci LM, Gallimore JR, Caligiuri G, Vitelli A, Altamura S, Ciliberto G, Rebuzzi AG, Crea F, Pepys MB, Maseri A. Enhanced inflammatory response to coronary angioplasty in patients with severe unstable angina. Circulation 1998;98:2370–2376.
67. Gaspardone A, Crea F, Versaci F, Tomai F, Pellegrino A, Chiariello L, Gioffre PA. Predictive value of C-reactive protein after successful coronary-artery stenting in patients with stable angina. Am J Cardiol 1998;82:515–518.
68. Casscells W, Hathorn B, David M, Krabach T, Vaughn WK, McAllister HA, Bearman G, Willerson JT. Thermal detection of cellular infiltrates in living atherosclerotic plaques: possible implications for plaque rupture and thrombosis. Lancet 1996;347:1447–1451.
69. Stefanadis C, Diamantopoulos L, Vlachopoulos C, Tsiamis E, Dernellis J, Toutouzas K, Stefanadi E, Toutouzas P. Thermal heterogeneity within human atherosclerotic coronary arteries detected in vivo: a new method of detection by application of a special thermography catheter. Circulation 1999;99:1965–1971.

70. Ridker PM, Glynn RJ, Hennekens CH. C-reactive protein adds to the predictive value of total and HDL cholesterol in determining risk of first myocardial infarction. Circulation 1998;97:2007–2011.
71. Ridker PM, Buring JE, Shih J, Matias M, Hennekens CH. Prospective study of C-reactive protein and the risk of future cardiovascular events among apparently healthy women. Circulation 1998;98:731–733.
72. Koenig W, Sund M, Frohlich M, Fischer HG, Lowel H, Doring A, Hutchinson WL, Pepys MB. C-Reactive protein, a sensitive marker of inflammation, predicts future risk of coronary heart disease in initially healthy middle-aged men: results from the MONICA (Monitoring Trends and Determinants in Cardiovascular Disease) Augsburg Cohort Study, 1984 to 1992. Circulation 1999;99:237–242.
73. Lagrand WK, Visser CA, Hermens WT, Niessen HW, Verheugt FW, Wolbink GJ, Hack CE. C-reactive protein as a cardiovascular risk factor: more than an epiphenomenon? Circulation 1999;100:96–102.
74. Toschi V, Gallo R, Lettino M, Fallon JT, Gertz SD, Fernandez-Ortiz A, Chesebro JH, Badimon L, Nemerson Y, Fuster V, Badimon JJ. Tissue factor modulates the thrombogenicity of human atherosclerotic plaques. Circulation 1997;95:594–599.
75. Pepys MB, Rowe IF, Baltz ML. C-reactive protein: binding to lipids and lipoproteins. Int Rev Exp Pathol 1985;27:83–111.
76. Volanakis JE. Complement activation by C-reactive protein complexes. Ann NY Acad Sci 1982;389:235–250.
77. Cermak J, Key NS, Bach RR, Balla J, Jacob HS, Vercellotti GM. C-reactive protein induces human peripheral blood monocytes to synthesize tissue factor. Blood 1993;82:513–520.
78. Rus HG, Niculescu F, Vlaicu R. Tumor necrosis factor-alpha in human arterial wall with atherosclerosis. Atherosclerosis 1991;89:247–254.
79. Horrevoets AJ, Fontijn RD, van Zonneveld AJ, de Vries CJ, ten Cate JW, Pannekoek H. Vascular endothelial genes that are responsive to tumor necrosis factor-alpha in vitro are expressed in atherosclerotic lesions, including inhibitor of apoptosis protein-1, stannin, and two novel genes. Blood 1999;93:3418–3431.
80. Ahmad M, Theofanidis P, Medford RM. Role of activating protein-1 in the regulation of the vascular cell adhesion molecule-1 gene expression by tumor necrosis factor-alpha. J Biol Chem 1998;273:4616–4621.
81. Morisaki N, Xu QP, Koshikawa T, Saito Y, Yoshida S, Ueda S. Tumour necrosis factor-alpha can modulate the phenotype of aortic smooth muscle cells. Scand J Clin Lab Invest 1993;53:347–352.
82. Weber C, Draude G, Weber KS, Wubert J, Lorenz RL, Weber PC. Downregulation by tumor necrosis factor-alpha of monocyte CCR2 expression and monocyte chemotactic protein-1-induced transendothelial migration is antagonized by oxidized low-density lipoprotein: a potential mechanism of monocyte retention in atherosclerotic lesions. Atherosclerosis 1999;145:115–123.
83. Barks JL, McQuillan JJ, Iademarco MF. TNF-alpha and IL-4 synergistically

increase vascular cell adhesion molecule-1 expression in cultured vascular smooth muscle cells. J Immunol 1997;159:4532–4538.
84. Libby P, Sukhova G, Lee RT, Galis ZS. Cytokines regulate vascular functions related to stability of the atherosclerotic plaque. J Cardiovasc Pharmacol 1995; 25:S9–S12.
85. Galis ZS, Muszynski M, Sukhova GK, Simon-Morrissey E, Unemori EN, Lark MW, Amento E, Libby P. Cytokine-stimulated human vascular smooth muscle cells synthesize a complement of enzymes required for extracellular matrix digestion. Circ Res 1994;75:181–189.
86. Rajavashisth TB, Xu XP, Jovinge S, Meisel S, Xu XO, Chai NN, Fishbein MC, Kaul S, Cercek B, Sharifi B, Shah PK. Membrane type 1 matrix metalloproteinase expression in human atherosclerotic plaques: evidence for activation by proinflammatory mediators. Circulation 1999;99:3103–3109.
87. Dosquet C, Weill D, Wautier JL. Cytokines and thrombosis. J Cardiovasc Pharmacol 1995;25:S13–S19.
88. Charles P, Elliott MJ, Davis D, Potter A, Kalden JR, Antoni C, Breedveld FC, Smolen JS, Eberl G, deWoody K, Feldmann M, Maini RN. Regulation of cytokines, cytokine inhibitors, and acute-phase proteins following anti-TNF-alpha therapy in rheumatoid arthritis. J Immunol 1999;163:1521–1528.
89. Biasucci LM, Liuzzo G, Fantuzzi G, Caligiuri G, Rebuzzi AG, Ginnetti F, Dinarello CA, Maseri A. Increasing levels of interleukin (IL)-1Ra and IL-6 during the first 2 days of hospitalization in unstable angina are associated with increased risk of in-hospital coronary events. Circulation 1999;99:2079–2084.
90. Miyao Y, Yasue H, Ogawa H, Misumi I, Masuda T, Sakamoto T, Morita E. Elevated plasma interleukin-6 levels in patients with acute myocardial infarction. Am Heart J 1993;126:1299–1304.
91. Kushner I, Ganapathi M, Schultz D. The acute phase response is mediated by heterogeneous mechanisms. Ann NY Acad Sci 1989;557:19–29.
92. Bevilacqua MP, Schleef RR, Gimbrone MA Jr, Loskutoff DJ. Regulation of the fibrinolytic system of cultured human vascular endothelium by interleukin 1. J Clin Invest 1986;78:587–591.
93. Youker K, Smith CW, Anderson DC, Miller D, Michael LH, Rossen RD, Entman ML. Neutrophil adherence to isolated adult cardiac myocytes. Induction by cardiac lymph collected during ischemia and reperfusion. J Clin Invest 1992;89:602–609.
94. Finkel MS, Oddis CV, Jacob TD, Watkins SC, Hattler BG, Simmons RL. Negative inotropic effects of cytokines on the heart mediated by nitric oxide. Science 1992;257:387–389.
95. Pannitteri G, Marino B, Campa PP, Martucci R, Testa U, Peschle C. Interleukins 6 and 8 as mediators of acute phase response in acute myocardial infarction. Am J Cardiol 1997;80:622–625.
96. Gerszten RE, Garcia-Zepeda EA, Lim YC, Yoshida M, Ding HA, Gimbrone MA Jr, Luster AD, Luscinskas FW, Rosenzweig A. MCP-1 and IL-8 trigger firm adhesion of monocytes to vascular endothelium under flow conditions. Nature 1999;398:718–723.

97. Yue TL, McKenna PJ, Gu JL, Feuerstein GZ. Interleukin-8 is chemotactic for vascular smooth muscle cells. Eur J Pharmacol 1993;240:81–84.
98. Folcik VA, Aamir R, Cathcart MK. Cytokine modulation of LDL oxidation by activated human monocytes. Arterioscler Thromb Vasc Biol 1997;17: 1954–1961.
99. Edgington TS, Mackman N, Brand K, Ruf W. The structural biology of expression and function of tissue factor. Thromb Haemost 1991;66:67–79.
100. Nie Q, Fan J, Haraoka S, Shimokama T, Watanabe T. Inhibition of mononuclear cell recruitment in aortic intima by treatment with anti-ICAM-1 and anti-LFA-1 monoclonal antibodies in hypercholesterolemic rats: implications of the ICAM-1 and LFA-1 pathway in atherogenesis. Lab Invest 1997;77: 469–482.
101. Mantovani A, Garlanda C, Introna M, Vecchi A. Regulation of endothelial cell function by pro- and anti-inflammatory cytokines. Transplant Proc 1998; 30:4239–4243.
102. Baeuerle PA. I-kappaB-NF-kappaB structures: at the interface of inflammation control. Cell 1998;95:729–731.
103. Mercurio F, Manning AM. Multiple signals converging on NF-kappaB. Curr Opin Cell Biol 1999;11:226–232.
104. Lee JI, Burckart GJ. Nuclear factor kappa B: important transcription factor and therapeutic target. J Clin Pharmacol 1998;38:981–993.
105. Barnes PJ, Karin M. Nuclear factor-kappaB: a pivotal transcription factor in chronic inflammatory diseases. N Engl J Med 1997;336:1066–1071.
106. Massi-Benedetti M, Federici MO. Cardiovascular risk factors in type 2 diabetes: the role of hyperglycaemia. Exp Clin Endocrinol Diabetes 1999;107: S120–S123.
107. Dichtl W, Nilsson L, Goncalves I, Ares MP, Banfi C, Calara F, Hamsten A, Eriksson P, Nilsson J. Very low-density lipoprotein activates nuclear factor-kappaB in endothelial cells. Circ Res 1999;84:1085–1094.
108. Brand K, Eisele T, Kreusel U, Page M, Page S, Haas M, Gerling A, Kaltschmidt C, Neumann FJ, Mackman N, Baeurele PA, Walli AK, Neumeier D. Dysregulation of monocytic nuclear factor-kappa B by oxidized low-density lipoprotein. Arterioscler Thromb Vasc Biol 1997;17:1901–1909.
109. Kranzhofer R, Browatzki M, Schmidt J, Kubler W. Angiotensin II activates the proinflammatory transcription factor nuclear factor-kappaB in human monocytes. Biochem Biophys Res Commun 1999;257:826–828.
110. Yerneni KK, Bai W, Khan BV, Medford RM, Natarajan R. Hyperglycemia-induced activation of nuclear transcription factor kappaB in vascular smooth muscle cells. Diabetes 1999;48:855–864.
111. Bustos C, Hernandez-Presa MA, Ortego M, Tunon J, Ortega L, Perez F, Diaz C, Hernandez G, Egido J. HMG-CoA reductase inhibition by atorvastatin reduces neointimal inflammation in a rabbit model of atherosclerosis. J Am Coll Cardiol 1998;32:2057–2064.
112. Ritchie ME. Nuclear factor-kappaB is selectively and markedly activated in humans with unstable angina pectoris. Circulation 1998;98:1707–1713.

113. Kopp E, Ghosh S. Inhibition of NF-kappa B by sodium salicylate and aspirin. Science 1994;265:956–959.
114. Weber C, Erl W, Pietsch A, Weber PC. Aspirin inhibits nuclear factor-kappa B mobilization and monocyte adhesion in stimulated human endothelial cells. Circulation 1995;91:1914–1917.
115. Mach F, Schonbeck U, Libby P. CD40 signaling in vascular cells: a key role in atherosclerosis? Atherosclerosis 1998;137(suppl):S89–S95.
116. Mohan C, Shi Y, Laman JD, Datta SK. Interaction between CD40 and its ligand gp39 in the development of murine lupus nephritis. J Immunol 1995; 154:1470–1480.
117. Larsen CP, Elwood ET, Alexander DZ, Ritchie SC, Hendrix R, Tucker-Burden C, Cho HR, Aruffo A, Hollenbaugh D, Linsley PS, Winn KJ, Pearson TC. Long-term acceptance of skin and cardiac allografts after blocking CD40 and CD28 pathways. Nature 1996;381:434–438.
118. Gerritse K, Laman JD, Noelle RJ, Aruffo A, Ledbetter JA, Boersma WJ, Claassen E. CD40-CD40 ligand interactions in experimental allergic encephalomyelitis and multiple sclerosis. Proc Natl Acad Sci USA 1996;93:2499–2504.
119. Mach F, Schonbeck U, Sukhova GK, Atkinson E, Libby P. Reduction of atherosclerosis in mice by inhibition of CD40 signalling. Nature 1998;394: 200–203.
120. Aukrust P, Muller F, Ueland T, Berget T, Aaser E, Brunsvig A, Solum NO, Forfang K, Froland SS, Gullestad L. Enhanced levels of soluble and membrane-bound CD40 ligand in patients with unstable angina: possible reflection of T lymphocyte and platelet involvement in the pathogenesis of acute coronary syndromes. Circulation 1999;100:614–620.
121. Plutzky J. Atherosclerotic plaque rupture: emerging insights and opportunities. Am J Cardiol 1999;84:15J–20J.
122. Ricote M, Li AC, Willson TM, Kelly CJ, Glass CK. The peroxisome proliferator-activated receptor-gamma is a negative regulator of macrophage activation. Nature 1998;391:79–82.
123. Nagy L, Tontonoz P, Alvarez JG, Chen H, Evans RM. Oxidized LDL regulates macrophage gene expression through ligand activation of PPARgamma. Cell 1998;93:229–240.
124. Tontonoz P, Nagy L, Alvarez JG, Thomazy VA, Evans RM. PPARgamma promotes monocyte/macrophage differentiation and uptake of oxidized LDL. Cell 1998;93:241–252.
125. Marx N, Sukhova G, Murphy C, Libby P, Plutzky J. Macrophages in human atheroma contain PPARgamma: differentiation-dependent peroxisomal proliferator-activated receptor gamma (PPARgamma) expression and reduction of MMP-9 activity through PPARgamma activation in mononuclear phagocytes in vitro. Am J Pathol 1998;153:17–23.
126. Chinetti G, Griglio S, Antonucci M, Torra IP, Delerive P, Majd Z, Fruchart JC, Chapman J, Najib J, Staels B. Activation of proliferator-activated receptors alpha and gamma induces apoptosis of human monocyte-derived macrophages. J Biol Chem 1998;273:25573–25580.

127. Jackson SM, Parhami F, Xi XP, Berliner JA, Hsueh WA, Law RE, Demer LL. Peroxisome proliferator-activated receptor activators target human endothelial cells to inhibit leukocyte-endothelial cell interaction. Arterioscler Thromb Vasc Biol 1999;19:2094–2104.
128. Marx N, Sukhova GK, Collins T, Libby P, Plutzky J. PPARalpha activators inhibit cytokine-induced vascular cell adhesion molecule-1 expression in human endothelial cells. Circulation 1999;99:3125–3131.
129. Delerive P, Martin-Nizard F, Chinetti G, Trottein F, Fruchart JC, Najib J, Duriez P, Staels B. Peroxisome proliferator-activated receptor activators inhibit thrombin-induced endothelin-1 production in human vascular endothelial cells by inhibiting the activator protein-1 signaling pathway. Circ Res 1999; 85:394–402.
130. Staels B, Koenig W, Habib A, Merval R, Lebret M, Torra IP, Delerive P, Fadel A, Chinetti G, Fruchart JC, Najib J, Maclouf J, Tedgui A. Activation of human aortic smooth-muscle cells is inhibited by PPARalpha but not by PPARgamma activators. Nature 1998;393:790–793.
131. Rubins HB, Robins SJ, Collins D, Fye CL, Anderson JW, Elam MB, Faas FH, Linares E, Schaefer EJ, Schectman G, Wilt TJ, Wittes J. Gemfibrozil for the secondary prevention of coronary heart disease in men with low levels of high-density lipoprotein cholesterol. Veterans Affairs High-Density Lipoprotein Cholesterol Intervention Trial Study Group. N Engl J Med 1999;341: 410–418.
132. Dubois RN, Abramson SB, Crofford L, Gupta RA, Simon LS, Van de Putte LB, Lipsky PE. Cyclooxygenase in biology and disease. FASEB J 1998;12: 1063–1073.
133. Cryer B, Dubois A. The advent of highly selective inhibitors of cyclooxygenase—a review. Prostaglandins Other Lipid Mediat 1998;56:341–361.
134. Xie WL, Chipman JG, Robertson DL, Erikson RL, Simmons DL. Expression of a mitogen-responsive gene encoding prostaglandin synthase is regulated by mRNA splicing. Proc Natl Acad Sci USA 1991;88:2692–2696.
135. Seibert K, Masferrer J, Zhang Y, Gregory S, Olson G, Hauser S, Leahy K, Perkins W, Isakson P. Mediation of inflammation by cyclooxygenase-2. Agents Actions Suppl 1995;46:41–50.
136. Baker CS, Hall RJ, Evans TJ, Pomerance A, Maclouf J, Creminon C, Yacoub MH, Polak JM. Cyclooxygenase-2 is widely expressed in atherosclerotic lesions affecting native and transplanted human coronary arteries and colocalizes with inducible nitric oxide synthase and nitrotyrosine particularly in macrophages. Arterioscler Thromb Vasc Biol 1999;19:646–655.
137. Schonbeck U, Sukhova GK, Graber P, Coulter S, Libby P. Augmented expression of cyclooxygenase-2 in human atherosclerotic lesions. Am J Pathol 1999;155:1281–1291.
138. Niiro H, Otsuka T, Tanabe T, Hara S, Kuga S, Nemoto Y, Tanaka Y, Nakashima H, Kitajima S, Abe M. Inhibition by interleukin-10 of inducible cyclooxygenase expression in lipopolysaccharide-stimulated monocytes: its underlying mechanism in comparison with interleukin-4. Blood 1995;85:3736–3745.

139. Arias-Negrete S, Keller K, Chadee K. Proinflammatory cytokines regulate cyclooxygenase-2 mRNA expression in human macrophages. Biochem Biophys Res Commun 1995;208:582–589.
140. Speir E, Yu ZX, Ferrans VJ, Huang ES, Epstein SE. Aspirin attenuates cytomegalovirus infectivity and gene expression mediated by cyclooxygenase-2 in coronary artery smooth muscle cells. Circ Res 1998;83:210–216.
141. Cockerill GW, Rye KA, Gamble JR, Vadas MA, Barter PJ. High-density lipoproteins inhibit cytokine-induced expression of endothelial cell adhesion molecules. Arterioscler Thromb Vasc Biol 1995;15:1987–1994.
142. Bishop-Bailey D, Burke-Gaffney A, Hellewell PG, Pepper JR, Mitchell JA. Cyclo-oxygenase-2 regulates inducible ICAM-1 and VCAM-1 expression in human vascular smooth muscle cells. Biochem Biophys Res Commun 1998; 249:44–47.
143. Sajadieh A, Wendelboe O, Hansen JF, Mortensen LS. Nonsteroidal anti-inflammatory drugs after acute myocardial infarction. DAVIT Study Group. Danish Verapamil Infarction Trial. Am J Cardiol 1999;83:1263–1265, A9.
144. Ridker PM, Cushman M, Stampfer MJ, Tracy RP, Hennekens CH. Inflammation, aspirin, and the risk of cardiovascular disease in apparently healthy men [published erratum appears in N Engl J Med 1997;337(5):356]. N Engl J Med 1997;336:973–979.
145. Sacks FM, Ridker PM. Lipid lowering and beyond: results from the CARE study on lipoproteins and inflammation. Cholesterol and Recurrent Events. Herz 1999;24:51–56.
146. Ridker PM, Rifai N, Pfeffer MA, Sacks FM, Moye LA, Goldman S, Flaker GC, Braunwald E. Inflammation, pravastatin, and the risk of coronary events after myocardial infarction in patients with average cholesterol levels. Cholesterol and Recurrent Events (CARE) Investigators. Circulation 1998;98: 839–844.
147. Vaughan CJ, Murphy MB, Buckley BM. Statins do more than just lower cholesterol. Lancet 1996;348:1079–1082.
148. McPherson R, Tsoukas C, Baines MG, Vost A, Melino MR, Zupkis RV, Pross HF. Effects of lovastatin on natural killer cell function and other immunological parameters in man. J Clin Immunol 1993;13:439–444.
149. Bellosta S, Via D, Canavesi M, Pfister P, Fumagalli R, Paoletti R, Bernini F. HMG-CoA reductase inhibitors reduce MMP-9 secretion by macrophages. Arterioscler Thromb Vasc Biol 1998;18:1671–1678.
150. Cheng JW, Ngo MN. Current perspective on the use of angiotensin-converting enzyme inhibitors in the management of coronary (atherosclerotic) artery disease. Ann Pharmacother 1997;31:1499–1506.
151. HOPE Investigators. Effects of an angiotensin-converting-enzyme inhibitor, ramapril, on death from cardiovascular causes, myocardial infarction, stroke in high-risk patients. N Engl J Med 2000. In press.
152. Faxon DP GR, Chronos NA, Gurbel PA, Martin JS. The effect of CD11/CD18 inhibitor (Hu23F2G) on infarct size following direct angioplasty: the HALT MI study. Circulation 1999;100:I-791.
153. Pasceri et al. Circulation 1999;100:2124–2126.

2

Vascular Biology of the Acute Coronary Syndromes

Peter Libby, Peter Ganz, Frederick J. Schoen, and Richard T. Lee

Brigham and Women's Hospital
and Harvard Medical School
Boston, Massachusetts

INTRODUCTION

Our everyday familiarity with and success in treating coronary artery disease as clinicians lulls us into the false belief that we understand this disease better than we actually do. Consider for example the enormous heterogeneity in the expression of this disease. Some individuals succumb at an advanced age of a noncardiac cause, only to be found on autopsy to have extensive coronary atherosclerotic disease, never having had a symptom or manifestation during life. Others may have chronic stable angina for decades without experiencing acute myocardial infarction or requiring hospitalization for unstable angina. In another, all too common scenario, often in relatively young individuals, coronary artery disease may first present as acute myocardial infarction. In approximately a third of cases of coronary artery disease, sudden cardiac death is the first manifestation. Angiography or an autopsy may reveal few and modestly occlusive atheroma in many of these patients.

How can we understand the dramatic difference between young individuals whose first manifestation of coronary artery disease may be sudden death but who have limited atherosclerosis, contrasted with elderly patients who die from noncardiovascular causes, but with extensive coronary atherosclerosis that may never have caused symptoms? This chapter will review the emerging vascular biology of the acute coronary syndromes (ACS) with the aim of providing a framework for understanding their pathogenesis.

FACTORS BOTH EXTRINSIC AND INTRINSIC TO THE ATHEROMATOUS PLAQUE INFLUENCE DEVELOPMENT OF ACS

The propensity to develop an acute coronary syndrome depends not only on the number, distribution, and severity of stenosis produced by the atheromatous lesions. We must also consider the complex balance of factors extrinsic to the plaque and aspects of the plaque not assessed by the angiogram. We will consider first the extrinsic factors that can trigger acute coronary events. We will then discuss the features of the plaque that may render it susceptible to the factors that may precipitate acute coronary syndromes. In particular, we will review some of the recent advances in the cell and molecular biology of the plaque which provide insight into the fundamental mechanisms that determine the propensity of a plaque to provoke an acute coronary syndrome. Finally, we will consider how clinically employed treatment strategies may affect these various fundamental pathogenic mechanisms underlying the acute coronary syndromes.

Triggering of ACS

The concept that thrombosis complicating an atheroma precipitates the acute coronary syndromes has gained wide acceptance. When such a thrombus does not occlude the artery or undergoes rapid lysis, it may precipitate an episode of rest angina pectoris. If the thrombus propagates such that it persistently occludes the vessel, it can cause acute myocardial infarction, particularly in the absence of adequate collateral circulation. We now understand that a disruption of the atherosclerotic plaque usually provides the thrombogenic stimulus. A number of factors extrinsic to the plaque itself can influence the development of such thrombi. These factors generally involve changes in the blood, including its formed elements, and hemodynamic variables.

A number of studies of the "triggering" of unstable coronary events such as acute myocardial infarction have appeared over the last decade. The work of Muller and colleagues has firmly established a diurnal variation in the incidence of acute myocardial infarction (1). These events tend to occur more in the morning hours than at other times of day. These workers and others have provided evidence that adrenergic stimulation associated with awakening may cause changes in platelet function that promote thrombosis. The finding that treatment with aspirin mitigates this morning peak in incidence of myocardial infarction lends further credence to the notion that augmented thrombotic potential, reflected by enhanced platelet aggregability, contributes to the morning peak in incidence of infarction.

Taken together, the results of these studies on triggers of acute myocardial infarction indicate that altered platelet function or adrenergic state can contribute to the precipitation of the acute coronary syndromes. Adrenergic stimulation such as that produced by unaccustomed effort or emotion, by altering local hydrodynamics impinging on the plaque, may influence the *timing* of "harvest" of vulnerable atherosclerotic lesions. However, the biological substrate of the potentially unstable plaque is the sine qua non of the thrombotic complications of atherosclerosis. The prevailing balance of thrombotic potential versus fibinolysis can determine whether an acute disruption of a plaque yields a disastrous total occlusion or an asymptomatic small mural or intramural thrombosis.

Potential Mechanisms of Triggering of ACS

In addition to altered platelet function, triggering of acute coronary syndromes may also occur because of altered hemodynamics that can increase the physical forces encountered by the atherosclerotic plaque and hence hasten its disruption and the consequent thrombosis. Bioengineering studies have firmly established a marked heterogeneity of physical stresses in different regions of atherosclerotic plaques that contribute to plaque rupture and subsequent thrombosis (2–7). Some of these studies have used an engineering technique known as finite element analysis in conjunction with measurements of the mechanical properties of the various types of human atherosclerotic plaques. The results have established that the thicker the fibrous portion of the plaque covering the thrombogenic lipid core, the less the circumferential wall stress. In addition, as the size of the soft lipid core of the plaque increases, the more circumferential stresses will increase, particularly in the "shoulder" region of an eccentric atheroma. Perhaps less intuitively, these measurements and calculations reveal that stenosis severity has little influence on plaque stresses. In fact, these studies show that the greater the degree of luminal stenosis a plaque causes, the lower the circumferential wall stress it will experience.

Aside from increases in the thrombogenic potential of platelets, adrenergic stimulation produced by awakening or by triggering events modeled by the Northridge earthquake could change the local hemodynamics in the coronary circulation, and thus the forces brought to bear on a potentially unstable plaque (8). Similar to Laplace's law, the circumferential wall stress varies directly with the luminal pressure. An increase in diastolic pressure, the maximum encountered by a coronary artery plaque, would augment circumferential stress and hence the propensity to rupture. An increased frequency or force of myocardial contraction elicited by adrenergic stimuli could augment the compressive forces on a plaque, also potentially precipitating disruption and consequent thrombosis, although direct evidence for such a hypothesis is lacking.

In addition to platelet function, a number of properties extrinsic to the plaque can influence the thrombotic potential. The concentration of fibrinogen in the blood varies directly with coronary risk independent of other factors (9). An elevated concentration of fibrinogen in the blood might augment the thrombus formation on a disrupted plaque. Many plaque disruptions do not provoke a clinically evident acute coronary syndrome (Table 1). Thus factors such as hyperfibrinogenemia that promote the growth of or promote the stability of a thrombus might tip the balance in favor of a clinically significant plaque disruption.

Quantitative and qualitative variations in plasminogen activator inhibitor 1 (PAI-1), an inhibitor of fibrinolysis, correlate with acute coronary events, particularly acute myocardial infarction in relatively young individuals (10,11). However, the role of specific mutations in the PAI-1 gene are controversial (12). Diminished fibrinolytic potential could stabilize clots and, like hyperfibrinogenemia, render it more likely that a plaque disruption would provoke an evident acute thrombotic event rather than remaining clinically silent.

An additional plasma factor correlated with coronary risk may influence fibrinolysis. Lipoprotein(a), Lp(a), is a form of low-density lipoprotein with apolipoprotein(a) bound to the characteristic protein of low-density lipoprotein, apolipoprotein B. Apolipoprotein(a) has many repeats of the fourth Kringle domain of plasminogen. Lp(a) can compete with plasminogen and thus inhibit its activation to the fibrinolytic enzyme plasmin, impairing the net fibrinolytic capacity of blood. Evidence regarding the importance of

Table 1 Factors That May Modulate the Consequences of Plaque Disruption

Thrombotic/coagulant balance
Platelet function, number
Fibrinogen levels
Tissue factor concentration in the plaque's core
Von Willebrand factor levels, multimerization
Fibrinolytic balance
Endogenous urokinase and tissue-type plasminogen activator levels
Plasminogen activator inhibitor levels and genotype
Lipoprotein(a) levels and genotype (?)

Lp(a) as a risk factor for the acute coronary syndromes is controversial (13). Certainly, the lack of a standardized laboratory method for assessing Lp(a) levels and the genetic heterogeneity of this putative risk factor render its evaluation challenging.

The foregoing factors extrinsic to the plaque potentially regulate the development of acute coronary syndromes by an effect on thrombosis, coagulation, or fibrinolysis. Other factors associated with the plasma may affect the intrinsic features of plaque stability to be discussed below. Such circulating factors that may alter intrinsic aspects of plaque stability include cytokinemia and endotoxemia. These circulating mediators of inflammation and the systemic response to microbial invasion may link a serious systemic illness, usually with fever caused by endotoxin and cytokine release, to development of acute coronary syndromes independent of direct effects on the clotting cascade (14,15).

One cytokine in particular, interleukin-6 (IL-6), can change the pattern of hepatic protein synthesis to one that favors production of the panel of proteins known as "acute phase reactants" (16). For example, IL-6 strongly induces the production of fibrinogen, a plasma protein associated with acute coronary syndromes (17). Consistent and strong clinical evidence link markers of the acute phase response (e.g., serum C-reactive protein or amyloid A levels) to both future risk for acute coronary syndromes and outcome in survivors (18,19). Thus, there exists a complex interplay between risk factors for acute coronary events extrinsic to the plaque and those intrinsic features discussed below.

The foregoing discussion of "triggering" events, and their influence on thrombotic and hemodynamic factors, illustrates how factors extrinsic to the plaque may contribute to the pathogenesis of the acute coronary syndromes. However, without a "vulnerable" atheroma as a substrate, no triggering stimulus would produce a coronary event. The subsequent section will discuss the factors intrinsic to the plaque that determine its susceptibility to these triggering events (Table 2).

Mechanisms of the ACS Intrinsic to the Plaque

Contemporary pathologic studies have firmly established the concept that physical disruption of atherosclerotic plaques most often underlies the thrombosis that produces acute coronary events (20–22). These physical disruptions can occur in two major ways. First, a superficial erosion of the blood vessel may occur uncovering the highly thrombogenic subendothelial basement membrane (Fig. 1) (23,24). The collagen thus exposed activates platelets, and Von Willebrand factor in the basal lamina underlying the endothelium promotes platelet aggregation by binding to glycoprotein Ib on

Table 2 Factors Determining Stability of Atherosclerotic Plaques

Factors extrinsic to the plaque itself regulating stability
Systemic arterial pressure
Intracoronary diastolic pressure
Heart rate
Factors intrinsic to the plaque regulating stability
Thickness of the plaque's fibrous cap
Amount of fibrillar collagen in the lesion's fibrous skeleton
Degree of luminal stenosis (greater stenoses produce less circumferential stress)
Size of the lipid-rich core
Content of macrophages
Level of inflammatory activation of resident cells

the platelet surface. This mechanism, superficial erosion of an atherosclerotic plaque, causes approximately a third of fatal coronary thromboses as shown by autopsy studies.

A frank rupture through the fibrous cap of the atheroma is another common route of plaque destabilization (Fig. 2) (25–27). Such a fracture permits contact of coagulation factors in the blood with highly thrombogenic substances in the plaque's central core. Tissue factor, a potent pro-coagulant, contributes substantially to the thrombotic material in the plaque lipid core (28,29). Tissue factor binds activated Factor VII in blood, markedly accelerating a cascade of events including formation of active Factor X and of the prothrombinase complex, leading to thrombus formation. Moreover, the disturbed flow field in the vicinity of a ruptured plaque may also favor

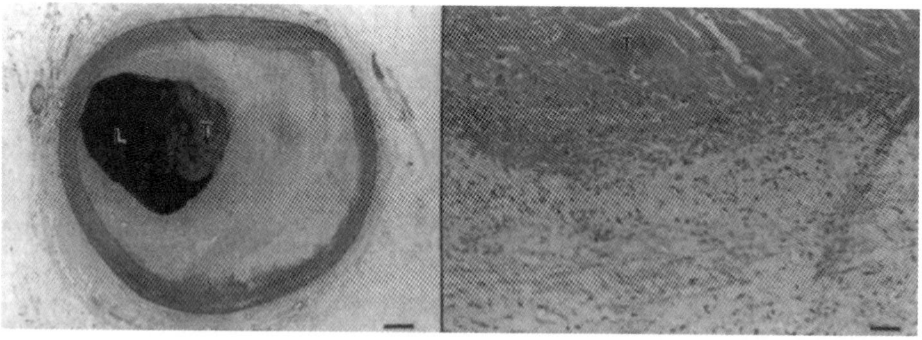

Figure 1 A superficial erosion. Low-power (right) and high-power (left) views of a fatal coronary artery thrombosis originating from a superficial erosion without rupture of the fibrous cap. (From Ref. 23.)

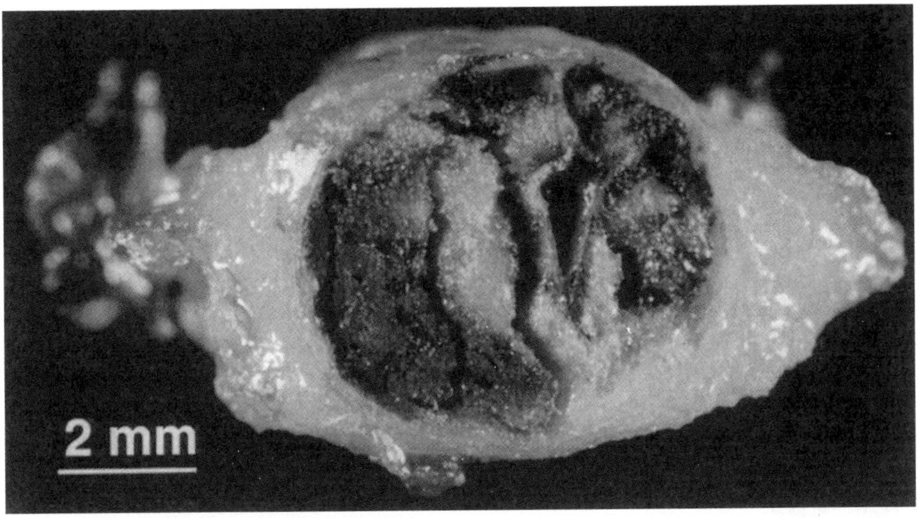

Figure 2 A ruptured plaque. Note the thrombus occluding the lumen (right side) and the intraplaque hemorrhage replacing the lipid core of the atheroma (left side). The fibrous cap separates these two compartments.

thrombosis. This type of plaque disruption accounts for approximately two-thirds of fatal coronary thromboses studied in autopsy series.

Sites of plaque disruption usually exhibit features of inflammation, especially in the case of rupture of the fibrous cap. Regions of atherosclerotic plaques prone to rupture characteristically have numerous macrophages, cells associated with multiple pro-inflammatory processes (2,30). These sites also have prominent accumulations of T lymphocytes (31). Moreover, cells in the vicinity of plaque disruptions frequently display a marker of activation (the histocompatibility molecule HLA-DR) (31). Studies from our laboratory and others have established that the product of activated T-cells, gamma interferon, likely leads to expression of HLA-DR by smooth muscle cells (32,33). Since gamma interferon can impair the ability of the smooth muscle cell to synthesize collagen required to maintain the integrity of the plaque's fibrous cap (34), the expression of this gamma interferon-inducible molecule HLA-DR at the site of disruption has particular importance (see below). Taken together, these findings indicate that the leukocytes at sites of plaque rupture are not merely innocent bystanders, but function in ways that can destabilize plaques.

Pathological studies have revealed several common characteristics of plaques that have ruptured and caused clinical events. These features include

1) a thin fibrous cap, 2) a large lipid core, 3) numerous macrophages, and 4) a relative paucity of smooth muscle cells compared with unruptured regions of plaques (Fig. 3) (35,36). The last several years have witnessed an explosion in knowledge of the molecular and cellular mechanisms which may influence these morphologic features, the functions of cells within the plaque, and their interaction with blood and blood elements. We will consider in turn the mechanisms that have emerged from this avenue of research. In particular, we will focus on the integrity of the plaque's fibrous cap as a

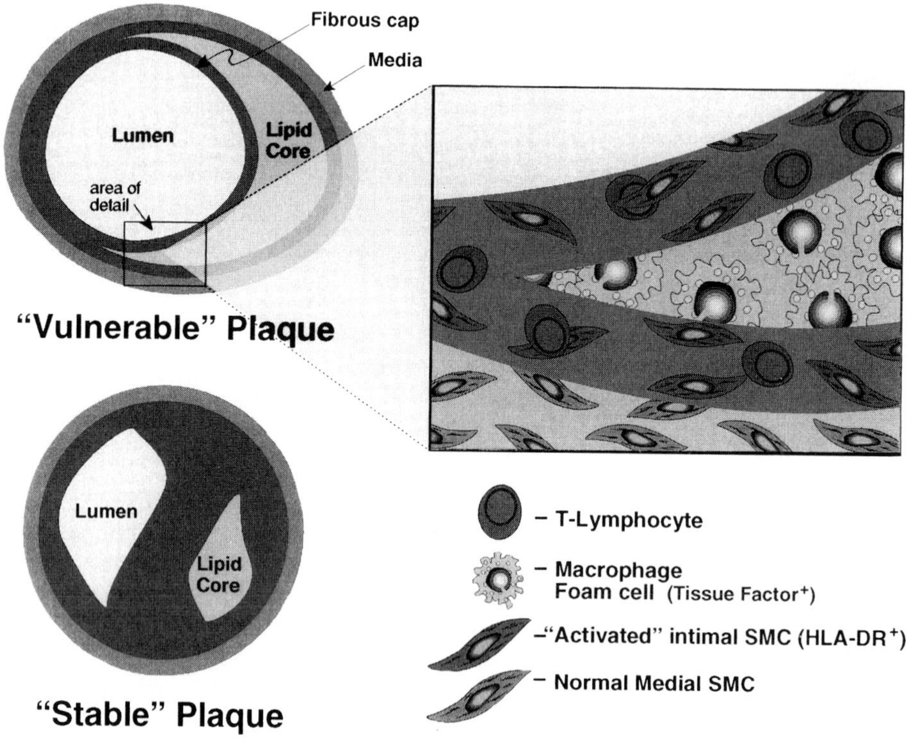

Figure 3 Comparison of the characteristics of "vulnerable" plaques and "stable" plaques. Vulnerable plaques often have a well-preserved lumen, as plaques grow outward initially. The vulnerable plaque typically has a substantial lipid core and a thin fibrous cap separating the thrombogenic macrophages bearing tissue factor from the blood. At sites of lesion disruption, smooth muscle cells are often activated as detected by their expression of the transplantation antigen HLA-DR. In contrast, the stable plaque has a relatively thick fibrous cap protecting the lipid core from contact with the blood. Clinical data suggest that stable plaques more often show luminal narrowing detectable by angiography than do vulnerable plaques. (From Ref. 21.)

crucial determinate of the vulnerability of a given plaque to disruption and hence thrombosis.

PLAQUE RUPTURE AS A PROBLEM OF EXTRACELLULAR MATRIX METABOLISM

The major constituent of the plaque's fibrous cap that confers resistance to rupture is interstitial collagen. Some dozen forms of collagen exist. Those most important in the structural integrity of the atheromatous plaque's fibrous cap include collagens type I and III. These triple helical molecules derive largely from smooth muscle cells found in the plaque. Ordinarily, interstitial collagen fibrils exhibit extraordinary stability. Three distinct mechanisms may alter this usual situation: reduced collagen synthesis, increased collagen breakdown, and loss of smooth muscle cells, the source of most arterial collagen. We will consider each of these mechanisms in turn. In addition, one must consider the biomechanical stresses that impinge upon the artery wall, and when focused on a vulnerable plaque can set the stage for disruption (Fig. 4).

Reduced Collagen Synthesis by Smooth Muscle Cells in Vulnerable Regions of Plaques

Smooth muscle cells under basal conditions produce the interstitial forms of collagen that make up much of the plaque's fibrous skeleton. A number of mediators thought to participate in atherogenesis can augment interstitial collagen production by smooth muscle cells. For example, active transforming growth factor beta or platelet-derived growth factor can stimulate de novo biosynthesis of interstitial forms of collagen by cultured human vascular smooth muscle cells (34). On the other hand, a cytokine known to be present in atherosclerotic plaques, gamma interferon, can inhibit collagen production by human smooth muscle cells in culture (34). Of the cells associated with atheroma, only T lymphocytes can synthesize gamma interferon. As alluded to above, gamma interferon can induce the expression of the activation marker HLA-DR on human smooth muscle cells. Smooth muscle cells bearing HLA-DR concentrate in regions of plaque rupture in association with T lymphocytes (31). Studies of the collagenous skeleton of atherosclerotic plaques have documented reduced levels of fibrillar collagens at sites of plaque rupture (22).

Taken together, these observations suggest the following scenario (Fig. 5). First, activated T cells elaborate the cytokine gamma interferon. Gamma interferon acts on neighboring smooth muscle cells to decrease their production of interstitial collagen. The expression of the gamma interferon-

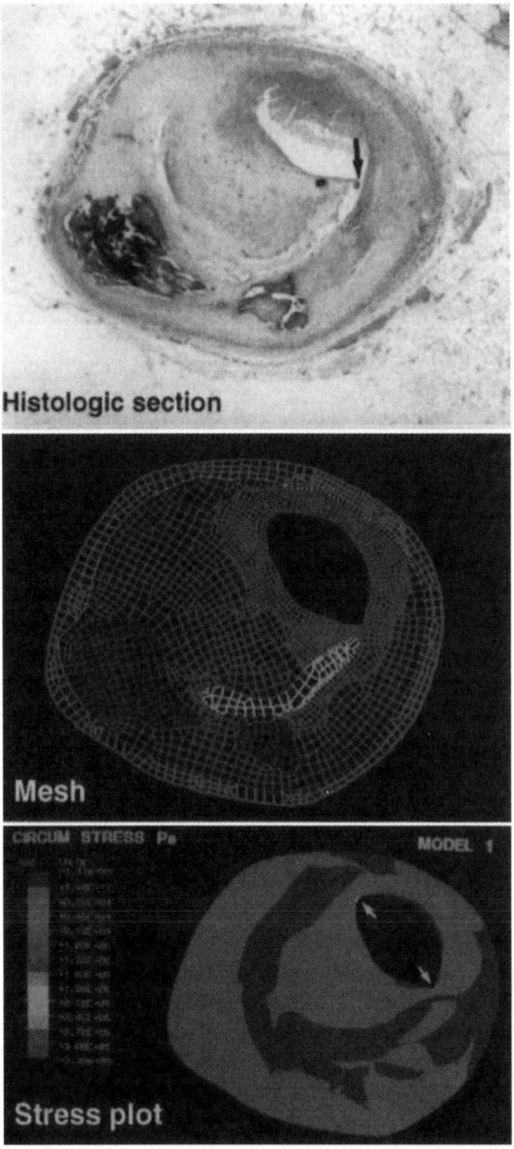

Figure 4 Biomechanical analysis of a human atherosclerotic plaque. The upper panel shows a histological section of the atheroma analyzed. A mesh diagram (middle panel) depicts the finite elements used by the computer to solve the stress equations. The bottom panel shows the stress diagram generated by the computer using the engineering technique denoted finite element analysis. The arrows (bottom panel) point to the "shoulder" region of the plaque, where the circumferential stress (in Pascals, P) as calculated to be maximal by this analysis. (From Ref. 84.)

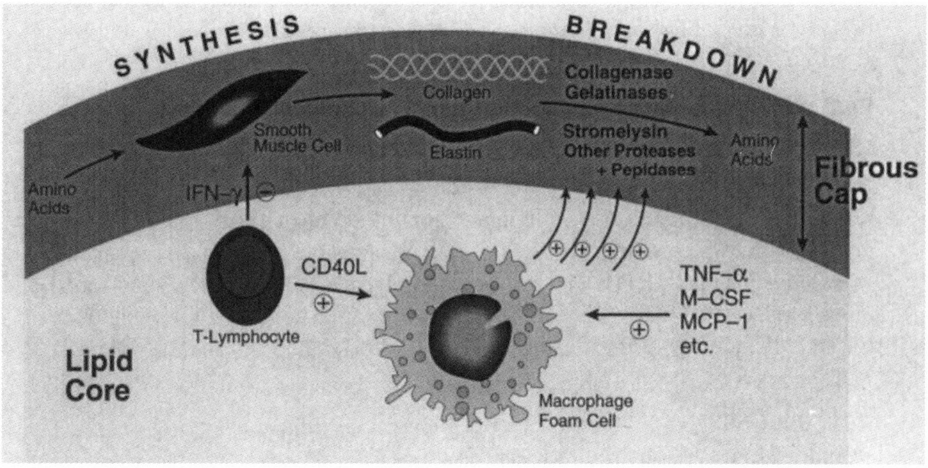

Figure 5 Molecular determinants of the collagen and elastin metabolism in the plaque's fibrous cap. The vascular smooth muscle cell synthesizes the extracellular matrix protein, collagen, and elastin from amino acids. In the unstable plaque, interferon-γ secreted by activated T cells may inhibit collagen synthesis, interfering with the maintenance and repair of the collagenous framework of the plaque's fibrous cap. The activated macrophage secretes proteinases that can break down both collagen and elastin to peptides and eventually amino acids. This breakdown of these structural molecules of the extracellular matrix can weaken the fibrous cap, rendering it particularly susceptible to rupture and precipitation of acute coronary syndromes. The macrophage in turn can be activated by interferon-γ secreted by the T lymphocytes, and by CD40 ligand expressed on the surface of these cells. Plaques also contain other activators of macrophages including tumor necrosis factor-α (TNF-α) macrophage-colony stimulating factor (M-CSF), macrophage chemoattractant protein-1 (MCP-1), and others. (From Ref. 21.)

inducible molecule HLA-DR on the surface of smooth muscle cells argues strongly that these cells have indeed encountered gamma interferon, the inhibitor of collagen synthesis. In this manner, chronic immune stimulation within the complicated atheroma, manifested by the activated T lymphocytes, can directly influence a function of the arterial smooth muscle cell that may determine the susceptibility of that particular region of the plaque to disruption.

Increased Degradation of Extracellular Matrix May Contribute to Weakening of the Plaque's Fibrous Skeleton

As noted above, fibrillar collagen resists breakdown by usual proteases. The initial proteolytic attack on fibrillar collagen molecules generally requires the action of a small family of highly specialized enzymes known as interstitial collagenases. These enzymes, like other members of the matrix metalloproteinase (MMP) family, require a zinc atom for their activity, hence their designation as metalloenzymes. Other members of this metalloproteinase family known as gelatinases carry on subsequent steps in the degradation of collagen fragments produced by the action of interstitial collagenase. Yet other members of the MMP family such as stromelysin can break down elastin, the core proteins of proteoglycans, and activate the precursor forms of other members of the MMP family, a step required for them to act enzymatically.

Under ordinary circumstances, cells within human arteries contain negligible amounts of the active forms of these specialized matrix-degrading enzymes. However, various cell types in vulnerable regions of human atherosclerotic plaques can express interstitial collagenase, gelatinases, and stromelysin (37–39). In particular, macrophage-derived foam cells express high levels of these MMPs (40). Substantial recent evidence suggests an important role for macrophage-derived metalloproteinases as contributors to a net increase in matrix-degrading activity in regions of inflammation within human and experimentally produced atherosclerotic plaques. For example, human macrophages elaborate activity that breaks down the collagen in fibrous caps isolated from actual human atheroma (41). Such data indicate a role for active breakdown of fibrillar collagen in the plaque fibrous cap as yet another mechanism that links the inflammatory response in vulnerable regions of atheroma with their susceptibility to rupture (Fig. 5).

Mere overexpression of MMP proteins, however, does not prove that an actual excess of enzymatic activity prevails. Like most protease systems involved in control of critical biological processes, a number of tightly regulated mechanisms control the MMPs. First, these enzymes exist first as inactive zymogen precursors. Serine proteases such as plasmin appear important in activating the MMPs to their catalytic forms from their enzymatically inactive zymogen precursors. Second, a series of endogenous inhibitors, the tissue inhibitors of metalloproteinases (TIMPs) hold in check the function of the enzymes following their conversion from the pro-enzyme to their active form. Arterial tissue and cells found within atheroma express all four known TIMPs (38,42–45). Hence, assessment of the importance of overexpression of MMP proteins requires more than immunostaining. The antibodies currently available do not distinguish the pro-enzyme from the active forms of MMPs. Weighing the balance between the MMPs and their inhibitors in tissues presents a daunting biochemical challenge.

To overcome this problem we have used several approaches. First, we have used gelatin zymography to demonstrate the existence of active forms of the gelatinolytic MMPs (MMP-2 and MMP-9) in extracts of atheroma

(38). The active forms of these enzymes have greater electrophoretic mobility than the zymogens. In contrast, normal arteries contain pro-MMP-2, but little MMP-9 or active form of MMP-2. We have used in situ zymographic approaches to demonstrate actual gelatinolytic or caseinolytic activity in frozen sections of vascular tissue. However, this technique lacks biochemical rigor, and may be confounded by artifacts (46).

We have recently used a novel approach to demonstrate the action of interstitial collagenase in advanced human atheroma. The interstitial collagenases make a stereotyped proteolytic attack at a single site on the intact collagen fibril, breaking it into fragments 1/4 and 3/4 of its native length. This limited cleavage uncovers a new carboxy terminus in the partially degraded molecule. Using an antibody that selectively recognizes this cleavage epitope, we have demonstrated the signature of the action of interstitial collagenase in a series of human atherosclerotic plaques (47). The collagen cleavage product in human plaques colocalizes with macrophages overexpressing MMPs 1 and 13, two of three mammalian enzymes thought capable of cleaving collagen fibrils (47). The third human interstitial collagenase, MMP-8, derives from neutrophils, a cell type not found in the human atherosclerotic intima before disruption.

Although much interest has recently focused on MMPs as contributors to extracellular matrix degradation in atheroma, increasing evidence suggests roles for nonmetalloenzymes in this process as well. For example, cells in human atheroma exhibit expression of a potent elastolytic enzyme, cathepsin S, that depends on a cysteinyl residue at the active site for catalytic activity rather than coordinated zinc atoms as in the case of the matrix metalloproteinases (48). Much of the elastolytic activity in extracts of human atheroma resembles cathepsin S, and does not depend on metal ions. Like the MMPs, these cysteinyl proteinases have endogenous inhibitors, constitutively expressed in normal arterial tissue. We have recently described a deficiency of a key inhibitor of cysteinyl elastases, cystatin C, in human atherosclerotic lesions (49). Thus, an excess of elastolytic activity may prevail in advanced human atheroma and aneurysmal tissue. These results establish that excess proteolysis in atheroma involves not only MMPs, but cysteine- and serine-dependent nonmetalloproteinses. Therefore attempts to prevent acute coronary syndromes with MMP antagonists may not inhibit the full spectrum of enzymes involved in remodeling of the arterial extracellular matrix.

Smooth Muscle Cell Cytostasis and Death as a Contributor to Plaque Vulnerability

Over recent decades, a great deal of research effort in atherosclerosis has focused on factors that augment smooth muscle proliferation, predicated on accumulation of smooth muscle cells as a prominent process in plaque growth. However, pathological studies of the characteristics of rupture-prone plaques have disclosed a relative paucity of smooth muscle cells at sites where plaques rupture and cause thrombosis (31,35). Indeed, many mature atherosclerotic plaques exhibit low degrees of cellularity in their fibrous portions. As noted above, the plaque's extracellular matrix derives almost entirely from the arterial smooth muscle cell. In this manner, smooth muscle cells almost certainly contribute to the formation of fibrous atherosclerotic plaques. The accumulation of extracellular matrix may occur relatively early in the life cycle of a plaque. Alternatively, smooth muscle proliferation and matrix elaboration may occur as a consequence of episodes of plaque disruption, with mural thrombosis. (Such events may occur rather commonly, and probably usually produce no clinical manifestations.) As such mural thrombi heal, smooth muscle cells may migrate into the scaffolding provided by the clot and elaborate a mature, crosslinked, collagenous matrix that replaces the provisional matrix afforded by the fibrin clot.

However, in the vulnerable plaque, the relative absence of smooth muscle cells may actually promote weakening of the fibrous cap by removing the very source of the interstitial collagen, elastin, and proteoglycan that make up the plaque matrix. According to this view, the smooth muscle cell may promote plaque growth at some point in the history of an atherosclerotic plaque. However this cell type also participates in the repair and maintenance of the matrix of the plaque's fibrous cap, as described above (50–52).

What mechanisms might lead to the relative lack of smooth muscle cells in vulnerable regions of human atheroma? Interestingly, gamma interferon, the same T cell-derived cytokine that can impede collagen synthesis by these cells, can also act as a cytostatic agent. Exposure of smooth muscle cells to gamma interferon in vitro or in vivo in experimental animals can inhibit smooth muscle cell replication (53,54). We have already reviewed the reasons to believe that T lymphocytes within vulnerable portions of atheroma secrete gamma interferon. Thus, inhibited growth of smooth muscle cells could contribute to their scarcity in regions of inflammation and increased propensity to rupture of human atheroma.

Smooth muscle cells within atheroma may die. Indeed, many of these cells may succumb to a form of programmed cell death know as apoptosis (50,55,56). Certain cytokines found in human atheroma, gamma interferon, tumor necrosis factor alpha, and interleukin-1 beta can act together to unleash the apoptotic pathway of cell death in cultured smooth muscle cells (57). Smooth muscle cells "primed" by exposure to these pro-inflammatory cytokines can undergo apoptosis when Fas, a cell surface receptor for a TNF-like ligand, is stimulated (58). We have moreover colocalized dying smooth muscle cells with interleukin-1 beta-converting enzyme (50). This specialized cysteine protease cleaves the inactive precursor form of interleukin-1 beta to its biologically active form. Interestingly, this enzyme belongs to a newly recognized family of proteinases that participate in the apoptotic cell death pathway. While the key substrates for these enzymes remain in general incompletely identified, the interleukin-1-beta-converting enzyme can activate IL-1 beta. Thus, inflammation, mediated by cytokines, can lead to smooth muscle death, another mechanism which may impair the integrity of the plaque's fibrous cap. Recent evidence has also implicated Fas-induced cell death in the extreme form of arterial remodeling encountered in aortic aneurysms (59).

MECHANISMS OF SUPERFICIAL EROSION OF PLAQUES

Pathologists generally agree that superficial erosion of the intima without frank fracture of the fibrous cap causes a substantial minority of acute coronary thromboses. Virmani's group has further presented evidence that this type of plaque disruption plays a particularly important role in sudden coronary death in women and diabetics, based on detailed and elegant study of selected referral cases from medical examiners (60,61). The endothelial lining of the intima usually displays a gamut of anticoagulant and pro-fibrinolytic functions which combat clotting. Desquamation of endothelium likewise uncovers a basement membrane rich in nonfibrillar collagens that can trigger thrombosis. Vitronectin in the subendothelial matrix binds plasminogen activator inhibitor 1 (PAI-1), a major inactivator of fibrinolytic enzymes (62,63). Hence, the loss of endothelium may promote thrombus accumulation in several ways.

Little direct evidence regarding the mechanisms of superficial erosion of plaques exists. However, the same fundamental processes involved in rupture of the fibrous cap may operate in this mode of thrombus formation as well: proteolysis and cell death (Fig. 6). Endothelial cells and inflammatory cells in atheroma alike can secrete precursors of the subclass of MMPs known as gelatinases. One of these gelatinases in particular, known as MMP-2, or gelatinase A, efficiently degrades type IV collagen, the principal collagen type in the subendothelial basement membrane. Moreover, when encountering inflammatory stimuli such as oxidized low-density lipoprotein or certain cytokines, endothelial cells can augment their expression of membrane-type MMP (MMP-14), which activates pro-MMP-2 into its catalytic form (64). Thus, in a pro-inflammatory environment, active gelatinases may be elaborated which can dissolve the matrix to which endothelial cells adhere, rendering them more susceptible to sloughing, and favoring local thrombus formation (Fig. 6).

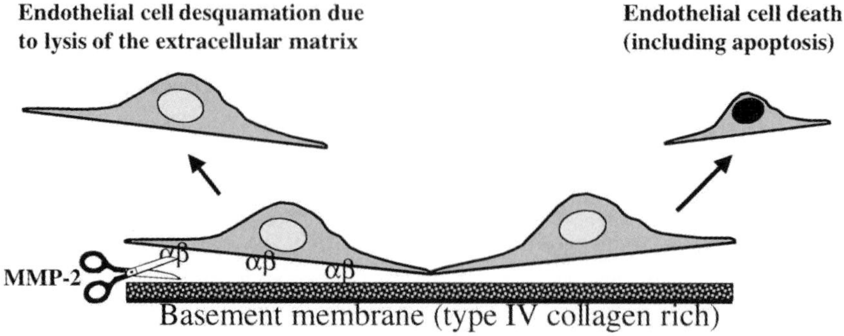

Figure 6 Potential mechanisms of superficial erosion causing coronary thrombosis. Death of endothelial cells, including apoptotic cell death, may lead to desquamation and promote thrombosis as platelets encounter subendothelial collagen pro-aggregatory apoptotic cells. Lysis of basement membrane (type IV) collagen by type IV collagenase (MMP-2) activated by inflammatory mediators may hasten endothelial apoptosis and desquamation as well. The endothelial cells bind to their subjacent matrix in part through membrane integrins, here depicted as alpha and beta.

Endothelial cells may also desquamate if they die. A number of proinflammatory mediators can promote endothelial cell death by apoptosis (65). Indeed, endothelial cells undergoing apoptosis can augment platelet adhesion, a critical step in arterial thrombosis (66). These examples illustrate how inflammation, now well accepted as a component of plaque rupture, may favor superficial erosion and thrombosis as well by stimulating local proteolysis and endothelial cell death.

CONCLUSIONS AND CLINICAL/THERAPEUTIC IMPLICATIONS

We have considered various mechanisms that may lead to the acute coronary syndromes. In particular, we have focused on factors external to the plaque which may trigger disruption and hence thrombosis. Moreover, we have examined some of the recent work that has increased our understanding of the mechanisms that determine the susceptibility of a given atherosclerotic plaque to disruption.

For the clinician, the importance of understanding these mechanisms relates to our ability to prevent acute coronary syndromes or treat them effectively. What preventive and therapeutic conclusion can we derive from the mechanistic work described above? Increased platelet aggregability seems important in the timing of thrombosis. The ability of aspirin treatment to mitigate the morning peak in the incidence of acute myocardial infarction indicates that interfering with platelet function can indeed inhibit acute coronary events (67,68). Aspirin treatment now enjoys wide application for this indication in secondary prevention of acute coronary syndromes. Many have adopted low-dose aspirin treatment as a therapeutic strategy in primary prevention, particularly of individuals at risk for coronary heart disease.

Another important aspect of the adrenergic stimulation associated with triggering of coronary events involves altered hemodynamics. Perhaps part of the benefit of beta blocker therapy in reducing reinfarction derives from an inhibition of some of the hemodynamic consequences of adrenergic stimulation that may impinge upon a potentially vulnerable plaque and provoke an acute coronary syndrome. Beta blockers should be employed in appropriately selected patients in secondary prevention of acute coronary syndromes. The penetration of this therapy into practice has lagged that of aspirin treatment (69).

With respect to some of the other extrinsic factors associated with increased risk for acute coronary events, specific therapies are either unavailable or seldom employed. Fibric acid derivatives used to treat certain dyslipidemias including hypertriglyceridemia, can also reduce fibrinogen concentration. The effectiveness of fibrates in reducing acute coronary events in trials such as the Helsinki Heart Study and the recent VA-HIT study could conceivably derive in part from a reduction in fibrinogen (70). Unfortunately, to date, therapeutic options effective for lowering Lp(a) are quite limited. This represents one area in which future drug development might prove productive in reducing acute coronary events. Likewise, no currently available therapeutic agents target plasminogen activator inhibitor 1, another risk factor for acute coronary events. This constitutes another potential target for intervention in the future.

With regard to the intrinsic aspects of plaque biology that govern susceptibility to disruption, the common theme is inflammation. One could envisage several strategies for interfering with this pathogenic cascade. One might target very distal mediators of this process such as the MMPs. Inhibitors of these enzymes do exist, and there is interest in exploring their utility as therapeutic agents in the context of the acute coronary syndromes. Experimental data suggest that MMP inhibition can delay neo-intima formation in various animal preparations (71,72). However, appropriate animal models for testing the effects of such agents in preventing plaque rupture do not yet exist.

Another therapeutic strategy might target the cytokines that mediate many of the aspects of plaque biology that can lead to vulnerability. A number of cytokine antagonists exist. Some have been employed in clinical trials designed to test their effectiveness in such systemic conditions as sepsis or adult respiratory distress syndrome. To date, these applications of cytokine antagonists have proven rather disappointing (73). The delivery of these agents to the arterial wall and the length of time that they might have to be administered render the indication of prevention or treatment of the acute coronary syndromes even more difficult than the "systemic" indications that have already been explored.

One can take one step back and try to imagine ways of removing the inflammatory stimulus to the cytokine production and thus of the distal effectors of plaque disruption such as MMPs. The current concepts of stimuli for inflammation in atherogenesis have concentrated on derivatives of lipoproteins. In particular, oxidized lipoproteins may elicit cytokine production and thus stimulate local inflammation within plaques. Lipid lowering strikingly reduces acute coronary events. We have proposed that reduction in LDL can act as an anti-inflammatory therapy in this regard (74). There is also currently interest in the concept of the HMG-CoA reductase inhibitors may reduce coronary events not only by lowering low-density lipoprotein but also by directly inhibiting pro-inflammatory pathways in the artery well. The reductase inhibitors indeed interfere with a number of biochemically important pathways such as prenylation of proteins important in certain types of signal transduction in smooth muscle cells, leukocytes, and other cells (75). In particular, excellent in vivo evidence documents an effect of HMG-CoA reductase inhibitors in cerebral ischemia reperfusion independent of lipid lowering (76). This effect derives in large part from augmented levels of endothelial nitric oxide synthase, the source of the vasodilatory and antiaggregatory nitric oxide radical.

Oxidation of lipoproteins represents a specific case of so-called "oxidative stress" which may trigger cytokine gene transcription, often through the common pathway of activation of a transcription factor known as nuclear factor κB (NFκB) (77). General antioxidant strategies might thus limit inflammation within plaques, although studies with carotenoids and with vitamin E have proven disappointing in this regard (78–80). Controlled prospective clinical trials with vitamin C have not yet emerged to support roles for this antioxidant vitamin in reducing coronary events. Other pharmacologic antioxidants might be expected to exert beneficial effects on plaque inflammation. However, one must bear in mind the disappointing results of the PQRST study of the potent lipid soluble antioxidant probucol in this context (81).

Another potential target for interrupting inflammatory activation in atheroma could involve inhibition of activation of the transcriptional pathway mediated by NFκB. Various strategies have been developed, including blocking the degradation of the endogenous inhibitor of this pathway IκB alpha (82). Interestingly, nitric oxide, the endogenous vasodilator mentioned above, also exerts anti-inflammatory effects on vascular wall cells by stabilizing IκB alpha (83). Thus, strategies that augment local NO production, or decrease its catabolism or inactivation, might limit vascular inflammation. One pathway of nitric oxide inactivation that operates in the vessel wall is reaction with superoxide anion (O_2^-). The oxidases that give rise to superoxide anion are currently the subject of intense scrutiny in a number of laboratories and may represent yet another pharmacologic target for limiting inflammation within atheroma (83). Indeed, as angiotensin II augments O_2^- production from vascular wall cells, angiotensin-converting enzyme (ACE) inhibitors may actually function as antioxidants. This effect, unrelated to the blood pressure-lowering actions of this class of drugs, might contribute to the consistent and unexpected benefit of ACE inhibitor therapy in regard to acute coronary events, most recently affirmed by the HOPE study (80).

Although the future prospects for identifying new pharmacologic targets and developing therapeutic strategies remain intriguing, we must use existing agents for the care of our patients at risk for acute coronary syndromes at present. The penetration of use of aspirin is quite satisfactory. The use of beta blockers among physicians could improve. The application of lipid-lowering strategies still lags considerably. We should strive as we evaluate and develop treatment and management plans for patients at risk for acute coronary syndromes to apply the results of recent clinical trials and increase the utilization of lipid-lowering treatment in appropriately selected patients. We need to employ our pharmaceutical armamentarium with the same alacrity that we have deployed our interventional skills in the past. A true mastery of the biology of the arterial wall may one day render less common the need for some of the end-stage interventions with which we have become so adept.

REFERENCES

1. Muller JE, Abela GS, Nesto RW, Tofler GH. Triggers, acute risk factors and vulnerable plaques: the lexicon of a new frontier. J Am Coll Cardiol 1994;23: 809–813.
2. Lendon CL, Davies MJ, Born GV, Richardson PD. Atherosclerotic plaque caps are locally weakened when macrophages density is increased. Atherosclerosis 1991;87:87–90.
3. Loree HM, Tobias BJ, Gibson LJ, Kamm RD, Small DM, Lee RT. Mechanical properties of model atherosclerotic lesion lipid pools. Arterioscler Thromb 1994;14:230–234.
4. Loree HM, Grodzinsky AJ, Park SY, Gibson LJ, Lee RT. Static circumferential tangential modulus of human atherosclerotic tissue. J Biomech 1994;27:195–204.

5. Loree HM, Kamm RD, Stringfellow RG, Lee RT. Effects of fibrous cap thickness on peak circumferential stress in model atherosclerotic vessels. Circ Res 1992;71:850–858.
6. Lee RT, Richardson SG, Loree HM, Grodzinsky AJ, Gharib SA, Schoen FJ, Pandian N. Prediction of mechanical properties of human atherosclerotic tissue by high-frequency intravascular ultrasound imaging. An in vitro study. Arterioscler Thromb 1992;12:1–5.
7. Lee R, Libby P. The unstable atheroma. Arterioscler Thromb Vasc Biol 1997; 17:1859–1867.
8. Leor J, Poole WK, Kloner RA. Sudden cardiac death triggered by an earthquake. N Engl J Med 1996;334:413–419.
9. Thompson SG, Kienast J, Pyke SD, Haverkate F, van de Loo JC. Hemostatic factors and the risk of myocardial infarction or sudden death in patients with angina pectoris. European Concerted Action on Thrombosis and Disabilities Angina Pectoris Study Group. N Engl J Med 1995;332:635–641.
10. Humphries SE, Green FR, Temple A, Dawson S, Henney A, Kelleher CH, Wilkes H, Meade TW, Wiman B, Hamsten A. Genetic factors determining thrombosis and fibrinolysis. Ann Epidemiol 1992;2:371–385.
11. Eriksson P, Kallin B, van't Hooft F, Bavenholm P, Hamsten A. Allele-specific increase in basal transcription of the plasminogen-activator inhibitor 1 gene is associated with myocardial infarction. Proc Natl Acad Sci USA 1995;92:1851–1855.
12. Ridker PM, Hennekens CH, Lindpaintner K, Stampfer MJ, Miletich JP. Arterial and venous thrombosis is not associated with the 4G/5G polymorphism in the promoter of the plasminogen activator inhibitor gene in a large cohort of US men. Circulation 1997;95:59–62.
13. Scanu AM. Atherothrombogenicity of lipoprotein(a): the debate. Am J Cardiol 1998;82:26Q–33Q.
14. Fleet JC, Clinton SK, Salomon RN, Loppnow H, Libby P. Atherogenic diets enhance endotoxin-stimulated interleukin-1 and tumor necrosis factor gene expression in rabbit aortae. J Nutr 1992;122:294–305.
15. Libby P, Egan D, Skarlatos S. Roles of infectious agents in atherosclerosis and restenosis: an assessment of the evidence and need for future research. Circulation 1997;96:4095–4103.
16. Gabay C, Kushner I. Acute-phase proteins and other systemic responses to inflammation [published erratum appears in N Engl J Med 1999 Apr 29; 340(17):1376]. N Engl J Med 1999;340:448–454.
17. Nijsten MWN, De Groot ER, Ten Duis HJ, Klasen HJ, Hack CE, Aarden LA. Serum levels of IL6 and acute phase responses. Lancet 1987;2:921.
18. Ridker PM, Cushman M, Stampfer MJ, Tracy RP, Hennekens CH. Inflammation, aspirin, and the risk of cardiovascular disease in apparently healthy men [published erratum appears in N Engl J Med 1997 Jul 31;337(5):356]. N Engl J Med 1997;336:973–979.
19. Ridker PM. C-reactive protein and risks of future myocardial infarction and thrombotic stroke. Eur Heart J 1998;19:1–3.

20. Falk E, Shah P, Fuster V. Coronary plaque disruption. Circulation 1995;92: 657–671.
21. Libby P. The molecular bases of the acute coronary syndromes. Circulation 1995;91:2844–2850.
22. Davies MJ. Stability and instability: the two faces of coronary atherosclerosis. The Paul Dudly White Lecture, 1995. Circulation 1996;94:2013–2020.
23. Farb A, Burke A, Tang A, Liang Y, Mannan P, Smialek J, Virmani R. Coronary plaque erosion without rupture into a lipid core. A frequent cause of coronary thrombosis in sudden coronary death. Circulation 1996;93:1354–1363.
24. Burke A, Farb A, Malcom G, Liang Y-H, Smialek J, Virmani R. Coronary risk factors and plaque morphology in men with coronary disease who died suddenly. N Engl J Med 1997;336:1276–1282.
25. Davies MJ, Thomas T. The pathological basis and microanatomy of occlusive thrombus formation in human coronary arteries. Phil Trans R Soc Lond (Biol) 1981;294:225–229.
26. Falk E. Plaque rupture with severe pre-existing stenosis precipitating coronary thrombosis characteristics of coronary atherosclerotic plaques underlying fatal occlusive thrombi. Br Heart J 1983;50:127–134.
27. Constantinides P. Plaque hemorrhages, their genesis and their role in supra-plaque thrombosis and atherogenesis. In: Glagov S, Newman WPI, Schaffer SA, eds. Pathobiology of the Human Atherosclerotic Plaque. New York: Springer-Verlag, 1989:393–412.
28. Wilcox JN, Smith KM, Schwartz SM, Gordon D. Localization of tissue factor in the normal vessel wall and in the atherosclerotic plaque. Proc Natl Acad Sci USA 1989;86:2839–2843.
29. Drake TA, Morrissey JH, Edgington TS. Selective cellular expression of tissue factor in human tissues. Implications for disorders of hemostasis and thrombosis. Am J Pathol 1989;134:1087–1097.
30. Moreno PR, Falk E, Palacios IF, Newell JB, Fuster V, Fallon JT. Macrophage infiltration in acute coronary syndromes. Implications for plaque rupture. Circulation 1994;90:775–778.
31. van der Wal AC, Becker AE, van der Loos CM, Das PK. Site of intimal rupture or erosion of thrombosed coronary atherosclerotic plaques is characterized by an inflammatory process irrespective of the dominant plaque morphology. Circulation 1994;89:36–44.
32. Pober JS, Collins T, Gimbrone MA, Jr., Libby P, Reiss CS. Inducible expression of class II major histocompatibility complex antigens and the immunogenicity of vascular endothelium. Transplantation 1986;41:141–146.
33. Warner SJC, Friedman GB, Libby P. Regulation of major histocompatibility gene expression in cultured human vascular smooth muscle cells. Arteriosclerosis 1989;9:279–288.
34. Amento EP, Ehsani N, Palmer H, Libby P. Cytokines positively and negatively regulate intersitial collagen gene expression in human vascular smooth muscle cells. Arteriosclerosis 1991;11:1223–1230.
35. Davies MJ, Richardson PD, Woolf N, Katz DR, Mann J. Risk of thrombosis

in human atherosclerotic plaques: role of extracellular lipid, macrophage, and smooth muscle cell content. Br Heart J 1993;69:377–381.

36. Davies M. The composition of coronary-artery plaques. N Engl J Med 1997; 336:1312–1314.
37. Henney AM, Wakeley PR, Davies MJ, Foster K, Hembry R, Murphy G, Humphries S. Localization of stromelysin gene expression in atherosclerotic plaques by in situ hybridization. Proc Natl Acad Sci USA 1991;88:8154–8158.
38. Galis Z, Sukhova G, Lark M, Libby P. Increased expression of matrix metalloproteinases and matrix degrading activity in vulnerable regions of human atherosclerotic plaques. J Clin Invest 1994;94:2493–2503.
39. Nikkari ST, O'Brien KD, Ferguson M, Hatsukami T, Welgus HG, Alpers CE, Clowes AW. Interstitial collagenase (MMP-1) expression in human carotid atherosclerosis. Circulation 1995;92:1393–1398.
40. Galis Z, Sukhova G, Kranzhöfer R, Clark S, Libby P. Macrophage foam cells from experimental atheroma constitutively produce matrix-degrading proteinases. Proc Natl Acad Sci USA 1995;92:402–406.
41. Shah PK, Falk E, Badimon JJ, Fernandez-Ortiz A, Mailhac A, Villareal-Levy G, Fallon JT, Regnstrom J, Fuster V. Human monocyte-derived macrophages induce collagen breakdown in fibrous caps of atherosclerotic plaques. Potential role of matrix-degrading metalloproteinases and implications for plaque rupture. Circulation 1995;92:1565–1569.
42. Galis Z, Muszynski M, Sukhova G, Simon-Morrisey E, Unemori E, Lark M, Amento E, Libby P. Cytokine-stimulated human vascular smooth muscle cells synthesize a complement of enzymes required for extracellular matrix digestion. Circ Res 1994;75:181–189.
43. Knox JB, Sukhova GK, Whittemore AD, Libby P. Evidence for altered balance between matrix metalloproteinases and their inhibitors in human aortic diseases. Circulation 1997;94.
44. Fabunmi RP, Sukhova GK, Sugiyama S, Libby P. Expression of tissue inhibitor of metalloproteinases-3 in human atheroma and regulation in lesion-associated cells: a potential protective mechanism in plaque stability. Circ Res 1998;83: 270–278.
45. Dollery CM, McEwan JR, Wang M, Sang QA, Liu YE, Shi YE. TIMP-4 is regulated by vascular injury in rats. Ann NY Acad Sci 1999;878:740–741.
46. Galis Z, Sukhova G, Libby P. Microscopic localization of active proteases by in situ zymography. Detection of matrix metalloproteinase activity in vascular tissue. FASEB J 1995;9:974–980.
47. Sukhova GK, Schonbeck U, Rabkin E, Schoen FJ, Poole AR, Billinghurst RC, Libby P. Evidence for increased collagenolysis by interstitial collagenases-1 and -3 in vulnerable human atheromatous plaques. Circulation 1999;99:2503–2509.
48. Sukhova GK, Shi GP, Simon DI, Chapman HA, Libby P. Expression of the elastolytic cathepsins S and K in human atheroma and regulation of their production in smooth muscle cells. J Clin Invest 1998;102:576–583.
49. Shi GP, Sukhova GK, Grubb A, Ducharme A, Rhode LH, Lee RT, Ridker PM,

Libby P, Chapman HA. Cystatin C deficiency in human atherosclerosis and aortic aneurysms. J Clin Invest 1999;104:1191–1197.
50. Geng Y-J, Libby P. Evidence for apoptosis in advanced human atheroma. Co-localization with interleukin-1 β-converting enzyme. Am J Pathol 1995;147: 251–266.
51. Lafont A, Libby P. The smooth muscle cell: sinner or saint in restenosis and the acute coronary syndromes? J Am Coll Cardiol 1998;32:283–285.
52. Weissberg PL, Clesham GJ, Bennett MR. Is vascular smooth muscle cell proliferation beneficial? Lancet 1996;347:305–307.
53. Hansson GK, Jonasson L, Holm J, Clowes MK, Clowes A. Gamma interferon regulates vascular smooth muscle proliferation and Ia expression in vivo and in vitro. Circ Res 1988;63:712–719.
54. Warner SJC, Friedman GB, Libby P. Immune interferon inhibits proliferation and induces 2′-5′-oligoadenylate synthetase gene expression in human vascular smooth muscle cells. J Clin Invest 1989;83:1174–1182.
55. Han D, Haudenschild C, Hong M, Tinkle B, Leon M, Liau G. Evidence for apoptosis in human atherogenesis and in a rat vascular injury model. Am J Pathol 1995;147:267–277.
56. Isner JM, Kearney M, Bortman S, Passeri J. Apoptosis in human atherosclerosis and restenosis. Circulation 1995;91:2703–2711.
57. Geng Y-J, Wu Q, Muszynski M, Hansson G, Libby P. Apoptosis of vascular smooth muscle cells induced by in vitro stimulation with interferon-gamma, tumor necrosis factor-alpha, and interleukin-1-beta. Arterioscler Thromb Vasc Biol 1996;16:19–27.
58. Geng Y-J, Henderson L, Levesque E, Muszynski M, Libby P. Fas is expressed in human atherosclerotic intima and promotes apoptosis of cytokine-primed humann vascular smooth muscle cells. Arterioscler Thromb Vasc Biol 1997; 17:2200–2208.
59. Henderson EL, Geng YJ, Sukhova GK, Whittemore AD, Knox J, Libby P. Death of smooth muscle cells and expression of mediators of apoptosis by T lymphocytes in human abdominal aortic aneurysms. Circulation 1999;99:96–104.
60. Burke AP, Farb A, Malcom GT, Liang Y, Smialek J, Virmani R. Effect of risk factors on the mechanism of acute thrombosis and sudden coronary death in women. Circulation 1998;97:2110–2116.
61. Virmani R, Farb A, Burke AP. Risk factors in the pathogenesis of coronary artery disease. Compr Ther 1998;24:519–529.
62. Loskutoff DJ, Curriden SA, Hu G, Deng G. Regulation of cell adhesion by PAI-1. Apmis 1999;107:54–61.
63. Robbie LA, Booth NA, Brown AJ, Bennett B. Inhibitors of fibrinolysis are elevated in atherosclerotic plaque. Arterioscler Thromb Vasc Biol 1996;16: 539–545.
64. Rajavashisth TB, Liao JK, Galis ZS, Tripathi S, Laufs U, Tripathi J, Chai NN, Xu XP, Jovinge S, Shah PK, Libby P. Inflammatory cytokines and oxidized low density lipoproteins increase endothelial cell expression of membrane type 1-matrix metalloproteinase. J Biol Chem 1999;274:11924–11929.

65. Slowik MR, Min W, Ardito T, Karsan A, Kashgarian M, Pober JS. Evidence that tumor necrosis factor triggers apoptosis in human endothelial cells by interleukin-1-converting enzyme-like protease-dependent and -independent pathways. Lab Invest 1997;77:257–267.
66. Bombeli T, Schwartz BR, Harlan JM. Endothelial cells undergoing apoptosis become proadhesive for nonactivated platelets. Blood 1999;93:3831–3838.
67. Physicians' Health Study Research Group. Final report on the aspirin component of the ongoing Physicians' Health Study. Steering Committee of the Physicians' Health Study Research Group. N Engl J Med 1989;321:129–135.
68. Antiplatelet Trialists' Collaboration. Collaborative overview of randomized trials of antiplatelet therapy. 1. Prevention of death, myocardial infarction, and stroke by prolonged antiplatelet therapy in various categories of patients. Br Med J 1994;308:81–106.
69. Soumerai SB, McLaughlin TJ, Spiegelman D, Hertzmark E, Thibault G, Goldman L. Adverse outcomes of underuse of beta-blockers in elderly survivors of acute myocardial infarction. JAMA 1997;277:115–121.
70. Rubins HB, Robins SJ, Collins D, Fye CL, Anderson JW, Elam MB, Faas FH, Linares E, Schaefer EJ, Schectman G, Wilt TJ, Wittes J. Gemfibrozil for the secondary prevention of coronary heart disease in men with low levels of high-density lipoprotein cholesterol. Veterans Affairs High-Density Lipoprotein Cholesterol Intervention Trial Study Group. N Engl J Med 1999;341:410–418.
71. Bendeck MP, Irvin C, Reidy MA. Inhibition of matrix metalloproteinase activity inhibits smooth muscle cell migration but not neointimal thickening after arterial injury. Circ Res 1996;78:38–43.
72. Prescott MF, Sawyer WK, Von Linden-Reed J, Jeune M, Chou M, Caplan SL, Jeng AY. Effect of matrix metalloproteinase inhibition on progression of atherosclerosis and aneurysm in LDL receptor-deficient mice overexpressing MMP-3, MMP-12, and MMP-13 and on restenosis in rats after balloon injury. Ann NY Acad Sci 1999;878:179–190.
73. Bone RC. Why sepsis trials fail. JAMA 1996;276:565–566.
74. Aikawa M, Rabkin E, Okada Y, Voglic S, Clinton S, Brinckerhoff C, Sukhova G, Libby P. Lipid lowering by diet reduces matrix metalloproteinase activity and increases collagen content of rabbit atheroma: a potential mechanism of lesion stabilization. Circulation 1998;97:2433–2444.
75. Laufs U, Marra D, Node K, Liao JK. 3-Hydroxy-3-methylglutaryl-CoA reductase inhibitors attenuate vascular smooth muscle proliferation by preventing rho GTPase-induced down-regulation of p27(Kip1). J Biol Chem 1999;274: 21926–21931.
76. Endres M, Laufs U, Huang Z, Nakamura T, Huang P, Moskowitz MA, Liao JK. Stroke protection by 3-hydroxy-3-methylglutaryl (HMG)-CoA reductase inhibitors mediated by endothelial nitric oxide synthase. Proc Natl Acad Sci USA 1998;95:8880–8885.
77. Thurberg B, Collins T. The nuclear factor-kappa B/inhibitor of kappa B autoregulatory system and atherosclerosis. Curr Opin Lipidol 1998;9:387–396.

78. Alpha-Tocopherol, Beta Carotene Cancer Prevention Study Group. The effect of vitamin E and beta carotene on the incidence of lung cancer and other cancers in male smokers. N Engl J Med 1994;330:1029–1035.
79. Gruppo Italiano per lo Studio della Sopravvivenza nell'Infarto Miocardico. Dietary supplementation with n-3 polyunsaturated fatty acids and vitamin E after myocardial infarction: results of the GISSI-prevenzione trial. Lancet 1999; 354:447–455.
80. Yusuf S, Sleight P, Pogue J, Bosch J, Davies R, Dagenais G. Effects of an angiotensin-converting-enzyme inhibitor, ramipril, on cardiovascular events in high-risk patients. The Heart Outcomes Prevention Evaluation Study Investigators. N Engl J Med 2000;342:145–153.
81. Walldius G, Erikson U, Olsson AG, Bergstrand L, Hadell K, Johansson J, Kaijser L, Lassvik C, Molgaard J, Nilsson S. The effect of probucol on femoral atherosclerosis: the Probucol Quantitative Regression Swedish Trial (PQRST). Am J Cardiol 1994;74:875–883.
82. Read MA, Neish AS, Luscinskas FW, Palombella VJ, Maniatis T, Collins T. The proteasome pathway is required for cytokine-induced endothelial-leukocyte adhesion molecule expression. Immunity 1995;2:493–506.
83. Peng HB, Libby P, Liao JK. Induction and stabilization of I kappa B alpha by nitric oxide mediates inhibition of NF-kappa B. J Biol Chem 1995;270:14214–14219.
84. Cheng GC, Loree HM, Kamm RD, Fishbein MC, Lee RT. Distribution of circumferential stress in ruptured and stable atherosclerotic lesions: a structural analysis with histopathologic correlation. Circulation 1993;87:1179–1187.

3

Plaque Rupture

Pathological and Anatomical Considerations

Ole Frøbert, Claus S. Jørgensen, and Erling Falk
*Skejby University Hospital
and Aarhus University
Aarhus, Denmark*

INTRODUCTION

Atherosclerosis in the coronary arteries is a very common autopsy finding, even in people not suffering from ischemic heart disease (1). Although ischemic heart disease is the leading cause of death in industrialized countries (2), more persons live with coronary atherosclerosis than die of it. Therefore, the key question is not why atherosclerosis develops but rather why a quiescent atherosclerotic plaque, after years of indolent growth, suddenly ruptures and becomes highly thrombogenic—the life-threatening event responsible for the great majority of the acute coronary syndromes (3,4).

The risk of plaque rupture is related to intrinsic properties within a plaque (its vulnerability) that predispose to rupture and extrinsic forces acting on the plaque (rupture triggers) that may precipitate rupture if the plaque is vulnerable (3). This chapter will review possible mechanisms responsible for the sudden conversion of a quiescent atherosclerotic plaque to an unstable, rapidly progressing, and highly thrombogenic lesion.

MATURE ATHEROSCLEROTIC PLAQUES

The distribution of atherosclerotic lesions is not random. Plaques tend to evolve at places of low shear stress and a high degree of flow oscillation—typically on the outer wall of bifurcations, along the inner wall of curved segments, and proximal to myocardial bridging (1,5–8). The diversity of atherosclerosis in different organs should be seen in the light of the fact that smooth muscle cells (SMC) are locally derived from individual organ parenchyma during embryogenesis in contrast to the embryonic endothelium which invades the organ (9). Although atherogenesis starts in early childhood, it takes decades to develop the mature plaques responsible for clinical diseases such as ischemic heart disease, ischemic stroke, aortic aneurysm, and claudication. As the name *atherosclerosis* implies, mature plaques consist typically of two main components: soft, lipid-rich *atheromatous* "gruel," and hard, collagen-rich *sclerotic* tissue (Fig. 1). The sclerotic component (fibrous tissue) is usually by far the most voluminous component of the plaque, constituting >70% of an average stenotic coronary plaque (3). Sclerosis is, however, relatively innocuous because fibrous tissue appears to stabilize plaques, protecting them against rupture. In contrast, the usually less

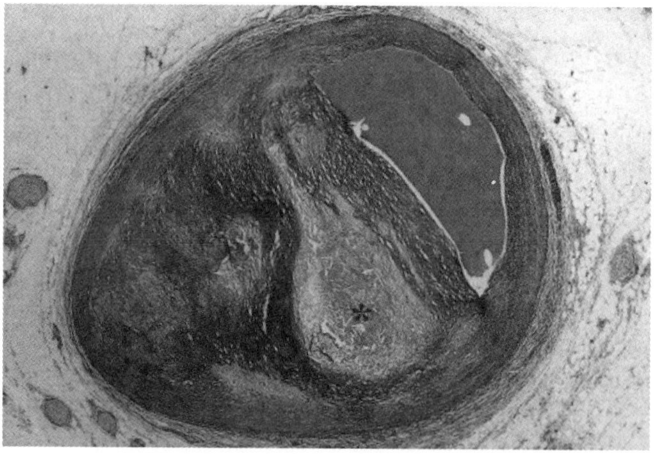

Figure 1 Atherosclerosis is characterized by two main components: atheromatous "gruel" and sclerotic tissue. The atheromatous component (asterisk) is lipid-rich and dangerous because it softens plaques, making them vulnerable to rupture with subsequent thrombosis. The sclerotic collagen-rich component is, as here, usually the most voluminous plaque component. Sclerosis, however, is rather innocuous; it may in fact, be good because it conveys stability to the lesion. (From Ref. 3. Copyright 1995, the American Heart Association.)

voluminous atheromatous component is the most dangerous component because the soft, lipid-rich gruel destabilizes plaques, making them vulnerable to rupture.

The lipid-rich core within a plaque is devoid of supporting collagen, avascular, hypocellular (except at the periphery of the core), rich in extracellular lipids, and soft like gruel (3). Macrophage foam cells surround the core and ceroid and macrophage-specific CD68 antigen and indicators of oxidant stress (F2-isoprostanes and hydroxyeicosatetraenoic acids), but not smooth muscle cell actin, are found within the gruel (10–12). This suggests that the death of lipid-laden macrophages contributes to gruel formation and thereby to core enlargement, which is why the core has been called the "graveyard of dead macrophages" (10,13). Another explanation to core formation is direct lipid trapping of LDL in the extracellular space of the arterial intima as a result of binding between insudating LDL and glycosaminoglycans, collagen, and fibrinogen (14–16). The relative contribution of cell necrosis versus direct lipid trapping in the development of the lipid-rich core is unclarified.

Plaque Size and Composition

Several pathoanatomical studies indicate that the lipid-rich atheromatous component enlarges with plaque growth, but the variability is great (3). A recent and probably the most detailed study, however, revealed no significant correlation between the size of a plaque and its composition (17). Thus, increased plaque thrombogenicity rather than increased vulnerability could explain the clinical observation that severely obstructive plaques are more prone to occlude and/or become culprit for myocardial infarction than are less obstructive plaques (18–23). Severely stenotic plaques at the carotid bifurcation frequently appear ulcerated and disrupted angiographically, and such lesions are indeed dangerous, being associated with a high risk of ipsilateral stroke (24).

Risk Factors and Plaque Composition

There is a remarkable and poorly understood variability in the way plaques evolve, and it is unclear how the various risk factors for clinical disease influence the development, composition, and vulnerability of atherosclerotic plaques. Age, male sex, hypercholesterolemia, hypertension, smoking, and diabetes correlate with the coronary plaque burden (extent of "plaquing") found at autopsy (25–28) and there is an increase in calcification with age and possibly male sex (29). Fibrous tissue seems to constitute the most voluminous component of mature coronary plaques, regardless of individual risk factors (3). In autopsy studies cigarette smoking is more often associated with acute coronary thrombosis than with stable plaque development (30,31). High total cholesterol to HDL cholesterol ratio in men (30) and total cholesterol in women (31) are associated with plaque rupture and age >50 years is associated with vulnerable plaques in women (31). A recent ultrasound study found that echolutency of carotid plaques was associated with high plasma levels of triglyceride-rich lipoproteins, which might predict a particularly vulnerable lipid-rich plaque type (32).

PLAQUE VULNERABILITY

Plaques containing a soft, lipid-rich core are vulnerable to rupture; i.e., the fibrous cap separating the core from the lumen may disintegrate, tear, or break, whereby the highly thrombogenic gruel is suddenly exposed to the flowing blood. Such disrupted plaques are found beneath about 75% of the thrombi responsible for acute coronary syndromes (33–37). Beneath the remaining thrombi, superficial plaque erosions without frank rupture (no deep injury) are usually found, often in combination with a severe atherosclerotic stenosis (33–35,38,39).

Pathoanatomical studies have identified three major determinants of a plaque's vulnerability to rupture: 1) size and consistency of the lipid-rich core; 2) thickness of the fibrous cap covering the core; and 3) inflammation and repair processes within the cap (40).

Atheromatous Core

The size and consistency of the lipid-rich core vary greatly and are critical for the stability of individual lesions. Gertz and Roberts reported the composition of plaques in 5-mm segments from 17 infarct-related arteries examined postmortem and found much larger cores in the 39 segments with plaque rupture than in the 229 segments with intact surface (32% and 5–12% of plaque area, respectively) (41). In aortic plaques, Davies et al. (42) found a similar relation between core size and plaque rupture, and they identified a critical threshold; intact aortic plaques containing a core occupying >40% of the plaque were considered particularly vulnerable and at high risk of rupture and thrombosis.

The consistency of the core depends on lipid composition and temperature; it is usually soft, like toothpaste, at room temperature postmortem, and it is even softer at body temperature in vivo. The semifluid cholesteryl esters soften plaques whereas the solid crystalline cholesterol has the opposite effect (43,44). Lipid-lowering therapy is expected to deplete plaque lipid, with an overall reduction in cholesteryl esters (liquid and mobile) and a relative increase in crystalline cholesterol (solid and inert), theoretically resulting in a stiffer and more stable plaque (43–45).

Cap Thickness

Fibrous caps vary widely in thickness, cellularity, matrix, strength, and stiffness, but they are often thinnest (and macrophage infiltrated) at their shoulder regions, where rupture most frequently occurs (33); the thinner the cap is, the greater risk of rupture (46,47). Loss of cells and calcification in fibrous caps are associated with increased stiffness (48), but the significance of cap stiffness for rupture propensity is unknown.

Cap Inflammation and Repair

Autopsy studies have shown that disrupted fibrous caps are usually heavily infiltrated by macrophage foam cells that are activated, indicating ongoing inflammation at the site of plaque rupture (34,35,49–51) (Fig. 2). For eccentric plaques, the shoulder regions are sites of predilection for both active inflammation and rupture (33,52,53), and in vitro mechanical testing of aortic fibrous caps indicates that foam cell infiltration indeed weakens caps locally, reducing their tensile strength (54). These postmortem findings have recently been confirmed by studies of plaque tissue retrieved by atherectomy. Coronary culprit lesions responsible for acute coronary syndromes contain significantly more macrophages than lesions responsible for stable angina pectoris (55), and lipoprotein(a) appears to be more massively engaged in coronary plaques from unstable than stable angina patients (56). Carotid, femoral, and aortic lipid-rich, rupture-prone plaques have an increased microvessel density and express increased levels of endothelial adhesion molecules (ICAM-1, VCAM-1, PECAM, E-selectin) compared with stable fibrous plaques (57).

Macrophages are capable of degrading extracellular matrix by phagocytosis or by secreting proteolytic enzymes such as plasminogen activators and a family of matrix metalloproteinases (MMPs: collagenases, gelatinases, and stromelysins) that may weaken the fibrous cap, predisposing it to rupture (58). Recent studies have demonstrated thermal heterogeneity in coronary and carotid plaques, indicating heat is released by activated macrophages (59,60). Activated mast cells are also present in disrupted caps (61) and they secrete powerful proteolytic enzymes such as tryptase and chymase that can activate proMMPs secreted by other cells. Their number is rather small, however, in comparison with macrophages (62).

Collagen is the main component of fibrous caps responsible for their tensile strength. Human monocyte-derived macrophages grown in culture are capable of degrading cap collagen, and they do, simultaneously, express MMP-1 (interstitial collagenase) and induce MMP-2 (gelatinolytic) activity in the culture medium (63). Several studies have now identified MMPs in human coronary plaques (64–66). Monocytes/macrophages could also play

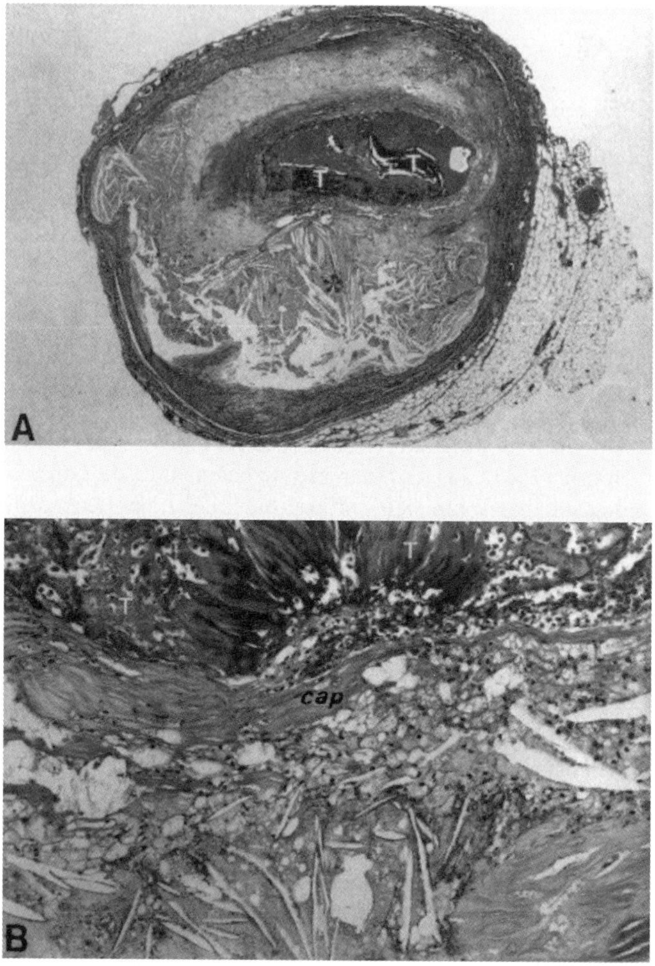

Figure 2 (A) A severely stenotic vulnerable plaque containing a huge atheromatous core (asterisk) that is separated from the narrowed lumen by only a thin fibrous cap. The lumen contains a nonoccluding thrombus (T). (B) Higher magnification of the plaque thrombus interface reveals that the fibrous cap beneath the thrombus is very thin and heavily foam cell infiltrated, indicating ongoing disease activity. The cap was ruptured nearby (the actual rupture site is not represented in this section), explaining why a luminal thrombus has evolved (From Falk E. Why do plaques rupture? Circulation 1992;86(suppl III):30–42. Copyright 1992, the American Heart Association.)

a detrimental role after plaque rupture, promoting thrombin generation and luminal thrombosis via tissue factor expression (67–71). Collagen is synthesized by vascular smooth muscle cells and it is likely that interferon-γ produced by T-lymphocytes decreases the ability of the smooth muscle cells to express the interstitial collagen genes in lipid-rich plaques (72). Several infectious agents have been suggested to play an active role in the development of cardiovascular diseases, particularly *C. pneumoniae* but also herpesviruses (including cytomegalovirus) and *Helicobacter pylori* (40,73,74). Chlamydia has been identified in atherosclerotic plaques (75); it contains lipopolysaccharide and heat shock protein 60, which are well-known strong inducers of many enzymes, among others MMPs (76).

Loss of SMCs and reduced collagen synthesis, resulting in impaired healing and repair, could also play a role in plaque destabilization and rupture, and disrupted caps contain indeed fewer SMCs and less collagen than intact caps (34,42,62,77,78). The cause of this potentially dangerous relative lack of SMCs in disrupted caps is unknown, but SMCs could vanish due to apoptotic cell death (13).

RUPTURE TRIGGERS

Coronary plaques are constantly stressed by a variety of mechanical and hemodynamic forces that may precipitate or "trigger" rupture of vulnerable plaques (79,80). Stresses imposed on plaques are usually concentrated at the weak points discussed above, namely, at points at which the fibrous cap is thinnest and tearing most frequently occurs (46). In theory, mechanical forces may act in the three principal directions: the circumferential, the longitudinal, and the radial. Below we will review the literature with respect to these principal directions and we will also consider shear, fatigue, and plaque configuration.

Circumferential Deformation

Stretching of the coronary artery wall results in a systolic-diastolic change in the circumferential length of about 10% in normal compliant arteries (79). The stiffness apparently increases with age (81,82) but there is no clear-cut relation between the degree of atherosclerosis and arterial stiffness (83–86). As could be anticipated, the less diseased arcs of the arterial wall are stretched more than diseased, often calcified arcs of the wall (87–89). The stress gradient in these zones—which usually coincide with the shoulder region of the plaque—from uneven circumferential stretching of the wall could partly explain why rupture frequently takes place here. In a population-based finite element analysis it was shown that the area of greatest stress in coronary atherosclerosis >20 years of age is at the shoulder region of the plaque and that age was strongly correlated with shoulder stress (90).

Cheng et al. (46) demonstrated that the maximal circumferential stress in plaques that ruptured and caused lethal myocardial infarction was almost three times higher than the maximum stress in stable control lesions. Moreover, in 7 of 12 lethal lesions rupture occurred in the region of maximum circumferential stress (46).

Longitudinal Deformation

The cyclic longitudinal stretching of the coronary arteries with each heart beat imposes equal tensile forces on the entire arterial wall where the direction of the deformation is in parallel with the artery. Where the artery curves, the deformation is nonparallel relative to the course of the artery, and some parts of the arterial wall are stretched more than others. At points of bending, some parts of the wall may even be in compression while the opposite segments are in tension. Angiographically, the angle of flexion during systole (an assessment of both longitudinal stretching and bending) has been found to be higher in lesions subsequently shown to progress than in lesions that did not progress (91). Furthermore, from a finite element mathematical stress model it was found that Von Mises stresses—a measure that may predict material failure—were higher within the subendothelium along the inner walls of curvatures compared to the outer walls (91).

Radial Deformation

Compressive forces acting from the lumen in the radial direction alone are unlikely to lead to plaque rupture. Lee et al. (48) applied uniaxial compression to atherosclerotic plaques from human abdominal aortas to study plaque stiffness. They were unable to produce evidence of fracture despite increase in stress to more than 20 atm. The authors explained the failure of the plaques to fracture from the fact that the specimens were not under circumferential or longitudinal tension in the testing apparatus.

In theory, plaque rupture may also occur in the opposite direction—from the plaque into the lumen. This kind of rupture requires that the intraplaque pressure supersedes the intraluminal pressure which could be caused by collapse of fragile stenoses, plaque edema, vasospasm, or bleeding from vasa vasorum.

With high-grade stenosis, a diseased artery may experience negative instead of positive transmural pressure around the stenotic region because of accelerated velocities in the throat of the stenosis. In a two-dimensional finite element model, Aoki and Ku (92) could demonstrate that the lateral edge of a stenotic cap may be subjected to high concentrations of compressive stresses. The stresses further increase with collapse of compliant stenoses, causing bending deformation from buckling of the wall.

Vasospasm has been suspected of "blowing" the fibrous cap off the plaque into the lumen (93,94). There is frequent coexistence of vasospasm and plaque rupture (95), but it is believed that the latter most often gives rise to the former rather than the other way around (95,96). Kaski and coworkers (97) found that drug-induced spasms seldom gave rise to myocardial infarction. By contrast, Noboyoshi et al. (18) found a strong positive correlation between ergonovine-induced coronary spasm and subsequent plaque progression, with or without infarct development.

Hemorrhage from fragile vasa vasorum into the plaque has been suggested to cause plaque rupture (98,99). The vasa vasorum blood flow has been shown to be up to 10 times as high in the coronary arteries of atherosclerotic monkeys compared with normal monkeys (100). However, it seems unlikely that the pressure generated by bleeding from capillary size vessels should exceed intracoronary blood pressure (101). Furthermore, in a study of 17 cases of fatal coronary thrombosis, Constantinides (49) was able to show that intraplaque haemorrhage could always be traced back to an entry of blood from the lumen through a crack in the plaque surface.

Shear Stress

In atherogenesis unsteady blood flow characteristics (turbulence and recirculation) rather than the magnitude of shear stress per se is considered the major determinant of hemodynamically induced endothelial cell turnover (102,103) and thereby possibly endothelial injury. Whereas the influence from shear stress on atherosclerotic lesion development is well accepted, it has been questioned whether shear alone may disrupt a stenotic plaque (41,80). A recent study of carotid plaques demonstrated that low shear areas downstream of plaques contain more SMCs and fewer macrophages than upstream high shear areas where fewer SMCs, more macrophages, and more plaque ruptures are found (78).

Shear stresses are generally considered an order of magnitude smaller than the stresses imposed on the plaque by the blood pressure (80). However, the stress in the cell membrane of an endothelial cell may be extremely high because of shear (104). In stenotic regions shear stress may shave the endothelium away (105), giving rise to plaque erosion rather than plaque rupture.

Fatigue and Turbulence

A stress may accentuate weaknesses in a material if applied repeatedly in the same way that a wire may eventually be broken by repetitive bending

(46). Fluttering of coronary stenoses between collapse and patency (92) and turbulent pressure fluctuations just distal to the stenoses could fatigue areas of the plaque surface, promoting plaque rupture (106).

The frequency of the applied stress, in terms of oscillating pressure, also changes the mechanical properties of a plaque (107,108). Regardless of the type of plaque (cellular, hypocellular, calcified), Lee et al. (48) demonstrated increased stiffness of fibrous caps with the frequency of the applied stress. From 0.5 to 2.0 Hz the increase in stiffness was approximately 15%. Loree and coworkers could demonstrate increased stiffness of model atherosclerotic lipid pools with increasing frequency of stress ranging from 0.1 to 3 Hz (43). One of the pathoanatomical consequences of the stiffness of plaque tissue may be that in stiff, calcified fibrous caps rupture may occur abruptly (as in a piece of glass), whereas cellular caps may fracture more gradually or ductilely (80).

ONSET OF CLINICAL DISEASE

Onset of acute coronary syndromes does not occur at random; a great fraction appears to be "triggered" by external factors or conditions (2,109,110). Myocardial infarction occurs at increased frequency in the morning (109,111–115), on Mondays (115,116), during winter months (117–119), and during emotional stress (120–123) and vigorous exercise (120,124–126). The pathophysiological mechanisms responsible for the nonrandom and apparently often triggered onset of infarction are unknown but probably related to: 1) *plaque rupture*, most likely caused by surges in sympathetic activity with a sudden increase in blood pressure, pulse rate, heart contraction, and coronary blood flow; 2) *thrombosis*, occurring on previously disrupted or intact plaques when the systemic thrombotic tendency is high because of platelet hyperaggregability, hypercoagulability, and/or impaired fibrinolysis; and 3) *vasoconstriction*, occurring locally around a coronary plaque or generalized (3).

PLAQUE RUPTURE: CLINICAL MANIFESTATIONS

Plaque rupture is common and probably asymptomatic in the great majority of cases; only when a flow-limiting thrombus evolves does plaque rupture manifest itself clinically (3,127). Autopsy data indicate that 9% of "normal" healthy persons have asymptomatic disrupted plaques in their coronary arteries, increasing to 22% in persons with diabetes or hypertension (128). Many persons who die of ischemic heart disease harbor both thrombosed and nonthrombosed disrupted plaques in their coronary arteries (129–131). In two studies of 47 and 83 persons who died of coronary atherosclerosis,

103 and 211 disrupted plaques, respectively, were identified (35,36); more than two disrupted plaques per person, and less than half (40 and 102, respectively) were associated with significant luminal thrombosis that caused critical flow obstruction. The majority of the other plaque ruptures were probably asymptomatic.

The most feared consequence of coronary plaque rupture is luminal thrombosis. The clinical presentation and outcome depend on the location, severity, and duration of myocardial ischemia. A nonocclusive or transiently occlusive thrombus most frequently underlies primary unstable angina with pain at rest and myocardial infarction without ST elevation, whereas a more stable and occlusive thrombus is most frequently seen in ST elevation infarction—overall, modified by vascular tone and available collateral flow (132). The lesion responsible for out-of-hospital cardiac arrest or sudden death is often similar to that of unstable angina: a disrupted plaque with superimposed nonocclusive thrombosis (129,133,134). It is noteworthy that many coronary arteries apparently occlude silently without causing myocardial infarction, probably because of a well-developed collateral circulation at the time of occlusion (20,135,136).

CONCLUSION

Coronary atherosclerosis is a common and often harmless finding. However, various mechanisms may convert a stable atherosclerotic plaque into an unstable highly thrombogenic lesion causing unstable angina, myocardial infarction, and/or sudden death. The risk of plaque rupture is related to plaque vulnerability and rupture triggers. The composition of the plaque, the location, and the different mechanical forces acting on it probably play a more important role for rupture than the size of the plaque. Rupture tends to occur in plaques with a large, lipid-rich core and a thin overlying cap at locations weakened by inflammation and at points of stress concentrations. The danger of vulnerable plaques is not the rupture itself but the resulting thrombotic response.

REFERENCES

1. Enos WF, Holmes RH, Beyer J. Coronary disease among United States soldiers killed in action in Korea. JAMA 1953;152:1090–1093.
2. Muller JE, Abela GS, Nesto RW, Tofler GH. Triggers, acute risk factors and vulnerable plaques: the lexicon of a new frontier. J Am Coll Cardiol 1994; 23:809–813.
3. Falk E, Shah PK, Fuster V. Coronary plaque disruption. Circulation 1995;92: 657–671.

4. Farb A, Tang AL, Burke AP, Sessums L, Liang Y, Virmani R. Sudden coronary death. Frequency of active coronary lesions, inactive coronary lesions, and myocardial infarction. Circulation 1995;92:1701–1709.
5. Ge J, Erbel R, Gorge G, Haude M, Meyer J. High wall shear stress proximal to myocardial bridging and atherosclerosis: intracoronary ultrasound and pressure measurements. Br Heart J 1995;73:462–465.
6. Ku DN, Giddens DP, Zarins CK, Glagov S. Pulsatile flow and atherosclerosis in the human carotid bifurcation. Positive correlation between plaque location and low oscillating shear stress. Arteriosclerosis 1985;5:293–302.
7. Asakura T, Karino T. Flow patterns and spatial distribution of atherosclerotic lesions in human coronary arteries. Circ Res 1990;66:1045–1066.
8. Kimura BJ, Russo RJ, Bhargava V, McDaniel MB, Peterson KL, DeMaria AN. Atheroma morphology and distribution in proximal left anterior descending coronary artery: in vivo observations. J Am Coll Cardiol 1996;27:825–831.
9. Schwartz SM, Heimark RL, Majesky MW. Developmental mechanisms underlying pathology of arteries. Physiol Rev 1990;70:1177–1209.
10. Ball RY, Stowers EC, Burton JH, Cary NR, Skepper JN, Mitchinson MJ. Evidence that the death of macrophage foam cells contributes to the lipid core of atheroma. Atherosclerosis 1995;114:45–54.
11. Mallat Z, Nakamura T, Ohan J, Leseche G, Tedgui A, Maclouf J, Murphy RC. The relationship of hydroxyeicosatetraenoic acids and F2-isoprostanes to plaque instability in human carotid atherosclerosis. J Clin Invest 1999;103:421–427.
12. Pratico D, Iuliano L, Mauriello A, Spagnoli L, Lawson JA, Rokach J, Maclouf J, Violi F, Fitzgerald GA. Localization of distinct F2-isoprostanes in human atherosclerotic lesions. J Clin Invest 1997;100:2028–2034.
13. Geng YJ, Libby P. Evidence for apoptosis in advanced human atheroma. Colocalization with interleukin-1 beta-converting enzyme. Am J Pathol 1995;147:251–266.
14. Guyton JR, Klemp KF. Development of the atherosclerotic core region. Chemical and ultrastructural analysis of microdissected atherosclerotic lesions from human aorta. Arterioscler Thromb 1994;14:1305–1314.
15. Witztum JL. The oxidation hypothesis of atherosclerosis. Lancet 1994;344:793–795.
16. Guyton JR, Klemp KF. Transitional features in human atherosclerosis. Intimal thickening, cholesterol clefts, and cell loss in human aortic fatty streaks. Am J Pathol 1993;143:1444–1457.
17. Mann JM, Davies MJ. Vulnerable plaque. Relation of characteristics to degree of stenosis in human coronary arteries. Circulation 1996;94:928–931.
18. Nobuyoshi M, Tanaka M, Nosaka H, Kimura T, Yokoi H, Hamasaki N, Kim K, Shindo T, Kimura K. Progression of coronary atherosclerosis: is coronary spasm related to progression? J Am Coll Cardiol 1991;18:904–910.
19. Giroud D, Li JM, Urban P, Meier B, Rutishauer W. Relation of the site of acute myocardial infarction to the most severe coronary arterial stenosis at prior angiography. Am J Cardiol 1992;69:729–732.

20. Alderman EL, Corley SD, Fisher LD, Chaitman BR, Faxon DP, Foster ED, Killip T, Sosa JA, Bourassa MG. Five-year angiographic follow-up of factors associated with progression of coronary artery disease in the Coronary Artery Surgery Study (CASS). CASS Participating Investigators and Staff. J Am Coll Cardiol 1993;22:1141–1154.
21. Chen L, Chester MR, Redwood S, Huang J, Leatham E, Kaski JC. Angiographic stenosis progression and coronary events in patients with "stabilized" unstable angina. Circulation 1995;91:2319–2324.
22. Ambrose JA, Tannenbaum MA, Alexopoulos D, Hjemdahl Monsen CE, Leavy J, Weiss M, Borrico S, Gorlin R, Fuster V. Angiographic progression of coronary artery disease and the development of myocardial infarction. J Am Coll Cardiol 1988;12:56–62.
23. Little WC, Constantinescu M, Applegate RJ, Kutcher MA, Burrows MT, Kahl FR, Santamore WP. Can coronary angiography predict the site of a subsequent myocardial infarction in patients with mild-to-moderate coronary artery disease? Circulation 1988;78:1157–1166.
24. Eliasziw M, Streifler JY, Fox AJ, Hachinski VC, Ferguson GG, Barnett HJ. Significance of plaque ulceration in symptomatic patients with high-grade carotid stenosis: North American Symptomatic Carotid Endaterectomy Trial. Stroke 1994;25:304–308.
25. Natural history of aortic and coronary atherosclerotic lesions in youth. Findings from the PDAY Study. Pathobiological Determinants of Atherosclerosis in Youth (PDAY) Research Group. Arterioscler Thromb 1993;13:1291–1298.
26. Solberg LA, Strong JP. Risk factors and atherosclerotic lesions: a review of autopsy studies. Arteriosclerosis 1983;3:187–198.
27. Reed DM, Strong JP, Resch J, Hayashi T. Serum lipids and lipoproteins as predictors of atherosclerosis: an autopsy study. Arteriosclerosis 1989;9:560–564.
28. Robertson WB, Strong JP. Atherosclerosis in persons with hypertension and diabetes mellitus. Lab Invest 1968;18:538–551.
29. Devries S, Wolfkiel C, Fusman B, Bakdash H, Ahmed A, Levy P, Chomka E, Kondos G, Zajac E, Rich S. Influence of age and gender on the presence of coronary calcium detected by ultrafast computed tomography. J Am Coll Cardiol 1995;25:76–82.
30. Burke AP, Farb A, Malcom GT, Liang Y, Smialek J, Virmani R. Coronary risk factors and plaque morphology in men with coronary disease who died suddenly. N Engl J Med 1997;336:1276–1282.
31. Burke AP, Farb A, Malcom GT, Liang Y, Smialek J, Virmani R. Effect of risk factors on the mechanism of acute thrombosis and sudden coronary death in women. Circulation 1998;97:2110–2116.
32. Gr¢nholdt MM, Nordestgaard BG, Wiebe BM, Wilhjelm JE, Sillesen H. Echo-lutency of computerized ultrasound images of carotid atherosclerotic plaques is associated with increased levels of triglyceride-rich lipoproteins as well as increased plaque lipid content. Circulation 1998;97:34–40.
33. Richardson PD, Davies MJ, Born GVR. Influence of plaque configuration and

stress distribution on fissuring of coronary atherosclerotic plaques. Lancet 1989;2:941–944.
34. van der Wal AC, Becker AE, van der Loos CM, Das PK. Site of intimal rupture or erosion of thrombosed coronary atherosclerotic plaques is characterized by an inflammatory process irrespective of the dominant plaque morphology. Circulation 1994;89:36–44.
35. Falk E. Plaque rupture with severe pre-existing stenosis precipitating coronary thrombosis. Characteristics of coronary atherosclerotic plaques underlying fatal occlusive thrombi. Br Heart J 1983;50:127–134.
36. Frink RJ. Chronic ulcerated plaques: new insights into the pathogenesis of acute coronary disease. J Invas Cardiol 1994;6:173–185.
37. Arbustini E, Dal Bello B, Morbini P, Burke AP, Bocciarelli M, Specchia G, Virmani R. Plaque erosion is a major substrate for coronary thrombosis in acute myocardial infarction. Heart 1999;82:269–272.
38. Farb A, Burke AP, Tang AL, Liang Y, Mannan P, Smialek J, Virmani R. Coronary plaque erosion without rupture into a lipid core. A frequent cause of coronary thrombosis in sudden coronary death. Circulation 1996;93:1354–1363.
39. Davies MJ. Stability and instability: two faces of coronary atherosclerosis. Paul Dudley White lecture 1995. Circulation 1996;94:2013–2020.
40. Ross R. Atherosclerosis—an inflammatory disease. N Engl J Med 1999;340: 115–126.
41. Gertz SD, Roberts WC. Hemodynamic shear force in rupture of coronary arterial atherosclerotic plaques. Am J Cardiol 1990;66:1368–1372.
42. Davies MJ, Richardson PD, Woolf N, Katz DR, Mann J. Risk of thrombosis in human atherosclerotic plaques: role of extracellular lipid, macrophage, and smooth muscle cell content. Br Heart J 1993;69:377–381.
43. Loree HM, Tobias BJ, Gibson LJ, Kamm RD, Small DM, Lee RT. Mechanical properties of model atherosclerotic lesion lipid pools. Arterioscler Thromb 1994;14:230–234.
44. Small DM. George Lyman Duff memorial lecture. Progression and regression of atherosclerotic lesions. Insights from lipid physical biochemistry. Arteriosclerosis 1988;8:103–129.
45. Wagner WD, St. Clair RW, Clarkson TB, Connor JR. A study of atherosclerosis regression in *Macaca mulatta*: III. Chemical changes in arteries from animals with atherosclerosis induced for 19 months and regressed for 48 months at plasma cholesterol concentrations of 300 or 200 mg/dl. Am J Pathol 1980;100:633–650.
46. Cheng GC, Loree HM, Kamm RD, Fishbein MC, Lee RT. Distribution of circumferential stress in ruptured and stable atherosclerotic lesions. A structural analysis with histopathological correlation. Circulation 1993;87:1179–1187.
47. Loree HM, Kamm RD, Stringfellow RG, Lee RT. Effects of fibrous cap thickness on peak circumferential stress in model atherosclerotic vessels. Circ Res 1992;71:850–858.

48. Lee RT, Grodzinsky AJ, Frank EH, Kamm RD, Schoen FJ. Structure-dependent dynamic mechanical behavior of fibrous caps from human atherosclerotic plaques. Circulation 1991;83:1764–1770.
49. Constantinides P. Plaque fissures in human coronary thrombosis. J Atheroscler Res 1966;6:1–17.
50. Friedman M. The coronary thrombus: its origin and fate. Hum Pathol 1971; 2:81–128.
51. Pasterkamp G, Schoneveld AH, van der Wal AC, Hijnen D, van Wolveren WJA, Plomp S, Teepen H, Borst C. Inflammation of the atherosclerotic cap and shoulder of the plaque is a common and locally observed feature in unruptured plaques of femoral and coronary arteries. Arterioscler Thromb Vasc Biol 1999;19:54–58.
52. Johnson Tidey RR, McGregor JL, Taylor PR, Poston RN. Increase in the adhesion molecule P-selectin in endothelium overlying atherosclerotic plaques. Coexpression with intercellular adhesion molecule-1. Am J Pathol 1994;144:952–961.
53. Poston RN, Haskard DO, Coucher JR, Gall NP, Johnson Tidey RR. Expression of intercellular adhesion molecule-1 in atherosclerotic plaques. Am J Pathol 1992;140:665–673.
54. Lendon CL, Davies MJ, Born GV, Richardson PD. Atherosclerotic plaque caps are locally weakened when macrophages density is increased. Atherosclerosis 1991;87:87–90.
55. Moreno PR, Falk E, Palacios IF, Newell JB, Fuster V, Fallon JT. Macrophage infiltration in acute coronary syndromes. Implications for plaque rupture. Circulation 1994;90:775–778.
56. Dangas G, Mehran R, Harpel, Sharma SK, Marcovina SM, Dube G, Ambrose JA, Fallon JT. Lipoprotein(a) and inflammation in human coronary atheroma: association with the severity of clinical presentation. J Am Coll Cardiol 1998; 32:2035–2042.
57. De Boor OJ, van der Wal AC, Teeling P, Becker AE. Leucocyte recruitment in rupture prone regions of lipid-rich plaques: a prominent role for neovascularization? Cardiovasc Res 1999;41:443–449.
58. Matrisian LM. The matrix degrading metalloproteinases. Bioessays 1992;14: 455–463.
59. Casscells W, Hathorn B, David M, Krabach T, Vaughn WK, McAllister HA, Bearman G, Willerson JT. Thermal detection of cellular infiltrates in living atherosclerotic plaques: possible implications for plaque rupture and thrombosis. Lancet 1996;347:1447–1449.
60. Stefanadis C, Diamantopoulos L, Vlachopoulos C, Tsiamis E, Dernellis J, Toutouzas K, Stefanadi E, Toutouzas P. Thermal heterogeneity within human atherosclerotic coronary arteries detected in vivo: a new method of detection by application of a special thermography catheter. Circulation 1999;99:1965–1971.
61. Kaartinen M, van der Wal AC, van der Loos CM, Piek JJ, Koch KT, Becker AE, Kovanen PT. Mast cell infiltration in acute coronary syndromes: implications for plaque rupture. J Am Coll Cardiol 1998;32:606–612.

62. Kovanen P, Kaartinen M, Paavonen T. Infiltrates of activated mast cells at the site of coronary atheromatous erosion or rupture in myocardial infarction. Circulation 1995;92:1084–1088.
63. Shah PK, Falk E, Badimon JJ, Fernandez Ortiz A, Mailhac A, Villareal Levy G, Fallon JT, Regnstrom J, Fuster V. Human monocyte-derived macrophages induce collagen breakdown in fibrous caps of atherosclerotic plaques. Potential role of matrix-degrading metalloproteinases and implications for plaque rupture. Circulation 1995;92:1565–1569.
64. Galis ZS, Sukhova GK, Lark MW, Libby P. Increased expression of matrix metalloproteinases and matrix degrading activity in vulnerable regions of human atherosclerotic plaques. J Clin Invest 1994;94:2493–2503.
65. Brown DL, Hibbs MS, Kearney M, Loushin C, Isner JM. Identification of 92-kD gelatinase in human coronary atherosclerotic lesions. Association of active enzyme synthesis with unstable angina. Circulation 1995;91:2125–2131.
66. Henney AM, Wakeley PR, Davies MJ, Foster K, Hembry R, Murphy G, Humphries S. Localization of stromelysin gene expression in atheroscleotic plaques by in situ hybridization. Proc Natl Acad Sci USA 1991;88:8154–8158.
67. Wilcox JN, Smith KM, Schwartz SM, Gordon D. Localization of tissue factor in the normal vessel wall and in the atherosclerotic plaque. Proc Natl Acad Sci USA 1989;86:2839–2843.
68. Palabrica T, Lobb R, Furie BC, Aronovitz M, Benjamin C, Hsu YM, Sajer SA, Furie B. Leukocyte accumulation promoting fibrin deposition is mediated in vivo by P-selectin on adherent platelets. Nature 1992;359:848–851.
69. Jude B, Agraou B, McFadden EP, Susen S, Bauters C, Lepelley P, Vanhaesbroucke C, Devos P, Cosson A, Asseman P. Evidence for time-dependent activation of monocytes in the systemic circulation in unstable angina but not in acute myocardial infarction or in stable angina. Circulation 1994;90:1662–1668.
70. Leatham EW, Bath PMV, Tooze JA, Camm AJ. Increased tissue factor expression in coronary disease. Br Heart J 1995;73:10–13.
71. Moreno PR, Bernadi VH, López-Cuéllar J, Murcia AM, Palacios IF, Gold HK, Mehran R, Sharma SK, Nemerson Y, Fuster V, Fallon JT. Macrophages, smooth muscle cells, and tissue factor in unstable angina. Implications for cell-mediated thrombogenicity in acute coronary syndromes. Circulation 1996;94:3090–3097.
72. Libby P. Molecular bases of the acute coronary syndromes. Circulation 1995; 91:2844–2850.
73. Danesh J, Collins R, Peto R. Chronic infections and coronary heart disease: is there a link? Lancet 1997;350:430–436.
74. Libby P, Egan D, Skarlatos S. Roles of infectious agents in atherosclerosis and restenosis: an assessment of the evidence and need for future research. Circulation 1997;96:4095–4103.
75. Muhlestein JB, Hammond EH, Carlquist JF, Radicke E, Thomson MJ, Karagounis LA, Woods ML, Anderson JL. Increased incidence of *Chlamydia*

species within the coronary arteries of patients with symptomatic atherosclerotic versus other forms of cardiovascular disease. J Am Coll Cardiol 1996; 27:1555–1561.
76. Kol A, Sukhova GK, Lichtman AH, Libby P. Chlamydial heat shock protein 60 localizes in human atheroma and regulates macrophage tumor necrosis factor-alpha and matrix metalloproteinase expression. Circulation 1998;98: 300–307.
77. Burleigh MC, Briggs AD, Lendon CL, Davies MJ, Born GV, Richardson PD. Collagen types I and III, collagen content, GAGs and mechanical strength of human atherosclerotic plaque caps: span-wise variations. Atherosclerosis 1992;96:71–81.
78. Dirksen MT, van der Wal AC, van den Berg FM, van der Loos CM, Becker AE. Distribution of inflammatory cells in atherosclerotic plaques relates to the direction of flow. Circulation 1998; 98:2000–2003.
79. Lee RT, Kamm RD. Vascular mechanics for the cardiologist. J Am Coll Cardiol 1994;23:1289–1295.
80. MacIsaac AI, Thomas JD, Topol EJ. Toward the quiescent coronary plaque. J Am Coll Cardiol 1993;22:1228–1241.
81. Alfonso F, Macaya C, Goicolea J, Hernandez R, Segovia J, Zamorano J, Bañuelos C, Zarco P. Determinants of coronary compliance in patients with coronary artery disease: an intravascular ultrasound study. J Am Coll Cardiol 1994;23:879–884.
82. Shimazu T, Hori M, Mishima M, Kitabatake A, Kodama K, Nanto S, Inoue M. Clinical assessment of elastic properties of large coronary arteries: pressure-diameter relationship and dynamic incremental elastic modulus. Int J Cardiol 1986;13:27–45.
83. Farrar DJ, Green HD, Wagner WD, Bond MG. Reduction in pulse wave velocity and improvement of aortic distensibility accompanying regression of atherosclerosis in the rhesus monkey. Circ Res 1980;47:425–432.
84. Cox RH, Detweiler DK. Arterial wall properties and dietary atherosclerosis in the racing greyhound. Am J Physiol 1979;236:H790–H797.
85. Pynadath TI, Mukherjee DP. Dynamic mechanical properties of atherosclerotic aorta. A correlation between the cholesterol ester content and the viscoelastic properties of atherosclerotic aorta. Atherosclerosis 1977;26:311–318.
86. Newman DL, Gosling RG, Bowden NL. Changes in aortic distensibility and area ratio with the development of atherosclerosis. Atherosclerosis 1971;14: 231–240.
87. Isner JM, Rosenfield K, Losordo DW, Rose L, Langevin RE Jr, Razvi S, Kosowsky BD. Combination balloon-ultrasound imaging catheter for percutaneous transluminal angioplasty. Validation of imaging, analysis of recoil, and identification of plaque fracture. Circulation 1991;84:739–754.
88. Baptista J, di Mario C, Ozaki Y, Escaned J, Gil R, de Feyter P, Roelandt JR, Serruys PW. Impact of plaque morphology and composition on the mechanisms of lumen enlargement using intracoronary ultrasound and quantitative angiography after balloon angioplasty. Am J Cardiol 1996;77:115–121.

89. de Korte CL, Cespedes EI, van der Steen AFW, Pasterkamp G, Bom N. Intravascular ultrasound elastography: assessment and imaging of elastic properties of diseased arteries and vulnerable plaque. Eur J Ultrasound 1998; 7:219–224.
90. Veress AI, Cornhill JF, Herderick EE, Thomas JD. Age-related development of atherosclerotic plaque stress: a population-based finite-element analysis. Coron Artery Dis 1998;9:13–19.
91. Stein PD, Hamid MS, Shivkumar K, Davis TP, Khaja F, Henry JW. Effects of cyclic flexion of coronary arteries on progression of atherosclerosis. Am J Cardiol 1994;73:431–437.
92. Aoki T, Ku DN. Collapse of diseased arteries with eccentric cross section. J Biomech 1993;26:133–142.
93. Leary T. Coronary spasm as a possible factor in producing sudden death. Am Heart J 1934;10:338–344.
94. Lin CS, Penha PD, Zak FG, Lin JC. Morphodynamic interpretation of acute coronary thrombosis, with special reference to volcano-like eruption of atheromatous plaque caused by coronary artery spasm. Angiology 1988;39:535–547.
95. Bogaty P, Hackett D, Davies G, Maseri A. Vasoreactivity of the culprit lesion in unstable angina. Circulation 1994;90:5–11.
96. Lam JY, Chesebro JH, Steele PM, Badimon L, Fuster V. Is vasospasm related to platelet deposition? Relationship in a porcine preparation of arterial injury in vivo. Circulation 1987;75:243–248.
97. Kaski JC, Tousoulis D, McFadden E, Crea F, Pereira WI, Maseri A. Variant angina pectoris. Role of coronary spasm in the development of fixed coronary obstructions. Circulation 1992;85:619–626.
98. Barger AC, Beeuwkes R 3d, Lainey LL, Silverman KJ. Hypothesis: vasa vasorum and neovascularization of human coronary arteries. A possible role in the pathophysiology of atherosclerosis. N Engl J Med 1984;310:175–177.
99. Paterson JC. Capillary rupture with intimal hemorrhage as a causative factor in coronary thrombosis. Arch Pathol 1938;25:474–487.
100. Williams JK, Armstrong ML, Heistad DD. Vasa vasorum in atherosclerotic coronary arteries: responses to vasoactive stimuli and regression of atherosclerosis. Circ Res 1988;62:515–523.
101. Jiang JP, Feldman CL, Stone PH. Models of the intracoronary pathogenesis of acute coronary heart disease. In: Willich SN, Muller JE, eds. Triggering of Acute Coronary Syndromes. Implications for Prevention. Dordrecht: Kluwer Academic Publishers, 1996:237–257.
102. Davies PF, Tripathi SC. Mechanical stress mechanisms and the cell. An endothelial paradigm. Circ Res 1993;72:239–245.
103. Davies PF, Remuzzi A, Gordon EJ, Dewey CF Jr, Gimbrone MA Jr. Turbulent fluid shear stress induces vascular endothelial cell turnover in vitro. Proc Natl Acad Sci USA 1986;83:2114–2117.
104. Fung YC. Biomechanics: Motion, Flow, Stress, and Growth. New York: Springer-Verlag, 1990.

105. Gertz SD, Uretzky G, Wajnberg RS, Navot N, Gotsman MS. Endothelial cell damage and thrombus formation after partial arterial constriction: relevance to the role of coronary artery spasm in the pathogenesis of myocardial infarction. Circulation 1981;63:476–486.
106. Loree HM, Kamm RD, Atkinson CM, Lee RT. Turbulent pressure fluctuations on surface of model vascular stenoses. Am J Physiol 1991;261:H644–H650.
107. Bergel DH. The dynamic elastic properties of the arterial wall. J Physiol 1961; 156:458–469.
108. Gow BS, Schonfeld D, Patel DJ. The dynamic elastic properties of the canine left circumflex coronary artery. J Biomech 1974;7:389–395.
109. Muller JE, Tofler GH, Stone PH. Circadian variation and triggers of onset of acute cardiovascular disease. Circulation 1989;79:733–743.
110. Willich SN, Maclure M, Mittleman MA, Arntz HR, Muller JE. Sudden cardiac death: support for a role of triggering in causation. Circulation 1993;87:1442–1450.
111. Goldberg RJ, Brady P, Muller JE, Chen ZY, de Groot M, Zonneveld P, Dalen JE. Time of onset of symptoms of acute myocardial infarction. Am J Cardiol 1990;66:140–144.
112. Quyyumi AA, Panza JA, Diodati JG, Lakatos E, Epstein SE. Circadian variation in ischemic threshold. A mechanism underlying the circadian variation in ischemic events. Circulation 1992;86:22–28.
113. Kono T, Morita H, Nishina T, Fujita M, Hirota Y, Kawamura K, Fujiwara A. Circadian variations of onset of acute myocardial infarction and efficacy of thrombolytic therapy. J Am Coll Cardiol 1996;27:774–778.
114. Willich SN, Collins R, Peto R, Linderer T, Sleight P, Schröder R, ISIS-2 (Second International Study of Infarct Survival) Collaborative Group. Morning peak in the incidence of myocardial infarction: experience in the ISIS-2 trial. Eur Heart J 1992;13:594–598.
115. Gnecchi-Ruscone T, Piccaluga E, Guzzeti S, Contini M, Montano N, Nicolis E. Morning and Monday: critical periods for the onset of acute myocardial infarction: the GISSI 2 Study experience. Eur Heart J 1994;15:882–887.
116. Willich SN, Lowel H, Lewis M, Hormann A, Arntz HR, Keil U. Weekly variation of acute myocardial infarction. Increased Monday risk in the working population. Circulation 1994;90:87–93.
117. Ornato JP, Siegel L, Craren EJ, Nelson N. Increased incidence of cardiac death attributed to acute myocardial infarction during winter. Coron Artery Dis 1990;1:199–203.
118. Douglas AS, al Sayer H, Rawles JM, Allan TM. Seasonality of disease in Kuwait. Lancet 1991;337:1393–1397.
119. Kloner RA, Poole KW, Perritt RL. When throughout the year is coronary death most likely to occur? A 12-year population-based analysis of more than 220,000 cases. Circulation 1999;100:1630–1634.
120. Gabbay FH, Krantz DS, Kop WJ, Hedges SM, Klein J, Gottdiener JS, Rozabski A. Triggers of myocardial ischemia during daily life in patients with coronary artery disease: physical and mental activities, anger and smoking. J Am Coll Cardiol 1996;27:585–592.

121. Mittleman MA, Maclure M, Sherwood JB, Mulry RP, Tofler GH, Jacobs SC, Friedman R, Benson H, Muller JE. Triggering of acute myocardial infarction by episodes of anger. Circulation 1995;92:1720–1725.
122. Leor J, Poole K, Kloner R. Sudden cardiac death triggered by an earthquake. N Engl J Med 1996;334:413–419.
123. Brown DL. Disparate effects of the 1989 Loma Prieta and 1994 Northridge earthquakes on hospital admissions for acute myocardial infarction: importance of superimposition of triggers. Am Heart J 1999;137:830–836.
124. Mittleman MA, Maclure M, Tofler GH, Sherwood JB, Goldberg RJ, Muller JE. Triggering of acute myocardial infarction by heavy physical exertion. Protection against triggering by regular exertion. Determinants of Myocardial Infarction Onset Study Investigators. N Engl J Med 1993;329:1677–1683.
125. Willich SN, Lewis M, Löwel H, Arntz HR, Schubert F, Schröder R. Physical exertion as a trigger of acute myocardial infarction. N Engl J Med 1993;329: 1684–1690.
126. Burke AP, Farb A, Malcom GT, Liang Y, Smialek J, Virmani R. Plaque rupture and sudden death related to exertion in men with coronary artery disease. JAMA 1999;281:921–926.
127. Mann J, Davies MJ. Mechanisms of progression in native coronary artery disease: role of healed plaque disruption. Heart 1999;82:265–268.
128. Davies MJ, Bland JM, Hangartner JR, Angelini A, Thomas AC. Factors influencing the presence or absence of acute coronary artery thrombi in sudden ischaemic death. Eur Heart J 1989;10:203–208.
129. Davies MJ, Thomas A. Thrombosis and acute coronary-artery lesions in sudden cardiac ischemic death. N Engl J Med 1984;310:1137–1140.
130. ElFawal MA, Berg GA, Wheatley DJ, Harland WA. Sudden coronary death in Glasgow: nature and frequency of acute coronary lesions. Br Heart J 1987; 57:329–335.
131. Qiao JH, Fishbein MC. The severity of coronary atherosclerosis at sites of plaque rupture with occlusive thrombus. J Am Coll Cardiol 1991;17:1138–1142.
132. Fuster V, Lewis A. Conner memorial lecture. Mechanisms leading to myocardial infarction: insights from studies of vascular biology. Circulation 1994; 90:2126–2146.
133. Lo YSA, Cutler JE, Blake K, Wright AM, Kron J, Swerdlow CD. Angiographic coronary morphology in survivors of cardiac arrest. Am Heart J 1988; 115:781–785.
134. Fuster V, Badimon L, Cohen M, Ambrose JA, Badimon JJ, Chesebro J. Insights into the pathogenesis of acute ischemic syndromes. Circulation 1988; 77:1213–1220.
135. Danchin N. Is myocardial revascularisation for tight coronary stenoses always necessary? Lancet 1993;342:224–225.
136. Bissett JK, Ngo WL, Wyeth RP, Matts JP, POSCH Group. Angiographic progression to total coronary occlusion in hyperlipidemic patients after acute myocardial infarction. Am J Cardiol 1990;66:1293–1297.

4

Embolization as a Pathological Mechanism

Deepak L. Bhatt and Eric J. Topol
The Cleveland Clinic Foundation
Cleveland, Ohio

INTRODUCTION

Spontaneous plaque rupture is the central event in the pathogenesis of acute coronary syndromes. Similarly, iatrogenic plaque rupture is induced in the cardiac catheterization laboratory during percutaneous coronary intervention. Plaque rupture leads to superimposed platelet adhesion, aggregation, and thrombus formation. Subsequent embolization of atherothrombotic material rich in platelets can lead to microvascular obstruction and dysfunction, and ultimately to myocardial necrosis (Fig. 1).

The real frequency and clinical significance of such distal embolization has only recently been appreciated. While other etiologies of microvascular obstruction such as tissue inflammation or edema exist, embolization has been increasingly recognized as having a major role in this process. Therapies that prevent embolization or minimize its impact in creating microvasculature obstruction are in evolution. Embolization and microvascular obstruction have a significant impact during both coronary interventional procedures and acute coronary syndromes. However, the impact and importance of distal embolization was first established for percutaneous coronary intervention. Initially, embolization was believed to be of little consequence unless it was manifest angiographically.

Accumulating evidence has revealed that embolization is not as benign a process as interventional cardiologists would like to believe. Using an

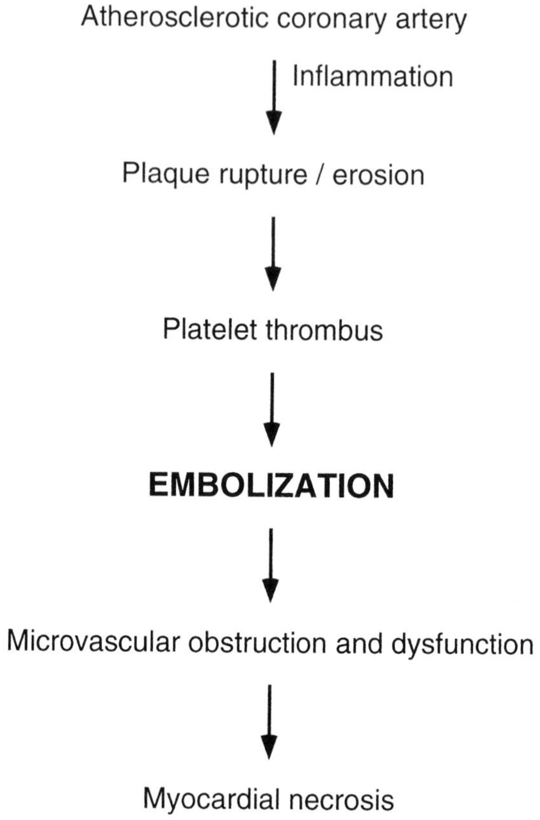

Figure 1 New paradigm for pathogenesis of acute coronary syndromes, highlighting the importance of distal embolization.

emboli capture device in routine stent and balloon coronary revascularization procedures, Yadav and colleagues (1) have shown that all patients undergoing coronary intervention have evidence of atheroembolic material. This observation provides a basis for interpretation of much of the pivotal data in the field.

PERIPROCEDURAL CREATINE KINASE ELEVATION

Measurement of periprocedural cardiac enzyme levels has provided insight into the occurrence of distal embolization. Even in the absence of clinically manifest myocardial necrosis, periprocedural cardiac enzyme elevation is associated with adverse long-term outcomes, including cardiac death (2–4).

There is a gradient of risk, with larger degrees of creatine kinase elevation being associated with a progressively worse prognosis. Initially, the importance of so-called infarctlets was debated within the interventional cardiology community. However, the EPIC 3-year data conclusively demonstrate the importance of periprocedural myocardial infarction (MI) and the long-term benefit of the glycoprotein IIb/IIIa inhibitor abciximab (5). In EPIC, the all-cause mortality for patients increased as a function of periprocedural creatine kinase elevation. At a creatine kinase elevation five times the upper limit of normal, the risk of death more than doubles. Only part of this elevated risk of death is attributable to death within 30 days of the periprocedural creatine kinase elevation, with the rest of the deaths occurring later, as can be appreciated from the EPIC survival curves (Fig. 2).

Other studies have corroborated the importance of even minimal cardiac enzyme elevation (6,7). The EPISTENT data show a reduction not only in periprocedural MI but also in 1-year all-cause mortality in patients treated with abciximab compared with placebo (8). Thus, agents that reduce embolization and prevent periprocedural MI ultimately also reduce mortality. The benefit of glycoprotein IIb/IIIa inhibitors in decreasing periprocedural MI, immediate ischemic complications, and long-term mortality supports the importance of distal embolization as a pathological entity, worthy of recognition and prevention.

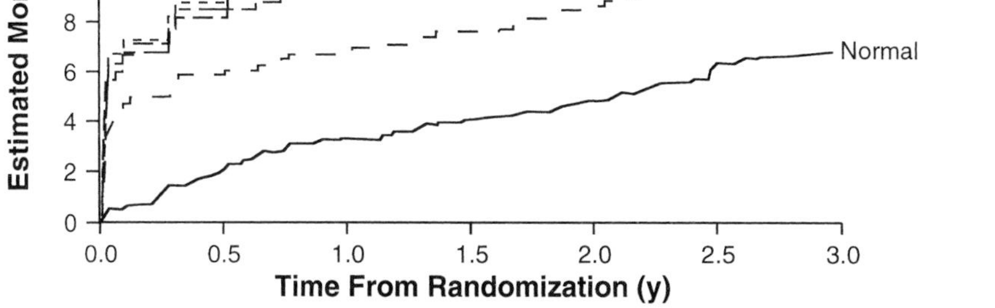

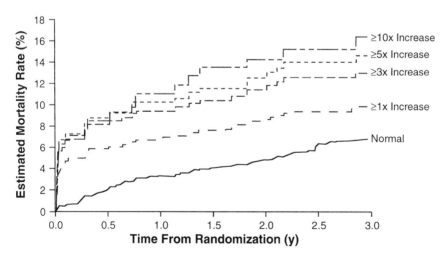

Figure 2 Long-term prognostic value of periprocedural creatine kinase elevation from the 3-year EPIC data. Mortality rises for patients with 1-fold to 10-fold increases in periprocedural CK levels as compared with patients without CK elevation. (From Ref. 5.)

ATHERECTOMY

Atherectomy is perhaps the ultimate in vivo model of distal embolization. Calcific atheroemboli have been documented in patients who have died after rotational atherectomy (9). Rotational atherectomy can also result in large amounts of creatine kinase elevation. Braden et al. (10) showed that abciximab can decrease the magnitude of creatine kinase elevation, and even its incidence. Rotational atherectomy often leads to transient perfusion defects on radionuclide imaging (Fig. 3), though abciximab markedly decreases such hypoperfusion (11). Interestingly, the patients who had elevation in cardiac enzymes associated with the procedure had larger perfusion defects than the patients without such injury. Again, distal embolization leads to ischemia, but antiplatelet therapy ameliorates the response of the microvasculature to the shower of atherothrombotic gruel.

Of note, directional coronary atherectomy (DCA) has the highest risk of periprocedural MI, compared with rotablation, stenting, or balloon (12,13). The CAVEAT trial found that DCA was associated with a higher rate of ischemic complications than PTCA (14). Directional atherectomy also caused significantly more non-Q-wave MI than did PTCA in the EPIC trial (15). The rate of non-Q-wave MI was 9.6% for DCA compared with 4.9% for PTCA, but use of abciximab in the DCA patients reduced the rate from 15.4% for placebo to 4.5% with treatment. Thus, much of the excess risk of DCA, due to platelet aggregation and embolization, can be minimized by abciximab use.

VEIN GRAFT EMBOLIZATION

The phenomenon of "no reflow," the lack of adequate blood flow despite epicardial patency, has been a perpetual concern with saphenous vein graft intervention. The embolization of atherothrombotic debris is widely accepted as responsible for no reflow. On histopathological examination, balloon angioplasty has been shown to be capable of causing extensive plaque rupture (16). This plaque rupture results in atheroembolization into the microvasculature. Percutaneous intervention of aged, degenerated atherosclerotic vein grafts is particularly plagued by such distal embolization (17). Atherectomy,

Figure 3 (a) Transient apical perfusion defect after rotational atherectomy of the LAD, as identified by SPECT imaging. Images were obtained before (preR), during (R), and 2 days after (postR) atherectomy. (b) Polar maps of the left ventricle of the same patient show relative tracer uptake values in the LAD territory. The highlighted regions indicate significantly reduced perfusion. (From Ref. 11.)

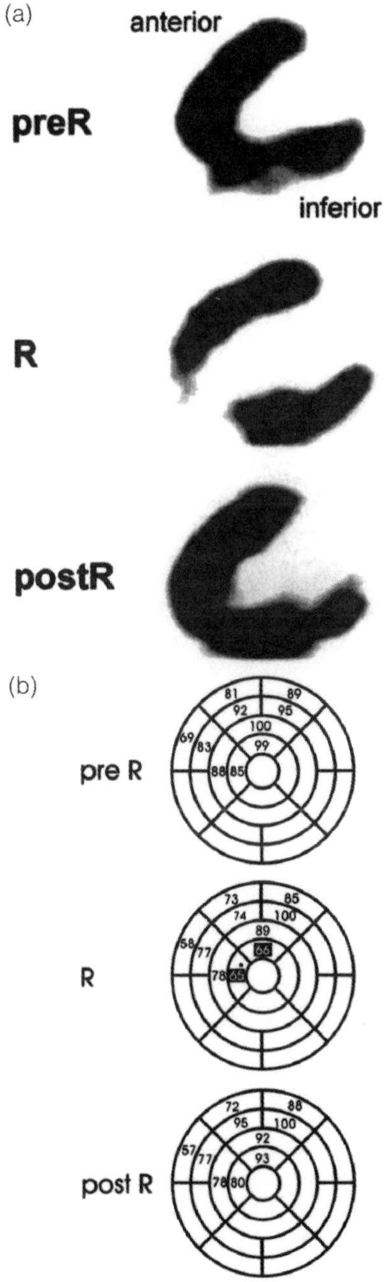
(a)
anterior
preR
inferior
R
postR
(b)
pre R
R
post R

as in native vessels, is especially prone to embolization. The CAVEAT II trial showed that the combination of directional coronary atherectomy and vein graft intervention was also associated with adverse outcomes (18). In the subset of patients from the EPIC trial who underwent vein graft intervention, 18% had distal embolization. Abciximab treatment decreased this rate to 2%. This reduction in distal embolization translated into a reduction in non-Q-wave MI.

An interesting observation was made by Trono et al. (19) in a study of patients undergoing percutaneous intervention of saphenous vein grafts. Autopsies of two patients revealed multiple atherosclerotic emboli to the distal epicardial coronary artery supplied by the vein graft upon which intervention was performed. Of course, this is not surprising. More importantly, there were multiple infarcts of varying ages, including some that clearly occurred prior to the time of intervention. Therefore, akin to the embolization caused by intervention, spontaneous embolization can occur in vein grafts as well.

Transluminal extraction atherectomy, initially proposed as a solution to distal embolization, is itself associated with a high rate of embolization (20). Furthermore, in patients who had distal embolization, the in-hospital mortality rate was 18.5%, versus 3.0% in those without distal embolization. Interestingly, a small study of transluminal extraction atherectomy for occluded vein grafts revealed that abciximab dramatically reduced the incidence of embolization, again highlighting the relevance of platelet aggregation to this process (21).

While atherectomy is not a solution for distal embolization in vein grafts, and in fact contributes to the problem, other technologies are in development to either capture or filter vein graft debris created at the site of intervention and prevent migration downstream into the microvasculature. In 21 out of 23 vein graft interventions, Webb et al. (22) were able to retrieve particulate matter. The average size of the atheromatous particles was 240 by 83 μm. Carlino et al. (23) have successfully used the PercuSurge GuardWire to mechanically prevent such distal embolization. Similar emboli protection devices will shortly be tested in the setting of acute myocardial infarction, potentially creating a marriage of mechanical and pharmacological therapies for prevention of embolization in acute coronary syndromes.

CORONARY ARTERY BYPASS GRAFTING

That atheroembolism can occur during bypass surgery has long been appreciated by cardiothoracic surgeons. In fact, it may occur on a much larger scale than with percutaneous intervention. Keon et al. (24) described thirteen cases of fatal perioperative myocardial infarction. Five of the cases involved emboli that originated from ulcerative atherosclerotic lesions in the aortic root at the site of the vein graft ostia. Embolization from coronary endarterectomy sites occurred in two cases. Two cases were due to mechanical disruption of plaque in the major epicardial coronary arteries during surgery. An additional four cases occurred during repeat bypass procedures and resulted from dislodgment of atheroma from previous vein grafts while they were being manipulated. If routine measurement of cardiac enzyme MB fractions were performed following surgery, the true incidence of distal embolization with microvascular obstruction could be appreciated. However, this practice was abandoned a number of years ago, owing to concerns of spurious laboratory results not reflective of actual myocardial necrosis (4,25–27).

THROMBOLYTIC THERAPY

The provocation of distal embolization, as with percutaneous intervention, can also occur after thrombolytic therapy. An autopsy study from the Mayo Clinic examined 32 patients who died within 3 weeks of either balloon angioplasty or thrombolytic therapy (28). Microemboli were seen in 81% of the patients. The majority of emboli were either thrombotic or atheromatous. The presence of emboli was significantly correlated with the development of new electrocardiographic abnormalities, new myocardial infarction, or extension of prior myocardial infarction after the procedure. The authors speculate that, in the living, recurrent ischemia can be due to microembolization. An earlier report had also provided histological evidence that thrombolytic therapy can lead to distal embolization of thrombus (29).

In addition, thrombolytic therapy can actually create a prothrombotic milieu. For example, activated platelets are capable of secreting plasminogen activator inhibitor-1 (30). In the future, the combination of thrombolytic therapy with glycoprotein IIb/IIIa inhibition will likely minimize the impact of distal embolization caused by platelet-rich thrombus (31). Numerous trials are already under way and are exploring the safety of this approach (32). Initial results suggest higher rates of TIMI 3 flow with this combination therapy (33). Adding mechanical intervention to this combination chemotherapy appears safe and may create the optimal reperfusion strategy (34). Catheter-directed ultrasound thrombolysis is another possible therapy that is being investigated for thrombus dissolution (35,36). However, as a standalone technique, it is unlikely that it will eliminate the problem of distal embolization of thrombus entirely, as embolization has been documented to occur with this device (37). It would seem that any device that has to be put into a diseased artery before being used or activated will always have a liability.

Thus, the wealth of data from the percutaneous coronary intervention literature supports the mechanistic importance of distal embolization and the value of minimizing its impact on the microvasculature. Furthermore, these data provide a conceptual framework for understanding spontaneous embolization that occurs during acute coronary syndromes.

EMBOLIZATION DURING ACUTE CORONARY SYNDROMES

In the setting of acute coronary syndromes, just as with percutaneous coronary intervention, distal embolization occurs and glycoprotein IIb/IIIa inhibitors improve outcomes (38). Numerous studies have documented the beneficial impact on death or MI that glycoprotein IIb/IIIa inhibitors have in acute coronary syndromes (39–42). Much of the benefit of glycoprotein IIb/IIIa inhibitors can be attributed to the effects they have on the occurrence of platelet embolization, as well as the microvasculature's response to this embolic burden (Table 1).

Platelet Embolization

A seminal contribution to the understanding of embolization in acute coronary syndromes was made by Davies et al. (43) in an autopsy study of ninety patients who suffered sudden cardiac death. Thirty percent of the patients had platelet aggregates found in small intramyocardial vessels (Fig. 4). In patients with unstable angina before death, 44.4% were found to have such

Table 1 Mechanisms of Myocyte Necrosis Due to Distal Embolization

Thrombosis
Platelet aggregation
Thrombin generation
Inflammation
Release of cytokines
Recruitment of monocytes and neutrophils
Apoptosis
Vasoconstriction
Endothelial dysfunction
Vasoactive amines, thromboxane A_2, serotonin
Compromised collateral flow
Infarct expansion

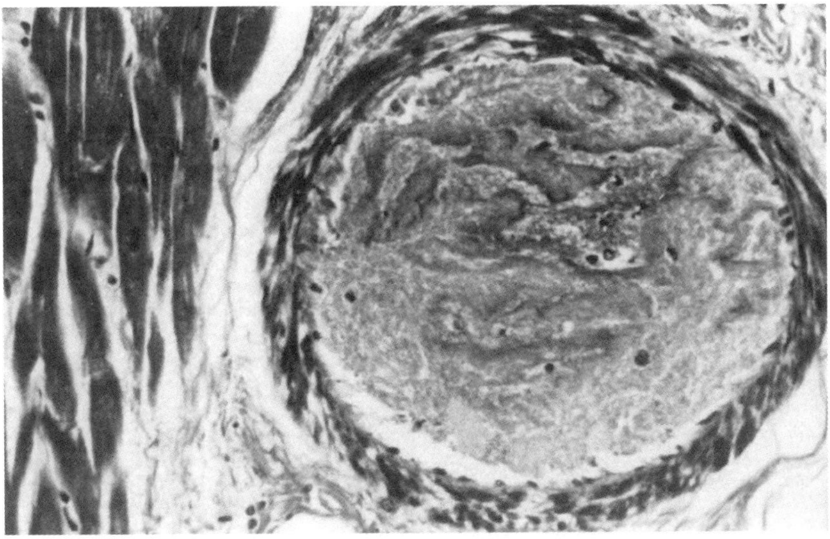

(a)

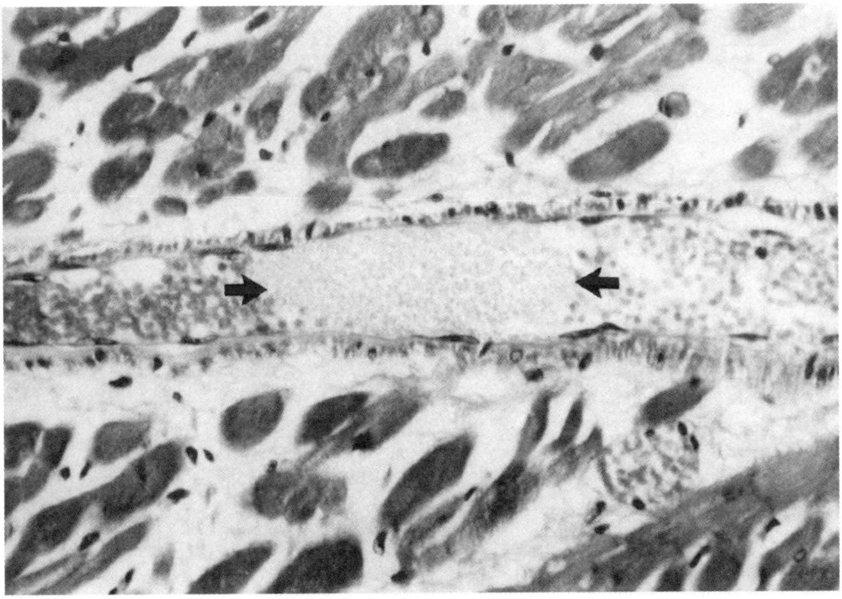

(b)

Figure 4 Deposition of platelet aggregates in the microvasculature, occupying the entire lumen of an intramyocardial artery, in cross section (a) and in longitudinal section (b). (From Ref. 43.)

platelet aggregates. Those patients with platelet emboli were much more likely to have multifocal microscopic necrosis involving the entire ventricular wall. The platelet aggregates were present in the myocardial territory subserved by an epicardial artery containing a ruptured plaque with overlying thrombus. Similarly, in a study of patients who died of acute myocardial infarction, 79% had platelet emboli found in the microcirculation (Fig.

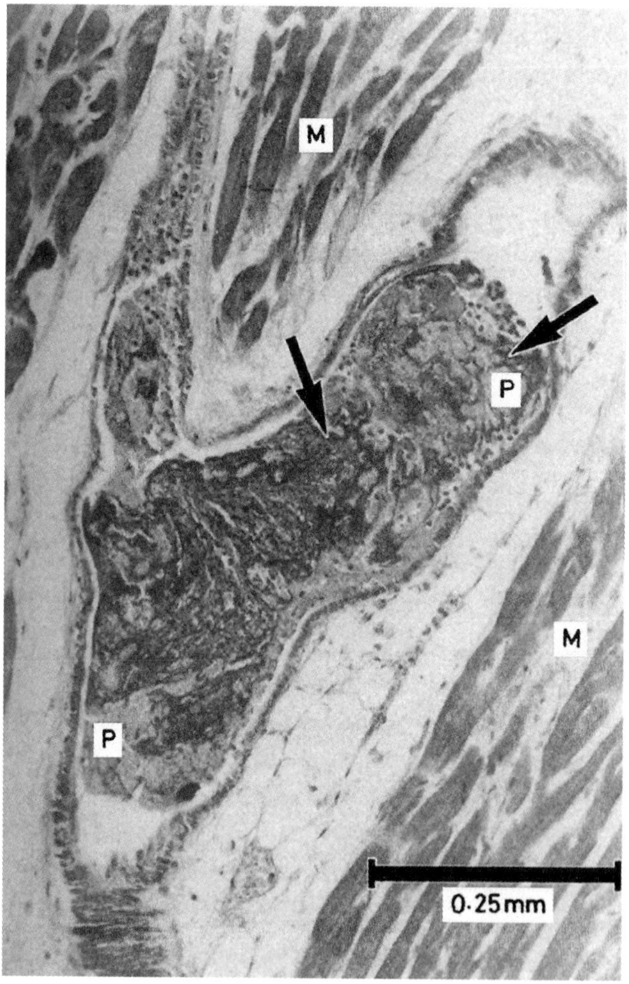

Figure 5 Intramyocardial arteriole containing a microembolus composed of platelets and fibrin. The arrows show fibrin strands forming islands of platelets; P, platelets; M, myocardium. (From Ref. 44.)

5) (44). Another autopsy study of 25 patients with sudden death revealed that 81% had epicardial thrombi with a layered structure, composed of thrombus material of differing ages (45). This important finding implies periodic growth of the epicardial thrombus, which was accompanied by intermittent fragmentation and embolization of thrombus in 73% of the cases, resulting in occlusion of small intramyocardial arteries with associated microscopic infarcts. Furthermore, during acute myocardial infarction, platelet microthrombi are not just confined to the infarct-related artery, but can be found in the circulation and are associated with infarct extension (46). Platelet and thrombin microthrombi are not found in normal hearts, only in patients with cardiac disease (47). In addition, platelet aggregation and embolization can lower the threshold for ventricular fibrillation (48). Thus, platelet embolization not only occurs, but also can lead to infarction of myocardial cells and even trigger sudden death.

Further indirect evidence of the importance of microvascular obstruction due to platelet aggregates comes from an analysis of patients with angiographically "insignificant" coronary artery disease in PURSUIT (49). Those patients presenting with acute coronary syndromes with <50% stenosis in any epicardial vessel nevertheless appeared to have modest benefit from eptifibatide therapy. Potentially, platelet embolization from the site of a ruptured plaque is minimized by glycoprotein IIb/IIIa blockade.

Role of the Endothelium

Concomitant endothelial dysfunction further aggravates the situation created by platelet embolization. Endothelial expression of P-selectin, capable of binding platelets and leukocytes, is upregulated distal to severe epicardial stenoses (50). In addition, endothelial integrity as assessed by electron microscopy can be disrupted. A study by Mutin et al. (51) found circulating endothelial cells in patients with acute myocardial infarction and unstable angina, but not in those with stable angina or in controls. It is also known that endothelial microparticles have both adhesive properties and procoagulant effects (52). Thus, embolization of endothelial cells in acute coronary syndromes does occur and can lead to further platelet activation and aggregation in the microvasculature, ultimately leading to obstruction and myocardial necrosis. An interesting hypothesis to explain part of the benefit of abciximab, in addition to its properties as a glycoprotein IIb/IIIa inhibitor, is its ability to bind the vitronectin receptor. This integrin is heavily expressed on activated endothelial cells. Potentially, by binding to this receptor on endothelial cells, endothelial microparticles are unable to bind to other tissue elements in the microvasculature.

Inflammation and Embolization

Inflammation and embolization are intimately intertwined. The inflamed artery contributes to plaque erosion, rupture, and the potential for subsequent distal embolization. The embolization of friable microparticulate atherosclerotic material, with or without platelet thrombus, likely promotes further inflammation. The CD40 ligand on activated platelets causes endothelial cells to express adhesion molecules and to secrete chemokines that attract leukocytes (53). Compared with control patients and those with stable angina, patients with unstable angina have elevated levels of CD40 ligand, in both its soluble and membrane-bound forms (54). Activated platelets can also cause endothelial cells to express tissue factor, generating a prothrombotic milieu (55). Platelet-leukocyte adhesion can occur via interaction between P-selectin on platelets and sialyl Lewis(x) on leukocytes (56,57). Compared with controls, patients with acute coronary syndromes have higher levels of platelet microparticles and greater degrees of platelet-leukocyte interaction (58). In patients with acute myocardial infarction, platelet-leukocyte adhesion is increased, leading to induction of IL-1 beta, IL-8, and MCP-1, and activation of nuclear factor kappa B (59). Thus, platelet embolization in acute coronary syndromes induces an inflammatory response that can lead to formation of a multicellular plug, composed of platelets, neutrophils, and endothelial cells, capable of occluding microvascular flow.

Prevention of platelet activation seems to be paramount in halting this deleterious cascade of events. However, it would be naïve to assume that the antiplatelet effect produced by glycoprotein IIb/IIIa therapy is the only operative mechanism. Abciximab binds to several other receptors in addition to the platelet glycoprotein IIb/IIIa receptor. It binds to the leukocyte integrin MAC-1, preventing binding of fibrinogen and ICAM-1 (60). Abciximab also binds to the vitronectin receptor and can lead to further reductions in thrombin generation, independent of the effects on glycoprotein IIb/IIIa inhibition (61). Blockade of the vitronectin receptor has other important biological effects and has resulted in a decrease in neointimal proliferation in animal models of arterial injury (62). Vitronectin can mediate platelet attachment to activated endothelium in the plasma of patients with acute myocardial infarction undergoing reperfusion (63). This nonspecific binding of abciximab to multiple receptors, in addition to promoting an antiplatelet and antithrombotic effect, produces simultaneous blockade of endothelial cells and leukocytes as well. These other actions may translate into further improvements in microvascular flow, beyond that exclusively due to antiplatelet effects.

Microvascular Function

Superimposed thrombus formation in the setting of distal embolization of atheromatous material further contributes to microvascular flow obstruction by triggering a cascade of biochemical events. Platelet activation and aggregation and vascular tone are intimately linked (64). Coronary stenosis and associated endothelial injury with subsequent platelet aggregation, dislodgment, and distal embolization lead to the now well recognized phenomenon of cyclic flow variation (65). Measures that reduce platelet aggregation reduce cyclic flow variation. This has been demonstrated for nitric oxide production (66), thrombin inhibition (67), and ADP receptor blockade (68).

Release of substances such as vasoactive amines from activated platelets leads to vasoconstriction and microcirculatory abnormalities. Intense microvascular constriction can occur due to release of such factors from platelets (69). Prostaglandin production can cause vasoconstriction (70). Platelet-activating factor can be released by either platelets or neutrophils and can lead to vasoconstriction in coronary arterioles (71,72). Thromboxane A_2 and serotonin, released from activated platelets, are potent vasoconstrictors (30). Thrombin, the production of which is accelerated by aggregated platelets, can also cause vasoconstriction (73). Agents that reverse this vasoconstriction, induced by multiple agonists, are potentially therapeutic in this situation. Taniyama et al. (74) showed that intracoronary verapamil at the time of primary PTCA leads to further improvements in microvascular flow. Similarly, Ito et al. (75) demonstrated that intravenous nicorandil, an adenosine triphosphate-sensitive potassium channel opener, further improves microvascular flow after apparently successful PTCA. Impaired flow even in nonculprit arteries during acute myocardial infarction has been demonstrated with the corrected TIMI frame count (76). Even with successful angioplasty of the culprit artery, flow in all arteries is still reduced compared to normal, likely due, at least in part, to abnormalities of microvascular flow (77). In addition to its effects on microvascular function, embolization may also compromise collateral flow and contribute to infarct expansion.

Embolization in Diabetic Patients

Diabetic patients with acute coronary syndromes have a higher rate of adverse outcomes (78–82). While this is due to multiple factors, diabetics are prone to distal embolization and are particularly ill suited to deal with its consequences. Diabetics have hyperreactivity of their platelets (83), making them more likely to adhere to the endothelium under conditions of shear stress (84). Their platelets are more prone to spontaneous aggregation (85). Even the prediabetic state is associated with increased platelet activation

(86). Diabetics with unstable angina are much more likely to have ulcerated plaque and intracoronary thrombus, as documented by angioscopy (87). Therefore, they are at much higher risk of embolization into the microvasculature. Their microvasculature is often diffusely diseased and dysfunctional, as reflected by a diminished coronary flow reserve (88,89), and an embolic shower is less likely to be tolerated and more likely to lead to microvascular obstruction and myocardial necrosis. Furthermore, the diabetic state leads to a heightened tendency for platelet-leukocyte interaction to occur (90). These findings may help explain the remarkable benefit of abciximab in reducing the increased rate of mortality in diabetic patients undergoing percutaneous coronary intervention (91). Thus, diabetic patients are particularly prone to distal embolization and more likely to suffer adverse clinical consequences as a result, but fortunately, therapy with abciximab can attenuate the adverse effect of embolization on their microvasculature.

MEASUREMENT OF EMBOLIZATION WITH TROPONINS

Troponin measurement is a sensitive indicator of distal embolization and resultant myocardial cellular damage (92). Troponins are found in myocytes in the troponin-tropomyosin complex. Troponins are much more sensitive than CK-MB at detecting myocardial damage and are useful in risk-stratifying patients with acute coronary syndromes (93–95). Elevated troponin levels are associated with an increased rate of adverse outcomes. This holds true even when the creatine kinase level is not elevated above normal limits. Hamm et al. (96) reported on the value of troponins in risk-stratifying patients with acute coronary syndromes and showed their usefulness in allocating patients to intravenous antiplatelet therapy in the CAPTURE trial (Fig. 6A,B). In fact, troponin elevation appears to be a more powerful tool for risk stratification and selection of patients for abciximab therapy than angiography in patients with unstable angina (97). In the PRISM trial as well, both troponin T and I were found to identify the group of patients with unstable angina who derived maximum benefit from glycoprotein IIb/IIIa blockade with tirofiban (98,99) (Fig. 6C,D). While the CAPTURE data documented the value of troponin measurement in risk stratification in a relatively high risk cohort of patients, the PRISM analysis extended this finding to a lower-risk cohort. In PRISM, tirofiban treatment in patients with positive troponins resulted in a significant decrease in mortality, both in patients who were medically managed and in those who subsequently underwent revascularization. In addition, the FRISC trial found that both troponin and C-reactive protein, a marker of inflammation, were independently able to predict cardiac death in a multivariable model (100). In FRISC II, long-term

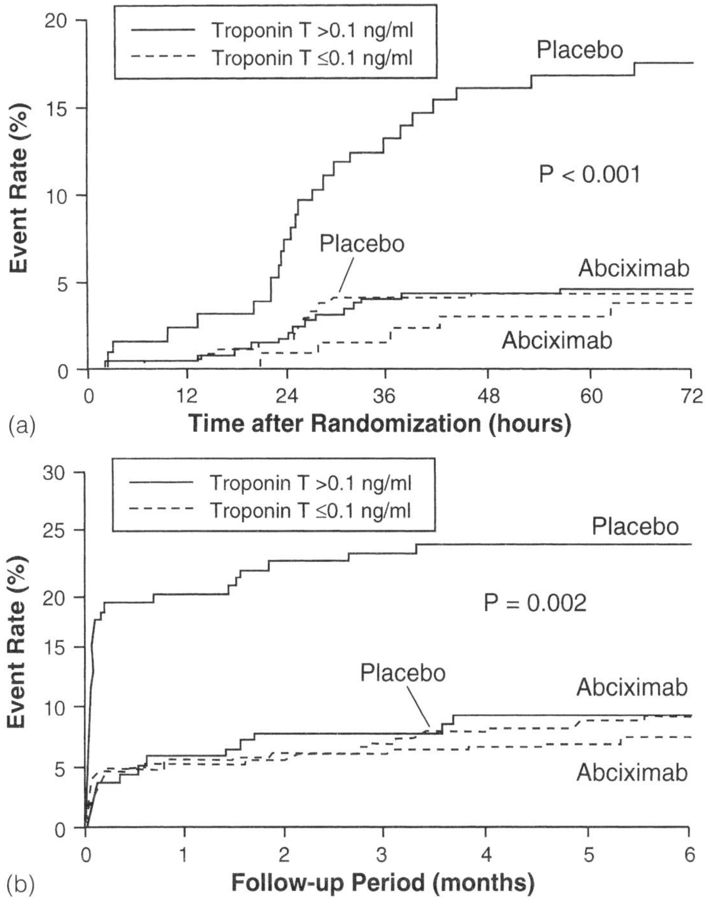

Figure 6 Data from the CAPTURE trial, showing the benefit of abciximab in reducing death and nonfatal MI in patients who are troponin positive in the initial 72 hours after randomization (a) and during 6 months of follow-up (b). (From Ref. 96.) The PRISM trial likewise showed a reduction in death and MI in patients who were troponin positive (c). This reduction was seen both in patients treated medically and with revascularization (d). (From Ref. 99.)

treatment with the low-molecular-weight heparin dalteparin in troponin-positive patients with unstable angina was also found to decrease cardiac events (101). Thus, measurement of troponins as a marker of distal embolization allows detection of levels of myocardial damage not previously possible. Measurements of C-reactive protein may add additional prognostic value.

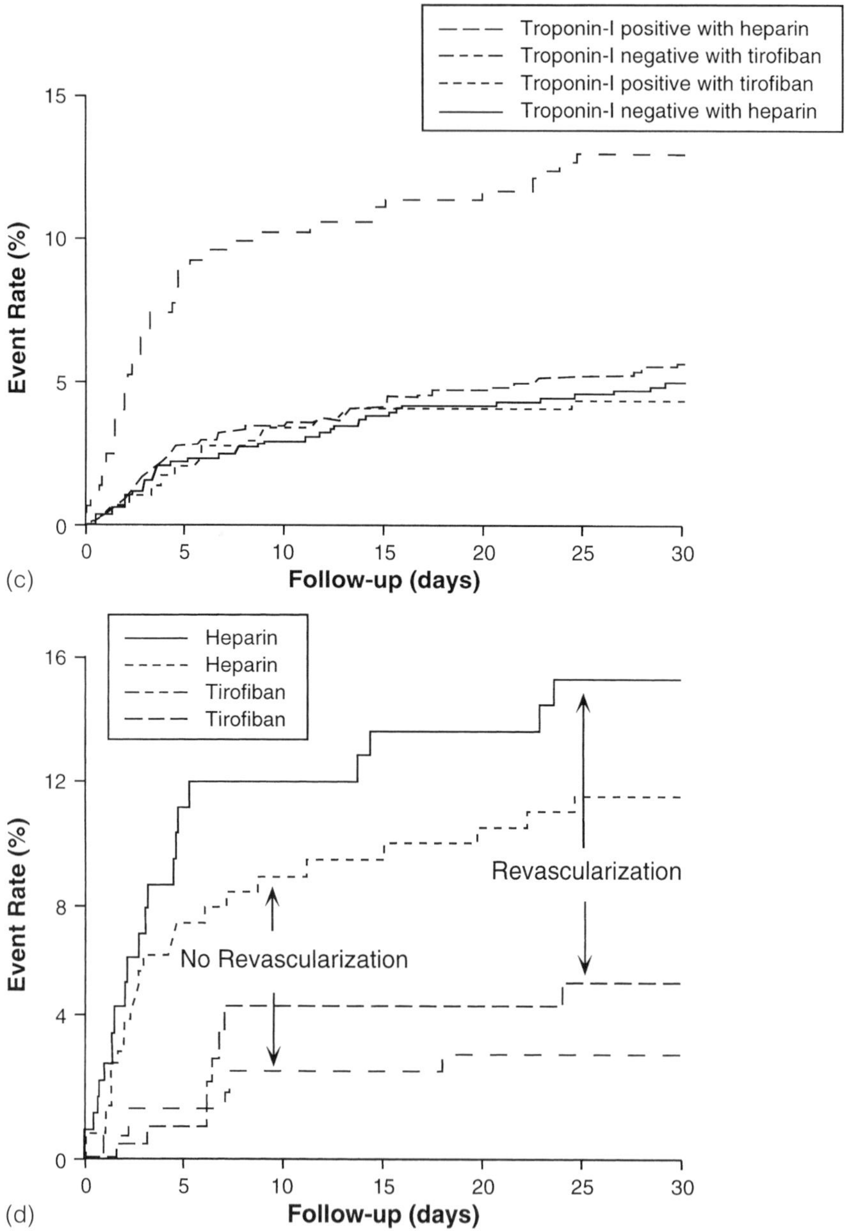

Figure 6 Continued

Furthermore, such information allows targeting of intravenous antiplatelet therapy or antithrombotic therapy to those patients most likely to have distal embolization.

IMAGING THE IMPACT OF EMBOLIZATION

The rapid evolution of imaging technology has allowed visualization of the importance of distal embolization on the microvasculature. Both contrast echocardiography and magnetic resonance imaging (MRI) are expanding our appreciation of embolization. Coronary flow measurements have also refined our understanding of microvasular function.

Contrast Echocardiography

Initially, Ito et al. (102) used intracoronary myocardial contrast echocardiography to study acute MI patients before and after revascularization. A sizable proportion of patients with TIMI 3 flow nevertheless had evidence of impaired microvascular perfusion, despite adequate epicardial patency; these patients did not have significant recovery of myocardial function as assessed by the ejection fraction. The ability of the left ventricle to remodel after acute MI was also adversely affected in those patients without adequate reflow on myocardial contrast echo, as reflected by increased left ventricular end-diastolic volumes (103). Contrast echo using intravenous perfluorocarbon-exposed sonicated dextrose albumin microbubbles has also been used to investigate reperfusion in acute MI (104). Of the patients with angiographic TIMI 3 flow, 29% had defects on contrast echocardiography (see Fig. 7). While the patients with reflow on contrast echocardiography had a significant decrease in end-systolic volume index, those with no reflow had a significant increase in this parameter. Determination of microvascular integrity by contrast echocardiography was also found useful for predicting subsequent clinical events (105). Myocardial contrast echo is thus poised to transition from being a research tool to being a clinically relevant method to assess embolization and microvascular flow.

Magnetic Resonance Imaging

Advances in MRI technology have also occurred at a rapid pace. Much like contrast echo, MRI can quantify microvascular obstruction and compares favorably with histopathologic methods (see Fig. 8) (106). MRI can quantify microvascular obstruction after myocardial infarction and correlates well with radioactive microsphere blood flow measurements (107). A study of 44 patients with acute MI by Wu et al. (108) examined cardiovascular outcomes at 2 years. Patients classified as having microvascular obstruction had a

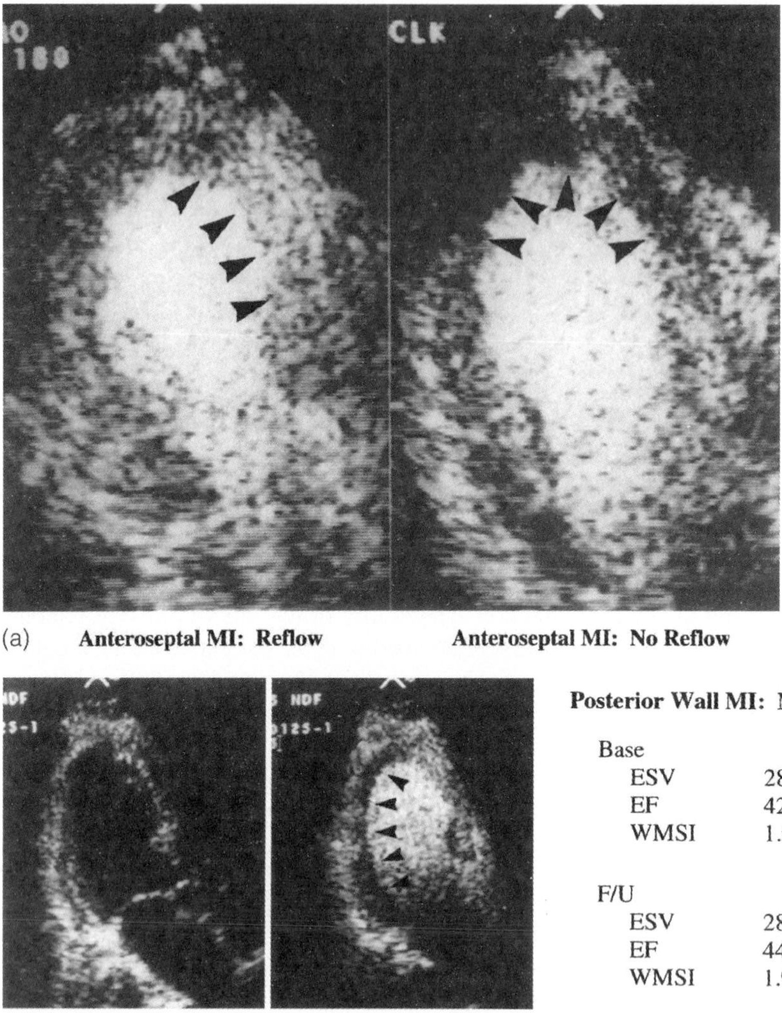

Figure 7 Contrast echocardiograms in two patients with restored epicardial flow in the LAD, one (a) showing reflow and the other showing no reflow during anteroseptal MI. In this patient with an acute left circumflex artery infarction, despite TIMI 3 flow on angiography, a microvascular perfusion defect as assessed by contrast echocardiography is seen in the posterior wall (b). (From Ref. 104.)

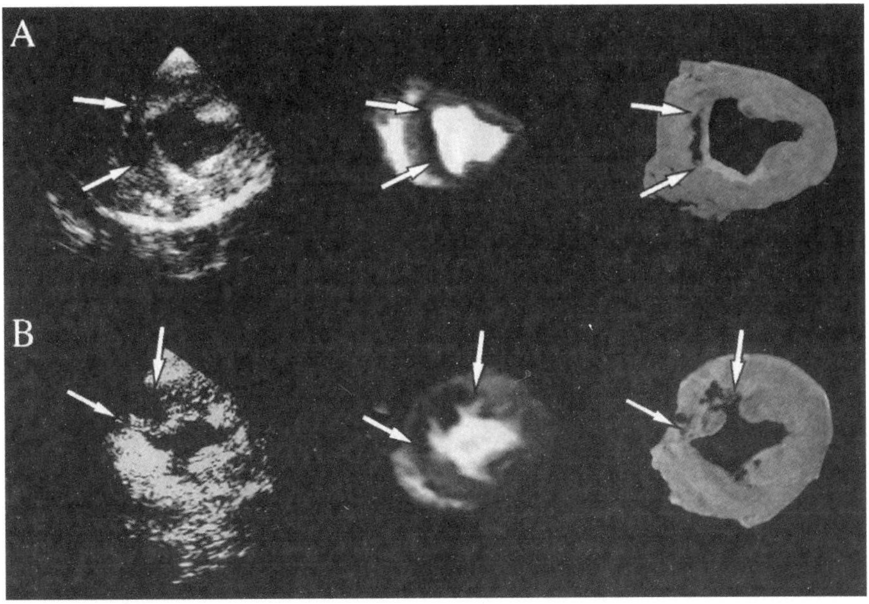

Figure 8 MRI showing two examples from separate animals (A and B) of microvascular obstruction and correlation with contrast echocardiography or postmortem thioflavin-S staining. (From Ref. 106.)

significantly higher rate of cardiovascular events than those without—45% versus 9%. Importantly, even after adjusting for infarct size, microvascular obstruction remained a statistically significant prognostic marker of complications. Among the 17 patients returning for follow-up MRI at 6 months, the presence of microvascular obstruction was associated with both fibrous scar formation and left ventricular remodeling. Therefore, although TIMI 3 flow on angiography has been the gold standard for reperfusion therapy, newer imaging modalities have conclusively demonstrated that TIMI 3 flow alone is not sufficient for demonstration of adequate tissue level perfusion. Furthermore, inadequate tissue perfusion leads to impaired left ventricular remodeling and function, as well as higher rates of cardiovascular events.

ECG ST SEGMENT RESOLUTION

While sophisticated imaging methodologies have been developed, the full potential of the standard electrocardiogram has still not been exhausted. Electrocardiographic resolution of ST segment elevation appears to be a powerful method to detect epicardial patency as well as tissue level reperfusion (109–111). Greater than or equal to 70% ST segment resolution in patients with acute myocardial infarction identified those who had preserved left ventricular function measured 1 week later (112). Continuous ST segment monitoring may provide a method to detect successful reperfusion or reocclusion (113–115). ST segment resolution may also provide insight into cyclic flow variation (116). The correlation of ST segment resolution with myocardial contrast echo is excellent (117). After either chemical or mechanical reperfusion, ST segment resolution is able to provide important prognostic information (118). An analysis of the TIMI 14 data examined the percent ST resolution in patients with angiographically demonstrated TIMI 3 flow (119). Patients who received abciximab in addition to reduced dose tPA had significantly greater ST segment resolution than patients who received standard tPA—69% complete resolution versus 44%, $P = .0002$. It is likely that improvements in the degree of ST segment resolution will translate into decreased mortality, and ongoing trials should provide this evidence. Thus, ECG ST segment resolution may be the gold standard to detect reperfusion at the tissue level and to identify therapies that enhance microvascular flow.

PREVENTING EMBOLIZATION—CLINICAL RELEVANCE

Potentially, impaired microvascular perfusion could be due to factors other than distal embolization, such as reperfusion injury, edema, or inflammation. While it is likely that the mechanism is multifactorial, there is direct evidence that therapies that target platelet aggregation (and possibly endothelial and neutrophil adhesion) improve tissue level perfusion. In an elegant analysis of patients undergoing stent implantation for acute MI, Neumann et al. (120) demonstrated that abciximab, in addition to its known beneficial effect on epicardial patency, improves microvascular perfusion. Compared with heparin, patients randomized to abciximab had higher peak flow velocity on Doppler wire measurements (see Fig. 9). Furthermore, the improvement in tissue level perfusion was associated with favorable left ventricular function, as the abciximab-treated group had a higher ejection fraction than the heparin-treated group—62% versus 56%, $P = .003$.

In an analysis of patients who received either thrombolytic therapy or primary angioplasty for a first-time acute MI, Agati et al. (121) assessed microvascular perfusion via intracoronary injection of sonicated microbubbles. In the subset of patients with TIMI 3 flow at 1 month, a perfusion defect occurred in 72% of the patients who received t-PA versus 31% of the patients who received primary angioplasty, $P = .00001$. The wall motion score index at 1 month was also significantly better in the patients treated with angioplasty. Again, improvements in tissue level reperfusion translate

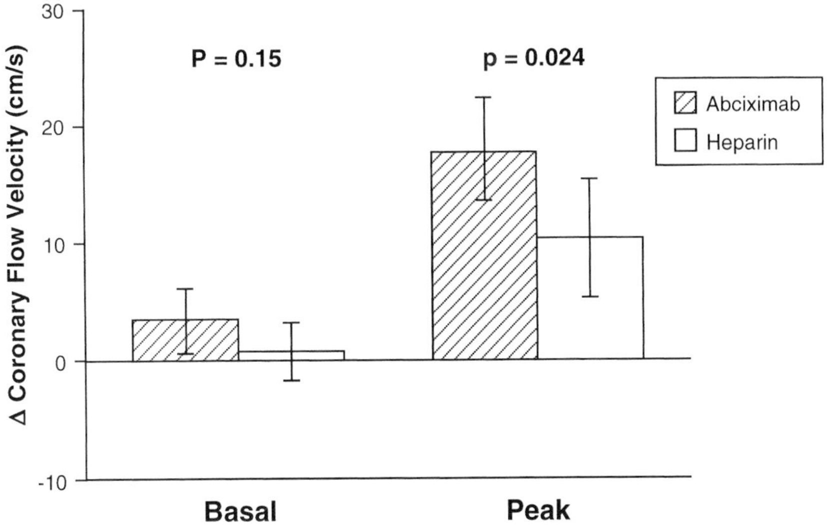

Figure 9 Differences in basal and peak coronary flow velocity for abciximab versus placebo. (From Ref. 120.)

into improved ventricular function. Furthermore, tissue level reperfusion can be enhanced both by pharmacological therapy with glycoprotein IIb/IIIa inhibition and by mechanical reperfusion therapy.

CONCLUSION

The great frequency with which embolization occurs is only now being appreciated. Filter devices that capture embolic debris, troponin measurements, and newer imaging modalities have each demonstrated that embolization is common and results in significant myocardial damage. Clearly, these recent data have shifted the focus in acute coronary syndromes from merely ensuring epicardial patency to reestablishing adequate microvascular perfusion. Methods of measuring embolization will continue to be refined (Table 2). Distal embolization is the major contributor to microvascular obstruction in the setting of ischemia, operating via a number of intertwined cellular and biochemical pathways. Successful mechanical, catheter-based approaches as well as pharmacological approaches have been developed to prevent embolization. However, the future lies in combining these previously divergent philosophies of reperfusion, and such efforts are under way with promising initial results. Thus, therapies that decrease embolization are effective in improving both short- and long-term outcomes of patients with

Table 2 Markers to Detect Embolization and Their Ability to Predict Outcome

Condition	Primary marker(s) of embolization	Outcome
Percutaneous coronary intervention	CK-MB	+++
Unstable angina	Troponin	++++
Acute MI	ECG ST resolution	++++ (?)
	Contrast echo	++
	MRI	++

acute coronary syndromes and represent a major advance in the field of cardiology.

REFERENCES

1. Yadav JS, Grube E, Rowold S, Kirchof N, Sedgewick J, Topol EJ. Detection and characterization of emboli during coronary intervention. Circulation 1999; 100:I–780.
2. Abdelmeguid AE, Topol EJ. The myth of the myocardial "infarctlet" during percutaneous coronary revascularization procedures. Circulation 1996;94: 3369–3375.
3. Abdelmeguid AE, Topol EJ, Whitlow PL, Sapp SK, Ellis SG. Significance of mild transient release of creatine kinase-MB fraction after percutaneous coronary interventions. Circulation 1996;94:1528–1536.
4. Califf RM, Abdelmeguid AE, Kuntz RE, Popma JJ, Davidson CJ, Cohen EA, Kleiman NS, Mahaffey KW, Topol EJ, Pepine CJ, Lipicky RJ, Granger CB, Harrington RA, Tardiff BE, Crenshaw BS, Bauman RP, Zuckerman BD, Chaitman BR, Bittl JA, Ohman EM. Myonecrosis after revascularization procedures. J Am Coll Cardiol 1998;31:241–251.
5. Topol EJ, Ferguson JJ, Weisman HF, Tcheng JE, Ellis SG, Kleiman NS, Ivanhoe RJ, Wang AL, Miller DP, Anderson KM, Califf RM. Long-term protection from myocardial ischemic events in a randomized trial of brief integrin beta-3 blockade with percutaneous coronary intervention. EPIC Investigator Group. Evaluation of Platelet IIb/IIIa Inhibition for Prevention of Ischemic Complication. JAMA 1997;278:479–484.
6. Simoons ML, van den Brand M, Lincoff M, Harrington R, van der Wieken R, Vahanian A, Rutsch W, Kootstra J, Boersma E, Califf RM, Topol E. Minimal myocardial damage during coronary intervention is associated with impaired outcome. Eur Heart J 1999;20:1112–1119.
7. Kong TQ, Davidson CJ, Meyers SN, Tauke JT, Parker MA, Bonow RO. Prognostic implication of creatine kinase elevation following elective coronary artery interventions. JAMA 1997;277:461–466.

8. Topol EJ. EPISTENT Trial: 1-year results. Presented at the 1998 Annual Meeting of the American Heart Association, Dallas, 1998.
9. Farb A, Roberts DK, Pichard AD, Kent KM, Virmani R. Coronary artery morphologic features after coronary rotational atherectomy: insights into mechanisms of lumen enlargement and embolization. Am Heart J 1995;129: 1058–1067.
10. Braden GA, Applegate RJ, Young TM, Love WW, Sane DC. Abciximab decreases both the incidence and magnitude of creatine kinase elevation during rotational atherectomy. J Am Coll Cardiol 1997;29:499A.
11. Koch KC, vom Dahl J, Kleinhans E, Klues HG, Radke PW, Ninnemann S, Schulz G, Buell U, Hanrath P. Influence of a platelet GPIIb/IIIa receptor antagonist on myocardial hypoperfusion during rotational atherectomy as assessed by myocardial Tc-99m sestamibi scintigraphy. J Am Coll Cardiol 1999; 33:998–1004.
12. Abdelmeguid AE, Ellis SG, Sapp SK, Whitlow PL, Topol EJ. Defining the appropriate threshold of creatine kinase elevation after percutaneous coronary interventions. Am Heart J 1996;131:1097–1105.
13. Kini A, Kini S, Marmur JD, Bertea T, Dangas G, Cocke TP, Sharma SK. Incidence and mechanism of creatine kinase-MB enzyme elevation after coronary intervention with different devices. Cathet Cardiovasc Intervent 1999; 48:123–129.
14. Topol EJ, Leya F, Pinkerton CA, Whitlow PL, Hofling B, Simonton CA, Masden RR, Serruys PW, Leon MB, Williams DO, et al. A comparison of directional atherectomy with coronary angioplasty in patients with coronary artery disease. The CAVEAT Study Group. N Engl J Med 1993;329:221–227.
15. Lefkovits J, Blankenship JC, Anderson KM, Stoner GL, Talley JD, Worley SJ, Weisman HF, Califf RM, Topol EJ. Increased risk of non-Q wave myocardial infarction after directional atherectomy is platelet dependent: evidence from the EPIC trial. Evaluation of c7E3 for the Prevention of Ischemic Complications. J Am Coll Cardiol 1996;28:849–855.
16. Saber RS, Edwards WD, Holmes DR, Jr., Vlietstra RE, Reeder GS. Balloon angioplasty of aortocoronary saphenous vein bypass grafts: a histopathologic study of six grafts from five patients, with emphasis on restenosis and embolic complications. J Am Coll Cardiol 1988;12:1501–1509.
17. Mak KH, Challapalli R, Eisenberg MJ, Anderson KM, Califf RM, Topol EJ. Effect of platelet glycoprotein IIb/IIIa receptor inhibition on distal embolization during percutaneous revascularization of aortocoronary saphenous vein grafts. EPIC Investigators. Evaluation of IIb/IIIa platelet receptor antagonist 7E3 in Preventing Ischemic Complications. Am J Cardiol 1997;80:985–988.
18. Lefkovits J, Holmes DR, Califf RM, Safian RD, Pieper K, Keeler G, Topol EJ. Predictors and sequelae of distal embolization during saphenous vein graft intervention from the CAVEAT-II trial. Coronary Angioplasty Versus Excisional Atherectomy Trial. Circulation 1995;92:734–740.
19. Trono R, Sutton C, Hollman J, Suit P, Ratliff NB. Multiple myocardial infarctions associated with atheromatous emboli after PTCA of saphenous vein grafts. A clinicopathologic correlation. Cleve Clin J Med 1989;56:581–584.

20. Moses JW, Moussa I, Popma JJ, Sketch MH Jr, Yeh W. Risk of distal embolization and infarction with transluminal extraction atherectomy in saphenous vein grafts and native coronary arteries. NACI Investigators. New Approaches to Coronary Interventions. Cathet Cardiovasc Intervent 1999;47:149–154.
21. Sullebarger JT, Dalton RD, Nasser A, Matar FA. Adjunctive abciximab improves outcomes during recanalization of totally occluded saphenous vein grafts using transluminal extraction atherectomy. Cathet Cardiovasc Intervent 1999;46:107–110.
22. Webb JG, Carere RG, Virmani R, Baim D, Teirstein PS, Whitlow P, McQueen C, Kolodgie FD, Buller E, Dodek A, Mancini GB, Oesterle S. Retrieval and analysis of particulate debris after saphenous vein graft intervention. J Am Coll Cardiol 1999;34:468–475.
23. Carlino M, De Gregorio J, Di Mario C, Anzuini A, Airoldi F, Albiero R, Briguori C, Dharmadhikari A, Sheiban I, Colombo A. Prevention of distal embolization during saphenous vein graft lesion angioplasty. Experience with a new temporary occlusion and aspiration system. Circulation 1999;99:3221–3223.
24. Keon WJ, Heggtveit HA, Leduc J. Perioperative myocardial infarction caused by atheroembolism. J Thorac Cardiovasc Surg 1982;84:849–855.
25. McGregor CG, Muir AL, Smith AF, Miller HC, Hannan WJ, Cameron EW, Wheatley DJ. Myocardial infarction related to coronary artery bypass graft surgery. Br Heart J 1984;51:399–406.
26. Roberts AJ, Combes JR, Jacobstein JG, Alonso DR, Post MR, Subramanian VA, Abel RM, Brachfeld N, Kline SA, Gay WA Jr. Perioperative myocardial infarction associated with coronary artery bypass graft surgery: improved sensitivity in the diagnosis within 6 hours after operation with 99mTc-glucoheptonate myocardial imaging and myocardial-specific isoenzymes. Ann Thorac Surg 1979;27:42–48.
27. Warren SG, Wagner GS, Bethea CF, Roe CR, Oldham HN, Kong Y. Diagnostic and prognostic significance of electrocardiographic and CPK isoenzyme changes following coronary bypass surgery: correlation with findings at one year. Am Heart J 1977;93:189–196.
28. Saber RS, Edwards WD, Bailey KR, McGovern TW, Schwartz RS, Holmes DR, Jr. Coronary embolization after balloon angioplasty or thrombolytic therapy: an autopsy study of 32 cases. J Am Coll Cardiol 1993;22:1283–1288.
29. Menke DM, Jordan MD, Aust CH, Storer W, Waller BF. Histologic evidence of distal coronary thromboembolism. A complication of acute proximal coronary artery thrombolysis therapy. Chest 1986;90:614–616.
30. Lefkovits J, Topol EJ. Role of platelet inhibitor agents in coronary artery disease. In: Topol EJ, ed. Textbook of Interventional Cardiology, 3rd ed. Philadelphia: W. B. Saunders, 1999:3–24.
31. Ohman EM, Kleiman NS, Gacioch G, Worley SJ, Navetta FI, Talley JD, Anderson HV, Ellis SG, Cohen MD, Spriggs D, Miller M, Kereiakes D, Yakubov S, Kitt MM, Sigmon KN, Califf RM, Krucoff MW, Topol EJ. Combined accelerated tissue-plasminogen activator and platelet glycoprotein IIb/IIIa in-

tegrin receptor blockade with Integrilin in acute myocardial infarction. Results of a randomized, placebo-controlled, dose-ranging trial. IMPACT-AMI Investigators. Circulation 1997;95:846–854.

32. Ohman EM, Lincoff AM, Bode C, Bachinsky W, Ardissino D, Pavia M, Betriu A, Schildcrout JS, Oliverio R, Barnathan E, Sherer J, Sketch MS, Topol EJ. Enhanced early reperfusion at 60 minutes with low-dose reteplase combined with full-dose abciximab in acute myocardial infarction. Preliminary results from the GUSTO IV (SPEED) dose-ranging trial. Circulation 1998;98:I-504.
33. Antman EM, Giugliano RP, Gibson CM, McCabe CH, Coussement P, Kleiman NS, Vahanian A, Adgey AA, Menown I, Rupprecht HJ, Van der Wieken R, Ducas J, Scherer J, Anderson K, Van de Werf F, Braunwald E. Abciximab facilitates the rate and extent of thrombolysis: results of the thrombolysis in myocardial infarction (TIMI) 14 trial. The TIMI 14 Investigators. Circulation 1999;99:2720–2732.
34. Herrmann HC, Moliterno DJ, Bode C, Betriu A, Lincoff AM, Ohman EM. Combination abciximab and reduced-dose reteplase facilitates early PCI in acute MI: results from the SPEED trial. Circulation 1999;100:I-188.
35. Rosenschein U, Bernstein JJ, DiSegni E, Kaplinsky E, Bernheim J, Rozenzsajn LA. Experimental ultrasonic angioplasty: disruption of atherosclerotic plaques and thrombi in vitro and arterial recanalization in vivo. J Am Coll Cardiol 1990;15:711–717.
36. Rosenschein U, Roth A, Rassin T, Basan S, Laniado S, Miller HI. Analysis of coronary ultrasound thrombolysis endpoints in acute myocardial infarction (ACUTE trial). Results of the feasibility phase. Circulation 1997;95:1411–1416.
37. Rosenschein U, Gaul G, Erbel R, Amann F, Velasguez D, Stoerger H, Simon R, Gomez G, Troster J, Bartorelli A, Pieper M, Kyriakides Z, Laniado S, Miller HI, Cribier A, Fajadet J. Percutaneous transluminal therapy of occluded saphenous vein grafts: can the challenge be met with ultrasound thrombolysis? Circulation 1999;99:26–29.
38. Kong DF, Califf RM, Miller DP, Moliterno DJ, White HD, Harrington RA, Tcheng JE, Lincoff AM, Hasselblad V, Topol EJ. Clinical outcomes of therapeutic agents that block the platelet glycoprotein IIb/IIIa integrin in ischemic heart disease. Circulation 1998;98:2829–2835.
39. PURSUIT Investigators. Inhibition of platelet glycoprotein IIb/IIIa with eptifibatide in patients with acute coronary syndromes. Platelet glycoprotein IIb/IIIa in unstable angina: receptor suppression using Integrilin therapy. N Engl J Med 1998;339:436–443.
40. PARAGON Investigators. International, randomized, controlled trial of lamifiban (a platelet glycoprotein IIb/IIIa inhibitor), heparin, or both in unstable angina. Platelet IIb/IIIa antagonism for the reduction of acute coronary syndrome events in a global organization network. Circulation 1998;97:2386–2395.
41. PRISM Investigators. A comparison of aspirin plus tirofiban with aspirin plus heparin for unstable angina. Platelet Receptor Inhibition in Ischemic Syndrome Management (PRISM) Study. N Engl J Med 1998;338:1498–1505.

42. PRISM-PLUS Investigators. Inhibition of the platelet glycoprotein IIb/IIIa receptor with tirofiban in unstable angina and non-Q-wave myocardial infarction. Platelet Receptor Inhibition in Ischemic Syndrome Management in Patients Limited by Unstable Signs and Symptoms (PRISM-PLUS). N Engl J Med 1998;338:1488–1497.
43. Davies MJ, Thomas AC, Knapman PA, Hangartner JR. Intramyocardial platelet aggregation in patients with unstable angina suffering sudden ischemic cardiac death. Circulation 1986;73:418–427.
44. Frink RJ, Rooney PA Jr, Trowbridge JO, Rose JP. Coronary thrombosis and platelet/fibrin microemboli in death associated with acute myocardial infarction. Br Heart J 1988;59:196–200.
45. Falk E. Unstable angina with fatal outcome: dynamic coronary thrombosis leading to infarction and/or sudden death. Autopsy evidence of recurrent mural thrombosis with peripheral embolization culminating in total vascular occlusion. Circulation 1985;71:699–708.
46. Mehta P, Mehta J. Platelet function studies in coronary artery disease. V. Evidence for enhanced platelet microthrombus formation activity in acute myocardial infarction. Am J Cardiol 1979;43:757–760.
47. El-Maraghi N, Genton E. The relevance of platelet and fibrin thromboembolism of the coronary microcirculation, with special reference to sudden cardiac death. Circulation 1980;62:936–944.
48. Kowey PR, Verrier RL, Lown B, Handin RI. Influence of intracoronary platelet aggregation on ventricular electrical properties during partial coronary artery stenosis. Am J Cardiol 1983;51:596–602.
49. Roe MT, Harrington RA, Ohman EM, Califf RM, Lincoff AM, Bhatt DL, Prosper DL, Topol EJ. Clinical and therapeutic profile of patients with acute coronary syndromes who do not have significant coronary artery disease. J Am Coll Cardiol 2000;35:347A.
50. Eguchi H, Ikeda H, Murohara T, Yasukawa H, Haramaki N, Sakisaka S, Imaizumi T. Endothelial injuries of coronary arteries distal to thrombotic sites: role of adhesive interaction between endothelial P-selectin and leukocyte sialyl LewisX. Circ Res 1999;84:525–535.
51. Mutin M, Canavy I, Blann A, Bory M, Sampol J, Dignat-George F. Direct evidence of endothelial injury in acute myocardial infarction and unstable angina by demonstration of circulating endothelial cells. Blood 1999;93: 2951–2958.
52. Combes V, Simon AC, Grau GE, Arnoux D, Camoin L, Sabatier F, Mutin M, Sanmarco M, Sampol J, Dignat-George F. In vitro generation of endothelial microparticles and possible prothrombotic activity in patients with lupus anticoagulant. J Clin Invest 1999;104:93–102.
53. Henn V, Slupsky JR, Grafe M, Anagnostopoulos I, Forster R, Muller-Berghaus G, Kroczek RA. CD40 ligand on activated platelets triggers an inflammatory reaction of endothelial cells. Nature 1998;391:591–594.
54. Aukrust P, Muller F, Ueland T, Berget T, Aaser E, Brunsvig A, Solum NO, Forfang K, Froland SS, Gullestad L. Enhanced levels of soluble and membrane-bound CD40 ligand in patients with unstable angina: possible reflection

of T lymphocyte and platelet involvement in the pathogenesis of acute coronary syndromes. Circulation 1999;100:614–620.
55. Slupsky JR, Kalbas M, Willuweit A, Henn V, Kroczek RA, Muller-Berghaus G. Activated platelets induce tissue factor expression on human umbilical vein endothelial cells by ligation of CD40. Thromb Haemost 1998;80:1008–1014.
56. Ikeda H, Ueyama T, Murohara T, Yasukawa H, Haramaki N, Eguchi H, Katoh A, Takajo Y, Onitsuka I, Ueno T, Tojo SJ, Imaizumi T. Adhesive interaction between P-selectin and sialyl Lewis(x) plays an important role in recurrent coronary arterial thrombosis in dogs. Arterioscler Thromb Vasc Biol 1999;19: 1083–1090.
57. Lefer AM, Campbell B, Scalia R, Lefer DJ. Synergism between platelets and neutrophils in provoking cardiac dysfunction after ischemia and reperfusion: role of selectins. Circulation 1998;98:1322–1328.
58. Katopodis JN, Kolodny L, Jy W, Horstman LL, De Marchena EJ, Tao JG, Haynes DH, Ahn YS. Platelet microparticles and calcium homeostasis in acute coronary ischemias. Am J Hematol 1997;54:95–101.
59. Neumann FJ, Marx N, Gawaz M, Brand K, Ott I, Rokitta C, Sticherling C, Meinl C, May A, Schomig A. Induction of cytokine expression in leukocytes by binding of thrombin-stimulated platelets. Circulation 1997;95:2387–2394.
60. Simon DI, Xu H, Ortlepp S, Rogers C, Rao NK. 7E3 monoclonal antibody directed against the platelet glycoprotein IIb/IIIa cross-reacts with the leukocyte integrin Mac-1 and blocks adhesion to fibrinogen and ICAM-1. Arterioscler Thromb Vasc Biol 1997;17:528–535.
61. Reverter JC, Beguin S, Kessels H, Kumar R, Hemker HC, Coller BS. Inhibition of platelet-mediated, tissue factor-induced thrombin generation by the mouse/human chimeric 7E3 antibody. Potential implications for the effect of c7E3 Fab treatment on acute thrombosis and "clinical restenosis." J Clin Invest 1996;98:863–874.
62. Coleman KR, Braden GA, Willingham MC, Sane DC. Vitaxin, a humanized monoclonal antibody to the vitronectin receptor, reduces neointimal hyperplasia and total vessel area after balloon injury in hypercholesterolemic rabbits. Circ Res 1999;84:1268–1276.
63. Gawaz M, Neumann FJ, Dickfeld T, Reininger A, Adelsberger H, Gebhardt A, Schomig A. Vitronectin receptor (alpha(v)beta3) mediates platelet adhesion to the luminal aspect of endothelial cells: implications for reperfusion in acute myocardial infarction. Circulation 1997;96:1809–1818.
64. Willerson JT, Golino P, Eidt J, Campbell WB, Buja LM. Specific platelet mediators and unstable coronary artery lesions. Experimental evidence and potential clinical implications. Circulation 1989;80:198–205.
65. Eidt JF, Ashton J, Golino P, McNatt J, Buja LM, Willerson JT. Thromboxane A2 and serotonin mediate coronary blood flow reductions in unsedated dogs. Am J Physiol 1989;257:H873–H882.
66. Yao SK, Ober JC, Krishnaswami A, Ferguson JJ, Anderson HV, Golino P, Buja LM, Willerson JT. Endogenous nitric oxide protects against platelet aggregation and cyclic flow variations in stenosed and endothelium-injured arteries. Circulation 1992;86:1302–1309.

67. Eidt JF, Allison P, Noble S, Ashton J, Golino P, McNatt J, Buja LM, Willerson JT. Thrombin is an important mediator of platelet aggregation in stenosed canine coronary arteries with endothelial injury. J Clin Invest 1989;84:18–27.
68. Yao SK, Ober JC, McNatt J, Benedict CR, Rosolowsky M, Anderson HV, Cui K, Maffrand JP, Campbell WB, Buja LM. ADP plays an important role in mediating platelet aggregation and cyclic flow variations in vivo in stenosed and endothelium-injured canine coronary arteries. Circ Res 1992;70:39–48.
69. Wilson RF, Laxson DD, Lesser JR, White CW. Intense microvascular constriction after angioplasty of acute thrombotic coronary arterial lesions. Lancet 1989;1:807–811.
70. Hirsh PD, Hillis LD, Campbell WB, Firth BG, Willerson JT. Release of prostaglandins and thromboxane into the coronary circulation in patients with ischemic heart disease. N Engl J Med 1981;304:685–691.
71. Ostrovsky L, King AJ, Bond S, Mitchell D, Lorant DE, Zimmerman GA, Larsen R, Niu XF, Kubes P. A juxtacrine mechanism for neutrophil adhesion on platelets involves platelet-activating factor and a selectin-dependent activation process. Blood 1998;91:3028–3036.
72. Huang Q, Wu M, Meininger C, Kelly K, Yuan Y. Neutrophil-dependent augmentation of PAF-induced vasoconstriction and albumin flux in coronary arterioles. Am J Physiol 1998;275:H1138–H1147.
73. Moliterno DJ. Anticoagulants and their use in acute coronary syndromes. In: Topol EJ, ed. Textbook of Interventional Cardiology, 3rd ed. Philadelphia: W.B. Saunders, 1999:25–51.
74. Taniyama Y, Ito H, Iwakura K, Masuyama T, Hori M, Takiuchi S, Nishikawa N, Higashino Y, Fujii K, Minamino T. Beneficial effect of intracoronary verapamil on microvascular and myocardial salvage in patients with acute myocardial infarction. J Am Coll Cardiol 1997;30:1193–1199.
75. Ito H, Taniyama Y, Iwakura K, Nishikawa N, Masuyama T, Kuzuya T, Hori M, Higashino Y, Fujii K, Minamino T. Intravenous nicorandil can preserve microvascular integrity and myocardial viability in patients with reperfused anterior wall myocardial infarction. J Am Coll Cardiol 1999;33:654–660.
76. Gibson CM, Cannon CP, Daley WL, Dodge JT Jr, Alexander B Jr, Marble SJ, McCabe CH, Raymond L, Fortin T, Poole WK, Braunwald E. TIMI frame count: a quantitative method of assessing coronary artery flow. Circulation 1996;93:879–888.
77. Gibson CM, Ryan KA, Murphy SA, Mesley R, Marble SJ, Giugliano RP, Cannon CP, Antman EM, Braunwald E. Impaired coronary blood flow in nonculprit arteries in the setting of acute myocardial infarction. The TIMI Study Group. Thrombolysis in myocardial infarction. J Am Coll Cardiol 1999; 34:974–982.
78. Gowda MS, Vacek JL, Hallas D. One-year outcomes of diabetic versus nondiabetic patients with non-Q-wave acute myocardial infarction treated with percutaneous transluminal coronary angioplasty. Am J Cardiol 1998;81:1067–1071.

79. Aronson D, Rayfield EJ, Chesebro JH. Mechanisms determining course and outcome of diabetic patients who have had acute myocardial infarction. Ann Intern Med 1997;126:296–306.
80. Barsness GW, Peterson ED, Ohman EM, Nelson CL, DeLong ER, Reves JG, Smith PK, Anderson RD, Jones RH, Mark DB, Califf RM. Relationship between diabetes mellitus and long-term survival after coronary bypass and angioplasty. Circulation 1997;96:2551–2556.
81. Mak KH, Moliterno DJ, Granger CB, Miller DP, White HD, Wilcox RG, Califf RM, Topol EJ. Influence of diabetes mellitus on clinical outcome in the thrombolytic era of acute myocardial infarction. GUSTO-I Investigators. Global Utilization of Streptokinase and Tissue Plasminogen Activator for Occluded Coronary Arteries. J Am Coll Cardiol 1997;30:171–179.
82. Gu K, Cowie CC, Harris MI. Diabetes and decline in heart disease mortality in US adults. JAMA 1999;281:1291–1297.
83. Tschoepe D, Roesen P. Heart disease in diabetes mellitus: a challenge for early diagnosis and intervention. Exp Clin Endocrinol Diabetes 1998;106:16–24.
84. Knobler H, Savion N, Shenkman B, Kotev-Emeth S, Varon D. Shear-induced platelet adhesion and aggregation on subendothelium are increased in diabetic patients. Thromb Res 1998;90:181–190.
85. Iwase E, Tawata M, Aida K, Ozaki Y, Kume S, Satoh K, Qi R, Onaya T. A cross-sectional evaluation of spontaneous platelet aggregation in relation to complications in patients with type II diabetes mellitus. Metabolism 1998;47:699–705.
86. Tschoepe D, Driesch E, Schwippert B, Lampeter EF. Activated platelets in subjects at increased risk of IDDM. DENIS Study Group. Deutsche Nikotinamid Interventionsstudie. Diabetologia 1997;40:573–577.
87. Silva JA, Escobar A, Collins TJ, Ramee SR, White CJ. Unstable angina. A comparison of angioscopic findings between diabetic and nondiabetic patients. Circulation 1995;92:1731–1736.
88. Akasaka T, Yoshida K, Hozumi T, Takagi T, Kaji S, Kawamoto T, Morioka S, Yoshikawa J. Retinopathy identifies marked restriction of coronary flow reserve in patients with diabetes mellitus. J Am Coll Cardiol 1997;30:935–941.
89. Yokayama I, Momomura SI, Ohtake T, Yonekura K, Nishikawa J, Sasaki Y, MO. Reduced myocardial flow reserve in non-insulin dependent diabetes mellitus. J Am Coll Cardiol 1997;30:1472–1477.
90. Tschoepe D, Rauch U, Schwippert B. Platelet-leukocyte cross-talk in diabetes mellitus. Horm Metab Res 1997;29:631–635.
91. Bhatt DL, Marso SP, Lincoff AM, Wolski KE, Ellis SG, Topol EJ. Abciximab reduces death in diabetics following percutaneous coronary intervention. Circulation 1999;100:I-67.
92. Antman EM, Grudzien C, Sacks DB. Evaluation of a rapid bedside assay for detection of serum cardiac troponin T. JAMA 1995;273:1279–1282.
93. Antman EM, Tanasijevic MJ, Thompson B, Schactman M, McCabe CH, Cannon CP, Fischer GA, Fung AY, Thompson C, Wybenga D, Braunwald E.

Cardiac-specific troponin I levels to predict the risk of mortality in patients with acute coronary syndromes. N Engl J Med 1996;335:1342–1349.
94. Hamm CW, Goldmann BU, Heeschen C, Kreymann G, Berger J, Meinertz T. Emergency room triage of patients with acute chest pain by means of rapid testing for cardiac troponin T or troponin I. N Engl J Med 1997;337:1648–1653.
95. Newby LK, Christenson RH, Ohman EM, Armstrong PW, Thompson TD, Lee KL, Hamm CW, Katus HA, Cianciolo C, Granger CB, Topol EJ, Califf RM. Value of serial troponin T measures for early and late risk stratification in patients with acute coronary syndromes. The GUSTO-IIa Investigators. Circulation 1998;98:1853–1859.
96. Hamm CW, Heeschen C, Goldmann B, Vahanian A, Adgey J, Miguel CM, Rutsch W, Berger J, Kootstra J, Simoons ML. Benefit of abciximab in patients with refractory unstable angina in relation to serum troponin T levels. c7E3 Fab Antiplatelet Therapy in Unstable Refractory Angina (CAPTURE) Study Investigators. N Engl J Med 1999;340:1623–1629.
97. Heeschen C, van Den Brand MJ, Hamm CW, Simoons ML. Angiographic findings in patients with refractory unstable angina according to troponin T status. Circulation 1999;100:1509–1514.
98. Hamm CW, Heeschen C, Goldmann BU, White HD. Benefit of Tirofiban in high-risk patients with unstable angina identified by troponins in the PRISM Trial. Circulation 1999;100:I-775.
99. Heeschen C, Hamm CW, Goldmann B, Deu A, Langenbrink L, White HD. Troponin concentrations for stratification of patients with acute coronary syndromes in relation to therapeutic efficacy of tirofiban. PRISM Study Investigators. Platelet Receptor Inhibition in Ischemic Syndrome Management. Lancet 1999;354:1757–1762.
100. Lindahl B, Toss H, Siegbahn A, Venge P, Wallentin L. Long-term mortality in unstable coronary artery disease in relation to markers of myocardial damage and inflammation. Circulation 1999;100:I-372.
101. Lindahl B, Diderholm E, Kontny F, Lagerqvist B, Husted S, Stahle E, Swahn E, Wallentin L. Long term treatment with low molecular weight heparin (dalteparin) reduces cardiac events in unstable coronary artery disease with troponin-T elevation: a FRISC II substudy. Circulation 1999;100:I-498.
102. Ito H, Okamura A, Iwakura K, Masuyama T, Hori M, Takiuchi S, Negoro S, Nakatsuchi Y, Taniyama Y, Higashino Y, Fujii K, Minamino T. Myocardial perfusion patterns related to thrombolysis in myocardial infarction perfusion grades after coronary angioplasty in patients with acute anterior wall myocardial infarction. Circulation 1996;93:1993–1999.
103. Ito H, Maruyama A, Iwakura K, Takiuchi S, Masuyama T, Hori M, Higashino Y, Fujii K, Minamino T. Clinical implications of the "no reflow" phenomenon. A predictor of complications and left ventricular remodeling in reperfused anterior wall myocardial infarction. Circulation 1996;93:223–228.
104. Porter TR, Li S, Oster R, Deligonul U. The clinical implications of no reflow demonstrated with intravenous perfluorocarbon containing microbubbles following restoration of Thrombolysis In Myocardial Infarction (TIMI) 3 flow

in patients with acute myocardial infarction. Am J Cardiol 1998;82:1173–1177.

105. Sakuma T, Hayashi Y, Sumii K, Imazu M, Yamakido M. Prediction of short- and intermediate-term prognoses of patients with acute myocardial infarction using myocardial contrast echocardiography one day after recanalization. J Am Coll Cardiol 1998;32:890–897.
106. Wu KC, Kim RJ, Bluemke DA, Rochitte CE, Zerhouni EA, Becker LC, Lima JA. Quantification and time course of microvascular obstruction by contrast-enhanced echocardiography and magnetic resonance imaging following acute myocardial infarction and reperfusion. J Am Coll Cardiol 1998;32:1756–1764.
107. Rochitte CE, Lima JA, Bluemke DA, Reeder SB, McVeigh ER, Furuta T, Becker LC, Melin JA. Magnitude and time course of microvascular obstruction and tissue injury after acute myocardial infarction. Circulation 1998;98:1006–1014.
108. Wu KC, Zerhouni EA, Judd RM, Lugo-Olivieri CH, Barouch LA, Schulman SP, Blumenthal RS, Lima JA. Prognostic significance of microvascular obstruction by magnetic resonance imaging in patients with acute myocardial infarction. Circulation 1998;97:765–772.
109. Fernandez AR, Sequeira RF, Chakko S, Correa LF, de Marchena EJ, Chahine RA, Franceour DA, Myerburg RJ. ST segment tracking for rapid determination of patency of the infarct-related artery in acute myocardial infarction. J Am Coll Cardiol 1995;26:675–683.
110. Schroder R, Dissmann R, Bruggemann T, Wegscheider K, Linderer T, Tebbe U, Neuhaus KL. Extent of early ST segment elevation resolution: a simple but strong predictor of outcome in patients with acute myocardial infarction. J Am Coll Cardiol 1994;24:384–391.
111. Schroder R, Wegscheider K, Schroder K, Dissmann R, Meyer-Sabellek W. Extent of early ST segment elevation resolution: a strong predictor of outcome in patients with acute myocardial infarction and a sensitive measure to compare thrombolytic regimens. A substudy of the International Joint Efficacy Comparison of Thrombolytics (INJECT) trial. J Am Coll Cardiol 1995;26:1657–1664.
112. Dissmann R, Schroder R, Busse U, Appel M, Bruggemann T, Jereczek M, Linderer T. Early assessment of outcome by ST-segment analysis after thrombolytic therapy in acute myocardial infarction. Am Heart J 1994;128:851–857.
113. Krucoff MW, Croll MA, Pope JE, Granger CB, O'Connor CM, Sigmon KN, Wagner BL, Ryan JA, Lee KL, Kereiakes DJ. Continuous 12-lead ST-segment recovery analysis in the TAMI 7 study. Performance of a noninvasive method for real-time detection of failed myocardial reperfusion. Circulation 1993;88:437–446.
114. Krucoff MW, Croll MA, Pope JE, Pieper KS, Kanani PM, Granger CB, Veldkamp RF, Wagner BL, Sawchak ST, Califf RM. Continuously updated 12-lead ST-segment recovery analysis for myocardial infarct artery patency as-

sessment and its correlation with multiple simultaneous early angiographic observations. Am J Cardiol 1993;71:145–151.

115. Langer A, Krucoff MW, Klootwijk P, Veldkamp R, Simoons ML, Granger C, Califf RM, Armstrong PW. Noninvasive assessment of speed and stability of infarct-related artery reperfusion: results of the GUSTO ST segment monitoring study. Global Utilization of Streptokinase and Tissue Plasminogen Activator for Occluded Coronary Arteries. J Am Coll Cardiol 1995;25:1552–1557.
116. Veldkamp RF, Green CL, Wilkins ML, Pope JE, Sawchak ST, Ryan JA, Califf RM, Wagner GS, Krucoff MW. Comparison of continuous ST-segment recovery analysis with methods using static electrocardiograms for noninvasive patency assessment during acute myocardial infarction. Thrombolysis and Angioplasty in Myocardial Infarction (TAMI) 7 Study Group. Am J Cardiol 1994;73:1069–1074.
117. Santoro GM, Valenti R, Buonamici P, Bolognese L, Cerisano G, Moschi G, Trapani M, Antoniucci D, Fazzini PF. Relation between ST-segment changes and myocardial perfusion evaluated by myocardial contrast echocardiography in patients with acute myocardial infarction treated with direct angioplasty. Am J Cardiol 1998;82:932–937.
118. van 't Hof AW, Liem A, de Boer MJ, Zijlstra F. Clinical value of 12-lead electrocardiogram after successful reperfusion therapy for acute myocardial infarction. Zwolle Myocardial Infarction Study Group. Lancet 1997;350:615–619.
119. De Lemos JA, Antman EM, Gibson M, McCabe CH, Giugliano RP, Murphy SA, Frey MJ, Van der Wieken R, Van de Werf F, Braunwald E. Abciximab improves both epicardial flow and myocardial reperfusion in ST elevation myocardial infarction: a TIMI 14 analysis. Circulation 1999;100:I-649.
120. Neumann FJ, Blasini R, Schmitt C, Alt E, Dirschinger J, Gawaz M, Kastrati A, Schomig A. Effect of glycoprotein IIb/IIIa receptor blockade on recovery of coronary flow and left ventricular function after the placement of coronary-artery stents in acute myocardial infarction. Circulation 1998;98:2695–2701.
121. Agati L, Voci P, Hickle P, Vizza DC, Autore C, Fedele F, Feinstein SB, Dagianti A. Tissue-type plasminogen activator therapy versus primary coronary angioplasty: impact on myocardial tissue perfusion and regional function 1 month after uncomplicated myocardial infarction. J Am Coll Cardiol 1998; 31:338–343.

5

Insights from Intravascular Ultrasound

Samir R. Kapadia,* E. Murat Tuzcu, and Steven E. Nissen
The Cleveland Clinic Foundation
Cleveland, Ohio

Over the past decade, intravascular ultrasound (IVUS) has made significant contributions to our understanding of acute coronary syndromes. The major advantage of intravascular ultrasound imaging is its ability to visualize the vessel wall in vivo, whereas angiography can only discern the effects of the atherosclerotic process on the vessel lumen (1,2). This chapter highlights technologic and methodological issues related to intravascular imaging in acute coronary syndrome as well as important intravascular ultrasound studies investigating key aspects of acute coronary syndromes.

IVUS IMAGING

Basic Principles

Unlike x-ray imaging, which generates shadows based on the atomic density of the tissues, ultrasound images are based on reflections from interfaces between tissues having different acoustic properties. Therefore, the strength and signal quality of the ultrasound beam returning to the transducer (backscatter) determines whether the ultrasound scanner visualizes a particular structure. The acoustic impedance of tissue determines the amplitude of the backscatter and the intensity of image. Acoustic properties of the tissues are

**Current affiliation*: University of Washington, Seattle, Washington.

determined by specific gravity, compressibility, and viscosity. Of these, the first two are of greatest importance in clinical imaging, and most of the differences in soft tissue are probably due to differences in specific gravity. In normal coronary arteries, collagen creates the strongest backscatter of the signal; thus, adventitia, with its high collagen content, strongly reflects ultrasound. On the other hand, the media of coronary arteries consists predominantly of smooth muscle cells and very little collagen; this layer thus reflects little of the ultrasound signal. The inner elastic membrane reflects ultrasound well due to its dense elastic tissue. Systematic interrogation of normal elastic, transitional, and muscular arteries reveals a linear correlation between integrated backscatter and both elastin and collagen content. The presence of smooth muscle cells has been inversely correlated with backscatter.

The blood within the vessel lumen exhibits a characteristic pattern in IVUS examinations. At frequencies >25 MHz, the lumen is characterized by blood flow seen as subtle, finely textured echoes moving in a characteristic swirling pattern. In many clinical situations, the presence of blood "speckle" can assist image interpretation by confirming the communication between a dissection plane and the lumen. The pattern of blood speckle is dependent upon the velocity of flow, exhibiting increased intensity and a coarser texture when flow is reduced. This latter property can represent a confounding variable if examination is carried out under slow-flow condition because the increased echogenicity of blood may interfere with delineation of the blood tissue interface. Increasing the frequency of the ultrasound to >40 MHz also increases blood contrast dramatically due to Rayleigh scattering.

In a normal coronary artery, the discrete echodense layer at the lumen-wall interface caused by the reflections of the internal elastic lamina, which is often referred to as intima. The tunica media is visualized as a distinct subintimal sonolucent layer, which is limited by an outer echodense media-adventitia interface. The outer or trailing edge of the adventitia is indistinct, as it merges into the surrounding perivascular connective tissue. The echodense intima and adventitia with the sonolucent medial layer in between give the arterial wall a trilaminar appearance. In young population, the internal elastic membrane is not dense enough to reflect ultrasound signal giving a typical monolayer appearance (3) (Fig. 1).

Equipment

The equipment required to perform intracoronary ultrasound consists of two major components, a catheter incorporating a miniaturized transducer, and a console containing the electronics necessary to reconstruct the image.

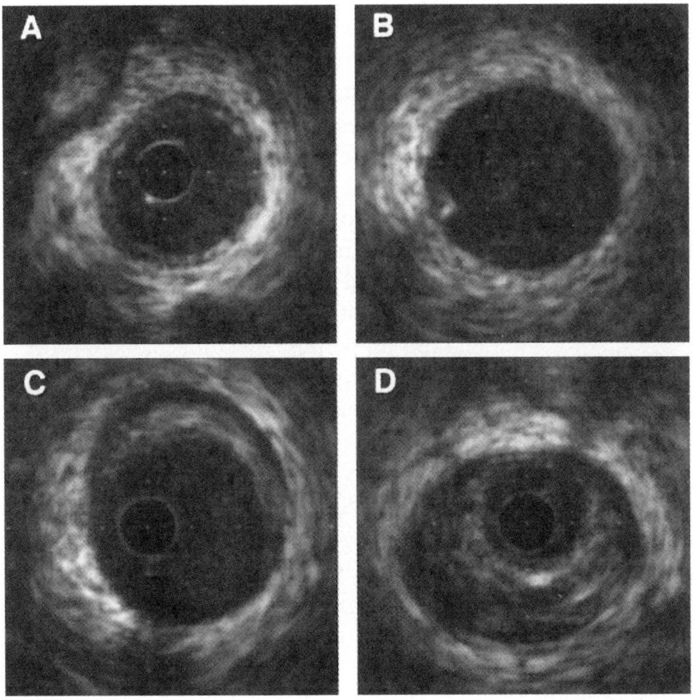

Figure 1 Intravascular ultrasound images from stable coronary artery disease. (A) Appearance of a coronary artery with minimal intimal thickening. In the center of the lumen is the IVUS catheter. Lumen of the artery shows blood speckles, which are more apparent on the real-time images. The lumen is separated from the sonolucent media by the minimally thickened intima. The media is separated from adventitia by the external elastic lamina (EEM). Adventitia merges with the surrounding connective tissue without clear demarcation. The scale superimposed on the image represents 1 mm between markers. Intimal thickness is measured from lumen to EEM and therefore includes the media. The area subtended by the EEM is also referred to as vessel area. Lumen area plus intimal area equals to the vessel area. (B) In young population the internal elastic membrane does not reflect ultrasound signal and therefore is not visualized. This gives a typical monolayer appearance with lumen area equal to EEM area. (C) A typical eccentric, noncircumferential plaque. (D) A typical advanced atherosclerotic plaque with 2×2 mm residual lumen.

Since the transducer is placed in close proximity to the vessel wall, high (20 to 50 MHz) ultrasound frequencies can be employed for high-resolution coronary imaging. At 30 MHz, the wavelength is approximately 50 μm, which permits axial resolution of approximately 100 μm. Determinants of lateral resolution are more complicated and are dependent on imaging depth and beam shape. Typically, lateral resolution for a 30 MHz device will average approximately 250 μm at typical distances in coronary imaging.

Two different technical approaches to transducer design have emerged—mechanically rotated devices and multielement electronic arrays. These two approaches exhibit significantly different characteristics, which can influence both image quality and handling properties. Most mechanical probes employ a drive cable running the length of the catheter that rotates a single piezoelectric transducer element mounted near the distal catheter tip. Typically a rotation rate of 1800 rpm is used, which corresponds to 30 full revolutions per second, yielding 30 images per second. In the electronic systems, an annular array of multiple (currently up to 64) piezoelectric transducer elements is activated sequentially to generate a tomographic image. The electronic signals are processed and multiplexed by several ultraminiaturized integrated circuits near the catheter tip. Image is generated by employing a reconstruction algorithm known as a synthetic aperture array. This approach provides a consistent focus and more uniform image quality throughout the near and far fields.

Tissue Characterization

One of the major advantages of the intravascular ultrasound over angiography is the ability to study the detailed morphology of arterial wall. Various investigators have attempted to define and validate ultrasound characteristics of plaque contents.

Typically a "soft" plaque is defined as a plaque with at least 80% area containing material with less echoreflectivity than the adventitia, and an arc of calcium $<10°$. A fibrous plaque is defined as the echoreflectivity as bright as or brighter than the adventitia of at least 80% of the plaque and mixed as plaque that contain both low and high echoreflective areas. Fibrous and mixed plaques are categorized as hard plaques.

Earlier studies have demonstrated the reliability of ultrasound imaging in predicting the composition of the atherosclerotic plaque. Gussenhoven et al. (4) compared the histology of the plaques in 1100 sections obtained from fresh human arteries to the corresponding ultrasound appearance. Lipid-laden lesions appeared as hypoechoic areas and "soft" echoes represented fibromuscular lesions. Dense fibrous or calcified tissues were recognized as bright echoes, the latter characterized by shadows obscuring the underlying internal elastic lamina (back shadow) (Fig. 2). Lesions containing lipid, fibromuscular tissue, and areas of calcification were described as shadows of variable echodensity. In lipid-laden or fibromuscular lesions with prominent overlying fibrous "caps," a more reflective structure separating the soft echoes from the lumen was identified. In a study of human coronary arteries, the plaque composition was accurately predicted by visual assessment of ultrasound images in 96% of 112 quadrants of 21 arteries (5). Fibrous and calcified plaque quadrants were correctly identified in almost all images (100/103, 97%), but only seven of nine quadrants (78%) with predominantly lipid deposits were correctly diagnosed (Fig. 3).

Ultrasound imaging has shown significant superiority over fluoroscopy or angiography in the detection of coronary calcification (Fig. 4). The severity of calcification has been quantified according to the angle subtended by the calcified arc of the vessel wall (6). In a clinical series of 110 patients undergoing transcatheter therapy, target lesion calcification was detected by ultrasound and fluoroscopy in 84 and 50 patients, respectively (76% vs. 14%, $P < .001$). There was a correlation between the severity of calcification by ultrasound and its detection by fluoroscopy; calcium in two or more quadrants ($\geq$180°), or $\geq$5 mm long increased the fluoroscopic detection rates to 74% and 86%, respectively (7).

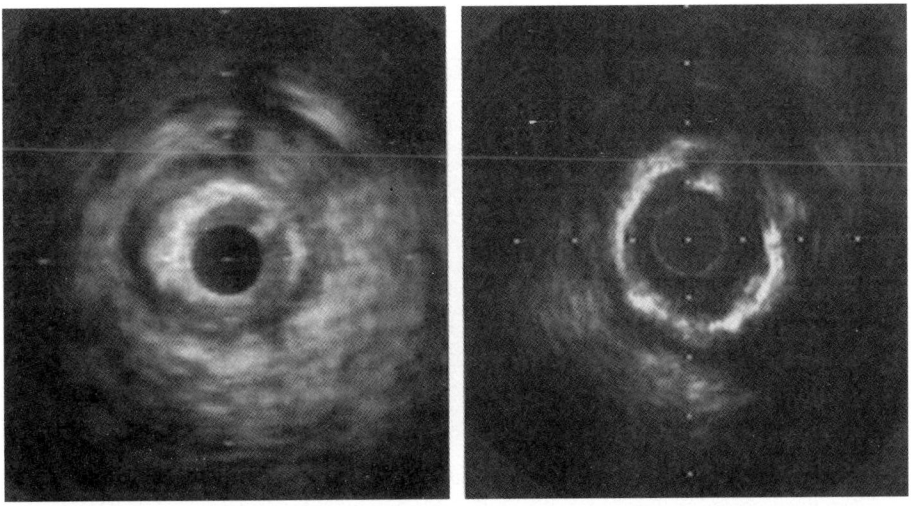

Figure 2 On the left panel the plaque has fibrous appearance between 7 and 2 o'clock with echodensity is equal to or greater than the surrounding adventitia. Note that there is no acoustic shadowing. On the right side is an example of a superficially calcified plaque with overt shadowing.

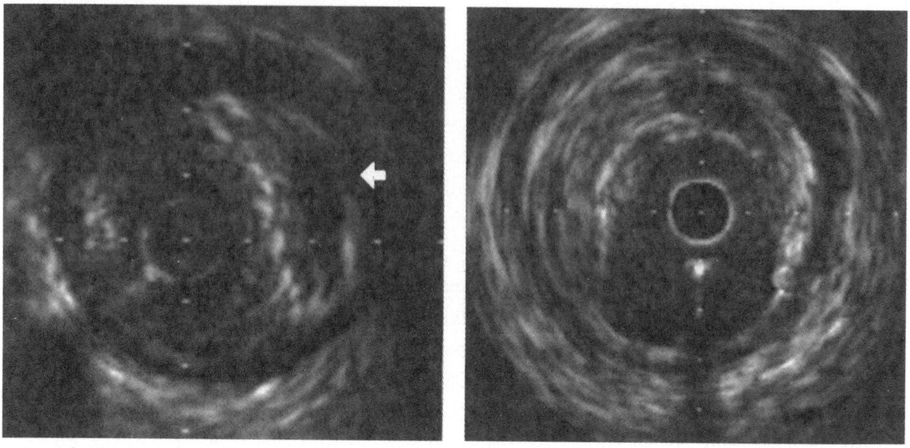

Figure 3 Image on the left shows echolucent area within the plaque (arrow) with intact, relatively thick fibrous cap. Image to the right shows thinning of the fibrous cap over the echolucent area (between 12 and 3 o'clock). Real-time image demonstrated independent movement of the thin fibrous cap suggestive of recent plaque rupture. Injection of the contrast was made to confirm communication of the echolucent area with the lumen.

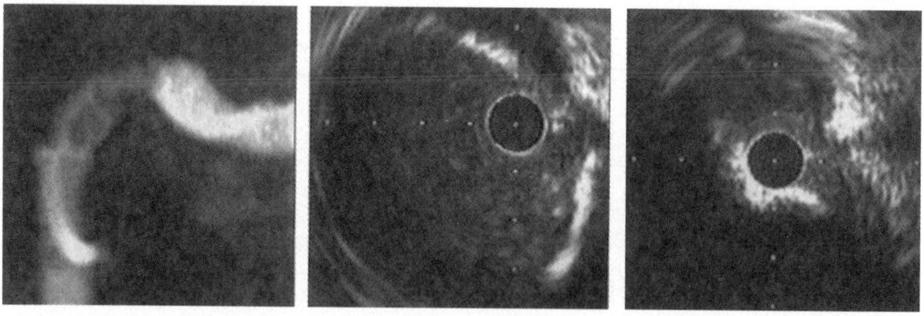

Figure 4 Some lesions with "classic" angiographic appearance of unstable plaque have unsuspected features by ultrasound. This patient presented with a non-Q-wave infarction and only angiographic finding was a large intraluminal filling defect in the proximal right coronary artery suggestive of thrombus. IVUS examination showed extensive, heavily calcified plaque (right panel) with a relatively disease-free proximal segment (middle panel).

The depth of calcification as determined by ultrasound also influences the recognition of calcification on fluoroscopy (8). In a retrospective analysis of the angiographic and ultrasound images of 183 consecutive interventional patients, calcification was detected in 138 patients by ultrasound and in 63 by fluoroscopy. The sensitivity and specificity of angiography were 46% and 82%, respectively. The assessment by the two techniques was concordant in 92 and discordant in 91 cases. The arc of calcium measured by ultrasound was greater in patients with angiographically visible calcification than in those without (175° ± 85° vs. 108° ± 71°, $P = .0001$). When calcium was detected angiographically, the calcification detected by ultrasound was likely >90° and superficial in location, whereas if no calcification could be visualized on the angiogram, the chance of detecting a large superficial arc of calcium by ultrasound was low (12%). Additionally, when calcification was angiographically detectable at remote sites and not at the target lesion, the probability of detection of target lesion calcification by ultrasound was high.

However, the accuracy of conventional videodensitometric analysis in identifying different atherosclerotic plaque types is limited to differentiating only three basic types of plaque: highly echoreflective regions with acoustic shadows often corresponding to calcified tissue; echodense areas representing fibrosis or microcalcification; and echolucent intimal thickening corresponding to fibrotic, thrombotic/hemorrhagic, or lipid tissue, or a mixture of these elements. More objective, quantitative texture analysis of videodensitometric data have not led to significant improvements in the ability to discriminate detailed plaque composition (9,10). Videodensitometric analysis uses gray scale values (typically black = 0 to white = 255) to describe the strength of the ultrasound signal on the image display. Although videodensitometric analysis is the most straightforward technique for quantifying IVUS data, these data are at the end of a long processing chain, including many nonlinear stages the purpose of which is to provide a pleasing image on the screen. The problem with using such data for further analysis is that their relation with the original acoustic signal has been highly distorted and can even be altered by display controls such as brightness and gain.

On the other hand, the analysis of the radiofrequency (RF) data results in an inherently more accurate and reproducible technique for measuring tissue properties. The RF signal is usually accessed very early on in the processing chain, before demodulation and scan conversion, and is directly related to the interaction of the ultrasound in the tissue wall. The analysis of RF data permits more reproducible measurement of the ultrasound signal and enables the application of more advanced signal processing techniques, such as frequency-based analyses (11). Studies on vessel wall (12,13) and thrombus (14) suggest that analysis of backscattered RF data may offer an objective and reproducible method of categorizing plaque components.

The backscattered ultrasonic energy and the attenuation suffered by the ultrasonic waves propagating through tissue are highly dependent on the angle of insonification with respect to the predominant fiber axis of the tissue. This property has been described by ultrasonic anisotropy. The magnitude of ultrasonic anisotropy can be quantified to provide a measure of the 3D organization of the tissue. It has been shown that backscatter from calcium is very dependent on the angle of insonification whereas this is less important for fibrous tissue. Recently, these properties have been explored for tissue characterization (15).

Remodeling

"Remodeling" refers to the changes in arterial dimensions associated with the development of disease. Initially, it was described as increase in arterial size that accommodates the deposition of atherosclerotic plaque material, frequently referred to as positive remodeling. In recent years, histopathologic and intravascular ultrasound studies have demonstrated a new dimension to arterial remodeling, the negative remodeling or arterial shrinkage. At diseased sites, the artery may actually shrink in size and contribute to, instead of compensate for, the degree of luminal stenosis.

Different methodologies have been utilized for investigating remodeling by intravascular ultrasound. Positive correlation between the plaque area and EEM area with no correlation between the plaque area and lumen area at the lesion site has been used as an evidence for positive remodeling. This method helps to study presence or absence of significant remodeling for a group lesions but does not allow quantification of remodeling for each lesion. Further, the negative remodeling cannot be studied with this methodology.

Remodeling ratio, a quantitative measure of extent and direction of remodeling can be calculated by comparing IVUS measurements of vessel area (EEM area) at lesion site with to the EEM area at the corresponding proximal and/or distal reference sites. Positive remodeling is typically defined as remodeling ratio >1.05 and negative remodeling as the ratio < 0.95. A 5% difference in the lesion and reference site is traditionally considered insignificant and represents variability of measurement (16). However, when this method is utilized for the quantification of remodeling, vessel tapering, obstruction of blood flow by IVUS catheter, and possible remodeling of the "reference site" can confound these measurements. Serial measurements of lumen, plaque, and vessel area at the lesion site can provide the most rigorous evidence for remodeling, but logistics of this type of studies and the practical difficulties in identifying the same exact site on follow-up examination limit the usefulness of this methodology (17).

Advantages of IVUS

Several characteristics inherent to intravascular ultrasound imaging have potential value in the precise quantification of atherosclerotic coronary disease (1,18–20). The tomographic orientation of ultrasound enables visualization of the full 360° circumference of the vessel wall, rather than a two-dimensional projection of the lumen. Accordingly, accurate measurement of lumen area can be accomplished by direct planimetry of a cross-sectional image, which unlike angiography is not dependent on the projection angle. In angiographic quantification, careful calibration of the analysis system is required to correct for radiographic magnification. However, ultrasound devices rely upon an internally generated electronic distance scale, which is overlaid upon the image. Because the velocity of sound within soft tissues is nearly constant, ultrasound measurements are inherently accurate and require no special calibration methods.

The tomographic perspective of ultrasound enables characterization of the extent of atherosclerotic disease in vessels that are typically difficult to assess by conventional angiographic techniques. These include diffusely diseased segments, lesions at bifurcation sites, ostial stenoses, and highly eccentric plaques (2) (Figs. 5, 6). In each of these circumstances, overlapping structures or foreshortening can preclude accurate angiographic imaging. However, intravascular ultrasound is unaffected by these factors, enabling accurate characterization of the lesion.

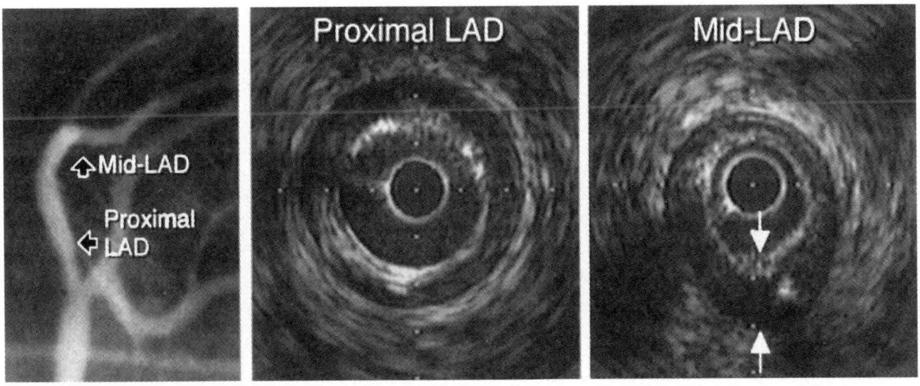

Figure 5 Angiography frequently underestimates the amount of atheroma present. This angiogram indicates a mild narrowing of the proximal left anterior descending (LAD) artery, but the ultrasound image (middle panel) demonstrates substantial atheroma. Further, in the mid-LAD there is minimal angiographic abnormality, but the ultrasound confirms a large atheroma, which is undetected angiographically due to the diffuse nature of the disease in the vessel and remodeling (arrows).

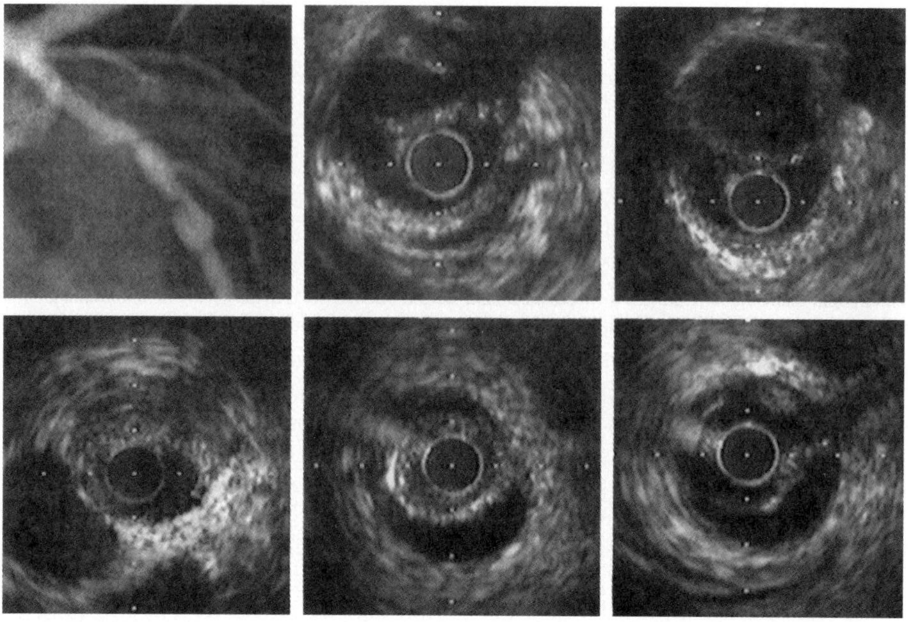

Figure 6 Occasionally a focal plaque rupture extends longitudinally along the vessel and results in spontaneous dissection of the coronary artery. In this example, the angiogram displayed a complex series of "focal" lesions extending over a 30-mm length of the vessel. However, ultrasound revealed diffuse disease with extensive dissection involving approximately 40 mm of the vessel.

Limitation of IVUS

The physical size of ultrasound catheters (currently about 1.0 mm) constitutes an important limitation in certain clinical applications. Although the operator may be able to reach to many critical stenoses with a 1.0-mm device, lesion morphology or quantitative measurements will be distorted by the distending effect of the catheter. Although reductions in transducer size will be feasible, there exist finite physical limitations to further transducer miniaturization. A smaller transducer reduces the "aperture" of the device, which limits available acoustic power, significantly reduces lateral resolution, and impairs the signal-to-noise ratio. The resolution limits at small apertures may be partially compensated by using higher-frequency transducers (40 to 50 MHz).

Geometric distortion can result from imaging in an oblique plane (not perpendicular to the long axis of the vessel). Noncoaxial alignment of the transducer within the artery results in an elliptical rather than circular cross-sectional imaging plane (21). This phenomenon can represent a significant confounding variable in application of intravascular ultrasound for quantitative plaque and lumen measurements. The maximum extent of obliquity is determined by the relative sizes of imaging catheter and lumen. Accordingly, this artifact can be more troublesome when imaging larger vessels such as the aorta or the peripheral vessels.

An important artifact, known as nonuniform rotational distortion (NURD), is present in all mechanical intravascular ultrasound systems. This artifact arises from uneven mechanical drag on the catheter drive shaft during the various portions of its rotational cycle, resulting in cyclical oscillations in rotational speed. Nonuniform speed variation, when severe, produces visible distortion of the ultrasound image. During the portion of the rotational cycle when velocity is high, the image exhibits circumferential "stretching" with "compression" of the contralateral vessel wall. NURD is most evident when the drive shaft is deformed into a small radius of curvature by either external manipulation or vessel tortuosity.

Ring-down artifact, a defect that appears in virtually all ultrasound devices, impairs the ability to image structures adjacent to the transducer surface. Ring-down artifacts are produced by acoustic oscillations in the piezoelectric transducer material resulting in high-amplitude ultrasound signals that preclude near field imaging. Inability to image structures immediately adjacent to the transducer results in an "acoustic" catheter size slightly larger than its physical size. Recent designs use carefully chosen transducer materials, ultrasound-absorbent backings, specialized coatings, and electronic filtering to suppress ring-down artifacts. In the electronic array design, the transducers are surface mounted, and ring-down must be reduced by digital subtraction.

ACUTE CORONARY SYNDROMES

Plaque Morphology

Intravascular ultrasound studies have shown that in patients with angiographically severe coronary disease, clinical symptoms correlate primarily with plaque characteristics rather than with the severity of stenosis (22,23). Ruptured plaques identified by IVUS correlate with clinical presentation of acute coronary syndrome (23) (Figs. 7, 8). Ruptured plaques are characterized by an echolucent zone within a plaque, with a thin ulcerated fibrous cap (type I), or by deep ulceration in the plaque (type II).

Morphological characteristics of a "vulnerable plaque" on IVUS examination have not been prospectively tested. However, various studies have described the morphology of culprit lesions in patients with unstable angina

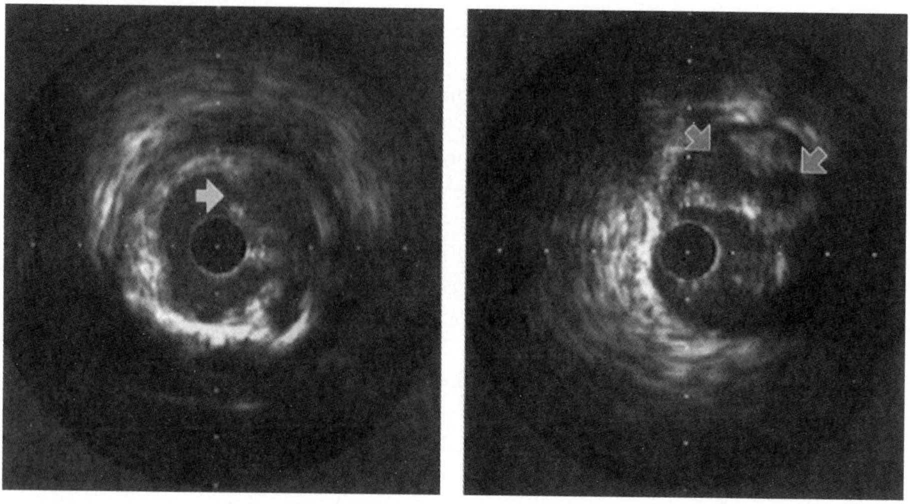

Figure 7 In the image on the left plaque rupture is demonstrated (arrow) involving lateral aspect of the plaque. The irregular margins of the ulcerated fibrous cap are well visualized. Panel on the right shows the same artery just distal to the site seen in the left panel. Intraplaque dissection with "excavation" of the plaque core is seen (arrows). Contrast injection proved communication of this echolucent area with the lumen.

and compared it to the morphology of lesions in patients with stable angina. Kearney et al. (24) reported the presence of a demarcated inner layer in unstable lesions, delimited by a fine circumferential line (Fig. 9); this pattern was noted in 77% (14/18) of unstable lesions and in 7% (1/15) of stable lesions. Rasheed et al. (25) performed multivariate analysis to identify independent predictors of plaque morphology and found stable angina, age >60 years, and location of a lesion in distal segments to be independent predictors of an echodense plaque. Gyongyosi et al. (26) studied the correlation between coronary atherosclerosis risk factors and plaque morphology in patients with unstable angina. In this study, hypercholesterolemia, smoking and male gender were associated with a higher frequency of thrombus. Diabetes mellitus and hypercholesterolemia were independent predictors for greater plaque volume.

Ge et al. (23) identified ruptured plaques (Fig. 10) with IVUS examination and compared the characteristics of these plaques with those without evidence of rupture. The area of the emptied plaque cavity (4.1 ± 3.2 mm^2) with rupture was larger than the echolucent zone in the plaques without rupture (1.32 ± 0.79 mm^2; $P = .001$). Authors suggested that a lipid core

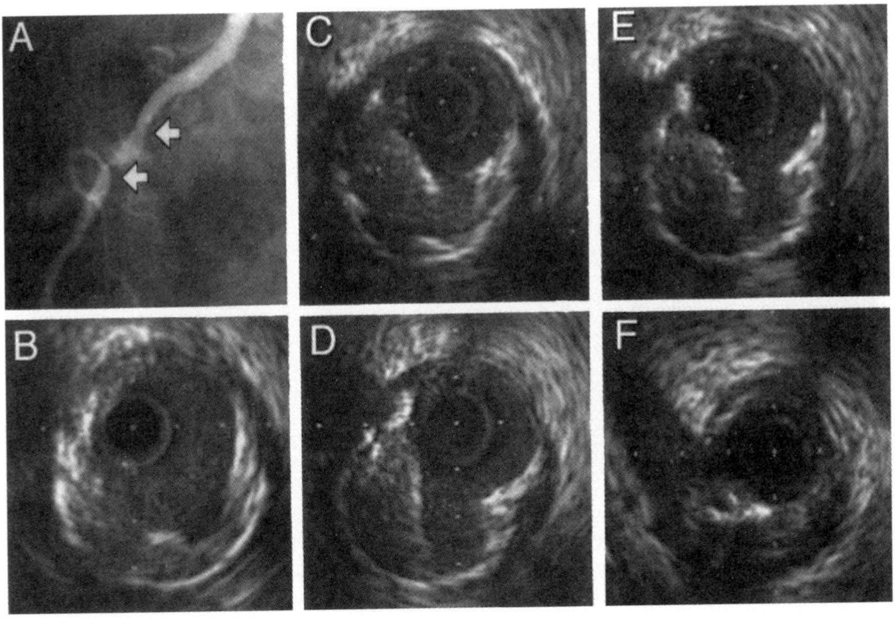

Figure 8 Study from a patient with new-onset angina demonstrating a severe lesion in the right coronary artery on angiography. Ultrasound revealed an extensive spontaneous plaque rupture with a large residual ulcer. Panels B through F indicate sequential ultrasound images obtained from the points indicated by the arrows. In panels B and F small defects in the fibrous cap are visible. In the images from the center of the plaque (C, D, E), a deep ulcer is evident.

larger than 1 mm^2 or a lipid core-to-plaque ratio of >20% and a fibrous cap thinner than 0.7 mm characterized a vulnerable plaque. This study also identified the site of plaque rupture and showed that shoulder region of the plaque is the most likely (55% in this study) site for rupture. Plaque erosion, where the underlying lipid core is not exposed to the lumen, is a recognized mechanism for acute coronary syndrome. However, in the study be Ge et al. (23), only 10% of the plaques had superficial ulceration. This may be due to the limited resolution of current intravascular ultrasound equipment.

As thrombus formation is the hallmark of unstable lesion, attempts have been made to characterize thrombus with IVUS examination (Fig. 11). Despite the high-frequency imaging provided by IVUS, it is still unreliable in differentiating acute thrombi from echolucent plaques, probably due to the similar echodensity of lipid and loose connective tissue within the plaque and stagnant blood forming the thrombus. In vitro comparison of ultrasound imaging to angioscopy revealed that it is less reliable for the diagnosis of

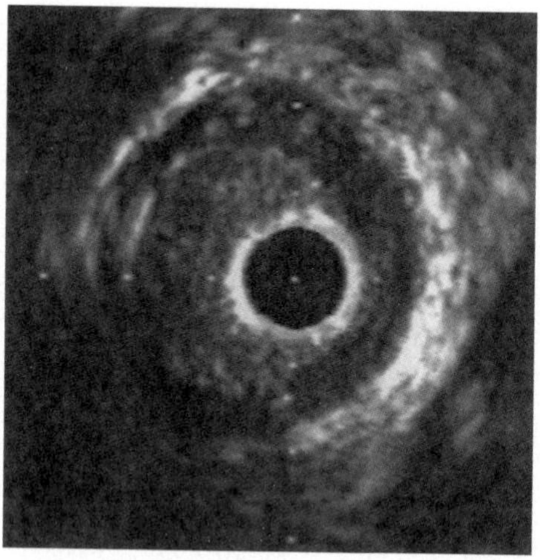

Figure 9 This IVUS image shows lumen filled with material that has echogenicity greater than surrounding plaque and on real-time images gives a scintillating appearance. The "line of demarcation" between this structure and atheromatous plaque is seen distinctly between 9 and 2 o'clock. This is consistent with thrombus as suggested by Kearney and colleagues.

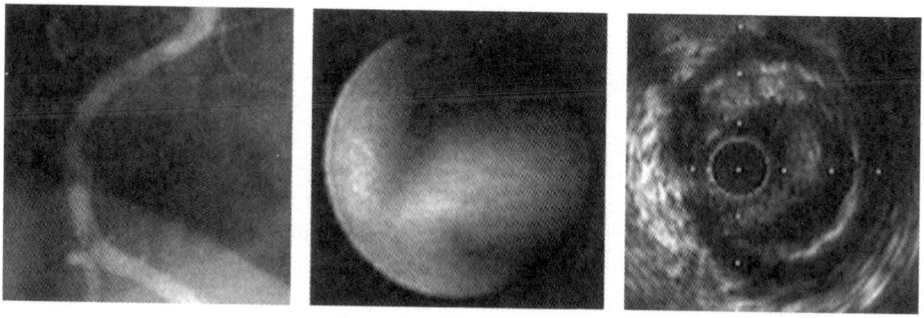

Figure 10 This is an example of acute plaque rupture seen with angiography, angioscopy, and intravascular ultrasound imaging. Intraluminal filling defect seen on coronary angiography could be interpreted as thrombus or ruptured plaque with dissection. The shape of the intraluminal structure on IVUS image helps to identify it as a ruptured plaque rather than a thrombus. This was verified to be the case as demonstrated by angioscopy in the middle panel.

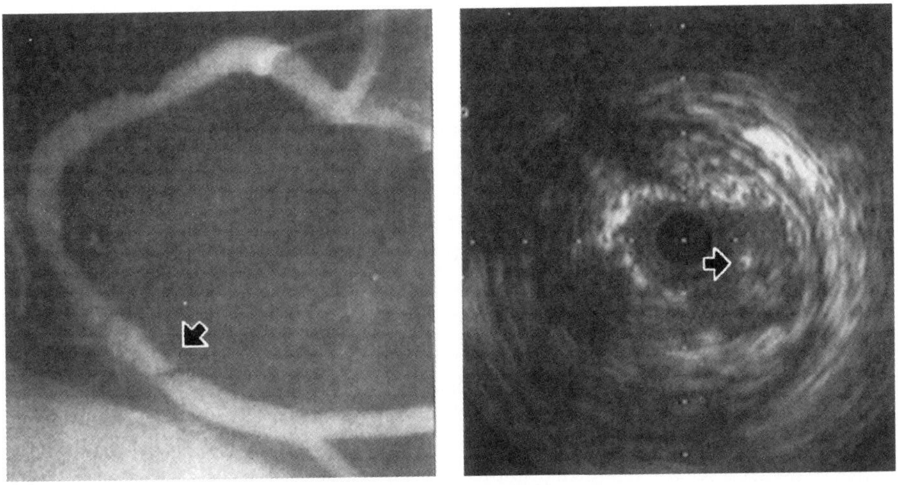

Figure 11 This angiogram and IVUS images were obtained from patient presenting with acute inferior wall MI after successful reperfusion with thrombolytic therapy. Angiogram suggests a flaplike intraluminal filling defect. IVUS imaging uncovers a complex ruptured plaque with irregular borders and evidence of thrombus (arrow) in the ulcer.

thrombi. The sensitivity of ultrasound was low (57%), although the specificity remained high (91%), but both were lower than angioscopy (sensitivity and specificity of 100%) (27).

Several small observational studies attempted to define the intravascular ultrasound appearance of a coronary thrombus. A thrombus was defined as low echogenic material within the lumen demonstrating slight synchronic pulsation, and significantly different acoustic impedance at the interface between it and the more echogenic plaque (24,28,29). Suspicion of thrombus according to ultrasound criteria was based on visualization of a structure with low signal intensity and very soft echoes, clearly separated from the adjacent vessel wall.

Chemarin-Alibelli et al. (61) studied ultrasound characteristics of thrombus in acute myocardial infarction patients undergoing directional atherectomy after thrombolytic therapy and confirmed the presence of thrombus with histology. The sensitivity of IVUS detection of thrombus compared to histology was 84% and specificity was 71%. All patients studied within first 5 days of acute MI (n = 12) had a thrombus protruding in the lumen that was characterized by bright, speckled, echogenic material that scintillated with movement. On the other hand, in patients undergoing IVUS examination after 5 days of acute MI (n = 18), echogenic thrombus protruding in the lumen was rarely found. The older thrombus was more difficult to identify as the speckled appearance was replaced with more echogenic linear pattern.

Bocksch et al. (28) performed intravascular ultrasound imaging in 50 patients with acute myocardial infarction within 6 hours after the onset of chest pain prior to percutaneous coronary angioplasty. Following angiographic documentation of a proximal occlusion, a 3.5 mechanical ultrasound catheter (30 MHz) was advanced successfully through the lesion in 42 of 50 patients (84%). Only 75 ± 22 sec was added to the total time of procedure, which was 42 min. In 37 (88%) patients, ultrasound differentiated between a thrombus characterized by a pulsatile, low echogenic, intraluminal material with a negative imprint of the IVUS catheter, and a highly echogenic atherosclerotic plaque. The plaque was eccentric in 32 (76%) patients with area stenosis of 48 ± 14%. Interestingly, contrary to other literature, the majority (76%) of the plaques were described as eccentric hard plaques with evidence of calcification in 83%.

Calcium is often considered a hallmark of "old" atherosclerotic lesions. Hodgson et al. (30) found that patients with unstable angina had more soft echolucent regions and fewer calcified plaques than patients with stable angina. De Servi et al. (31) suggested that ultrasound images consistent with focal calcification are actually common in plaques that cause acute coronary syndromes. In 43 patients with unstable angina, 54% had either mild or heavily calcific deposits at the suspected culprit lesion site. Interestingly, patient in Braunwald class IB were more likely to have focal calcific deposits than patients in class II or IIIB, in whom soft, noncalcified lesions were most common. In a much larger series (n = 1442), the independent predictors of the arc of target lesion calcium included patient age, stable angina and lesion site, and reference segment plaque burden (32). However, the vast majority of patients with acute coronary syndromes and at least moderate angiographic disease have identifiable coronary calcium by ultrafast CT. Patients with no calcium are younger and tend to be active cigarette smokers (33). In patients with acute coronary syndromes but no angiographically critical stenoses, the number of segments with calcified plaques increases linearly with increase in number of diseased segments (34).

Culprit Lesion Severity

Angiographic studies have demonstrated that the severity of coronary stenosis alone is inadequate to accurately predict the time or location of a subsequent coronary occlusion that will produce a myocardial infarction. Little and colleagues (35) found that 66% of the patients had <50% maximal narrowing in the infarct vessel prior to infarction, 17% had <50% stenosis, yet all had at least luminal irregularities. Further, patients with uncomplicated stable angina have more severe and extensive atherosclerosis compared with those with unheralded AMI, also underscoring the absence of correlation between angiographic severity of disease and clinical presentation.

It has been postulated that progression of a lesion occurs with repeated plaque rupture and plaque stabilization cycles with few or no symptomatic episodes until the stenosis reaches a significant level (36–38). This theory provides one explanation for greater severity of stenosis in patients with stable plaques compared with the stenosis in patients with unstable plaques. Ge et al. (23) reported intravascular imaging data from 139 studies in 144 consecutive patients with angina. Ruptured plaques, characterized by a plaque cavity and a tear on the thin fibrous cap, were identified in 31 patients. Culprit lesion stenosis in patients with evident plaque rupture (n = 31) was more than in patients without intravascular ultrasound evidence of plaque rupture (n = 108) (56 ± 16% vs. 68 ± 13%; $P = .001$) Of note, the plaque area was not significantly different between the groups.

Some other studies have reported a larger plaque burden in patients with unstable coronary artery disease compared to those with stable coronary syndrome. However, almost uniformly the area stenosis of ruptured plaques is less than the stable plaques (22,39). These findings underscore the importance of remodeling in unstable atherosclerotic plaques (vide infra).

Infrequently, patients with acute coronary syndrome have angiographically normal coronary arteries. It has been hypothesized that the mechanism of acute myocardial infarction in these patients is temporary occlusion of the infarct-related vessel by spasm or thrombus or a combination of the two. In these patients, IVUS examination may help to uncover the mechanism for MI. Mild disease with large thrombus, spontaneous dissection, posttraumatic dissections, and at times moderate or even severe disease can be unraveled by IVUS examination (40–42).

Myocardial bridging is usually asymptomatic but has been associated with acute MI in patients in the absence of risk factors for coronary artery disease. Although a common postmortem finding, myocardial bridging is manifest in up to 5% of patients undergoing diagnostic angiography. As coronary arterial blood flow is primarily diastolic, the relevance of bridging in clinical practice has been debated. However, deep muscle bridges can twist the coronary artery and compromise diastolic blood flow and this disturbance in flow at the site of the bridge might increase the propensity for intimal damage or platelet aggregation.

De Winter et al. (43) recently reported a case of recurrent AMI caused by a soft atheromatous plaque within a myocardial bridge. This plaque was invisible during coronary angiography and could only be imaged using intravascular ultrasound. In symptomatic patients with myocardial bridging,

IVUS examination may be useful to rule out a significant atherosclerotic lesion within the bridged segment. Myocardial bridging is characterized by a specific, echolucent half-moon phenomenon over the bridge segment, which exists throughout the cardiac cycle; systolic compression of the bridge segment; accelerated flow velocity in early diastole (finger-tip phenomenon); no or reduced systolic antegrade flow; and retrograde flow in the proximal segment, which is provoked and enhanced by nitroglycerin injection (44).

Remodeling

Coronary artery remodeling was described as a compensatory mechanism to prevent lumen loss in the early stages of atherosclerosis. However, recent studies have demonstrated the relationship between arterial remodeling and clinical presentation of acute coronary syndrome.

Schoenhagen et al. (16) studied culprit lesions in 76 patients with unstable angina and acute infarction and compared them to lesions in 40 patients presenting with stable angina. Positive and negative remodeling at the lesion sites were defined as remodeling ratio of >1.05 and <0.95, respectively. In the unstable patients, EEM area, plaque area, and remodeling ratio were significantly larger than the corresponding measurements in the stable patients. Positive remodeling was more prevalent in the unstable group (51% vs. 18%, $P = .002$) and negative remodeling was more prevalent in the stable group (58% vs. 33%, $P = .002$).

Smits et al. (45) reported identical results from a similarly designed study. In another study, Gyongyosi et al. (46) reported their data from 60 of 95 consecutively admitted patients with unstable angina where positive remodeling was more frequent than negative remodeling (37% vs. 23%). Patients with adaptive remodeling showed more thrombi and plaque disruption, and larger plaque and vessel cross-sectional areas. Patients with constrictive remodeling were significantly older and had a higher angina score. Nakamura et al. (47) also reported more frequent (74% vs. 37%) positive remodeling of the culprit lesion in patients with acute coronary syndrome compared to patients with stable angina pectoris. The extent of remodeling was also greater in patients with unstable symptoms (remodeling ratio of 1.13 ± 0.10 vs. 0.0.96 ± 0.13).

The direction and extent of remodeling also depend on the plaque composition and patient characteristics. Arc of calcium has been identified as an independent negative predictor of adequate remodeling, whereas hard plaques were defined as an independent predictor of negative remodeling (48–50). Age has also been thought to play an important role in direction of remodeling in patients with unstable angina (26).

The relation of remodeling to unstable plaque may be pathophysiologically linked. Interestingly, histologic markers of plaque vulnerability have been correlated to positive remodeling in peripheral arteries (51). In a study of 50 femoral arteries, 1521 sections were stained for the presence of macrophages (CD68), T-lymphocytes (CD45R), smooth muscle cells (alpha-actin), and collagen. Significantly more macrophages, more lymphocytes, less collagen, and less alpha actin staining were observed with larger plaque and vessel areas. These histologic markers of cellularity and inflammation, traditionally associated with vulnerable plaque, were more prevalent in larger and more remodeled plaques (51). Further, human vascular cells can produce the matrix metalloproteinases that may play a crucial role in vascular remodeling during development, growth, and rupture of an atherosclerotic plaque (52,53). These may provide an explanation for positive remodeling seen in large lipid-laden plaques with activated macrophages encountered in unstable angina. Further studies are needed to examine whether the extent and direction of remodeling can predict clinical outcome.

Future Developments

Advances in the intravascular ultrasound technology will allow for smaller devices with better resolution and more accurate tissue characterization. The ability to perform three-dimensional reconstruction may add to the accuracy of measurement and localization of sites for serial studies.

Tissue Characterization

Analysis of unprocessed radiofrequency backscatter signals to perform "tissue characterization" of coronary plaques is under investigation. Identification of a vulnerable plaque from tissue composition and morphology may become feasible with the availability of improved data collection and analyzer systems. High-frequency (40 to 50 MHz) catheters may also become available in the future and will likely yield significantly improved spatial resolution, although issues like greater backscatter from blood cells and possible lesser penetration need to be overcome. These improvements in the imaging catheter may further enhance our ability in tissue characterization.

Three-Dimensional Reconstruction

Three-dimensional (3D) reconstruction of intravascular ultrasound has been proposed as a means to facilitate understanding of the spatial relationship between the structures within different tomographic cross sections (54–57). A prerequisite for 3D reconstruction is the use of a motorized pullback, allowing the acquisition of successive cross sections separated by known distance. The current algorithms applied for 3D reconstruction do not consider the presence of curvatures of the vessel and assume that the catheter passes in a straight line through the center of consecutive cross sections. The systolic expansion of the coronary vessel and the movements of the catheter within the vessel during the cardiac cycle also generate characteristic artifacts. Accordingly, the reconstructed images are not faithful representations of the vessel. Simultaneous digitization of biplane fluoroscopic tracking of the radiopaque transducer and catheter tip may overcome some of these limitations (58–60).

REFERENCES

1. Ziada KM, Kapadia SR, Tuzcu EM, Nissen SE. The current status of intravascular ultrasound imaging. Curr Probl Cardiol 1999;24:541–566.
2. Topol EJ, Nissen SE. Our preoccupation with coronary luminology. The dissociation between clinical and angiographic findings in ischemic heart disease. Circulation 1995;92:2333–2342.
3. Fitzgerald PJ, St.Goar FG, Connolly AJ, Pinto FJ, Billingham ME, Popp RL, Yock PG. Intravascular ultrasound imaging of coronary arteries. Is three layers the norm? Circulation 1992;86:154–158.
4. Gussenhoven EJ, Essed CE, Lancee CT, Mastik F, Frietman P, van Egmond FC, Reiber J, Bosch H, van Urk H, Roelandt J. Arterial wall characteristics determined by intravascular ultrasound imaging: an in vitro study. J Am Coll Cardiol 1989;14:947–952.
5. Potkin BN, Bartorelli AL, Gessert JM, Neville RF, Almagor Y, Roberts WC, Leon MB. Coronary artery imaging with intravascular high-frequency ultrasound. Circulation 1990;81:1575–1585.
6. Honye J, Mahon DJ, Jain A, White CJ, Ramee SR, Wallis JB, al-Zarka A, Tobis JM. Morphological effects of coronary balloon angioplasty in vivo assessed by intravascular ultrasound imaging. Circulation 1992;85:1012–1025.
7. Mintz GS, Douek P, Pichard AD, Kent KM, Satler LF, Popma JJ, Leon MB. Target lesion calcification in coronary artery disease: an intravascular ultrasound study. J Am Coll Cardiol 1992;20:1149–1155.
8. Tuzcu EM, Berkalp B, De Franco AC, Ellis SG, Goormastic M, Whitlow PL, Franco I, Raymond RE, Nissen SE. The dilemma of diagnosing coronary calcification: angiography versus intravascular ultrasound. J Am Coll Cardiol 1996;27:832–838.
9. Rasheed Q, Dhawale PJ, Anderson J, Hodgson JM. Intracoronary ultrasound-defined plaque composition: computer-aided plaque characterization and correlation with histologic samples obtained during directional coronary atherectomy. Am Heart J 1995;129:631–637.
10. Peters RJ, Kok WE, Bot H, Visser CA. Characterization of plaque components with intracoronary ultrasound imaging: an in vitro quantitative study with videodensitometry. J Am Soc Echocardiogr 1994;7:616–623.
11. Linker DT, Yock PG, Gronningsaether A, Johansen E, Angelsen BA. Analysis of backscattered ultrasound from normal and diseased arterial wall. Int J Card Imaging 1989;4:177–185.

12. Landini L, Sarnelli R, Picano E, Salvadori M. Evaluation of frequency dependence of backscatter coefficient in normal and atherosclerotic aortic walls. Ultrasound Med Biol 1986;12:397–401.
13. Barzilai B, Saffitz JE, Miller JG, Sobel BE. Quantitative ultrasonic characterization of the nature of atherosclerotic plaques in human aorta. Circ Res 1987; 60:459–463.
14. Ramo MP, Spencer T, Kearney PP, Shaw ST, Starkey IR, McDicken WN, Fox KA. Characterisation of red and white thrombus by intravascular ultrasound using radiofrequency and videodensitometric data-based texture analysis. Ultrasound Med Biol 1997;23:1195–1199.
15. Hiro T, Leung CY, Karimi H, Farvid AR, Tobis JM. Angle dependence of intravascular ultrasound imaging and its feasibility in tissue characterization of human atherosclerotic tissue. Am Heart J 1999;137:476–481.
16. Schoenhagen P, Ziada KM, Nissen SE, Tuzcu EM. Arterial remodeling in stable versus unstable coronary syndromes: an intravascular ultrasound study. Circulation 1998;98:I-368. Abstract.
17. Ziada KM, Kapadia SR, Crowe TD. Adaptive coronary remodeling is evident in later stages of transplant vasculopathy: a serial intravascular ultrasound study. J Am Coll Cardiol 1999;33:90A.
18. Nissen SE, Gurley JC, Grines CL, Booth DC, McClure R, Berk M, Fischer C, DeMaria AN. Intravascular ultrasound assessment of lumen size and wall morphology in normal subjects and patients with coronary artery disease. Circulation 1991;84:1087–1099.
19. Nissen SE, Gurley JC. Application of intravascular ultrasound for detection and quantitation of coronary atherosclerosis. Int J Card Imaging 1991;6:165–177.
20. Nissen SE, Gurley JC, Booth DC, DeMaria AN. Intravascular ultrasound of the coronary arteries: current applications and future directions. Am J Cardiol 1992;69:18H–29H.
21. Di Mario C, Gorge G, Peters R, Kearney P, Pinto F, Hausmann D, von Birgelen C, Colombo A, Mudra H, Roelandt J, Erbel R. Clinical application and image interpretation in intracoronary ultrasound. Study Group on Intracoronary Imaging of the Working Group of Coronary Circulation and of the Subgroup on Intravascular Ultrasound of the Working Group of Echocardiography of the European Society of Cardiology. Eur Heart J 1998;19:207–229.
22. Erbel R, Ge J, Gorge G, Baumgart D, Haude M, Jeremias A, von Birgelen C, Jollet N, Schwedtmann J. Intravascular ultrasound classification of atherosclerotic lesions according to American Heart Association recommendation. Coron Artery Dis 1999;10:489–499.
23. Ge J, Chirillo F, Schwedtmann J, Haude M, Baumgart D, Shah V, von Birgelen C, Sack S, Boudoulas H, Erbel R. Screening of ruptured plaques in patients with coronary artery disease by intravascular ultrasound. Heart 1999;81:621–627.
24. Kearney P, Erbel R, Rupprecht HJ, Ge J, Koch L, Voigtlander T, Stahr P, Gorge G, Meyer J. Differences in the morphology of unstable and stable coronary

lesions and their impact on the mechanisms of angioplasty. An in vivo study with intravascular ultrasound. Eur Heart J 1996;17:721–730.

25. Rasheed Q, Nair R, Sheehan H, Hodgson JM. Correlation of intracoronary ultrasound plaque characteristics in atherosclerotic coronary artery disease patients with clinical variables. Am J Cardiol 1994;73:753–758.
26. Gyongyosi M, Yang P, Hassan A, Weidinger F, Domanovits H, Laggner A, Glogar D. Coronary risk factors influence plaque morphology in patients with unstable angina. Coron Artery Dis 1999;10:211–219.
27. Siegel RJ, Ariani M, Fishbein MC, Chae JS, Park JC, Maurer G, Forrester JS. Histopathologic validation of angioscopy and intravascular ultrasound. Circulation 1991;84:109–117.
28. Bocksch WG, Schartl M, Beckmann SH, Dreysse S, Paeprer H. Intravascular ultrasound imaging in patients with acute myocardial infarction: comparison with chronic stable angina pectoris. Coron Artery Dis 1994;5:727–735.
29. Bocksch W, Schartl M, Beckmann S, Dreysse S, Fleck E. Intravascular ultrasound imaging in patients with acute myocardial infarction. Eur Heart J 1995; 16(suppl):46–52.
30. Hodgson JM, Reddy KG, Suneja R, Nair RN, Lesnefsky EJ, Sheehan HM. Intracoronary ultrasound imaging: correlation of plaque morphology with angiography, clinical syndrome and procedural results in patients undergoing coronary angioplasty. J Am Coll Cardiol 1993;21:35–44.
31. De Servi S, Arbustini E, Marsico F, Bramucci E, Angoli L, Porcu E, Costante AM, Kubica J, Boschetti E, Valentini P, Specchia G. Correlation between clinical and morphologic findings in unstable angina. Am J Cardiol 1996;77:128–132.
32. Mintz GS, Pichard AD, Popma JJ, Kent KM, Satler LF, Bucher TA, Leon MB. Determinants and correlates of target lesion calcium in coronary artery disease: a clinical, angiographic and intravascular ultrasound study. J Am Coll Cardiol 1997;29:268–274.
33. Schmermund A, Baumgart D, Gorge G, Seibel R, Gronemeyer D, Ge J, Haude M, Rumberger J, Erbel R. Coronary artery calcium in acute coronary syndromes: a comparative study of electron-beam computed tomography, coronary angiography, and intracoronary ultrasound in survivors of acute myocardial infarction and unstable angina. Circulation 1997;96:1461–1469.
34. Schmermund A, Baumgart D, Adamzik M, Ge J, Gronemeyer D, Seibel R, Sehnert C, Gorge G, Haude M, Erbel R. Comparison of electron-beam computed tomography and intracoronary ultrasound in detecting calcified and noncalcified plaques in patients with acute coronary syndromes and no or minimal to moderate angiographic coronary artery disease. Am J Cardiol 1998;81:141–146.
35. Little WC, Constantinescu M, Applegate RJ, Kutcher MA, Burrows MT, Kahl FR, Santamore WP. Can coronary angiography predict the site of a subsequent myocardial infarction in patients with mild-to-moderate coronary artery disease? Circulation 1988;78:1157–1166.
36. Davies MJ. Stability and instability: two faces of coronary atherosclerosis. Paul Dudley White Lecture 1995. Circulation 1996;94:2013–2020.

37. Mann J, Davies MJ. Mechanisms of progression in native coronary artery disease: role of healed plaque disruption. Heart 1999;82:265–268.
38. Ge J, Haude M, Gorge G, Liu F, Erbel R. Silent healing of spontaneous plaque disruption demonstrated by intracoronary ultrasound. Eur Heart J 1995;16: 1149–1151.
39. Weissman NJ, Sheris SJ, Chari R, Mendelsohn FO, Anderson WD, Breall JA, Tanguay JF, Diver DJ. Intravascular ultrasonic analysis of plaque characteristics associated with coronary artery remodeling. Am J Cardiol 1999;84:37–40.
40. Williams MJ, Restieaux NJ, Low CJ. Myocardial infarction in young people with normal coronary arteries. Heart 1998;79:191–194.
41. Morocutti G, Spedicato L, Vendrametto F, Bernardi G. [Intravascular echocardiography (ICUS) diagnosis of post-traumatic coronary dissection involving the common trunk. A case report and review of the literature.] G Ital Cardiol 1999;29:1034–1037.
42. Kearney P, Erbel R, Ge J, Zamorano J, Koch L, Gorge G, Meyer J. Assessment of spontaneous coronary artery dissection by intravascular ultrasound in a patient with unstable angina. Cathet Cardiovasc Diagn 1994;32:58–61.
43. De Winter RJ, Kok WE, Piek JJ. Coronary atherosclerosis within a myocardial bridge, not a benign condition. Heart 1998;80:91–93.
44. Ge J, Jeremias A, Rupp A, Abels M, Baumgart D, Liu F, Haude M, Görge G, Von Birgelen C, Sack S, Erbel R. New signs characteristic of myocardial bridging demonstrated by intracoronary ultrasound and Doppler. Eur Heart J 1999; 20:1707–1716.
45. Smits PC, Pasterkamp G, Quarles van Ufford MA, Eefting FD, Stella PR, de Jaegere PP, Borst C. Coronary artery disease: arterial remodelling and clinical presentation. Heart 1999;82:461–464.
46. Gyongyosi M, Yang P, Hassan A, Weidinger F, Domanovits H, Laggner A, Glogar D. Arterial remodelling of native human coronary arteries in patients with unstable angina pectoris: a prospective intravascular ultrasound study. Heart 1999;82:68–74.
47. Nakamura M, Nishikawa H, Mukai S, Setsuda M, Tamada H, Suzuki H, Ohnishi T, Kakuta Y, Lee DP, Yeung AC. Comparison of coronary remodeling in the culprit lesion in the acute coronary syndrome and stable angina pectoris. J Am Coll Cardiol 1999;33(suppl A):18A.
48. Tauth J, Pinnow E, Sullebarger JT, Basta L, Gursoy S, Lindsay J Jr, Matar F. Predictors of coronary arterial remodeling patterns in patients with myocardial ischemia. Am J Cardiol 1997;80:1352–1355.
49. Mintz GS, Kent KM, Pichard AD, Satler LF, Popma JJ, Leon MB. Contribution of inadequate arterial remodeling to the development of focal coronary artery stenoses. An intravascular ultrasound study. Circulation 1997;95:1791–1798.
50. Sabate M, Kay IP, de Feyter PJ, van Domburg RT, Deshpande NV, Ligthart JM, Gijzel AL, Wardeh AJ, Boersma E, Serruys PW. Remodeling of atherosclerotic coronary arteries varies in relation to location and composition of plaque. Am J Cardiol 1999;84:135–140.
51. Pasterkamp G, Schoneveld AH, van der Wal AC, Haudenschild CC, Clarijs RJ, Becker AE, Hillen B, Borst C. Relation of arterial geometry to luminal nar-

rowing and histologic markers for plaque vulnerability: the remodeling paradox. J Am Coll Cardiol 1998;32:655–662.
52. Rajavashisth TB, Xu XP, Jovinge S, Meisel S, Xu XO, Chai NN, Fishbein MC, Kaul S, Cercek B, Sharifi B, Shah PK. Membrane type 1 matrix metalloproteinase expression in human atherosclerotic plaques: evidence for activation by proinflammatory mediators. Circulation 1999;99:3103–3109.
53. Galis ZS, Sukhova GK, Lark MW, Libby P. Increased expression of matrix metalloproteinases and matrix degrading activity in vulnerable regions of human atherosclerotic plaques. J Clin Invest 1994;94:2493–2503.
54. Bom N, Li W, van der Steen AF, Lancee CT, Cespedes EI, Slager CJ, de Korte CL. New developments in intravascular ultrasound imaging. Eur J Ultrasound 1998;7:9–14.
55. Di Mario C, von Birgelen C, Prati F, Soni B, Li W, Bruining N, de Jaegere PP, de Feyter PJ, Serruys PW, Roelandt JR. Three dimensional reconstruction of cross sectional intracoronary ultrasound: clinical or research tool? Br Heart J 1995;73:26–32.
56. Gil R, von Birgelen C, Prati F, Di Mario C, Ligthart J, Serruys PW. Usefulness of three-dimensional reconstruction for interpretation and quantitative analysis of intracoronary ultrasound during stent deployment. Am J Cardiol 1996;77:761–764.
57. Prati F, Di Mario C, Gil R, von Birgelen C, Camenzind E, Montauban van Swijndregt WJ, de Feyter PJ, Serruys PW, Roelandt JR. Usefulness of on-line three-dimensional reconstruction of intracoronary ultrasound for guidance of stent deployment. Am J Cardiol 1996;77:455–461.
58. Evans JL, Ng KH, Wiet SG, Vonesh MJ, Burns WB, Radvany MG, Kane BJ, Davidson CJ, Roth SI, Kramer BL, Meyers SN, McPherson DD. Accurate three-dimensional reconstruction of intravascular ultrasound data. Spatially correct three-dimensional reconstructions. Circulation 1996;93:567–576.
59. Krams R, Wentzel JJ, Oomen JA, Vinke R, Schuurbiers JC, de Feyter PJ, Serruys PW, Slager CJ. Evaluation of endothelial shear stress and 3D geometry as factors determining the development of atherosclerosis and remodeling in human coronary arteries in vivo. Combining 3D reconstruction from angiography and IVUS (ANGUS) with computational fluid dynamics. Arterioscler Thromb Vasc Biol 1997;17:2061–2065.
60. Pellot C, Bloch I, Herment A, Sureda F. An attempt to 3D reconstruct vessel morphology from x-ray projections and intravascular ultrasounds modeling and fusion. Comput Med Imaging Graph 1996;20:141–151.
61. Chemarin-Alibelli MJ, Pieraggi MT, Elbaz M, Carrie D, Fourcade J, Puel J, Tobis J. Identification of coronary thrombus after myocardial infarction by intracoronary ultrasound compared with histology of tissues sampled by atherectomy. Am J Cardiol 1996;77:344–349.

6

Differences Between Unstable Angina and Acute Myocardial Infarction

The Pathophysiological and Clinical Spectrum

David J. Moliterno
The Cleveland Clinic Foundation
Cleveland, Ohio

Christopher B. Granger
Duke University Medical Center
Durham, North Carolina

INTRODUCTION

It has been recognized that acute coronary syndromes are a diagnostic and pathophysiologic continuum ranging from unstable angina to Q-wave myocardial infarction. At the interface between unstable angina and myocardial infarction, these entities become nearly indistinct as most features are shared. Indeed, the phrase "unstable angina" was first used by Conti (1) and Fowler (2) in the early 1970s to specifically describe symptom complexes intermediate in severity between stable angina pectoris and myocardial infarction. Other terms used to describe unstable angina also show its close apposition to myocardial infarction: intermediate coronary syndrome and preinfarction angina (2–5). On the other hand, a number of features distinguish unstable angina from acute myocardial infarction. These differences are seen in the pathophysiologic as well as the clinical spectrum of acute coronary syndromes, and they affect the diagnosis, treatment, and outcome. This chapter will review the shared features and distinguishing characteristics of unstable angina and acute myocardial infarction regarding etiology, pathology, and clinical course.

The first distinction bewteen unstable angina and acute myocardial infarction can be seen when considering their definitions or classifications. Whereas unstable angina has a broad, less distinct definition, the definition of acute myocardial infarction is specific. The diversity of clinical conditions which cause unstable angina, its varying intensity and frequency of pain, and its unpredictability have made classification difficult (6). Braunwald (7) suggested a classification scheme based upon angina severity, clinical circumstances, presence of electrocardiographic changes, and intensity of antianginal therapy (Table 1). Patients in class I have new or accelerated *exertional* angina, whereas those in class II have subacute (>48 hours since last pain) or class III acute ($\leq$48 hours since last pain) *rest* angina. Among $\sim$3000 consecutive 1996 hospital admissions for unstable angina in the United States, the Global Unstable Angina Registry and Treatment Evaluation (GUARANTEE) study reported that one-third of patients had new or accelerated symptoms associated with exertion, whereas two-thirds presents with symptoms at rest (8). The clinical circumstances associated with unstable angina are categorized as type A, secondary (e.g., anemia, fever, hypoxia); B, primary; or C, postinfarction (<2 weeks after infarction). Intensity of antianginal therapy is subclassified as 1, no treatment; 2, usual oral therapy; and 3, intense therapy, such as intravenous nitroglycerin. A patient with atherosclerotic heart disease and acute chest pain during minimal activity or at rest while taking usual medical therapy would be categorized as class

Table 1 Braunwald Classification of Unstable Angina

Severity	I	Symptoms with exertion
	II	Symptoms at rest: subacute (2–30 days prior)
	III	Symptoms at rest: acute (within prior 48 hours)
Precipitant	A	Secondary
	B	Primary
	C	Postinfarction
Therapy presented during symptoms	1	No treatment
	2	Usual angina therapy
	3	Maximal therapy

Table 2 Braunwald Classification of Patients in the GUARANTEE Study

	Severity			
Precipitant	I Exertional	II Rest: subacute	III Rest: acute	Total %
A Secondary	1%	1%	3%	5%
B Primary	31%	13%	50%	94%
C Postinfarction	<1%	<1%	<1%	<1%
Total	33%	14%	53%	100%

Data based on 2948 consecutive hospital admissions in the United States for unstable angina in the Global Unstable Angina Registry and Treatment Evaluation (GUARANTEE) study (8).

$IIIB_2$. This is by far the most common presentation. The categorical breakdown of the patients from the GUARANTEE study according to the Braunwald classification is presented in Table 2. In contrast, acute myocardial infarction is commonly separated into two distinct categories solely by electrocardiographic criteria: non-Q-wave and Q-wave.

PATHOPHYSIOLOGY

Supply/Demand Mismatch

The myocardial ischemia of unstable angina and myocardial infarction, like all causes of tissue ischemia, results from excessive demand or inadequate supply of oxygen and nutrients. *Excess demand* from increased myocardial workload (heart rate systolic pressure product) is responsible for nearly all cases of stable angina, approximately one-third of unstable angina episodes, and, very rarely, cases of myocardial infarction. For example, in Braunwald class I unstable angina, stable symptoms accelerate and become more intense, more frequent, or more easily provoked, and this is from heightened demands outstripping myocardial blood supply. Conversely, *inadequate supply* alone is responsible for few cases of stable angina, two-thirds of unstable angina episodes, and almost all myocardial infarctions. The etiology of the supply/demand mismatch can be further classified as primary or secondary. Primary causes of ischemia are from obstructive coronary lesions. Secondary causes are varied, extrinsic to the coronary arterial bed, and are more often seen in unstable angina than acute infarction. These precipitants of myocardial ischemia usually increase myocardial demands in the presence of un-

Table 3 Secondary Cause of Myocardial Ischemia

Increased myocardial oxygen demand
Fever
Tachyarrhythmias
Malignant hypertension
Thyrotoxicosis
Pheochromocytoma
Cocaine
Amphetamines
Aortic stenosis
Supravalvular aortic stenosis
Obstructive cardiomyopathy
Aortovenous shunts
High output states
Congestive failure
Decreased oxygen supply
Anemia
Hypoxemia
Polycythemia

Source: Ref. 28.

derlying non-critical coronary artery stenoses. Listed in Table 3 are common examples of secondary disorders which increase myocardial oxygen demand (e.g., fever, thyrotoxicosis, cocaine) or decrease oxygen supply (e.g., hypoxemia, anemia) and lead to the transient ischemia of unstable angina or rarely infarction.

Plaque Disruption

Braunwald class II and III unstable angina and nearly all cases of myocardial infarction are the result of reduction in coronary arterial perfusion associated with atherosclerotic plaque disruption and thrombosis. As the lipid-rich plaque grows, production of macrophage proteases (9) and neutrophil elastases (10) within the plaque cause thinning of the overlying fibromuscular cap. This, in combination with circumferential wall stress and blood flow shear stress, can lead to endothelial erosion, plaque fissuring, or plaque rupture, especially at the junction of the cap and the vessel wall (Chap. 3). The extent of plaque disruption occurs over a spectrum with endothelial erosion and most minor fissuring being occult and moderate to large disruptions leading to acute infarction. Minor plaque ulceration with relatively small areas of exposed subendothelium explains some cases of unstable angina.

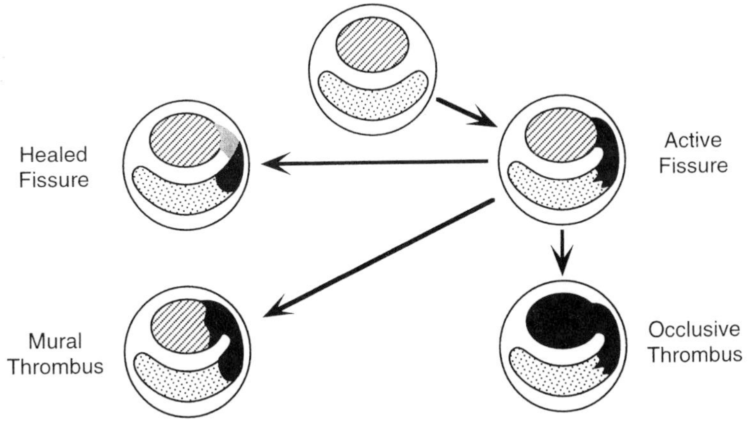

Figure 1 Schematic diagram of an atherosclerotic plaque rupture leading to UAP vs. AMI. Several outcomes follow plaque rupture including uneventful healing if the fissure is small and no clinically siginficant thrombus forms. If plaque rupture is extensive or the thromus formed is significant, partial or transient vessel occlusion may occur with resultant unstable angina or non-Q-wave myocardial infarction. If complete occlusion occurs and remains present, myocardial necrosis may occur leading to Q-wave myocardial infarction.

Because the area of damage is limited, coronary flow remains brisk, accumulation of thrombus does not occur, and the lesion heals uneventfully (Fig. 1). Falk and others have histologically (11) and angiographically (12) demonstrated that coronary stenoses of unstable angina are the result of repeated episodes of plaque ulceration and healing with a resultant gradual increase in plaque volume. During vessel wall repair, the lesion may increase its fibrous content (thrombus organization), thereby limiting the extent of future disruptions. In contrast, in acute myocardial infarction the extent of plaque disruption is larger, thrombus accumulation is occlusive, and tissue infarction results. In several reports of acute myocardial infarction, the underlying plaque was found to be immature—i.e., a recently developed, soft, underlying stenosis of only moderate lumen diameter narrowing. Whether or not vessel occlusion occurs depends on many factors including the extent of vessel disruption, rheology of blood (vessel diameter, lesion geometry, and distal vasoconstriction), platelet aggregability, and the balance of endogenous hemostatic and thrombolytic factors.

Thrombosis

The thrombotic process following plaque rupture is multistaged and begins with the exposure of subendothelial constituents such as collagen, von Willebrand factor, fibronectin, and vitronectin. These matrix components are recognized by platelet surface receptors (primarily glycoprotein Ib), and platelet attachment to the vessel wall (adhesion) occurs. As platelets adhere to the vessel wall, they become activated. During activation platelets secrete a host of substances from their alpha granules which lead to vasoconstriction, chemotaxis, mitogenesis, and activation of neighboring platelets (13) (Fig. 2). The released substances include thromboxane A_2, serotonin, fibrinogen, plasminogen activator inhibitor (PAI-1), and growth factors. Platelet activation leads to the recruitment and "functionalization" of glycoprotein IIb/IIIa integrins or specialized surface receptors which mediate aggregation

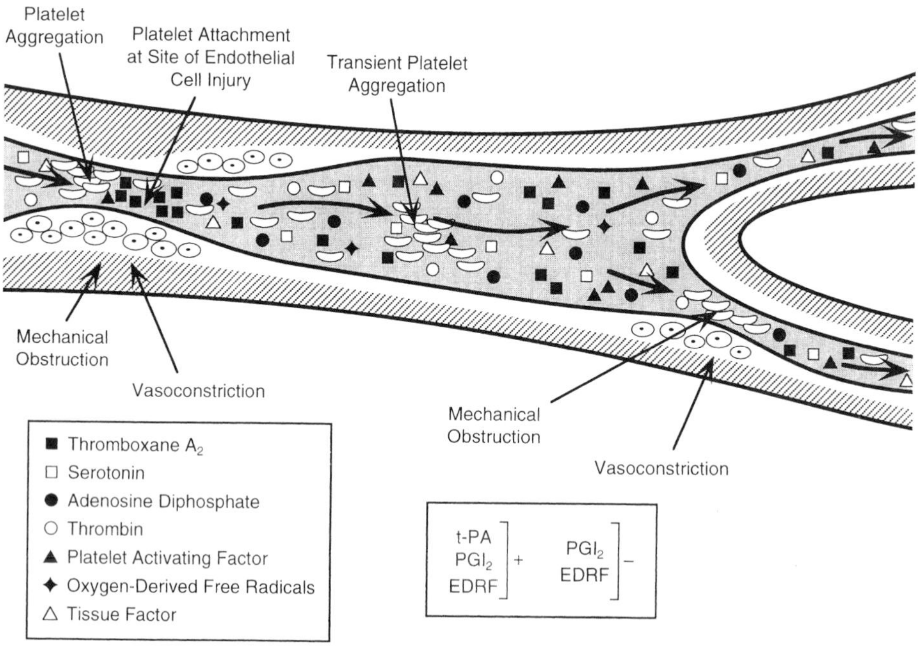

Figure 2 Schematic diagram of mechanism underlying primary acute coronary syndromes. At the site of atheorsclerotic plaque (anatomic obstruction) endothelial injury is present. This in combination with the release of vasoactive and platelet-activating substances such as thromboxane A2, serotonin, thrombin, and adenosine diphosphate (ADP) causes a physiologic obstruction superimposed on the anatomic obstruction. Platelet activation and aggregation can occur as a result of these substances or in response to exposure of the subendothelial matrix following plaque fissuring or rupture. Platelets release additional vasoactive factors and fibrinogen which, in turn, leads to further vasoconstriction, platelet activation, thrombin formation, and potentially vessel obstruction. (From Ref. 27.)

(platelet-platelet binding). Aggregated platelets accelerate the production of thrombin by providing the surface for the binding of cofactors required for the conversion of prothrombin to thrombin. In a reciprocating fashion, thrombin is a potent agonist for further platelet activation, and it stabilizes the thrombus by converting fibrinogen to fibrin. Sherman et al. (14) performed angioscopy in 10 patients with unstable angina. Distinctive intimal abnormalities were observed in all patients, four of whom had complex plaque morphology and seven (70%) had identifiable thrombus. Patients with accelerating symptoms had complex plaque morphology while those with rest angina consistently had intracoronary thrombus. Similar findings are seen by intravascular ultrasound (Fig. 3). In contrast to the nonocclusive thrombus of unstable angina, the thrombus associated with myocardial infarction is transiently or persistently occlusive. Depending on the extent and duration of occlusion, the presence of collateral vessels, and the area of myocardium perfused, non-Q-wave or Q-wave infarction results. Infarction in the absence of atherothrombosis is rare and may be secondary to disorders such as those producing secondary unstable angina. In addition, unsual conditions, such as nonthrombotic embolism, myocardial contusion, and aortic dissection, may lead to myocardial infarction (Table 4).

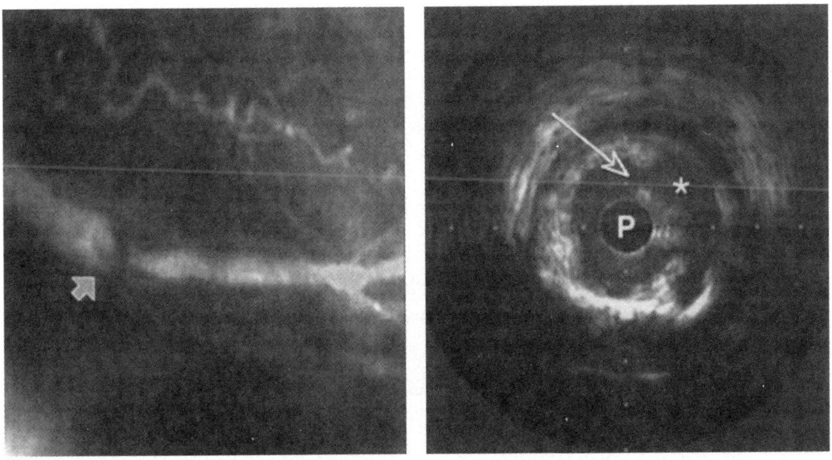

Figure 3 (Left) Angiographic image of cornary artery at the site of atherosclerotic plaque rupture in a patient presenting with unstable angina. The plaque appears irregular, and frank thrombus can be seen (arrowhead). (Right) Intravascular utlrasound at the corresponding site reveals rupture of the fibromuscular cap (arrow) which overlies the lipid-rich plaque (*). The ultrasound probe (P) is in the true lumen.

Table 4 Causes of Myocardial Infarction Without Atherothrombosis

Nonatherosclerotic coronary arterial narrowing or compression	
	Spasm (Prinzmetal's angina)
	Dissection of the aorta with coronary ostium compression
	Dissection of coronary artery
	Anomalous coronary artery origin
Emboli	
	Endocarditis
	Atheroma or air associated with invasive coronary artery procedures
	Cardiac myxoma
	Thromboembolism from prosthetic valve
	Thromboembolism from left atrium or ventricle
Excessive myocardial oxygen demand	
	Aortic stenosis
	Aortic insufficiency
	Thyrotoxicosis
	Cocaine or amphetamines
Inadequate myocardial oxygen supply	
	Carbon monoxide poisoning
	Hypoxemia
	Sustained hypotension
Miscellaneous	
	Chest wall or myocardial trauma
	Radiation-induced coronary fibrosis
	Arteritis

Since thrombus is believed responsible for the vast majority of cases of acute coronary syndromes, several investigations have been performed to assess serologic factors associated with hemostasis and endogenous thrombolysis. Wilensky and colleagues (15) measured fibrinopeptide A among 70 patients with stable angina, unstable angina, or noncardiac chest pain. Fibrinopeptide A is the polypeptide fragment cleaved from fibrinogen when thrombin converts it to fibrin. Compared to patients with stable angina or noncardiac chest pain, those with unstable angina on average had substantially higher levels ($P < .002$). Merlini et al. (16) showed elevations in prothrombin fragment 1+2 and fibrinopeptide A among patients with unstable angina and myocardial infarction compared to a healthy control group (Fig. 4). Interestingly, when studied months following the acute coronary syndrome persistent elevations in F 1+2 were still present while the fibrinopeptide A levels normalized.

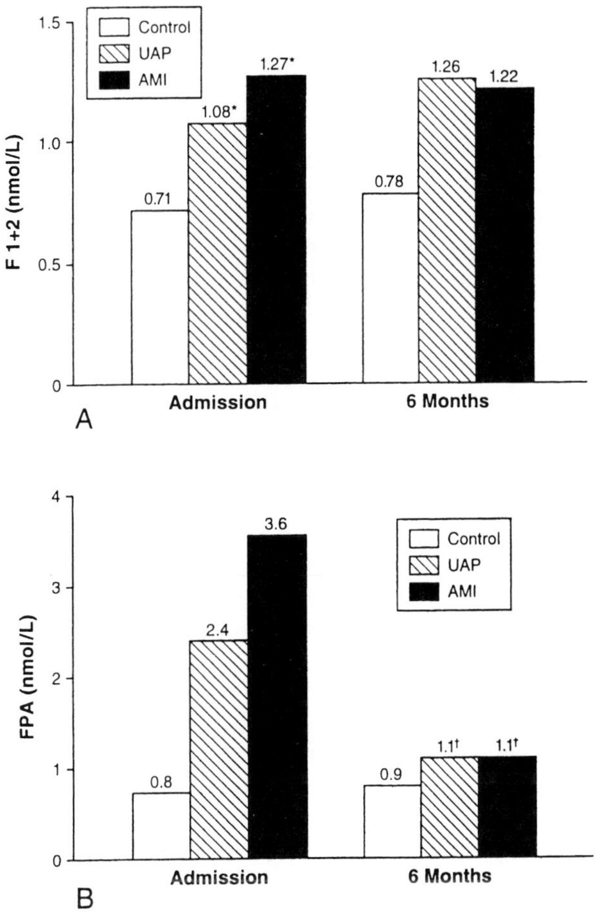

Figure 4 Plasma concentrations of prothrombin fragment 12 (F 1+2) (panel A) and fibrinopepetide A (FPA) (panel B) in healthy control volunteers (control, n = 32), patients with unstable angina (UAP, n = 80), and acute myocardial infarction (AMI, n = 32) measured at hospital admission and at 6-month follow-up. Patients with an acute coronary syndrome had elevations in both F 1+2 and FPA at admission compared to the control group (*$P < .01$). At follow-up, levels of FPA "normalized" ($^{\dagger} = P < .01$ compared to admission level), whereas the F 1+2 levels remained elevated. (From Ref. 16.)

Théroux et al. (17) also reported acutely elevated fibrinopeptide A in unstable angina; Kruskal et al. (18) found increased levels of D-dimer; and Zalewski et al. (19) reported increased levels of PAI-1 activity. These observations support the concept that thrombin activity is heightened in some patients with unstable angina. On the other hand, other investigations have not found heightened levels or activities of hemostatic factors in patients with unstable angina. Explanations for these seemingly inconsistent findings include the heterogeneous population of patients with unstable angina, the relatively small thrombus burden present in some lesions, and the transient nature to these hemostatic factors. For example, Alexopoulos et al. (20) reported no difference in D-dimer or PAI-1 levels among patients with unstable angina compared to control when measured within 24 hours of the last episode of pain. In contrast, the positive findings for D-dimer reported by Kruskal (18) were from samples collected within minutes of symptoms. Finally, in many patients heightened platelet activity may be more etiologically important than fibrin formation.

As mentioned, in acute coronary syndromes platelets adhere to the exposed vessel wall and aggregate in response to exposed vessel wall collagen or local aggregants (thromboxane, adenosine diphosphate). Platelets may bind to the vessel wall or to other platelets via von Willebrand factor (vWF). Montalescot and colleagues (21) measured vWF among 64 patients in the ESSENCE trial (22) (which randomized ACS patients to low-molecular-weight heparin or unfractionated heparin). From baseline to 48 hours after hospital admission, the vWF antigen rose from 180% to 228% (normal range 60% to 110%) in the overall cohort. The rise in vWF from baseline independently predicted outcome at 14 days, rising 75% ± 15% among those with an ischemic event as compared with 34% ± 11% among those free of events (Fig. 5). Thus, acute-phase events associated with platelet activation can also be seen to delineate a spectrum of ACS outcome. Furthermore, when activated, platelets release vasoactive substances which promote vasoconstriction (thromboxane, platelet factor 4) and thrombosis (plasminogen activator inhibitor [PAI-1]) (19). Fitzgerald et al. (23) measuring levels of thromboxane metabolites among subjects with coronary artery disease found the highest levels in those with unstable angina. Eighty-four percent of episodes of chest pain were associated with phasic increases in excretion of thromboxane, suggesting a close temporal relation between platelet activation and clinical events. Heightened platelet activation occurs to some extent in all patients with thrombus-related unstable angina or acute infarction.

Vasocontriction and Cyclic Flow Variation

Continuous monitoring in patients with unstable angina at rest has revealed that many first display a decrease in coronary sinus blood flow. This is

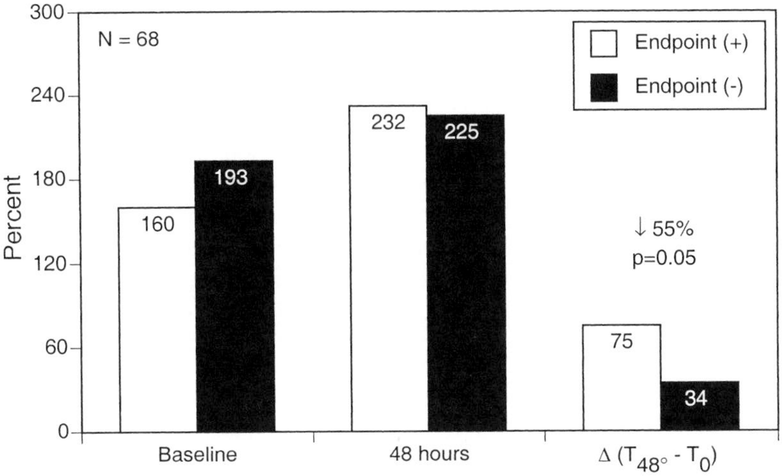

Figure 5 Plasma von Willebrand (vWF) factor levels measured at baseline and at 48 hours after randomization in the ESSENCE trial (22). Patients having an ischemic event by 14-day follow-up had a significantly higher increase in vWF from basline. (From Ref. 21.)

followed by typical electrocardiographic changes of ischemia and then chest discomfort. Therefore, in response to chest pain, heart rate and systolic arterial pressure may rise (24,25). These episodes of ischemia, as well as those documented by Holter monitoring (26), resolve minutes later and may recur cyclically during disease instability. Episodic platelet aggregation at the site of coronary stenoses have been shown responsible for the cyclic flow reduction and transient myocardial ischemia in animal models (27). In short, most subjects with rest angina have recurrent, transient reduction in coronary blood supply secondary to vasoconstriction and thrombus formation at the site of atherosclerotic plaque rupture. These events occur as a complex interaction among the vascular wall, leukocytes, platelets, and atherogenic lipoproteins. Among patients with myocardial infarction these events may also occur as prodromal angina or during early recanalization of the infarct-related artery.

CLINICAL SPECTRUM

Epidemiology

Clinically, the acute coronary syndromes are the leading causes of hospitalizations for adults in the United States. The incidence of unstable angina is increasing, and approximately 800,000 hospitalizations each year are with a primary diagnosis of unstable angina. A similar number of unstable angina episodes likely occur outside the hospital setting and are unrecognized or managed in the outpatient setting. With heightened public awareness, improved survival following acute myocardial infarction, and an increasing proportion of the population being of advanced age, this number should continue to rise despite primary and secondary prevention measures. Approximately 1.5 million myocardial infarctions occur annually, and of these approximately one-sixth will die before hospitalization. Several studies have suggested that the incidence of unstable angina has steadily increased to exceed that of acute myocardial infarction (28).

Demographics

The demographics of acute coronary syndromes mainly reflect the risk factors associated with atherosclerosis. Most patients hospitalized are between ages 50 and 70 years, with patients having unstable angina being slightly older. Since the Global Use of Strategies to Open Occluded Coronary Arteries (GUSTO) IIb study (29) simultaneously enrolled patients across the spectrum of ACS, its data are particularly relevant. In GUSTO IIb, of the 12,142 patients studied, the median ages for those with acute myocardial infarction and unstable angina were 63 and 66 years, respectively (Fig. 6). Perhaps because females represent a greater percentage of the elderly population, they have a relatively greater presence in the unstable angina population. While men more commonly have acute coronary syndromes than women, the ratio of men to women with unstable angina (2:1) is lower than for acute myocardial infarction (3:1). Coronary artery disease risk factors—hypertension, hypercholesterolemia, and tobacco—are each present in 30% to 40% of patients with an acute coronary syndrome, whereas diabetes is usually present in 15% to 20% (Table 5). Again, perhaps because of somewhat older age, those with unstable angina are more likely to have diabetes, hypertension, and hypercholesterolemia compared to patients with myocardial infarction. Finally, for several reasons including more advanced age, more extensive coronary artery disease, and a higher representation of vessel reocclusion, patients with unstable angina are more likely to have had a prior infarction or myocardial revascularization procedure.

Physical and Laboratory Assessment

The symptoms and physical findings of unstable angina compared to stable angina primarily differ in that the pain of unstable angina is usually less predictable, more intense, and easily provoked. Patients with acute infarction may have pain or associated signs and symptoms (nausea, dyspnea, diapho-

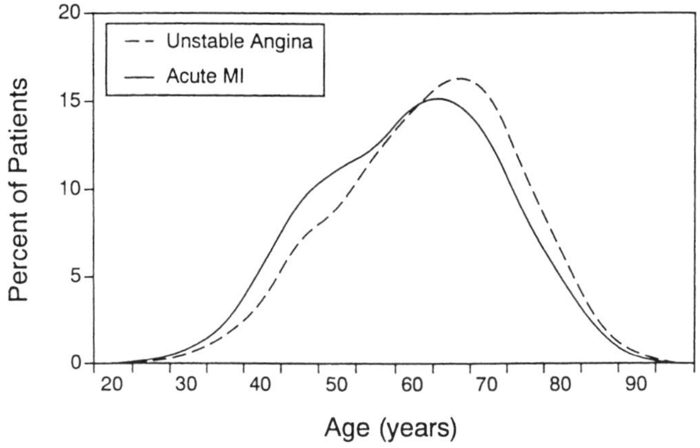

Figure 6 Histogram of the age of patients enrolled in the Global Use of Strategies to Open Occluded Coronary Arteries (GUSTO) IIb study (29) separated by diagnosis of non-ST-segment elevation (unstable angina and non-Q-wave myocardial infarction) or ST-segment elevation (Q-wave myocardial infarction). The median ages for those with acute myocardial infarction and unstable angina were 63 and 66 years, respectively.

Table 5 Baseline Characteristics of Patients with Acute Coronary Syndromes in GUSTO-IIb

Characteristic	Unstable angina (n = 8011)	Myocardial infarction (n = 4131)
Age (years)	66	63
Systolic blood pressure (mm Hg)	139	130
Female gender (%)	33	24
Diabetes (%)	19	16
Hypertension (%)	48	40
Hypercholesterolemia (%)	41	36
Current smoker (%)	27	41
Prior myocardial infarction (%)	32	17
Prior CABG (%)	12	5
Prior PTCA (%)	11	6

Source: Ref. 29.

Data for continuous variables are median values. CABG, coronary artery bypass grafting; PTCA, percutaneous transluminal coronary angioplasty.

resis) of greater severity than that of unstable angina, but may be of similar hemodynamic stability. For example, in the GUSTO-IIb study, the percent of patients in Killip class I, II, and III-IV (88%, 11%, and 1%, repectively) was identical for patients whether presenting with ST-segment depression or elevation. Reasons for this lack of difference in Killip class may stem from the study's relatively homogeneous population shaped by the inclusion and exclusion criteria. Patients who were critically ill (e.g., cardiogenic shock) were not enrolled for logistic reasons. On the other hand, all patients had to have significant ST-segment abnormalities associated with chest pain. These criteria exluded patients at the ends of the spectrum, i.e., those with less severe unstable angina or those with massive infarctions. In general, several percent of patients with acute myocardial infarction present in cardiogenic shock, whereas this occurs even less frequently among patients with unstable angina. Thus, in many respects patients with unstable angina may be indistinguishable from those with myocardial infarction (especially non-Q-wave infarction). Diagnostic hallmarks for acute myocardial infarction are ischemic ST-segment elevation on 12-lead electrocardiography or serologic evidence for myocardial necrosis.

Elevation of the ST-segments are interpreted as transmural myocardial ischemia, as opposed to subendocardial ischemia associated with ST-segment depression of unstable angina or non-Q-wave infarction. Interestingly, continuous electrocardiographic recordings by Holter monitoring in subjects with unstable angina reveal frequent episodes of ST-segment abnormalities without associated symptoms, (i.e., silent ischemia), and this may be related to cyclic flow variation in the culprit lesion. Gottlieb et al. (26) found that >50% of unstable angina patients in the intensive care unit had silent ischemia during aggressive medical therapy, and this portended a worse prognosis. The recent development of more sensitive markers of myocardial cell injury (Chap. 12), such as troponin-T or myosin, has provided evidence of cell necrosis in some subjects with unstable angina (30,31). Hamm et al. (30) observed circulating cardiac troponin-T, an intracellular contractile protein not normally found in blood, in 39% of subjects with acute angina at rest (Braunwald class III). Among these subjects with detected troponin-T, 30% manifested a myocardial infarction (i.e., electrocardiographic changes and elevated levels of creatine kinase MB activity) days later. In contrast, no subject with accelerated (class I) or subacute (class II) unstable angina had detectable troponin-T. These data nicely demonstrate the pathophysiologic continuum of acute myocardial ischemia such that subjects with the most severe unstable angina have minimal but detectable myocardial cell necrosis thereby bordering the conventional definition of myocardial infarction. The hallmark of unstable angina is unpredictability, but specific prognostic indicators, such as silent ischemia on Holter monitoring or detected circulating cardiac troponin-T, may be helpful to stratify patients with unstable angina into groups who need early angiography and revascularization versus conservative medical therapy.

Coronary Anatomy

Angiographic studies in patients with unstable angina have differed greatly regarding the observed presence and severity of coronary atherosclerosis, thrombosis, and irregular lesion morphology. The seeming inconsistency of these reports, which has fueled disagreement among investigators, is also understandable when considering the diversity of patients falling under the definition of unstable angina as well as the timing and limitations of arteriography. Data from some series of unstable angina patients (32–34) suggest the distribution of diseased coronary vessels among those with severe coronary stenoses is approximately 15%, 35%, and 50% for one, two, and three-vessel, respectively.

Compared to subjects with stable angina or first myocardial infarction, these data suggest there is more extensive coronary artery disease in patients with unstable angina. Autopsy studies in patients with unstable angina support the finding from angiography that these subjects have more extensive coronary artery disease (35) and eccentrically located stenoses (36) compared to those with stable angina. Histopathologic studies from severe cases of unstable angina with resultant sudden death provide interesting support for the pathophysiologic role of intracoronary thrombi and embolization. In contrast, the Thrombolysis in Myocardial Infarction (TIMI) IIIA study (37), which evaluated the effects of thrombolytic therapy on culprit lesions in subjects with ischemia at rest, found one-, two-, and three-vessel disease in 35%, 39%, and 26%, respectively. These data are more similar to those found in subjects with chronic stable angina. When considering all patients undergoing angiography for unstable chest pain, the reported incidence of left main artery disease is roughly 5% to 10% while on average 10% to 15% have no or insignificant residual stenosis (34,37).

The reported presence of thrombus at coronary angiography in patients with unstable angina has ranged widely, from <10% (38) among those with chest pain within the previous month, to >50% (39–41) among those with rest angina within the preceding 24 hours. Twenty-nine percent of unstable angina subjects in the TIMI IIIA angiographic trial were found to have apparent thrombus while an additional group was categorized as having possible thrombus. Considering patients with acute myocardial infarction, important angiographic studies by DeWood et al. demonstrated occlusive coronary thrombi in the acute setting of both Q-wave (42) and non-Q-wave (43) infarctions. These and similar studies have also shown the incidence of angiographically demonstrable thrombus to steadily decrease in the hours to days following myocardial infarction, remaining evident in 40% to 50% of subjects at 2 weeks. It is not surprising, therefore, that thrombus is present in many patients with Braunwald class C unstable angina (i.e., that occurring within 2 weeks of infarction) and in others spontaneous thrombolysis may occur. In most subjects with acute coronary syndromes, the inciting pathophysiologic event is an occlusive coronary arterial thrombus, but in some of these individuals endogenous thrombolysis occurs within minutes thereby avoiding myocardial cell necrosis. In addition to rapid endogenous lysis of the thrombus, additional reasons that a number of unstable angina subjects do not have angiographic evidence of thrombus, is likely due to the limitations of angiography and the mulifaceted etiology of this syndrome.

Noninvasive Cardiac Assessment

In addition to routine 12-lead electrocardiography to discern the presence of previous infarction, ST-segment or T-wave abnormalities, continuous electrocardiographic observation by Holter monitoring may provide helpful information. Depending on the criteria of ST-segment deviation, the timing of monitoring relative to disease instability, and the intervening medical therapy, abnormal ST-segment shifts can be observed in roughly one-third of patients. Exercise electrocardiographic testing is a helpful tool in the diagnosis of angina in patients without ST-segment abnormalities as baseline. Exercise testing should not be performed in the acute phase of unstable angina or in subjects with recent rest angina. However, subjects in whom disease activity becomes controlled after several days of medical therapy may safely undergo stress testing before hospital discharge (44–46). Predischarge testing is preferential to testing weeks to months following discharge since no prognostic value is lost with early testing and a high proportion of the adverse cardiac events occur during this interval (47). Among men, shorter exercise duration, lower maximal rate-pressure product, and exercise-induced angina or ST-segment depression have correlated with unfavorable outcome (44,45). In multivariable analysis, Wilcox et al. (48) found predischarge exercise tests added independent prognostic information to known important clinical descriptors (e.g., recurrent rest pain and evolutionary T-wave changes). The positive predictive value for future ischemic events with routine exercise testing, however, is low, even among patients with recent myocardial injury (49). This is among the reasons why some physicians prefer to have nearly all unstable angina patients directly undergo nuclear imaging or cardiac catheterization.

Nuclear scintigraphy, assessing regional myocardial perfusion using thallium-201, can be performed at rest, i.e., between anginal episodes, or in combination with physiologic or pharmacologic stress. Pooling data from several studies (46,50–53) the sensitivity of thallium-201 imaging at rest alone for the detection of severe coronary artery stenoses averages <60%. With the addition of dypyridamole, a pharmacologic "stress," thallium-201 imaging in patients with unstable angina has increased sensitivity to 90% while maintaining a specificity of approximately 80% (54). When present, perfusion defects can provide prognostic information; Wackers et al. (50) observed perfusion defects in 76% of subjects who had a complicated clinical course compared to 32% of those who had an uncomplicated outcome following an acute coronary syndrome. Assessing myocardial tissue metabolism with positron emission tomography (PET) using 5-fluordeoxyglucose in patients with unstable angina demonstrates increased glucose consumption at rest compared to subjects with stable angina. This occurs in the absence of symptoms or electrocardiographic evidence of myocardial ischemia and also suggests a state of prolonged or chronic hypoperfusion. Thus, nuclear myocardial studies can detect and localize severe coronary stenoses with a moderate to high sensitivity; however, a substantial percentage of subjects who have an untoward outcome may not be prospectively identified. These imaging modalities can be similarly useful following episodes of unstable angina or postinfarction.

Invasive Assessment

Since numerous studies have demonstrated ≥80% of subjects with unstable angina have important atherosclerotic coroanry artery disease and this percentage is higher postinfarction, some physicians feel it is prudent to directly define the extent and severity of disease in these patients during index hospitalization. Indeed, among 1457 consecutive hopsital admissions with unstable angina in the GUARANTEE study (8) who underwent angiography, 82% had significant coronary artery diesease. Others reasons cited for early angiographic assessment include evidence that roughly half of these subjects have left main or three-vessel CAD and may benefit from prompt surgical revascularization. These points, combined with an overall moderate positive predictive value of noninvasive assessments, suggest a significant percentage of important coronary lesions may be initially unappreciated without angiography.

Finally, a small percentage of patients presenting with unstable angina will have angiographically normal coronary arteries. For these patients and for those with minimal coronary arterial lesions following myocardial infarction, their prognosis is very good and this provides reassurance to patient and physician alike. In large-scale studies such as GUSTO-IIb, GUARANTEE, and PURSUIT (8,29,55), approximately 60% to 80% of patients undergo coronary angiography during the initial hospitalization. This percent is similar for those with unstable angina and acute myocardial infarction.

TREATMENT AND OUTCOME

Medical Therapy

Since there is signifcant overlap in the pathophysiology of unstable angina and acute myocardial infarction, there are many similarities in treatment strategies. As mentioned, the pathophysiologic cornerstone of unstable angina and acute myocardial infarction is the formation of thrombus which involves platelets and a number of plasma and tissue factors. Treatment of this thrombotic process, therefore, can be directed at platelets, thrombin, fibrin, and other coagulation factors. The respective categories of therapy are: 1) antiplatelet agents (Chaps. 15 and 16), such as aspirin, ticlopidine, and potent platelet glycoprotein IIb/IIIa inhibtors; 2) antithrombins (Chap. 18), such as heparin and hirudin; 3) fibrinolytic agents or plasminogen activators (Chaps. 9 and 10); and 4) inhibitors of vitamin K-dependent coagulation proteins, such as warfarin. Since inhibitors of the vitamin K-dependent factors usually take days to become effective, they are not clinically important in the unstable phase of acute coronary syndromes. Rather, most patients presenting with unstable angina or infarction will receive a combination of rapid-acting anticoagulant therapies, such as intravenous heparin and oral aspirin.

Antiplatelets

The benefit of aspirin, thienopyridines, and platelet glycoprotein IIb/IIIa inhibitors alone or in combination with heparin in the treatment of unstable angina has been proven in many randomized trials. Such trials of antiplatelet therapies in ACS are detailed in Chapters 15 and 16. In general, several observations can be made when assessing the relative benefit of oral antiplatelet therapies in the spectrum of ACS. Pooling data from >2000 patients with unstable angina (56–59), the occurrence of infarction or death in the early weeks was reduced from 11.8% (control) to 6.0% (aspirin).

In the setting of an acute ST-elevation MI, aspirin was shown to reduce mortality by 23% in the second International Study of Infarct Survival (ISIS-2) (60). More recently, aspirin's role in achieving infarct artery patency is suggested by a smaller study suggesting that when chewed aspirin alone is taken in the hyperacute phase of a myocardial infarction, stable reperfusion can be achieved in nearly 50% of patients, compared with 25% in controls (61). The ability of aspirin to reduce the risk of recurrent cardiovascular complications in patients who have survived a myocardial infarction has been studied in eight trials involving nearly 16,000 patients (62). Collectively, these eight studies demonstrate a one-third reduction in the risk of nonfatal myocardial infarction and a one-fourth decrease in the occurrence of myocardial (re)infarction, stroke, or vascular death. In brief, because of the platelet-centric etiology of most acute coronary syndromes, aspirin plays a fundamental role in the treatment of both unstable angina and acute myocardial infarction.

Ticlopidine and clopidogrel (thienopyridines) reduce secondary ischemic events of ACS similar to aspirin (63,64) but are not commonly used in the hyperacute phase of ischemia since they take hours to become effective. The newest, and most potent antiplatelet agents are the glycoprotein IIb/IIIa receptor inhibitors. These agents have become standard therapy in patients undergoing PCI and as empiric therapy for ACS patients without ST elevation. Four such large clinical trials, the so-called 4 P's were recently published: the Platelet IIb/IIIa Antagonism for the Reduction of Acute Coronary Syndrome Events in a Global Organization Network (PARAGON) trial (65); the Platelet Receptor Inhibition in Ischemic Syndrome Management (PRISM) study (66); the Platelet Receptor Inhibition in Ischemic Syndrome Management in Patients Limited by Unstable Signs and Symptoms (PRISM-PLUS) study (67); and the Platelet IIb/IIIa in Unstable Angina: Receptor Suppression Using Integrilin Therapy (PURSUIT) trial (55). Overall, these trials show a reduction in death or MI at 30 days of 10% to 15% beyond that of standard therapy. Importantly, several posthoc analyses have shown that patients most likely to receive benefit are those with non-Q-wave MI at presentation (elevated troponin levels) as compared with those with unstable angina (no evidence for myocardial necrosis at entry). For example, in PRISM there was no reduction in the 30-day death or MI composite by tirofiban among those who were troponin-I negative (heparin 4.9% vs. tirofiban 5.7%). In contrast, those who were troponin-I positive had a 67% reduction in 30-day events with tirofiban (13.0% vs. 4.3%, $P < .001$) (Fig. 7) (68).

In the setting of ST-elevation MI, phase II studies have also been completed using conjunctive IIb/IIIa antagonists with fibrinolytic therapy. In the Thrombolysis and Angioplasty in Myocardial Infarction (TAMI) 8 study (69), patients received m7E3 (murine form of c7E3, abciximab) hours following administration of t-PA. In the treatment group, ischemic events were reduced and major bleeding occurred at a similar rate to the control group. The second trial, Integrilin to Manage Platelet Aggregation to Prevent Coronary Thrombosis in Acute Myocardial Infarction (IMPACT-AMI) (70), studied eptifibatide given at the same time as front-loaded t-PA. The primary endpoint, angiographic TIMI grade 3 flow at 90 min, was present in 39% of the control group, 52% of the overall eptifibatide group, and 66% of those receiving the highest dose of eptifibatide.

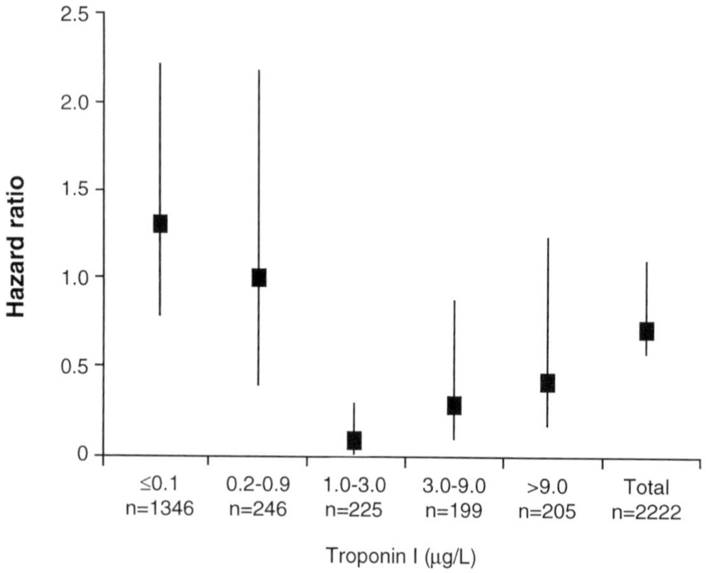

Figure 7 PRISM outcome: adjusted hazard ratios (decrease 30-day death or MI) and 95% confidence intervals for treatment with tirofiban by troponin quartiles. Hazard ratios below 1.0 favor treatment with tirofiban. (From Ref. 68.)

Although there was an early effect on reperfusion, at late (30-day) follow-up a composite of death, myocardial infarction, revascularization, or new heart failure, occurred in 45% of the treatment group and 42% of the control group. The PARADIGM group studied lamifiban in combination with streptokinase or accelerated t-PA. The primary clinical endpoint was the absence of TIMI grade 3 flow by angiography, continuous electrocardiography, or a clinical indication of inadequate coronary perfusion (death, MI, recurrent ST-segment elevation). By continuous electrocardiography, those receiving lamifiban had faster and more stable initial reperfusion and fewer episodes of recurrent ischemia during drug infusion. The ischemic composite event occurred in 40% of the lamifiban-treated patients and 42% of those receiving placebo. Each of these AMI studies showed the combination of IIb/IIIa antagonists to thrombolytic strategies to be feasible and safe. Each also showed promise for the improvement of myocardial reperfusion, but alone or in combination, there was no demonstration of a reduction in 30-day mortality. The Strategies for Patency Enhancement in the Emergency Department (SPEED) (71) and TIMI 14A (72) studies randomized patients to abciximab alone, fibrinolytic alone, or the combination of abciximab with reduced-dose fibrinolytic therapy to assess 60- to 90-min TIMI grade flow.

The INTRO-AMI (73) was performed similarly using eptifibatide and reduced-dose t-PA. Collectively, these studies show an approximately 15% absolute increase in 60- to 90-min TIMI-3 flow (55% in the fibrinolytic alone group vs. 70% in the abciximab plus *reduced-dose* fibrinolytic groups). Each trial has a planned or ongoing Phase III corresponding trial testing IIb/IIIa therapy in combination with a half-dose fibrinolytic agent versus standard fibrinolysis to assess the impact on 30-day mortality.

Antithrombins

Thrombin, the end product of the coagulation mechanism, initiates transformation of fibrinogen to a fibrin clot and activates platelets. Its antagonist, antithrombin III, is the major endogenous inhibitor of the coagulation cascade and is the essential cofactor for heparin. Heparin is a mucopolysaccharide which forms a heparin-antithrombin III complex increasing antithrombin activity several thousandfold. Clinically, many trials have been performed using heparin in unstable angina and in conjunction with thrombolytic therapy for acute myocardial infarction. These are detailed in Chapter 18. Oler and colleagues performed a meta-analysis of six trials with >1300 patients who were treated with heparin (aPTT 1.5-2x control) in addition to 75 to 650 mg aspirin per day for patients with unstable angina. With the addition of heparin there was a trend (P = .06) for a lower rate of the composite of death or myocardial infarction during inpatient therapy (relative risk = .67) though this was lost at follow-up weeks to months later (relative risk = .82) (74). When more potent antiplatelet therapy is utilized, such as the IIb/IIIa inhibitors studied in PARAGON and PRISM, the modest benefit of heparin therapy is likely further attenuated.

The antithrombin effect of heparin is lost when thrombin is bound to fibrin or the endothelium, and heparin can be inactivated by platelet factor 4 and heparinases. Low-molecular-weight or fractionated heparins have more inhibitory activity against factor Xa and are less inactivated by platelet factor 4. New antithrombins, such as hirudin and hirulog, differ from heparin in that they are effective against free as well as bound thrombin, and they do not require antithrombin III as a cofactor. Both LMWH and hirudin have been studied in acute coronary syndromes and shown to be effective. Examples include the Efficacy and Safety of Subcutaneous Enoxaparin in Non-Q-Wave Coronary Events (ESSENCE) study (22), which randomized 3171 patients with unstable angina or non-Q-wave myocardial infarction to LMWH (enoxaparin) or unfractionated heparin for 2 to 8 days. At 30-day follow-up the rate of death, (re)infarction, and recurrent ischemia was reduced 15% (23.3% to 19.8%, P = .017) by enoxaparin; the rate of death or (re)infarction was reduced 20% (P = .081). Similarly, when hirudin was compared to heparin for all acute coronary syndromes in the GUSTO-IIb study among 12,142 patients the rate of death or (re)infarction was slightly reduced (9.8% to 8.9%, OR = 0.89, $P = .058$). Similar to the IIb/IIIa inhibitor studies of unstable angina, patients in these LMWH trials who were troponin positive appear to derive particular benefit. At 40-day follow-up in the Fragmin in Unstable Coronary Artery Disease (FRISC) study, dalteparin reduced the incidence of death or MI by 48% as compared with placebo among patients who were troponin positive. For patients who were troponin negative no reduction in events was seen (4.7% placebo vs. 5.7% dalteparin) (75). In summary, the similarly important benefit provided to the outcome of unstable angina, non-Q-wave, and Q-wave myocardial infarction by antiplatelet and antithrombin therapies cements the common underlying pathophysiology and acute pharmacologic management. On the other hand, the spectrum of disease acuity and the importance of underlying thrombus are evidenced by those studies showing that most of the benefit of potent antiplatelet and antithrombin therapy is extended to patients who are troponin positive.

Fibrinolytic Therapy

Since coronary thrombus formation is known to be pathophysiologically responsible for unstable angina, as it is in MI, and fibrinolytic therapy is of clear benefit in the setting of ST-elevation MI, fibrinolysis for unstable angina seems intuitive. The earliest trials of fibrinolytic agents in unstable angina were without control populations and demonstrated little benefit. These were followed by angiographic trials of intracoronary thrombolysis in acute coronary syndromes and revealed angiographic improvement—however, without substantial clinical benefit. A number of placebo-controlled trials have been performed with intravenous thrombolytic agents used in conjunction with aspirin and heparin (76–89) (Table 6). The results from these trials, assessing the incidence of nonfatal infarctions and death, vary substantially. Three of the four largest trials did observe a tendency for more nonfatal infarctions among subjects receiving thrombolytic therapy. While none of these differences was strongly powered, a formal meta-analysis (90) of nearly 2500 patients demonstrated a paradoxically higher ($P < .05$) rate of nonfatal infarction or the combination of death and infarction (12.4% vs. 11.0%) among subjects receiving thrombolysis. The risk of major bleeding events was also higher among patients receiving thrombolytic therapy.

The worsened outcomes for unstable angina patients receiving thrombolysis are in striking contrast to patients with acute myocardial infarction who gain unarguable survival benefit from thrombolytic therapy (Table 6). These points can be evidenced by data from the Fibrinolytic Therapy Trialists' Collaborative Group (91). This study group combined nine large-scale international thrombolytic trials, reported data from 58,600 patients treated with thrombolytic therapy, including 32,346 with ST-segment elevation and

Table 6 Thrombolytic Therapy in Acute Coronary Syndromes (UAP and AMI)

				Death (%)		MI (%)		Major bleed (%)	
Study	Year	N	Agent	TTx	Placebo	TTx	Placebo	TTx	Placebo
Unstable angina trials									
Gold (80)	1987	24	tPA	0	0	0	8.3	33.3	0
Nicklas (83)	1989	40	tPA	10.0	0	10.0	10.0	25.0	0
Schreiber (86)	1989	149	UK	0	0	8.3	3.8	0	1.9
Ardissino (76)	1990	24	tPA	0	8.3	8.3	16.7	8.3	8.3
Neri Seneri (82)	1990	39	tPA	5.0	0	0	0	0	0
Roberts (84)	1990?	80	tPA	12.5	10.0	47.5	45.0	2.5	2.5
Saran (85)	1990	48	SK	0	12.5	4.2	16.7	0	0
Williams (89)	1990	68	tPA	0	0	6.7	4.3	15.6	8.7
Scrutino (87)	1991	60	tPA	0	13.3	3.3	3.3	0	0
Bär (77)	1992	159	APSAC	3.8	1.3	36.3	26.6	7.5	1.3
Charbonnier (78)	1992	50	tPA	0	4.0	20	8.0	4.0	4.0
Freeman (79)	1992	70	tPA	2.9	2.9	5.7	2.9	2.9	0
Karlsson (81)	1992	205	tPA	3.0	1.9	8.0	9.5	0	0
TIMI-IIIB (88)	1994	1473	tPA	2.3	2.6	6.5	4.4	0.5	0
Pooled UAP		2489		2.5	3.0	9.9	8.0	2.3	0.6
Myocardial infarction trials									
Fibrinolytic therapy trialists' group (91)	1994	32,346		10.4	12.8			1.2	0.4

4,237 with ST-segment depression. Whereas those with ST-segment elevation had a 19% higher survival rate if treated with thrombolytic therapy, there was a 10% lower survival rate among those with ST-segment depression receiving thrombolysis compared to placebo. This translated into 14 excess deaths per 1000 ST-segment depression patients treated. Not surprisingly, there was also an excess of serious bleeding events and stroke among those receiving thrombolytic therapy. In short, among the many areas of similar pharmacologic therapies for treatment of acute coronary syndromes, thrombolytic therapy is a clear exception and should be reserved for patients with ST-segment elevation or bundle branch morphology.

Antianginals

The obvious goal of antianginal therapy is to reverse the oxygen supply/demand mismatch by minimizing requirements and maximizing delivery of tissue nutrients. Secondary precipitants, such as anemia, hypoxemia, and thyroid dysfunction, are more common in unstable angina than infarction and should be sought after and corrected. Specific therapy for primary causes of ischemia should be directed at each pathophysiologic origin. Nitrates, the century-old category of antianginals, remain the therapeutic mainstay for patients with ACS. Whether given topically, sublingually, orally, or intravenously, they ameliorate several pathways of angina (92). Recent study of platelet function in whole blood found intravenous nitroglycerin to inhibit aggregation, an effect that was substantial and rapidly reversible (93). Other possible beneficial effects or nitroglycerin include an increase in coronary collateral blood flow (94) and a favorable redistribution of regional flow (95). Important caveats to nitrate therapy include rapid (<24 hour) development of drug tolerance with continuous therapy (i.e., without a nitrate-free interval) and reported induction of heparin resistance (96,97). Long-acting forms of oral nitrates have become popular recently, but should be reserved for patients with stable symptoms.

Beta-adrenergic blocking agents, like nitrates, serve a number of important roles in the treatment of myocardial ischemia. Their main function, blocking adrenergic receptors, serves to blunt heart rate increases which occur in response to physical exertion, chest pain, or as a reflex to vasodilators. In addition, beta-blockers decrease blood pressure and myocardial contractility, thereby lowering myocardial oxygen demands. Clinical trials of beta-adrenoreceptor blockers in the setting of stable and unstable angina have shown decrease in both ischemic symptoms and occurrence of myocardial infarctions (98). Another potential benefit of beta-adrenergic blocking agents is inhibition of platelet aggregation, which has been observed in several in vitro studies (99,100). Infrequent situations of angina where beta-blocker therapy should be avoided include nonischemic exacerbation of heart failure, cocaine-induced coronary vasoconstriction (101), and vasospastic angina (102). Beta-blockers should be used cautiously or avoided in those susceptible to reactive (bronchospastic) airway disease. Cardioselective beta-blockers, such as metoprolol and atenolol, are preferred to the nonnselective beta-blockers since they produce fewer unwanted (noncardiac) effects.

Calcium channel antagonists are effective in lowering blood pressure and decreasing chest pain frequency among patients with stable angina. They are generally considered safe as long as the patient does not have important systolic ventricular dysfunction. The use of short-acting calcium channel antagonists in the treatment of unstable angina has produced mixed results, which is not surprising considering similarly diverse results found in the treatment of postinfarction subjects. By partially blocking the flux of calcium ions into muscle cells, calcium channel blockers cause relaxation of vascular smooth muscle and the myocardium. Like other vasodilators, these effects intuitively decrease myocardial oxygen consumption. Some calcium channel blockers, such as verapamil and diltiazem, cause reduction in heart rate, whereas nifedipine may actually lead to a reflex increase in heart rate.

The Holland Interuniversity Nifedipine/metoprolol Trial (HINT) (98) was a double-blind, placebo-controlled, randomized study of medical therapies in 515 subjects with unstable angina. Among subjects receiving nifedipine without pretreatment or concomitant beta-blocker therapy, the event ratio of recurrent ischemia or infarction was 1.15 relative to placebo. When nifedipine was used in combination with metoprolol or initiated among patients already receiving beta-blockade, respective cardiac event ratios were 0.80 and 0.68 compared to placebo. Diltiazem, on the other hand, was shown to be equally effective to propranolol in reducing episodes of symptomatic ischemia and produced a similar long-term outcome regarding cardiovascular events (103). The newest calcium channel antagonists, nicardipine and amlodipine, reportedly have minimal to no cardiodepressant or chronotropic effects, so they can more safely be used in combination with beta-blockers or used in patients with known chronic heart failure (104).

Because patients with acute myocardial infarction often have more ischemia, they are more likely to receive a fuller or more aggressive antianginal regimen. For example in the GUSTO-IIb study nearly all patients were treated with beta-blockers, though patients with myocardial infarction were more likely to receive them intravenously (25% vs. 13%). Patients suffering infarction are also more likely to receive angiotensin-converting enzyme (ACE) inhibtors to reduce afterload and favorably affect ventricular remodeling. In summary, nitrates, beta-adrenergic antagonists, and calcium channel blockers are each able to lower myocardial oxygen demands, weakly inhibit platelet aggregation, and reduce the frequency of chest pain in stable and acute coronary syndromes. There are no marked distinctions among the acute coronary syndromes strongly favoring a particular therapy though most patients receive nitroglycerin first line. As a monotherapy, nifedipine appears to increase the risk of nonfatal myocardial infarction in the early hours of angina instability, likely due to reflex sympathetic stimulation. Beta-blockers, alone or in combination with other agents, have been shown to reduce the relative risk of myocardial infarction by 10% to 15% (105,106). Combinations of these classes of antianginals are reportedly similar or superior to monotherapy (98,107) and likely for patients with an acute coronary syndrome, a combination of all three agents is optimal.

Invasive Procedures

As mentioned, the percentages of patients with unstable angina or myocardial infarction who undergo cardiac catheterization are similar. Also consistent between unstable angina and acute myocardial infarction is that approximately 30% to 40% of patients undergo coronary revascularization in the days to weeks following presentation. Uniquely different between these coronary syndromes is that patients with acute myocardial infarction are more likely to undergo percutaneous angioplasty, whereas those with unstable angina undergo percutaneous and surgical revascularization with a similar frequency. This is likely due to the ability of angioplasty to restore coronary perfusion promptly and with relative safety compared to emergent bypass surgery in the setting of infarction. An early aggressive versus initially conservative strategy regarding angiography and revascularization (Chap. 14) has been tested among patients presenting with unstable angina and non-Q-wave MI (108–110). While results from these trials have been debated, like potent antiplatelet and antithrombin therapies, an initially aggressive approach with PCI appears to improve outcome among patients presenting with evidence for myocardial necrosis (troponin positive) (111).

OUTCOME

Bleeding Events

Considering outcome in ACS, the safety of therapies employed can usually be judged by the incidence of bleeding complications since much of the pharmacologic armamentarium targets platelets and the coagulation cascade. Transfusions are given to 5% to 10% of hospitalized patients with ACS. Among patients with electrocardiographic evidence of ischemia at rest, either Braunwald class II-III unstable angina or acute myocardial infarction, transfusions are consistenly seen used in ~10% of patients (29). Severe bleeding, usually defined as >5 g hemoglobin loss or bleeding that results in hemodynamic compromise, occurs in a similarly low frequency (1% to 1.5%) between groups with unstable angina and myocardial infarction. The incidence of all strokes (hemorrhagic and nonhemorrhagic) is roughly similar among the acute coronary syndromes. Key determinants of stroke may differ in frequency among patients with unstable angina and myocardial infarction. Patients with acute infarction are more likely to receive thrombolytic therapy, and this is associated with a higher hemorrhagic stroke rate. On the other hand, patients with unstable angina are more likely to be elderly and have slightly higher systolic blood pressure; these are also known risk factors for intracranial hemorrhage. Thus, the rate of all strokes ranges from 0.7% to 1.2% with a slightly higher occurrence among those with myocardial infarction due to the higher rate of hemorraghic stroke.

Death and (Re)Infarction

Because the course of unstable angina can be unpredictable and potentially life threatening, the level of care or aggressiveness of approach needs to be prudently established. In the late 1980s studies reported the incidence of MI in the early weeks following non-ST-elevation ACS to be approximately 10% and the incidence of death 4%. Using then-contemporary strategies, the TIMI IIIB investigators in the early 1990s (88) reported a 6-week rate of nonfatal myocardial infarction of 5.4% and death of 2.4%. Similarly, the overall rate of death or myocardial infarction at 30 days in GUSTO-IIb was 9.4% and the rate of stroke was 1% (29). The most contemporary ACS studies, with strict guidelines for monitoring CK elevations, definitions of myocardial infarctions, and blinded adjudication of events, report a 30-day composite of death or nonfatal myocardial infarction of ~12% (112). With these important adverse cardiac events in mind, an assertive approach should be initially taken in all patients to ameliorate ongoing or recurrent myocardial ischemia. The outcome for unstable angina patients found to be troponin positive or with electrocardiographic ST-segment depression plus T-wave inversion have an outcome similar to patients with acute infarction (Fig. 8).

Savonitto and colleagues (113) showed among the 12,142 GUSTO-IIb patients that the 30-day death or MI rate was 5.5% for those with T-wave inversion, 9.4% with ST-segment elevation, 10.5% with ST-segment depression, and 12.4% for those with ST-segment elevation and depression. Other predictors for long-term outcome for those with unstable angina include age, baseline hemodynamics, and underlying left ventricular systolic function. For patients with acute myocardial infarction the 30-day mortality is approximately 7% depending on the initial strategy employed for perfusion restoration. The 30-day incidence of recurrent infarction is 5% and the risk of stroke is approximately 1%. Independent predictors of mortality and

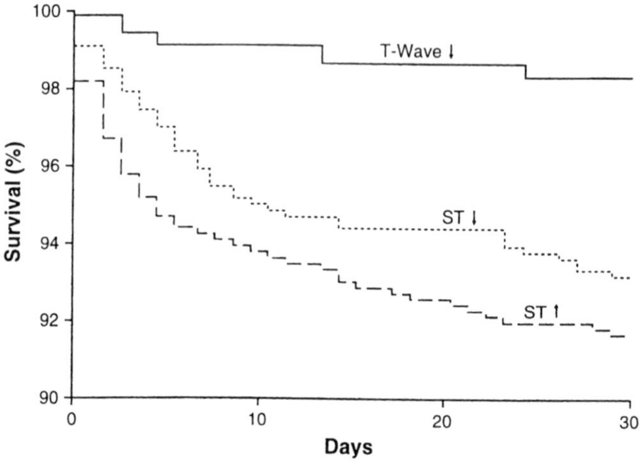

Figure 8 Correlation of 30-day mortality and electrocardiogram on presentation in the Global Use of Strategies to Open Occluded Coronary Arteries (GUSTO) IIa study. A dichotomous outcome for patients with unstable angina could be seen when separated according to the presenting electrocardiogram. Patients presenting with isolated T-wave inversion (T-wave↓) had a relatively low mortality. In contrast, patients with ST-segment depression (ST↓) had a significantly worse outcome which paralelled that of patients with acute myocardial infarction (ST↑). (From Ref. 115.)

(re)infarction for patients with unstable angina and non-Q-wave MI and mortality for patients with Q-wave MI (114) have been statistically determined and are compared in Table 7.

SUMMARY

The continuum of the acute coronary syndromes exists because of shared pathophysiology, evaluation, and treatments for unstable angina, non-Q-wave and Q-wave myocardial infarction. Despite many similarities, unique differences separate unstable angina and myocardial infarction. In general, patients with unstable angina are older and more likely to have comorbidities, mulitvessel coronary artery disease, and previous myocardial revascularization. While the etiology and definition of unstable angina can be broad, these are narrow for myocardial infarction. An atherothrombotic coronary arterial lesion is present in almost every case of myocardial infarction while it is present in many but not necessarily a large majority of cases of unstable angina. For this reason, the electrocardiogram of infarction is frank ST elevation while it may be subtle ST depression or T-wave inversion in unstable

Table 7 Independent Predictors of 30-Day Adverse Ischemic Events[a] (Death or MI)

GUSTO-I	GUSTO-IIb	PURSUIT
Age	Age	Age
Systolic blood pressure	MI at enrollment	MI at enrollment
Killip class	Heart failure	Geographic region
Heart rate	ST depression	ST depression
MI location	Tachycardia	Female gender
Prior MI	Diabetes	Heart failure

[a] 30-day outcome modeling from GUSTO-I (ST elevation MI patients) are for independent predictors of death; data from Lee et al. (114). Outcome from both GUSTO-IIb and PURSUIT (non-ST-elevation patients) are independent predictors for death or (re)infarction at 30 days. Data are from Refs. 29 and 55. These leading six predictors supply >90% of the independent predictive value for outcome. MI, myocardial infarction.

angina. Indeed, patients with unstable angina may present with a normal electrocardiogram, whereas this would be most unusual for the patient with acute infarction.

Among patients presenting with unstable angina and dynamic electrocardiographic changes, one-third will have subsequent evidence for myocardial necrosis, thus crossing the line into infarction. With this, unstable angina patients have inconsistent results with thrombolytic therapy, but the majority of these patients have a more negative outcome than those not receiving thrombolysis. This is in contrast to the patient with acute infarction who receives substantial benefit from thrombolysis.

Outside of thrombolysis, the antianginal, anticoagulant, and revascularization strategies are often the same. The short-term survival for patients with unstable angina is generally better than for those with myocardial infarction, except for unstable angina patients with ST-segment depression with T-wave inversion upon presentation, who have a similarly guarded outcome. In the ACS spectrum, unstable angina patients who become troponin positive receive particular benefit from aggressive antiplatelet, antithrombin, and revascularization strategies. Because the outcome for both unstable angina and acute myocardial infarction can still be substantially improved, efforts continue to further define the similarities and difference within the acute coronary syndrome continuum. With this knowledge, further development and tailoring of diagnostic tests as well as antiplatelet, antithrombin, antianginal, and revascularization strategies can be extended to these syndromes.

REFERENCES

1. Conti CR, Greene B, Pitt B, Griffith L, Humphries O, Brawley R, Taylor D, Bender H, Gott V, Ross RS. Coronary surgery in unstable angina pectoris. Circulation 1971;44(suppl II):II-154.
2. Fowler NO. Preinfarction angina: a need for an objective definition and for a controlled clinical trial of its management. Circulation 1971;44:755–758.
3. Wood P. Acute and subacute coronary insufficiency. Br Med J 1961;I:1779–1782.
4. Vakil RJ. Preinfarction syndrome: management and follow-up. Am J Cardiol 1964;14:55–63.
5. Scanlon PJ, Nemickas R, Moran JF, Talano JV, Amirparviz F, Pifarre R. Accelerated angina pectoris: clinical hemodynamic, arteriographic, and therapeutic experience in 85 patients. Circulation 1973;47:19–26.
6. Fuster V, Chesebro JH. Mechanisms of unstable angina. N Engl J Med 1986; 315:1023–1024.
7. Braunwald E. Unstable angina. A classification. Circulation 1989;80:410–414.
8. Moliterno DJ, Aguirre FV, Cannon CP, Every NP, Granger CB, Sapp SK, Booth JE, Fergsuon JJ, for the GUARANTEE Investigators. The Global Unstable Angina Registry and Treatment Evaluation. Circulation 1996;94:I.
9. Aceti A, Taliani G, de Bac C, Sebastiani A. Monocyte activation and increased procoagulant activity in unstable angina. Lancet 1990;336:1444–1446.
10. Dinerman JL, Mehta JL, Saldeen TGP, Emerson S, Wallin R, Davda R, Davidson A. Increased neutrophil elastase release in unstable angina pectoris and acute myocardial infarction. J Am Coll Cardiol 1990;15:1559–1563.
11. Falk E. Unstable angina with fatal outcome: dynamic coronary thrombosis leading to infarction and/or sudden death. Circulation 1985;71:699–708.
12. Moise A, Théroux P, Taeymans Y, Descoings B, Lespérnace J, Waters DD, Pelletier GB, Bourasa MG. Unstable angina and progression of coronary atherosclerosis. N Engl J Med 1983;309:685–689.
13. Coller BS. The role of platelets in arterial thrombosis and the rationale for blockade of platelet GP IIb/IIIa receptors as antithrombotic therapy. Eur Heart J 1995;16:11–15.
14. Sherman CT, Litvack F, Grundfest W, Lee M, Hickey A, Chaux A, Kass R, Blanche C, Matloff J, Morgenstern L, Ganz W, Swan HJC, Forrester J. Coronary angioscopy in patients with unstable angina pectoris. N Engl J Med 1986;315:913–919.
15. Wilensky RL, Bourdillon P, Vix VA, Zeller JA. Intracoronary artery thrombus formation in unstable angina: a clinical, biochemical and angiographic correlation. J Am Coll Cardiol 1993;21:692–699.
16. Merlini PA, Bauer KA, Oltrona L, Ardissino D, Cattaneo M, Belli C, Mannucci PM, Rosenberg RD. Persistent activation of coagulation mechanism in unstable angina and myocardial infarction. Circulation 1994;90:61–68.
17. Théroux P, Latour J, Leger-Gauthier C, DeLara J. Fibrinopeptide A and platelet factor levels in unstable angina pectoris. Circulation 1987;75:156–162.

18. Kruskal JB, Commerford PJ, Franks JJ, Kirsch RE. Fibrin and fibrinogen-related antigens in patients with stable and unstable coronary artery disease. N Engl J Med 1987;309:1361–1365.
19. Zalewski A, Shi Y, Nardone D, Bravette B, Weinstock P, Fischman D, Wilson P, Goldberg S, Levin DC, Bjornsson TD. Evidence for reduced fibrinolytic activity in unstable angina at rest. Circulation 1991;83:1685–1691.
20. Alexopoulos D, Ambrose JA, Stump D, Borrico S, Gorlin R, Deshmukh P, Fisher EA. Thrombosis-related markers in unstable angina pectoris. J Am Coll Cardiol 1991;17:866–871.
21. Montalescot G, Philippe F, Ankri A, Vicaut E, Bearez E, Poulard JE, Carrie D, Flammang D, Dutoit A, Carayon A, Jardel C, Chevrot M, Bastard JP, Bigonzi F, Thomas D, for the French Investigators of the ESSENCE Trial. Early increase of Von Willebrand factor predicts adverse outcome in unstable coronary artery disease. Circulation 1999;98:294–299.
22. Cohen M, Demers C, Gurfinkel EP, Turpie A, Fromell GJ, Goodman S, Langer A, Califf RM, Fox KA, Premmereur J, Bigonzi F. A comparison of low-molecular-weight heparin with unfractionated heparin for unstable coronary artery disease. N Engl J Med 1997;337:447–452.
23. Fitzgerald DJ, Roy L, Catella F, Fitzgerald GA. Platelet activation in unstable coronary disease. N Engl J Med 1986;315:983–989.
24. Chierchia S, Brunelli C, Simonetti I, Lazzari M, Maseri A. Sequence of events in angina at rest: primary reduction in coronary flow. Circulation 1980;61: 759–768.
25. Davies GJ, Bencivelli W, Fragasso G, Chierchia S, Crea F, Crow J, Crean PA, Pratt T, Morgan M, Maseri A. Sequence and magnitude of ventricular volume changes in painful and painless myocardial ischemia. Circulation 1988;78:310–319.
26. Gottlieb SO, Weisfeldt ML, Ouyang P, Mellits ED, Gerstenblith G. Silent ischemia as a marker for early unfavorable outcomes in patients with unstable angina. N Engl J Med 1986;314:1214–1219.
27. Willerson JT, Golino P, Eidt J, Campbell WB, Buja LM. Specific platelet mediators and unstable coronary artery lesions experimental evidence and potential clinical implications. Circulation 1989;80:198–205.
28. Théroux P, Liddon R-M. Unstable angina: pathogenesis, diagnosis and treatment. Curr Prob Cardiol 1993;18:157–231.
29. Global Use of Strategies to Open Occluded Coronary Arteries (GUSTO) IIb Investigators. A comparison of recombinant hirudin with heparin for the treatment of acute coronary syndromes. N Engl J Med 1996;335:775–782.
30. Hamm C, Ravkilde J, Gerhardt W, Jorgensen P, Peheim E, Ljungdahl L, Goldman B, Katus H. The prognostic value of serum troponin T in unstable angina. New Engl J Med 1992;327:146–150.
31. Katus HA, Diederich KW, Hoberg E, Kubler W. Circulating cardiac myosin light chains in patients with angina at rest: identification of a high risk subgroup. J Am Coll Cardiol 1988;11:487–493.
32. Luchi RJ, Scott SM, Deupree RH, and the Principal Investigators and Their Associates of Veterans Administration Cooperative Study No. 28. Comparison

of medical and surgical treatment for unstable angina pectoris. N Engl J Med 1987;316:977–984.
33. CASS Principal Investigators. Myocardial infarction and mortality in the Coronary Artery Surgery Study (CASS) randomized trial. N Engl J Med 1984; 310:750–758.
34. Alison HW, Russell ROJ, Mantle JA, Kouchoukos NT, Moraski RE, Rackley CE. Coronary anatomy and arteriography in patients with unstable angina pectoris. Am J Cardiol 1978;41:204–209.
35. Roberts W. Qualitative and quantitative comparison of amounts of narrowing by atherosclerotic plaques in the major epicardial coronary arteries at necropsy in sudden coronary death, transmural acute myocardial infarction, transmural healed myocardial infarction and unstable angina pectoris. Am J Cardiol 1989;64:324–328.
36. Saner GE, Gobel FL, Salomonowitz E, et al. The disease-free wall in coronary atherosclerosis: its relation to the degree of obstruction. J Am Coll Cardiol 1985;6:1096.
37. TIMI IIIA Investigators. Early effects of tissue-type plasminogen activator added to conventional therapy on the culprit coronary lesion in patients presenting with ischemic cardiac pain at rest: results of the Thrombolysis in Myocardial Ischemia (TIMI IIIA) Trial. Circulation 1993;87:38–52.
38. Vetrovec GW, Cowley MJ, Overton H, Richardson DW. Intracoronary thrombus in syndromes of unstable myocardial ischemia. Am Heart J 1981;102: 1202.
39. Freeman MR, Williams AE, Chisholm RJ, Armstrong PW. Intracoronary thrombus and complex morphology in unstable angina. Circulation 1989;80: 17–23.
40. Capone G, Wolf NM, Meyer B, Meister SG. Frequency of intracoronary filling defects by angiography in angina pectoris at rest. Am J Cardiol 1985;56: 403–406.
41. Gotoh K, Minamino T, Katoh O, Hamano Y, Fukui S, Hori M, Kusuoka H, Mishima M, Inoue M, Kamada T. The role of intracoronary thrombus in unstable angina: angiographic assessment and thrombolytic therapy during ongoing anginal attacks. Circulation 1988;77:526–534.
42. DeWood MA, Spores J, Notske R, Mouser LT, Burroughs R, Golden MS, Lang HT. Prevalence of total coronary occlusion during the early hours of transmural myocardial infarction. 1980;303:897–902.
43. DeWood MA, Stifter WF, Simpson CS, Spores J, Eugster GS, Judge TP, Hinnen ML. Coronary arteriographic findings soon after non-Q-wave myocardial infarction. N Engl J Med 1986;315:417–423.
44. Swahn E, Areskog M, Berglund U, et al. Predictive importance of clinical findings and a predischarge exercise test in patients with suspected unstable coronary artery disease. Am J Cardiol 1987;59:208.
45. Butman SM, Olson HG, Butman LK. Early exercise testing after stabilization of unstable angina: correlation with coronary angiographic findings and subsequent cardiac events. Am Heart J 1986;111:11–18.

46. Freeman MR, Chisholm RJ, Armstrong PW. Usefulness of exercise electrocardiography and thallium scintigraphy in unstable angina pectoris in predicting the extent and severity of coronary artery disease. Am J Cardiol 1988; 62:1164–1170.
47. Larson H, Areskog M, Areskog NH, Nylander E, Nyman I, Swahn E, Wallentin L. Should the exercise test (ET) be performed at discharge or one month later after an episode of unstable angina or non-Q-wave myocardial infarction? Int J Card Imaging 1991;7:7–14.
48. Wilcox I, Freedman B, Allman KC, Collins FL, Leitch JW, Kelly DT, Harris PJ. Prognostic significance of a predischarge exercise test in risk stratification after unstable angina pectoris. J Am Coll Cardiol 1991;18:677–683.
49. Pitt B. Evaluation of the postinfarct patient. Circulation 1995;91:1855–1860.
50. Wackers FJT, Lie KI, Liem KL, Sokole EB, Samson G, Van de Shoot JB, Durrer D. Thallium-201 scintigraphy in unstable angina pectoris. Circulation 1978;57:738–741.
51. Brown KA, Okada RD, Boucher CA, Phillips HR, Strauss HW, Pohost GM. Serial thallium-201 imaging at rest in patients with unstable and stable angina pectoris: relationship of myocardial perfusion at rest to presenting clinical syndrome. Am Heart J 1983;106:70–77.
52. Berger BC, Watson DD, Burwell LR, Crosby IK, Wellons HA, Teates CD, Beller GA. Redistribution of thallium at rest in patients with stable and unstable angina and the effects of coronary artery bypass surgery. Circulation 1979;60:1114–1125.
53. Gerwitz H, Beller GA, Strauss HW, Dinsmore RE, Zir LM, McKusick K, Pohost GM. Transient defects of resting thallium scans in patients with coronary artery disease. Circulation 1979;59:707–713.
54. Zhu YY, Chung WS, Botvinick EH, Dae MW, Lim AD, Ports TA, Danforth JW, Wolfe CL, Goldschlager N, Chatterjee K. Dipyridamole perfusion scintigraphy: the experience with its application in one hundred seventy patients with known or suspected unstable angina. Am Heart J 1991;121:33–43.
55. PURSUIT Trial Investigators. Inhibition of platelet glycoprotein IIb/IIIa with eptifibatide in patients with acute coronary syndromes. N Engl J Med 1998; 339:436–463.
56. Cairns JA, Gent M, Singer J, Finnie KJ, Frogatt GM, Holder DA, Jablonsky G, Kostuk WJ, Melendez LJ, Myers MG, Sackett DL, Sealey BJ, Tanser PH. Aspirin, sulfinpyrazone, or both in unstable angina. N Engl J Med 1985;313: 1369–1375.
57. Lewis HDJ, Davis JW, Archibald DG, Steinke WE, Smitherman TC, Doherty JE, Schnaper HW, LeWinter MW, Linares E, Pouget JM, Sabharwal SC, Chesler E, DeMots H. Protective effects of aspirin against acute myocardial infarction and death in men with unstable angina. N Engl J Med 1983;309: 396–403.
58. Théroux P, Ouimet H, McCans J, Latour J, Joly P, Levy G, Pelletier E, Juneau M, Stasiak J, de Guise P, Pelletier GB, Rinzler D, Waters DD. Aspirin, heparin, or both to treat acute unstable angina. N Engl J Med 1988;319:1105–1111.

59. Wallentin LC, and the Research Group on Instability in Coronary Artery Disease in Southeast Sweden. Aspirin (75 mg/day) after an episode of unstable coronary artery disease: long-term effects on the risk for myocardial infarction, occurrence of severe angina and the need for revascularization. J Am Coll Cardiol 1991;18:1587–1593.
60. ISIS-2 (Second International Study of Infarct Survival) Collaborative Group. Randomized trial of intravenous streptokinase, oral aspirin, both, or neither among 17,187 cases of suspected acute myocardial infarction; ISIS-2. Lancet 1988;II:349.
61. Freifeld A, Rabinowitz B, Kaplinsky E, Benderly M, Scheinowitz M, Agranat O, Freimark D, Hod H. Aspirin-induced reperfusion in acute myocardial infarction. J Am Coll Cardiol 1995;310A.
62. Antiplatelet Trialists' Collaboration. Collaborative overview of randomised trials of antiplatelet therapy. I. Prevention of death, myocardial infarction, and stroke by prolonged antiplatelet therapy in various categories of patients. Br Med J 1994;308:81–106.
63. Balsano F, Rizzon P, Violi F, Scrutinio D, Cimminiello C, Aguglia F, Pasotti C, Rudelli G, and the Studio della Ticlopidina nell'Angina Instabile Group. Antiplatelet treatment with ticlopidine in unstable angina. A controlled multicenter clinical trial. Circulation 1990;82:17–26.
64. CAPRIE Steering Commitee. A randomised, blinded, trial of clopidogrel versus aspirin in patients at risk of ischaemic events (CAPRIE). Lancet 1996;348: 1329–1339.
65. PARAGON Investigators. An international, randomized, controlled trial of lamifiban, a platelet glycoprotein IIb/IIIa inhibitor, heparin, or both in unstable angina. Circulation 1998;97:2386–2395.
66. Platelet Receptor Inhibition in Ischemic Syndrome Management (PRISM) Study Investigators. A comparison of aspirin plus tirofiban with aspirin plus heparin for unstable angina. N Engl J Med 1998;338:1498–1505.
67. Platelet Receptor Inhibition in Ischemic Syndrome Management in Patients Limited by Unstable Signs and Symptoms (PRISM-PLUS) Study Investigators. Inhibition of the platelet glycoprotein IIb/IIIa receptor with tirofiban in unstable angina and non-Q-wave myocardial infarction. N Engl J Med 1998; 338:1488–1497.
68. Heeschen C, Hamm CW, Goldmann B, Deu A, Langenbrink L, White HD, for the PRISM Study Investigators. Troponin concentrations for stratification of patients with acute coronary syndromes in relation to therapeutic efficacy of tirofiban. Lancet 1999;354:1757–1762.
69. Kleiman NS, Ohman EM, Califf RM, George BS, Kereiakes D, Aguirre FV, Weisman H, Schaible T, Topol EJ. Profound inhibition of platelet aggregation with monoclonal antibody 7E3 Fab after thrombolytic therapy: results of the Thrombolysis and Angioplasty in Myocardial Infarction (TAMI) 8 Pilot Study. J Am Coll Cardiol 1993;22:381–389.
70. Ohman EM, Kleinman NS, Gacioch G, Worley SJ, Navetta FI, Talley JD, Anderson HV, Ellis SG, Cohen MD, Spriggs D, Miller M, Kereiakes D, Yakubov S, Kitt MM, Sigmon KN, Califf RM, Krucoff MW, Topol EJ, for the

IMPACT-AMI Investigators. Combined accelerated tissue-plasminogen activator and glycoprotein IIb/IIIa integrin receptor blockade with Integrilin in acute myocardial infarction: results of a randomized, placebo-controlled, dose-ranging trial. IMPACT-AMI Investigators. Circulation 1997;95:846–854.

71. Strategies for Patency Enhancement in the Emergency Department (SPEED) Group. Randomized trial of abciximab with and without low-dose reteplase for acute myocardial infarction. Circulation 2000.
72. Antman EM, Giugliano RP, Gibson CM, McCabe CH, Coussement P, Kleiman NS, Vahanian A, Adgey AAJ, Menown I, Rupprecht HJ, Van der Wieken R, Ducas J, Scherer J, Anderson K, Van de Werf F, Braunwald E, for the TIMI 14 Investigators. Abciximab facilitates the rate and extent of thrombolysis: results of the thrombolysis in myocardial infarction (TIMI) 14 trial. Circulation 1999;99:2720–2732.
73. Brener S. The INTRO-AMI study preliminary results. Am Heart J 1999.
74. Oler A, Whooley MA, Oler J, Grady D. Adding heparin to aspirin reduces the incidence of myocardial infarction and death in patients with unstable angina: a meta-analysis. JAMA 1996;2276:811–815.
75. Lindahl B, Venge P, Wallentin L. Troponin T identifies patients with unstable coronary artery disease who benefit from long-term antithrombotic protection. Fragmin in Unstable Coronary Artery Disease (FRISC) Study Group. J Am Coll Cardiol 1997;29:43–48.
76. Ardissino D, Barberis P, De Servi S, Mussini A, Rolla A, Visani L, Specchia G. Recombinant tissue-type plasminogen activator followed by heparin compared with heparin alone for refractory unstable angina pectoris. Am J Cardiol 1990;66:910–914.
77. Bär F, Verheugt F, Materne P, Monassier J, Geslin P, Metzger J, Raynaud P, Foucault J, de Zwaan C, Vermeer F. Thrombolysis in patients with unstable angina improves the angiographic but not the clinical outcome: Results of UNASEM, a multicenter, randomized, placebo-controlled, clinical trial with anistreplase. Circulation 1992;86:131–137.
78. Charbonnier B, Bernadet P, Schiele F, Thery C, Bauters C. Intravenous thrombolysis by recombinant plasminogen activator (rt-PA) in unstable angina. A multicenter study versus placebo. Arch Mal Coeur Vaiss 1992;85:1471–1477.
79. Freeman MR, Langer A, Wilson RF, Morgan CD, Armstrong PW. Thrombolysis in unstable angina. Randomized double-blind trial of t-PA and placebo. Circulation 1992;85:150–157.
80. Gold HK, Coller BS, Yasuda T, Saito T, Fallon JT, Guerrero JL, Leinbach RC, Ziskind AA, Collen D. Rapid and sustained coronary artery recanalization with combined bolus injection of recombinant tissue-type plasminogen activator and monoclonal antiplatelet GP IIb/IIIa antibody in a canine preparation. Circulation 1988;77:670–677.
81. Karlsson J, Berglund U, Bjorkholm A, Ohlsson J, Swahn E, Wallentin L, for the TRIC Study Group. Thrombolysis with recombinant human tissue-type plasminogen activator during instability in coronary artery disease—effect on myocardial ischemia and need for coronary revascularization. Am Heart J 1992;124:1419–1426.

82. Neri Serneri G, Gensini GF, Poggesi L, Trotta F, Modesti PA, Boddi M, Ieri A, Margheri M, Casolo GC, Bini M, Rostagno C, Carnovali M, Abbate R. Effect of heparin, aspirin, or alteplase in reduction of myocardial ischaemia in refractory unstable angina. Lancet 1990;335:615–618.
83. Nicklas J, Topol E, Kander N, O'Neill W, Walton J, Ellis S, Gorman L, Pitt B. Randomized, double-blind, placebo-controlled trial of tissue plasminogen activator in unstable angina. J Am Coll Cardiol 1989;13:434–441.
84. Roberts MJ, McNeil AJ, Dalzell GW, Wilson CM, Webb SW, Khan MM, Patterson GC, Adgey AA. Double-blind randomized trial of alteplase versus placebo in patients with chest pain at rest. Eur Heart J 1993;14:1536–1542.
85. Saran RK, Bhandari K, Narain VS, Ahuja RC, Puri VK, Thakur R, Dwivedi S, Hasan M. Intravenous streptokinase in the management of a subset of patients with unstable angina: a randomized controlled trial. Int J Cardiol 1990;28:209–213.
86. Schreiber T, Rizik D, White C, Sharma G, Cowley M, Macina G, Reddy P, Kantounis L, Timmis G, Margulis A, Bunnell P, Barker W, Sasahara A. Randomized trial of thrombolysis versus heparin in unstable angina. Circulation 1992;86:1407–1414.
87. Scrutinio D, Biasco MG, Rizzon P. Thrombolysis in unstable angina: results of clinical studies. Am J Cardiol 1991;68:99B-104B.
88. TIMI IIIB Investigators. Effects of tissue-type plasminogen activator and a comparison of early invasive and conservative strategies in unstable angina and non-Q-wave myocardial infarction: results of the TIMI IIIB trial. Circulation 1994;89:1545–1556.
89. Williams DO, Topol EJ, Califf RM, Roberts R, Mancini GBJ, Joelson JM, Ellis SG, Kleiman NS. Intravenous recombinant tissue-type plasminogen activator in patients with unstable angina pectoris. Circulation 1990;82:376–383.
90. Moliterno D, Sapp S, Topol E. The paradoxical effect of thrombolytic therapy for unstable angina: meta-analysis. J Am Coll Cardiol 1994;23:288A.
91. Fibrinolytic Therapy Trialists' (FTT) Collaborative Group. Indications for fibrinolytic therapy in suspected acute myocardial infarction: collaborative overview of early mortality and major morbidity results from all randomised trials of more than 1000 patients. Lancet 1994;343:311–322.
92. Curfman GD, Heinsimer JA, Lozner EC, Fung H-L. Intravenous nitroglycerin in the treatment of spontaneous angina pectoris: a prospective, randomized trial. Circulation 1983;67:276–282.
93. Diodati J, Theroux P, Latour JG, Lacoste L, Lam JYT, Waters D. Effects of nitroglycerin at therapeutic doses on platelet aggregation in unstable angina pectoris and acute myocardial infarction. Am J Cardiol 1990;66:683–688.
94. Cohen MV, Downey JM, Sonnenblick EH, Kirk ES. The effects of nitroglycerin on coronary collaterals and myocardial contractility. J Clin Invest 1973; 52:2836–2847.
95. Bache RJ, Ball RM, Cobb FR, Rembert JC, Greenfield JC. Effects of nitroglycerin on transmural myocardial blood flow in the unanesthetized dog. J Clin Invest 1975;55:1219–1228.

96. Becker RC, Corrao JM, Bovill EG, Gore JM, Baker SP, Miller ML. Intravenous nitroglycerin-induced heparin resistance: a qualitative antithrombin III abnormality. Am Heart J 1990;119:1254–1261.
97. Habbab MA, Haft JI. Heparin resistance induced by intravenous nitroglycerin. Arch Intern Med 1987;147:857–860.
98. Lubsen J, Tijssen JGP, for the HINT Research Group. Efficacy of nifedipine and metoprolol in the treatment of unstable angina in the coronary care unit: findings from the Holland Interuniversity Nifedipine/Metoprolol Trial (HINT). Am J Cardiol 1987;60:18A–25A.
99. Gasser JA, Betterridge DJ. Comparison of the effects of carvedilol, propranolol, and verapamil on in vitro platelelt function in healthy volunteers. J Cardiovasc Pharm 1991;18(suppl 4):S29–S34.
100. Ondriasova E, Ondrias K, Stasko A, Nosal R, Csollei J. Comparison of the potency of five potential beta-adrenergic blocking drugs and eight calcium channel blockers to inhibit platelet aggregation and to perturb liposomal membranes prepared from platelet lipids. Physiol Res 1992;41:267–272.
101. Lange RA, Cigarroa RG, Flores ED, Hillis LD. Potentiation of cocaine-induced coronary vasoconstriction by beta-adrenergic blockade. Ann Intern Med 1990;112:897–903.
102. Robertson RM, Wood AJJ, Vaughn WK, et al. Exaccerbation of vasotonic angina pectoris by propranolol. Circulation 1982;65:281–285.
103. Théroux P, Taeymans Y, Morissette D, Bosch X, Pelletier GB, Waters DD. A randomized study comparing propranolol and diltiazem in the treatment of unstable angina. J Am Coll Cardiol 1985;5:717–722.
104. Packer M, O'Connor C, Ghali J, Pressler M, Carson P, Belkin R, Miller A, Neuberg G, Frid D, Wertheimer J, Cropp A, DeMets D. Effect of amlodipine on morbidity and mortality in severe chronic heart failure. N Engl J Med 1996;335:1107–1114.
105. Yusuf S, Wittes J, Friedman L. Overview of results of randomized trials in heart disease. II. Unstable angina, heart failure, primary prevention with aspirin, and risk factor modification. JAMA 1988;260:2259–2263.
106. Tijssen JG, Lubsen J. Early treatment of unstable angina with nifedipine and metoprolol—the HINT trial. J Cardiovasc Pharm 1988;12(suppl 71).
107. Lubsen J. Medical management of unstable angina. What have we learned from the randomized trials. Circulation 1990;82:82–87.
108. Anderson HV, Cannon CP, Stone PH, et al. One-year results of the Thrombolysis in Myocardial Infarction (TIMI) IIIB clinical trial. A randomized comparison of tissue-type plasminogen activator versus placebo and early invasive versus early conservative strategies in unstable angina and non-Q-wave myocardial infarction. J Am Coll Cardiol 1995;26:1643–1650.
109. Boden WE, O'Rourke RA, Crawford MH, Blaustein AS, Deedwania PC, Zoble RG, Wexler LF, Kleiger RE, Pepine CJ, Ferry DR, Chow BK, Lavori PW. Outcomes in patients with acute non-Q-wave myocardial infarction randomly assigned to an invasive as compared with a conservative management strategy. Veterans Affairs Non-Q-Wave Infarction Strategies in Hospital (VANQWISH) Trial Investigators. N Engl J Med 1998;338:1785–1792.

110. Fragmin and Fast Revascularization During Instability in Coronary Artery Disease (FRISC) II Investigators. Invasive compared with non-invasive treatment in unstable coronary-artery disease: FRISC II prosepective randomised multicentre study. Lancet 1999;354:708–715.
111. Fuchs S, Kornowski R, Mehran R, Satler LF, Pichard AD, Kent KM, Hong MK, Slack S, Stone GW, Leon MB. Cardiac troponin I levels and clinical outcome in patients with acute coronary syndromes. J Am Coll Cardiol 1999; 34:1704–1710.
112. Moliterno DJ, White HD. Unstable angina: PARAGON, PURSUIT, PRISM, and PRISM-PLUS. In: Lincoff AM, Topol EJ, eds. Contemporary Cardiology: Platelet Glycoprotein IIb/IIIa Inhibitors in Cardiovascular Disease. Totowa, NJ: Humana Press, 1999: 201–227.
113. Savonitto S, Ardissino D, Granger C, Morando G, Prando M, Mafrici A, Cavallini C, Melandri G, Thompson T, Vahanian A, Ohman E, Califf R, Van de Werf F, Topol E. Prognostic value of the admission electrocardiogram in acute coronary syndromes. JAMA 1999;281:707–713.
114. Lee KL, Woddlief LH, Topol EJ, Weaver WD, Betriu A, Col J, Simoons M, Aylward P, Van de Werf F, Califf RM. Predictors of 30-day mortality in the era of reperfusion for acute myocardial infarction. Results from an international trial of 41,021 patients. GUSTO-I Investigators. Circulation 1995;91: 1659–1668.
115. Moliterno D, Sgarbossa E, Armstrong P, Granger C, Van de Werf F, Califf R, Topol E, for the GUSTO IIa Investigators. A major dichotomy in unstable angina outcome: ST depression vs. T-wave inversion—GUSTO II results. J Am Coll Cardiol 1996;27:182A.

7

Acute ST-Segment Elevation Myocardial Infarction

The Open Artery and Tissue Reperfusion

Steven Vanderschueren and Frans Van de Werf

Gasthuisberg University Hospital
and University of Leuven
Leuven, Belgium

INTRODUCTION

Two considerations have had a tremendous impact on the modern management of ST-segment elevation acute myocardial infarction (AMI). First, occlusive thrombosis superimposed on a ruptured atheroma in an epicardial coronary artery was firmly established as the usual proximate cause of AMI (1,2). Coronary artery occlusion sets off a wave front of myocardial necrosis spreading from endocardium to epicardium, with an inverse relation between the time to reperfusion and the ultimate size and extent of transmurality of the infarct (3). Transmural AMI, as opposed to subendocardial AMI, is characterized pathologically by necrosis involving not only the inner half but also significant amounts of the outer half of the ventricular wall, and electrocardiographically by the ST-segment elevation/Q-wave pattern. However, it was shown recently that even in a so-called transmural AMI functional recovery of subepicardial fibers occurs after successful reperfusion, contributing to the late improvement in left ventricular function (4). Secondly, restoration of coronary artery patency was found to correlate with survival.

Recanalization can be achieved by pharmacological dissolution of the coronary clot (thrombolysis). Current thrombolytic therapy consists of intravenous infusion of plasminogen activators that dissolve the fibrin matrix of a thrombus. Alternatively, mechanical interventions within the occluded coronary artery, mainly involving percutaneous transluminal coronary angioplasty (PTCA), or "balloon angioplasty," supplemented or not by coronary stenting, may restore patency. Although the link between patency and survival is intuitively appealing and was firmly supported by laboratory animal experiments, only in the early 1990s did the GUSTO-I study convincingly establish the "open-artery hypothesis" (Fig. 1).

GUSTO-I AND THE OPEN ARTERY

The GUSTO-I trial enrolled 41,021 patients within 6 hours after the onset of ST-segment elevation AMI to one of four different thrombolytic regimens: streptokinase with either intravenous or subcutaneous heparin; front-loaded rt-PA with intravenous heparin; or a combination of streptokinase and rt-PA with intravenous heparin (5). Before GUSTO-I the open-artery hypothesis was challenged. Whereas earlier patency studies demonstrated that rt-PA recanalized vessels more efficiently than streptokinase (6,7), no significant survival difference emerged from large-scale mortality trials, such as the GISSI-2/International Study Group (8) and ISIS-3 (9) trials, that compared rt-PA with streptokinase in patients with suspected AMI.

Two alternative explanations for this apparent discrepancy were put forward: thrombolytic agents improve clinical outcome largely by mechanisms other than early coronary artery recanalization (implying that the open-artery hypothesis is not valid), or alternatively, the administration scheme of rt-PA in the GISSI-2/International Study Group and ISIS-3 trials was suboptimal, thereby masking the superiority of this agent (implying that the open-artery theory may still hold true). GUSTO-I was designed to clarify this controversy. To explore the relation between coronary artery patency status and clinical outcome, a subset of 2431 patients were evaluated angiographically (10). Moreover, to optimize the frequency, speed, and durability of rt-PA-induced reperfusion, the administration of rt-PA was accelerated or "front-loaded," implying infusion of two-thirds of the dose over the first 30 min and of the total dose (maximally 100 mg) over 90 min instead of 3 hours (11), and combined with immediate intravenous heparin (12).

As in most patency studies, angiographic characterization of coronary flow relied on the scoring system introduced by the Thrombolysis in Myocardial Infarction (TIMI) study group (Table 1) (13). The regimen inducing the greatest perfusion benefit at 90 min—i.e., accelerated or front-loaded rt-PA in conjunction with aspirin and immediate intravenous heparin—also

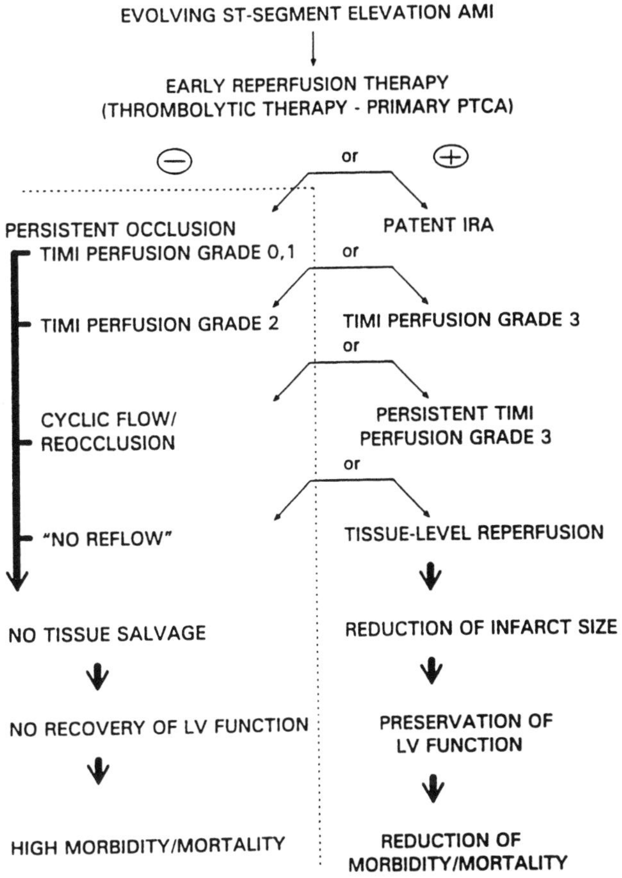

Figure 1 Time-dependent benefits of reperfusion for evolving ST-segment elevation myocardial infarction. The ideal chain of events is depicted on the right, the alternative scenario (left panel) is associated with a worse outcome. Besides this time-dependent effect ("early open artery"), less time-dependent effects account for the clinical benefit associated with reperfusion (see text). AMI; acute myocardial infarction; IRA; infarct-related artery; LV; left ventricular.

produced the greatest survival benefit: 30-day mortality rates were 6.3% after accelerated rt-PA versus 7.3% after streptokinase-only strategies ($P = .001$). The survival benefit with rt-PA was already apparent at 24 hours. TIMI flow grade 3 rates following accelerated rt-PA were significantly higher at 90 min than the streptokinase regimens (54% vs. 31%; $P < .001$), but not at 180 min (43% vs. 38%; P = NS) or later. The failure of this angiographic "catch-

Table 1 TIMI Flow Grades

0	No penetration of contrast beyond the point of obstruction.
1	Contrast penetrates the point of obstruction but does not completely opacify the entire distal vessel.
2	Complete contrast opacification of the infarct-related vessel but either contrast opacification or washout is delayed.
3	Brisk, "normal" flow.

up phenomenon" by streptokinase to equalize survival rates indirectly underscores the relative importance of early reperfusion over late patency.

Figure 2 relates TIMI flow grades at 90 min to 30-day mortality. Mortality in patients with TIMI flow grade 2 at 90 min was not significantly different from the mortality with TIMI flow grades 0 or 1 at 90 min and approximately twice the mortality with TIMI flow grade 3. A meta-analysis of the GUSTO-I and four other angiographic studies elaborated these findings: the odds ratio for early mortality following TIMI grade 3 perfusion at 90 min was 0.45 (95% confidence interval [CI], 0.34 to 0.61; $P < .0001$) versus

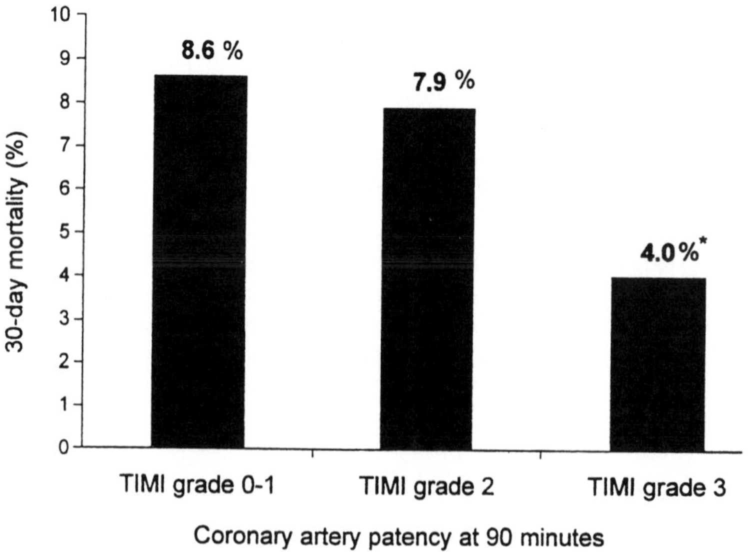

Figure 2 Coronary artery patency at 90 min and 30-day mortality in GUSTO-I (all thrombolytic regimens combined). $*P < .05$ relative to TIMI grades 0–1. (Modified from Ref. 15.)

TIMI grade <3, and 0.54 (95% Cl, 0.37 to 0.78; *P* = .001) versus TIMI grade 2 (14).

The 30-day mortality differences among the four thrombolytic strategies compared in the main GUSTO-I Trial (all 41,021 patients) could be predicted very accurately (R^2 = 0.92) from differences in 90-min TIMI 3 flow rates in the angiographic substudy (recorded in 1210 patients) (15). This close match between mortality differences predicted from early patency data and actual mortality supports the paradigm that early and complete coronary artery reperfusion is a critical mechanism underlying the life-saving potential of thrombolytic therapy.

Patency of the IRA was also associated with longer-term benefits. Among 12,864 patients enrolled in GUSTO-I who underwent coronary angiography and who had no previous mechanical or surgical intervention, 1-year mortality was significantly lower in patients with patent IRA than in patients with occluded IRA: 3.3% versus 8.5% in medically treated patients; 2.5% versus 8.5% in patients who underwent PTCA; and 4.2% versus 9.6% in patients who underwent coronary artery bypass surgery (16). The survival benefit of 1% of accelerated rt-PA over streptokinase observed after 30 days was unchanged at 1 year (17), and the survival benefit of early TIMI grade 3 flow, regardless of the lytic given, was amplified at 2 years (18) (Fig. 3).

Successful thrombolysis also resulted in improved left ventricular function. Irrespective of treatment assignment, left ventricular ejection fraction at 90 min was significantly better in patients with than without TIMI grade 3 flow (62% vs. 55%, respectively; *P* < .001). The aforementioned meta-analysis confirmed the relation between early IRA patency and cardiac morbidity: acute and convalescent ejection fraction, regional wall motion, and risk of heart failure were each significantly less in patients achieving TIMI grade 3 than TIMI grade 2 (or lower) perfusion (14). Although differences were small, patients treated with rt-PA in GUSTO-I had better left ventricular function than patients given streptokinase (10). Accordingly, cardiac complications associated with poor left ventricular function were less frequent in the rt-PA group, supporting previous observations in placebo-controlled trials of a lower cardiac morbidity in the thrombolysis arm. Indeed, the incidence of major cardiac in-hospital events including serious arrhythmias and congestive heart failure is consistently lower with thrombolytic regimens that establish higher rates of early and adequate reperfusion (Table 2). Thus, early reperfusion results not only in better survival but also in less morbidity among survivors.

Reocclusion eliminated the advantages of initially successful thrombolysis. The 30-day mortality for patients with documented reocclusion in the angiographic substudy of GUSTO-I was 12%, compared with 1.1% for

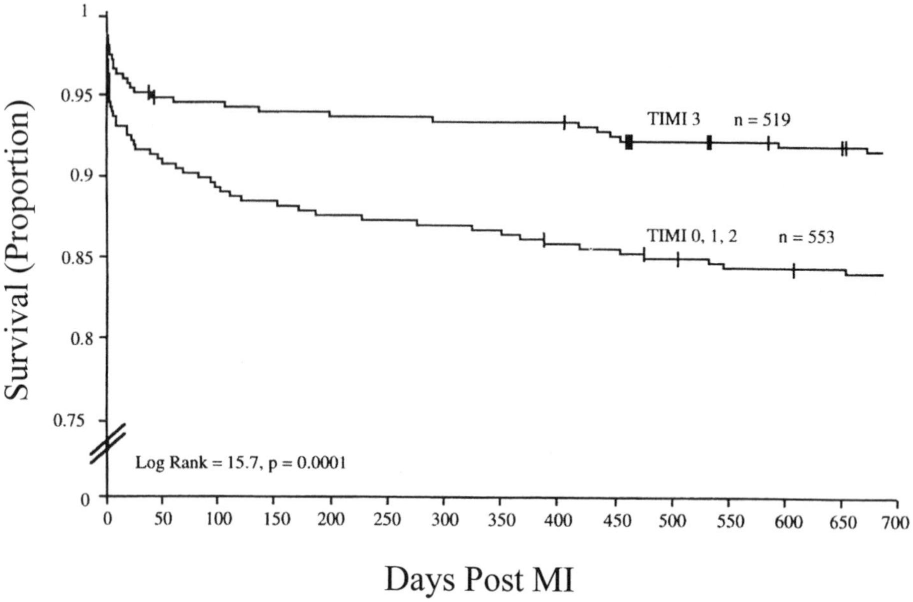

Figure 3 Two-year survival curves for patients with 90-min TIMI flow. (Modified from Ref. 18.)

patients with persistently patent coronary arteries ($P < .001$), and 8.9% for patients with initially closed IRAs (20).

PROMPT, COMPLETE, SUSTAINED CORONARY RECANALIZATION

GUSTO-I thus convincingly demonstrated that the potential of thrombolytic agents to save myocardium and lives, depends primarily on their ability to induce *prompt, complete*, and *sustained* coronary artery recanalization.

First, the benefits conferred by thrombolytic therapy are time dependent. Even without thrombolytic therapy, endogenous fibrinolysis assures high late coronary artery patency rates (>54% overall patency at 3 weeks) (21). The rate by which infused plasminogen activators speed up this natural process determines their impact on morbidity and mortality. Although administering thrombolytic agents up to 12 hours after the onset of symptoms may be beneficial (22), every minute that reperfusion is postponed will inevitably entail more extensive necrosis. Early in the course of AMI, the thrombus may be smaller and easier to lyse. In a meta-analysis, the proportional mortality reduction following thrombolytic therapy was calculated to

Table 2 Early Patency and Selected In-Hospital Cardiac Events after Thrombolysis with Agents that Establish Different Rates of Reperfusion

	GUSTO-I			INJECT		
	SK[a]	rt-PA[b]	*P*	SK	Reteplase	*P*
n	17,929	9,235		3,006	3,004	
Heart failure	17.2	15.2	<.001	26.3	23.6	<.05
Cardiac shock	6.6	5.1	<.001	6.0	4.7	<.05
Atrioventricular block[c]	9.1	7.3	<.001	4.2	3.8	NS
Ventricular tachycardia	6.7	5.6	.001	8.1	7.8	NS
Ventricular fibrillation	7.0	6.3	.02	5.5	4.8	NS
Asystole	6.2	5.3	.003	NR	NR	
Atrial fibrillation[d]	9.9	8.6	.001	8.8	7.2	<.05

Cardiac event rates (in %) are derived from GUSTO-I (4) and INJECT (International Joint Efficacy Comparison of Thrombolytics (19). Thrombolytic therapy was started within 6 h of symptom onset in GUSTO-I and within 12 h in INJECT.
[a] Both streptokinase arms (with intravenous and subcutaneous heparin) combined.
[b] Accelerated infusion of recombinant tissue-type plasminogen activator (rt-PA).
[c] Second- or third-degree block in GUSTO-I; third-degree block in INJECT.
[d] Includes atrial flutter in GUSTO-I.
Abbreviations: SK = streptokinase; NS = not significant; NR = not reported.

be 44% (95% CI, 32% to 53%) in patients treated within 2 hours versus 20% (95% CI, 15% to 25%) in those treated later ($P = .001$) (23).

Secondly, coronary reflow has to be brisk to substantially improve prognosis. Conventionally, persistently occluded IRAs (comprising TIMI flow grades 0 and 1) were regarded as thrombolytic failures, whereas patent IRAs (TIMI flow grade 2 or 3) denoted thrombolytic successes. GUSTO-I and other recent studies demonstrated that TIMI grade 2 flow is associated with a clearly worse clinical outcome than TIMI grade 3 flow (15,24–27). Irrespective of the question whether TIMI grade 2 flow is the cause or consequence of impaired tissue reperfusion, the immediate goal of coronary thrombolysis should be the rapid and persistent restoration of TIMI grade 3 flow. Interestingly, 67% of patients in GUSTO-I with TIMI grade 2 flow at 90 min had improved to TIMI grade 3 flow at day 5 to 7. These patients had significantly better left ventricular function than patients with persistent TIMI grade 0, 1, or 2 flow (28).

Thirdly, angiographically documented acute coronary reocclusion occurs in 5% to 10% of patients, resulting in a significant deterioration of left ventricular function and a steep increase in in-hospital mortality. Late reocclusions are also frequent, occurring in up to 20% to 30% of previously patent infarct-related vessels (29,30). Rethrombosis may be mediated by the interaction of vasospasm, aggregating platelets, clot-bound thrombin, the thrombogenicity of partially lysed clot and ruptured atheroma, the persistence of a flow-limiting stenosis and high shear stress, and paradoxical procoagulant and platelet-activating effects of thrombolytic agents.

CORONARY ARTERY PATENCY RATES AS A MARKER FOR SUCCESS

The direct correlation between coronary artery patency and survival, derived from the open-artery theory, validates patency trials for assessing the clinical value of reperfusion strategies. Traditionally, TIMI flow at 60 or 90 min has been the primary endpoint of these trials. Yet, this evaluation carries possible flaws and some caveats must be considered (31).

First, patency may have resulted from successful pharmacological dissolution of the occlusive thrombus by the thrombolytic drug, but may also have occurred spontaneously or may even have been present before drug infusion. Recanalization (as opposed to patency) studies include a pretreatment angiogram to confirm baseline occlusion of the IRA. Forceful injection of contrast dye directly into the occluded IRA may mechanically promote recanalization in the absence of any pharmacological dissolution of thrombus.

Secondly, patency of the large epicardial vessels does not equal reestablishment of tissue-level perfusion, the ultimate goal of thrombolysis. Recent studies on the coronary microcirculation with contrast echocardiography (32,33) positron emission tomography (PET) (34) suggest that impaired myocardial tissue perfusion persists in over one-third of patients despite restoration of TIMI grade 3 perfusion. This "low-reflow" or "no-reflow" phenomenon may be a consequence of extensive cellular necrosis and, most importantly, microcirculatory damage. Clot dislodgment with downstream migration of microemboli and "reperfusion injury" (see Chap. 23) may be implicated. On the basis of myocardial tissue flow measurements by PET within the first 24 hours of acute myocardial infarction, patients with TIMI flow grade 3 of the IRV at 90 min could be divided in three groups. Patients with severely impaired regional myocardial flow (<50% of normally perfused myocardium) despite successful thrombolysis had no recovery of left ventricular function at 3 months. Patients with high flow (>75% of normal) showed preserved regional contractile function at 3 months. Patients with intermediate flow (50% to 75% of normal) showed functional improvement only when a PET mismatch, indicative of viable but ischemically compromised myocardium, was present and an additional revascularization procedure was performed (34). PET may thus be helpful in selecting patients for additional revascularization. The new concepts of microcirculation damage and impaired tissue perfusion have introduced new important tools for evaluating the microcirculation and tissue perfusion such as resolution of ST-segment elevation (35), intracoronary Doppler wire measurements (36), magnetic resonance imaging (37), and TIMI myocardial perfusion grades (38) (Table 3).

Thirdly, as stated before, the angiographic definition of successful pharmacological reperfusion has recently been narrowed: not overall patency (TIMI perfusion grades 2 and 3) but rather complete patency (TIMI perfusion grade 3) predicts improved clinical outcome. Moreover, the conventional categorical TIMI flow classification is hampered by high interobserver variability. TIMI frame counting has been advocated as a continuous, more reproducible, objective, and quantitative index of coronary reperfusion than conventional TIMI flow grading (39). TIMI frame count represents the number of cineframes needed for contrast dye to reach standardized distal coronary landmarks. The longer left anterior descending coronary artery TIMI frame counts are divided by 1.7 to correct for the disparities in vessel length between the left anterior descending artery and the circumflex or right coronary artery (corrected TIMI frame count). Only a third of patients with an open IRV (TIMI 2 or 3) at 90 min after thrombolytic therapy were found to achieve flow truly within the normal range (corrected TIMI frame count <28). TIMI frame counting, has been validated and its relationship to major clinical endpoints after thrombolysis has been established (40).

Fourthly, 60 or 90 min is an arbitrary time point and may be too late to appreciate the true efficacy of a thrombolytic regimen in view of the time-dependent benefits of thrombolytic therapy. Conversely, reopening of the IRA beyond 60 or 90 min is more beneficial than a persistent occlusion (28,41). The finding that mortality benefits produced by thrombolytics frequently exceeded their impact on systolic left ventricular function has evoked the postulation that even late recanalization may improve outcome by other mechanisms than myocardial salvage and infarct size reduction

Table 3 Evaluation of Myocardial Tissue Reperfusion

Resolution of ST-segment elevation (35)
Contrast-echocardiography (32,33)
TIMI (angiographic) myocardial perfusion grades (38)
Intracoronary Doppler guidewire (36)
Magnetic resonance imaging (37)
Positron emission tomography (34)

(42–44). These mechanisms include enhanced provision of a conduit for augmentation of collateral flow (45,46), electrical stability (47,48), reduction of left ventricular wall stress and aneurysm formation, and attenuation of left ventricular remodeling and dilatation (49,50). Acute reperfusion therapy has been consistently shown to reduce ventricular volume, even beyond the time frame for myocardial salvage (51).

At least two studies have confirmed that IRA patency is a significant predictor of late survival independent of late ventricular function (52,53). The open-artery hypothesis has thus been expanded to include not only time-dependent but also less time-dependent effects of IRA recanalization. Furthermore, a single angiogram at 60 or 90 min only provides a snapshot, neglecting the dynamic processes involved in the formation and dissolution of a coronary thrombus. Cyclic flow and frank reocclusion often follow initially successful recanalization. Angiographic trials sometimes incorporate an angiogram at 24 hours to assess (early) reocclusion. As mentioned earlier, later reocclusions frequently occur.

A final limitation regards the invasive nature and the logistical challenge of the angiographic assessment of early coronary patency. Noninvasive and reliable reperfusion markers, readily available for routine use, are being validated. Despite these caveats, the frequency of inducing early and sustained coronary artery TIMI flow grade 3 remains a standard measure of reperfusion efficacy. It is, however, likely that in the future other measurements, more focusing on the microcirculation and on tissue perfusion (Table 3) will be increasingly used not only in trials but also in clinical practice.

PATENCY RECORD AND ASSOCIATED CLINICAL BENEFIT OF CURRENT THROMBOLYTIC STRATEGIES

How close do conventionally available thrombolytics come to this goal of rapid and stable normalization of epicardial coronary flow? The most effective thrombolytic regimen in GUSTO-I (i.e., accelerated rt-PA combined with aspirin and immediate intravenous heparin) achieved TIMI flow 3 in the IRV at 90 min in only just over half of patients, and streptokinase-based regimens in but one-third (10). Failure of thrombolysis may be related to clot composition: platelet-rich clots exhibit an intrinsic resistance to lysis with conventional agents. Hemorrhage within the plaque may mechanically prevent pharmacological coronary artery recanalization. Also, inhibitors may neutralize the action of exogenously administered plasminogen activators (e.g., preformed anti-SK antibodies for SK and APSAC, and plasminogen activator inhibitor-1 [PAI-1] for rt-PA and urokinase).

On average, the onset of restoration of antegrade coronary blood flow is delayed for 30 to 45 min with intravenous infusions of conventional thrombolytic agents. Frequent reocclusions undo the initial gain. This high incidence of primary and secondary treatment failures, together with the appreciation that even sustained TIMI 3 flow, does not equal restoration of tissue perfusion, as discussed before, may account for the modest mean salvage of left ventricular function following thrombolysis in placebo-controlled trials (21,42). The same mechanisms may explain why large patency differences do not consistently translate into equally large mortality and morbidity differences and why extra gain from thrombolytic therapy after hospital discharge is usually absent (54). Indeed, in GUSTO-I, a 65% increase in TIMI 3 patency with rt-PA relative to streptokinase accounted for only a 15% mortality reduction. In GUSTO-I, as in most other trials, survival curves after hospital discharge did not diverge further but ran parallel for 1 to 4 years. The presumption that thrombolytic therapy in patients with a very poor residual left ventricular function only postpones death by some weeks to months, may contribute to this phenomenon. Likewise, the (very) low ejection fractions of these early reperfused patients may mask the gain in ejection fraction obtained in other reperfused patients and therefore distort the comparison with surviving patients not treated with thrombolytic agents or treated with less potent agents.

In the aggregate, only a minority of patients with ST-segment elevation AMI eventually appear to achieve significant myocardial salvage and true sustained benefit from therapy with current thrombolytic strategies (30). Moreover, patients with non-Q-wave AMI or unstable angina do not appear to profit from standard thrombolytic therapy (55,56). A retrospective subgroup analysis of the LATE (Late Assessment of Thrombolytic Efficacy) trial, however, suggests that thrombolytic therapy may be beneficial in some patients with AMI and ST-segment depression, and calls for more prospective studies (57). Fibrinolytic agents when given in association with potent antiplatelet agents may have a role in some patients with unstable angina. This needs to be studied in new trials.

IMPROVING CORONARY ARTERY PATENCY AND MYOCARDIAL TISSUE PERFUSION

Various strategies have been developed to improve the efficacy and benefit-to-risk ratios of current thrombolytic agents (reviewed in 58–60). Infusion times, particularly of rt-PA, have been gradually shortened from 180 to 90 min, to accelerated and, finally to (double) bolus administration. A large comparative trial did not indicate that double-bolus administration will replace accelerated infusion as the standard administration scheme for rt-PA (61). Also, combinations of fibrinolytic agents have been investigated, without clear evidence that the benefit-to-risk ratio will outperform that of present standard regimens. Novel plasminogen activators have been designed or purified from natural sources (62). Much sought-after properties include long half-life (which allows bolus administration), enhanced fibrin specificity, and resistance to natural inhibitors (e.g., plasminogen-activator inhibitor-1). Plasminogen activators, which possess one or more of these properties and which have entered or completed clinical testing, include genetically engineered variants of rt-PA such as reteplase (r-PA), lanoteplase (n-PA) and tenecteplase (TNK-t-PA), *Desmodus* salivary plasminogen activator-a_1 (DSPAa1; derived from the saliva of the vampire bat *Desmodus rotundus*), and recombinant staphylokinase, produced by *Staphylococcus aureus*. Reteplase has already been marketed and the large Phase III trials with lanoteplase and tenecteplase have been recently completed. The results indicate that bolus fibrinolytics are not better than accelerated infusion of rt-PA in reducing 30-day mortality. In the total population studied in ASSENT-2, tenecteplase, however, was associated with a significant reduction in noncerebral bleeds and less need for blood transfusions (63). Moreover, in high-risk populations such as elderly, female, and low-weight patients tenecteplase induced fewer intracranial hemorrhages and other major bleeding complications. These advantages have been attributed to its higher fibrin selectivity.

To accelerate coronary thrombolysis, overcome resistance to lysis, and prevent reocclusion, various new antithrombotic agents such as direct antithrombins, low-molecular-weight heparins, and novel antiplatelet agents are undergoing preclinical or clinical evaluation (reviewed in 64,65). Present clinical evidence in particular favors the concomitant use of glycoprotein IIb/IIIa antagonists, such as abciximab, a humanized, monoclonal antibody that blocks the final pathway of platelet activation, as an important new approach (66).

The TIMI 14, SPEED, and INTRO-AMI, trials all indicate that abciximab with half a dose of a fibrinolytic (rt-PA or r-PA) not only enhances recanalization of the culprit epicardial vessel but also improves tissue reperfusion (as evaluated by the amount of ST-segment resolution) and facilitates coronary interventions if needed (67). The clinical benefit of this combination therapy will be tested in large Phase III trials (GUSTO-IV AMI and ASSENT-3). Similar benefits of concomitant abciximab have also been observed with primary PTCA/stenting trials (RAPPORT, ADMIRAL, CADILLAC) (68). Other GPIIb/IIIa inhibitors such as tirofiban and eptifibatide will also be studied in conjunction with a reduced dose of a fibrinolytic (tenecteplase). The search for newer and better tools for pharmacological and also mechanical reperfusion continues to be active and inspired and, in the near future, will inevitably lead to new standards of care and further improve the morbidity and mortality rates of patients with AMI.

SECONDARY ANGIOPLASTY

Thrombolytic therapy at best lyses the occlusive coronary thrombosis, but it does not treat the underlying stenosis. It thus seems a logical approach to supplement—even successful—thrombolytic therapy with elective angioplasty, in an attempt to improve further myocardial perfusion. Surprisingly, trials comparing routine immediate angioplasty following thrombolysis with more conservative treatment, in the absence of continued or recurrent ischemia, showed that the invasive approach was associated with a higher complication rate, including abrupt artery closure, reinfarction, and death (69–71). One explanation for this unexpected finding is that current fibrinolytic agents activate platelets and the coagulation system, promoting thrombotic complications in the setting of angioplasty. It is likely that the reduced dose of the fibrinolytic and the coadministration of more potent antiplatelet agents like the glycoprotein IIb/IIIa inhibitors may significantly reduce the risk of early interventions. The PACT trial has shown that, even in the absence of a GPIIb/IIIa antagonist, coronary interventions can be safely performed immediately following a single bolus of 50 mg rt-PA (72). Furthermore, this approach was associated with a better left ventricular function when compared with (primary) PTCA alone. A strategy of early pharmacological reperfusion followed by mechanical intervention will be intensively studied in the near future.

At present, patients with continuing chest pain or with severe left ventricular failure or signs of cardiogenic shock despite therapy are considered to be good candidates for rescue coronary interventions.

PRIMARY ANGIOPLASTY

Pooled analysis of data from all randomized controlled trials including a total of 2606 patients with ST-segment elevation AMI, indicates that 30-day mortality after primary angioplasty is significantly lower (4.4%) than after thrombolytic therapy (6.5%; OR 0.66; 95% CI, 0.46–0.94; $P = .02$) (73). On the other hand, most registry studies indicate that there is no striking (long-term) benefit of primary angioplasty, suggesting that in the randomized studies a selection bias in terms of patients and operators may have played a role. Anyhow, offering the opportunity of direct angioplasty represents a major logistical challenge and requires permanent availability of experienced interventional cardiologists, technical and paramedical support, and skilled surgical backup. In patients with a high risk for intracranial hemorrhage and in patients with cardiogenic shock, primary angioplasty is clearly the treatment of choice. A recent study indicates that with successful primary angioplasty a significant number of patients also did not show signs of adequate tissue perfusion (74). These data suggest that concomitant therapy to protect the microcirculation will also be beneficial with primary angioplasty and stenting. Primary angioplasty and stenting will be discussed in greater detail in Chapter 10.

CONCLUSION

Prompt, complete, and sustained recanalization of the IRA is a prerequisite for tissue reperfusion and is mandatory to reduce mortality and morbidity of patients with ST-segment elevation AMI. In recent years we have witnessed a vast expansion of the "coronary reperfusion arsenal." Different pharmacological and mechanical revascularization strategies have been compared with reference to efficacy, safety, and cost, frequently evoking vigorous debate. Taken together, newer, often more expensive approaches offer a small benefit over older strategies that is only marginal, compared with the benefit of any timely reperfusion therapy over placebo or merely supportive therapy. In other words, rapid treatment aimed at reperfusion is more important than the actual choice of a treatment modality. In practice, the best choice will depend on on-the-spot availability. If an important time delay before hospital arrival is anticipated (e.g., transport time >90 min), prehospital thrombolysis must be considered. The new (single) bolus fibrinolytics seem to be very appropriate in this regard. Patients with AMI and ST-segment elevation or (presumably new) left bundle branch block who present to centers with immediate access to angioplasty, are good candidates for primary angioplasty. The majority of these patients, however, are admitted to hospitals without facilities for emergency angioplasty. These patients, if eligible, should be offered pharmacological reperfusion as soon as possible. Present evidence does not support routine acute transfer to centers with angioplasty facilities. Adjunctive therapy, unless contraindicated, should include aspirin, heparin (when fibrin-selective thrombolytic agents such as rt-PA are given), beta-adrenergic antagonists, and oral angiotensin-converting enzyme inhibitors, as reviewed elsewhere (75). Very likely immediate IV administration of a GPIIb/IIIa antagonist will also become standard therapy in the near future. Whether LMW heparins or direct antithrombins will have a role will become more clear when the results of large trials like HERO-2 and ASSENT-3 will be presented.

Undoubtedly, research will continue to refine and optimize methods to detect and to achieve myocardial tissue reperfusion and to reset the standards of care for AMI. Also in the future, prompt diagnosis and restoration of tissue flow will remain the cornerstone of successful therapy for ST-segment elevation AMI.

REFERENCES

1. DeWood MA, Spores J, Notske R, et al. Prevalence of total coronary occlusion during the early hours of transmural myocardial infarction. N Engl J Med 1980; 303:897–902.
2. Davies MJ, Thomas AC. Plaque fissuring—the cause of acute myocardial infarction, sudden ischaemic death, and crescendo angina. Br Heart J 1985;53: 363–373.
3. Reimer KA, Lowe JE, Rasmussen MM, Jennings RB. The wavefront phenomenon of ischemic cell death. 1. Myocardial infarct size vs duration of coronary occlusion in dogs. Circulation 1977;56:786–794.
4. Bogaert J, Maes A, Van de Werf F, et al. Functional recovery of subepicardial myocardial tissue in transmural myocardial infarction after successful reperfusion. Circulation 1999;99:36–43.
5. GUSTO Investigators. An international randomized trial comparing four thrombolytic strategies for acute myocardial infarction. N Engl J Med 1993;329: 673–682.
6. TIMI Study Group. The Thrombolysis in Myocardial Infarction(TIMI) Trial: Phase I findings. N Engl J Med 1985;312:932–936.
7. Verstraete M, Bernard R, Bory M, et al. Randomised trial of intravenous recombinant tissue-type plasminogen activator versus intravenous streptokinase in acute myocardial infarction. Report from the European Cooperative Study Group for Recombinant Tissue-type Plasminogen Activator. Lancet 1985;1: 842–847.
8. International Study Group. In-hospital mortality and clinical course of 20,891 patients with suspected acute myocardial infarction randomised between alteplase and streptokinase with and without heparin. Lancet 1990;336:71–75.
9. ISIS-3 (Third International Study of Infarct Survival) Collaborative Group. ISIS-3: a randomised comparison of streptokinase vs tissue plasminogen activator vs anistreplase and of aspirin plus heparin vs aspirin alone among 41,299 cases of suspected acute myocardial infarction. Lancet 1992;339:753–770.
10. GUSTO Angiographic Investigators. The effects of tissue plasminogen activator, streptokinase, or both on coronary-artery patency, ventricular function, and survival after acute myocardial infarction. N Engl J Med 1993;329:1615–1622.
11. Neuhaus KL, Feuerer W, Jeep-Tebbe S, Niederer W, Vogt A, Tebbe U. Improved thrombolysis with a modified dose regimen of recombinant tissue-type plasminogen activator. J Am Coll Cardiol 1989;14:1566–1569.
12. Bleich SD, Nichols TC, Schumacher RR, Cooke DH, Tate DA, Teichman SL. Effect of heparin on coronary arterial patency after thrombolysis with tissue plasminogen activator in acute myocardial infarction. Am J Cardiol 1990;66: 1412–1417.
13. Chesebro JH, Knatterud G, Roberts R, et al. Thrombolysis in Myocardial Infarction (TIMI) Trial, Phase I: a comparison between intravenous tissue plasminogen activator and intravenous streptokinase. Clinical findings through hospital discharge. Circulation 1987;76:142–154.

14. Anderson JL, Karagounis LA, Califf RM. Meta-analysis of five reported studies on the relation of early coronary patency grades with mortality and outcomes after acute myocardial infarction. Am J Cardiol 1996;78:1–8.
15. Simes RJ, Topol EJ, Holmes DR Jr, et al. Link between the angiographic substudy and mortality outcomes in a large randomized trial of myocardial reperfusion. Importance of early and complete infarct artery reperfusion. Circulation 1995;91:1923–1928.
16. Puma JA, Sketch MH Jr, Simes RJ, Morris DC, Topol EJ, Califf RM. Long-term impact of a patent infarct-related artery: 1-year survival in the GUSTO trial. J Am Coll Cardiol 1995;Special Issue 130A.
17. Califf RM, White HD, Van de Werf F, et al. One year results from the Global Utilization of Streptokinase and TPA for Occluded Coronary Arteries (GUSTO-1) trial. Circulation 1996;94:1233–1238.
18. Ross AM, Coyne KS, Moireyra A, et al. Extended mortality benefit of early postinfarction reperfusion. Circulation 1998;97:1549–1556.
19. International Joint Efficacy Comparison of Thrombolytics. Randomized, double-blind comparison of reteplase double-bolus administration with streptokinase in acute myocardial infarction (INJECT): trial to investigate equivalence. Lancet 1995;346:329–336.
20. Reiner JS, Lundergan CF, Rohrbeck SC, et al. The impact on left ventricular function of coronary reocclusion after successful thrombolysis for acute myocardial infarction. J Am Coll Cardiol 1994;23:13A.
21. Granger CB, White HD, Bates ER, Ohman EM, Califf RM. A pooled analysis of coronary arterial patency and left ventricular function after intravenous thrombolysis for acute myocardial infarction. Am J Cardiol 1994;74:1220–1228.
22. Fibrinolytic Therapy Trialists' (FTT) Collaborative Group. Indications for fibrinolytic therapy in suspected acute myocardial infarction: collaborative overview of early mortality and major morbidity results from all randomised trials of more than 1000 patients. Lancet 1994;343:311–322.
23. Boersma E, Maas ACP, Deckers JW, Simoons ML. Early thrombolytic treatment in acute myocardial infarction: reappraisal of the golden hour. Lancet 1996;348:771–775.
24. Clemmensen P, Ohman EM, Sevilla DC, et al. Importance of early and complete reperfusion to achieve myocardial salvage after thrombolysis in acute myocardial infarction. Am J Cardiol 1992;70:1391–1396.
25. Vogt A, von Essen R, Tebbe U, Feuerer W, Appel KF, Neuhaus KL. Impact of early perfusion status of the infarct-related artery on short-term mortality after thrombolysis for acute myocardial infarction: retrospective analysis of four German multicenter studies. J Am Coll Cardiol 1993;21:1391–1395.
26. Kennedy JW. Optimal management of acute myocardial infarction requires early and complete reperfusion. Circulation 1995;91:1905–1907.
27. Lenderink T, Simoons ML, Van Es GA, et al. Benefit of thrombolytic therapy is sustained throughout five years and is related to TIMI perfusion grade 3 but not grade 2 flow at discharge. Circulation 1995;92:1110–1116.

28. Reiner JS, Lundergan CF, Fung A, et al. Evolution of early TIMI 2 flow after thrombolysis for acute myocardial infarction. Circulation 1996;94:2441–2446.
29. Brouwer MA, Böhncke JR, Veen G, Meijer A, Van Eenige MJ, Verheugt FWA. Adverse long-term effects of reocclusion after coronary thrombolysis. J Am Coll Cardiol 1995;26:1440–1444.
30. White HD, French JK, Hamer AW, et al. Frequent reocclusion of patent infarct-related arteries between 4 weeks and 1 year: effects of antiplatelet therapy. J Am Coll Cardiol 1995;25:218–223.
31. Lincoff AM, Topol EJ. Illusion of reperfusion. Does anyone achieve optimal reperfusion during acute myocardial infarction? Circulation 1993;88:1361–1374.
32. Ito H, Tomooka T, Sakai N, et al. Lack of myocardial perfusion immediately after successful thrombolysis. A predictor of poor recovery of left ventricular function in anterior myocardial infarction. Circulation 1992;85:1699–1705.
33. Ito H, Okamura A, Iwakura K, et al. Myocardial perfusion patterns related to thrombolysis in myocardial infarction perfusion grades after coronary angioplasty in patients with acute anterior wall myocardial infarction. Circulation 1996;93:1993–1999.
34. Maes A, Van de Werf F, Nuyts J, Bormans G, Desmet W, Mortelmans L. Impaired myocardial tissue perfusion early after successful thrombolysis. Impact on myocardial flow, metabolism, and function at late follow-up. Circulation 1995;92:2072–2078.
35. Schröder R, Wegscheider K, Schröder K, Dissmann R, Meyer-Sabellek W. Extent of early ST-segment elevation resolution: a strong prediction of outcome in patients with acute myocardial infarction and a sensitive measure to compare thrombolytic regimens. J Am Coll Cardiol 1995;26:1657–1664.
36. Kawamoto T, Yoshida K, Akasada T, et al. Can coronary blood flow velocity pattern after primary percutaneous transluminal coronary angiography predict recovery of regional left ventricular function in patients with acute myocardial infarction? Circulation 1999;100:339–345.
37. Wu KC, Zerhouni EA, Judd RM, et al. Prognostic significance of microvascular obstruction by magnetic resonance imaging in patients with acute myocardial infarction. Circulation 1998;97:765–772.
38. Gibson MC, Cannon CP, Murphy SA, et al. Relationship of TIMI myocardial perfusion grade to mortality after administration of thrombolytic drugs. Circulation 2000;101:125–130.
39. Gibson CM, Cannon CP, Daley WL, et al. TIMI frame count: a quantitative method of assessing coronary artery flow. Circulation 1996;93:879–888.
40. Gibson CM, Murphy SA, Rizzo MJ, et al. Relationship between TIMI frame count and clinical outcomes after thrombolytic administration. Circulation 1998;99:1945–1950.
41. Schröder R, Neuhaus K-L, Linderer T, Brüggeman T, Tebbe U, Wegscheider K. Impact of late coronary reperfusion on left ventricular function one month after acute myocardial infarction (results of the ISAM study). Am J Cardiol 1989;64:878–884.

42. Van de Werf F. Discrepancies between the effects of coronary reperfusion on survival and left ventricular function. Lancet 1989;1:1367–1369.
43. Kim CB, Braunwald E. Potential benefits of late reperfusion of infarcted myocardium. The open artery hypothesis. Circulation 1993;88:2426–2436.
44. Nash J. The open infarct-related artery: theoretical and practical considerations. Coron Artery Dis 1995;6:739–749.
45. Braunwald E. Myocardial reperfusion, limitation of infarct size, reduction of left ventricular dysfunction and improved survival. Should the paradigm be expanded? Circulation 1989;79:441–444.
46. Califf RM, Topol EJ, Gersh BJ. From myocardial salvage to patient salvage in acute myocardial infarction: the role of reperfusion therapy. J Am Coll Cardiol 1989;14:1382–1388.
47. Gang ES, Lew AS, Hong M, Wang FZ, Siebert CA, Peter T. Decreased incidence of ventricular late potentials after successful thrombolytic therapy for acute myocardial infarction. N Engl J Med 1989;321:712–716.
48. Sager PT, Perlmutter RA, Rosenfeld LE, McPherson CA, Wackers FJ, Batsford WP. Electrophysiologic effects of thrombolytic therapy in patients with a transmural anterior myocardial infarction complicated by left ventricular aneurysm formation. J Am Coll Cardiol 1988;12:19–24.
49. Hochman JS, Choo H. Limitation of myocardial infarct expansion by reperfusion independent of myocardial salvage. Circulation 1987;75:299–306.
50. Lavie CJ, O'Keefe JH Jr, Chesebro JH, Clements IP, Gibbons RJ. Prevention of late ventricular dilatation after acute myocardial infarction by successful thrombolytic reperfusion. Am J Cardiol 1990;66:31–36.
51. Pfeffer MA, Braunwald E. Ventricular remodeling after myocardial infarction. Experimental observations and clinical implications. Circulation 1990;81:1161–1172.
52. White HD, Cross DB, Elliot JM, Norris RM, Yee TW. Long term prognostic importance of patency of the infarct related coronary artery after thrombolytic therapy for acute myocardial infarction. Circulation 1994;89:61–67.
53. Lamas GA, Flaker GC, Mitchell G, et al. Effect of infarct artery patency on prognosis after acute myocardial infarction. The Survival and Ventricular Enlargement Investigators. Circulation 1995;92:1101–1109.
54. Van de Werf F. Thrombolysis for acute myocardial infarction. Why is there no extra benefit after hospital discharge? Circulation 1995;91:2862–2864.
55. TIMI IIIB Investigators. Effects of tissue plasminogen activator and a comparison of early invasive and conservative strategies in unstable angina and non-Q-wave myocardial infarction. Results of the TIMI IIIB trial. Thrombolysis in Myocardial Ischemia. Circulation 1994;89:1545–1556.
56. Waters D, Lam JY. Is thrombolytic therapy striking out in unstable angina? Circulation 1992;86:1642–1644.
57. Langer A, Goodman SG, Topol EJ, et al. Late assessment of the thrombolytic efficacy (LATE) study: prognosis in patients with non-Q wave myocardial infarction (LATE Study Investigators). J Am Coll Cardiol 1996;27:1327–1332.
58. Collen D, Lijnen HR. Basic and clinical aspects of fibrinolysis and thrombolysis. Blood 1991;78:3114–3124.
59. Verstraete M, Lijnen HR, Collen D. Thrombolytic agents in development. Drugs 1995;50:29–42.

60. White HD, Van de Werf F. Thrombolysis for acute myocardial infarction. Circulation 1998;97:1632–1646.
61. COBALT Investigators. A comparison of continuous infusion or alteplase with double bolus administration for acute myocardial infarction. N Engl J Med 1997;337:1124–1130.
62. Van de Werf F. New fibrinolytics. In: Topol EJ, ed. Textbook of Cardiovascular Medicine Updates. Vol. 2. New York: Lippincott Williams & Wilkins, 1999: 1–11.
63. ASSENT-2 Investigators. Single-bolus tenecteplase compared with frontloaded alteplase in acute myocardial infarction: the ASSENT-2 double-blind randomized trial. Lancet 1999;354:716–722.
64. Verstraete M, Zoldhelyi P. Novel antithrombotic drugs in development. Drugs 1995;49:856–884.
65. Weitz JI, Califf RM, Ginsberg JS, Hirsch J, Théroux P. New antithrombotics. Chest 1995;108:471S–485S.
66. Lefkovits J, Topol EJ. Platelet glycoprotein IIb/IIIa receptor antagonists in coronary artery disease. Eur Heart J 1996;17:9–18.
67. Antman EM, Giugliano RP, Gibson CM, et al. Abciximab facilitates the rate and extent of thrombolysis: results of the thrombolysis in myocardial infarction (TIMI) 14 trial. Circulation 1999;99:2720–2732.
68. Brener SJ, Barr LA, Burchenal JE, et al. Randomized, placebo-controlled trial of platelet glycoprotein IIb/IIIa blockade with primary angioplasty for acute myocardial infarction (RAPPORT). Circulation 1998;98:734–741.
69. TIMI Study Group. Comparison of invasive and conservative strategies after treatment with intravenous tissue plasminogen activator in acute myocardial infarction. Results of the Thrombolysis in Myocardial Infarction (TIMI) Phase II trial. N Engl J Med 1989;320:618–627.
70. Topol EJ, Califf RM, George BS, et al. A randomized trial of immediate versus delayed elective angioplasty after intravenous tissue plasminogen activator in acute myocardial infarction. N Engl J Med 1987;317:581–588.
71. Simoons ML, Arnold AE, Betriu A, et al. Thrombolysis with tissue plasminogen activator in acute myocardial infarction: no additional benefit from immediate percutaneous coronary angioplasty. Lancet 1988;1:197–203.
72. Ross AM, Coyne KS, Reiner JS, et al. A randomized trial comparing primary angioplasty with a strategy of short-acting thrombolysis and immediate planned rescue angioplasty in acute myocardial infarction: the PACT trial. J Am Coll Cardiol 1999;34:1954–1962.
73. Weaver WD, Simes RJ, Betriu A, et al. Comparison of primary coronary angioplasty and intravenous thrombolytic therapy for acute myocardial infarction: a quantitative review. JAMA 1997;278:2093–2098.
74. Claeys MJ, Bosmans J, Veenstra L, Jorens P, De Raedt H, Vrints CJ. Determinants and prognostic implications of persistent ST-segment elevation after primary angioplasty for acute myocardial infarction: importance of microvascular reperfusion injury on clinical outcome. Circulation 1999;99:1972–1977.
75. ACC/AHA Guidelines for the management of patients with acute myocardial infarction. Executive summary and recommendations. Circulation 1999;100: 1016–1030.

8

Prehospital Treatment of Acute Myocardial Infarction

Kevin J. Beatt
Imperial College Medical School
and Hammersmith Hospital
London, England

INTRODUCTION

The concept of prehospital management of myocardial infarction (MI) was introduced in the mid-1960s in recognition of the very substantial loss of life occurring before patients could be admitted to the hospital. At a time when there was no effective treatment for the majority of patients with this condition, 60% of patients died within the first hour and many failed to reach the hospital within the first 12 hours (1). Recent surveys suggest that up to 50% of the deaths from myocardial infarction (MI) are still within the first hour and perhaps as high as 80% within the first 24 hours (2). Forty percent of patients wait 4 hours or more before seeking help (3), and a significant number still fail to reach hospital within 12 hours. In the United States, an estimated 300,000 patients die each year prior to reaching the hospital. This suggests that despite the recognized improvement in mortality of those reaching the hospital there has been little or no change in the overall prehospital mortality.

The importance of ventricular fibrillation as an early cause of death and the ability of resuscitation and cardioversion to have an impact on mortality were the factors that initially drove the development of prehospital programs for treatment of acute MI. The logistic difficulties of providing the service were such that any benefits were confined to a relatively small proportion of the overall MI population, bringing into question the value of this type of care. However, the recent recognition of the value of thrombolysis and, in particular, the realization that the initiation of very early treatment before 90% of patients are seen in the hospital may be more beneficial than previously thought, have led to renewed interest in prehospital management of myocardial infarction. The cost-benefit arguments are now more compelling because of the larger number of patients who stand to benefit, although many of the logistic problems remain.

CARDIOPULMONARY RESUSCITATION

For almost 30 years, it has been recognized that prehospital resuscitation and prompt treatment of life-threatening arrhythmias can be effective at reducing mortality (4). Ventricular fibrillation is the only important cause of death in patients who die in the first hour following the onset of MI and may be 25 times more common in this early period than the in-hospital occurrence (2). In the majority of cases, provided that treatment is immediate, DC cardioversion will successfully terminate the arrhythmia. Many studies have shown that trained nonmedical personnel are able to deliver effective treatment (5). The principal limitation of prehospital resuscitation as a treatment strategy is the inability to provide trained personnel to cover every event, a situation made particularly difficult as patients may not seek medical help or consider asking for it until the moment of collapse, despite having the pain of an evolving myocardial infarction.

Targeting Levels of Expertise

Initial attempts to resuscitate patients in the community relied primarily on the expertise of trained ambulance staff. However, it soon became clear that even a prompt ambulance response was unable to arrive soon enough in many cases, and there was a need to have a larger, more responsive, body of personnel trained in cardiopulmonary resuscitation (CPR). Observations in Seattle prior to the introduction of thrombolytic therapy showed that 28% of those found in a state of cardiac arrest were eventually discharged from the hospital. If cardioversion was performed by the first responder to a call for help, the survival was 38%; if performed by someone witnessing the arrest, survival was 70%. The ability of a witness to perform resuscitation rather than having to wait the extra time for a paramedic team to arrive was estimated to result in an additional 100 lives saved per 1000 patients treated. These observations led to the concept and subsequently the development of a two-tier system, the first, early-response tier consisting of personnel more likely to be in the vicinity, trained in resuscitation, and, if possible, equipped with defibrillators. Groups targeted for training include firemen, police, railway personnel, selected individuals in large establishments, and relatives of patients who are at risk for MI. In Seattle this approach has achieved a response time of 3.1 min for the first tier (generally without defibrillators) and 6.2 min for the more experienced, highly trained second tier (6).

The impact of such services is difficult to evaluate. Randomized trials are clearly not possible within the same community, and sequential outcomes analyses are of limited value because of the changing rate of cardiac mortality in most communities. A 62% reduction in prehospital mortality in patients $\leq$70 years old was observed after the introduction of a prehospital CPR program (7). Just over a third of the patients with acute MI who were attended by the unit had experienced a cardiac arrest. One-third of these died despite resuscitative measures, 18% during ambulance transport. These observations, which are free from the influence of thrombolytic agents, were used to crudely estimate a benefit of 15 lives saved per 100,000 population each year. Data from Belfast, comparing two similar communities in the same city, one with a mobile coronary care unit and one without, supported these findings. Community mortality was 63% where there was no specific prehospital service and 50% where there was, the difference being most marked in younger patients (8). The median delay from onset of symptoms to hospital admission was 135 min with the prehospital service and 256 min without.

There is little doubt that with concerted efforts, resources, and dedication it is possible to develop services that provide an effective means of resuscitating a significant number of patients. A degree of benefit can be achieved by concentrating resources for training and the provision of equipment, particularly portable defibrillators, on paramedical staff. However, a far more substantial benefit can be achieved by having a more widespread body of expertise, people who are able to perform cardiopulmonary resuscitation and cardioversion. In contrast, the focusing of resources on individuals who will be called upon to resuscitate infrequently may be unrewarding. A survey among 200 primary care physicians who were supplied portable defibrillators as part of a British Heart Foundation initiative showed that over a 1-year period 53 attempts at resuscitation were made. However, only 19 arrests occurred in the near vicinity of a physician, with 13 patients being successfully cardioverted and nine surviving to hospital discharge. On average, a primary physician will use the defibrillator only once every 4 years in this setting.

Automated external defibrillators (AEDs) were developed through the 1980s. These devices have now become more portable and simpler to use. The latest device measures $6 \times 22 \times 20$ cm and weigh 2 kg. This device is designed to make possible the use of defibrillation by individuals other than paramedics and hospital staff. Recent trial demonstrated that during mock cardiac arrest, the speed of AED use by untrained children was only slightly slower than that of professionals (9). Ease of use and widespread availability will allow many more patients to be treated effectively by cardioversion.

PREHOSPITAL THROMBOLYSIS

Rationale for Prehospital Thrombolysis

The benefit of thrombolytic therapy is greatest when it is given early after the onset of symptoms. Early animal studies have demonstrated a temporal relationship between the extent of myocardial damage and duration of coronary artery occlusion (9). In the dog model, 64% of involved myocardium is salvageable after 40 min of coronary artery occlusion, whereas after 3 hours only 11% is salvageable (10). In determining the optimal use of thrombolysis, it is crucial to establish whether *substantial* additional benefit can be achieved by administering thrombolysis in the first 1 or 2 hours after the onset of pain. Mortality reduction in those treated within 1 hour of symptom onset in the International Study of Infarct Survivals (ISIS 2) (11) was 56% and in the Gruppo Italiano per lo Studio della Streptochinasi nell'Infarcto Miocardico (GISSI 1) (12) was 46%, whereas the mortality reduction in those treated between 3 and 6 hours was 17% in the latter study (Fig. 1). In the Global Utilization of Streptokinase and Tissue Plasminogen Activator for Occluded Coronary Arteries (GUSTO 1) study (13), 30-day mortality rate in patients treated within 2 hours of onset of symptoms was 5.5%, and 9.0% in those treated after 4 hours (Fig. 1). In the Myocardial Infarction Triage and Intervention (MITI) prehospital thrombolytic trial (14), the mortality rate in those treated within 70 min of symptom onset was as low as 1.2%, compared with 8.7% in those who were treated after that time. There was no detectable evidence of myocardial damage in 40% of cases who were treated early using quantitative thallium tomography. Close examination of the effect of time to thrombolysis on outcome following an acute MI has shown that in the first 1 to 2 hours after the onset of chest pain the relationship between time of treatment and survival is more exponential (15,16) (Fig. 2). However, the relationship becomes more linear after this period. This analysis suggests that the benefit of thrombolytic therapy was 65, 37, 26, and 29 lives saved per 1000 treated patients in the 0–1, 1–2, 2–3, and 3–6 hour interval, respectively (15). Proportional mortality reduction was significantly higher in patients treated within 2 hours than in those treated later (44% vs. 20%; $P = .001$) (Figs. 2, 3).

Although the importance of time to treatment may be influenced by factors such as the presence or absence of collaterals, myocardial workload,

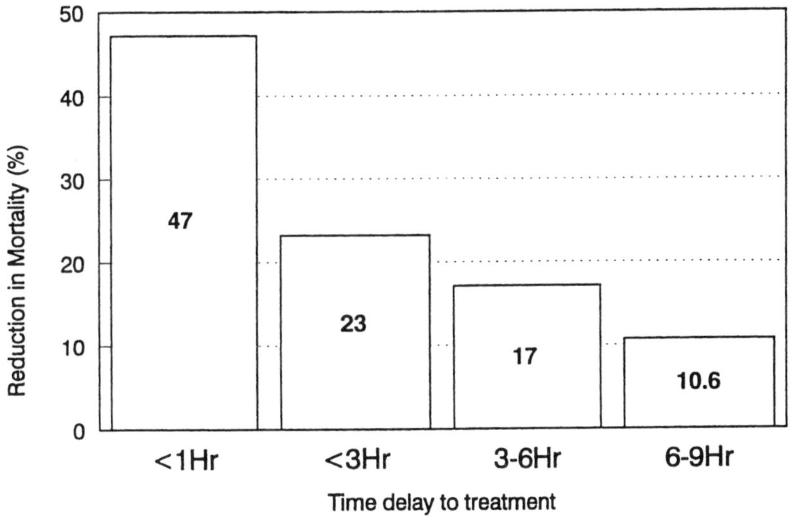

Figure 1 Percentage mortality reduction in thrombolysis versus placebo group according to treatment delay. (From Ref. 12.)

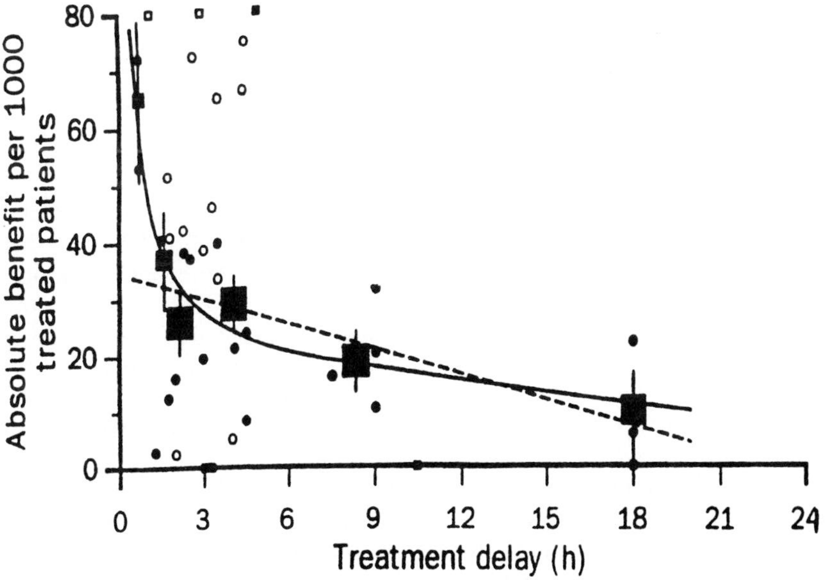

Figure 2 Absolute 35-day mortality reduction versus treatment. (From Ref. 15.)

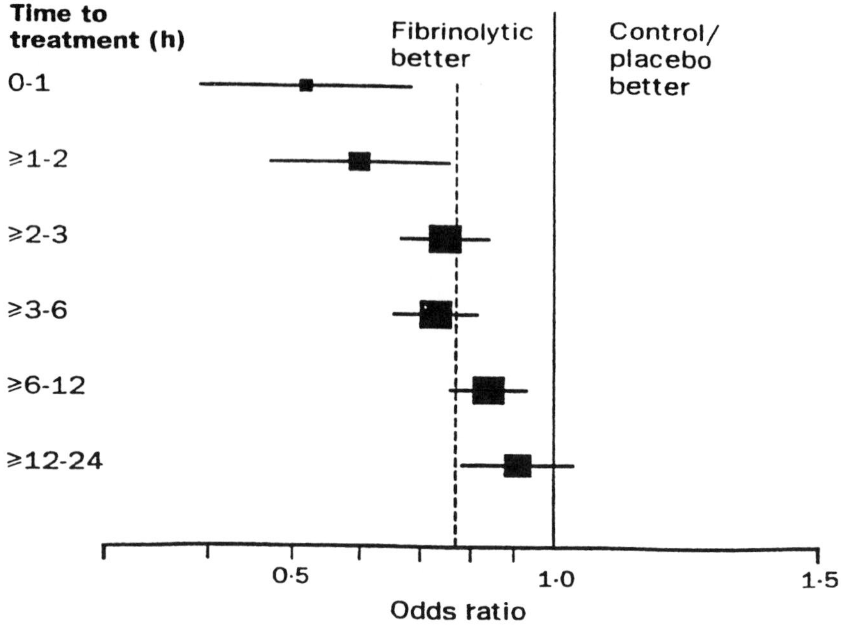

Figure 3 Proportional effect of fibrinolytic therapy on 35-day mortality according to treatment delay. (From Ref. 15.) Odds ratios, plotted with 95% Cl on a log scale, are significantly different over the six groups (P = .001).

preconditioning, and episodes of flow and no-flow which may occur during a stuttering infarct, studies have now confirmed that early, complete, and sustained reperfusion of the infarct-related artery remains the most crucial factor in preventing death and impairment of cardiac function following MI in most patients. A major confounding factor limiting the benefit of thrombolytic therapy is the failure to initiate treatment in the first 1 to 1.5 hours after symptom onset. The different components in the delay to administration of thrombolytic therapy have been documented (17). These include:

1. Failure of most patients to react rapidly and appropriately to symptoms.
2. Long time delays from summoning help to hospital arrival, the median time from onset of chest pain and hospital admission in most hospitals being from 81 to 160 min.
3. Delays from hospital arrival to treatment, with a median delay time of 31 to 80 min (18).

A logical step to reducing the prehospital delay is for thrombolytic therapy to be brought and administered to the patient whether in his or her home or out in the community.

Clinical Trials of Prehospital Thrombolysis

The first study of prehospital thrombolysis was published by Koren et al. in 1985 (19). In this study, nine patients received prehospital streptokinase at home given by a physician attached to a mobile coronary care unit (MCCU), and 44 received hospital treatment. Patients treated <1.5 hours after the onset of pain had a significantly higher global ejection fraction (56% ± 15 vs. 47% ± 14; $P < .05$) and a lower QRS score (5.6 ± 4.9 vs. 8.6 ± 5.5; $P < .01$) than patients receiving treatment between 1.5 and 4 hours after the onset of chest pain. Patients treated earlier by the MCCU also had better left ventricular function than patients treated in the hospital. There are now several trials confirming the feasibility and safety of prehospital thrombolysis in widely varying circumstances and settings (20–25).

Having established the feasibility and safety of prehospital thrombolysis, randomized studies comparing prehospital with hospital thrombolysis were required to determine if a reduction in mortality could be achieved. There are now eight such studies published (13,26–32). Design characteristics of these studies are shown in Table 1. The number of patients recruited ranged from 57 to 5469. Six studies (13,26–29,31) required presence of diagnostic ST-segment elevation whereas two studies (30,32) recruited all patients with a suspected infarct. The time saved by giving prehospital thrombolysis varied from 34 to 130 min, depending on the setting in which the trial was carried out, with the greatest saving achieved in patients living in rural areas (Table 2).

Table 1 Design Characteristics of Randomized Trials of Prehospital Thrombolysis

McNeil	DB	t-PA	Urban	Dr	<4	<75
Castaigne	Open	APSAC	Urban	Dr	<3	<75
Barbash	Open	t-PA	Urban	Dr	<4	<72
Schofer	DB	Urokinase	Urban	Dr	<4	<70
GREAT	DB	APSAC	Rural	GP	<4	No limit
McAleer	Open	SK	Rural	Dr	<6	No limit
EMIP	DB	APSAC	MC	Dr	<6	No limit
MITI	Open	t-PA	MC	Remote Dr	<6	<75

DB, double blind; MC, multicenter; GP, general practitioner.

Table 2 Time Saving on Prehospital Thrombolysis

Study	Median time to prehospital Rx (min)	Median time to hospital Rx (min)	Time saving (min)
McNeil	119	187	68
Castaigne	131	180	60
Barbash	96	132	40
Schofer	85	137	43
GREAT	101	240	130
McAleer	138	172	34
EMIP	130	190	55
MITI	77	110	33

The European Myocardial Infarction Project (EMIP) study (32) has been the largest of randomized studies (n = 5469). In this multicenter study, enrollment was carried out by MCCU staff from 163 centers in 15 European countries and Canada. There was a nonsignificant trend toward a lower mortality in the prehospital treated group (9.7% vs. 11.1%; $P = .08$).

Partly because of the small number of patients involved, these studies individually did not show a significant reduction in in-hospital or 30-day mortality in the prehospital-treated group (33,33a). However, analysis of pooled data from these studies shows a significantly lower mortality in favor of the prehospital-treated group (34). In this overview, the mortality was 9% in the prehospital- and 10.8% in hospital-treated group ($P = .01$). This represents a reduction in mortality of 16.7%, translating into 18 extra lives saved per 1000 patients treated in the community (Table 3; Fig. 4). In addition, it has been shown that early diagnosis of MI at home reduces the time to administration of thrombolytic therapy in the hospital by mobilization of the hospital team for immediate evaluation and treatment on the patient's arrival (13).

Which Patients Are Suitable for Prehospital Therapy?

As the feasibility and safety of prehospital thrombolysis have now been confirmed, the criteria for prehospital administration should be the same as for patients who are treated in the hospital. It is crucial to take a brief history and to perform an ECG to establish the diagnosis and suitability of patients to receive thrombolytic therapy. Several studies have now shown that only

Table 3 Overview of Mortality Data from Randomized Trials of Prehospital Thrombolysis

	No. of deaths/total no.		
Study	Prehosp	Hosp	*P* value
McNeil	2/27	3/30	.7
Castaigne	3/50	2/50	.6
Barbash	1/43	3/44	.35
Schofer	1/40	2/38	.5
GREAT	11/163	17/148	.14
McAleer	1/43	12/102	.07
EMIP	266/2750	303/2719	.08
MITI	10/175	15/185	.4
Pooled	295/3291	357/3316	.01

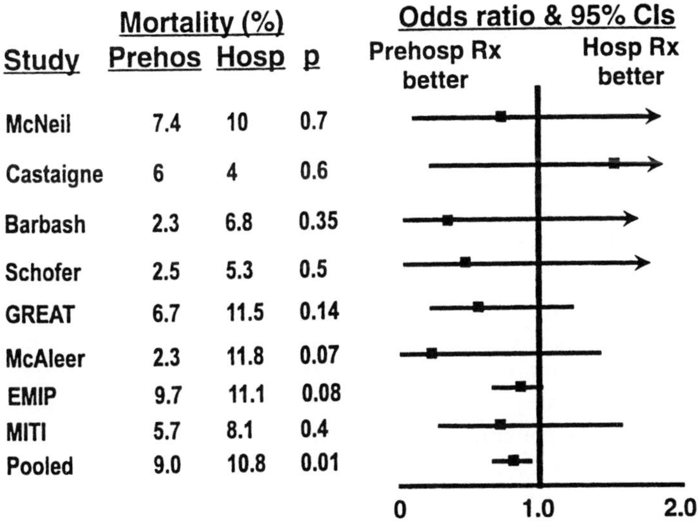

Figure 4 Overview of randomized trials prehospital versus hospital thrombolysis. Mortality rates, odds ratio, and 95% CI for the individual studies and the pooled data are shown.

patients with ST elevation or new bundle branch block benefit from thrombolytic therapy (14). Moreover, in the two prehospital thrombolysis studies where ST elevation was not a criterion for recruitment, diagnosis of MI was only correct in 78% or 88% of cases (30,32). This meant that up to 20% of patients in these two studies were inappropriately treated. In studies where ST elevation was required, the diagnosis was correct for 96% to 100% of the cases. There should be no age limit.

In What Setting Should Prehospital Thrombolysis Be Used?

As discussed above, the greatest benefit of thrombolytic therapy is achieved when it is given within 1 to 1.5 hours after onset of chest pain. Prehospital thrombolysis should therefore be considered in locations where achieving this goal would not otherwise be possible. In particular, it should be considered in places where the transfer time from home to hospital is >90 min. In the Grampian Region Early Anistreplase Trial (GREAT) study, there was a 42% reduction in 3 months mortality in the prehospital-treated group ($P = .04$) where the time saved by giving prehospital thrombolysis was >90 min (30). Similarly, in the EMIP study (32), there was a significant 42% ($P = .05$) reduction in mortality in the prehospital subgroup who received treatment >90 min sooner than the hospital group. Settings that would therefore be most suited for prehospital thrombolysis are those where the distance between home and hospital is >10 km, such as rural areas and regions where MCCUs with a fast response rate have already been established, in particular in cities where traffic jams may be a major problem.

Adverse Events

In the prehospital-treated group of the EMIP study (32) there was a small but significantly greater rate of ventricular fibrillation (2.5% vs. 1.6%; $P = .02$) and shock (including cardiogenic and allergic shock and those with symptomatic hypotension [6.3% vs. 3.9%; $P < .001$]) in the period between the arrival of the emergency medical team and hospital admission. However, a greater rate of ventricular fibrillation and shock following admission in the hospital-treated group meant that the overall rates of these two complications were similar in the two groups. There were no significant differences in the incidence of other major complications including cardiac arrest, acute pulmonary edema, and stroke up until the time of hospital discharge.

Which Thrombolytic Agent Should Be Used?

Several agents have been used in the prehospital trials. The ease of administration (bolus injection over 5 min) of anistreplase has meant that it is most commonly used in the community. However, it must be kept at 2 to 8°C and not frozen. It is rendered ineffective by exposure to normal temperature for more than 2 or 3 hours and it has a relatively short shelf life. In addition, the ultimate aim of early thrombolysis is to establish earlier and complete reperfusion of the infarct-related artery. In the GUSTO-1 study (12), irrespective of the thrombolytic therapy used, patients with a fully patent artery (referred to as TIMI grade 3) 90 min after commencement of treatment had the lowest mortality rate (4.4%), compared with 8.9% in those with an occluded artery at 90 min. In an overview of 4687 patients with MI who underwent coronary angiography 90 min following thrombolysis, the mortality rate was lowest in patients with TIMI grade 3 flow (3.7%) and significantly lower than in those with TIMI 2 (6.6%; $P = .0003$), or TIMI 0/1 (9.2%; $P < .0001$) flow (36). In view of the importance of very early reperfusion, it makes sense to optimize the benefit of prehospital treatment by giving an agent that achieves the highest early patency rate.

Accelerated t-PA has been shown to be associated with a >90-min TIMI 3 flow compared with both streptokinase (37) and APSAC (38). However, it has the disadvantage of requiring a more complicated infusion regimen. Although this agent could be given as bolus injections, this may be associated with an increased risk of hemorrhagic complications (39). Recently a recombinant form of t-PA called reteplase has been approved for use in MI. Results indicate that this agent is at least as effective as accelerated t-PA without compromising safety (40,41). In addition, this drug has the advantage of ease of administration. The usual regimen for this drug is two bolus injections of 10 units, given 30 min apart. This enables the first injection to be given in the community and the second in the hospital following reassessment of the patient. In this way, should the diagnosis be wrong or side effects develop, the second dose could be withheld.

Who Should Be Giving the Agent?

Studies detailed above have shown that thrombolytic therapy can be safely given in the community in different settings by primary care physicians, doctors on board an MCCU, and trained paramedics. The most effective staffing and structure of units will depend on preexisting services and the structure and finance of medical services. Trained paramedics are able to effectively screen patients and administer thrombolysis. In most countries, including the United States, this seems to be the most practical and cost-effective system. The ability to administer thrombolysis within the first 2 hours is crucial, and the overall service needs to incorporate a trained group of very early responders. In more isolated areas the primary care physician may provide the earliest response.

What Skills and Equipment Are Required?

Cardiac arrest and ventricular fibrillation are common during the first few hours after the onset of myocardial infarction. Whoever attends the patient at home should be properly trained and proficient in performing defibrillation and CPR. They should be able to manage the complications of MI and thrombolytic therapy such as shock, including cardiogenic and allergic shock, and symptomatic hypotension.

Since the diagnosis of MI and the decision to give thrombolysis depend on ECG findings, personnel should be able to perform and correctly interpret the ECG findings. In the study by Gemmill et al. (42), primary care physicians were equipped with an ECG machine and asked to undertake a home recording in 69 patients with suspected MI. Only 75% of ECGs were successfully completed; of these, the recording was satisfactory in only 60%. In McCrea and Saltissi's study (43) primary care physicians were asked to interpret a series of different ECGs. Although 82% of primary care physicians were able to recognize a normal ECG, recognition of an acute abnormality was less reliable. Between 33% and 66% correctly identified acute transmural ischemia or infarction depending on the specific trace presented. Accurate localization of the site of the infarct was achieved by 8% to 30% of participants, while only 22% to 25% correctly interpreted nonacute abnormalities. Clearly, if primary care physicians are going to be involved in any prehospital thrombolysis program, they need proper training in all aspects of managing an acute MI. Although there is no substitute for proper training, technology such as ECGs equipped with a computer algorithm may be particularly useful. Such programs have been shown to have high sensitivity (about 80%) and specificity (about 98%) for identifying patients with acute MI and ST-segment elevation (44). Another, potentially important technology, as used in the MITI trial (14), is the ability to transmit ECG information by cellular telephone.

ADJUVANT THERAPY

Aspirin

Aspirin has been shown to be beneficial in patients with unstable angina or acute MI (11,45). In ISIS-2 study, 5-week vascular mortality was reduced by 23% when aspirin was given alone and by 42% when it was given together with streptokinase within 24 hours of the onset of chest pain (11). There is no study that examines the role of early prehospital aspirin on mortality, but subgroup analysis from ISIS-2 study (11) showed that there was a nonsignificant trend of 16% reduction in mortality in patients who received aspirin within 2 hours of the onset of chest pain compared with patients who received treatment within 5 to 12 hours. Furthermore, experimental studies have shown that effective inhibition of platelet activity can be achieved within 1 hour of administration of aspirin (46). Aspirin is very cheap and is easily administered, with a very low adverse-effect profile, especially as a single dose. Patients with both unstable angina and acute MI benefit from aspirin. The risk of side effects in those with chest pain from noncardiac causes is very small. Aspirin is therefore an ideal agent for early prehospital use and should be given to any patient with chest pain suspected to be cardiac in origin without a need to perform an ECG, unless there is a major bleeding contraindication. Despite this favorable profile, there is evidence that many patients with acute MI or unstable angina do not receive this therapy even when they are seen at home by a physician (21,47). In the study by Round and Marshall (47), 89% of primary care physicians stated that they gave aspirin routinely to patients with acute MI. However, examination of the records of patients referred to the hospital by the same primary care physicians revealed that aspirin was given in only 29% of cases.

A >325-mg dose of aspirin does not substantially increase platelet inhibition, but it increases the risk of bleeding (48). Most experts therefore advocate an initial loading dose of 325 mg and a maintenance dose of between 75 and 325 mg.

β-Blockers

The only study that has examined the use of β-blockers in a prehospital setting is the Thrombolysis Early in Acute Heart Attack Trial (TEAHAT) (49). In this study, 352 patients with acute MI were randomized to receive placebo or t-PA. All patients with no contraindications also received intravenous metoprolol. In 29% of patients, intravenous metoprolol was started prior to hospital admission, and only patients with chest pain of <2 hours 45 min were recruited. Thirty-seven percent of patients had contraindications to β-blockers, the most frequent of which were a heart rate of <60 beats per minute or hypotension. No side effects of metoprolol either alone or in combination with t-PA was observed during the prehospital phase. Patients treated with metoprolol had lower incidence of Q-wave infarction, congestive cardiac failure, and ventricular fibrillation. There was also a reduction in infarct size, as assessed by cardiac enzymes, in patients who had a β-blocker in addition to t-PA. The Thrombolysis in Myocardial Infarction (TIMI) IIB trial (50) compared immediate intravenous metoprolol within 6 hours of onset of chest pain (a mean of 42 min after initiation of t-PA administration) to delayed oral metoprolol (on day 6). Subgroup analysis showed that very early treatment was associated with significant benefit compared with delayed treatment with a reduction in 6-week mortality or reinfarction of 61% ($P = .01$) when metoprolol was given within 2 hours of onset of symptom. A similar marked benefit was also observed in patients treated with intravenous β-blocker within the first 2 hours in the ISIS-1 study (51). Whenever possible, intravenous β-blockers should be given to patients with acute MI in the community—in particular, in those with high blood pressure and ongoing chest pain.

Analgesia

During acute myocardial infarction, severe pain and stress increase sympathetic nerve activity and catecholamine release. This leads to increased blood pressure and heart rate and therefore increased afterload, myocardial workload, myocardial wall stress, and oxygen consumption. Increased sympathetic activity also leads to reduced myocardial blood flow during diastole, and mobilization of free fatty acids which may have a direct toxic effect (52–55). These changes during myocardial ischemia may lead to infarct extension, cardiac arrhythmias, and death (54,55). In addition to their high efficacy in relieving pain and therefore blunting the heightened sympathetic activity, narcotic analgesic agents such as morphine and diamorphine have venodilatory properties and reduce cardiac preload. These agents are therefore an essential part of the prehospital management of the patients. Despite their beneficial effect, analgesics are generally underused in prehospital settings.

Antiarrhythmics

Patients with acute MI are at risk of ventricular fibrillation, cardiac arrest, and sudden death within the first hours after the onset of chest pain. These findings prompted several trials of prophylactic antiarrhythmic drug administration following acute myocardial infarction, with disappointing results. A meta-analysis of trials of prophylactic lidocaine has shown a significant (35%) reduction in ventricular fibrillation but a nonsignificant (38%) increase in mortality (56). The increased mortality could be a result of an increased risk of bradyarrhythmias, atrioventricular block, and asystole with the use of lidocaine. Similarly, class la and lc drugs may lead to increased mortality following acute MI (57,58). Trials with amiodarone, a class III agent, have been more promising. However, its effect very early after the onset of infarction has not been assessed. Recent trial suggest that amiodarone injection during cardiac arrest may increase the numbers of survivals to hospital admission (58). The routine use of antiarrhythmic drugs following acute MI is therefore not recommended, but in view of the increased incidence of arrhythmic events in the prehospital phase with the use of prehospital thrombolysis, the ability to administer antiarrhythmics appropriately and safely is desirable, particularly if the journey time to the hospital is prolonged.

LOGISTIC PROBLEMS

The principal arguments against the widespread use of prehospital thrombolysis concern the logistics of implementing this service in a comprehensive manner. Chest pain is common and whereas many patients may seek medical attention, the number with acute MI who are eligible for thrombolysis is relatively small. In any prehospital thrombolysis program, the service will be called upon to screen a large number of patients, where only a few will benefit. In the MITI study (14), during a 3-year period, 8863 patients with chest pain were examined by five paramedic units operating in Seattle. Of these, 1973 (22%) fulfilled the criteria for a history of acute MI, but only 483 had ST-segment elevation on ECG and only 360 (4%) were eligible for thrombolysis according to the trial's inclusion criteria.

On average, each paramedic unit administered prehospital thrombolytics only 24 times a year. The involvement of individual paramedics was even less, as each unit was manned by several paramedics covering a 24-hour rota. In a similar study combining the prehospital experience of units in Nashville and Cincinnati (59), only 27 (4.8%) of 562 screened for chest pain were candidates for thrombolytic therapy. In that study a decline in paramedic skills was noted because of lack of experience resulting from the infrequent administration of a thrombolytic agent. The majority of patients with MI who did not receive thrombolysis were >75 years old, which was considered an exclusion criterion. Eliminating the age limit may increase the proportion of patients receiving prehospital thrombolysis up to 32% (32), but the number of patients treated per individual paramedic per year will remain relatively small. The situation is worse when a primary care physician is involved in giving prehospital thrombolysis. In the United Kingdom, a primary care physician has on average about 1000 patients in his practice and, although many patients with chest pain will be seen each year, only 2 to 8 of them will have MIs (60). Similarly, only 5% of cardiac arrest events are witnessed by a primary care physician. This underlines a central problem in any thrombolysis or resuscitation program in the community, something that is not properly addressed in the randomized trials, as only the relatively few patients suitable for prehospital treatment are included in the analysis. Interpretation of the randomized trials should be performed with a full understanding of how limited and selected the sample populations are.

It is difficult to maintain a high level of training and skill in administering thrombolytic therapy and dealing with a life-threatening situation when the events occur so infrequently in any individual's experience. Is it appropriate to provide the very considerable resources necessary to screen so many patients in order to treat a few? The cost-benefit analysis of prehospital thrombolysis is difficult and controversial, as any individual assessment can only apply to the region surveyed and may vary dramatically with differing regions. For example, the benefit in regions where there is a longer time to transport to the hospital will be greater (31,32). Prehospital thrombolysis would be cheaper in settings where there is already an established paramedic system.

Clearly, there is a difference in cost depending on the level of staffing, whether the program is run by primary care physicians, or by a doctor or a paramedic manning an MCCU. Other issues that need to be considered in any such assessment are the cost of ECG communication, drug cost, and medicolegal risks for physicians and other prehospital providers. There are few studies examining this issue. In one setting, in a city in Virginia, it has been estimated that to equip all ambulances for the diagnosis of MI and administration of thrombolytic therapy would cost $70,000 to save a life (61). However, adding only a defibrillator to all ambulances would cost $3000 per life saved.

SUMMARY

There is now strong scientific support for the very early treatment of patients with acute myocardial infarction. In clinical studies, early resuscitation and the administration of prehospital thrombolysis have been shown to be safe and feasible in the community when administered by trained paramedics with ECG transmission facilities, physician-staffed MCCUs, or primary care physicians. An overview of randomized trials has shown that on average such a program may lead to saving of 18 extra lives per 1000 patients treated. However, introducing a prehospital thrombolysis program is logistically difficult, and presenting a favorable cost-benefit argument is a challenge, largely because of regional variations in geography, patient populations, and medical facilities, and the difficulty of acquiring pertinent data. A general national policy of prehospital thrombolysis therefore cannot be recommended (62).

A clear distinction must be made between early treatment, within the first few hours, and very early treatment, within the first hour. The greatest benefit of prehospital treatment is in settings where the transfer time to the hospital is >90 min. Attempts at establishing a prehospital thrombolysis service should therefore be considered if the predicted time to transfer to the hospital is likely to be greater than this, where the prehospital delay cannot be shortened, or where there is already an established infrastructure for providing such a service. Even in the absence of a prehospital thrombolysis service, it is important to reach every patient with suspected MI as early as possible. Early attendance in the community results in more successful resuscitation and a shorter time to thrombolysis administered in the hospital. It also allows prompt identification of potential complications and the administration of other beneficial drugs such as aspirin, analgesia, and nitrates.

REFERENCES

1. Bainton CR, Peterson DR. Deaths from coronary heart disease in persons fifty years of age and younger. A community-wide study. N Engl J Med 1963;268: 569–575.
2. Tunstall-Pedoe H, Kuulasmaa K, Amouyel P, Arveiler D, Rajakangas A-M, Pajak A. Myocardial infarction and coronary deaths in the World Health Organisation MONICA project. Registration procedures, event rates, and case-fatality rates in 38 populations from 21 countries in four continents. WHO MONICA project. Circulation 1994;90:583–612.
3. Weaver WD, for the National Registry of Myocardial Infarction Investigators (NRMI). Factors influencing the time to hospital administration of thrombolytic therapy: results from a large national registry. Circulation 1992; 86(suppl):11–16. Abstract.
4. Pantridge JF, Geddes JS. A mobile intensive-care unit in the management of myocardial infarction. Lancet 1967;ii:271–273.
5. National Heart, Lung and Blood Institute. Patient/Bystander Recognition and Action: Rapid Identification and Treatment of Acute Myocardial Infarction. National Heart Attack Alert Program (NHAAP). Bethesda, MD: National Institutes of Health, 1993. NIH Publication No. 93-3303.
6. Weaver WD, Cobb LA, Hallstrom AP, Fahrenbruch C, Copass MK, Ray R. Factors influencing survival after out-of-hospital cardiac arrest. J Am Coll Cardiol 1986;7:752–757.
7. Crampton RS, Aldrich RF, Gascho JA, Miles JR, Stillerman R. Reduction in prehospital, ambulance, and community coronary death rates by the community-wide emergency cardiac care system. Am J Med 1975;58:151–165.
8. Mathewson ZM, McCloskey BG, Evans AE, Russell CJ, Wilson C. Mobile coronary care and community mortality from myocardial infarction. Lancet 1985;I:441–444.
9. Gundry JW, Comess KA, DeRook FA, Jorgenson D, Bardy GH. Comparison of naïve sixth grade childern with trained professionals in the use of an automated external defibrillator. Circulation 1999;100:1703–1707.
10. Reimer KA, Lowe JE, Rasmussen MM, Jennings RB. The wavefront phenomenon of ischemic cell death: myocardial infarct size versus duration of coronary occlusion in dogs. Circulation 1977;56:786–794.
11. ISIS-2 (Second International Study of Infarct Survival) Collaboration Group. Randomised trial of intravenous streptokinase, oral aspirin, both, or neither among 17187 cases of acute myocardial infarction. Lancet 1988;ii:349–360.

12. Gissi (Gruppo Italiano per lo Studio della Streptochinasi nell'Infarto Miocardico). Effectiveness of intravenous thrombolytic treatment in acute myocardial infarction. Lancet 1986;i:397–401.
13. GUSTO Investigators. An international randomised trial comparing four thrombolytic strategies for acute myocardial infarction. N Engl J Med 1993;329: 673–682.
14. Cerqueira M, Hallstrom AP, Litwin PE, et al. Prehospital-initiated vs hospital-initiated thrombolytic therapy. JAMA 1993;270:1211–1216.
15. Boersma E, Mass ACP, Deckers JW, Simoons ML. Early thrombolytic therapy in acute myocardial infarction: reappraisal of the golden hour. Lancet 1996; 348:771–775.
16. Fath-Ordoubadi F, Beatt KJ. Fibrinolytic therapy in suspected acute myocardial infarction (letter). Lancet 1994;343:912.
17. Weaver WD. Time to thrombolytic treatment: factors affecting delay and their influence on outcome. J Am Coll Cardiol 1995;25:3S–9S.
18. Birkhead J, on behalf of the joint audit committee of the British Cardiac Society and a cardiology committee of Royal College of Physicians of London. Time delays in provision of thrombolytic treatment in six district hospitals. BMJ 1992;305:445–448.
19. Keron G, Weiss AT, Hasin Y, et al. Prevention of myocardial damage in acute myocardial ischemia by early treatment with intravenous streptokinase. N Engl J Med 1985;313:1384–1389.
20. Kereiakes DJ, Weaver D, Anderson JL, et al. Time delays in the diagnosis and treatment of acute myocardial infarction: a tale of eight cities. Report from the prehospital study group and the Cincinnati heart project. Am Heart J 1990;120:773–779.
21. Weaver WD, Eisenberg MS, Martin JS, et al. Myocardial Infarction Triage and Intervention project—phase I. Patient characteristics and feasibility of prehospital initiation of thrombolytic therapy. J Am Coll Cardiol 1990;15: 925–931.
22. Thrombolysis Early in Acute Heart Attack Trial Study Group. Very early thrombolysis therapy in suspected acute myocardial infarction. Am J Cardiol 1990;65:401–407.
23. Roth A, Barbash GI, Hod H, et al. Should thrombolytic therapy be administered in the mobile intensive care unit in patients with evolving myocardial infarction? A pilot study. J Am Coll Cardiol 1990;15:932–936.
24. BEPS Collaborative group. Prehospital thrombolysis in acute myocardial infarction: the Belgian Eminase Prehospital Study (BEPS). Eur Heart J 1991; 12:965–967.
25. Bouten MJM, Simoon ML, Hartman JAM, et al. Prehospital thrombolysis with alteplase (rt-PA) in acute myocardial infarction. Eur Heart J 1992;13: 925–931.
26. McNeill AJ, Cunningham SR, Flannery DJ, et al. A double blind placebo controlled study of early and late administration of recombinant tissue plasminogen activator in acute myocardial infarction. Br Heart J 1989;61:316–326.

27. Castaigne AD, Herve C, Duval-Moulin A, et al. Prehospital use of APSAC: results of a placebo-controlled study. Am J Cardiol 1989;64(suppl A):30–33.
28. Barbash Gl, Roth A, Hod H, et al. Improved survival but not left ventricular function with early and prehospital treatment with tissue plasminogen activator in acute myocardial infarction. Am J Cardiol 1990;66:261–266.
29. Schofer J, Buttner J, Geng G, et al. Prehospital thrombolysis in acute myocardial infarction. Am J Cardiol 1990;66:1429–1433.
30. GREAT Group. Feasibility, safety, and efficacy of domicilliary thrombolysis by general practitioners; Grampian region early anistreplase trial. Br Med J 1992;305:548–553.
31. McAleer B, Ruane B, Burke E, et al. Prehospital thrombolysis in a rural community: short and long-term survival. Cardiovasc Drugs Ther 1992;6: 369–372.
32. European Myocardial Infarction Project Group. Prehospital thrombolytic therapy in patients with suspected acute myocardial infarction. N Engl J Med 1993;329:383–389.
33. Fath-Ordoubadi F. Prehospital thrombolytic therapy for myocardial infarction. N Engl J Med 1994;330:290–291.
33a. Fath-Ordoubadi F, Al-Mohammad A, Huehns TY, Beatt KJ. Meta-analysis of randomised trials of prehospital versus hospital thrombolysis. Circulation 1994;90(4):I-325.
34. Fibrinolytic Therapy Trialists' (FTT) Collaborative Group. Indication for fibrinolytic therapy in suspected acute myocardial infarction: collaborative overview of early mortality and major morbidity results from all randomised trials of more than 1000 patients. Lancet 1994;343:311–322.
35. Fath-Ordoubadi F, Al-Mohammad A, Huehns TY, Beatt KJ. Significance of the Thrombolysis in myocardial infarction scoring system in assessing infarct-related artery reperfusion and mortality rates after acute myocardial infarction. Am Heart J 1997;134:62–68.
36. GUSTO Angiographic Investigators. The effects of tissue plasminogen activator, streptokinase, or both on coronary-artery patency, ventricular function, and survival after acute myocardial infarction. N Engl J Med 1993;329:673–682.
37. Neuhaus KL, Essen RV, Tebbe U, Vogt A, Roth M, Riess M. Improved thrombolysis in acute myocardial infarction with front-loaded administration of alteplase: results of the rt-PA-APSAC patency study (TAPS). J Am Coll Cardiol 1992;19:885–891.
38. Continuous Infusion versus Double-Bolus Administration of Alteplase (COBALT) Investigators. A comparison of continuous infusion of alteplase with double-bolus administration for acute myocardial infarction. N Engl J Med 1997;337(16):1124–1130.
39. Bode C, Smalling RW, Berg G, et al. Randomized comparison of coronary thrombolysis achieved with double bolus reteplase (r-PA) and front-loaded accelerated alteplase (rt-PA) in patients with acute myocardial infarction. Circulation 1996;94:891–898.

40. International Joint Efficacy Comparison of Thrombolytics. Randomised, double-blind comparison of reteplase double-bolus administration with streptokinase in acute myocardial infarction (INJECT): trial to investigate equivalence. Lancet 1995;346:329–336.
41. Gemmill JD, Lifson WK, Rae AP, Hillis SW, Dunn FG. Assessment by general practitioners of suitability of thrombolysis in patients with suspected acute myocardial infarction. Br Heart J 1993;70:503–506.
42. McCrea WA, Saltissi S. Electrocardiogram interpretation in general practice: relevance to prehospital thrombolysis. Br Heart J 1993;70:219–225.
43. Kudenchuk PJ, Ho MT, Weaver WD, et al. Accuracy of computer-interpreted electrocardiography in selecting patients for thrombolytic therapy. MITI Project Investigators. J Am Coll Cardiol 1991;17:1486–1491.
44. Lewis HD Jr, Davis JW, Archibald DG, et al. Protective effects of aspirin against acute myocardial infarction and death in men with unstable angina: results of a Veterans Administration co-operative study. N Engl J Med 1983; 309:396–403.
45. Hirsh J, Dalen JE, Fuster V, Harker LB, Salzman EW. Aspirin and other platelet-active drugs: the relationship between dose, effectiveness, and side effects. Chest 1992;102(suppl):327S–336S.
46. Round A, Marshall AJ. Survey of general practitioners' prehospital management of suspected acute myocardial infarction. BMJ 1994;309:375.
47. Willard JE, Lange RA, Hillis LD. The use of aspirin in ischemic heart disease. N Engl J Med 1992;327:175–181.
48. Risenfors M, Herlitz J, Berg CH, et al. Early treatment with thrombolysis and beta-blockade in suspected acute myocardial infarction: results from the TEAHAT study. J Intern Med 1991;229(suppl 1):35–42.
49. Roberts R, Rogers WJ, Mueller HS, et al. Immediate versus deferred b-blockade following thrombolytic therapy in patients with acute myocardial infarction: results of the thrombolysis in myocardial infarction (TIMI) II-B study. Circulation 1991;83:422–437.
50. ISIS-l Study Group. Randomised trial of intravenous atenolol among 16027 cases of suspected acute myocardial infarction: ISIS-I. Lancet 1986;ii:57–65.
51. Valori C, Thomas M, Shillingford J. Free noradrenaline and adrenaline excretion in relation to clinical syndromes following myocardial infarction. Am J Cardiol 1967;20:605.
52. Gupta DK, Jewitt DE, Young R. Increased plasma free fatty acid concentrations and their significance in patients with acute myocardial infarction Lancet 1969;2:1209.
53. Oliver MF, Opie LH. Effects of glucose and fatty acids on myocardial ischaemia and arrhythmias. Lancet 1994;343:155–158.
54. Oliver MF, Kurien VA, Greenwood TW. Relation between serum free fatty acids and arrhythmias and death after acute myocardial infarction. Lancet 1968;1:710–714.
55. MacMahon S, Collins R, Peto R, Koster RW, Yusuf S. Effects of prophylactic lidocaine in suspected acute myocardial infarction. An overview of results from the randomized, controlled trials. JAMA 1988;260:1910–1916.

56. Echt DS, Liebson PR, Mitchell LB, et al. Mortality and morbidity in patients receiving encainide, flecainide, or placebo. Cardiac Arrhythmia Suppression Trial. N Engl J Med 1991;324:781–788.
57. Cardiac Arrhythmia Suppression Trial II Investigators. Effect of the antiarrhythmic agentmoricizine on survival after myocardial infarction. N Engl J Med 1992;327:227–233.
58. Kudenchuk PJ, Cobb LA, Copass MK, Cummins RO, Doherty AM, Fahrenbruch CE, Hallstrom AP, Murray WA, Olsufka M, Walsh T. Amiodarone for resuscitation after out-of-hospital cardiac arrest due to ventricular fibrillation. N Engl J Med 1999;341(12):871–878.
59. Gibler WB, Kereiakes DJ, Dean EN, et al. Prehospital diagnosis and treatment of acute myocardial infarction: a north-south perspective. The Cincinnati Heart Project and the Nashville Prehospital TPA Trial. Am Heart J 1991;121: 1–10.
60. Fath-Ordoubadi F, Dana A, Tork A, Huehns TY, Beatt KJ. Prehospital thrombolysis: a survey of UK's general practitioners' views and skills in two different settings (urban vs rural). Eur Heart J 1996;17:569. Abstract.
61. Short R. Benefit and cost of prehospital thrombolysis. Br J Hosp Med 1990; 44(5):366.
62. Ryan TJ, Anderson JL, Antman EM, et al. ACC/AHH guidelines for the management of patients with acute myocardial infarction. A report of the American College of Cardiology/American Heart Association task force on practice guidelines (Committee on Management of Acute Myocardial Infarction). J Am Coll Cardiol 1996;28:1328–1428.

9

Thrombolysis for Acute Myocardial Infarction

First- and Second-Generation Agents

Eric R. Bates
University of Michigan
Ann Arbor, Michigan

INTRODUCTION

The development of thrombolytic therapy for acute myocardial infarction (MI) stands as a paradigm for cooperation among basic science, clinical research, and industry. The result has been the elucidation of the pathogenesis of acute MI, the development of an important new class of pharmacological agents, and the legitimization of multicenter randomized trials as the standard for proving clinical utility. Most importantly, thrombolytic therapy has been shown to restore infarct artery patency, reduce infarct size, preserve left ventricular function, and decrease mortality in patients with acute MI.

Three seminal events ushered in the "thrombolytic era." First, DeWood and colleagues (1) performed coronary angiography in patients with acute MI and showed that as many as 85% had thrombotic coronary artery occlusion in the early hours of transmural MI. Second, Rentrop and coworkers (2) demonstrated acute reperfusion of occluded infarct arteries with streptokinase. Third, Reimer et al. (3) demonstrated in a dog model that myocardial necrosis after coronary artery occlusion spread from the endocardial surface to the epicardial surface over a period of hours and that restoration of arterial patency before 3 hours preserved an epicardial rim of viable muscle.

The Western Washington randomized trial of intracoronary streptokinase (4) and the Netherlands Interuniversity Cardiology Institute trial (5) stimulated intense interest in the potential of thrombolytic therapy which resulted in an unprecedented explosion in clinical research activity. It is beyond the scope of this review to accurately document the many invaluable accomplishments and observations made by the efforts of so many talented investigators. Nevertheless, the cumulative contributions of the Thrombolysis and Angioplasty in Myocardial Infarction (TAMI) investigators (6–15) (Table 1), the Thrombolysis in Myocardial Infarction (TIMI) investigators (16–26) (Table 2), the European Cooperative Study Group (ECSG) investigators (27–32) (Table 3), the Gruppo Italiano per lo Studio Della Sopravvivenza nell'Infarto Miocardico (GISSI) investigators (33–35) (Table 4), the International Study of Infarct Survival (ISIS) investigators (36–39) (Table 5), and the Global Utilization of Strategies to Open Occluded Coronary Arteries (GUSTO) investigators (40–43) (Chap. 24) are noteworthy.

This review will summarize information on the first- and second-generation thrombolytic agents including streptokinase, alteplase, duteplase, anistreplase, urokinase, and saruplase. Characteristics of the three drugs available in the United States are shown in Table 6.

STREPTOKINASE

Tillet and Garner (44) discovered in 1933 that a filtrate of b-hemolytic strains of *Streptococcus* could dissolve human thrombus. Streptokinase is a single-chain nonenzyme protein which forms a 1:1 stoichiometric complex with plasminogen. The streptokinase-plasminogen activator complex then converts plasminogen to plasmin which initiates fibrinolysis. Intravenous streptokinase was initially used in the late 1950s for acute MI (45) and was tested in several multicenter trials in the 1960s and 1970s (46). Unfortunately, improvement in left ventricular function and mortality were inconsistently found because of inadequate doses and late implementation of therapy. Immediate arteriographic recanalization following intracoronary injection of streptokinase during acute MI was first reported by Chazov (47) and later in the English literature by Rentrop et al. (2). These observations legitimized thrombolytic therapy for acute MI and initiated the angiographic evaluation of mechanisms and clinical benefit.

Coronary Patency, Infarct Size, and Left Ventricular Function

The conventional dose of 1.5 million units over 60 min for intravenous streptokinase was derived empirically by Schroeder and colleagues (48). Sixty- and 90-min patency rates are approximately 50% and 2 to 3 hour patency rates are 70% (49) (Table 7).

Table 1 Thrombolysis and Angioplasty in Myocardial Infarction (TAMI) Trials

Trial	Syndrome	Comparison	No. of patients	Major findings
TAMI-1	Acute MI <4–6 h	t-PA plus immediate vs. delayed PTCA	386	No advantage for immediate PTCA
TAMI-2	Acute MI <4–6 h	Combination thrombolysis with t-PA and UK	146	Safe and may reduce reocclusion after rescue PTCA
TAMI-3	Acute MI <4–6 h	t-PA plus immediate vs. 90″ delayed IV heparin	134	No difference
TAMI-4	Acute MI <6 h	t-PA ± prostacyclin	50	Negative pharmacokinetic interaction
TAMI-UK	Acute MI <6 h	High-dose UK	102	Safe and effective monotherapy
TAMI-5	Acute MI <6 h	1. t-PA vs. UK vs. combination 2. Immediate vs. delayed cardiac catheterization	575	1. Combination reduced in-hospital events 2. Early catheterization may benefit
TAMI-6	Acute MI 6–24 h	Late t-PA vs. placebo	197	t-PA improves patency and prevents cavity dilation
TAMI-7	Acute MI <6 h	Accelerated t-PA regimes ± UK	232	No regimen better than Neuhaus front-loading
TAMI-8	Acute MI <6 h	t-PA plus platelet GP IIb/IIIa inhibition	70	↑ Patency with potent platelet inhibition
TAMI-9	Acute MI <6 h	t-PA plus fluosol vs. placebo	430	No difference

Table 2 Thrombolysis in Myocardial Infarction (TIMI) Trials

Trial	Syndrome	Comparison	No. of patients	Major findings
TIMI-I	Acute MI <7 h	t-PA vs. SK	290	↑ Reperfusion with t-PA
TIMI-IIA	Acute MI <4 h	t-PA plus immediate PTCA vs. delayed PTCA	586	No benefit from immediate PTCA
TIMI-IIB	Acute MI <4 h	1. t-PA plus routine PTCA vs. PTCA for recurrent ischemia	3262	1. No benefit from routine PTCA
		2. Intravenous vs. delayed beta blockade		2. ↓ Reinfarction, ischemia with early B-blocker
TIMI-IIIA	UA/non-Q MI	t-PA vs. placebo	306	Small benefit for t-PA in stenosis severity
TIMI-IIIB	UA/non-Q MI	1. t-PA vs. placebo 2. Early invasive vs. conservative strategy	1473	1. No benefit t-PA, possible harm 2. Minimal benefit early PTCA; no difference death or MI
TIMI-4	Acute MI <6 h	Accelerated t-PA vs. APSAC vs. combination	382	Better 60″ patency with t-PA, ↓ 6-week mortality
TIMI-5	Acute MI <6 h	Hirudin vs. heparin with t-PA	246	↑ Patency with hirudin 18–36 h, ↓ death and recurrent MI
TIMI-6	Acute MI <6 h	Hirudin vs. heparin with SK	193	Trend for ↓ recurrent MI, ↓ CHF, ↑ EF with hirudin
TIMI-7	UA	Dose finding for bivalirudin	410	Higher doses more effective
TIMI-8	UA/non-Q MI	Bivalirudin vs. heparin	132	Canceled by sponsor
TIMI-9A	Acute MI <12 h	Hirudin vs. heparin with thrombolytics	757	Excessive bleeding
TIMI-9B	Acute MI <12 h	Hirudin vs. heparin with thrombolytics	3002	No difference
TIMI-10A	Acute MI <12 h	Dose finding for TNK	113	Higher patency with 30–50 mg
TIMI-10B	Acute MI <12 h	Accel t-PA vs. TNK	886	Equivalent patency

TIMI-11A	UA/non-Q MI	Dose finding for Enoxaparin	629	Feasible and safe
TIMI-11B	UA/non-Q MI	Enoxaparin vs. heparin	3910	Enoxaparin superior
TIMI-12	Post ACS	Dose finding for oral sibrafiban	329	Safe, effective platelet inhibition
TIMI-14	Acute MI <12 h	Full-dose lytic vs. abciximab plus reduced dose SK, rt-PA, r-PA	888	Higher patency with abciximab plus reduced dose lytic
TIMI-15A	ACS	Dose finding for IV klerval	62	Higher doses more effective
TIMI-15B	ACS	IV/PO klerval vs. placebo	192	↑ Platelet inhibition, ↑ thrombocytopenia
TIMI-16 (OPUS)	ACS	Orbofiban vs. placebo	10,302	↑ Bleeding and mortality with orbofiban
TIMI-17 (INTIME-II)	Acute MI <6 h	Accel rt-PA vs. lanoteplase	15,078	No difference
TIMI-18 (TACTICS)	UA/non-Q MI	Tirobifan, early invasive vs. tirobifan, early conservative	2222	In progress
ER-TIMI-19	Acute MI	Feasibility of prehospital r-PA	—	In progress
TIMI-20 (INTEGRITI)	Acute MI <6 h	TNK vs. ↓ TNK/eptifibatide	—	In progress
TIMI-21 (A2Z)	ACS	1. Tirofiban/enoxaparin vs. tirofiban/heparin 2. Aggressive vs. standard simvistatin	—	In progress
TIMI-22 (PROVE-IT)	ACS	1. Pravastatin vs. atorvastatin 2. Antibiotic vs. placebo	—	In progress
TIMI-23 (ENTIRE)	Acute MI <6 h	1. TNK vs. ↓ TNK/abciximab 2. Enoxaparin vs. heparin	—	In progress
TIMI-24 (FASTER)	Acute MI <6 h	TNK vs. ↓ TNK/tirofiban	—	In progress

Table 3 European Cooperative Study Group (ECSG) Trials

Trial	Syndrome	Comparison	No. of patients	Major findings
ECSG-1	Acute MI <6 h	t-PA vs. SK	129	↑ Patency with t-PA
ECSG-2	Acute MI <6 h	t-PA vs. placebo	129	↑ Patency with t-PA
ECSG-3	Acute MI <4 h	6h t-PA infusion vs. placebo in patent infarct artery	123	No difference in late reocclusion
ECSG-4	Acute MI <5 h	t-PA ± PTCA at 2 h	367	PTCA detrimental
ECSG-5	Acute MI <5 h	t-PA vs. placebo	721	↓ Infarct size, trend ↓ mortality
ECSG-6	Acute MI <6 h	t-PA ± heparin	652	Better patency with heparin

Table 4 Gruppo Italiano per lo Studio della Sopravvivenza nell'Infarto Miocardico (GISSI) Trials

Trial	Syndrome	Comparison	No. of patients	Major findings
GISSI-1	Acute MI <12 h	SK vs. placebo	11,806	↓ Mortality with SK
GISSI-2	Acute MI <6 h	1. t-PA vs. SK 2. SQ heparin vs. placebo	12,490	1. No mortality difference 2. No mortality difference
GISSI-3	Acute MI <24 h	1. Nitrate vs. placebo 2. Lisinopril vs. placebo	19,394	1. No mortality difference 2. Mild mortality benefit

Table 5 International Study of Infarct Survival (ISIS) Trials

Trial	Syndrome	Comparison	No. of patients	Major findings
ISIS-1	Suspected MI <12 h	Atenolol vs. placebo	16,027	↓ Mortality with atenolol
ISIS-2	Suspected MI <24 h	SK vs. placebo ± ASA	17,187	↓ Mortality with SK, ASA; lowest with both
ISIS-3	Suspected MI <24 h	1. Duteplase vs. SK vs. APSAC 2. SQ heparin vs. placebo	39,713	1. No mortality difference 2. No mortality difference
ISIS-4	Suspected MI <24 h	1. Magnesium vs. placebo 2. Nitrate vs. placebo 3. Captopril vs. placebo	58,050	1. No mortality difference 2. No mortality difference 3. Mild mortality benefit

Table 6 Characteristics of Thrombolytic Drugs

	Streptokinase	Alteplase	Anistreplase
Plasma clearance time (min)	15–25	4–8	50–90
Fibrin specificity	Minimal	Moderate	Minimal
Plasminogen binding	Indirect	Direct	Indirect
Potential allergic reaction	Yes	No	Yes
Typical dose	1.5×10^6 units	100 mg	30 units
Administration (min)	60	90	5
Cost ($)	310	2200	1930

Enzymatic estimation of infarct size in the Netherlands Interuniversity Cardiology Institute study (50) of intracoronary streptokinase demonstrated a 51% decrease in infarct size in patients treated within 1 hour of onset of symptoms, of 31% of those treated between 1 and 2 hours, and of 13% treated between 2 and 4 hours. The Intravenous Streptokinase in Acute Myocardial infarction (ISAM) trial (51) measured a lower enzymatic infarct size in patients treated within 3 hours after onset of pain, but no difference in patients treated later.

Likewise, early treatment is associated with preservation of approximately six ejection fraction points (52,53). End-systolic volume measurements are smaller in treated patients (52,54).

Mortality Trials

The Western Washington intracoronary streptokinase trial (4) randomized 134 patients to streptokinase and 116 patients to control. Recanalization was achieved in 68% of the streptokinase-treated group and 30 day mortality was significantly reduced (3.7% vs. 11.2%).

The Netherlands Intrauniversity Cardiology Institute trial (5) allocated 264 patients to conventional treatment and 269 to intracoronary streptokinase, the last 117 of which were first treated with 500,000 units of intravenous streptokinase. Time to treatment was 80 min faster than in the Western Washington trial and the recanalization rate was higher (79%). Mortality rates at 28 days were significantly reduced with streptokinase (5.9% vs. 11.7%).

The ISAM trial (51) randomized 1741 patients to intravenous streptokinase or control within 6 hours of symptom onset. Mortality at 21 days was lower than expected in the control group, rendering the trial underpowered to detect a treatment difference. However, the insignificant relative re-

Table 7 Infarct Artery Patency Results[a]

Time	Control	Streptokinase	Alteplase (3h)	Alteplase (90 min)	Anistreplase	Urokinase
60 min	15 (6–24)	48 (41–56)	57 (52–61)	74 (70–77)	61 (55–67)	—
90 min	21 (11–31)	51 (48–55)	70 (68–72)	84 (82–87)	70 (66–74)	60 (55–64)
2–3 h	24 (14–35)	70 (65–75)	73 (65–80)	—	74 (68–80)	58 (48–68)
1 day	21 (9–32)	86 (82–89)	84 (82–86)	86 (82–90)	80 (77–83)	—
3–21 days	61 (57–64)	73 (70–78)	80 (78–81)	89 (85–94)	85 (81–89)	72 (63–81)

[a]Percent (95% confidence interval).
Source: Ref. 52.

duction in mortality associated with streptokinase therapy (6.3% vs. 7.1%) was similar to that seen in the GISSI-1 trial.

The GISSI-1 trial (33) randomized 11,806 patients to either intravenous streptokinase or control within 12 hours of symptom onset. Mortality at 21 days was 10.7% in the streptokinase group versus 13% in the control group, an 18% reduction. The largest reduction (47%) was seen when treatment was initiated within 1 hour of symptom onset.

The ISIS-2 trial (37) randomized 17,187 patients within 24 hours of the onset of symptoms of suspected MI to either streptokinase, aspirin, both, or neither. Streptokinase alone reduced 5-week vascular mortality (9.2% vs. 12%) and the combination of aspirin plus streptokinase additionally reduced mortality (8% vs. 13.2%).

The Estudio Multicentrico Estreptoquinasa Republicas de America del Sur (EMERAS) trial (55) found an insignificant 14% reduction (11.7% vs. 13.2%) in hospital mortality in 2080 patients randomized to streptokinase or placebo 6 to 12 hours after symptom onset, but no benefit in patients presenting after 13 to 24 hours.

ALTEPLASE

Tissue plasminogen activator is a naturally occurring single-chain serine protease normally secreted by vascular endothelium. It was first obtained from the Bowes melanoma cell line and is now produced by recombinant DNA techniques. Native t-PA and alteplase (rt-PA) have a binding site for fibrin which causes a great affinity for attaching to thrombus and preferentially lysing it, although systemic plasminogen activation occurs at clinical doses.

Coronary Patency, Infarct Size, and Left Ventricular Function

The TIMI-I (16) and ECSG-1 (27) studies established higher 90-min patency rates for rt-PA than streptokinase. The TIMI-II trial (18) began with a dose of 150 mg over 6 hours, but this was reduced to 100 mg over 3 hours because of an unacceptable rate of intracerebral hemorrhage. Numerous studies established a 90-min patency rate of 70% with this dose (49), a success rate equal to that achieved with streptokinase 2 to 3 hours after initiation of therapy (Table 7).

Neuhaus and colleagues (56) accelerated the dosing, infusing the total dose of 100 mg before the 90-min angiogram and achieved a 90-min patency rate of 91%. Purvis and coworkers (57) tested double-bolus (two 50-mg injections 30 min apart) alteplase and demonstrated 93% patency rates at 90 min. Subsequent testing has established that a weight-adjusted accelerated or front-loaded dose (15-mg bolus, 0.75 mg/kg over 30 min, 0.5 mg/kg over 60 min) is superior to double-bolus dosing and achieves 90-min patency rates of approximately 82% (41,49).

The ECSG-5 trial (31) was a double-blind placebo-controlled trial in 721 patients treated within 5 hours of symptom onset. The cumulative myocardial enzyme release over 72 hours was 20% lower in patients treated with alteplase. Three small trials (58–60) had previously revealed a 6% to 7% higher ejection fraction in patients treated with alteplase. The ECSG-5 (31) trial measured a 2.2% higher ejection fraction and lower end-diastolic and end-systolic volumes in patients randomized to alteplase.

Mortality Trials

The Anglo-Scandinavian Study of Early Thrombolysis (ASSET) (61) randomized 5011 patients with <5 hours of symptoms to alteplase or placebo. Although patients received intravenous heparin, aspirin was not given. At 1 month, mortality was reduced by 26% with alteplase (7.2% vs. 9.8%).

The Late Assessment of Thrombolytic Efficacy (LATE) study (62) randomized 5711 patients with symptoms between 6 and 24 hours from onset to alteplase or placebo. A significant 26% reduction in 35-day mortality (8.9% vs. 12%) was found in the 6- to 12-hour group, but no difference was seen between 12 and 24 hours.

The ECSG-5 trial (31) randomized 721 patients with <5 hours of symptoms to alteplase or placebo. Despite only small differences in ejection fraction, the 14-day mortality was reduced with alteplase (2.8% vs. 5.7%).

There have been two comparative trials of alteplase versus streptokinase (Table 8). The GISSI-II trial (34) tested a 3-hour alteplase infusion and found no treatment advantage. The 12,490 patients from GISSI-II were added

Table 8 Study Design of Thrombolytic Megatrials

	International[a]	ISIS-III	GUSTO-1
Sample size	20,891	41,299	41,021
Thrombolytic regimen	1. Streptokinase 2. Alteplase (3 h)	1. Streptokinase 2. Duteplase (4 h) 3. Anistreplase	1. Streptokinase 2. Alteplase (90 min) 3. Streptokinase/alteplase
Heparin regimen	12,500 IU sc bid or placebo	12,500 IU sc bid or placebo	12,500 IU sc bid or 1000–1200 IU/h
Delay in heparin Rx	12 h	4 h	4 h sc, 0 h IV

[a]Includes 12,490 patients from GISSI-2 trial.

to 8401 recruited elsewhere to form the International Study (63), with no mortality difference between alteplase and streptokinase (8.9% vs. 8.5%). In contrast, the GUSTO-I trial (40) tested the accelerated dose combined with intravenous heparin and found a significant mortality reduction (6.3% vs. 7.3%).

Finally, the Continuous Infusion vs. Double Bolus Administration of Alteplase (COBALT) trial (64), comparing double-bolus dosing with the accelerated dose in 7169 patients, was prematurely stopped when no mortality benefit (8.0% vs. 7.5%) was seen during an interim analysis.

The TAMI Trials

The TAMI Study Group (Table 1) completed 10 studies (6–15) of various therapeutic regimens in acute MI with alteplase and urokinase, focusing on dosing and adjunctive therapies. Angiography was used to assess infarct artery patency and left ventricular function. Ten different doses of alteplase were given, with an accelerated dose similar to the dose used by Neuhaus et al. having the highest patency rate (13,59). Treating patients 6 to 24 hours after symptom onset improved early patency (65% vs. 27%) and preserved end-diastolic volume (TAMI-6) (12). The strategy of immediate PTCA after successful thrombolysis offered no clinical benefit (TAMI-1) (6), but acute angiography and rescue PTCA as necessary were feasible and potentially useful [(TAMI-1 (6), TAMI-5 (11)]. Immediate heparin administration did not facilitate thrombolysis (TAMI-3) (8), as suggested in animal studies, but more potent platelet inhibition with a monoclonal antibody directed against the platelet GP IIb/IIIa receptor did improve patency (TAMI-8) (14). Preclinical studies suggesting that prostacyclin and fluosol decreased reperfusion injury, by inhibiting free radicals and neutrophil activity, and improved left ventricular function were not confirmed in the TAMI-4 (9) and TAMI-9 (15) studies, respectively. Furthermore, the TAMI dataset was analyzed in a number of publications to examine patient selection, clinical outcomes, and prognosis (65).

The TIMI Trials

In parallel with the TAMI investigators, the TIMI investigators were also studying thrombolysis with alteplase and adjunctive strategies (16–26) (Table 2). After demonstrating superior recanalization rates for rt-PA compared with streptokinase in TIMI-1 (16), the TIMI-2 (17,18) trial showed no advantage for PTCA immediately or 18 to 48 hours after thrombolysis versus a selective strategy of treating postinfarction ischemia. The TIMI-3 trial (19,20) examined patients with unstable angina and non-Q-wave MI. Patients treated with alteplase instead of placebo had a higher rate of MI (8.3%

vs. 4.6%) and a 0.55% risk of intracerebral hemorrhage. An early invasive strategy with angiography rather than an early conservative strategy with routine medical care and risk stratification was associated with no difference in death or MI, but fewer patients were rehospitalized or taking antianginal medications at 6 weeks. In TIMI-4 (21), accelerated alteplase had higher earlier patency rates and improved clinical benefit compared with anistreplase or combination thrombolytic therapy. Hirudin, a direct thrombin inhibitor, achieved a more consistent level of anticoagulation than heparin when tested with alteplase in TIMI-5 (22) and streptokinase in TIMI-6 (23). Clinical endpoints were also improved. However, a high dose was associated with an unacceptable rate of intracerebral hemorrhage in TIMI-9 (25) and a lower dose had no survival advantage (26). Bivalirudin, also a direct thrombin inhibitor, appeared to be a promising adjunct (TIMI-7, TIMI-8) (24), but further development was terminated by the sponsor. Several additional trials by this productive group have been performed or are in progress (Table 2) (66–74). The TIMI dataset has also produced a number of important publications (75).

DUTEPLASE

Duteplase is a nearly pure two-chain form of rt-PA. It differs from alteplase only in the substitution of methionine for valine at position 245 in the amino acid sequence in the kringle 2 region. Duteplase produced a 90-min patency rate of 69% in 488 patients when given over 4 hours, with 0.4 megaunits/kg given in the first hour (including a 10% bolus) and 0.2 megaunits/kg given over the subsequent 3 hours (76). As with the conventional alteplase dose of 100 mg over 3 hours used in the GISSI-II trial (34), two-thirds the dose was administered by 90 min. This dose was used in the ISIS-III trial (38) where no mortality difference was seen between streptokinase (10.6%), duteplase (10.3%), and anistreplase (10.5%). Patency results and the mortality data from GISSI-II and ISIS-III suggest that duteplase and alteplase are clinically equivalent. Duteplase was withdrawn from further development after loss of a patent infringement legal suit to the manufacturer of alteplase.

ANISTREPLASE

Anistreplase (anisoylated plasminogen streptokinase activator complex, APSAC) is a stoichiometric combination of streptokinase and human lys-plasminogen. An anisoyl group reversibly bound to the catalytic center of the plasminogen moiety slowly undergoes deacylation prior to direct plasminogen activation. The delayed onset of action permits the agent to be administered over a few minutes.

Coronary Patency, Infarct Size, and Left Ventricular Function

A dose of 30 mg injected over 5 minutes contains approximately 1 million units of streptokinase. Patency rates are equivalent to those seen with the 3-hour alteplase dose, with a 70% 90-min patency rate (49).

The APSAC Multicenter Trial Group (77) found no difference in peak creatine kinase activity although the time to peak activity was shorter with anistreplase than with placebo. In contrast, Bassand et al. (78) demonstrated a 31% decrease in infarct size measured by single-photon emission computed tomography. Similarly, the former trial (77) showed no difference in left ventricular function, whereas the latter trial (78) found a 6% higher mean left ventricular ejection fraction with anistreplase.

Mortality Trials

The APSAC Intervention Mortality Study (AIMS) (79) randomized 1258 patients to anistreplase or placebo within 6 hours from symptom onset. The trial was stopped prematurely owing to the 47% mortality reduction seen with anistreplase (6.4% vs. 12.1%).

There have been five comparative trials involving anistreplase, streptokinase, and rt-PA. The Second Thrombolytic Trial of Eminase in Acute Myocardial Infarction (TEAM-2) (80) compared anistreplase and streptokinase, showing comparable patency and mortality (5.9% vs. 7.1%) results in 370 patients. The TEAM-3 trial (81) documented equivalent patency rates and mortality (6.2% vs. 7.9%) between anistreplase and standard alteplase in 325 patients. The ISIS-3 study (38) showed no difference in mortality between streptokinase, duteplase, and anistreplase. The rt-PA-APSAC Patency Study (TAPS) (82) showed higher patency and lower mortality (2.4% vs. 8.1%) for accelerated alteplase versus anistreplase in 435 patients. Similarly, TIMI-4 (21) showed the same mortality advantage (2.2% vs. 8.8%) for accelerated alteplase compared with anistreplase in 382 patients.

UROKINASE

Urokinase is a double-chain serine protease derived initially from urine and subsequently from neonatal renal parenchymal cell cultures. It directly activates plasminogen without forming an activator complex, like alteplase, but like streptokinase, it is not specific for fibrin-bound thrombus.

Urokinase can be given as a bolus, like alteplase, or infused over 60 to 90 min. Mathey and coworkers (83) injected a bolus of 2 million units and documented a 60% patency rate at 60 min in 50 patients. Four other trials had similar patency rates at 90 min with 3 million unit infusion protocols (10,11,84,85). Mortality trials have not been performed, and intravenous urokinase (unlike intracoronary urokinase) is not formally approved by the Food and Drug Administration for use in acute MI.

Urokinase has been used in combination with alteplase (7,11,13,86), producing an improved 90-min patency rate of 72% and low reocclusion rates. However, other trials (21,40) of combination thrombolytic therapy have not demonstrated clinical benefit, and there may be an increased risk of intracerebral hemorrhage. The production of urokinase was suspended in 1999 because the manufacturer could not prove the absence of risk in transmitting infectious agents in a drug derived from human source material.

SARUPLASE

Saruplase is a recombinant unglycosylated form of single-chain urokinase (pro-urokinase). It exhibits relative fibrin specificity, a short half-life, and concomitant need for adjunctive heparin infusion. Saruplase has generally been administered as a 20-mg bolus and a 60-mg infusion over 60 min. In the Pro-Urokinase in Myocardial Infarction (PRIMI) trial (87), saruplase patency rates were superior to streptokinase and equivalent to those seen with standard alteplase and anistreplase. The Comparative Trial of Saruplase versus Streptokinase (COMPASS) trial (88) showed that 30-day mortality rates were at least as low with saruplase as with streptokinase (5.7% vs. 6.7%). The Study in Europe of Saruplase and Alteplase in Myocardial Infarction (SESAM) trial (89) found equivalent patency, reocclusion, and complication rates compared with standard alteplase.

COMPLICATIONS

The major complication of thrombolytic therapy is bleeding. Although fibrin-specific agents were expected to result in fewer bleeding complications, the large comparative trials found no difference in bleeding or transfusion rates (33,36,40). The true incidence of bleeding has been difficult to determine because of underreporting in larger trials of streptokinase, the subjective nature of the events, and the variable use of invasive procedures. In GUSTO-I (40), the transfusion rate was 10%. Concomitant use of heparin increases bleeding risk, particularly when the aPTT exceeds 100 sec (90). Therefore, therapeutic heparin is not recommended with the longer-acting agents streptokinase and anistreplase, although it is given with alteplase and saruplase to prevent infarct artery reocclusion.

Many patients have conditions which increase the risk of serious bleeding and which are absolute contraindications for thrombolytic therapy (91,92). These include aortic dissection, acute pericarditis, active bleeding, previous cerebral hemorrhage, intracerebral vascular or neoplastic disease, and major surgery, organ biopsy, or trauma in the preceding 2 weeks. Relative contraindications include blood pressure >180/110 mm Hg, history of stroke, prolonged or traumatic cardiopulmonary resuscitation, puncture of a noncompressible vessel, and major surgery or trauma in the preceding 2 to 4 weeks. When life-threatening bleeding occurs, heparin should be discontinued. Therapeutic interventions include protamine to normalize the aPTT, cryoprecipitate to increase fibrinogen levels, fresh-frozen plasma to replace clotting factors, platelet transfusions if the bleeding time is prolonged, and packed red blood cells to restore hemoglobin mass (93). A computerized tomographic scan of the head should be performed to document suspected intracranial hemorrhage.

The most devastating complication of thrombolytic therapy is intracerebral hemorrhage. Data from clinical trials and unselected populations suggest that the risk is 0.5% to 1% (94). At least half the patients die, and severe disability occurs in an additional 25%. Increased risk is associated with age >65 years, hypertension, and low body weight (95). More potent thrombolytic agents increase risk. In GUSTO-I (40), an excess of two intracerebral hemorrhages per 1000 patients was seen with alteplase compared with streptokinase. It is important to note, however, that thrombolytic therapy decreases late, presumably thrombotic, stroke so there is no overall excess in stroke.

Streptokinase and anistreplase are antigenic. Because of antibody formation, retreatment should not be given after 4 days of the initial exposure to avoid neutralization of streptokinase activity (96). Moreover, mild allergic reactions (fever, rash, rigor, bronchospasm) occur in 5%, including anaphylactic shock in 0.2%, and release of bradykinin produces hypotension in 5% to 10% (37).

Early reports suggested that reocclusion rates were higher with alteplase (14%) than with streptokinase, anistreplase, or urokinase (8%) (94). However, no differences were seen in GUSTO-I (40), perhaps due to the use of monitored intravenous heparin with alteplase. Additionally, there does not appear to be any difference between agents in rates of recurrent ischemia (20%) or reinfarction (4%).

The incidence of atrial and ventricular arrhythmias, congestive heart failure, and cardiogenic shock were each reduced by an absolute 1% with alteplase versus streptokinase in GUSTO-1 (40).

CONCLUSION

First-generation thrombolytics including streptokinase, anistreplase, and urokinase are not fibrin specific and activate plasminogen systemically. Second-generation thrombolytics including alteplase, duteplase, and saruplase preferentially activate plasminogen at the fibrin clot. Accelerated or front-loaded alteplase administered with intravenous heparin for 24 to 48 hours has proven to be the best thrombolytic strategy tested to date. Its superior ability to restore early normal blood flow to the infarct artery has been associated with improved left ventricular function and lower mortality and morbidity rates than the other agents. Neither bolus administration of alteplase nor combination therapy with alteplase and streptokinase, anistreplase, or urokinase has proven to be a superior strategy. The standard 3-hour infusion of alteplase appears to produce clinical outcomes similar to streptokinase, anistreplase, and saruplase. Anistreplase is the easiest to administer and streptokinase is the least expensive agent. Long-term follow-up demonstrates that the short-term reduction in mortality is maintained for at least 1 year (97–100).

The link between normal infarct artery blood flow, preserved left ventricular function, and mortality reduction documented in GUSTO-I (40,41) has stimulated new efforts to develop superior lytic agents (Chap. 10) and new adjunctive strategies (Chaps. 15, 16, 18). The wealth of information provided by the studies summarized in this review have clearly established the benchmarks against which new strategies will be tested.

REFERENCES

1. DeWood MA, Spores J, Notske R, Mouser LT, Burroughs R, Golden MS, Lang HT. Prevalence of total coronary occlusion during the early hours of transmural infarction. N Engl J Med 1980;303:897–902.
2. Rentrop KT, Blanke H, Karsch KR, Weigand V, Kostering H. Acute myocardial infarction: intracoronary application of nitroglycerine and streptokinase. Clin Cardiol 1979;2:354–363.
3. Reimer KA, Lowe JE, Rasmussen MM, Jennings RB. The wave-front phenomenon of ischemic death. I. Myocardial infarct size vs duration of coronary occlusion in dogs. Circulation 1977;56:786–794.
4. Kennedy JW, Ritchie JL, Davis KB, Fritz JK. Western Washington randomized trial of intracoronary streptokinase in acute myocardial infarction. N Engl J Med 1983;309:1477–1482.
5. Simoons M, Van den Brand M, De Zwaan C, Verheugt FWA, Remme WJ, Serruys PW, Bär F, Res J, Krauss XH, Vermeer F, Lubsen J. Improved survival after early thrombolysis in acute myocardial infarction: a randomized trial of the Interuniversity Cardiology Institute in the Netherlands. Lancet 1985;2:578–582.
6. Topol EJ, Califf RM, George BS, Kereiakes DJ, Abbottsmith CW, Candela RJ, Lee KL, Pitt B, Stack RS, O'Neill WW. A randomized trial of immediate versus delayed elective angioplasty after intravenous tissue plasminogen activator in acute myocardial infarction. N Engl J Med 1987;317:581–588. (TAMI-1)

7. Topol EJ, Califf RM, George BS, Kereiakes DJ, Rothbaum D, Candela RJ, Abbottsmith CW, Pinkerton CA, Stump DC, Collen D, Lee KL, Pitt B, Kline EM, Boswick JM, O'Neill WW, Stack RS. Coronary arterial thrombolysis with combined infusion of recombinant tissue-type plasminogen activator and urokinase in patients with acute myocardial infarction. Circulation 1988;77: 1100–1107. (TAMI-2)
8. Topol EJ, George BS, Kereiakes DJ, Stump DC, Candela RJ, Abbottsmith CW, Aronson L, Pickel A, Boswick JM, Lee KL, Ellis SG, Califf RM. A randomized controlled trial of intravenous tissue plasminogen activator and early intravenous heparin in acute myocardial infarction. Circulation 1989; 79:281–286. (TAMI-3)
9. Topol EJ, Ellis SG, Califf RM, George BS, Stump DC, Bates ER, Nabel EG, Walton JA, Candela RJ, Lee KL, Kline EM, Pitt B. Combined tissue-type plasminogen activator and prostacyclin therapy for acute myocardial infarction. J Am Coll Cardiol 1989;14:877–884. (TAMI-4)
10. Wall TC, Phillips HR, Stack RS, Mantell S, Aronson L, Boswick J, Sigmon K, DiMeo M, Chaplin D, Whitcomb D, Pasi D, Zawodniak M, Hajisheik M, Hegde S, Barker W, Tenney R, Califf RM. Results of high dose intravenous urokinase for acute myocardial infarction. Am J Cardiol 1990;65:124–131. (TAMI-UK)
11. Califf RM, Topol EJ, Stack RS, Ellis SG, George BS, Kereiakes DJ, Samaha JK, Worley SJ, Anderson JL, Harrelson-Woodlief L, Wall TC, Phillips HR, Abbottsmith CW, Candela RJ, Flanagan WH, Sasahara AA, Mantell SJ, Lee KL. Evaluation of combination thrombolytic therapy and timing of cardiac catheterization in acute myocardial infarction. Results of Thrombolysis and Angioplasty in Myocardial Infarction—Phase 5 randomized trial. Circulation 1991;83:1543–1556. (TAMI-5)
12. Topol EJ, Califf RM, Vandormael M, Grines CL, George BS, Sanz ML, Wall T, O'Brien M, Schwaiger M, Aguirre FV, Young S, Popma JJ, Sigmon KN, Lee KL, Ellis SG. A randomized trial of late reperfusion therapy for acute myocardial infarction. Circulation 1992;85:2090–2099. (TAMI-6)
13. Wall TC, Califf RM, George BS, Ellis SG, Samaha JK, Kereiakes DJ, Worley SJ, Sigmon K, Topol EJ. Accelerated plasminogen activator dose regimens for coronary thrombolysis. J Am Coll Cardiol 1992;19:482–489. (TAMI-7)
14. Kleiman NS, Ohman EM, Califf RM, George BS, Kereiakes D, Aguirre FV, Weisman H, Schaible T, Topol EJ. Profound inhibition of platelet aggregation with monoclonal antibody 7E3 fab after thrombolytic therapy: results of the Thrombolysis and Angioplasty in Myocardial Infarction (TAMI) 8 pilot study. J Am Coll Cardiol 1993;22:381–389. (TAMI-8)
15. Wall TC, Califf RM, Blankenship J, Talley JD, Tannenbaum M, Schwaiger M, Gacioch G, Cohen MD, Sanz M, Leimberger JD, Topol EJ. Intravenous fluosol in the treatment of acute myocardial infarction: Results of the Thrombolysis and Angioplasty in Myocardial Infarction 9 trial. Circulation 1994;90: 114–120. (TAMI-9)
16. TIMI Study Group. The Thrombolysis in Myocardial Infarction (TIMI) trial. Phase 1 findings. N Engl J Med 1985;312:932–936. (TIMI-1)

17. Rogers WJ, Baim DS, Gore JM, Brown BG, Roberts R, Williams DO, Chesebro JH, Babb JD, Sheehan FH, Wackers FJT, Zaret BL, Robertson TL, Passamani ER, Ross R, Knatterud GL, Braunwald E, for the TIMI II-A Investigators. Comparison of immediate invasive, delayed invasive, and conservative strategies after tissue-type plasminogen activator. Results of the Thrombolysis in Myocardial Infarction (TIMI) Phase II-A trial. Circulation 1990;81:1457–1476. (TIMI-IIA)
18. TIMI Study Group. Comparison of invasive and conservative strategies after treatment with intravenous tissue plasminogen activator in acute myocardial infarction. Results of the Thrombolysis in Myocardial Infarction (TIMI) Phase II trial. N Engl J Med 1989;320:618–627. (TIMI-IIB)
19. TIMI IIIA Investigators. Early effects of tissue-type plasminogen activator added to conventional therapy on the culprit lesion in patients presenting with ischemic cardiac pain at rest. Results of the Thrombolysis in Myocardial Ischemia (TIMI-IIIA) trial. Circulation 1993;87:38–52. (TIMI-IIIA)
20. TIMI IIIB Investigators. Effects of tissue plasminogen activator and a comparison of early invasive and conservative strategies in unstable angina and non-Q-wave myocardial infarction: results of the TIMI IIIB trial. Circulation 1994;89:1545–1556. (TIMI-IIIB)
21. Cannon CP, McCabe CH, Diver DJ, Herson S, Greene RM, Shah PK, Sequeira RF, Leya F, Kirshenbaum JM, Magorien RD, Palmeri ST, Davis V, Gibson CM, Poole WK, Braunwald E. Comparison of front-loaded recombinant tissue-type plasminogen activator, anistreplase and combination thrombolytic therapy for acute myocardial infarction: results of the Thrombolysis in Myocardial Infarction (TIMI) 4 trial. J Am Coll Cardiol 1994;24:1602–1610. (TIMI-4)
22. Cannon CP, McCabe CH, Henry TD, Schweiger M, Gibson RS, Mueller HS, Becker RC, Kleiman NS, Haugland JM, Anderson JL, Sharaf BL, Edwards S, Rogers W, Williams DO, Braunwald E. A pilot trial of recombinant desulfatohirudin compared with tissue-type plasminogen activator and aspirin for acute myocardial infarction: results of the Thrombolysis in Myocardial Infarction (TIMI) 5 trial. J Am Coll Cardiol 1994;23:993–1003. (TIMI-5)
23. Lee LV. Initial experience with hirudin and streptokinase in acute myocardial infarction: results of the Thrombolysis in Myocardial Infarction (TIMI) 6 trial. Am J Cardiol 1995;75:7–13. (TIMI-6)
24. Fuchs J, Cannon CP. Hirulog in the treatment of unstable angina: results of the Thrombin Inhibition in Myocardial Ischemia (TIMI) 7 trial. Circulation 1995;92:727–733. (TIMI-7)
25. Antman EM. Hirudin in acute myocardial infarction: safety report from the Thrombolysis and Thrombin Inhibition in Myocardial Infarction (TIMI) 9A trial. Circulation 1994;90:1624–1630. (TIMI-9A)
26. Antman EM. Hirudin in acute myocardial infarction. Thrombolysis and Thrombin Inhibition in Myocardial Infarction (TIMI) 9B trial. Circulation 1996;94:911–921. (TIMI-9B)
27. Verstraete M, Bernard R, Bory M, Brower RW, Collen D, de Bono DP, Erbel R, Huhmann W, Lennane RJ, Lubsen J, Mathey D, Meyer J, Michels HR,

Rutsch W, Schartl M, Schmidt W, Uebis R, von Essen R. Randomised trial of intravenous recombinant tissue-type plasminogen activator versus intravenous streptokinase in acute myocardial infarction. Lancet 1985;1:842–847. (ECSG-1)

28. Verstraete M, Bleifeld W, Brower RW, Charbonnier B, Collen D, de Bono DP, Dunning AJ, Lennane RJ, Lubsen J, Mathey DG, Michel PL, Raynaud PH, Schofer J, Vahanian A, Vanheke J, van de Kley GA, Van de Werf F, von Essen R. Double-blind randomised trial of intravenous tissue-type plasminogen activator versus placebo in acute myocardial infarction. Lancet 1985;2: 965–969. (ECSG-2)
29. Verstraete M, Arnold AER, Brower RW, Collen D, de Bono DP, De Zwaan C, Erbel R, Hillis WS, Lennane RJ, Lubsen J, Mathey D, Reid DS, Rutsch W, Schartl M, Schofer J, Serruys PW, Simoons ML, Uebis R, Vahanian A, Verheugt FWA, von Essen R. Acute coronary thrombolysis with recombinant human tissue-type plasminogen activator: initial patency and influence of maintained infusion on reocclusion rate. Am J Cardiol 1987;60:231–237. (ECSG-3)
30. Simoons ML, Betriu A, Col J, von Essen R, Lubsen J, Michel PL, Rutsch W, Schmidt W, Thery C, Vahanian A, Willems GM, Arnold AER, DeBono DP, Dougherty PC, Lambertz H, Meier B, Raynaud P, Sanz GA, Uebis R, Van de Werf F, Wood D, Verstraete M. Thrombolysis with tissue plasminogen activator in acute myocardial infarction: no additional benefit from immediate percutaneous coronary angioplasty. Lancet 1988;1:197–202. (ECSG-4)
31. Van de Werf F, Arnold AER. Intravenous tissue plasminogen activator and size of infarct, left ventricular function, and survival in acute myocardial infarction. Br Med J 1988;297:1374–1379. (ECSG-5)
32. de Bono DP, Simoons ML, Tijssen J, Arnold AE, Betriu A, Burgersdijk C, Lopez Bescos L, Mueller E, Pfisterer M, Zijlstra F, Verstraete M, Van de Werf F. Effect of early intravenous heparin on coronary patency, infarct size, and bleeding complications after alteplase thrombolysis: results of a randomised double blind European Cooperative Study Group trial. Br Heart J 1992;67: 122–128. (ECSG-6)
33. Gruppo Italiano per lo Studio della Streptochinasi nell'Infarto Miocardico (GISSI). Effectiveness of intravenous thrombolytic treatment in acute myocardial infarction. Lancet 1986;1:397–401. (GISSI-1)
34. Gruppo Italiano per lo Studio Della Sopravvivenza nell'Infarto Miocardico. GISSI-2: a factorial randomised trial of alteplase versus streptokinase and heparin versus no heparin among 12,490 patients with acute myocardial infarction. Lancet 1990;336:65–71. (GISSI-2)
35. Gruppo Italiano per lo Studio della Sopravvivenza nell'Infarto Miocardico. GISSI-3: effects of lisinopril and transdermal glyceryl trinitrate singly and together on 6-week mortality and ventricular function after acute myocardial infarction. Lancet 1994;343:1115–1122. (GISSI-3)
36. ISIS-1 (First International Study of Infarct Survival) Collaborative Group. Randomised trial of intravenous atenolol among 16,027 cases of suspected acute myocardial infarction: ISIS-1. Lancet 1986;2:57–66. (ISIS-1)

37. ISIS-2 (Second International Study of Infarct Survival) Collaborative Group. Randomised trial of intravenous streptokinase, oral aspirin, both, or neither among 17,187 cases of suspected acute myocardial infarction: ISIS-2. Lancet 1988;2:349–360. (ISIS-2)
38. ISIS-3 (Third International Study of Infarct Survival) Collaborative Group. ISIS-3: a randomized comparison of streptokinase vs tissue plasminogen activator vs anistreplase and of aspirin plus heparin vs aspirin alone among 41,299 cases of suspected acute myocardial infarction. Lancet 1992;339:753–770. (ISIS-3)
39. ISIS-4 (Fourth International Study of Infarct Survival) Collaborative Group. ISIS-4: a randomized factorial trial assessing early oral captopril, oral mononitrate, and intravenous magnesium sulphate in 58,050 patients with suspected acute myocardial infarction. Lancet 1995;345:669–685. (ISIS-4)
40. GUSTO Investigators. An international randomized trial comparing four thrombolytic strategies for acute myocardial infarction. N Engl J Med 1993;329: 673–682.
41. GUSTO Angiographic Investigators. The effects of tissue plasminogen activator, streptokinase, or both on coronary-artery patency, ventricular function, and survival after acute myocardial infarction. N Engl J Med 1993;329:1615–1622.
42. GUSTO IIa Investigators. Randomized trial of intravenous heparin versus recombinant hirudin for acute coronary syndromes. Circulation 1994;90:1631–1637.
43. GUSTO-IIb Investigators. A comparison of recombinant hirudin versus heparin for the treatment of acute coronary syndromes. N Engl J Med 1996;335:775–782.
44. Tillet WS, Garner RI. The fibrinolytic activity of hemolytic streptococci. J Exp Med 1933;58:485–502.
45. Fletcher AP, Alkjaersig N, Smyrniotis FE, Sherry S. The treatment of patients suffering from early myocardial infarction with massive and prolonged streptokinase therapy. Trans Assoc Am Physicians 1958;71:287–296.
46. Yusuf S, Collins R, Peto R, Furberg C, Stampfer MJ, Goldhaber SZ, Hennekens CH. Intravenous and intracoronary fibrinolytic therapy in acute myocardial infarction: overview of results on mortality, reinfarction, and side-effects from 33 randomized controlled trials. Eur Heart J 1985;6:556–585.
47. Chazov EI, Mateeva LS, Mazaev AV, Sargin KE, Sadovskaia GV. Intracoronary administration of fibrinolysis in acute myocardial infarction. Ter Arkh 1976;48:8–19.
48. Schröder, Biamino G, von Leitner ER, Linderer T, Brueggeman T, Heitz J, Vohringer HF, Wegscheider K. Intravenous short-term infusion of streptokinase in acute myocardial infarction. Circulation 1983;67:536–548.
49. Granger CB, White H, Bates ER, Ohman EM, Califf RM. Patency profiles and left ventricular function after intravenous thrombolysis: a pooled analysis. Am J Cardiol 1994;74:1220–1228.
50. Simoons ML, Serruys PW, van den Brand M, Res J, Verheugt FWA, Krauss XH, Remme WJ, Bär F, de Zwaan C, van der Laarse A, Vermeer F, Lubsen

J. Early thrombolysis in acute myocardial infarction: limitation of infarct size and improved survival. J Am Coll Cardiol 1986;7:717–728.
51. ISAM Study Group. A prospective trial of intravenous streptokinase in acute myocardial infarction (I.S.A.M.). Mortality, morbidity and infarct size at 21 days. N Engl J Med 1986;314:1465–1471.
52. Serruys PW, Simoons ML, Suryapranata H, Vermeer F, Wijns W, van den Brand M, Bär F, de Zwaan C, Krauss XH, Remme WJ, Res J, Verheugt FWA, Van Domburg R, Lubsen J, Hugenholtz PG. Preservation of global and regional left ventricular function after early thrombolysis in acute myocardial infarction. J Am Coll Cardiol 1986;7:729–742.
53. White HD, Norris RM, Brown MA, Takayama M, Maslowski A, Bass NM, Ormiston JA, Whitlock T. Effect of intravenous streptokinase on left ventricular function and early survival after acute myocardial infarction. N Engl J Med 1987;317:850–855.
54. White HD, Norris RM, Brown MA, Brandt P, Whitlock R, Wild CJ. Left ventricular end-systolic volume as the major determinant of survival after recovery from myocardial infarction. Circulation 1987;76:41–51.
55. EMERAS (Estudio Multicentrico Estreptoquinasa Republica de America de Sur) Collaborative Group. Randomised trial of late thrombolysis in patients with suspected acute myocardial infarction. Lancet 1993;342:767–772.
56. Neuhaus K-L, Feuerer W, Jeep-Tebbe S, Niederer W, Vogt A, Tebbe U. Improved thrombolysis with a modified dose regimen of recombinant tissue-type plasminogen activator. J Am Coll Cardiol 1989;14:1556–1559.
57. Purvis JA, McNeill AJ, Rizwan A, Siddiqui RA, Roberts MJD, McClements BM, McEnearney D, Campbell NPS, Kahn MM, Webb SW, Wilson CM, Adgey AAJ. Efficacy of 100 mg of double-bolus alteplase in achieving complete perfusion in the treatment of acute myocardial infarction. J Am Coll Cardiol 1994;23:6–10.
58. Guerci AD, Gerstenblith G, Brinker JA, Chandra NC, Gottlieb SO, Bahr RD, Weiss JL, Shapiro EP, Flaherty JT, Bush DE, Chew PH, Gottlieb SH, Halperin HR, Ouyang P, Walford GD, Bell WR, Fatterpaker AK, Llewellyn M, Topol EJ, Healy B, Siu CO, Becker LC, Weisfeldt ML. A randomized trial of intravenous tissue plasminogen activator for acute myocardial infarction with subsequent randomization to elective coronary angioplasty. N Engl J Med 1987; 317:1613–1618.
59. O'Rourke M, Baron D, Keogh A, Kelly R, Nelson G, Barnes C, Raftos J, Rivers J, Graham K, Hillman K, Newman H, Healey J, Woolridge J, Rivers J, White H, Whitlock R, Norris R. Limitation of myocardial infarction by early infusion of recombinant tissue-type plasminogen activator. Circulation 1988;77:1311–1315.
60. National Heart Foundation of Australia Coronary Thrombolysis Group. Coronary thrombolysis and myocardial salvage by tissue plasminogen activator given up to 4 hours after onset of myocardial infarction. Lancet 1988;1:203–207.
61. Wilcox RG, von der Lippe G, Olsson CG, Jensen G, Skene AM, Hampton JR. Trial of tissue plasminogen activator for mortality reduction in acute myo-

cardial infarction: The Anglo-Scandinavian Study of Early Thrombolysis (ASSET). Lancet 1988;2:525–530.
62. LATE Study Group. Late Assessment of Thrombolytic Efficacy (LATE) study with alteplase 6–12 hours after onset of acute myocardial infarction. Lancet 1993;342:759–766.
63. International Study Group. In-hospital mortality and clinical course of 20,891 patients with suspected acute myocardial infarction randomized between alteplase and streptokinase with or without heparin. Lancet 1990;336:71–75.
64. COBALT Investigators. A comparison of continuous infusion of alteplase with double-bolus administration for acute myocardial infarction. The continuous infusion versus double bolus administration of alteplase (rt-PA): the COBALT trial. N Engl J Med 1997;337:1124–1130.
65. Barseness GW, Ohman EM, Califf RM, Kereiakes DJ, George BS, Topol EJ. The Thrombolysis and Angioplasty in Myocardial Infarction (TAMI) trials: a decade of reperfusion strategies. J Intervent Cardiol 1996;9:89–115.
66. Cannon CP, McCabe CH, Gibson CM, Ghali M, Sequeira RF, McKendall GR, Breed J, Modi NB, Fox NL, Tracy RP, Love TW, Braunwald E, and the TIMI-10A Investigators. TNK-tissue plasminogen activator in acute myocardial infarction: results of the thrombolysis in myocardial infarction (TIMI) 10A dose-ranging trial. Circulation 1997;95:351–356. (TIMI-10A)
67. Cannon CP, Gibson CM, McCabe CH, Adgey AAJ, Schweiger MJ, Sequeira RF, Grollier G, Giugliano RP, Frey M, Meuller HS, Steingart RM, Weaver WD, Van de Werf F, Braunwald E, for the Thrombolysis in Myocardial Infarction (TIMI) 10B Investigators. TNK-tissue plasminogen activator compared with front-loaded alteplase in acute myocardial infarction: results of the TIMI 10B trial. Circulation 1998;98:2805–2814. (TIMI-10B)
68. Thrombolysis in Myocardial Infarction (TIMI) 11A Investigators. Dose-ranging trial of enoxaparin for unstable angina: results of TIMI-11A. J Am Coll Cardiol 1997;29:1474–1482 (TIMI-11A)
69. Antman EM, McCabe C, Garfinkel E, Turpie AGG, Bernik PJLM, Salein D, Bayes deLuna A, Fox K, Lablanche JM, Radley D, Premmereur J, Braunwald E. Enoxaparin prevents death and cardiac ischemia events in unstable angina/non-Q-wave myocardial infarction. Results of the Thrombolysis in Myocardial Infarction (TIMI-11B) trial. Circulation 1999;100:1593–1601. (TIMI-11B)
70. Cannon CP, McCabe CH, Borzak S, Henry TD, Tischler MD, Mueller HS, Feldman R, Palmeri ST, Ault K, Hamilton SA, Rothman JM, Novotny WF, Braunwald E, for the TIMI 12 Investigators. Randomized trial of an oral platelet glycoprotein IIb/IIIa antagonist, sibrafiban, in patients after an acute coronary syndrome. Results of the TIMI 12 trial. Circulation 1998;97:340–349. (TIMI-12)
71. Antman EM, Giugliano RP, Gibson CM, McCabe CH, Coussement P, Kleiman NS, Vahanian A, Adgey AAJ, Menown I, Rupprecht H-J, Van der Wieken R, Ducas J, Scherer J, Anderson K, Van de Werf F, Braunwald E, for the TIMI 14 Investigators. Abciximab facilitates the rate and extent of throm-

bolysis: results of the Thrombolysis in Myocardial Infarction (TIMI) 14 trial. Circulation 1999;99:2720–2732. (TIMI-14)
72. Giugliano RP, McCabe CH, Sequeira RF, Henry TD, Piana RN, Schweiger MJ, Mueller HS, Borzak S, Tischler MD, Tamby J, Ramsey KE, Jacoski MV, Wise RJ, Braunwald E. Dose ranging study of intravenous RPR 109891 in patients with acute coronary syndromes—results of TIMI 15A. J Am Coll Cardiol 1998;31(suppl A):93A. (TIMI-15A)
73. Giugliano RP, McCabe CH, Frey M, Mueller HS, Tamby J-F, Jensen BK, Nicholas SB, Jennings LK, Wise RJ, Braunwald E. First report of an intravenous and oral GP IIb/IIIa inhibitor administered in patients—results of TIMI 15B. Eur Heart J 1999;20:376. (TIMI-15B)
74. Morris DC. Results from late-breaking clinical trials sessions at ACCIS '99 and ACC '99. J Am Coll Cardiol 1999;34:1–8. (TIMI-16, TIMI-17)
75. Cannon CP, Braunwald E, McCabe CH, Antman EM. The Thrombolysis in Myocardial Infarction (TIMI) trials: the first decade. J Intervent Cardiol 1995; 8:117–135.
76. Kalbfleisch JM, Kurnik PB, Thadani U, DeWood MA, Kent R, Magorien RD, Jain AC, Spaccavento LJ, Morris DL, Taylor GJ, Perry JM, Kutcher MA, Gorfinkel HJ, Littlejohn JK. Myocardial infarct artery patency and reocclusion rates after treatment with duteplase at the dose used in the International Study of Infarct Survival-3. Am J Cardiol 1993;71:386–392.
77. Meinertz T, Kasper W, Schumacher M, Just H. The German multicenter trial of anisoylated plasminogen streptokinase activator complex versus heparin for acute myocardial infarction. Am J Cardiol 1988;62:347–351.
78. Bassand JP, Machecourt J, Cassagnes J, Anguenot T, Lusson R, Borel E, Peycelow P, Wolf E, Ducellier D. Multicenter trial of intravenous anisoylated plasminogen streptokinase activator complex (APSAC) in acute myocardial infarction: effects on infarct size and left ventricular function. J Am Coll Cardiol 1989;13:988–997.
79. AIMS Trial Study Group. Effect of intravenous APSAC on mortality after acute myocardial infarction: preliminary report of a placebo-controlled clinical trial. Lancet 1988;1:545–549.
80. Anderson JL, Sorenson S, Moreno F, Hackworthy R, Browne K, Dale HT, Leya F, Dangoisse V, Eckerson H, Marder V. Multicenter patency trial of intravenous APSAC compared with streptokinase in acute myocardial infarction. Circulation 1991;88:126–140.
81. Anderson JL, Becker LC, Sorenson SG, Karagounis LA, Browne KF, Shah PK, Morris DC, Fintel DJ, Mueller HS, Ross AM, Hall SM, Askins JK, Doorey AJ, Grines CL, Moreno FL, Marder VJ. APSAC versus alteplase in acute myocardial infarction: comparative effects on left ventricular function, morbidity and 1-day coronary artery patency. J Am Coll Cardiol 1992;20: 753–766.
82. Neuhaus K-L, Von Essen R, Tebbe U, Vogt A, Roth M, Riess M, Niederer W, Forycki F, Wirtzfeld A, Maeurer W, Limbourg P, Merx W, Haerten K. Improved thrombolysis in acute myocardial infarction with front-loaded ad-

ministration of alteplase: Results of the rt-PA-APSAC Patency Study (TAPS). J Am Coll Cardiol 1992;19:885–891.

83. Mathey DG, Schofer J, Sheehan FH, Becher H, Tilsner V, Dodge HT. Intravenous urokinase in acute myocardial infarction. Am J Cardiol 1985;55:878–882.
84. Neuhaus KL, Tebbe U, Gotwik M, Weber M, Feurer W, Niederer W, Haerer W, Praetorius F, Grosser KD, Huhmann W, Hoepp HW, Alber G, Sheikhzadeh A, Schneider B. Intravenous recombinant tissue plasminogen activator (rt-PA) and urokinase in acute myocardial infarction: results of the German Activator Urokinase Study (GAUS). J Am Coll Cardiol 1988;12:581–587.
85. Whitlow PL, Bashore TM. Catheterization/Rescue Angioplasty Following Thrombolysis (CRAFT) study. Acute myocardial infarction treated with recombinant tissue plasminogen activator versus urokinase (abstr). J Am Coll Cardiol 1991;17:276A.
86. Urokinase and Alteplase in Myocardial Infarction Collaborative Group (URALMI). Combination of urokinase and alteplase in the treatment of myocardial infarction. Coron Artery Dis 1991;2:225–235.
87. PRIMI Trial Study Group. Randomized double-blind trial of recombinant prourokinase against streptokinase in acute myocardial infarction. Lancet 1989;1:863–868.
88. Tebbe U, Michels R, Adgey J, Boland J, Caspi AVI, Charbonnier B, Windeler J, Barth H, Groves R, Hopkins GR, Fennell W, Betriu A, Ruda M, Milczoch J. Randomized, double-blind study comparing saruplase with streptokinase therapy in acute myocardial infarction: the COMPASS equivalence trial. J Am Coll Cardiol 1998;31:487–493.
89. Bär FW, Meyer J, Vermeer F, Michels R, Charbonnier B, Haerten K, Spiecker M, Macaya C, Hanssen M, Heras M, Boland JP, Morice M-C, Dunn FG, Uebis R, Hamm C, Ayzenberg O, Strupp G, Withagen AJ, Klein W, Windeler J, Hopkins G, Barth H, von Fisenne MJM, for the SESAM Study Group. Comparison of saruplase and alteplase in acute myocardial infarction. Am J Cardiol 1997;79:727–732.
90. Granger CB, Hirsh J, Califf RM, Col J, White HD, Betriu A, Woodlief LH, Lee KL, Bovill EG, Simes RJ, Topol EJ. Activated partial thromboplastin time and outcome after thrombolytic therapy for acute myocardial infarction. Results from the GUSTO-I trial. Circulation 1996;93:870–878.
91. Cairns JA, Kennedy JW, Fuster V. Coronary thrombolysis. Chest 1998; 114(suppl):634S–657S.
92. Ryan TJ, Antman EM, Brooks NH, Califf RM, Hillis LD, Hiratzka LF, Rapaport E, Riegel BJ, Russell RO, Smith EE III, Weaver WD. 1999 update: ACC/AHA guidelines for the management of patients with acute myocardial infarction: a report of the American College of Cardiology/American Heart Association Task Force on Practice Guidelines (Committee on Management of Acute Myocardial Infarction). J Am Coll Cardiol 1999;34:890–911.
93. Sane DC, Califf RM, Topol EJ, Stump DC, Mark DB, Greenberg CS. Bleeding during thrombolytic therapy for acute myocardial infarction: mechanisms and management. Ann Intern Med 1989; 111:1010–1022.

94. Granger CB, Califf RM, Topol EJ. Thrombolytic therapy for acute myocardial infarction. Drugs 1992;44:293–325.
95. Simoons ML, Maggioni AP, Knatterud G, Leimberger JD, de Jaegere P, van Domburg R, Boersma E, Franzosi MG, Califf R, Schroeder R, Braunwald E. Individual risk assessment for intracranial hemorrhage during thrombolytic therapy. Lancet 1993;342:1523–1528.
96. White HD. Thrombolytic treatment for recurrent myocardial infarction. Avoid repeating streptokinase or anistreplase. Br Med J 1991;302:429–430.
97. Gruppo Italiano per lo Studio della Streptochinasi nell 'Infarto Miocardico (GISSI). Long-term effects of intravenous thrombolysis in acute myocardial infarction. Final report of the GISSI study. Lancet 1987;2:871–877.
98. AIMS Trial Study Group: Long-term effects of intravenous anistreplase in acute myocardial infarction: Final report of the AIMS study. Lancet 1990; 335:427–431.
99. Wilcox RG, von der Lippe C, Olsson CG, Jensen G, Skene AM, Hampton JR. Effects of alteplase in acute myocardial infarction: 6-month results from the ASSET study. Lancet 1990;335:1175–1178.
100. Califf RM, White HD, van de Werf F, Sadowski Z, Armstrong PW, Vahanian A, Simoons ML, Simes RJ, Lee KL, Topol EJ. One-year results from the Global Utilization of Streptokinase and TPA for Occluded Coronary Arteries (GUSTO-1) trial. Circulation 1996;94:1233–1238.

10

Third-Generation Thrombolytic Agents for Acute Myocardial Infarction

Sorin J. Brener
The Cleveland Clinic Foundation
Cleveland
and Ohio State University
Columbus, Ohio

Eric J. Topol
The Cleveland Clinic Foundation
Cleveland, Ohio

INTRODUCTION

Fibrinolytic therapy remains the most widely utilized reperfusion strategy in acute myocardial infarction around the world. After two decades of intense research and improved application in ever expanding groups of patients, we are still faced with the challenge of surpassing the initial results obtained with recombinant native t-PA (1), understanding the complex interactions between thrombin and platelets, translating improvements in arterial patency (2), into survival advantage, and limiting the devastating consequences of major bleeding, particularly intracranial hemorrhage. The current chapter will focus on the new, third-generation fibrinolytic agents. A comprehensive review of the structure and action of the first- and second-generation fibrinolytics is provided in Chapter 9.

The key obstacles to a more pronounced effect of fibrinolysis with t-PA center around four issues:

1. Inability to deaggregate the platelet core of the thrombus formed at the site of plaque rupture and the susceptibility to inhibition by platelet-derived PAI-1.
2. Creation of a pro-coagulant milieu due to liberation of fibrin-bound thrombin after fibrinolysis, which further accentuates platelet aggregation and rethrombosis.
3. Lack of tissue perfusion despite epicardial vessel patency in a substantial proportion of patients.
4. Despite substantial fibrin-selectivity, nearly 1% of treated patients experience intracerebral hemorrhage, responsible for an important number of fatalities and severe morbidity.

Recently, three large randomized clinical trials using the third generation fibrinolytic agents derived from t-PA have been performed. In each, the novel agent was tested against the benchmark of pharmacological reperfusion—the accelerated t-PA regimen. The objective in each was to compare the two agents with respect to mortality at 30 days from enrollment. It is sobering to see that despite important efforts to streamline the process of reperfusion, including public education regarding the importance of time in myocardial infarction, the duration from chest pain onset to lytic administration has been unaffected in the last decade, remaining at 2.7 to 3.1 hours (3). Since door-to-needle time has been optimized in most institutions, it is clear that better and faster-acting drugs are needed to achieve similar or better results in an aging and more disease-ridden population presenting with acute myocardial infarction. We will review these landmark trials in detail and highlight the important messages relevant to patient care and future research.

RETEPLASE (r-PA)

Recombinant plasminogen activator (reteplase, r-PA; Fig. 1) is a nonglycosylated deletion mutant of wild-type t-PA, expressed in *Escherichia coli* (4). It maintains the kringle-2 and protease domains, but lacks the kringle 1, finger and epidermal growth factor domains. It becomes active after in vitro refolding. In comparison with t-PA, these modifications result in preferential activation of fibrin bound plasminogen; a longer half-life in animals, healthy volunteers, and patients (5); enhanced fibrinolytic potency; and lower affinity for endothelial cells (4). The profile of plasma reteplase activity is monophasic ($t_{1/2}$ = 11.2 min), while the reteplase antigen activity displays a biphasic curve with an initial $t_{1/2}$ of 13.9 min and a terminal $t_{1/2}$ of almost 3 hours. These observations, made in healthy volunteers (6), suggested that there exists a dissociation between the antigenic and lytic activity of rete-

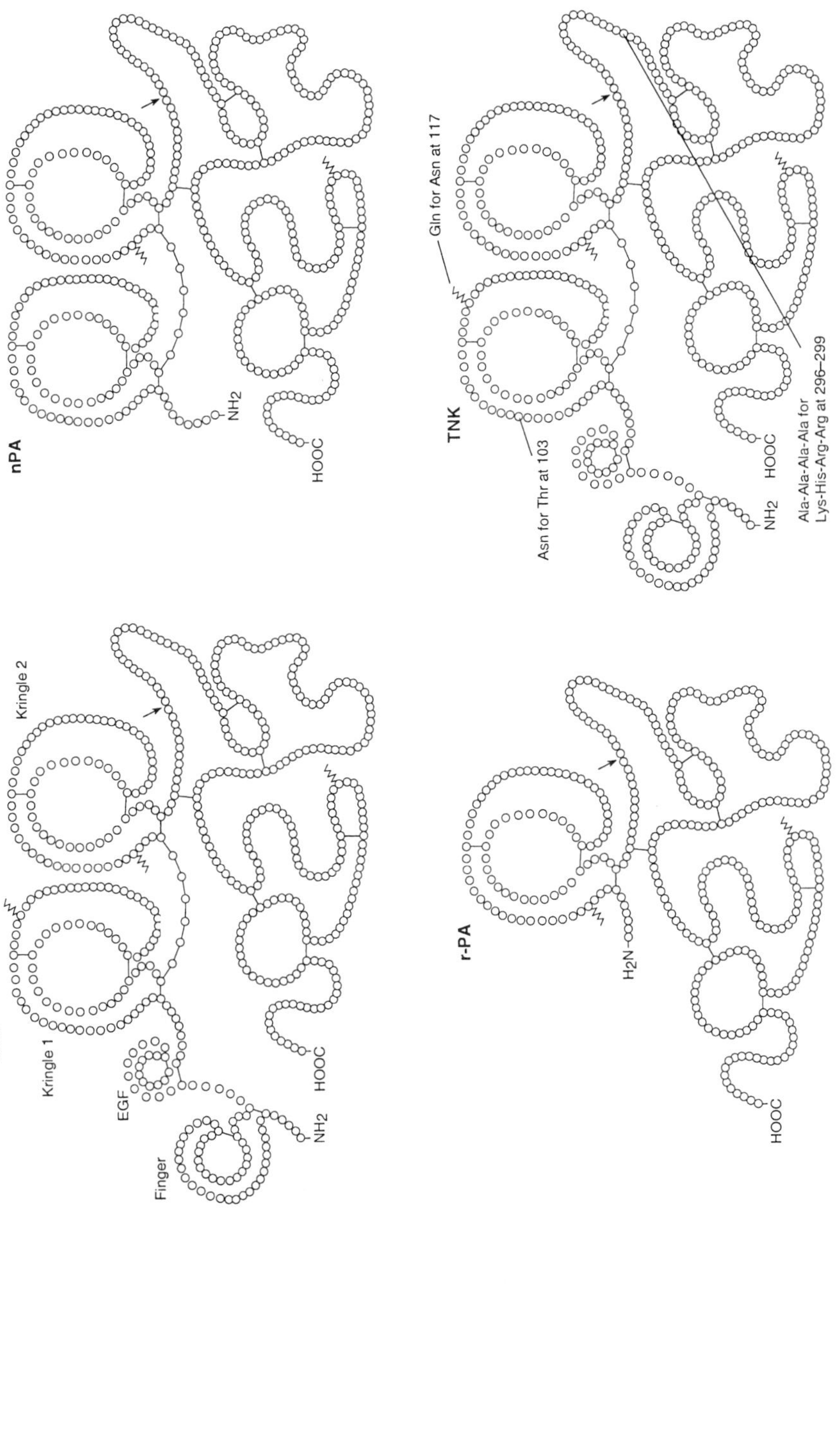

Figure 1 Schematic representation of the molecular structure of t-PA, r-PA, n-PA, TNK-PA.

plase. Reteplase-specific antibodies were not detected in 2400 patients treated initially with this drug.

Some of the initial dose-finding studies were performed by Neuhaus and colleagues in 1993 and 1994 (7).

The RAPID Trials

The RAPID I Investigators (8) compared the efficacy and safety of various doses of r-PA with t-PA and concomitant heparin in 606 patients presenting within 6 hours of the onset of an acute myocardial infarction. Reteplase was given as a single 15 MU bolus, a 10 + 5 MU double bolus, or a 10 + 10 MU double bolus, 30 min apart. The t-PA arm consisted of the 3-hour rather than the 90-min accelerated dosing regimen. Angiographic assessment (verified by a core laboratory) was obtained at 30, 60, and 90 min, and before hospital discharge. Efficacy and safety endpoints were monitored for 30 days. The four groups were similar in terms of baseline characteristics, location of infarct, and time to treatment. The double-bolus dose of 10+10 MU of r-PA had significantly higher rates of TIMI 3 flow than the t-PA arm at 60 and 90 min and at hospital discharge (Fig. 2), as well as a statistically significant improvement in the global and regional wall motion function.

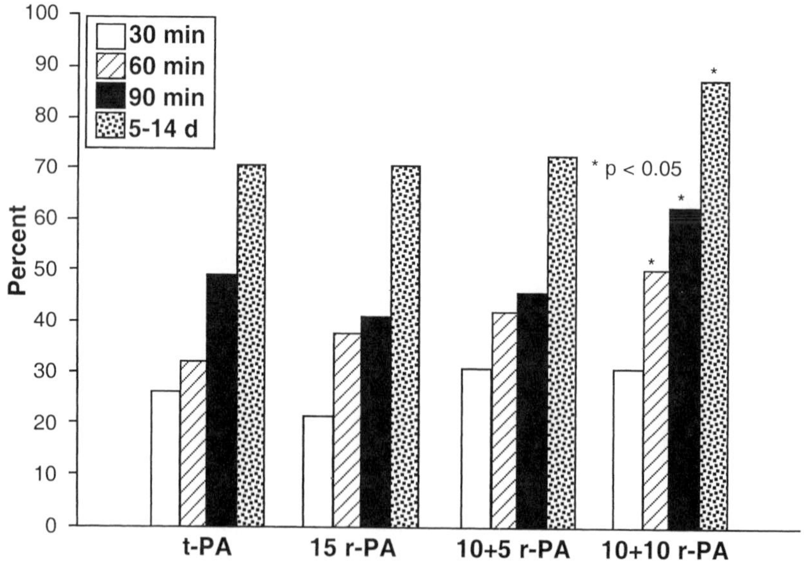

Figure 2 Incidence of TIMI 3 flow in the RAPID I trial at 60 and 90 min and at hospital discharge.

There was an insignificant trend towards lower rates of reocclusion in the r-PA group. The bleeding complications and major adverse clinical events were not different among the groups.

The RAPID 2 trial was designed to compare the most effective dose of double-bolus r-PA with an "accelerated" t-PA regimen in evolving myocardial infarction of <12 hours' duration. Bode et al. (2) randomly assigned 169 patients to r-PA (10+10 MU, 30 minutes apart) and 155 patients to t-PA (accelerated regimen). The primary endpoint, TIMI 3 flow in the infarct-related artery at 90 min, was achieved in 59.9% and 45.2%, respectively, $P < .05$. This difference in complete patency rates was even more pronounced at 60 min (51.2% vs. 37.4%; $P = .01$) (Fig. 3). Interestingly, a limited number of patients had angiography within 30 min of administration of fibrinolytic therapy. The rate of TIMI 3 flow was 27% in the r-PA (n = 55) and 39% in the t-PA (n = 41) groups. The important endpoints are displayed in Table 1. As compared with the t-PA group, the reteplase treated patients required less coronary interventions over the ensuing 6 hours in response to persistent ischemia (26.5% vs. 13.3%, respectively; $P = .01$). There was a trend toward decreased mortality at 35 days (4.1% for r-PA vs. 8.4% for t-PA), while the incidence of severe bleeding and hemorrhagic stroke was similar in the two groups (12.4% vs. 9.7%, and 1.2% vs. 1.8%,

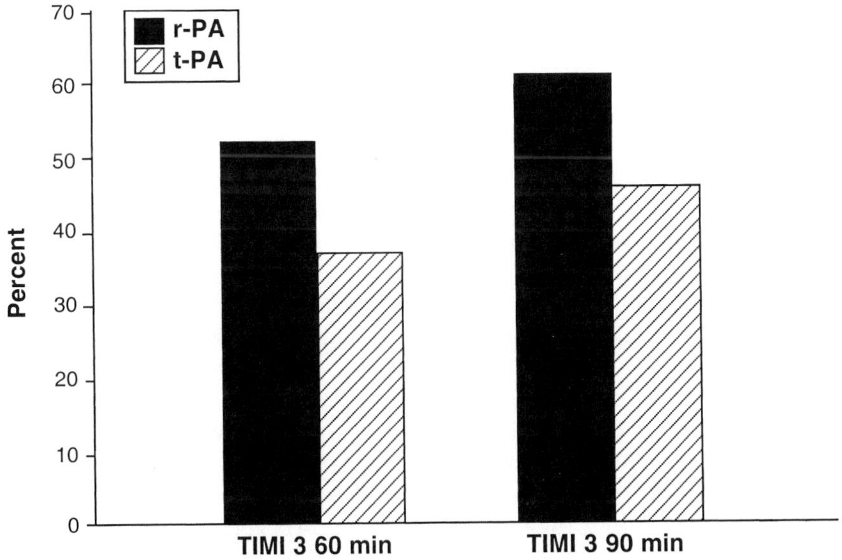

Figure 3 Incidence of TIMI 3 flow in the RAPID II trial at 60 and 90 min. (From Ref. 32.)

Table 1 Major Clinical Endpoints in the RAPID II Trial

Endpoint	Accelerated t-PA (n = 155)	r-PA (n = 169)	*P*
Rescue PTCA within 6 h, %	26.5	13.3	.01
35-day mortality, %	8.4	4.1	.11
Severe bleeding, %	12.4	9.7	.42
Reinfarction, %	4.7	4.5	>.5

PTCA, percutaneous transluminal coronary angioplasty; r-PA, reteplase; t-PA, tissue plasminogen activator.
Source: Ref. 2.

respectively). The same favorable trend was observed in the incidence of congestive heart failure (9.5% vs. 12.3%) and recurrent ischemia (29.0% vs. 34.2%). Reinfarction occurred in 4.7% and 4.5% of the two groups, respectively. The conclusion was that reteplase achieves 60- and 90-min patency rates superior to the most effective regimen of t-PA, without a demonstrable increase in significant adverse events. The curves of cumulative patency seemed to intersect at 30 min, with t-PA being superior to r-PA in the early phase of treatment.

INJECT

This much larger European Cooperative study (9) compared the efficacy and safety of 10 + 10 MU of r-PA versus 1.5 MU of streptokinase with concomitant heparin in 6010 patients with an acute myocardial infarction of <12 hours' duration. Thirty-five days and 6 months clinical outcomes were monitored. As prespecified by the investigators, the goal of the trial was to demonstrate equivalency of the two treatments, i.e., that the 35-day mortality of reteplase does not exceed by more that 1% that observed with streptokinase. This concept evolved from the results of the GUSTO I trial, which showed a similar difference between t-PA and the combined streptokinase arm.

As shown in Table 2, the two groups were equivalent at baseline. At 35 days, the survival in the reteplase group was slightly improved (9.02% vs. 9.53%), which by the statistical specifications of the trial indicated at least equivalency to streptokinase. This difference increased to a full absolute 1% advantage by 6 months (Table 2; Fig. 4). There was no evidence for a preferential effect in any subgroup of patients. The incidence of stroke and other bleeding events was similar among the two treatment arms (Table 2).

Table 2 Baseline Characteristics and Major Endpoints in the INJECT Trial

	Reteplase (n = 3004)	Streptokinase (n = 3006)
Baseline characteristics		
Age, years (±SD)	61.8 ± 12	61.9 ± 12
Male sex, %	71.8	72.9
Previous MI, %	14.5	14.7
Anterior MI, %	41.4	44.0
Time to therapy, h (±SD)	4.2 ± 2.8	4.1 ± 2.4
Major endpoints		
35 days mortality, %	9.02	9.53
6 months mortality, %	11.02	12.05
Reinfarction,[a] %	5.0	5.4
Cardiogenic shock,[a] %	4.7	6.0*
Hemorrhagic stroke,[a] %	0.77	0.37
Any stroke,[a] %	1.23	1.00
Major bleeding,[a] %	4.6	4.7

*$P < .05$.
[a]In-hospital events.
Source: Ref. 9.

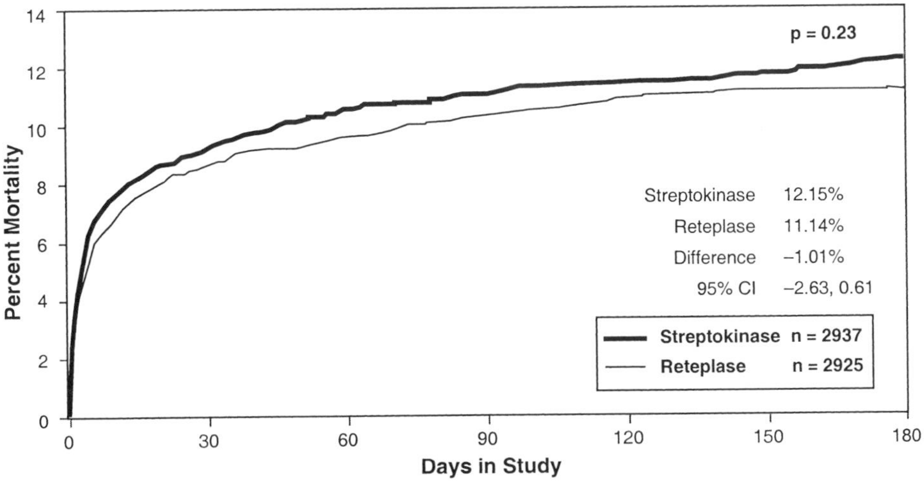

Figure 4 Six-month survival in the INJECT trial. (From Ref. 9.)

GUSTO III

This large-scale Phase III study (3) of 15,059 patients compared the effects of r-PA and t-PA on 30-day mortality of patients with acute myocardial infarction presenting within 6 hours of symptom onset. All patients received aspirin 160 mg and heparin 5000 U bolus followed by a 1000 U/hr infusion (lowered to 800 U/hr for patients weighing <80 kg) adjusted to maintain the aPTT at 50 to 70 sec. The first adjustment of the heparin dose was made 6 hours after lytic administration. Patients were randomly allocated in a 2:1 ratio to either r-PA 10 MU in two bolus doses given 30 min apart, or to weight-adjusted t-PA (maximum 100 mg given in an accelerated fashion over 90 min). Important endpoints included 30-day mortality, freedom from death, and nondisabling stroke, as well as the other common indices of efficacy and safety. The study had an 85% power to detect a 20% relative reduction in mortality with r-PA compared with t-PA.

Important baseline characteristics of the patients are shown in Table 3. Death occurred by 30 days in 7.47% of the r-PA and 7.24% of the t-PA patients (Fig. 5), odds ratio 1.03 (95% confidence interval 0.91 to 1.18), $P = .61$, covariate-adjusted $P = .54$. The 95% confidence intervals for the difference in 30-day mortality were −1.11% to 0.66%. Prespecified subgroup analyses based on age, infarct location, region of treatment, and time to treatment did not indicate any heterogeneity in outcome. At 1 year the two groups continued to have nearly identical rates of death, 11.19% for r-PA and 11.06% for t-PA, $P = .66$ (Fig. 6).

Table 3 Baseline Characteristics of the Patients Enrolled in GUSTO III

	r-Pa (n = 10,038)	t-PA (n = 4,921)
Median age (years)[a]	63 (53, 71)	63 (53, 72)
Age >75 years, %	14	14
Male gender, %	73	73
Previous MI, %	18	18
Diabetes mellitus, %	16	16
Hypertension, %	40	39
Smoking, %	41	41
Median time to therapy, hours[a]	2.7 (1.8, 3.8)	2.7 (1.9, 3.9)
Median heart rate, bpm[a]	73 (62, 86)	73 (62, 86)
Median systolic BP, mm Hg[a]	135 (119, 150)	134 (119, 150)
Anterior MI, %	47	48

[a]25th–75th interquartile range.
Source: Ref. 3.

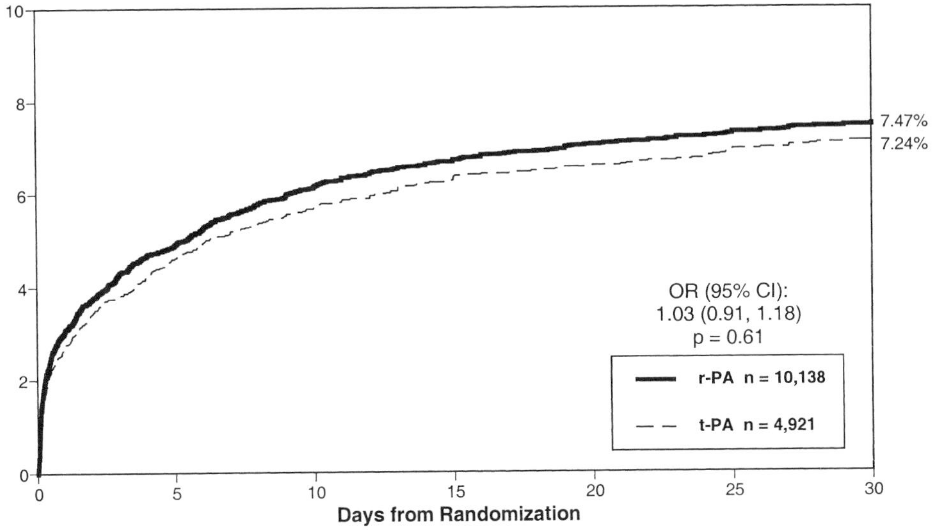

Figure 5 Thirty-day rates of death in the GUSTO III trial.

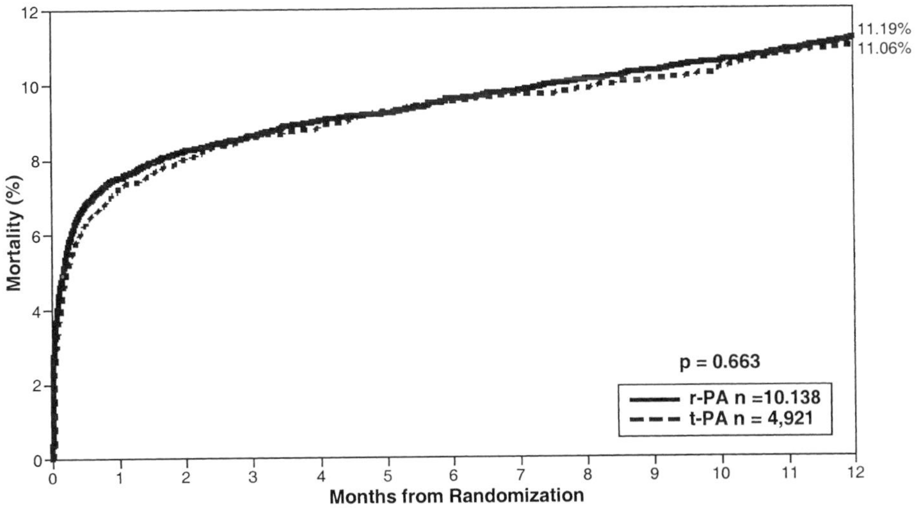

Figure 6 One-year rates of death in the GUSTO III trial.

Table 4 Incidence of Adjudicated Stroke in GUSTO III[a]

Endpoint	r-PA	t-PA
All stroke, %	1.64 (1.39–1.89)	1.79 (1.42–2.16)
Hemorrhagic, %	0.91 (0.73–1.09)	0.87 (0.61–1.13)
Nonhemorrhagic, %	0.60 (0.40–0.75)	0.75 (0.51–0.99)

[a]Percent and 95% confidence intervals.
Source: Ref. 3.

The incidence of stroke was very similar in the two groups (Table 4). Among older patients (>75 years), the incidence of hemorrhagic stroke was insignificantly higher in the r-PA group, 2.5% vs. 1.7%, $P = .21$. The incidence of death or disabling stroke was 7.89% for r-PA and 7.91% for t-PA. The rate of major bleeding was 0.95% and 1.2%, respectively, while the need for blood transfusion was 5.9% and 6.2%, respectively. There was no statistically significant difference in any clinical outcome between the two groups.

Although the trial did not demonstrate superiority of r-PA over t-PA, its favorable safety profile and ease of administration have secured its approval for use in patients with acute myocardial infarction. Possible explanations for the dissociation between improved angiographic patency with r-PA and lack of reduction in mortality include: the lower fibrin-specificity translating in a lower rate of TIMI 3 flow at 30 min compared with t-PA (2); higher rates of reocclusion; overestimation of the angiographic advantage in the Phase II trials; a higher rate and intensity of platelet activation by r-PA; or simply the play of chance.

A prospective evaluation of platelet activation and aggregation following fibrinolysis has been reported by Gurbel et al. (10). At 24 hours after therapy, patients treated with r-PA had a significantly higher rate of aggregation in response to various concentrations of ADP, thrombin, and collagen than patients treated with t-PA. Furthermore, the r-PA patients also had a significantly higher expression of the glycoprotein receptor IIb/IIIa and the platelet-endothelial cell adhesion molecule 1(PECAM-1). However, a more recent and comprehensive evaluation of the effect of r-PA and t-PA on early platelet aggregation showed a higher suppression of platelet activation with r-PA than with t-PA (11). These observations highlight the uncertainty regarding the effect of plasminogen activators on platelet biology and the need for prolonged antiplatelet therapy, particularly 24 hours after r-PA, in preventing late ischemic events.

n-PA (LANOTEPLASE)

n-PA (Fig. 1), a wild-type t-PA mutant, resembles r-PA, and was developed specifically with the intent to allow single bolus administration while enhancing fibrinolytic potency. This molecule lacks the finger and epidermal growth factor domains and has a nonglycosylated moiety at position 117 to enhance fibrin binding (12). Its plasma half-life is 30 to 45 min. In comparison with t-PA, lanoteplase is associated with a lower increase in serum PAI-1 activity, which may contribute to its efficacy, both in vitro and in vivo (13). In animal studies, n-PA demonstrated a 8.8-fold higher potency on a mg/kg basis, compared with t-PA, without a decrease in the degree of fibrin specificity. It caused 20% and 30% reduction in fibrinogen and α_2-antiplasmin, respectively, at doses producing 50% thrombolysis. There was no evidence for immunogenic response to this compound in various animal models.

InTIME I

The Intravenous n-PA for Treating Infarcting Myocardium Early (InTIME I) compared the efficacy and safety of a single bolus of four escalating doses of n-PA (15, 30, 60, and 120 kU/kg) with t-PA (weight-adjusted, accelerated dosing) in 603 patients presenting within 6 hours of onset of an acute myocardial infarction (14). Angiography was performed at 60 and 90 min and on day 3 to 5, and rescue angioplasty was allowed after 90 min, if patency (TIMI 2 or 3 flow) was not achieved. The primary endpoint was the demonstration of a graded dose response relationship with respect to 60 min TIMI 3 flow in the infarct-related artery. The composite clinical endpoint included freedom from death, reinfarction, heart failure, moderate or major bleeding, and revascularization. Patients were treated at an average of 3 hours from symptom onset. As shown in Figure 7, there was a graded response in the incidence of TIMI 3 flow at both 60 and 90 min. The rates of complete and overall patency were superior for the highest dose of n-PA, as compared with accelerated t-PA.

Moderate and major bleeding occurred in 5.7%, 7.3%, 4.9%, and 8.1%, respectively, of the 4 n-PA groups, as compared with 10.5% in the t-PA patients. At 30 days, the composite endpoint was achieved in 87%, 96.3%, 86%, and 89% of the 4 n-PA groups, respectively. These data were not statistically different from the 76% rate observed in the t-PA group.

InTIME II

Based on these promising results, the InTIME 2 study (preliminary results, American College of Cardiology 1999) enrolled 15,078 patients with typical

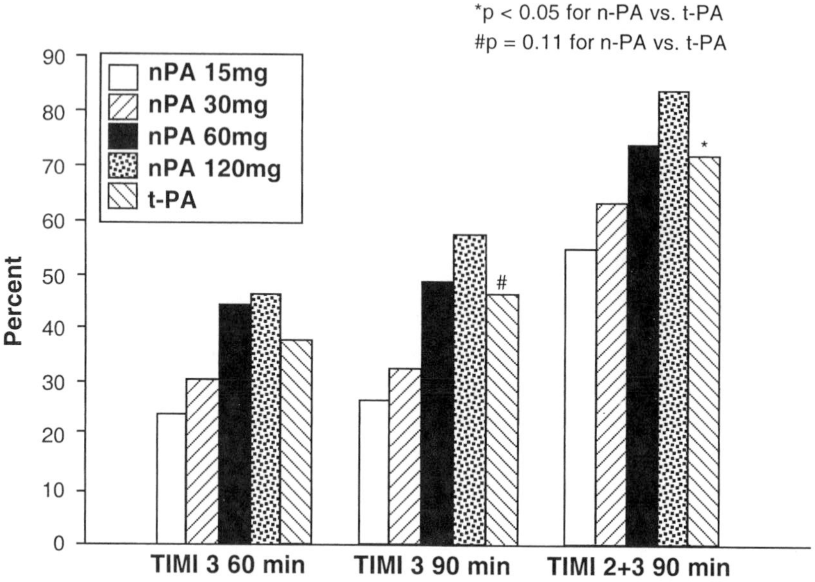

Figure 7 Incidence of TIMI 3 and TIMI 2+3 flow at 60 and 90 min in InTIME I. #*P* = .11 for n-PA vs. t-PA; **P* < .05 for n-PA vs. t-PA.

ST segment elevation acute myocardial infarction within 6 hours of symptom onset in a double-blind randomized trial designed to demonstrate equivalence of n-PA to t-PA with regard to 30-day all-cause mortality. Assuming a mortality of 7.5% in the t-PA arm and accepting a relative risk of <1.196, the study had a 89% power to demonstrate equivalence with one-tailed α of 0.05.

Patients were allocated to n-PA bolus 120 kU/kg or t-PA 100 mg over 90 min, in a 2:1 ratio. All patients received aspirin ≥150 mg and heparin at 70 U/kg (maximum 4000 U) followed by an infusion of 15 U/kg/hr (maximum 1000 U/hr), to maintain the aPTT at 1.5 to 2.0 times the upper limit of normal. Importantly, the adjustment of the aPTT started 6 hours after lytic administration, and halfway through the study this interval was lowered to 3 hours.

Key baseline characteristics of the patients, which were well balanced between the groups, are shown in Table 5. The 30-day mortality of patients in the two groups was very similar at 6.60% (95% confidence interval 5.91 to 7.29) for t-PA and 6.77% (6.28 to 7.36) for n-PA with a relative risk (n-PA/t-PA) of 1.03 (0.91 to 1.17), fulfilling the predetermined criteria for noninferiority (Fig. 8). The 24-hour mortality rates were 2.49% and 2.39%,

Table 5 Baseline Characteristics of the Patients Enrolled in InTIME-II

	n-Pa (n = 10,051)	t-PA (n = 5027)
Mean age, years	61	61.1
Male gender, %	75	75
Previous MI, %	16	15
Diabetes mellitus, %	14	15
Hypertension, %	30	31
Smoking, %	45	45
Mean time to therapy, h	3.1	3.1
Mean heart rate, bpm	76	76
Mean systolic BP, mm Hg	139	139
Anterior MI, %	42	41
Aspirin before MI, %	20	20
Beta-blocker before MI, %	16	15

respectively. The 30-day death rates among patients not suffering intracranial hemorrhage were 6.11% and 6.20%, respectively.

The incidence of total stroke and its components is shown in Table 6. As noted, although the total incidence of stroke was not statistically different between the two lytic agents, a substantially higher incidence of intracranial hemorrhage was noted in the n-PA group, coupled with a lower than usual rate of this event in the t-PA patients. The net clinical benefit, comprising

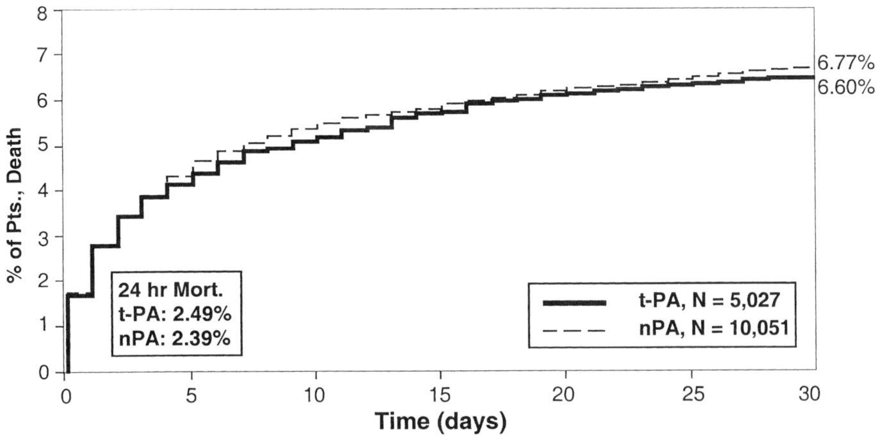

Figure 8 Thirty-day rates of death in InTIME II.

Table 6 Incidence of Adjudicated Stroke in InTIME II

Endpoint	n-PA	t-PA	*P*
All stroke, %	1.89	1.52	.103
Intracranial hemorrhage, %	1.13	0.62	.003
Ischemic infarction, %	0.53	0.62	.490
Hemorrhagic conversion, %	0.14	0.12	.231

death and disabling stroke at 30 days, was 7.00% (6.29 to 7.70) for t-PA and 7.23% (6.72 to 7.73) for n-PA with a relative risk (n-PA/t-PA) of 1.04 (0.92 to 1.17), $P = .61$ (Fig. 9).

Intracranial hemorrhage (ICH) was substantially more common in both lytic groups among patients >75 years, 1.48% and 2.81% for t-PA and n-PA respectively, as compared with 0.48% and 0.86% among patients <75 years. There was no statistical interaction between age and the type of lytic with respect to ICH. Lightweight patients also had a higher rate of ICH than heavier subjects (1.42% and 1.64% vs. 0.39% and 0.99%, respectively). There was a strong trend towards a statistical interaction between weight and type of lytic, $P = .073$.

Major (0.6% in both groups) and minor bleeding (2.3% and 2.4%) were similar in the two groups, as was the need for and extent of blood transfusion. There was statistical significant excess of minor bleeding in the n-PA group, 19.6% vs. 14.7%, $P < .0001$.

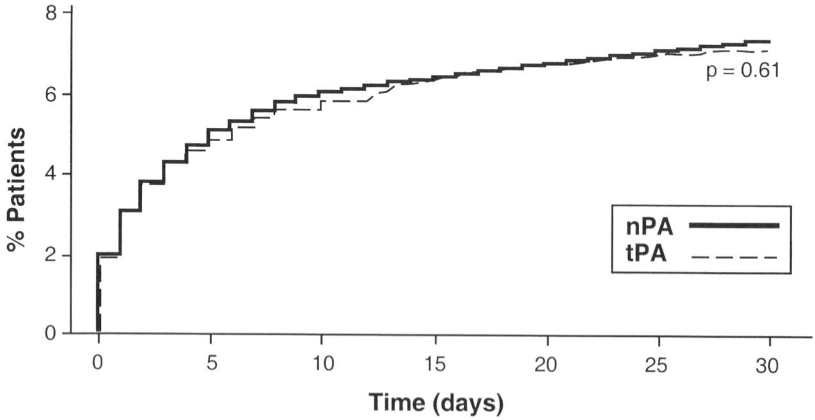

Figure 9 Thirty-day rates of death and/or disabling stroke in InTIME II.

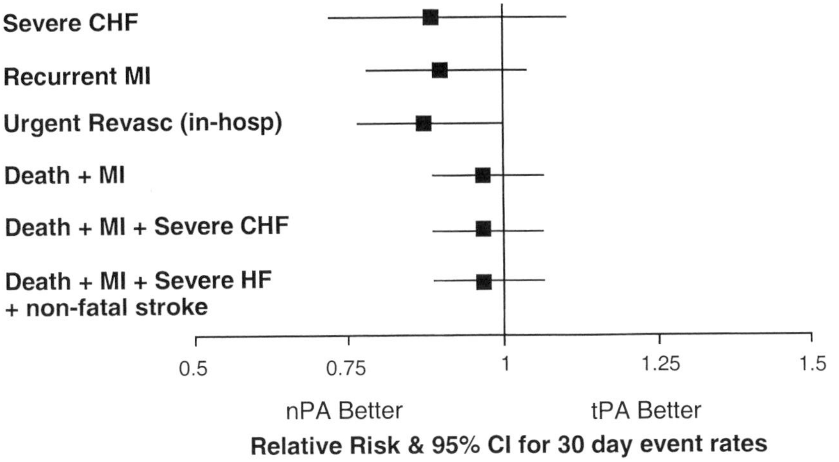

Figure 10 Thirty-day clinical outcome in InTIME II.

All secondary clinical endpoints were insignificantly less frequent in the n-PA group, as shown in Figure 10. There was no significant difference in 30-day mortality among patients with anterior versus inferior infarct, males versus females, smokers versus nonsmokers, younger versus older patients, or those with or without prior infarction (Fig. 11). At 6 months,

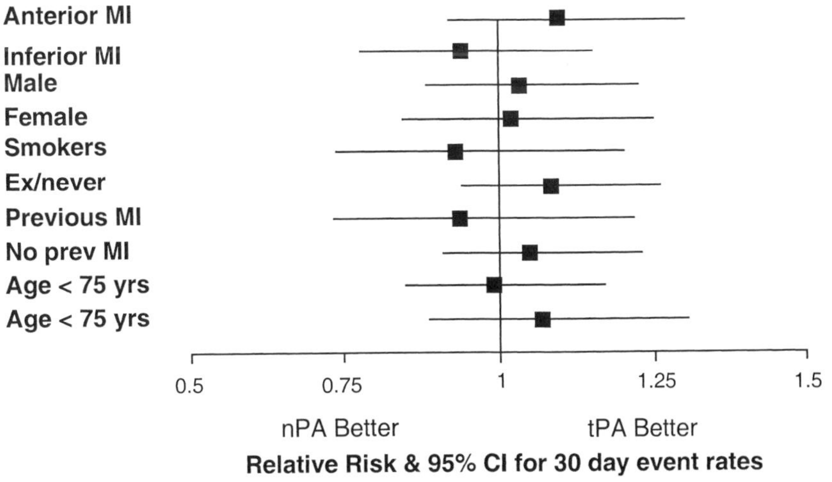

Figure 11 Analysis of 30-day mortality by prespecified subgroups in InTIME II.

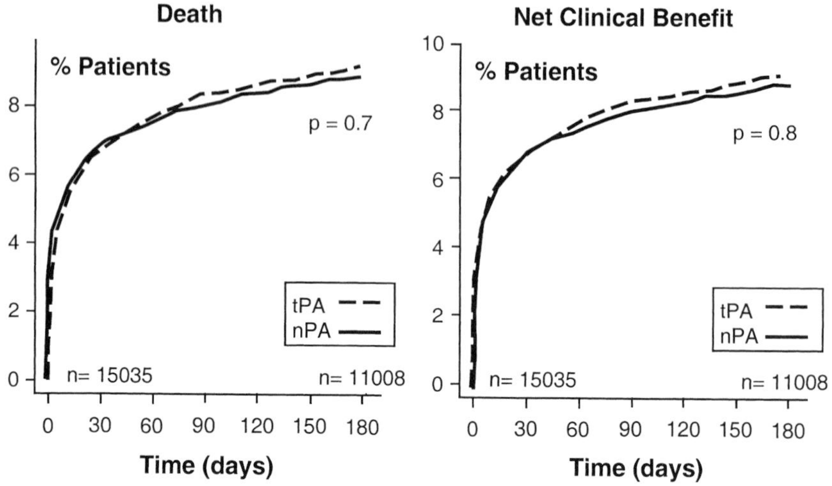

Figure 12 Six months death and death/disabling stroke in InTIME II.

the incidence of death and death and/or disabling stroke remained statistically indistinguishable, $P = .7$ and .8, respectively (Fig. 12).

The InTIME II investigators conducted a registry (InTIME IIb) in which patients received n-PA and had had earlier adjustment of heparin drip. Intracerebral hemorrhage occurred in only 0.68% of patients, compared with 1.00% of those receiving heparin bolus and having first infusion adjustment at 3 hours and 1.22% in those with first adjustment at 6 hours ($P < .001$). Even in the t-PA group, earlier heparin adjustment was associated with a lower intracranial hemorrhage rate (0.51% for 3 hours vs. 0.74% for 6 hours). Because of these results, particularly the heightened incidence of ICH, the further commercial development of lanoteplase remains uncertain at this time.

TNK-tPA (TENECTEPLASE)

The need to improve the pharmacokinetics of t-PA and to reduce its susceptibility to circulating inhibitors led to a systematic approach to submolecular modifications of t-PA and the development of a triple mutant, TNK-t-PA (Fig. 1). It is remarkable for its decreased plasma clearance, increased resistance to PAI-1, and improved fibrin specificity. A threonine (T) at position 103 was substituted by asparagine and added a glycosylation site. An asparagine (N) at position 117 was replaced by glutamine, removing a glycosylation site at that position, slowing plasma clearance and increasing fibrin binding. Finally, lysine, histidine, and two arginines (K) at positions 296 to 299 were replaced by four alanines, which increased fibrin specificity and enhanced resistance to PAI-1 80-fold (15,16). The lack of susceptibility to inactivation by PAI-1 is an important attribute, because it combats the increased levels of PAI-1 secreted by platelets activated by the lytic agent. This compound was tested by Collen et al. (17) in various experimental thrombosis models, and subsequently in clinical studies.

The TIMI 10A Trial

The TIMI (Thrombolysis in Myocardial Infarction) 10A study was a Phase I study designed to find the optimal dose of TNK-t-PA (18). One hundred thirteen patients within 12 hours of the onset of an acute myocardial infarction were allocated to increasing doses of TNK-t-PA (5 to 50 mg), administered as a bolus over 5 to 10 sec. Heparin was used to maintain the activated prothrombin time at 55 to 85 sec for 48 to 72 hours. Angiography at 60 to 90 min was performed in all patients. The important endpoints were the rate of TIMI 3 flow at 90 min, pharmacokinetics, serious bleeding, and standard clinical endpoints. The mean time to treatment was 3.0 hours. The plasma half-life of TNK-t-PA varied from 11 $\pm$ 5 to 20 $\pm$ 6 min, as compared to 3.5 min for t-PA. The patients treated with 30 to 50 mg had a 59% to 64% rate of TIMI 3 flow, significantly higher than those treated with lower doses (0% to 60%; P = .032). Two-thirds of those achieving TIMI 3 flow already demonstrated it by 60 min. There was remarkably little consumption of fibrinogen (3%) and plasminogen (13%), even at the higher doses of TNK-t-PA. The death rate was 3.5%, the reinfarction rate was 4.4%, and serious bleeding was noted in 6.2%. There were no instances of intracranial bleeding or development of antibodies to TNK-t-PA.

TIMI 10B

In view of these promising results, the efficacy of TNK-t-PA was compared directly with accelerated t-PA in the angiographic TIMI 10B trial (19). Eight hundred eighty-six patients with acute ST-elevation myocardial infarction were randomly allocated to an accelerated t-PA regimen, TNK-t-PA 30 mg bolus or TNK-t-PA 50 mg bolus, followed by 90-min angiogram. Due to the high rate of intracranial hemorrhage in the 50-mg arm, the higher dose was reduced to 40 mg, heparin dose was reduced, and dose adjustments were begun at 6 hours. T-PA and TNK-t-PA 40 mg produced nearly identical rates of TIMI 3 flow at 90 min, 62.7% and 62.8%. At 60 min, the respective rates were 48.2% and 48.9%. The patients receiving only 30 mg TNK-t-PA had a significantly lower patency rate at both time points. The overall rate of intracranial hemorrhage was 1.9% for the 40-mg TNK-t-PA and t-PA groups.

A pharmacokinetic susbstudy confirmed the substantially longer elimination half-life of TNK-t-PA and its marked fibrin specificity, causing less than half the depletion in fibirinogen and plasminogen caused by t-PA.

ASSENT I

In Europe, Van de Werf and colleagues enrolled 3235 patients with acute ST segment elevation myocardial infarction of <12 hours duration in a safety and efficacy study of TNK-t-PA, using 30- and 40-mg single-bolus administration. The primary endpoint of the study was the rate of intracranial hemorrhage (ICH) (20). The incidence of ICH was 0.94% for the 30-mg group and 0.62% in the 40-mg group. The slightly higher rate of ICH in the 30-mg group can be attributed in part to the higher dose of heparin given to the first 248 patients, of whom 1.62% had a hemorrhagic stroke, compared with 0.82% in the low-heparin cohort. Death occurred in 6.4% of all patients and major bleeding was noted in 2.8%.

ASSENT-2

In view of its safety and efficacy, as demonstrated in the above-mentioned trials, TNK-t-PA was compared with t-PA in a large, double-blind mortality trial entitled Assessment of the Safety and Efficacy of a New Thrombolytic (ASSENT-2) (21). At 1021 hospitals a total of 16,949 patients presenting within 6 hours of the onset of ST-segment elevation acute myocardial infarction were randomized to weight-adjusted accelerated t-PA (maximum 100 mg) over 90 min (8488 patients) or weight-adjusted TNK-t-PA (30 to 50 mg) as a bolus over 5 to 10 sec (8461 patients). All patients received aspirin 150 to 325 mg and weight-adjusted heparin 4000 and 5000 U bolus followed by an infusion of 800 to 1000 U/hr adjusted to maintain the aPTT at 50 to 75 sec, for 48 to 72 hours. The primary endpoint was 30-day all-cause mortality. A secondary endpoint defined as net clinical benefit measured the incidence of lack of death or nondisabling stroke at 30 days.

The study was designed as an equivalence trial with a 80% power to reject the null hypothesis that TNK-t-PA has a risk of death greater by 1% (absolute) or 14% (relative) than t-PA, assuming a 7.2% event rate in the t-PA group and using a one-sided significance level of 0.05. The primary analysis was non-parametric, covariate-adjusted for age, Killip class, heart rate, systolic blood pressure, and infarct location.

Key baseline characteristics are shown in Table 7, demonstrating adequate randomization. The primary endpoint was achieved in 6.18% and 6.15% of the TNK-t-PA and t-PA groups, fulfilling the criteria for equivalency (Fig. 13).

Table 7 Baseline Characteristics of the Patients Enrolled in ASSENT-2

	TNK-t-PA (n = 8461)	t-PA (n = 8488)
Median age, years[a]	61 (52, 70)	61 (52, 70)
Age >75 years, %	12	13
Male gender, %	77	77
Previous MI, %	16	16
Diabetes mellitus, %	14	15
Hypertension, %	38	39
Smoking, %	45	44
Median time to therapy, hours[a]	2.7 (1.9, 3.8)	2.8 (1.9, 3.9)
Median heart rate, bpm[a]	72 (62, 85)	73 (62, 85)
Median systolic BP, mm Hg[a]	133 (120, 150)	133 (119, 150)
Anterior MI, %	40	40

[a]25th–75th interquartile range.
Source: Ref. 21.

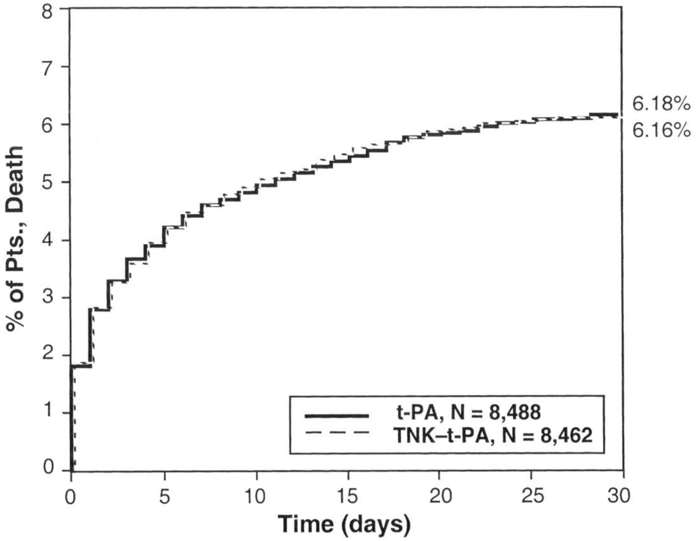

Figure 13 Thirty-day rates of death in ASSENT-2.

Table 8 Incidence of Adjudicated Stroke in ASSENT-2

Endpoint	TNK-t-PA	t-PA	*P*
All stroke, %	1.78	1.66	.555
Intracranial hemorrhage, %	0.93	0.94	1.000
Ischemic infarction, %	0.72	0.64	.514
Hemorrhagic conversion, %	0.07	0.09	.790

Source: Ref. 21.

The incidence of all strokes and its components is shown in Table 8. The incidence of death or nonfatal stroke was 7.11% for TNK-t-PA and 7.04% for t-PA, relative risk 1.01 (0.91 to 1.13). Major noncerebral bleeding was 4.66% and 5.94%, respectively, $P = .0002$ and the total incidence of noncerebral bleeding was 26.4% and 29.0%, respectively, $P = .0003$, resulting in lower incidence and intensity of blood transfusion ($P = .0002$).

There was no significant difference between the groups with respect to in-hospital clinical events or need for percutaneous revascularization, with the exception of the development of heart failure (Killip class >1), which occurred in 6.1% and 7.0%, respectively, $P = .03$. There was a significantly lower incidence of CABG in TNK-t-PA patients, 5.5% versus 6.2%, $P = .05$.

Multiple univariate analyses for death at 30 days were performed with respect to age, gender, time to treatment, infarct location, Killip class, diabetes, hypertension, and previous CABG or MI. Only patients randomized more than 4 from symptom onset demonstrated a lower (unadjusted) mortality for TNK-t-PA compared with t-PA (7.0% vs. 9.2%; $P = .018$). There were no significant differences in outcome in any of the other subgroups.

The demonstrated efficacy of TNK-t-PA coupled with its enhanced safety and ease of administration have led to its approval by the FDA for treatment of patients with acute myocardial infarction.

RECOMBINANT STAPHYLOKINASE

The other third-generation lytic agent to reach human clinical investigation is staphylokinase. Staphylokinase is a 136-amino-acid protein produced by certain strains of *Staphylococcus aureus*. Its thrombolytic properties were initially tested in vitro and in vivo in the 1950s and 1960s (22). At that time it appeared to be of little clinical value due to low efficacy and profound depletion of plasma plasminogen. Renewed interest in staphylokinase emerged after the successful cloning of its gene in 1980, followed by its expression in *Escherichia coli* (23).

Elucidation of its molecular interactions revealed a most interesting mechanism of fibrin selectivity, with great potential for clinical application. Like streptokinase, staphylokinase binds in a 1:1 stochiometric complex with plasminogen. In contrast to streptokinase, the staphylokinase-plasminogen complex is inactive, requiring the transformation to staphylokinase-plasmin to expose its active site and become an effective plasminogen activator. In the absence of fibrin, this latter complex is quickly inactivated by α_2-antiplasmin (a process greatly retarded by fibrin), while its predecessor is not. Furthermore, staphylokinase is released for recycling to other plasminogen molecules after the inactivation occurs.

The interactions described above confer staphylokinase a unique mechanism for fibrin selectivity. First, the agent is not activated in the absence of fibrin. In contrast, where fibrin is present, small amounts of plasmin on the fibrin surface form an active staphylokinase-plasmin complex, bound to fibrin via the lysine binding sites of plasmin, and protected from rapid inhibition by α_2-antiplasmin. Later on, after the thrombus undergoes dissolution, the staphylokinase-plasmin complex is released and inactivated, effectively interrupting further plasminogen activation.

Collen and Van de Werf (24) reported the initial clinical experience with recombinant staphylokinase (STAR) in 1993. Five patients presenting with an acute myocardial infarction of <6 hours' duration, received a 10-mg infusion of STAR over 30 min. At 40 min, TIMI 3 flow had been reestablished in four of the five patients. Reocclusion had occurred in one patient by 24 hours, while the patient with persistent infarct artery occlusion at the initial angiogram demonstrated delayed recanalization. No bleeding complications were observed.

Three other important aspects were clarified by this pilot study. First, there was no appreciable decrease in the levels of fibrinogen and α_2-antiplasmin (5% to 10% from baseline), confirming the agent's remarkable fibrin selectivity. Second, there was a gradual, time-dependent elevation in the fibrin fragment D-dimer, suggesting detectable fibrin digestion in vivo. Finally, it could be determined that STAR-related antigen is cleared from the plasma in a biphasic mode, with a terminal half-life of 37 ± 15 min. At 14 to 35 days after the infusion, antibody-mediated STAR-neutralizing activity could be detected in plasma, which did not crossreact with streptokinase. Collen et al. (25) reported on two new staphylokinase variants, SakSTAR$_{[K74]}$, which has a single substitution of lysine at position 74 with alanine, and SakSTAR$_{[K74ER]}$, which, in addition, has glutamine at position 75 and arginine at position 77 also substituted with alanine. These two mutants show significantly less neutralizing antibody induction, as compared to the unaltered SakSTAR. Larger scale, controlled studies were required to confirm these findings.

The Staphylokinase Versus t-PA Trial

Vanderschueren et al. (26) enrolled 100 patients with an evolving myocardial infarction in an open trial comparing 10 mg (23 patients), or 20 mg (25 patients) of STAR given over 30 min with an accelerated dosing regimen of weight-adjusted t-PA (52 patients). Angiography was performed at baseline, 90 min, and 24 hours. PTCA or additional thrombolysis was undertaken if patency (TIMI flow > grade 1) was not restored. TIMI 3 flow at 90 min was achieved in 62% and 58% of the STAR and t-PA groups, respectively. There was a trend toward higher patency rates in patients treated with the higher versus lower dose of STAR (74% vs. 50%). There was no statistical difference in the incidence of bleeding events (21% for STAR vs. 31% for t-PA), most of which were minor. No allergic reactions or intracerebral hemorrhage were observed. The study population was too small to effectively compare the rate of reinfarction, or death. As compared with t-PA, STAR significantly reduced the consumption of fibrinogen, plasminogen, and α_2-antiplasmin, and the prolongation of the activated prothrombin time (aPTT). The majority of patients treated with staphylokinase demonstrated neutralizing antibodies one week after treatment.

CAPTORS

A modified SAKSTAR, SAK 42D was tested recently in the Collaborative Angiographic Patency Trial of Recombinant Staphylokinase (CAPTORS) (27). Eighty-two patients (43% anterior infarct, presenting at an average of 2.7 hours from chest pain onset) were randomized to 15, 30, or 45 mg SAK 42D, given as a 20% bolus and an 80% infusion over 30 min. The primary endpoint, TIMI 3 flow at 90 min, occurred in 62%, 65%, and 63% of the three groups, respectively (*P* not significant). There were no intracerebral hemorrhages and no severe bleeding episodes.

In order to reduce the agent's clearance and enable bolus administration, the molecule of SAKSTAR was combined with polyethyleneglycol (28). This compound has demonstrated absolute fibrin specificity and in a small trial achieved TIMI 3 flow at 60 min in 14 of 18 patients treated (78%). Further investigation is planned.

KEY MESSAGES FROM THIRD-GENERATION FIBRINOLYTIC COMPARATIVE TRIALS

Two important concepts have evolved from these three large clinical trials. The first refers to the design of studies comparing two strategies with similar

Table 9 Anticoagulation and Hemorrhagic Stroke in t-PA Patients

Study	Heparin bolus	Heparin infusion	Target aPTT	1s aPTT change	ICH
GUSTO I	5000 U	1000/1200 U/h[a]	60–85 sec	12 h	0.72%
GUSTO III	5000 U	800/1000 U/h[a]	50–70 sec	6 h	0.87%
ASSENT-2	5000/4000 U[b]	1000/800 U/h[b]	50–75 sec	6 h	0.94%
InTIME-II	≤4000 U	≤1000 U/h	50–60 sec	6 h	0.71%
InTIME-II	≤4000 U	≤1000 U/h	50–70 sec	3 h	0.52%

[a]Weight >80 kg.
[b]Weight <67 kg.
Source: Ref. 30.

outcome. When GUSTO III failed to show superiority of r-PA over t-PA, despite positive angiographic and clinical results from small Phase II trials, it became evident that equivalence trials are better able to fulfill statistical requirements, while preserving a clinically meaningful endpoint and a reasonable sample size. The difficult decision was to identify an acceptable difference between the control and experimental arms that would still be viewed as clinically insignificant. Such a "confidence interval" was mostly derived from the difference in outcome between t-PA and streptokinase in the GUSTO I trial.

The second important lesson was the safety aspects of new lytic agents. The incidence of intracranial hemorrhage has not declined despite refinements in therapy, and has even increased in some of the trials. Table 9 synthesizes the relation between intensity of concomitant anticoagulation and hemorrhagic stroke. Weight-adjusted heparin bolus and infusion rate and early adjustment of the heparin dose based on aPTT appear to be important in minimizing the incidence of stroke. Caution should be exerted in reducing the intensity of anticoagulation in view of the potential relation between mortality and aPTT (29).

THE IDEAL FIBRINOLYTIC AGENT

The properties required from the perfect fibrinolytic agent have not changed and are listed in Table 10. Ideally, the agent would restore TIMI 3 flow in 100% of patients, within a few minutes of its administration. To ensure these properties, enhanced lytic potency, combined with slow plasma clearance (allowing bolus administration) are vital. It would be directed exclusively against the coronary thrombus, by virtue of its marked fibrin specificity, and display significant resistance against plasminogen activator inhibitors present

Table 10 Main Characteristics of the Ideal Fibrinolytic Agent

Characteristic	Goal
Enhanced potency	TIMI 3 flow in ~100% of patients
Rapid onset of action	Clot lysis in 5–15 min
Improved tissue perfusion	Prevent or reduce microvascular obstruction
Slow plasma clearance	Bolus administration, sustained action
Fibrin specificity	No or minimal fibrinogen degradation
Decreased bleeding tendency	0–0.2% intracerebral hemorrhage
Lysis of platelet-rich thrombi	
Low cost	

in the clot vicinity. This specificity can be achieved either by immunologically mediated targeting (antifibrin antibody), or by linking its action to a factor present only in fibrin. By activating only fibrin-bound plasminogen, the ideal fibrinolytic agent would minimize the depletion of the circulating plasminogen activator inhibitors and prevent widespread fibrinogen degradation. Preservation of adequate plasma fibrinogen levels would lead to continuous replenishment of the thrombus milieu with fresh fibrinogen, the substrate for plasmin-induced lysis. Enhanced fibrin specificity would reduce the hazards of reocclusion and intracerebral hemorrhage, currently observed with moderately specific lytics.

The drug should incorporate the ability to penetrate and dissolve platelet-rich thrombi, especially since this component exists universally at the site of plaque rupture and to minimize platelet activation after lysis. Lack of an immunogenic response is required to permit repeat administration for reinfarction, and the cost for such an agent should promote its use for most patients with an acute ST-segment elevation myocardial infarction.

Importantly, these structural and physiologic properties should translate into clinical benefit, with respect to mortality, left ventricular dysfunction (improvement of tissue perfusion), and major bleeding complications.

CONCLUSIONS

Intravenous fibrinolytic therapy is the most widely applied and investigated therapy for acute myocardial infarction. Since its initial introduction in the mid-1980s, significant strides have been taken to widen its application, enhance its efficacy, and reduce its complications. Yet, there remains considerable room for improvement. Currently, only slightly better than half of the infarct-related arteries achieve complete and sustained patency with the weight-adjusted, accelerated regimen of t-PA and adjunctive aspirin and heparin therapy, while mortality and morbidity remain at a suboptimal level.

Abundant evidence links the immediate infarct artery patency with early and late mortality and morbidity after an acute myocardial infarction. Emerging data emphasize not only the importance of epicardial patency—a prerequisite for tissue perfusion—but also the existence of downstream flow into the myocytes as a marker for good prognosis. The ability to detect microvascular obstruction with ECG, contrast myocardial echocardiography, and magnetic resonance should enable better assessment of the true efficacy of the new agents.

Of the new plasminogen activators described in this chapter, r-PA is the first of the third-generation fibrinolytic agents to be established as an alternative to accelerated t-PA therapy. TNK-t-PA is an excellent fibrinolytic agent with unique pharmacokinetic properties and less bleeding complications than t-PA. Staphylokinase possesses a unique mechanism of action, and awaits confirmation of its clinical utility. Nevertheless, none of the new agents to date have provided improved efficacy compared with t-PA.

Importantly, the focus of fibrinolytic therapy has to shift from an angiographic one to an "end-organ" approach dedicated to better perfusion at the tissue level. This transition is based on the understanding of the factors governing tissue perfusion, the interaction of the thrombus and vessel wall with platelets and the maintenance of arterial patency after initial reperfusion. As described elsewhere, combination fibrin and platelet lysis promises to facilitate this shift.

REFERENCES

1. GUSTO Angiographic Investigators. The effects of tissue plasminogen activator, streptokinase, or both on coronary-artery patency, ventricular function, and survival after acute myocardial infarction. N Engl J Med 1993;329:1615–1621.
2. Bode C, Smalling RW, Berg G, Burnett C, Lorch G, Kalbfleisch JM, Chernoff R, Christie LG, Feldman RL, Seals AA, Weaver WD. Randomized comparison of coronary thrombolysis achieved with double-bolus reteplase (recombinant plasminogen activator) and front-loaded, accelerated alteplase (recombinant tissue plasminogen activator) in patients with acute myocardial infarction. The RAPID II Investigators. Circulation 1996;94:891–898.
3. Investigators TGI. A comparison of reteplase and alteplase for acute myocardial infarction. N Engl J Med 1997;337:1118–1123.
4. Hu CK, Kohnert U, Wilhelm O, Fischer S, Llinas M. Tissue-type plasminogen activator domain-deletion mutant BM 06.022: modular stability, inhibitor binding, and activation cleavage. Biochemistry 1994;33:11760–11766.
5. Martin U, Sponer G, Strein K. Evaluation of thrombolytic and systemic effects of the novel recombinant plasminogen activator BM 06.022 compared with

alteplase, anistreplase, streptokinase and urokinase in a canine model of coronary artery thrombosis. J Am Coll Cardiol 1992;19:433–440.
6. Martin U, van Mollendorf E, Akpan W, et al. Pharmacokinetic and hemostatic properties of the recombinant plasminogen activator BM 06.022 in healthy volunteers. Thromb Haemost 1991;66:569–574.
7. Neuhaus KL, von Essen R, Vogt A, Tebbe U, Rustige J, Wagner HJ, Appel KF, Stienen U, Konig R, Meyer-Sabellek W. Dose finding with a novel recombinant plasminogen activator (BM 06.022) in patients with acute myocardial infarction: results of the German Recombinant Plasminogen Activator Study. A study of the Arbeitsgemeinschaft Leitender Kardiologischer Krankenhausarzte (ALKK). J Am Coll Cardiol 1994;24:55–60.
8. Smalling RW, Bode C, Kalbfleisch J, Sen S, Limbourg P, Forycki F, Habib G, Feldman R, Hohnloser S, Seals A. More rapid, complete, and stable coronary thrombolysis with bolus administration of reteplase compared with alteplase infusion in acute myocardial infarction. RAPID Investigators. Circulation 1995; 91:2725–2732.
9. INJECT Investigators. International Joint Efficacy Comparison of Thrombolytics. Randomized, double-blind comparison of reteplase double-bolus administration with streptokinase in acute myocardial infarction (INJECT): trial to investigate equivalence. Lancet 1995;346:329–336.
10. Gurbel PA, Serebruany VL, Shustov AR, Bahr RD, Carpo C, Ohman EM, Topol EJ. Effects of reteplase and alteplase on platelet aggregation and major receptor expression during the first 24 hours of acute myocardial infarction treatment. GUSTO-III Investigators. Global Use of Strategies to Open Occluded Coronary Arteries. J Am Coll Cardiol 1998;31:1466–1473.
11. Moser M, Nordt T, Peter K, Ruef J, Kohler B, Schimttner M, Smalling R, Kubler W, Bode C. Platelet function during and after thrombolytic therapy for acute myocardial infarction with reteplase, alteplase, or streptokinase. Circulation 1999;100:1858–1864.
12. Hansen L, Blue Y, Barone K, Collen D, Larsen GR. Functional effects of asparagine-linked oligosaccharide on natural and variant human tissue-type plasminogen activator. J Biol Chem 1988;263:15713–15719.
13. Ogata N, Ogawa H, Ogata Y, Numata Y, Morigami Y, Suefuji H, Soejima H, Sakamoto T, Yasue H. Comparison of thrombolytic therapies with mutant tPA (lanoteplase/SUN9216) and recombinant tPA (alteplase) for acute myocardial infarction. Jpn Cir J 1998;62:801–806.
14. den Heijer P, Vermeer F, Ambrosioni E, Sadowski Z, Lopez-Sendon JL, von Essen R, Beaufils P, Thadani U, Adgey J, Pierard L, Brinker J, Davies RF, Smalling RW, Wallentin L, Caspi A, Pangerl A, Trickett L, Hauck C, Henry D, Chew P. Evaluation of a weight-adjusted single-bolus plasminogen activator in patients with myocardial infarction: a double-blind, randomized angiographic trial of lanoteplase versus alteplase. Circulation 1998;98:2117–2125.
15. Paoni T, Keyt B, Refino C, Chow A, Nguyen H, Berleau L, Badillo J, Pena L, Brady K, Wurm F, Ogez G, Bennett W. A slow clearing, fibrin-specific, PAI-1 resistant variant of t-PA. (T103N, KHRR 296-299 AAAA). Thromb Haemost 1993;70:307–312.

16. Refino C, Paoni N, Keyt B, Pater C, Badillo J, Wurm F, Ogez G, Bennett W. A variant of t-PA (T103N, KHRR 296-299 AAAA) that, by bolus, has increased potency and decreased systemic activation of plasminogen. Thromb Haemost 1993;70:313–319.
17. Collen D, Stassen JM, Yasuda T, Refino C, Paoni N, Keyt B, Roskams T, Guerrero JL, Lijnen HR, Gold HK, et al. Comparative thrombolytic properties of tissue-type plasminogen activator and of a plasminogen activator inhibitor-1-resistant glycosylation variant, in a combined arterial and venous thrombosis model in the dog. Thromb Haemost 1994;72:98–104.
18. Cannon C, McCabe C, Gibson M, Ghali M, Sequeira R, McKendall G, Breed J, Modi N, Fox N, Tracy R, Lowe T, Braunwald E, Investigators ftTA. TNK-tissue pasminogen activator in acute myocardial infarction. Results of the Thrombolysis in Myocardial Infarction (TIMI) 10A dose-ranging study. Circulation 1997;95:351–356.
19. Cannon CP, Gibson CM, McCabe CH, Adgey AA, Schweiger MJ, Sequeira RF, Grollier G, Giugliano RP, Frey M, Mueller HS, Steingart RM, Weaver WD, Van de Werf F, Braunwald E. TNK-tissue plasminogen activator compared with front-loaded alteplase in acute myocardial infarction: results of the TIMI 10B trial. Circulation 1998;98:2805–2814.
20. Van de Werf F, Cannon CP, Luyten A, Houbracken K, McCabe CH, Berioli S, Bluhmki E, Sarelin H, Wang-Clow F, Fox NL, Braunwald E. Safety assessment of single-bolus administration of TNK tissue plasminogen activator in acute myocardial infarction: the ASSENT-1 trial. Am Heart J 1999;137:786–791.
21. ASSENT-2 Investigators. Single-bolus tenecteplase compared with front-loaded alteplase in acute myocardial infarction: the ASSENT-2 double-blind randomized trial. Lancet 1999;354:716–722.
22. Collen D, Lijnen HR. Staphylokinase, a fibrin-specific plasminogen activator with therapeutic potential? Blood 1994;84:680–686.
23. Schlott B, Hartmann M, Guhrs KH, Birch-Hirschfeid E, Pohl HD, Vanderschueren S, Van de Werf F, Michoel A, Collen D, Behnke D. High yield production and purification of recombinant staphylokinase for thrombolytic therapy. Bio/Technology 1994;12:185–189.
24. Collen D, Van de Werf F. Coronary thrombolysis with recombinant staphylokinase in patients with evolving myocardial infarction. Circulation 1993;87: 1850–1853.
25. Collen D, Stockx L, Lacroix H, Suy R, Vanderschueren S. Recombinant staphylokinase variants with altered immunoreactivity. IV. Identification of variants with reduced antibody induction but intact potency. Circulation 1997;95: 463–472.
26. Vanderschueren S, Barrios L, Kerdsinchai P, Van den Heuvel P, Hermans L, Vrolix M, De Man F, Benit E, Muyldermans L, Collen D. A randomized trial of recombinant staphylokinase versus alteplase for coronary artery patency in acute myocardial infarction. Circulation 1995;92:2044–2049.
27. Armstrong PW, Burton JR, Palisaitis D, Thompson CR, Van de Werf F, Rose BF, Collen D, Teo KK. Collaborative Angiographic Patency Trial of Recombinant Staphylokinase (CAPTORS). Circulation 199;100:I-650. Abstract.

28. Sinnaeve P, Janssens S, Van deWerf F, Collen D. Single bolus administration of polyethilene glycol-derivated cysteine substitution variants of recombinant staphylokinase in acute myocardial infarction. Circulation 1999;100:I-650. Abstract.
29. Granger CB, Hirsch J, Califf RM, Col J, White HD, Betriu A, Woodlief LH, Lee KL, Bovill EG, Simes RJ, Topol EJ. Activated partial thromboplastin time and outcome after thrombolytic therapy for acute myocardial infarction: results from the GUSTO-I trial. Circulation 1996;93:870–878.
30. Giugliano RP, Cutler SS, Llevadot J. Risk of intracranial hemorrhage with accelerated t-PA: importance of the heparin dose. Circulation 1999;100:I-650. Abstract.

11

Combination Fibrinolysis and Platelet IIb/IIIa Antagonism for Acute Myocardial Infarction

Sorin J. Brener
The Cleveland Clinic Foundation
Cleveland
and Ohio State University
Columbus, Ohio

INTRODUCTION

Despite impressive advances in the treatment of acute myocardial infarction, we continue to face important challenges. While there is abundant evidence that rapid, complete, and durable epicardial artery patency is associated with improved survival and left ventricular function (1,2), it is increasingly obvious that tissue perfusion is less predictably achieved (3,4) and plays a key role in translating flow into myocardial salvage. Strategies directed at improving it are currently lacking or suboptimal.

The paradigm of rapid arterial reperfusion with intravenous fibrinolysis has reached a ceiling of efficacy that can not be surpassed by the currently available, third-generation agents (see Chap. 10). More than 50% of treated patients do not achieve full reperfusion within 60 min of therapy, and a full 40% have less than Thrombolysis in Myocardial Infarction (TIMI) 3 flow (5) at 90 min. Some of the limitations of this therapy flow from its potential to activate platelets and "rev up" the coagulation cascade by liberating clot-bound thrombin. While efficacy is suboptimal, safety considerations preclude the administration of these agents to patients at high risk for intracranial hemorrhage, particularly elderly patients with poorly controlled hypertension and previous manifestations of cerebrovascular disease. Even when the therapy is successful, early (6,7) and late reocclusion (8–10) minimize its effectiveness.

The alternative approach to pharmacological reperfusion—direct angioplasty—is very effective (11) in restoring epicardial artery flow but is limited by a lack of timely availability, high cost, and significant potential for restenosis. Recently, coronary stents have gained popularity and acceptance as the preferred strategy of revascularization in acute myocardial infarction. Yet, the microvascular dysfunction associated with stent insertion may be more severe than that observed with balloon angioplasty alone because of more pronounced thrombus and plaque embolization. Indeed, the rate of TIMI 3 flow following stenting is slightly inferior to that with angioplasty (12).

New pathophysiologic insight into the biology of acute plaque rupture unequivocally places platelet activation and aggregation at the center of the events surrounding the formation of coronary thrombus (13). As it became clear that inhibition of platelet aggregation with aspirin is insufficient, the pivotal discovery of the glycoprotein IIb/IIIa receptor has speared the synthesis of potent inhibitors of this final common pathway of platelet function. Furthermore, experimental evidence in animals and humans pointed to the ability of platelet inhibitors to cause "dethrombosis," or reverse the process of fibrin deposition on a biological template provided by the cellular membrane of aggregating platelets (14).

Because of these challenges and considerations, combination fibrin and platelet lysis has the following theoretical advantages:

1. It can arrest and modify the process of coronary thrombosis, thus promoting faster and more complete restoration of flow in a larger proportion of patients.
2. It can improve tissue perfusion by minimizing the deleterious effects of thrombus embolization, which are often related to platelet degranulation and activation.
3. It can obviate the need for, or facilitate the performance of immediate percutaneous revascularization in patients who fail to reperfuse or are selected for immediate mechanical revascularization on clinical grounds.
4. By employing a lower dose of fibrinolytics, it can reduce the most severe complications of full-dose lytics, particularly intracranial hemorrhage.

I will review in this chapter the early results of combination full-dose fibrin and platelet lysis and summarize in detail three contemporary trials of platelet inhibition with reduced-dose fibrinolysis. Finally, the ongoing efforts designed to solidify a new paradigm of reperfusion centered on the inhibition of the platelet GP IIb/IIIa receptor will be presented together with the remaining areas of investigation.

EARLY TRIALS OF COMBINATION FIBRIN AND PLATELET LYSIS

The initial efforts of combining these two antithrombotic therapies were directed mostly at preventing reocclusion following initial patency, and revolved around a plasminogen activator-based regimen, to which GP IIb/IIIa inhibition was added. This approach was based on the assumption that a large amount of plasminogen activator is needed and on the lack of appreciation of the prothrombotic effect of these agents.

Thrombolysis and Angioplasty in Myocardial Infarction (TAMI) 8

Kleiman et al. (15) conducted a pilot study in 60 patients treated with t-PA, aspirin, and heparin (control group) and ascending doses of the monoclonal antibody 7E3 (abciximab precursor) initiated at various intervals after fibrinolysis (3 to 15 hours). Arterial patency (TIMI 2 and 3 flow) was detected in 56% of the control group and 92% of the 7E3 patients without an increase in major bleeding complications. Optimal platelet inhibition was obtained at a bolus dose of 0.25 mg/kg.

IMPACT AMI

The IMPACT-AMI investigators (16) extended this concept to a dose-ranging trial in which 180 patients with acute myocardial infarction were treated with accelerated full-dose t-PA and a peptide inhibitor of the GP IIb/IIIa receptor, eptifibatide, given in escalating doses. The primary endpoint was the rate of TIMI 3 flow at 90 min. The highest dose eptifibatide used—180 μg/kg bolus and 0.75 μg/kg/min infusion for 24 hours—achieved TIMI 3 flow in 66%, compared with 39% in t-PA alone patients ($P = .006$). Importantly, the time to complete ST segment deviation resolution was markedly reduced in the optimal eptifibatide group, from a median of 116 min to 65 min ($P = .05$), indicating better and faster tissue perfusion. Severe bleeding complications occurred in 4% of the high-dose eptifibatide (one patient had intracranial hemorrhage) and 5% of t-PA control patients, while severe thrombocytopenia was found in 4% and 6%, respectively. Platelet inhibition appeared to be consistently above 70% in the highest dose of eptifibatide, but subsequent studies have demonstrated a much lower inhibition with this dose when calcium-rich plasma is tested (17).

Eptifibatide and Streptokinase in Acute MI

In Europe, eptifibatide was tested in a similar study in combination with streptokinase (18). One hundred eighty-one patients with acute myocardial infarction received aspirin, heparin, and full-dose streptokinase, 1.5 million units, as well as eptifibatide or placebo. The doses of eptifibatide tested were 180 μg/kg bolus followed by an infusion of 0.75 (IMPACT-AMI dose), 1.33 or 2.0 (PURSUIT doses) (19) μg/kg/min. The primary endpoint—TIMI 3 flow at 90 min—was achieved in 38% of the streptokinase-alone group and 53%, 44% and 52% of the eptifibatide groups, respectively. The two higher doses of the platelet inhibitor were associated with an incidence of moderate or severe bleeding (1) of 40%, compared with 16% and 3% for the low-dose eptifibatide and streptokinase-alone groups, respectively. The lack of a significant dose-effect response in arterial patency and the high rate of bleeding led to the discontinuation of the enrollment in the high-dose group.

PARADIGM

The Platelet Aggregation Receptor Antagonist Dose Investigation and Reperfusion Gain in Myocardial Infarction (PARADIGM) investigators enrolled 353 patients with acute MI of <12 hours in three phases of a dose-finding study (20). All patients received aspirin and heparin; t-PA (75% of patients) or streptokinase (25%) was administered in the usual fashion. Placebo or lamifiban (a highly selective nonpeptide inhibitor of the GP IIb/IIIa receptor) in escalating doses of 300 to 400 μg/kg bolus and infusions of 1.0, 1.5, or 2.0 μg/kg/min for 24 hours was added. The primary efficacy endpoint was achievement of ≥85% platelet inhibition in response to ADP (10 μmol/L) and thrombin receptor agonist peptide (TRAP). At the highest dose (400/2.0), lamifiban induced marked platelet inhibition both after the bolus (86% and 63% for ADP and TRAP, respectively) and at steady state (91% and 78%, respectively). The effects of lamifiban were more pronounced in the streptokinase-treated patients. As in IMPACT-AMI, time to steady-state recovery of the ST-segment deviation was shortened by lamifiban from 122 to 88 min (P = .003). The patients enrolled in this study did not undergo systematic angiography, precluding the correlation between ST-segment recovery and angiographically documented arterial patency. Adverse clinical events occurred insignificantly less often in the patients treated with lamifiban than placebo, and major bleeding was noted in 3.0% and 1.7%, respectively.

GP IIb/IIIa INHIBITION AND REDUCED-DOSE FIBRINOLYSIS

The early trials described above have demonstrated the feasibility of combining platelet and fibrin antagonists. A consistent outcome appeared to be a more rapid normalization of the ECG, suggesting less microvascular dysfunction after reperfusion. There was a higher rate of TIMI 3 flow in IMPACT-AMI, although the improvement did not constitute a major breakthrough beyond the effect of full-dose t-PA alone, considering the fact that the 39% rate of TIMI 3 flow in the t-PA group was significantly lower than previous reports for this agent. The combination of eptifibatide and streptokinase did not substantially improve arterial patency, and resulted in high bleeding rates hinting to the "incompatibility" of platelet antagonists and non-fibrin-specific plasminogen activators. Thus, the next phase in developing a viable new strategy of reperfusion focused on truly breaking the "efficacy ceiling" of lytic agents without excess bleeding, maximizing tissue perfusion and facilitating percutaneous revascularization, when necessary. Three trials, described below, addressed these challenges.

Thrombolysis in Myocardial Infarction (TIMI) 14

Between March 1997 and June 1998, 888 patients <75 years with an acute myocardial infarction of <12 hours were enrolled at 63 centers in North America and Europe in a multiphase reperfusion trial (21). The protocol is depicted in Figure 1. Essentially, patients were randomized to either t-PA alone with standard-dose heparin, abciximab alone with low-dose heparin,

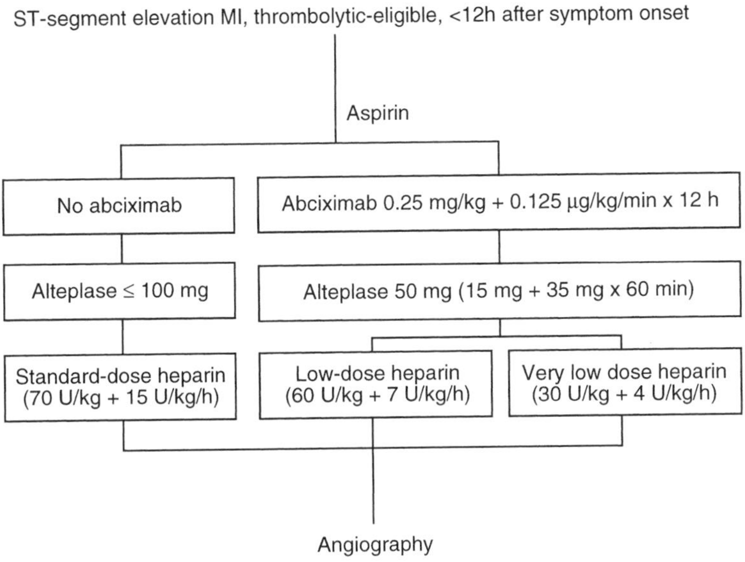

Figure 1 Protocol of the TIMI 14 trial. (From Ref. 21.)

or a variety of regimens comprising reduced-dose streptokinase or t-PA with low-dose heparin. This is the first trial to base reperfusion therapy on platelet antagonism rather than fibrinolysis. All patients underwent control angiography at 60 and 90 min and rescue angioplasty, when feasible and indicated, for TIMI flow <3 at 90 min. The baseline characteristics of the patients are summarized in Table 1. The majority were current smokers and a third had an anterior infarct. The median time from symptom onset to therapy was 3 hours.

The highest rate of TIMI 3 flow at 60 and 90 min was achieved by the combination of half-dose t-PA (15-mg bolus and 35 mg over 1 hour) and full-dose abciximab for 12 hours. The combination of streptokinase and abciximab was inferior to t-PA alone and caused more bleeding. Representative rates of TIMI 3 flow in the best regimens are shown in Figure 2. The most potent independent predictors of achieving TIMI 3 flow at 90 min are shown in Figure 3, highlighting that neither infarct location nor time to treatment was as important as the use of abciximab. Importantly, the choice of lytic (comparing t-PA with r-PA in a subsequent extension of the trial) did not affect significantly angiographic patency.

At both 60 and 90 min the median corrected TIMI frame count (cTFC) was significantly lower in patients receiving abciximab and t-PA compared with either alone, as shown in Table 2. This aspect of facilitated reperfusion was supported by observations from the ECG ST-segment resolution study incorporated in TIMI 14. Complete ST-segment resolution (>70% from baseline) was significantly more common in all patients treated with the combination regimen than with t-PA alone (59% vs. 37%; $P = .001$) and even among those who achieved TIMI 3 flow at 90 minutes (69% vs. 44%, respectively, $P = .001$) (22).

Table 1 Baseline Characteristics of Patients in TIMI 14

Characteristic	Value[a]
Number	888
Age, years	58 (50, 67)
Male gender	684 (77)
Diabetes mellitus	111 (13)
Hypertension	233 (26)
Prior infarct	110 (13)
Index anterior infarct	330 (37)
Current smoker	461 (52)
Symptom onset to therapy, h	3 (2, 5)

[a]Number (%) or median with 25th to 75th interquartile range.

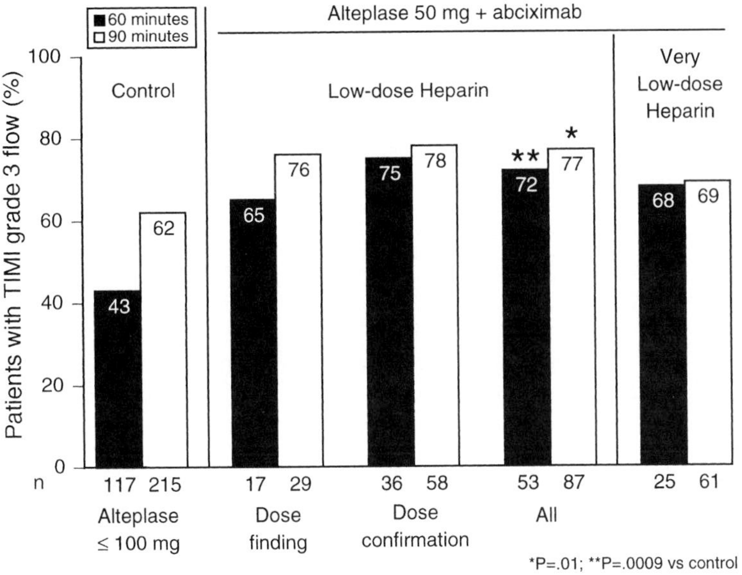

Figure 2 TIMI 3 flow at 60 and 90 min in TIMI 14. (From Ref. 21.)

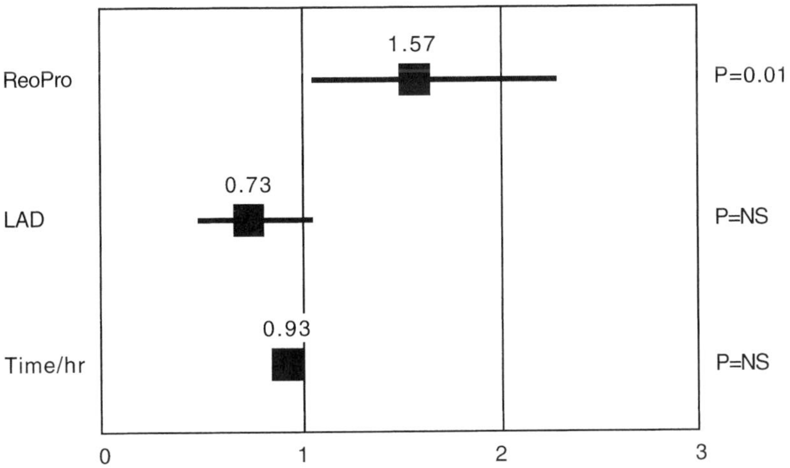

Figure 3 Predictors of TIMI 3 flow at 90 min in TIMI 14 (odds ratio and 95% confidence intervals). (From Ref. 21.)

Table 2 Median cTFC in Selected Reperfusion Regimens in TIMI 14

Group	60 min*	90 min**
Abciximab alone	100	100
t-PA alone	50	46
50 mg t-PA + abciximab	34	28

*P = .001 for trend.
**P = .005 for trend.

The incidence of important efficacy and safety endpoints is shown in Table 3. Rescue angioplasty and recurrent ischemia leading to revascularization was most common among patients treated with abciximab alone (41% and 59%, respectively), compared with the other regimens of reperfusion. The incidence of major hemorrhage was commensurate with other studies of immediate angiography in acute MI (11). Approximately two-thirds of the major bleeding episodes were related to instrumentation for angiography. The overall rate of intracranial hemorrhage was 1.1%.

Two other important conclusions were gleaned from this trial. Firstly, fibrinolysis, even at a reduced dose, needs to be sustained. Patients receiving 50 mg t-PA as a bolus had a lower rate of 90 min TIMI 3 flow than those treated with an infusion over 30 and, particularly, 60 min (49% vs. 62% vs. 74%; P = .002). Secondly, the use of very low dose heparin (30 U/kg bolus and 4 U/kg/hr infusion) resulted in a slightly lower rate of 90 min TIMI 3 flow (69% vs. 77% for low-dose heparin), but in a lower incidence of major hemorrhage and even death (1% vs. 7%, and 0% vs. 5%, respectively). These data, derived from small groups of patients, need to be interpreted cautiously and further explored.

Table 3 Key Efficacy and Safety Endpoints in TIMI 14

Endpoint	Incidence
Death	4%
Reinfarction	3%
Severe congestive heart failure	1%
Recent ischemia leading to revascularization	31%
Rescue angioplasty	19%
TIMI major hemorrhage[a]	7%
Intracranial hemorrhage	1.1%

[a]Defined as intracranial hemorrhage or a decline in hemoglobin >5 g/dL.

Strategies for Patency Enhancement in the Emergency Department (SPEED)

As a preamble to a large mortality trial to assess the efficacy of combination fibrinolysis and platelet antagonism in acute myocardial infarction (GUSTO IV), the SPEED investigators (23) conducted a randomized clinical pilot study to test this strategy. Similar to TIMI 14, the study encompassed dose finding and confirmation phases. Patients presenting within 6 hours of symptom onset and typical ST elevation acute MI were randomized to full-dose r-PA alone, abciximab alone, or a variety of regimens combining the two drugs. Unlike in TIMI 14, angioplasty was allowed and encouraged (when feasible and indicated) even if there was TIMI 3 flow at the 60- to 90-minute control angiogram. The primary endpoint was the rate of TIMI 3 flow (assessed by an independent core laboratory) at 60 to 90 min from therapy and the usual efficacy and safety parameters constituted secondary endpoints.

Between October 1997 and December 1998, 528 patients were enrolled at 61 centers and their baseline characteristics are shown in Table 4. The highest rate of TIMI 3 flow was obtained in patients treated with half-dose r-PA (5 + 5 MU) and full-dose abciximab for 12 hours, as shown in Figure 4. Essentially, these rates pertain to 60 min from therapy, since the median time to angiography was 62 min (60, 70 interquartile range) and 88% of patients underwent angiography between 55 and 80 min from therapy. Immediate angioplasty was performed in 71% (of whom 77% received a stent). Procedural success was significantly higher in patients with an initially patent (TIMI 2 or 3 flow) than in those with an occluded infarct artery (93% vs. 81%; $P = .001$), which was associated with better clinical outcome. Death (3.0% vs. 4.1%), reinfarction (0.5% vs. 2.4%), severe recurrent ischemia (1.5% vs. 1.6%), and their composite (4.6% vs. 7.3%, $P < .05$) were less

Table 4 Baseline Characteristics of Patients in SPEED

Characteristic	Value[a]
Number	528
Age, years	59 (52, 70)
Male gender	388 (73)
Diabetes mellitus	97 (18)
Hypertension	174 (33)
Prior infarct	63 (12)
Index anterior infarct	203 (38)
Symptom onset to therapy, h	2.7 (2.0, 3.9)

[a]Number (%) or median with 25th to 75th interquartile range.

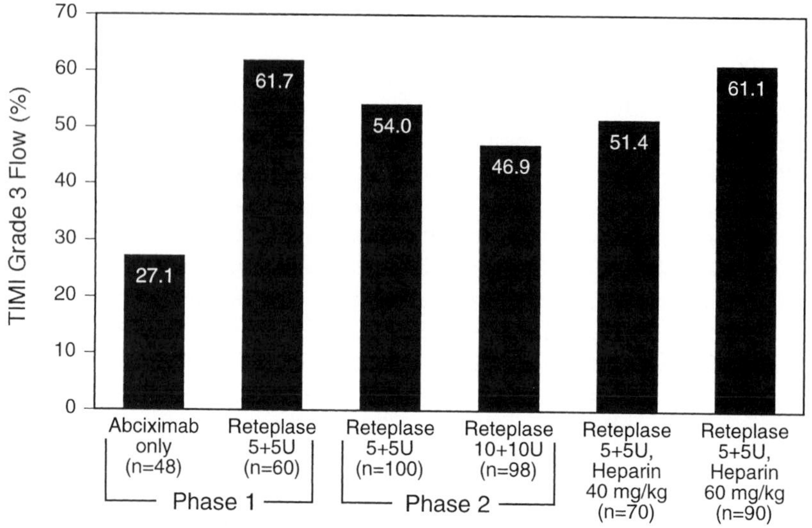

Figure 4 TIMI 3 flow at 60 to 90 min in SPEED. (From Ref. 23.)

frequent in patients with a patent artery before revascularization. The very favorable results of immediate angioplasty echoed the results of rescue angioplasty in the GUSTO III study, in which patients receiving abciximab after failed reperfusion with r-PA or t-PA had a lower adjusted 30-day mortality (3.7% vs. 9.8%; $P = .04$) than those undergoing the intervention without platelet inhibition (24). The synergism was particularly prominent in patients pretreated with r-PA.

Major efficacy and safety endpoints are shown in Table 5. There was a trend for a higher rate of severe bleeding in the combination groups (9.2%) compared with either abciximab alone (3.3%) or r-PA alone (3.7%).

This study confirmed the trends observed in TIMI 14: better reperfusion can be achieved with sustained fibrinolysis (46% vs. 62% for single bolus 10 MU and 5 + 5 MU, respectively) and with a slightly higher dose of heparin (51% for very low dose heparin vs. 61% for low dose-heparin).

Integrilin and Reduced dose of Thrombolytics for Acute Myocardial Infarction (INTRO AMI)

The third trial to combine reduced-dose fibrinolysis (t-PA) with a GP IIb/IIIa receptor antagonist (eptifibatide) has recently completed the enrollment of 344 patients in the dose-finding phase (25). A confirmation phase, including a control arm of full-dose t-PA, is under way. Patients with an acute

Table 5 Key Efficacy and Safety Endpoints in SPEED

Endpoint	Incidence
Death	3.8%
Reinfarction	2.5%
Urgent revascularization	5.9%
Severe congestive heart failure	4%
GUSTO severe hemorrhage[a]	7.5%
Intracranial hemorrhage	0.6%

[a]Defined as intracranial hemorrhage or bleeding associated with hemodynamic instability and requiring transfusion.

MI of <6 hours' duration and without previous surgical revascularization were assigned to escalating doses of the two drugs in a sequential fashion, as shown in Table 6. The primary efficacy endpoint was the incidence of TIMI 3 flow (adjudicated by a central angiographic laboratory) at 60 min from t-PA bolus. The key baseline characteristics of the study population are shown in Table 7 and are typical of low-risk patients enrolled in reperfusion studies. The rates of TIMI 3 flow at 60 and 90 min are shown in Figure 5. Eptifibatide given as double bolus (180 + 90 μg/kg 30 min apart) and infusion of 1.33 μg/kg/min in conjunction with 50 mg t-PA over 1 hour achieved the highest rate of TIMI 3 flow—65% at 60 min and 78% at 90 min, very similar to TIMI 14 and SPEED. Importantly, this group of patients also achieved the highest rate of complete ST-segment resolution at 3 hours (83%). Efficacy and safety secondary endpoints are detailed in Table 8.

Table 6 INTRO-AMI Study Groups

Group	N	t-PA	Bolus	Infusion
A	35	25 mg	180 μg/kg	1.33 μg/kg/min
B	37	25 mg	180 + 90 μg/kg	1.33 μg/kg/min
E	33	50 mg[a]	180 μg/kg	1.33 μg/kg/min
F	53	50 mg[a]	180 + 90 μg/kg	1.33 μg/kg/min
G	33	50 mg[a]	180 μg/kg	2.0 μg/kg/min
I	49	50 mg[a]	180 + 90 μg/kg	2.0 μg/kg/min
N	56	50 mg[a]	180 + 180 μg/kg	1.33 μg/kg/min
O	48	50 mg[a]	180 + 180 μg/kg	2.0 μg/kg/min

[a]Administered as 15-mg bolus and 35-mg infusion over 60 min.

Table 7 Baseline Characteristics of Patients in INTRO-AMI

Characteristic	Value[a]
Number	344
Age, years	61 ± 11
Male gender	261 (76)
Diabetes mellitus	62 (18)
Hypertension	141 (41)
Prior infarct	38 (11)
Index anterior infarct	119 (35)

[a]Number (%) or mean ± SD.

Supporting the observations from the other combination fibrin and platelet lysis studies, the INTRO-AMI investigators (26) reported a higher rate of TIMI 3 flow with 50 vs. 25 mg t-PA (63% vs. 48%; $P = .04$). Furthermore, patients with TIMI 3 flow before immediate angioplasty had a higher rate of TIMI 3 flow at the end of procedure (94% vs. 69%; $P < .001$) and demonstrated a trend towards lower mortality (3.3% vs. 5.4%) than patients with suboptimal flow before intervention (27).

ADVANTAGES OF REPERFUSION REGIMENS BASED PRINCIPALLY ON PLATELET INHIBITION

While the three trials described above provided the mechanistic proof of concept regarding the enhanced ability of combination fibrin and platelet lysis to restore full epicardial flow, the additional benefits of this therapy beyond flow resumption have far-reaching implications for acute MI patients.

As far as efficacy is concerned, two aspects of platelet inhibition in acute MI merit special attention. The first is reocclusion after successful reperfusion. Numerous studies (28,29) have shown that mortality increases two- to threefold when the infarct-related artery reoccludes before hospital discharge, while survivors have a higher incidence of significant heart failure. Recently, Ross et al. (30) evaluated the contribution of half-dose t-PA, antiplatelet monotherapy with aspirin and heparin before emergency angiography in acute MI in the Plasminogen-activator Angioplasty Compatibility Trial (PACT) (30). While 50 mg t-PA promoted arterial patency, the rate of TIMI 3 flow before angioplasty was only 33% (15% for placebo), very similar to that produced by abciximab alone (without t-PA) in TIMI 14. Preangiography reduced-dose fibrinolysis did not reduce reocclusion (5.9% vs. 3.7% for placebo), reinfarction (3.0% vs. 2.6%, respectively), or urgent

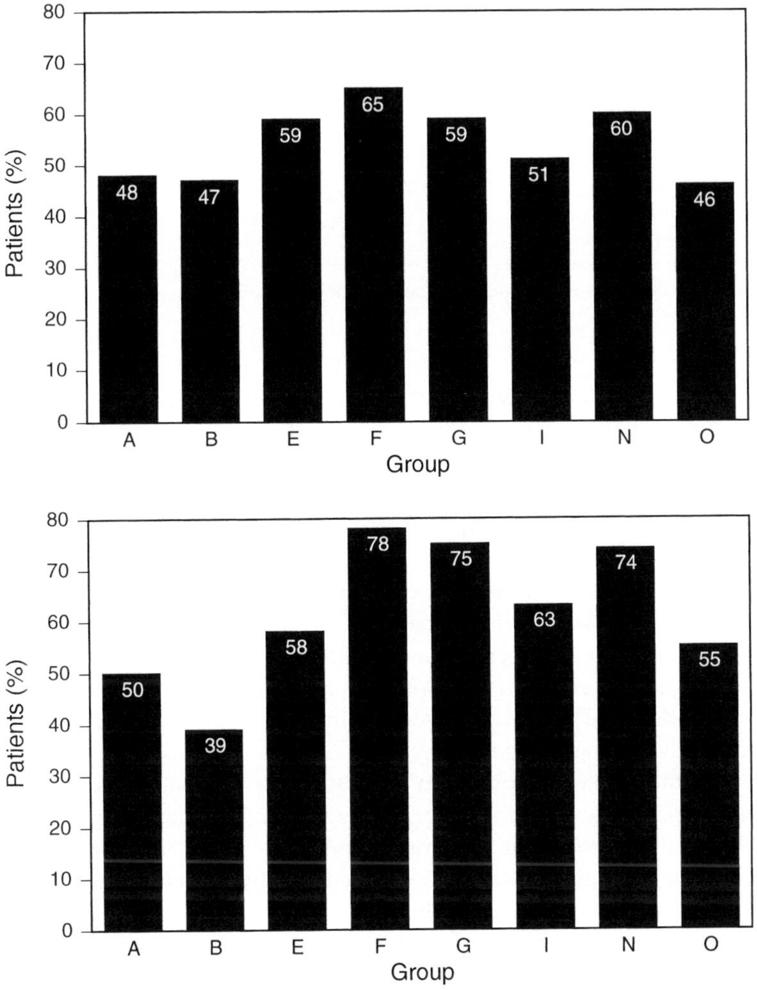

Figure 5 TIMI 3 flow at (top) 60 and (bottom) 90 min in INTRO-AMI. For group legend see Table 6. (From Ref. 25.)

angioplasty in those with initial TIMI 3 flow (7.9% vs. 5.6%, respectively). In contrast, all trials of platelet IIb/IIIa receptor blockade have shown a 60% to 70% reduction in the incidence of urgent target vessel (31,32), which constitutes a logical surrogate for reocclusion. Although urgent coronary intervention prevents or attenuates reinfarction, the fact that it is needed attests to the instability of the plaque and the tendency to rethrombose.

Table 8 Key Efficacy and Safety Endpoints in INTRO-AMI

Endpoint	Incidence
Death	2.9%
Reinfarction	2.3%
Any revascularization	52%
TIMI major bleeding[a]	18%
Intracranial hemorrhage	1.1%

[a]Defined as intracranial hemorrhage or a decline in hemoglobin >5 g/dL.

Indeed, in the confirmation phase of SPEED, urgent revascularization was needed in 2.6% of the patients treated with combination therapy and 3.7% of those receiving full-dose r-PA. Reinfarction occurred in 0.87% and 2.8%, respectively. In INTRO-AMI, where all patients received the platelet inhibitor eptifibatide, the rate of reinfarction was only 2.3%. These results were obtained in patients in whom immediate angioplasty after control angiography was encouraged. The lesser rate of reocclusion after platelet inhibition stems in part from the attenuation of cyclical flow observed in arteries after percutaneous intervention or reperfusion (33–35). Activated platelets (36) at the site of plaque rupture secrete vasoactive substances, which affect vasomotor tone, both at the epicardial level and in the microcirculation.

The electrocardiographic manifestation of reocclusion is frequently recurrent ST-segment elevation observed in the first few hours after fibrinolysis or primary angioplasty, which is dramatically reduced by platelet inhibition (16,20,22). As demonstrated in PARADIGM and IMPACT-AMI, the time to stabilization of the ST-segment was markedly reduced by the administration of lamifiban and eptifibatide, respectively.

The prevention of reocclusion and stabilization of the ruptured plaque tie in with the second component of the benefit associated with platelet inhibition, the lessening of microvascular dysfunction. This phenomenon is an amalgamation of various factors, such as destruction of the capillary network by necrosis, embolization of plaque and thrombus from the epicardial artery following pharmacological or mechanical reperfusion, and the response of the microvasculature to this "showering" of atherothrombotic material. While the first component is likely irreversible, platelet IIb/III receptor inhibition eliminates the principal component of rethrombosis at the epicardial level and the platelet-thrombus response to embolization in the smaller vessels.

The consequences of microvascular damage are extremely serious, as demonstrated by the evaluation of myocardial perfusion with magnetic resonance or contrast echocardiography. In a small series of 44 patients with acute MI, MRI-detected microvascular obstruction at 10 days after the event was associated with a fivefold increase in future cardiac events at 1 to 2 years of follow-up (45% vs. 9%; $P = .016$) (37). Microvascular damage was an independent predictor of adverse outcome even after correcting for infarct size. Similarly, microvascular dysfunction detected by contrast-enhanced echocardiography was a powerful predictor of persistent regional and global left ventricular dysfunction, even after successful epicardial reperfusion (3,38). Even using a simpler method of assessing myocardial perfusion, such as ST-segment elevation resolution after primary angioplasty, Matetzki et al. (39) showed that early ST segment normalization is associated with improved predischarge left ventricular function and a lower in-hospital and long-term rate of major adverse cardiac events. Most likely, the lack of early ST-segment normalization in the presence of a patent epicardial artery is the electrical manifestation of the "no-reflow" phenomenon demonstrated by Ito (40), Santoro (41), and their collaborators.

Platelet antagonism with the IIb/IIIa receptor blocker abciximab decreases these manifestations of presumed plaque and thrombus embolization. In a study of primary angioplasty with and without abciximab, Neumann et al. (42) found a higher flow velocity after stenting in patients treated with the active drug compared to placebo, suggesting better tissue perfusion. This physiologic observation correlated with better convalescent regional and global left ventricular function. The ReoPro and Primary PTCA Organization and Randomized Trial (RAPPORT) investigators (43) showed a faster rate of reperfusion after primary angioplasty with adjunctive abciximab, compared with placebo, as evidenced by a shorter time to peak creatine kinase, despite a similar frequency of TIMI 3 flow. The SPEED investigators (23) showed, like the TIMI 14 group, that abciximab and r-PA achieve faster coronary flow than either component alone, using the corrected TIMI frame counts (34 [25th to 75th interquartile range 24 to 100] for the combination therapy vs. 44 [24,100] for r-PA and 100 [40,100] for abciximab).

From the safety standpoint, three large trials of new fibrinolytic agents comparing reteplase (r-PA) (44), lanoteplase (n-PA) (preliminary results, American College of Cardiology 1999), or tenecteplase (TNK-t-PA) (45) with accelerated-dose t-PA have highlighted the high rate of intracranial hemorrhage with third-generation fibrinolytics (0.91%, 0.94%, and 1.13% for r-PA, TNK-t-PA, and n-PA, respectively). Even for t-PA, the rate of ICH has increased from 0.71% in GUSTO I to 0.94% in ASSENT II. This is due mostly to changing demographics for patients participating in acute MI trials, particularly age and coexisting illnesses predisposing to stroke (44). In contrast, platelet IIb/IIIa receptor blockade is associated with a very low rate of stroke. When these agents are used in conjunction with aspirin and heparin, the incidence of stroke among patients enrolled in randomized trials of percutaneous coronary intervention or acute coronary syndromes was 0.073% to 0.14% for the active drug and 0.063% to 0.091% for the control patients, nearly 10 times lower than the incidence observed in fibrinolytic trials (46). So far, in the combination trials, with many fewer patients enrolled than in the IIb/IIIa receptor blockade trials, the rate of ICH has varied from 0.6% to 1.1%, suggesting that even half the dose of fibrinolysis may be sufficient to induce this complication. Even small decrements in the incidence of ICH are important in view of the fact that the in-hospital mortality associated with it is 50% to 60% (47).

THE FUTURE OF REPERFUSION THERAPY FOR ACUTE MI

The better understanding of the structure of the coronary thrombus and the important role of platelets in its formation has led to a new paradigm of reperfusion therapy for all acute coronary syndromes. In this model, powerful platelet inhibition via blockade of the GP IIb/IIIa receptor serves as the platform on which adjunctive therapy is supplemented in a targeted approach. In the case of ST-elevation MI, in which an important component of fibrin deposition exists following deep arterial wall injury, reduced-dose fibrinolysis is added to facilitate dethrombosis and heparin is directed toward the thrombin liberated from the thrombus. Antithrombin agents with more upstream action, or direct thrombin inhibitors, are likely to replace it. In general, this "cocktail" is well tolerated and improves not only flow in the epicardial artery, but also tissue perfusion. This important advantage of such a strategy promises to shift our attention from infarct artery patency to its effects on the end organ, the myocardium. Finally, basing reperfusion therapy on platelet inhibition rather than on fibrinolysis appears to facilitate early mechanical reperfusion in all patients, and particularly in those who failed to respond to pharmacologically induced lysis.

Before this model of platelet preeminence (48) becomes the new standard of therapy in acute coronary syndromes, its superiority over established strategies with respect to mortality and other ischemic complications needs to be established. To this end, the GUSTO IV trial is currently enrolling patients in two large protocols. In the ST-elevation MI, 16,600 patients are randomized to full-dose r-PA or half-dose r-PA with abciximab, while in the unstable angina/non-ST-elevation MI, nearly 8000 patients are assigned to abciximab or placebo in conjunction with standard aspirin and heparin therapy. The safety and efficacy of these strategies will be definitively evaluated in these trials.

Additional investigation is needed to assess the effect of combination fibrin and platelet lysis on microvascular reperfusion. The role and timing of facilitated percutaneous revascularization after such therapy await confirmation and need to be compared with the existing benchmark of direct angioplasty with adjunctive GP IIb/IIIa blockade.

REFERENCES

1. GUSTO I Angiographic Investigators. The effects of tissue plasminogen activator, streptokinase, or both on coronary-artery patency, ventricular function, and survival after acute myocardial infarction. N Engl J Med 1993;329:1615–1621.
2. Antiplatelet Trialists' Collaboration. Collaborative overview of randomized trials of antiplatelet therapy. I. Prevention of death, myocardial infarction, and stroke by prolonged antiplatelet therapy in various categories of patients. Br Med J 1994;308:81–106.
3. Ito H, Okamura A, Iwakura K, Masuyama T, Hori M, Takiuchi S, Negoro S, Nakatsuchi Y, Taniyama Y, Higashino Y, Fujii K, Minamino T. Myocardial perfusion patterns related to thrombolysis in myocardial infarction perfusion grades after coronary angioplasty in patients with acute anterior wall myocardial infarction. Circulation 1996;93:1993–1999.
4. Iliceto S, Galiuto L, Marchese A, Cavallari D, Colonna P, Biasco G, Rizzon P. Analysis of microvascular integrity, contractile reserve, and myocardial viability after acute myocardial infarction by dobutamine echocardiography and myocardial contrast echocardiography. Am J Cardiol 1996;77:441–445.
5. TIMI Study Group. The Thrombolysis in Myocardial Infarction I (TIMI) trial: Phase I findings. N Engl J Med 1985;312:932.
6. Lincoff AM, Topol EJ. Illusion of reperfusion. Does anyone achieve optimal reperfusion during acute myocardial infarction? [corrected and republished article originally printed in Circulation 1993;87(6):1792–1805]. Circulation. 1993;88:1361–1374.
7. Hsia J, Kleiman N, Aguirre F, Chaitman BR, Roberts R, Ross AM. Heparin-induced prolongation of partial thromboplastin time after thrombolysis: relation to coronary artery patency. HART Investigators. J Am Coll Cardiol 1992;20:31–35.
8. Brouwer MA, Bohncke JR, Veen G, Meijer A, van Eenige MJ, Verheugt FW. Adverse long-term effects of reocclusion after coronary thrombolysis. J Am Coll Cardiol 1995;26:1440–1444.
9. Meijer A, Verheugt FW, van Eenige MJ, Werter CJ. Left ventricular function at 3 months after successful thrombolysis. Impact of reocclusion without reinfarction on ejection fraction, regional function, and remodeling. Circulation 1994;90:1706–1714.
10. Nijland F, Kamp O, Verheugt FW, Veen G, Visser CA. Long-term implications of reocclusion on left ventricular size and function after successful thrombolysis for first anterior myocardial infarction. Circulation 1997;95:111–117.
11. Weaver WD, Simes RJ, Betriu A, Grines CL, Zijlstra F, Garcia E, Grinfeld L, Gibbons RJ, Ribeiro EE, DeWood MA, Ribichini F. Comparison of primary

coronary angioplasty and intravenous thrombolytic therapy for acute myocardial infarction: a quantitative review. JAMA 1997;278:2093–2098.

12. Stone GW, Brodie B, Griffin J, Morice M-C, St. Goar FG, Costantini C, Overlie PA, Jones D, Grines C. A prospective, multicenter trial of primary stenting in acute myocardial infarction—the PAMI Stent Pilot Study. Circulation 1996;94: I-570. Abstract.
13. Weinberger I, Fuchs J, Davidson E, Rotenberg Z. Circulating aggregated platelets, number of platelets per aggregate, and platelet size during acute myocardial infarction. Am J Cardiol 1992;70:981–983.
14. Gold HK, Garabedian HD, Dinsmore RE, Guerrero LJ, Cigarroa JE, Palacios IF, Leinbach RC. Restoration of coronary flow in myocardial infarction by intravenous chimeric 7E3 antibody without exogenous plasminogen activators. Observations in animals and humans. Circulation 1997;95:1755–1759.
15. Kleiman NS, Ohman ME, Califf RM, George BS, Kereiakes D, Aguirre FV, Weisman H, Schaible T, Topol EJ. Profound inhibition of platelet aggregation with monoclonal antibody 7E3 fab after thrombolytic therapy. Results of the thrombolysis and angioplasty in myocardial infarction (TAMI) 8 pilot study. J Am Coll Cardiol 1993;22:381–389.
16. Ohman EM, Kleiman NS, Gacioch G, Worley SJ, Navetta FI, Talley JD, Anderson HV, Ellis SG, Cohen MD, Spriggs D, Miller M, Kereiakes D, Yakubov S, Kitt MM, Sigmon KN, Califf RM, Krucoff MW, Topol EJ, for the IMPACT-AMI Investigators. Combined accelerated tissue-plasminogen activator and platelet glycoprotein IIb/IIIa integrin receptor blockade with Integrilin in acute myocardial infarction. Results of a randomized, placebo-controlled, dose-ranging trial. Circulation 1997;95:846–854.
17. Phillips DR, Teng W, Arfsten A, Nannizzi-Alaimo L, White MM, Longhurst C, Shattil SJ, Randolph A, Jakubowski JA, Jennings LK, Scarborough RM. Effect of Ca^{2+} on GP IIb-IIIa interactions with integrilin: enhanced GP IIb-IIIa binding and inhibition of platelet aggregation by reductions in the concentration of ionized calcium in plasma anticoagulated with citrate. Circulation 1997;96: 1488–1494.
18. Ronner E, van Kesteren HAM, Zijnen P, Tebbe U, Molhoek P, Cuffie C, Veltri E, Lorenz T, Neuhaus K-L, Simoons ML. Combined therapy with streptokinase and Integrilin. J Am Coll Cardiol 1998;31:191A. Abstract.
19. PURSUIT Trial Investigators. Inhibition of platelet glycoprotein IIb/IIIa with eptifibatide in patients with acute coronary syndromes. Platelet Glycoprotein IIb/IIIa in Unstable Angina: Receptor Suppression Using Integrilin Therapy. N Engl J Med 1998;339:436–443.
20. PARADIGM Investigators. Combining thrombolysis with the platelet glycoprotein IIb/IIIa inhibitor lamifiban: results of the Platelet Aggregation Receptor Antagonist Dose Investigation and Reperfusion Gain in Myocardial Infarction (PARADIGM) trial. J Am Coll Cardiol 1998;32:2003–2010.
21. Antman EM, Giugliano RP, Gibson CM, McCabe CH, Coussement P, Kleiman NS, Vahanian A, Adgey AA, Menown I, Rupprecht HJ, Van der Wieken R, Ducas J, Scherer J, Anderson K, Van de Werf F, Braunwald E. Abciximab facilitates the rate and extent of thrombolysis: results of the Thrombolysis in

Myocardial Infarction (TIMI) 14 trial. The TIMI 14 Investigators. Circulation 1999;99:2720–2732.
22. De Lemos JA, Antman EM, Gibson CM, McCabe CH, Giugliano RP, Murphy SA, Frey MJ, Van der Wieken LR, Van de Werf F, Braunwald E. Abciximab improves both epicardial flow and myocardial reperfusion in ST elevation myocardial infarction: a TIMI 14 analysis. Circulation 1999;100:I-650(3429). Abstract.
23. SPEED Investigators. Randomized trial of abciximab with and without low-dose reteplase for acute myocardial infarction. J Am Coll Cardiol 2000. In press.
24. Miller JM, Ohman EM, Schildcrout JS, Smalling RW, Betriu A, Califf RM, Topol EJ. Survival benefit of abciximab administration during early rescue angioplasty: analysis of 387 patients from the GUSTO-III trial. J Am Coll Cardiol. 1998;31:191A. Abstract.
25. Brener SJ, Vrobel TR, Lopez JF, L'Allier PL, Strony JS, Van der Wieken LR, Topol EJ. INTRO AMI: marked enhancement of arterial patency with eptifibatide and low-dose t-PA in acute myocardial infarction. Circulation 1999;100:I-649(3423). Abstract.
26. Brener SJ, L'Allier PL, Ivanc T, Strony JS. Critical need for sufficient fibrinolysis in combination with platelet-lysis for reperfusion in acute myocardial infarction: the INTRO AMI study. Circulation 1999;100:I-511(2695). Abstract.
27. L'Allier PL, Lopez JF, Vrobel TR, Strony JS, Brener SJ. Favorable results with immediate coronary intervention after low-dose t-PA and eptifibatide for acute MI: results from the INTRO-AMI trial. Circulation 1999;100:I-359(1885). Abstract.
28. Ohman E, Califf R, Topol E, Candela R, Abottsmith C, Ellis S, Sigmon K, Kereiakes D, George B, Stack R, Group TS. Consequences of reocclusion after successful reperfusion therapy in acute myocardial infarction. Circulation 1990; 82:781–791.
29. Lundergan CF, Reiner JS, McCarthy WF, Coyne KS, Califf RM, Ross AM. Clinical predictors of early infarct-related artery patency following thrombolytic therapy: importance of body weight, smoking history, infarct-related artery and choice of thrombolytic regimen: the GUSTO-I experience. Global Utilization of Streptokinase and t-PA for Occluded Coronary Arteries. J Am Coll Cardiol 1998;32:641–647.
30. Ross AM, Coyne KS, Reiner JS, Greenhouse SW, Fink C, Frey A, Moreyra E, Traboulsi M, Racine N, Riba AL, Thompson MA, Rohrbeck S, Lundergan CF, for the PACT Investigators. A randomized trial comparing primary angioplasty with a strategy of short-acting thrombolysis and immediate planned rescue angioplasty in acute myocardial infarction: the PACT trial. Plasminogen-activator Angioplasty Compatibility Trial. J Am Coll Cardiol 1999;34:1954–1962.
31. Brener SJ, Barr LA, Burchenal JE, Katz S, George BS, Jones AA, Cohen ED, Gainey PC, White HJ, Cheek HB, Moses JW, Moliterno DJ, Effron MB, Topol EJ, for the ReoPro and Primary PTCA Organization and Randomized Trial (RAPPORT) Investigators. Randomized placebo-controlled trial of platelet gly-

coprotein IIb/IIIa blockade with primary angioplasty for acute myocardial infarction. Circulation 1998;98:734–741.
32. Kong DF, Califf RM, Miller DP, Moliterno DJ, White HD, Harrington RA, Tcheng JE, Lincoff AM, Hasselblad V, Topol EJ. Clinical outcomes of therapeutic agents that block the platelet glycoprotein IIb/IIIa integrin in ischemic heart disease. Circulation 1998;98:2829–2835.
33. Kern M, Donahue T, Bach R, Aquirre F, Bell C. Monitoring cyclical coronary blood flow alterations after coronary angioplasty for stent restenosis with a Doppler guide wire. Am Heart J 1993;125:1159–1169.
34. Kern MJ, Aguirre FV, Donohue TJ, Bach RG, Caracciolo EA, Flynn MS. Coronary flow velocity monitoring after angioplasty associated with abrupt reocclusion. Am Heart J 1994;127:436–438.
35. Kern MJ, Aguirre FV, Donohue TJ, Bach RG, Caracciolo EA, Flynn MS, Wolford T, Moore JA. Continuous coronary flow velocity monitoring during coronary interventions: velocity trend patterns associated with adverse events. Am Heart J 1994;128:426–434.
36. Iwabuchi M, Haruta S, Taguchi A, Ichikawa Y, Genda T, Katai S, Imaoka T, Shimuzu Y, Owa M. Intravascular ultrasound findings after successful primary angioplasty for acute myocardial infarction: predictors of abrupt occlusion. J Am Coll Cardiol 1997;30:1437–1444.
37. Wu KC, Zerhouni EA, Judd RM, Lugo-Olivieri CH, Barouch LA, Schulman SP, Blumenthal RS, Lima JA. Prognostic significance of microvascular obstruction by magnetic resonance imaging in patients with acute myocardial infarction. Circulation 1998;97:765–762.
38. Iliceto S, Galiuto L, Marchese A, Colonna P, Oliva S, Rizzon P. Functional role of microvascular integrity in patients with infarct-related artery patency after acute myocardial infarction. Eur Heart J 1997;18:618–624.
39. Matetzky S, Novikov M, Gruberg L, Freimark D, Feinberg M, Elian D, Novikov I, Di Segni E, Agranat O, Har-Zahav Y, Rabinowitz B, Kaplinsky E, Hod H. The significance of persistent ST elevation versus early resolution of ST segment elevation after primary PTCA. J Am Coll Cardiol 1999;34:1932–1938.
40. Ito H, Maruyama A, Iwakura K, Takiuchi S, Masuyama T, Hori M, Higashino Y, Fujii K, Minamino T. Clinical implications of the 'no reflow' phenomenon. A predictor of complications and left ventricular remodeling in reperfused anterior wall myocardial infarction. Circulation 1996;93:223–228.
41. Santoro GM, Valenti R, Buonamici P, Bolognese L, Cerisano G, Moschi G, Trapani M, Antoniucci D, Fazzini PF. Relation between ST-segment changes and myocardial perfusion evaluated by myocardial contrast echocardiography in patients with acute myocardial infarction treated with direct angioplasty. Am J Cardiol 1998;82:932–937.
42. Neumann FJ, Blasini R, Schmitt C, Alt E, Dirschinger J, Gawaz M, Kastrati A, Schomig A. Effect of glycoprotein IIb/IIIa receptor blockade on recovery of coronary flow and left ventricular function after the placement of coronary-artery stents in acute myocardial infarction. Circulation 1998;98:2695–2701.

43. Brener SJ, Barr LA, Burchenal JE, Wolski KE, Effron MB, Topol EJ, for the RAPPORT investigators. Effect of abciximab on the pattern of reperfusion in patients with acute myocardial infarction treated with primary angioplasty. ReoPro And Primary PTCA Organization and Randomized Trial. Am J Cardiol 1999;84:728–730.
44. GUSTO-III Investigators. A comparison of reteplase and alteplase for acute myocardial infarction. N Engl J Med 1997;337:1118–1123.
45. ASSENT-2 Investigators. Single-bolus tenecteplase compared with front-loaded alteplase in acute myocardial infarction: the ASSENT-2 double-blind randomized trial. Lancet 1999;354:716–722.
46. Blankenship JC. Bleeding complications of glycoprotein IIb-IIIa receptor inhibitors. Am Heart J 1999;138:287–296.
47. Gore JM, Granger CB, Simoons ML, Sloan MA, Weaver WD, White HD, Barbash GI, Van de Werf F, Aylward PE, Topol EJ. Stroke after thrombolysis. Mortality and functional outcomes in the GUSTO-I trial. Global Use of Strategies to Open Occluded Coronary Arteries. Circulation 1995;92:2811–2818.
48. Topol EJ. Toward a new frontier in myocardial reperfusion therapy: emerging platelet preeminence. Circulation 1998;97:211–218.

12

Diagnosis of Acute Coronary Syndromes in the Emergency Department

Evolution of Chest Pain Centers

W. Brian Gibler
University of Cincinnati College of Medicine and University of Cincinnati Hospital Cincinnati, Ohio

Andra L. Blomkalns
University of Cincinnati College of Medicine Cincinnati, Ohio

INTRODUCTION

The diagnosis of acute coronary syndrome (ACS) in patients presenting to the emergency department (ED) with chest discomfort is challenging. An estimated 8 million ED visits are related to complaints of chest pain or other symptoms suggesting potential cardiac ischemia (1), 5 million of which are admitted to the hospital each year in the United States for possible ACS. Of these patients, about 300,000 will suffer sudden death and 1.2 million will ultimately receive the diagnosis of acute myocardial infarction (AMI). More than 2 million patients presenting to emergency departments with chest pain are found to have a noncardiac cause for their symptoms. For the emergency physician, the challenge is to accurately diagnose and admit the patient with potentially life-threatening ACS, while avoiding the inappropriate release of patients to home who have AMI because of the potential for these individuals to suffer morbidity and mortality.

Over the last 20 years, the diagnosis and treatment of patients with possible myocardial ischemia or infarction has evolved significantly. In the 1970s, patients with electrocardiographically proven AMI, unstable angina, or possible myocardial ischemia were admitted to a coronary care unit for close observation and therapy. Fibrinolytic therapy and interventional techniques, such as percutaneous transluminal coronary angioplasty (PTCA) or placement of intracoronary stents, have become standard treatment for patients with AMI having ST-segment elevation by 12-lead electrocardiography (ECG). Traditionally, in the attempt to identify every patient with ACS presenting to the ED, clinicians often admit many patients with noncardiac causes of chest pain. These patients can occupy expensive and sometimes scarce intensive care beds, generating nearly $600 million per year in unnecessary inpatient costs (2). Despite such a vigorous effort by clinicians to identify patients with ACS, of the 40% of patients from the ED with chest pain that are discharged to home, 1% to 2% actually have an MI (2–4). Subsequently, 20% of the dollars lost in malpractice litigation for emergency physicians are related to the diagnosis and treatment of AMI (1,5).

Early diagnosis, as well as rapid treatment, represents an important goal for the clinician in the emergency setting. In recent years, great strides have been made to improve both the diagnostic evaluation and treatment of patients with potential ACS. Further clinical investigation continues to help define subsets of patients with AMI having a nondiagnostic ECG who might benefit from earlier intervention or minimize the likelihood of releasing the patient with ACS from the ED. Out of necessity, the development of chest pain centers, or rapid diagnosis and treatment units, have increased the efficiency while decreasing the cost of evaluating and treating patients presenting to the ED with chest pain (6–16).

INITIAL EVALUATION

Emergency physicians demonstrate impressive sensitivity in identifying patients with ACS. Using the patient's history, physical examination, and initial 12-lead ECG, 92% to 98% of patients presenting to EDs with AMI and approximately 90% of patients with unstable angina are admitted to the hospital (17–24). Conversely, only 30% to 40% of patients admitted to hospitals throughout the United States for possible ischemic chest discomfort will be ultimately found to have ACS (25,26). The challenge for clinicians and researchers is to have diagnostic sensitivity approach 100% for ACS while also decreasing hospital admission for patients with noncardiac causes of chest pain.

History

Chest discomfort considered to be ACS is approached through a careful history, physical exam, 12-lead ECG, and determination of risk factors. Clinical history still remains the basis for making an accurate diagnosis of ACS. Several studies have specifically evaluated patient symptoms on ED presentation, compared to ultimate hospital discharge diagnosis (27–29). Ischemic chest pain is often described by the patient as squeezing, pressure, or suffocating pain which is substernal in location. Other descriptions include dull, cramping, aching, burning, tightness, severe, or hard pain which is unaffected by respiration. Radiation of the pain to either shoulder, the neck, jaw, or left or right arm with extension to the fingertips may be elicited from the patient. Involvement of the medial arm and forearm, with ulnar distribution of the pain to the hand may also be present (30).

Patients with fixed coronary artery lesions of 50% or greater may describe chest discomfort with exercise or emotional stress. Increased myocardial oxygen demand in a patient with a fixed coronary artery lesion can produce ischemia and pain. In patients with unknown coronary artery anatomy or no known history of cardiac disease, a history of exercise-induced chest discomfort is a cause for concern and may indicate a need for admission to observe and for further evaluation. In some individuals, silent myocardial ischemia is present as indicated through ambulatory monitoring of ST segments, and has been demonstrated to have the same morbidity and mortality as painful ischemia (31).

Patients having acute ischemic coronary syndromes often present with other symptoms in addition to chest discomfort. One-third of patients with AMI have shortness of breath as an associated symptom, while almost 10% of patients with AMI present only with dyspnea. Acute cardiac ischemia should therefore be considered by the emergency clinician in any patient of appropriate age with risk factors for coronary artery disease presenting with shortness of breath. Vomiting and diaphoresis have been found to occur in 40% and 50%, respectively, in patients with AMI (28,32). These expressions of autonomic hyperactivity in a patient with chest pain should alert the clinician to the increased likelihood of ACS as the underlying cause of the patient's complaints.

A significant concern for many emergency physicians is the patient with an atypical presentation of ACS. Nearly 25% of patients with an ultimate diagnoses of AMI have an unusual initial presentation. The Framingham Study and Western Collaborative Group Study found that 25% to 30% of all myocardial infarctions are clinically unrecognized (33–35). Approximately half of these unrecognized infarctions are truly silent, while the other half of patients will remember an atypical symptom complex which likely represented the myocardial infarction.

In patients having AMI without chest or epigastric discomfort, atypical symptoms can include dyspnea, syncope, confusion, stroke, fatigue or generalized weakness, or nausea/vomiting. Increasing patient age reduces the likelihood of chest pain as the chief complaint in AMI. In patients >75, the clinician should anticipate the atypical presentation of AMI rather than expect typical descriptions of chest pain. In these patients, central nervous system complaints of stroke, confusion, and syncope become more prevalent. Diaphoresis and nausea/vomiting appear less often. Younger patients, particularly women, may also have atypical presentations of ACS. Diabetes mellitus, possible secondary to ablation of the autonomic nervous system sympathetic cardiac afferent nerve fibers, can result in atypical presentations of AMI. Uretsky et al. (36) noted that patients with atypical AMI presentations averaged 10 years older, smoked less, and rarely described a history of angina, compared to patients with typical presentations. As improved myocardial salvage with fibrinolytic therapy and percutaneous coronary intervention (PCI) is time dependent, the clinician must consider atypical AMI presentations in high-risk groups such as the elderly or diabetics to decrease time to intervention.

The characteristics of patients released to home from the ED with ACS or AMI are of great interest to clinicians working in the emergency setting. Four percent of patients with AMI released from the ED in a Chest Pain Study Group Protocol were significantly younger, had atypical symptomatology, and were less likely than a control group of patients with AMI to have ECG evidence of ischemia or infarction (4). Overall, younger patients and individuals without previous hospitalization for cardiac disease were more likely to be refused admission. It has been postulated that improved ECG reading skills could decrease the number of patients with AMI released from the ED (3,4). Atypical or obscure presentation was cited as the major reason for incorrect diagnosis in a review of closed claim data from insurance companies. In addition, patients responsible for the care of these patients with missed AMI tended to have less experience in the ED, document histories less clearly, admitted fewer patients to the hospital, and had difficulty interpreting ECGs (5).

Physical Examination

The physical examination, while often crucial in many life-threatening disease processes, is often not helpful in distinguishing patients with ACS. Congestive heart failure and cardiogenic shock provide the best evidence of significant cardiac injury. Change in mental status, poor peripheral perfusion, diaphoresis, rales, jugular venous distension, and S3 and S4 heart sounds can also provide evidence of significant myocardial involvement in AMI.

Villanueva et al. (37) noted that patients with evidence of myocardial dysfunction including a third heart sound, fourth heart sound, or rales on ED presentation were at much greater risk for adverse cardiovascular events including nonfatal MI, death, stroke, life-threatening arrhythmia, and cardiac injury. The physician may be falsely reassured when the patient's pain is reproducible by palpation or movement. Tierney et al. (28) noted that 15% of patients with AMI complained of tenderness on chest wall palpation. Careful questioning of the patient may reveal that the pain caused by chest wall palpation is different from the sensation that initially brought the patient to the hospital.

Serial physical examinations should be performed on patients with chest discomfort. As acute ischemic coronary disease is a dynamic process, evolution of frank cardiac dysfunction may become apparent to the clinician prior to patient release from the ED or, just as importantly, prior to transfer in-hospital for a prolonged period without physician reexamination.

Initial 12-Lead ECG

The ECG can be used for multiple purposes by the clinician. First, the ECG serves as a screen for AMI in patients with atypical presentations for ACS such as in the individual with diabetes or the elderly patient. Second, the ECG can assist in the diagnosis of nonischemic diagnoses such as pericarditis or pulmonary embolus. Third, risk stratification in patients presenting to the ED with chest discomfort can partly be accomplished with ECG. For instance, a normal ECG in the young patient with pleuritic chest discomfort has a low risk of ischemic disease. Finally, ST-segment elevation in patients presenting to the ED with clinical presentations consistent with AMI has been the principal indication for the use of fibrinolytic therapy (38). Delivery of fibrinolytic therapy early in the course of AMI has been unequivocally demonstrated to decrease mortality. If delivered within the first 70 min after symptom onset, fibrinolytic therapy may abort the infarction, leaving the patient with no perceptible evidence of myocardial injury (39).

The ECG is helpful for diagnosis and treatment of patients only when positive, and should not be used by the physician to exclude a presentation of ACS or to release the patient home from an acute-care setting. In the Chest Pain Study Group, Rouan et al. (40) demonstrated that an ECG on presentation that is normal or has minimal nonspecific changes carries a collective 3% rate of AMI with a mortality of 6% versus a 12% mortality in patients with ECG elevation. Comparison of the initial ECG obtained on patient presentation to the ED with previous ECGs is important in terms of determining patient risk and prognosis. Fesmire et al. (41) demonstrated that patients with ischemic changes on the presentation ECG when compared to previous ECGs, even if nondiagnostic for AMI, are at greater risk for interventions, life-threatening complications, and AMI.

Serial 12-Lead Electrocardiography

Nearly 50% of patients with AMI present to the ED with a normal or nondiagnostic standard 12-lead ECG, yet early in the course of hospitalization, up to 20% of these patients will develop electrocardiographic changes consistent with transmural injury (25,26). In the patient presenting to the ED with continuous chest pain, serial acquisition of a 12-lead ECG every 30 min can improve diagnostic accuracy. In particular, serial ECGs can identify the diagnostic evolution of ST-segment elevation, identifying a candidate for treatment with fibrinolytic therapy. Just as importantly, minor ECG changes indicative of ischemia may prompt the clinician to admit a patient with ACS who otherwise may have been released.

Serial 12-lead ECG tracings obtained every 20 sec, with computer interpretation and comparison, have been developed for the continuous monitoring of ST segments in patients with AMI. ST-segment trend monitoring in multiple investigations has proven to be effective for noninvasive evaluation of reperfusion after delivery of fibrinolytic therapy (39,42–48). Serial 12-lead ECG can also provide surveillance of patients presenting to the ED with chest pain and nondiagnostic ECGs on presentation (46,49). Such ST-segment trend monitoring could provide the earliest evidence of coronary occlusion in patients presenting with preinfarction angina and is more sensitive and specific than the initial ECG in such scenarios (50). In addition, such evaluation may provide evidence of painless or silent ischemia. Transient elevation or depression of ST segments, without chest discomfort, may identify high-risk patients who otherwise would have been released from the ED.

It is important for the clincian to understand that ACS is a continuum and not a static event. Serial physical and electrocardiographic examinations are necessary for the accurate and expedient diagnosis. Furthermore, repeat or continuous evaluations can help identify patients with already known acute coronary syndromes in need of different or more aggressive treatment.

EARLY SERUM MARKERS OF ACS

The elevation of cardiac biomarkers in the serum over several days of hospitalization has been the standard method for diagnosing AMI over the past 25 years (25,26,51–129). Creatine phosphokinase-MB (CK-MB) is the typical marker used by most clinical laboratories to indicate myocardial necrosis. In the past, detection of AMI by characteristic enzyme elevation over a

48- to 72-hour period was sufficient to establish the diagnosis of AMI. Due to the evolution of fibrinolytic therapy and acute mechanical intervention, significant pressure now exists to identify patients with AMI early after ED presentation. In the patients presenting to the ED with a nondiagnostic ECG, early serum markers of myocardial cell necrosis have the potential for identifying candidates for fibrinolytic therapy or PCI.

Rapid immunochemical testing for CK-MB has evolved over the past 15 years with the development of monoclonal and polyclonal antibody technology. Current immunochemical methods for CK-MB determination require 10 min to perform and can be automated. Real-time testing for serum markers while the patient undergoes clinical evaluation in the ED has radically altered the diagnostic process for patients with possible AMI in many centers. The diagnosis of AMI in patients having nondiagnostic ECGs is now possible less than 4 hours after symptom onset (122). This has the potential for reducing the numbers of patients with AMI unintentionally released from the ED and identifying patients for intervention while myocardial salvage remains feasible. Gibler et al. (25) demonstrated serial CK-MB sampling to have a sensitivity and specificity of >90% within 3 hours after ED presentation using immunochemical methodology. The sensitivity for detecting all patients with AMI approaches 100% within 11 hours after symptom onset (26). Serial sampling for CK-MB in the ED provides important diagnostic information for the clinician in the evaluation of the patient with chest pain. A positive CK-MB determination in the patient with a nondiagnostic ECG and suspected MI alerts the clinician to the potentially unstable patient. Triage of this patient to an intensive-care setting should be considered as elevated ED CK-MB levels have been associated with an increased complication rate in patients with nondiagnostic ECGs (125). These patients should also be evaluated by the cardiologist for early mechanical intervention. Serial ECGs and ST-segment trend monitoring may subsequently identify individuals who are candidates for administration of fibrinolytic therapy.

While CK-MB is a logical cardiac protein for serial determination in the ED due to its high sensitivity and specificity, other serum markers have release kinetics that may improve diagnostic capabilities in the very early period after coronary artery occlusion. Myoglobin is attractive as an indicator for myocardial injury. It is a much smaller protein with a molecular weight of 17,000 daltons compared to 82,000 daltons of CK-MB. Gibler et al. (130) noted that myoglobin levels are elevated in the serum within 1 to 2 hours after symptom onset, peaking 4 to 5 hours after AMI in patients presenting to the ED with AMI. Sensitivity improved from 62% on ED presentation to 100% 3 hours later, compared to 50% and 95%, respectively, for CK-MB analysis. Myoglobin was found to have a 100% negative predictive value for AMI. Polanczyk et al. (131) showed that in patients who presented within 4 hours of symptom onset, myoglobin levels 2 to 3 hours later had the highest yield for detecting myocardial infarction. Myocardial myoglobin, however, is not distinguishable immunologically from skeletal muscle myoglobin, reducing its specificity to approximately 80% compared to 94% for immunochemical CK-MB determination 3 hours after ED presentation (130,132,133). Determination of serum levels of carbonic anhydrase III, an enzyme specific to skeletal muscle, has been suggested as an adjunct to myoglobin analysis to increase specificity. Myoglobin is elevated in patients with renal failure due to decreased clearance, making this marker alone less useful in a patient population that tends to be at high risk for ACS (134). Myoglobin levels as markers of reperfusion define another important potential role for this protein (135,136).

The myocardial-specific proteins troponin I and troponin T have release kinetics similar to CK-MB. Troponin T with a molecular weight of 39,000 daltons, and troponin I with a molecular weight of 23,000 daltons appear to slightly precede release of the less specific CK-MB into the serum (137–154). While CK-MB is located only in the cytosol, the troponins both have a cytosolic component and are entwined with the actual contractile apparatus of the myocardial cell. CK-MB may disappear from the serum within 2 to 3 days after an AMI, whereas slow destruction of the myocardial cell contractile proteins provides a sustained release of the troponins for up to 7 to 11 days. Also, the troponins demonstrate increased myocardial specificity when compared to CK-MB. Some clinicians are suggesting replacing the traditional CK-MB definition of AMI with troponin (155). The cardiac troponins seem to be of most benefit when evaluating AMI >6 hours after presentation (156) (Table 1).

Many of the studies surrounding cTnI and cTnT involve using these markers for both short- and long-term prognosis in patients with already

Table 1 Characteristics of Important Cardiac Markers for Emergency Department Use

Cardiac marker	Cardiac specificity	First rise	Duration elevation	Renal function dependent
Myoglobin	No	1–3 h	12–24 h	Yes
Total CK	No	4–8 h	36–48 h	No
CK-MB mass	++	3–4 h	24–36 h	Yes
CKMB subtypes	++	2–4 h	16–24 h	No
Cardiac TnT	++++	3–4 h	10–14 d	?
Cardiac Tnl	++++	4–6 h	10–14 d	?

Source: Ref. 158.

known cardiac disease (157–160). Ottani et al. (161) demonstrated that elevations of troponin I and T identify myocardial damage in patients with unstable angina and those patients with elevations had a worse short-term outcome. Benamer et al. (162) prospectively studied 195 patients with UA and determined that the rate of major in-hospital cardiac events, such as death, myocardial infarction, or emergency revascularization, was higher in patients with elevations of cTnI in the first 24 hours. Antman et al. (163) found that in patients with acute coronary syndromes, each increase in 1 ng/mL of troponin I correlated with a significant increase in the risk ratio of death.

Studies using troponin I and T in the heterogenous group of patients presenting to emergency departments are less clear. Polanczyk et al. (164) collected serial cTnI and CK-MB measurements on 1047 patients admitted for chest pain. Among those patients who ruled out for AMI, cTnI was elevated in 26% who had major cardiac complication, in comparison to only 5% for CK-MB. However, in patients without AMI or unstable angina, cTnI levels did not correlate with complications. The positive predictive value of abnormal cTnI was only 8%. Sayre et al. (165) prospectively evaluated 667 patients presenting to the emergency department with symptoms suggestive of ACS. The sensitivity and specificity of cTnT for AMI within 24 hours of ED arrival were 97% and 92%, respectively. Additionally, patients with cTnT levels of 0.2 μg/L or greater were 3.5 times more likely to have a cardiac complication within 60 days of ED arrival. The data suggest that bedside troponin assays can identify those patients at higher risk for mortality, adverse cardiac events, and more complicated hospital stays (166,167).

Ultimately, serum protein testing will likely include a panel of multiple markers that provide a spectrum of information regarding ACS (168). An early sensitive marker such as myoglobin, when combined with CK-MB and troponin I or T, could provide the clinician with critical information necessary to make decisions in the emergency setting. The National Academy of Clinical Biochemistry (NACB) has prepared recommendations on the use of cardiac markers for patient triage in the emergency setting. They recommend a two-marker system for evaluation: 1) an early marker which is reliably increased the blood within 6 hours of symptoms and 2) a more definitive marker which is increased in the blood after 6 hours of symptoms and remains elevated for several days. As fibrinolytic therapy and acute mechanical intervention for AMI have proven beneficial up to 12 hours after symptom onset, serum marker testing could become the mainstay in the diagnosis of AMI and ACS in patients from the ED with nondiagnostic ECGs. Such serum testing, if positive, could drive appropriate further testing and treatment, and ultimately provide information about prognosis. Additionally, in

AMI treated with fibrinolytics, measurements of cardiac enzymes can accurately predict reperfusion (169).

GRADED EXERCISE TESTING

Relatively few studies have evaluated the effectiveness and safety of graded exercise testing in patients presenting to the ED with chest discomfort. Stress testing in patients presenting with acute unstable angina or AMI has been in the past considered hazardous due to the potential for ischemic complications such as arrythmias and infarction extension (170–178). Several studies have evaluated the role of exercise testing in patients presenting to the ED with chest discomfort (179–181). These patients were considered to be low risk, with normal or nondiagnostic ECGs. Stress testing was found to be safe and effective in the evaluation for myocardial ischemia in these low-risk populations and suggested a substantial benefit in the cost of caring for these patients. Further evidence that exercise testing was safe in this low- to moderate-risk cohort was presented by Gibler et al. (16), who evaluated 384 patients through an ED chest pain evaluation unit protocol without ischemic complication. Immediate exercise testing has also been shown to be a safe and effective means of stratifying low-risk patients with known CAD into groups that can safely be discharged and those who require hospital admission (182). In a prospective study of 613 outpatients with suspected coronary artery disease, a prognostic score based on results of treadmill testing accurately predicted patients who would expire during the next 4 years (183).

Graded exercise testing has a sensitivity of 60% to 70% for identifying patients with exercise-induced ischemia and underlying coronary artery disease. False-positive tests in female patients tend to decrease the usefulness of graded exercise testing in young women. Fixed lesions of the circumflex artery are also difficult to identify by graded exercise testing, as is complete thrombosis of this artery by standard 12-lead ECG in patients with AMI. Patients with underlying baseline ECG abnormalities such as bundle branch block or digitalis effect may require referral for outpatient exercise sestamibi or thallium testing. Patients unable to exercise due to amputation or underlying pulmonary disease can undergo dipyridamole thallium testing, dobutamine echocardiography, or other radionuclide testing.

ECHOCARDIOGRAPHY IN ACS

Two-dimensional echocardiography is a noninvasive imaging method that has been demonstrated to be an effective tool for detecting regional wall abnormality associated with myocardial ischemia and AMI in the emergency setting (184–191). Impaired myocardial contractility can be observed echocardiographically in patients with myocardial ischemia and AMI, often following a progressive course from hypokinesis to akinesis. Impaired myocardial relaxation during diastole results in decreased ventricular distensibility. After AMI, paradoxical wall motion observed during systole indicates the subsequent loss of muscle tone secondary to necrosis. Decreased ejection fraction may also result from these ventricular wall motion abnormalities.

Studies evaluating patients presenting to the ED with chest pain have correlated regional wall motion abnormality with the presence of myocardial ischemia and AMI. Horowitz et al. (189) demonstrated a 94% sensitivity in detecting regional wall motion abnormality in AMI patients presenting within 12 hours of symptom onset to a coronary care unit using two-dimensional echocardiography. In two investigations performed in the ED, two-dimensional echocardiography was shown to be effective in detecting myocardial ischemia and AMI (187,188). Technical limitations restrict the use of echocardiography in the emergent diagnosis of AMI and myocardial ischemia. These limitations include the quality of the study, which is proportional to the experience of the operator and expertise of the reader performing the test at the patient's bedside. It has been reported that nondiagnostic echocardiograms occur in 10% to 27% of patients (192). In addition, the inability of two-dimensional echocardiogram to distinguish among ischemia, AMI, or old infarctions can further limit the usefulness of two-dimensional echocardiography. Levitt et al. (193) found that when combined with a cardiac marker approach, two-dimensional echocardiography does not appear to add to the evaluation of AMI in the ED.

Echocardiography is typically less expensive than radionuclide testing and offers more anatomic detail. Decisions to use two-dimensional echocardiography versus other available testing should be based on institution availability, patient population, and risk assessment level.

RADIONUCLIDE SCANNING

Radionuclide perfusion imaging has emerged as an important tool in assessing patients with known cardiovascular disease, and also in evaluating the patient presenting to the ED with possible ACS. Myocardial perfusion imaging has been shown to be a valuable diagnostic tool for detecting coronary artery disease with a sensitivity of >90%. In addition, normal perfusion images, even when present in patients with known disease, are associated with a favorable prognosis (194).

Thallium-201 has been used as a predominant perfusion agent for over 20 years. Several studies suggest that thallium scintigraphy may be useful in detecting AMI in patients presenting to the ED with chest pain. Areas of decreased thallium uptake by myocardium, seen as negative scintigraphic images, indicate regions of severely ischemic or infarcted myocardium within the first 6 hours after symptom onset. Mace et al. (195) reported a small study in which 6 of 20 patients with AMI were detected by thallium scanning. Although thallium imaging appears to be reliable in detecting AMI, its rapid redistribution is a major limitation in intermittent episodes of chest pain such as unstable angina.

Technitium-99 sestamibi tomographic imaging is currently being used in patients presenting to the ED with suspected acute ischemic coronary syndromes (196,197) (Table 2). Studies have shown that positive rest perfusion imaging accurately identifies patients at high risk for adverse cardiac events (198). Tatum et al. (200) demonstrated in a large study comprising 1187 patients, that an initially abnormal sestamibi scan was associated with a 1-year event rate of 42%, with 11% infarctions and 8% deaths. On the other hand, a normal perfusion study was associated with a 3% event rate and no myocardial infarctions or deaths. Furthermore, Iskander and Iskandrian (199) analyzed published reports on risk assessment using Tc-99m perfusion tracers. Data from 12,000 patients in 14 studies demonstrated that patients with stable symptoms and normal stress SPECT sestamibi studies had a very low risk of death or nonfatal MI (199). Kontos et al. (201) compared early sestamibi imaging with cTnI in patients with low to moderate risk of ACS. They found that while cTnI and perfusion imaging had comparable sensitivities for identifying AMI (90% and 92%, respectively), perfusion imaging identified more patients who underwent revascularization or who had significant coronary artery disease. This suggested that cTnI and sestamibi imaging could provide complementary information for identifying pa-

Table 2 Sensitivity, Specificity, and Predictive Value of Sestamibi Myocardial Perfusion Imaging with Acute Chest Pain

Study	Year	Sample size	Sensitivity (%)	Specificity (%)	PPV (%)	NPV (%)	Endpoint
Bilodeau et al.	1991	45	96	79	86	94	CAD
Varetto et al.	1993	64	100	9	90	100	CAD
Hilton et al.	1994	102	94	83	44	99	Event
Varetto et al.	1994	27	100	93	—	—	CAD
Stowers et al.	1995	187	97	78	—	—	Event
Tatum et al.	1997	438	100	78	7	100	MI

Source: Ref. 196.

tients at risk for ACS (200,201). It appears that the previously difficult patient, the individual with symptoms of typical angina and a nondiagnostic ECG, can be safely and cost-effectively evaluated on an outpatient basis if a normal initial SPECT perfusion scintigram is obtained during symptoms (202,203).

The diagnostic sensitivity of myocardial perfusion imaging is theoretically in part dependent on the timing of injection in relation to chest pain. Bilodeau et al. (204) and Stowers et al. (205) showed a decrease in sensitivity for CAD from 96% to 65% and 97% to 33%, respectively, when the agent was injected after the resolution of pain (Fig. 1). However, for ongoing chest pain symptoms exceeding 30 min within 12 hours of time of evaluation, sestamibi imaging performs with a sensitivity of 100% (202).

Sestamibi imaging is emerging as an alternative to traditional methods of observation and patient care. Kontos et al. (206) suggested that because AMI is an infrequent cause of cocaine-related chest pain, early perfusion imaging may offer an effective alternative for evaluating patients with cocaine-related cardiac symptoms.

The major obstacles for radionuclide studies have traditionally included cost and accessibility. The perfusion agents have a 6- to 12-hour shelf life, and thus have to be prepared several times a day to be available for acute imaging. It has been shown that use of ED myocardial perfusion imaging resulted in more appropriate use of coronary catheterization (207). Current protocols that include sestamibi imaging in the evaluation of patients with ongoing chest pain and a nondiagnostic ECG appear to be highly cost-effective (7,205,208,209). While accessibility will always largely be institution dependent, more frequent accepted indications and growing evidence for cost-effectiveness should fuel the demand for these studies.

CURRENT MODELS OF CHEST PAIN CENTERS

The University of Cincinnati Center for Emergency Care "Heart ER" has evaluated over 2600 patients since its inception in October 1991 (210). Patients presenting with chest pain or other symptoms suggestive of ACS are initially evaluated using standard techniques of history, physical examination, and initial 12-lead ECG. Hemodynamically unstable patients are treated with fibrinolytics or PCI and admitted to the intensive-care unit. Patients with ECG findings indicative of AMI or myocardial ischemia are directly admitted to the hospital after initial ED therapy and stabilization. Patients with ongoing chest pain consistent with unstable angina are admitted for therapy with heparin and nitroglycerin.

Patients admitted to the Heart ER program are considered to be a low- to moderate-risk cohort for ACS. Evaluation consists of serial CK-MB, my-

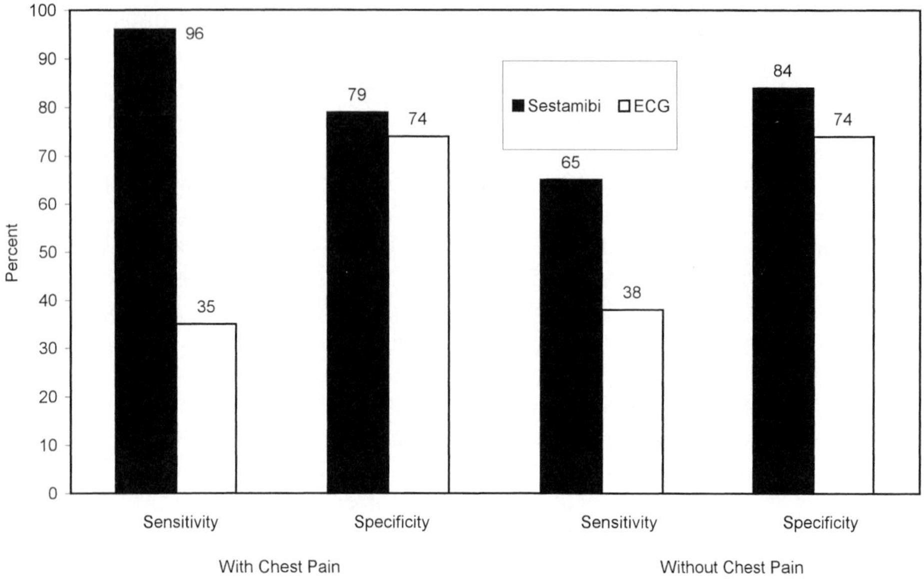

Figure 1 Comparative diagnostic accuracy of ECG and acute Tc-99m sestamibi perfusion imaging in patients who presented to an ED with chest pain. (From Ref. 204.)

oglobin, and cTnT levels drawn at 0, 3, and 6 hours while undergoing continuous ST-segment trend monitoring. Graded exercise testing or Tc-99m sestamibi radionuclide scanning is performed depending on a patient's functional status and test availability. Patients having negative evaluations in the Heart ER are released to home with careful follow up as an outpatient.

The Heart ER concept has proved to be a safe and cost-effective means for the evaluation of patients presenting to the Emergency Department with chest pain and possible ACS. Low-risk patients undergoing a systematic evaluation protocol tend to have more efficient resource utilization including fewer unnecessary admissions and catheterizations (6). Kontos et al. (7) demonstrated that implementation of an evaluation and triage protocol in all patients presenting with chest pain reduced costs approximately \$1000 per patient. At the University of Cincinnati (Fig. 2), in the first 2131 consecutive patients evaluated over a 6-year period, 309 (14.5%) required admission and 1822 (85.5%) were released to home from the ED. Of admitted patients, 94 (30%) were found to have a cardiac cause for their chest pain. Follow-up of 1696 patients discharged from the Heart ER to home yielded nine cardiac events (0.53%, CI 0.24% to 1.01%; 7 PTCA, 1 CABG, 1 death) (210). These

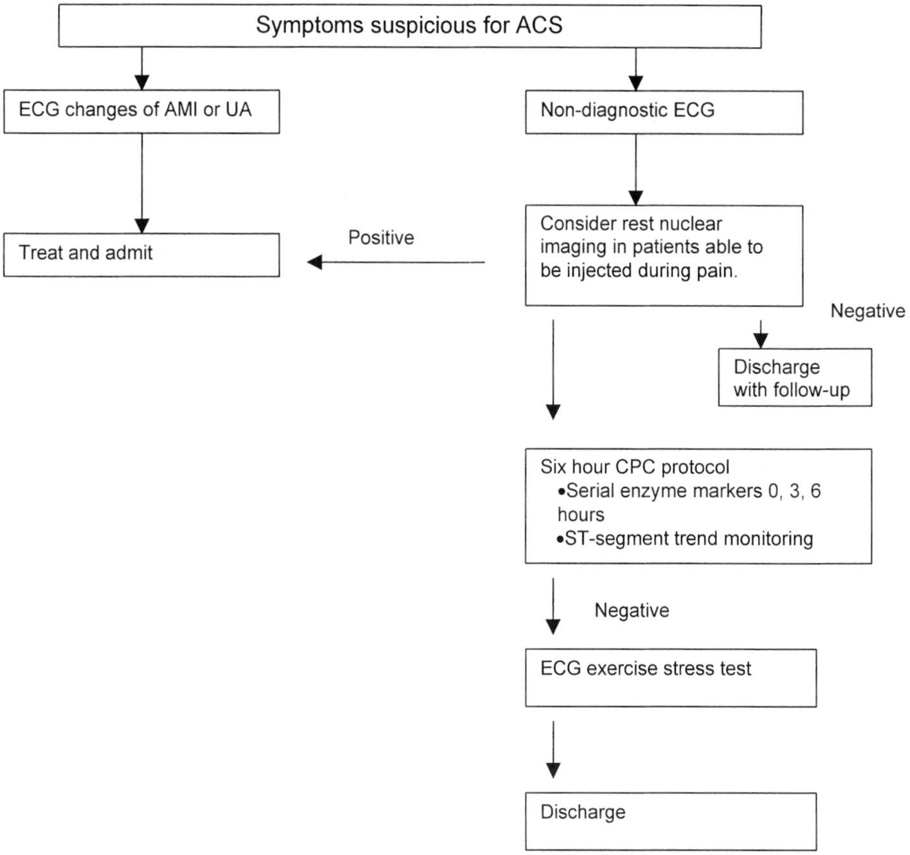

Figure 2 University of Cincinnati Heart ER Strategy. (From Ref. 210.)

data concluded that the Heart ER program provides a safe and effective means for evaluating low- to moderate-risk patients with possible ACS presenting to the ED.

Other institutions have refined effective chest pain center strategies. For instance, the Mayo Clinic separates patients into low-, intermediate-, and high-risk categories according to Agency for Health Care Policy Research (AHCPR) guidelines (211). Intermediate risk patients are evaluated with CK-MB levels at 0, 2, and 4 hours while undergoing continuous ST-segment monitoring and 6-hour observation. If this evaluation in negative, an ECG exercise test, a nuclear stress test, or an echocardiographic stress test is performed. Patients with positive or equivocal evaluations are admitted while patients with negative evaluations are discharged to home with a 72-hour follow-up. The Medical College of Virginia triages chest pain patients into five distinct levels: level 1 patients have ECG criteria for AMI while level 5 patients have clearly noncardiac chest discomfort. Triage level severity dictates treatment and further diagnostic measures (212,213). Intermediate-level patients include individuals with variable probability of unstable angina. The patient is admitted to the CCU for the diagnosis of acute angina while less acute patients undergo serial biomarker determination and Tc-99m sestamibi radionuclide imaging. Lastly, Brigham and Women's Hospital (Fig. 4) divides patients into three groups: UA or AMI, possible ischemia, and nonischemic. Patients with unstable angina or AMI are admitted while definitively nonischemic chest pain patients are discharged. The intermediate, or "possible ischemia," group either undergoes exercise treadmill testing with a 6-hour period of observation or a 12-hour period of observation. At the end of the observation period, stable patients are discharged to home (Fig. 3). Nichol et al. (214) evaluated the impact of this pathway approach in a retrospective cohort of 4585 patients and found that a 17% reduction in admissions and an 11% reduction in length of stay would occur if even <50% of eligible patients for observation and exercise testing had participated. Each institution has tailored CPC protocols to its patient population and resources to meet the growing demands of chest pain evaluation.

COMPUTER-AIDED DECISION MAKING

Computer-assisted diagnostic algorithms provide an interesting approach to evaluating the patient with chest pain and possible myocardial ischemia or AMI. Models such as logistic regression, classification tree, and neural network can provide very good predictive performance of medical-outcomes clinical-decision aids. Improving physician risk estimates for patients with chest discomfort presenting to the ED, and increasing the preevaluation likelihood of the patient having ACS, will ultimately increase the likelihood of the patients admitted to the hospital having coronary artery disease while decreasing the likelihood of patients being released from the ED with ACS (215–224).

Several reports indicate that retrospectively validated computer programs can prospectively match the sensitivity and specificity of the clinician. Goldman et al. (217) have attempted to define a high-risk group for AMI of ≥7%. Initial data suggested a protocol sensitivity of 92% and specificity of 70%, which was equivalent to clinicians not using the protocol. In revising the initial protocol as part of the Chest Pain Study Group, the algorithm was used prospectively on 4770 patients presenting with chest pain to six study hospitals. While sensitivity did not increase beyond the clinician's impres-

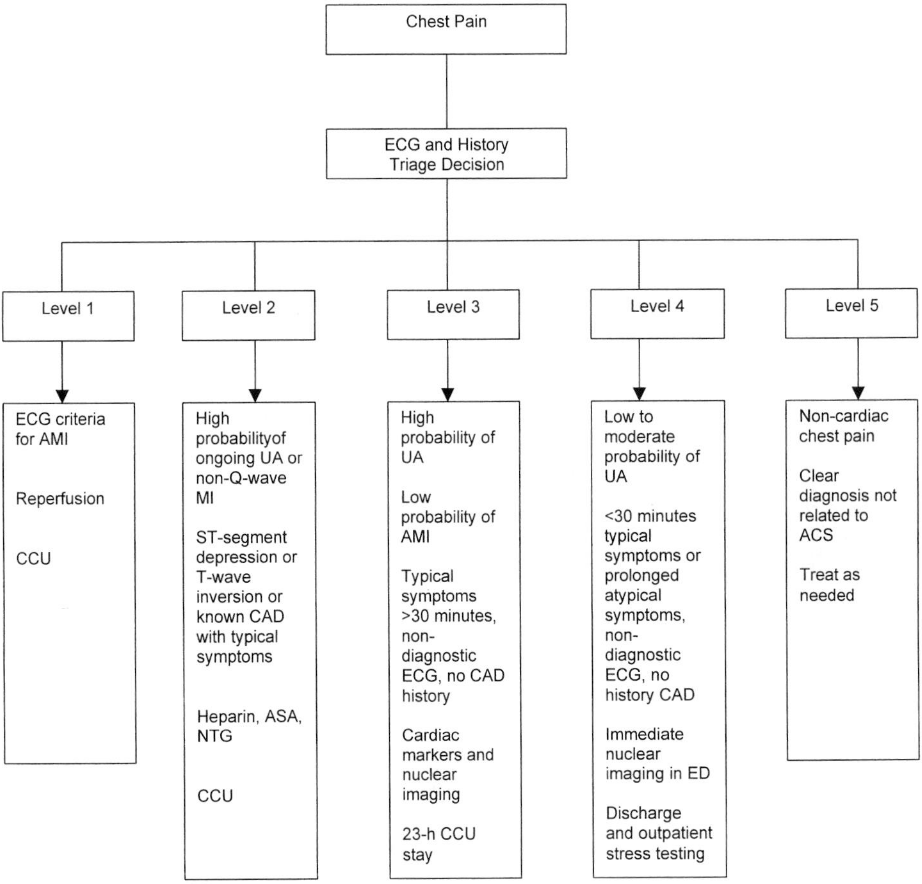

Figure 3 Medical College of Virginia clinical pathways "track" strategy. (From Refs. 212, 213.)

sion, 88% based on CCU admission of patients with AMI, specificity was significantly better when using the algorithm (74% vs. 71%). If the algorithm had been used by the clinicians, it would have reduced CCU admissions by 11.5% in patients without AMI while admitting the same number of patients with AMI (223). Pozen et al. (222), using multivariant logistic regression analysis, have developed predictive instruments that give clinicians an estimate of a patient's likelihood of acute ischemia, not only AMI. In the regression model, ECG findings are combined with patient description of chest pain, abdominal pain or nausea, dyspnea, and dizziness or lightheadedness. In prospective, controlled trial using the algorithm, CCU admissions decreased from 51% to 33%, while CCU admissions for patients with acute ischemic coronary syndromes did not increase (218). In a prospective controlled trial of 2320 patients presenting to the ED, when the physician was given the predicted probability of ischemia in half the cases, the predictive instrument used maintained a high diagnostic sensitivity of 95% for acute ischemia while increasing specificity from 73% to 78% (P = .002) (222). Diagnostic accuracy was therefore increased from 74% to 89% (P = .002) with the device. A 30% decrease in CCU admissions for patients without acute ischemia was obtained while no decrease was seen for patients with acute ischemic coronary syndromes.

Lastly, Selker et al. (225) showed in a multicenter controlled trial with nearly 11,000 patients that use of acute cardiac ischemia time-insensitive predictive instrument (ACI-TIPI) was associated with fewer hospitalizations among ED patients without cardiac ischemia without affecting appropriate admissions for patients with unstable angina or AMI. An innovative software approach for detecting acute ischemic coronary syndromes describes the training of a neural network. A neural network differs from conventional software analysis in that the network consists of a neuronlike system that has the ability to sum inhibitory and excitatory stimuli to produce a discrete output that in turn may synapse with other similar outputs. The network can also be "taught" to make informed decisions by providing it with sets of input data and pairing these input data with their associated outputs. Over time, the discriminatory capability of a neural network should improve. The neural network is considered free of the many biases and random errors that may influence the busy clinician.

The neural network has been prospectively validated in a trial of 331 consecutive ED patients with the chief complaint of anterior chest pain (215). Thirty-six of these patients were ultimately diagnosed as having AMI. The network performed with a sensitivity of 97.2% and a specificity of 96.2% in this patient cohort; the physicians caring for the study patients performed with a sensitivity of 77.7% and a specificity of 84.7%. In an extension of this original study, 1070 patients were evaluated with a similar neural network. The network performed with a diagnostic sensitivity and specificity of 96.0% and 96.0%, respectively. Seven percent of the patients ultimately had a diagnosis of AMI (216). Such sophisticated computer modeling may provide a powerful tool for the evaluation of patients with chest discomfort in the ED as well as the outpatient office setting.

EVOLUTION OF NEW DIAGNOSTIC MODALITIES

Interventions for AMI such as fibrinolytic therapy and PCI have intensified the interest of clinicians in the early diagnosis and treatment of patients.

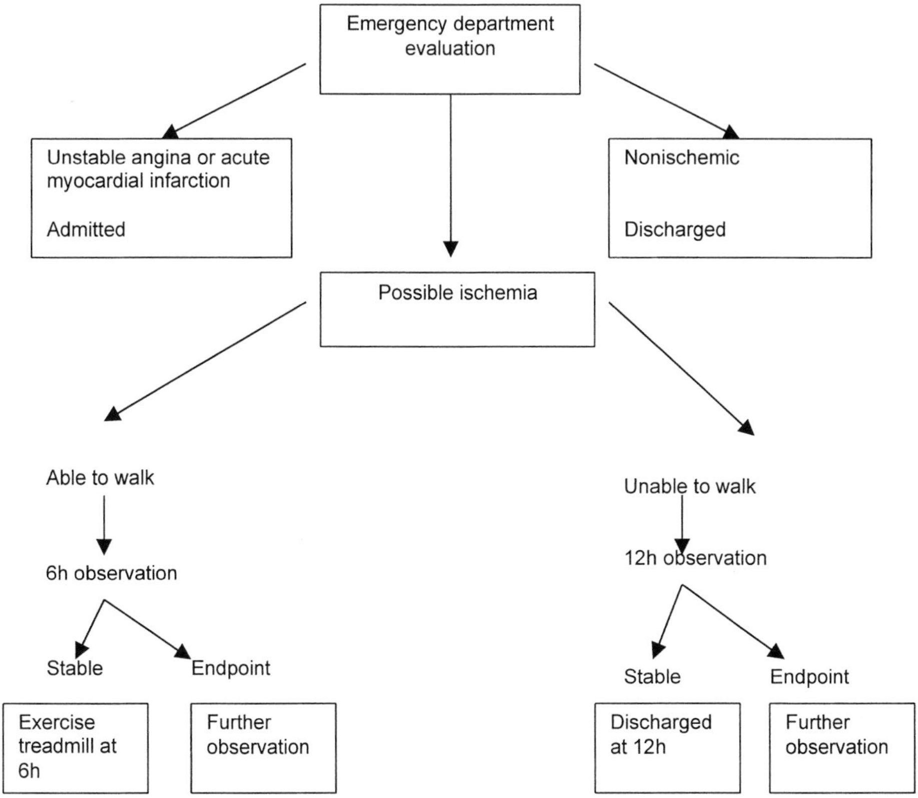

Figure 4 Brigham and Women's Hospital critical pathway for the management of patients presenting with acute chest pain who are at low risk for AMI. (From Ref. 214.)

While standard methods for evaluating the patient with chest pain and suspected ACS remain the foundation for the diagnostic evaluation of these patients in the emergency setting, new techniques are now available which can augment clinical judgment. Recent advances in early diagnostic strategies may improve clinical sensitivity as well as specificity for detecting ACS including AMI early in the ED, while decreasing costs associated with admitting a large number of patient with noncardiac disease (226).

Improved methods for ECG acquisition and computerized interpretation have improved the usefulness of this standard method for assessing the cardiac electrical signal. Sophisticated computer processing of the ECG signal, particularly for the ST segment, allows continuous ST-segment trend monitoring over prolonged periods in patients with chest pain. Serial rapid determinations of serum markers for myocardial necrosis, ideally in a point-of-care environment, now allow detection of AMI in the ED or acute-care setting more rapidly than ever before.

New modalities and methodologies continue to surface for the evaluation and treatment of patients with possible ACS or AMI. For instance, electron beam (ultrafast) CT is an imaging technique that detects the presence of calcium in the coronary vessels. Laudon et al. (227) recently demonstrated that electron beam computed tomography (EBCT) was a rapid and efficient screening tool for patients presenting to the ED with symptoms suggestive of angina, normal cardiac enzymes, nondiagnostic ECGs, and no previous history of coronary artery disease. This small study of 105 patients suggested that a negative EBCT scan allows a patient to be safely discharged from the ED without further testing or observation. Like CT, MRI also produces excellent resolution of cardiac structures. The role of these advanced imaging techniques has yet to be determined.

Changes in ED management of patients with known ACS is evolving as well, incorporating the diagnostic evaluation to identify patients at high risk for appropriate treatment with new therapies such as glycoprotein IIb/IIIa inhibitors and low-molecular-weight heparins. Hamm et al. (228) suggest identifying a high-risk subgroup of patients with unstable angina and elevated serum cTnT levels who will particularly benefit from antiplatelet therapy with abciximab. Patients with elevated cTnT may also represent a subgroup in whom prolonged antithrombotic treatment with dalteparin is beneficial (229). Antman et al. (230) showed that enoxaparin was more effective than unfractionated heparin for reducing death and serious cardiac ischemic events during the acute management of unstable angina and non-Q-wave MI without significant increase in the rate of major hemorrhage.

Continued study in two-dimensional echocardiography, radionuclide imaging, and computer algorithm-driven neural networks may provide powerful mechanisms for evaluating patients with possible ACS or AMI in the future. Research on the inflammatory nature of coronary atherosclerosis may create new avenues for the diagnosis and management of patients with cardiovascular disease (231).

CONCLUSION

Early identification of patients with ACS is the primary goal for any clinician working in the acute-care setting. There has been a recent shift in focus from just simply ruling out myocardial infarction to risk assessment and appropriate treatment of all patients presenting with symptoms suggestive of ACS. Multiple techniques, some undergoing only recent evaluation on patients presenting with possible ACS to the ED, will likely improve the identification and treatment of such patients in the future. Serial electrocardiography with ST-segment monitoring, early serum marker analysis, two-dimensional echocardiography, graded exercise testing, radionuclide scanning, and computer algorithms are available to assist the physician's clinical judgment. Incorporation of these new diagnostic methods into a coordinated CPC protocol should improve the evaluation of patients with possible ACS. Rapid identification and treatment of patients with ACS should improve patient outcome, and increased efficiency should decrease costs.

REFERENCES

1. Dunn J. ACEP Foresight: Chest Pain. Dallas. ACEP Publications, 1986:1–3.
2. Jesse RL, Kontos MC. Evaluation of chest pain in the emergency department. Curr Probl Cardiol 1997;22(4):149–236.
3. McCarthy BD, Beshansky JR, D'Agostino RB, Selker HP. Missed diagnoses of acute myocardial infarction in the emergency department: results from a multicenter study. Ann Emerg Med 1993;22:579–582.
4. Lee TH, Rouan GW, Weisberg MC, Brand DA, et al. Clinical characteristics and natural history of patients with acute myocardial infarction sent home from the emergency room. Am J Cardiol 1987;60:219–224.
5. Rusnak RA, Stair TO, et al. Litigation against the emergency physician: common features in cases of missed myocardial infarction. Ann Emerg Med 1989; 18:1029–1034.
6. Jesse RL, Kontos MC, Ornato JP, et al. A systematic evaluation protocol results in more appropriate resource utilization for low risk chest pain patients. Circulation 1999;100:I317. Abstract.
7. Kontos MC, Jesse RL, Ornato JP, et al. Cost effectiveness of a comprehensive strategy for the evaluation and triage of the chest pain patient. Circulation 1999;100:I290.
8. Bahr RD. Concept of community chest pain centers in emergency departments. Clinician 1996;14:5–6.
9. Joseph AJ. Chest pain centers: an emerging model for the emergency evaluation of chest pain and treatment of acute myocardial infarction. Clinician 1996;14:56–58.
10. Sayre MR, Gibler WB. The evolution of chest pain centers: the impact of technological advances on the evaluation of patients with possible acute ischemic coronary syndrome. Clincian 1996;14:47–52.
11. DeLeon AC, Farmer CA, King G, et al. Chest pain evaluation unit: a cost effective approach for ruling out acute myocardial infarction. South Med J 1989;82:1083–1089.
12. Gibler WB, Runyon JP, Levy RC, et al. A rapid diagnostic and treatment center for patients with chest pain in the emergency department. Ann Emerg Med 1995;25:1–8.

13. Gomez MA, Anderson JL, Karagounis LA, et al. An emergency department-based protocol for rapidly ruling out myocardial ischemia reduces hospital time and expense: results of a randomized study (ROMIO). J Am Coll Cardiol 1996;28:25–33.
14. Zalenski RJ, Rydman RJ, McCarren M, et al. Feasibility of a rapid diagnostic protocol for an emergency department chest pain unit. Ann Emerg Med 1997; 29:99–108.
15. Bahr RD. State-of-the-art in community coronary care. Maryland State Med J 1983;32:516–520.
16. Gibler WB, Walsh RA, Levy RC, Runyon JP. Rapid diagnostic and treatment centers in the emergency department for patients with chest pain. Circulation 1992;86:1–15.
17. Howell JM, Hedges JR. Differential diagnosis of chest discomfort and general approach to myocardial ischemia decision making. Am J Emerg Med 1991; 9:571–579.
18. Lee TH, Rouan GW, Weisberg MC, et al. Sensitivity of routine clinical criteria for diagnosing myocardial infarction within 24 hours of hospitalization. Ann Intern Med 1987;106:181–186.
19. Lee TH. Chest pain in the emergency department: Uncertainty and the test of time. Mayo Clin Proc 1991;66:963–965.
20. Eagle KA. Medical decision making in patients with chest pain. N Engl J Med 1991;324:1282–1283.
21. Tierney WM, Fitzgerald J, McHenry R, et al. Physicians' estimates of the probability of myocardial infarction in emergency room patients with chest pain. Med Decis Making 1986;6:12–17.
22. McCarthy BD, Wong JB, Selker HP. Detecting acute cardiac ischemia in the emergency department: a review of the literature. J Gen Intern Med 1990;5: 365–373.
23. Hedges JR, Kobernick MS. Detection of myocardial ischemia/infarction in the emergency department patient with chest discomfort. Emerg Med Clin North Am 1988;6:317–340.
24. Villanueva FS, Sabia PJ, Afrooktch A, et al. Value and limitations of current methods of evaluating patients presenting to the emergency room with cardiac-related symptoms for determining long-term prognosis. Am J Cardiol 1992;69:746–750.
25. Gibler WB, Lewis LM, Erb RE, et al. Early detection of acute myocardial infarction in patients presenting with chest pain and non-diagnostic ECGs: serial CK-MB sampling in the emergency department. Ann Emerg Med 1990; 19:1359–1366.
26. Gibler WB, Young GP, Hedges JR, et al. Acute myocardial infarction in chest pain patients with nondiagnostic ECGs: serial CK-MB sampling in the emergency department. Ann Emerg Med 1992;21:504–512.
27. Lee TH, Rouan GW, Weisberg MC, et al. Sensitivity of routine clinical criteria for diagnosing myocardial infarction within 24 hours of hospitalization. Ann Intern Med 1987;106:181–186.

28. Tierney WM, Fitzgerald J, McHenry R, et al. Physicians' estimates of the probability of myocardial infarction in emergency room patients with chest pain. Med Decis Making 1986;6:12–17.
29. Lee TH, Cook FE, Weisberg M, et al. Acute chest pain in the emergency room: identification and examination of low risk patients. Arch Intern Med 1985;145:65–69.
30. Sawe U. Pain in acute myocardial infarction—a study of 137 patients in a coronary care unit. Acta Med Scand 1971;190:79–81.
31. Myerburg RJ, Kessler KM, Mallon SM. Life-threatening ventricular arrhythmias in patients with silent myocardial ischemia due to coronary artery vasospasm. N Engl J Med 1992;326:1451–1455.
32. Ingram DA, Fulton RA, Portal RW, P'Aber C. Vomiting as a diagnostic aid in acute ischemic cardiac pain. Br Med J 1980;281:636–637.
33. Margolis JR, Kannel WB, Feinlab M, et al. Clinical features of unrecognized myocardial infarction—silent and symptomatic. Eighteen years follow-up: the Framingham Study. Am J Cardiol 1973;32:1–7.
34. Kannel WB, Abbott RD. Incidence and prognosis of unrecognized myocardial infarction: an update on the Framingham Study. N Engl J Med 1984;311: 1144–1147.
35. Rosenman RH, Friedman M, Jenkins CD, et al. Clinically unrecognized myocardial infarction in the Western Collaborative Group Study. Am J Cardiol 1967; 19(6):776–782.
36. Uretsky BF, Farquhar DS, Berezin AF, et al. Symptomatic myocardial infarction without chest pain: prevalence and clincial course. Am J Cardiol 1977; 40:498–503.
37. Villanueva FS, Sabia PJ, Afrooteh A, et al. Value and limitations of current methods of evaluating patients presenting to the emergency room with cardiac-related symptoms for determining long-term prognosis. Am J Cardiol 1992;69:746–750.
38. Hedges JR, Kobernick MS. Detection of myocardial ischemia/infarction in the emergency department patient with chest discomfort. Emerg Med Clin North Am 1988;6:317–340.
39. Weaver WD, Cerqueira M, Hallstrom AP, et al. Prehospital-initiated vs hospital-initiated thrombolytic therapy: The myocardial infarction triage and intervention trial. JAMA 1993;270:1211–1216.
40. Rouan GW, Lee TH, Cook EF, et al. Clinical characteristics and outcome of acute myocardial infarction in patients with initially normal or nonspecific electrocardiogram. Am J Cardiol 1989;64:1087–1092.
41. Fesmire FM, Percy RF, Wears RL. Diagnostic and prognostic importance of comparing the initial to the previous electrocardiogram in patients admitted for suspected acute myocardial infarction. South Med J 1991;84:941–946.
42. Krucoff MW, Pope JE, Bottner RK, et al. Computer-assisted ST-segment monitoring: experience during and after brief coronary occlusion. J Electrocardiol (suppl) October 1987.
43. Krucoff MW, Green CE, Satler LF, et al. Noninvasive detection of coronary

artery patency using continuous ST-segment monitoring. Am J Cardiol 1986; 57:916–922.
44. Krucoff MW, Parente AR, Bottner RK et al. Stability of multilead ST-segment "fingerprints" over time after percutaneous transluminal coronary angioplasty and its usefulness in detecting reocclusion. Am J Cardiol 1988;61:1232–1237.
45. Krucoff MW, Wagner NB, Pope JE, et al. The portable programmable microprocessor-driven real-time 12-lead electrocardiographic monitor: a preliminary report of a new device for the non-invasive detection of successful reperfusion or silent coronary reocclusion. Am J Cardiol 1990;65:143–148.
46. Fesmire FM, Smith EE. Continuous 12-lead electrocardiograph monitoring in the emergency department. Am J Emerg Med 1993;11:54–60.
47. Hogg KJ, Hornung RS, Howie CA, et al. Electrocardiographic prediction of coronary artery patency after thrombolytic treatment in acute myocardial infarction: use of the ST-segment as a non-invasive marker. Br Heart J 1988; 60:275–280.
48. McQueen MJ, Holder D, El-Maraghi RH. Assessment of the accuracy of serial electrocardiograms in the diagnosis of myocardial infarction: correlation with technetium-99m stannous pyrophosphate myocardial scintigraphy. Am J Med 1980;68:405–413.
49. Gibler WB, Sayre MR, Levy RC, et al. Serial 12-lead electrocardiographic monitoring in patients presenting to the emergency department with chest pain. J Electrocardiol 1994;26(suppl):238–243.
50. Fesmire FM, Percy RF, Bardoner JB, et al. Usefulness of automated serial 12-lead ECG monitoring during the initial emergency department evaluation of patients with chest pain. Ann Emerg Med 1998;31:3–11.
51. Sobel BE, Bresnahan GF, Shell WE, Yoder RD. Estimation of infarct size in many and its relation to prognosis. Circulation 1972;46:640–648.
52. Grenadier E, Keidar S, Kahana L, et al. The roles of serum myoglobin, total CPK, and CK-MB isoenzyme in the acute phase of myocardial infarction. Am Heart J 1983;105:408–416.
53. Varat MA, Mercer DW. Cardiac specific creative phosphokinase isoenzyme in the diagnosis of acute myocardial infarction. Circulation 1975;51:855–859.
54. Grande P, Hansen BG, Christiansen C, Naestoft J. Estimation of acute myocardial infarct size in many by serum CK-MB measurements. Circulation 1982;65:756–764.
55. Roe CR, Limbird LE, Wagner GS, Nerenberg ST. Combined isoenzyme analysis in the diagnosis of myocardial injury: application of electrophoretic methods for the detection and quantitation of the creatine phosphokinase MB isoenzyme. J Lab Clin Med 1972;80:577–589.
56. Gerhardt W, Hofvendahl S, Ljungdahl L, Waldenstrom J. S-CK and S-CKB in suspected acute myocardial infarction. Upsala J Med Sci 1983;88:193–199.
57. Wu AHB, Gornet TG, Harker CC, Chen H-L. Role of rapid immunoassays for urgent ("stat") determinations of creatine kinase isoenzyme MB. Clin Chem 1989;35:1752–1756.

58. Shell WE, Kligerman M, Rorke MP, Burnam M. Sensitivity and specificity of MB creatine kinase activity determined with column chromatography. Am J Cardiol 1979;44:67–75.
59. Thompson WG, Mahr RG, Yohannan WS, Pinens MR. Use of creatine kinase MB isoenzyme for diagnosing myocardial infarction when total creatine kinase activity is high. Clin Chem 1988;34:2208–2210.
60. Eisenberg PR, Shaw D, Schaab C, Jaffe AS. Concordance of creatine kinase-MB activity and mass. Clin Chem 1989;35:440–443.
61. Bernstein LH, Good IJ, Holtzman GI, Deaton ML, Babb J. Diagnosis of acute myocardial infarction from two measurements of creatine kinase MB with use of nonparametric probability estimation. Clin Chem 1989;35:444–447.
62. Blomberg DT, Kimber WD, Burke MD. Creatine kinase isoenzymes: predictive value in the early diagnosis of acute myocardial infarction. Am J Med 1975;59:464–469.
63. Irvin RG, Cobb FR, Roe CR. Acute myocardial infarction and MB creatine phosphokinase: relationship between onset of symptoms of infarction and appearance and disappearance of enzyme. Arch Intern Med 1980;140:329–334.
64. Shell We, Kligerman M, Rorke MP, Burnam M. Sensitivity and specificity of MB creatine kinase activity determined with column chromatography. Am J Cardiol 1979;44:67–75.
65. Jockers-Wreton E, Pfleiderer G. Quantitation of creatine kinase isoenzymes in human tissues and sera by an immunological method. Clin Chim Acta 1975;58:223–232.
66. Brush JE, Brand DA, Acampora D, Goldman L, Cabin HS. Relation of peak creatine kinase levels during acute myocardial infarction to presence or absence of previous manifestations of myocardial ischemia (angina pectoris or healed myocardial infarction). Am J Cardiol 1988;62:534–537.
67. Lee RT, Lee TH, Poole K, Gustafson N, Stone PH, et al. Rate of disappearances of creatine kinase-MB after acute myocardial infarction: clinical determinants of variability. Am Heart J 1988;116:1493–1497.
68. Stein EA, Kaplan LA. Serum enzymes, isoenzymes, myoglobin, and contractile proteins in acute myocardial infarction: non-invasive diagnostic methods in cardiology. Cardiovasc Clin 1983;13:355.
69. Roark SF, Wagner GS, Izlar HL, Roe CR. Diagnosis of acute myocardial infarction in a community hospital: significance of CPK-MB determination. Circulation 1976;53:965–969.
70. Herlitz J, Hjalmarson A, Waldenstrom J. Estimated appearance of raised serum enzyme activity in relation to onset of symptoms in acute myocardial infarction. Acta Cardiol 1985;40:461–476.
71. Wagner GS. Optimal use of serum enzyme levels in the diagnosis of acute myocardial infarction. Arch Intern Med 1980;140:317–319.
72. Quale J, Kimmelstiel C, Lipschik G, Schrem S. Use of sequential cardiac enzyme analysis in stratification of risk for myocardial infarction in patients with unstable angina. Arch Intern Med 1988;148:1277–1279.

73. Morison IM, Cayson KJ, Fine JS. Effect of creatine kinase-mm subtype composition on a CK-MB immunoinhibition assay. Clin Chem 1988;34:535–538.
74. El Allaf M, Chapelle J-P, El Allaf D, et al. Differentiating muscle damage from myocardial injury by means of the serum creatine kinase (CK) isoenzyme MB mass measurement/total CK activity ratio. Clin Chem 1986;32: 291–295.
75. Lott JA. Serum enzyme determinations in the diagnosis of acute myocardial infarction: an update. Hum Pathol 1984;706–716.
76. Lee TH, Weisberg MC, Cook EF, et al. Evaluation of creatine kinase and creatine kinase-MB for diagnosing myocardial infarction: clinical impact in the emergency room. Arch Intern Med 1987;147:115–121.
77. Hong RA, Licht JD, Wei JY. Elevated CK-MB with normal total creatine kinase in suspected myocardial infarction: associated clinical findings and early prognosis. Am Heart J 1986;111:1041–1047.
78. Heller GV, Blanstein AS, Wei JY. Implications of increased myocardial isoenzyme level in the presence of normal creatine kinase activity. Am J Cardiol 1983;51:24–27.
79. Jay DW. Macro-creatine kinase co-immigrating with CK-MB on electrophoresis. Clin Chem 1988;34:1920.
80. Dillon MC, Calbreath DF, Dixon AM, et al. Diagnostic problem in acute myocardial infarction: CK-MB in the absence of abnormally elevated total creatine kinase levels. Arch Intern Med 1982;142:33–38.
81. Galen RS. The enzyme diagnosis of myocardial infarction. Hum Pathol 1975; 6:141–155.
82. Galen RS, Reiffel JA, Gambino SR. Diagnosis of acute myocardial infarction. JAMA 1975;232:145–147.
83. Roberts R, Sobel BE. Creatine kinase isoenzymes in the assessment of heart disease. Am Heart J 1978;95:521–528.
84. Konttinen A, Somer H. Determination of serum creatine kinase isoenzymes in myocardial infarction. Am J Cardiol 1972;29:817–820.
85. Wagner GS, Roe CR, Limbird LE, Rosati RA, Wallace AG. The importance of identification of the myocardial-specific isoenzyme of creatine phosphokinase (MB form) in the diagnosis of acute myocardial infarction. Circulation 1973;47:263–269.
86. Fisher ML, Carliner NH, Becker LC, Peters RW, Piotnick GD. Serum creatine kinase in the diagnosis of acute myocardial infarction: optimal sampling frequency. JAMA 1983;249:393–394.
87. Ma KW, Brown DC, Steele BW, From AHL. Serum creatine kinase MB isoenzyme activity in long-term hemodialysis patients. Arch Intern Med 1981; 141:164–166.
88. Lott JA, Stang JM. Serum enzymes and isoenzymes in the diagnosis and differential diagnosis of myocardial ischemia and necrosis. Clin Chem 1980; 26:1241–1250.
89. Lee TH, Goldman L. Serum enzyme assays in the diagnosis of acute myocardial infarction: recommendations based on a quantitative analysis. Ann Intern Med 1986;105:221–233.

90. Collinson PO, Rosalki SB, Flather M, Wolman R, Evans T. Early diagnosis of myocardial infarction by timed sequential enzyme measurements. Ann Clin Biochem 1988;25:376–382.
91. Jaffe AS, Ritter C, Mettzer V, Harter H, Roberts R. Unmasking artifactual increases in creatine kinase isoenzymes in patients with renal failure. J Lab Clin Med 1984;104:193–202.
92. Kwong TC, Arran DA. How many creatine kinase "isoenzymes" are there and what is their clinical significance? Clin Chim Acta 1981;115:3–8.
93. D'Souza JP, Sine HE, Horvitz RA, et al. The significance of the MB isoenzyme in patients with acute cardiovascular disease with abnormal or borderline total CPK activity. Clin Biochem 1978;11:204–209.
94. Roberts R, Herman C. An improved, rapid radioimmunoassay for individual human CK isoenzymes. Am J Cardiol 1980;45:400. Abstract.
95. Nordbeck H, Kahles H, Preussi C-J, Spieckermann PG. Enzymes in cardiac lymph and coronary blood under normal and pathophysiological conditions. J Mol Med 1977;2:255–263.
96. Mego DM, Pupa LE, Bailey SR. Clinical evaluation of a rapid immunoinhibition assay for creatine kinase-MB in suspected myocardial infarction. Mil Med 1993;158:651–654.
97. Quale J, Kimmelstiel C, Lipschik G, Schrem S. Use of sequential cardiac enzyme analysis in stratification of risk for myocardial infarction in patients with unstable angina. Arch Intern Med 1988;148:1277–1279.
98. Sharkey SW, Apple FS, Elsperger J, et al. Early peak of creatine kinase-MB in acute myocardial infarction with a non-diagnostic electrocardiogram. Am Heart J 1988;116:1207–1211.
99. Apple FS, Preese L, Bennett R, Fredrickson A. Clinical and analytical evaluation of two immunoassays for direct measurement of creatine kinase MB with monoclonal anti-CK-MB antibodies. Clin Chem 1988;34:2364–2367.
100. Chan K-W, Ladenson JH, Pierce GF, Jaffe AS. Increased creatine kinase-MB in the absence of acute myocardial infarction. Clin Chem 1986; 32:2044–2051.
101. Chapelle J-P, El Allaf M, Heusghem C. Serum CK-MB after myocardial infarction and coronary bypass surgery: superiority of mass concentration measurement over determination of catalytic activity. Adv Clin Enzymol 1987;5: 94–102.
102. Dufour DR, LaGrenade A, Guerra J. Rapid serial enzyme measurements in evaluation of patients with suspected myocardial infarction. Am J Cardiol 1989;63:652–655.
103. Seager SB. Cardiac enzymes in the evaluation of chest pain. Ann Emerg Med 1980;9:346–349.
104. Hedges JR, Young GP, Henkel GF, Gibler WB, Green TR, Swanson JR. Serial ECGs are less accurate than serial CK-MB results for emergency department diagnosis of myocardial infarction. Ann Emerg Med 1992;21:1445–1450.
105. Landt Y, Vaidya HC, Porter SE, et al. Semi-automated direct colorimetric measurement of creatine kinase isoenzyme MB activity after extraction from

serum by use of a CK-MB-specific monoclonal antibody. Clin Chem 1988; 34:575–581.
106. Al-Sheikh W, Heal AV, Petkaros KC, et al. Evaluation of an immunoradiometric assay specific for the CK-MB isoenzyme for detection of acute myocardial infarction. Am J Cardiol 1984;54:269–273.
107. Clyne CA, Medeiros LJ, Marton KI. The prognostic significance of immunoradiometric CK-MB assay (IRMA) diagnosis of myocardial infarction in patients with low total CK and elevated MB isoenzymes. Am Heart J 1989; 118:901–906.
108. Green GB, Hanse KN, Chan DW, et al. The potential utility of a rapid CK-MB assay in evaluating emergency department patients with possible myocardial infarction. Ann Emerg Med 1991;20:954–960.
109. Nanji AA. Serum creatine kinase isoenzymes: a review. Muscle Nerve 1983; 6:83–90.
110. Puleo PR, Guadagno PA, Roberts R, Perryman MB. Sensitive, rapid assay of subforms of creatine kinase MB in plasma. Clin Chem 1989;35:1452–1455.
111. Wu AHB. Creatine kinase MM and MB isoforms. Lab Med 1992;23:303–305.
112. Apple FS. Acute myocardial infarction and coronary reperfusion: serum cardiac markers for the 1990's. Am J Clin Pathol 1992;97:217–226.
113. Collins DR, Wright DJ, Rinsler MG, et al. Early diagnosis of acute myocardial infarction with use of a rapid immunochemical assay of creatine kinase MB isoenzyme. Clin Chem 1993;39:1725–1728.
114. Tsung SH. Several conditions causing elevation of serum CK-MB and CK-BB. Am J Clin Pathol 1981;75:711–715.
115. Collinson PO, Ramhamadany EM, Rosalki SB, et al. Diagnosis of acute myocardial infarction from sequential enzyme measurements obtained within 12 hours of admission to hospital. J Clin Pathol 1989;42:1126–1131.
116. Collinson PO, Rosalki SB, Kuwana T, et al. Early diagnosis of acute myocardial infarction by CK-MB mass measurements. Ann Clin Biochem 1992; 29:43–47.
117. Lewis F, Jishi F, Sissons CE, Baker JT, Child DF. Value of emergency cardiac enzymes: audit in a coronary care unit. J R Soc Med 1991;84:398–399.
118. Ellis AK. Serum protein measurements and the diagnosis of acute myocardial infarction. Circulation 1991;83:1107–1109.
119. Apple FS. Creatine kinase-MB. Lab Med 1992;23:298–302.
120. Lang H, Wurzburg U. Creatine kinase, an enzyme of many forms. Clin Chem 1982;28:1439–1447.
121. Norregaard-Hansen K, Egstrup K, Nielsen JR, et al. Lack of indication of myocardial cell damage after myocardial ischemia in patients with severe stable angina. Eur Heart J 1992;13:188–193.
122. Young GP, Gibler WB, Hedges JR, et al. For the EMCREG Study Group. Acad Emerg Med 1997;4:869–877.
123. Wu AHB, Gornet TG, Bretandiere J-P, Panfill PR. Comparison of enzyme immunoassay and immunoprecipitation for creatine kinase MB in diagnosis of acute myocardial infarction. Clin Chem 1985;31:470–474.

124. Grande P, Granborg J, Clemmenson P, et al. Indices of reperfusion in patients with acute myocardial infarction using characteristics of the CK-MB time-activity curve. Am Heart J 1991;122:400–408.
125. Hoekstra JW, Hedges JR, Gibler WB, et al. Emergency department CK-MB—a predictor of ischemic complications. Acad Emerg Med 1994;1:17–28.
126. Lange RA, Cigarroa RG, Yancy CW. Cocaine-induced coronary-artery vasoconstriction. N Engl J Med 1989;321:1557–1562.
127. Nademanee K, Gorelick DA, Josephson MA, et al. Myocardial ischemia during cocaine withdrawal. Ann Intern Med 1989;111:876–880.
128. Tokarski GF, Paganussi P, Urbanski R. An evaluation of cocaine-induced chest pain. Ann Emerg Med 1990;19:1088–1092.
129. Puleo PR, Guadagno PA, Roberts R, et al. Early diagnosis of acute myocardial infarction based on assay for subforms of creatine kinase-MB. Circulation. 1990;82:759–764.
130. Gibler WB, Gibler CD, Weinshenker E, et al. Myoglobin as an early indicator of acute myocardial infarction. Ann Emerg Med 1987;16:851–856.
131. Polanczyk CA, Lee TH, Cook EF, Walls R, Wybenga D, Johnson PA. Value of additional two-hour myoglobin for the diagnosis of myocardial infarction in the emergency department. Am J Cardiol 1999;83:525–529.
132. Vaidga HC. Myoglobin. Lab Med 1992;23:306–310.
133. Ohman EM, Casey C, Bengston JR, et al. Early detection of acute myocardial infarction: additional diagnostic information from serum concentrations of myoglobin in patients without ST-elevation. Br Heart J 1990;63:335–338.
134. Vuori J, Huttunen K, Vuotikka P, Vaananen HK. The use of myoglobin/carbonic anhydrase III ratio as a marker for myocardial damage in patients with renal failure. Clin Chim Acta 1997;265:33–40.
135. Plebani M, Zaninotto M. Diagnostic strategies using myoglobin measurement in myocardial infarction. Clin Chim Acta 1998;272:69–77.
136. Christenson RH, Ohman EM, Topol EJ, et al. for the TAMI-7 Study Group. Assessment of coronary reperfusion after thrombolysis with a model combining myoglobin, creatine kinase, and clinical variables. Circulation 1997;86: 1776–1782.
137. Bodor GS, Porter S, Landt Y, Ladenson JH. Development of monoclonal antibodies for an assay of cardiac troponin-I and preliminary results in suspected cases of myocardial infarction. Clin Chem 1992;38:2203–2214.
138. Katus HA, Schoeppenthau M, Tanzeem A, et al. Non-invasive assessment of perioperative myocardial cell damage by circulating cardiac troponin T. Br Heart J 1991;65:259–264.
139. Katus HA, Remppis A, Scheffold T, Diederich KW, Kuebler W. Intracellular compartmentation of cardiac troponin T and its release kinetics in patients with reperfused and nonreperfused myocardial infarction. Am J Cardiol 1991; 67:1360–1367.
140. Katus HA, Scheffold T, Remppis A, Zehlein J. Proteins of the troponin complex. Lab Med 1992;23:311–317.
141. Katus HA, Looser S, Hallermayer K, et al. Development and in vitro char-

acterization of a new immunoassay of cardiac troponin T. Clin Chem 1992; 38:386–393.
142. Katus HA, Remppis A, Nuemann FJ, et al. Diagnostic efficiency of troponin T measurements in acute myocardial infarction. Circulation 1991;83:902–912.
143. Hamm CW, Ravkilde J, Gerhardt W, et al. The prognostic value of serum troponin T in unstable angina. N Engl J Med 1992;327:146–150.
144. Adams JE, Bodor GS, Davila-Roman VG, et al. Cardiac troponin I: a marker with high specificity for cardiac injury. Circulation 1993;88:101–106.
145. Braunwald E. Unstable angina: a classification. Circulation 1989;80:410–414.
146. Gerhardt W, Katua HA, Rarkilde J, et al. S-troponin T in suspected ischemic myocardial injury compared with mass and catalytic concentrations of s-creatine kinase isoenzyme MB. Clin Chem 1991;37:1405–1411.
147. Van der Werf F. Cardiac troponins in acute coronary syndromes. N Engl J Med 1996;335:1388–1389.
148. Katus HA, Remppis A, Looser S, et al. Enzyme linked immuno assay of cardiac troponin T for the detection of acute myocardial infarction in patients. J Mol Cell Cardiol 1989;21:1349–1353.
149. Katagiri T, Kobayashi Y, Sasai Y, Toba K, Niitani H. Alterations in cardiac troponin subunits in myocardial infarction. Jpn Heart J 1981;22:653–664.
150. Falk E. Unstable angina with fatal outcome: dynamic coronary thrombosis leading to infarction and/or sudden death. Circulation 1985;71:699–708.
151. Talasz H, Genser N, Mair J, et al. Side-branch occlusion during percutaneous transluminal coronary angioplasty. Lancet 1992;339:1380–1382.
152. Chesebro JH, Fuster V. Thrombosis in unstable angina. N Engl J Med 1992; 327:192–194.
153. Larue C, Calzolari C, Bertinchant J-P, et al. Cardiac-specific immunoenzymometric assay of troponin I in the early phase of acute myocardial infarction. Clin Chem 1993;39:972–979.
154. Ohman EM, Armstrong PW, Christenson RH, et al. Cardiac troponin T levels for risk stratification in acute myocardial ischemia. N Engl J Med 1996;335: 1333–1341.
155. Falahati A, Sharkey SW, Christensen D, McCoy M, Miller E, Murakami MA, Apple FS. Implementation of serum cardiac troponin I as marker for detection of acute myocardial infarction. Am Heart J 1999;137:332–337.
156. Tucker JF, Collins RA, Anderson AJ, Hauser J, Kalas J, Apple FS. Early diagnostic efficiency of cardiac troponin I and troponin T for acute myocardial infarction. Acad Emerg Med 1997;4:13–21.
157. Galvani M, Ottani F, Ferrini D, Ladenson JH, Destro A, Baccos D, et al. Prognostic influence of elevated values of cardiac troponin I in patients with unstable angina. Circulation 1997;95:2053–2059.
158. Christenson RH, Duh SH, Newby K, Ohman EM, Califf RM, Granger CB, et al. Cardiac troponin T and cardiac troponin I: relative value in short-term risk stratification of patients with acute coronary syndromes. Clin Chem 1998; 44:494–501.

159. Wu AH, Lane PL. Metaanalysis in clinical chemistry: validation of cardiac troponin T as a marker for ischemic heart disease. Clin Chem 1995;41:1228–1233.
160. Stubbs P, Collinson P, Moseley D, Greenwood T, Noble M. Prognostic significance of admission troponin T concentrations in patients with myocardial infarction. Circulation 1996;94:1291–1297.
161. Ottani F, Galvani M, Ferrini D, Ladenson JH, Puggioni R, Destro A, et al. Direct comparison of early elevations of cardiac troponin T and I in patients with clinical unstable angina. Am Heart J 1999;137:284–291.
162. Benamer H, Steg PG, Benessiano J, Vicaut E, Gaultier C, Boccara A, et al. Comparison of the prognostic value of C-reactive protein and troponin I in patients with unstable angina pectoris. Am J Cardiol 1998;82:845–850.
163. Antman EM, Tanasijevic MJ, Thompson B, Schactman M, McCabe CH, Cannon CP, et al. Cardiac-specific troponin I levels to predict the risk of mortality in patients with acute coronary syndromes. N Engl J Med 1996;335:1342–1349.
164. Polanczyk CA, Lee TH, Cook EF, Walls R, Wybenga D, Printy-Klein G, et al. Cardiac troponin I as a predictor of major cardiac events in emergency department patients with acute chest pain. J Am Coll Cardiol 1998;32:8–14.
165. Sayre MR, Kaufmann KH, Chen IW, Sperling M, Sidman R, Diercks DB, et al. Measurement of cardiac troponin T is an effective method for predicting complications among emergency department patients with chest pain. Ann Emerg Med 1998;31:539–549.
166. Antman EM, Sacks DB, Rifai N, McCabe CH, Cannon CP, Braunwald E. Time to positivity of a rapid bedside assay for cardiac-specific troponin T predicts prognosis in acute coronary syndromes. J Am Coll Cardiol 1998;31:326–330.
167. Adams JE, Bodor GS, Davila-Roman VG, et al. Cardiac troponin I: a marker with high specificity for cardiac injury. Circulation 1993;88:101–106.
168. Collinson PO. Troponin T or I or CK-MB (or none?). Eur Heart J 1998;19(suppl N):N16–N24.
169. Stewart JT, French JK, Theroux P, Ramanathan K, Solymoss BC, Johnson R, White HD. Early noninvasive identification of failed reperfusion after intravenous thrombolytic therapy in acute myocardial infarction. J Am Coll Cardiol 1998;31:1499–1505.
170. Ascoop CA, Simoons ML, Egmond WG, Bruschke AVG. Exercise test, history, and serum lipid levels in patients with chest pain and normal electrocardiogram at rest: comparison to findings of coronary arteriography. Am Heart J 1971;82:609–617.
171. Weiner DA, Ryan TJ, McCabe CH. Correlations among history of angina, ST-segment response, and prevalence of coronary-artery disease in the Coronary Artery Surgery Study (CASS). N Engl J Med 1979;301:230–235.
172. Cumming GR, Dufresne C, Kich L, Samm J. Exercise electrocardiographic patterns in normal women. Br Heart J 1973;35:1055–1061.

173. Bartel AG, Behar VS, Peter RH, Orgain ES, Kong Y. Graded exercise stress tests in angiographically documented coronary artery disease. Circulation 1974;49:348–356.
174. Redwood DR, Epstein SE. Uses and limitations of stress testing in the evaluation of ischemic heart disease. Circulation 1972;46:1115–1131.
175. Pratt CM, Francis MJ, Divine GW, Young JB. Exercise testing in women with chest pain: are there additional exercise characteristics that predict true positive test results? Chest 1989;95:139–144.
176. Mark DB, Shaw L, Harrell FE, et al. Prognostic value of a treadmill exercise score in outpatients with suspected coronary artery disease. N Engl J Med 1991;325:849–853.
177. Goldschlager N, Selzer A, Cohn K. Treadmill stress tests indicators of presence and severity of coronary artery disease. Ann Intern Med 1976;85:277–286.
178. Sheffield LT, Reeves TJ. Graded exercise in the diagnosis of angina pectoris. Mod Concepts Cardiovasc Dis 1965;34:1–6.
179. Kerns JR, Shaub TF, Fontanarosa PB. Emergency cardiac stress testing in the evaluation of emergency department patients with atypical chest pain. Ann Emerg Med 1993;22:794–798.
180. Tsakonis JS, Shesser R, Rosenthal R, et al. Safety of immediate treadmill testing in selected emergency department patients with chest pain. Am J Emerg Med 1991;9:557–559.
181. Kirk JD, Turnipseed S, Lewis WR, Amsterdam EA. Evaluation of chest pain in low-risk patients presenting to the emergency department: the role of immediate exercise testing. Ann Emerg Med 1998;32:1–7.
182. Lewis WR, Amsterdam EA, Turnipseed S, Kirk JD. Immediate exercise testing of low risk patients with known coronary artery disease presenting to the emergency department with chest pain. J Am Coll Cardiol 1999;33:1843–1847.
183. Mark DB, Shaw L, Harrell FE, et al. Prognostic value of a treadmill exercise score in outpatients with suspected coronary artery disease. N Engl J Med 1991;325:849–853.
184. Sabia P, Abbott RD, Afrookteh A, Keller MW, Touchstone DA, Kaul S. Importance of two-dimensional echocardiographic assessment of left ventricular systolic function in patients presenting to the emergency room with cardiac-related symptoms. Circulation 1991;84:1615–1624.
185. Sasaki H, Charuzi Y, Beeder C, et al. Utility of echocardiography for the early assessment of patients with non-diagnostic chest pain. Am Heart J 1986;112:494–497.
186. Berthe C, Pierard LA, Hiernaux M, et al. Predicting the extent and location of coronary artery disease in acute myocardial infarction by echocardiography during dobutamine infusion. Am J Cardiol 1986;58:1167–1172.
187. Sabia P, Afrookteh A, Touchstone DA, et al. Value of regional wall motion abnormality in the emergency room diagnosis of acute myocardial infarction: a prospective study using two dimensional echocardiography. Circulation 1991;84:85–92.

188. Peels CH, Visser CA, FunkeKupper AJ, Visser FC, Roos JP. Usefulness of two-dimensional echocardiography for immediate detection of myocardial ischemia in the emergency room. Am J Cardiol 1990;65:687–691.
189. Horowitz RS, Morganroth J, Parrotto C, et al. Immediate diagnosis of acute myocardial infarction by two dimensional echocardiography. Circulation 1982;65:323–329.
190. Loh IK, Charuzi Y, Breeder C, Marshall CA, Ginsburg JH. Early diagnosis of nontransmural myocardial infarction by two-dimensional echocardiography. Heart J Am 1982;104:963–968.
191. Oh JK, Shub C, Miller FA, Evans WE, Tajik AJ. Role of two-dimensional echocardiography in the emergency room. Echocardiography 1985;2:217–226.
192. Hoffman R, Lethen H, Kleinhaus E, et al. Comparative evaluation of bicycle and dobutamine stress echocardiography and perfusion scintigraphy and bicycle electrocardiogram for identification of coronary artery disease. Am J Cardiol 1993;74:987–990.
193. Levitt MA, Promes SB, Bullock S, Disano M, Young GP, Goe G, Peaslee D. Combined cardiac marker approach with adjunct two-dimensional echocardiography to diagnose acute myocardial infarction in the emergency department. Ann Emerg Med 1996;27:1–7.
194. Zaret BL, Wackers FJT. Nuclear cardiology. N Engl J Med 1993;329:775–783,855–863.
195. Mace SE. Thallium myocardial scanning in the emergency department evaluation of chest pain. Am J Emerg Med 1989;7:321–328.
196. Kim SC, Adams SL, Hendel RC. Role of nuclear cardiology in the evaluation of acute coronary syndromes. Ann Emerg Med 1997;30:210–218.
197. Hilton TC, Thompson RC, Williams HJ, et al. Technitium-99m sestamibi myocardial perfusion imaging in the emergency room evaluation of chest pain. J Am Coll Cardiol 1994;23:1016–1022.
198. Kontos MC, Jesse RL, Schmidt KL, Ornato JP, Tatum JL. Value of acute rest sestamibi perfusion imaging for evaluation of patients admitted to the emergency department with chest pain. J Am Coll Cardiol 1997;30:976–982.
199. Iskander S, Iskandrian AE. Risk assessment using single-photon emission computed tomographic technitium-99m sestamibi imaging. J Am Coll Cardiol 1998;32:57–62.
200. Tatum JL, Jesse RL, Kontos MC, et al. Comprehensive strategy for the evaluation and triage of the chest pain patient. Ann Emerg Med 1997;116–125.
201. Kontos MC, Jesse RL, Anderson P, Schmidt KL, Ornato JP, Tatum JL. Comparison of myocardial perfusion imaging and cardiac troponin I in patients admitted to the emergency department with chest pain. Circulation 1999;99: 2073–2078.
202. Varetto T, Cantalupi D, Altieri A, et al. Emergency room technitium-99m sestamibi imaging to rule out acute myocardial ischemic events in patients with nondiagnostic electrocardiograms. J Am Coll Cardiol 1993;22:1804–1808.
203. Hilton TC, Fulmer H, Abuan T, Thompson RC, Stowers SA. Ninety-day follow-up of patients in the emergency department with chest pain who undergo

initial single-photon emission computed tomographic perfusion scintigraphy with technitium 99m-labeled sestamibi. J Nucl Cardiol 1996;3:308–311.
204. Bilodeau L, Theroux P, Gregoire J, et al. Technitium-99m sestamibi tomography in patients with spontaneous chest pain. J Am Coll Cardiol 1991;18: 1684–1691.
205. Stowers SA, Abuan TH, Szymanski TJ, et al. Technitium-99m sestamibi SPECT and technitium-99m tetrofosmin SPECT in prediction of cardiac events in patients injected during chest pain and following resolution of pain. J Nucl Med 1995;36:88P–89P. Abstract.
206. Kontos MC, Schmidt KL, Nicholson CS, Ornato JP, Jesse RL, Tatum JL. Myocardial perfusion imaging with technitium-99m sestamibi in patients with cocaine-associated chest pain. Ann Emerg Med 1999;33:639–645.
207. Kontos MC, Alimard R, Krishnaswami A, et al. Use of acute emergency department perfusion imaging results in more appropriate ise of coronary angiography. Circulation 1999;100:I584. Abstract.
208. Radensky PW, Stowers SA, Hilton TC, et al. Cost-effectiveness of acute myocardial perfusion imaging with Tc-99m sestamibi for risk stratification of emergency strategies in unstable angina and non-Q-wave myocardial infarction. Circulation 1994;90:I-528. Abstract.
209. Weismann IA, Dickinson CZ, Dworkin HJ, et al. Cost-effectiveness of myocardial perfusion imaging with SPECT in the emergency department evaluation of patients with unexplained chest pain. Radiology 1996;199:353–357.
210. Storrow AB, Gibler WB, Walsh RA, et al. An emergency department chest pain rapid diagnosis and treatment unit: results from a six year experience. Circulation 1998;98:I425. Abstract.
211. Christain TF, Clements JP, Gibbons RJ. Non-invasive identification of myocardium at risk in patients with acute myocardial infarction and non-diagnostic electrocardiograms with Tc-99m sestamibi. Circulation 1991;83:1615–1620.
212. Peberdy MA, Ornato JP. Improving triage with chest pain. Contemp Intern Med 1997;9:53–62.
213. Ornato JP. Critical pathways for triage and treatment of chest pain patients in the emergency department. Clinician 1996;14:53–55.
214. Nichol G, Walls R, Goldman L, et al. A critical pathway for management of patients with acute chest pain who are at low risk for myocardial ischemia: recommendations and potential impact. Ann Intern Med 1997;127:996–10005.
215. Baxt WB. Use of an artificial neural network for the diagnosis of myocardial infarction. Ann Intern Med 1991;115:906–907.
216. Baxt WG, Skora J. Prospective validation of artificial neural network trained to identify acute myocardial infarction. Lancet 1996;347:12–15.
217. Goldman L, Weinberg M, Weisberg M, et al. A computer-delivered protocol to aid in the diagnosis of emergency room patients with acute chest pain. N Engl J Med 1982;307:588–596.
218. Willems JL, Cassiano A-L, Arnaud P, et al. The diagnostic performance of computer programs for the interpretation of electrocardiograms. N Engl J Med 1991;325:1767–73.

219. Pozen MW, D'Agostino RB, Mitchell JB, et al. The usefulness of a predictive instrument to reduce inappropriate admissions to the coronary care unit. Ann Intern Med 1980;92:238–242.
220. Sawe U. Pain in acute myocardial infarction—a study of 137 patients in a coronary care unit. Acta Med Scand 1971;190:79–81.
221. McNutt RA, Selker HP. How did the acute ischemic heart disease predictive instrument reduce unnecessary coronary care unit admissions? Med Decis Making 1988;8:90–94.
222. Pozen MW, D'Agostino RB, Selker HP, et al. A predictive instrument to improve coronary-care-unit admission practices in acute ischemic heart disease. N Engl J Med 1984;310:1273–1278.
223. Goldman L, Cook EF, Brand DA, et al. A computer protocol to predict myocardial infarction in emergency department patients with chest pain. N Engl J Med 1988;318:797–803.
224. National Heart Attack Alert Program Coordinating Committee 60 Minutes to Treatment Working Group. Rapid identification and treatment of acute myocardial infarction in the emergency department. Ann Emerg Med 1994;23: 311–329.
225. Selker HP, Beshansky JR, Griffith JL, et al. Use of the acute cardiac ischemia time-insensitive predictive instrument (ACI-TIPI) to assist with triage of patients with chest pain or other symptoms suggestive of acute cardiac ischemia. A multicenter, controlled clinical trial. Ann Intern Med 1998;129:845–855.
226. Selker HP, Zalenski RJ, Antman EM, et al. An evaluation of technologies for identifying acute cardiac ischemia in the emergency department: a report from a National Heart Attack Alert Program Working Group. Ann Emerg Med 1997;29:13–87.
227. Laudon DA, Vukov LF, Breen JF, et al. Use of electron-beam computed tomography in the evaluation of chest pain patients in the emergency department. Ann Emerg Med 1999;33:15–21.
228. Hamm CW, Heeschen C, Goldmann B, Vahanian A, Adgey J, Miguel CM, Rutsch W, Berger J, Kootstra J, Simoons ML. Benefit of abciximab in patients with refractory unstable angina in relation to serum troponin T levels. c7E3 Fab antiplatelet therapy in unstable refractory angina (CAPTURE) study investigators. N Engl J Med 1999;340:1623–1629.
229. Lindahl B, Venge P, Wallentin L. Troponin T identifies patients with unstable coronary artery disease who benefit from long-term antithrombotic protection. J Am Coll Cardiol 1997;29:43–48.
230. Antman EM, McCabe CH, Gurfinkel EP, Turpie A, Bernink P, Salein D, deLuna AB, Fox K, Lcblanche JM, Radley D, Premmereur J, Braunwald E, for the TIMI 11B investigators. Enoxaparin prevents death and cardiac ischemic events in unstable angina/non-Q-wave myocardial infarction. Circulation 1999;100:1593–1601.
231. Ross R. Atherosclerosisan inflammatory disease. N Engl J Med 1999;340: 115–126.

13

The Role of the Troponins and Other Markers of Myocardial Necrosis in Risk Stratification

L. Kristin Newby and E. Magnus Ohman
Duke University Medical Center and Duke Clinical Research Institute Durham, North Carolina

Robert H. Christenson
University of Maryland School of Medicine and University of Maryland Medical Center Baltimore, Maryland

INTRODUCTION

The acute coronary syndromes (ACS) represent a pathological, diagnostic, and risk continuum from unstable angina through myocardial infarction (MI) with or without ST-segment elevation. The management strategies and outcomes of patients who present with symptoms of acute coronary ischemia depend upon where they fall within this spectrum. The ability to accurately diagnose and risk-stratify this group of patients at presentation and to provide continuous risk evaluation thereafter is critical, not only for patient outcome but also for efficiency of care. As the health care environment evolves, our focus must also evolve from traditional categorical diagnosis to baseline and long-term risk stratification and to methods that allow continuous risk assessment. Unfortunately, as shown by Lee and colleagues in 1986, the ability of physicians to accurately risk-stratify patients based on clinical factors alone is limited and subject to wide variability among physicians (1). Neither experience nor practice setting of the physician significantly affects predictions of outcome (2).

For the group of patients who undergo thrombolysis for ST-segment elevation MI, the rapid reestablishment of arterial patency, in particular Thrombolysis in Myocardial Infarction (TIMI) grade 3 flow, is related to outcome. In patients in whom thrombolysis is unsuccessful, one would like to intervene early to establish reperfusion, yet it would be impractical to use angiography to determine infarct-artery patency in all patients who undergo thrombolysis. There are clinical signs (such as relief of pain and 50% or greater resolution of ST-segment elevation) that suggest successful reperfusion, but the diagnostic criteria and accuracy of these clinical markers of reperfusion have differed.

The past 10 years have seen extensive investigations into the use of various cardiac markers to establish the diagnosis and prognosis in acute coronary syndromes and to evaluate perfusion after thrombolysis. This chapter will examine the characteristics of the various serum markers of myocardial necrosis that are available today, and focus on their current use in practice as well as the evidence supporting these practices.

SERUM MARKERS OF MYOCARDIAL NECROSIS

The Ideal Marker

To be useful for diagnosis in the clinical setting, a serum marker of myocardial necrosis should be rapidly released early after the onset of ischemic symptoms and remain elevated for 12 to 24 hours in the serum, but not so long as to preclude detection of recurrent myocardial injury after an index event. It should be released in proportion to the degree of myocardial injury and should be very specific for myocardial cell damage versus skeletal muscle or other tissue damage (that is, found in cardiac muscle but not in other tissues). To have a very sensitive, rapid, quantitative assay for the marker would be ideal, but semiquantitative or qualitative whole-blood bedside assays are particularly useful in emergency departments, where online decisions can facilitate rapid identification and triage of ACS patients. Finally, for use in short- and long-term risk stratification, there should be a correlation between outcome and the presence or absence of a marker in the serum or the degree of elevation of the marker above "normal."

Available Cardiac Markers

The available markers of myocardial necrosis include myoglobin, creatine kinase (CK), its myocardial band isoenzyme fraction (CK-MB) and its subforms (MB1 and MB2), cardiac troponins I and T (cTnI and cTnT), and lactate dehydrogenase (LDH). Characteristics of the commonly used cardiac markers are shown in Table 1, and their time courses in Figure 1. Table 2 shows the sensitivity and specificity of the currently used cardiac markers for myocardial infarction by time from symptom onset. With the development of the CK-MB mass assay and assays that are specific for the cardiac troponins, the use of LDH has become largely of historic interest and will not be discussed further in this chapter.

Myoglobin

Myoglobin is a 17.8-kDa heme protein that is found in all striated muscle, including cardiac tissue. It is released early after the onset of ischemia, is usually elevated at between 1 and 2 hours, peaks at 6 to 12 hours, and returns to baseline by 12 to 24 hours because of rapid renal clearance. Because it is found in all striated muscle, it is not specific for cardiac injury and may be "falsely" elevated in skeletal muscle trauma or skeletal myopathies. Further, because it is excreted renally, it may be falsely positive in patients with renal failure. However, the diagnostic sensitivity and predictive value of a negative result are high in the first hours after MI (3). Although sensitive, rapid commercial assays are available, as a marker for cardiac muscle necrosis, it suffers from its lack of specificity and rapid renal clearance. Therefore, even though it may be positive very early after injury, it cannot provide a sole basis for a decision.

Creatine Kinase

Creatine kinase (~85 kDa molecular weight) is a ubiquitous enzyme in the cytosol of striated muscle (and many other tissues) that catalyzes the phosphorylation of creatine to creatine phosphate. There are three isoenzymes of creatine kinase, each composed of two subunits (M and B) that, in dimeric form, constitute the functional enzyme. CK-MM is found predominantly in striated muscle (skeletal and cardiac), CK-MB predominantly in the heart, and CK-BB in the brain. With myocardial necrosis, total CK is detectable above the reference range 4 to 6 hours after the onset of ischemic symptoms. Total CK is not specific for cardiac muscle, however, and the normal reference interval varies by age, race, muscle mass, and sex (4). It may be elevated in a variety of pathological and other conditions. Therefore CK alone has limited utility in the diagnosis of myocardial necrosis.

Creatine Kinase-MB

Creatine kinase-MB (CK-MB) is the myocardial-specific isoenzyme of CK, composed of one M and one B subunit. It is found in small amounts in skeletal muscle, where further production can be induced by stress or injury (5,6). CK-MB can be quantified by both activity and mass assays, although

Table 1 Characteristics of Various Biochemical Markers of Myocardial Necrosis

	Myoglobin	Total CK	CK-MB (mass)	MB2/MB1	cTnT	cTnI	LDH
Molecular weight (kDa)	17.8	85	85	NA	33	23.5	135
Cardiac-specific	No	No	++	++	+++	+++	No
Affected by renal function	Yes	No	Yes	No	Yes	Yes	No
Initial detection	1–3 h	4–8 h	3–4 h	3–4 h	4–6 h	4–6 h	8–12 h
Duration of elevation	18–24 h	12–24 h	24–36 h	Unknown	10–14 d	7–10 d	10 d
Rapid laboratory assay	Yes	Yes	Yes	Yes	Yes	Yes	Yes
Bedside assay	Yes	Yes	Yes	No	Yes	Yes	No

CK, creatine kinase; cTnT, cardiac troponin T; cTnI, cardiac troponin I; LDH, lactate dehydrogenase; NA, not available; h, hours; d, days; ++, very specific; +++, extremely specific.

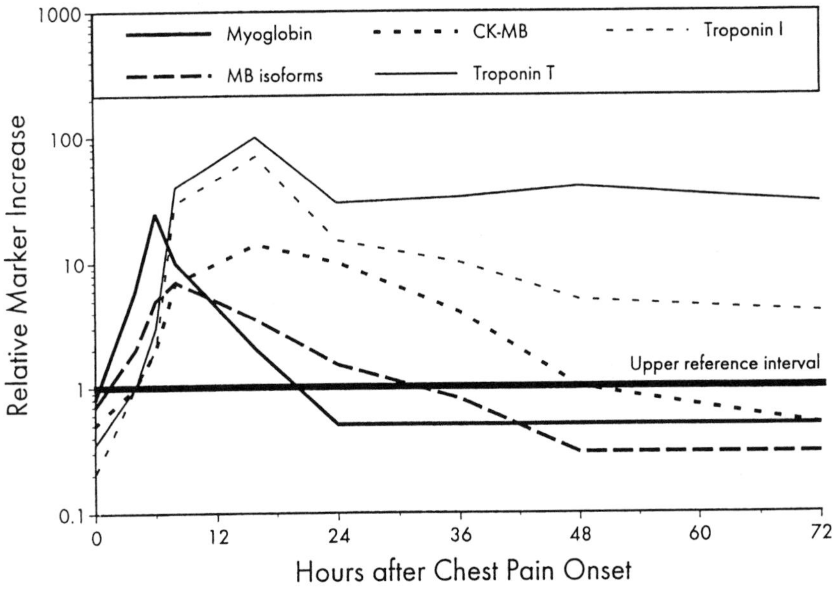

Figure 1 Time course after symptom onset for various biochemical markers of myocardial necrosis. CK-MB = creatine kinase-MB isoenzyme.

the latter is more sensitive and favored for early detection of myocardial necrosis. By mass assay, CK-MB is detectable above the reference range in the serum within 4 hours after the onset of ischemia and remains elevated for 24 to 36 hours. Because of its fairly rapid rise and fall, it can be used to detect reinfarction after an initial MI. Like myoglobin and total CK, the use of CK-MB is limited somewhat in conditions resulting in skeletal muscle damage, because about 5% of skeletal muscle CK is of the MB isoform. Table 3 summarizes conditions in which CK and CK-MB may be elevated with no myocardial ischemia (7).

CK-MB Subforms

Although four CK-MB isoforms can occur in the serum, CK-MB exists predominantly in two forms—MB2, the predominant form in tissue, and MB1, the seroconverted form. CK-MB is released as the MB2 subform at myocardial cell death and is converted in the serum by carboxypeptidase to MB1 through cleavage of the terminal lysine on the M subunit (Fig. 2). With acute myocardial necrosis, more MB2 is released than normal, increasing the amount of MB2 relative to MB1. When the ratio of MB2 to MB1 exceeds 1.5 and the absolute value for the MB2 subfraction is ≥1.0 U/L, the

Table 2 Diagnostic Sensitivity and Specificity of Markers for Myocardial Infarction Based on Time from Onset of Chest Pain

	Early diagnosis (%)			Late diagnosis (%)			
Marker	2 h	4 h	6 h	10 h	14 h	18 h	22 h
CK-MB subforms							
Sensitivity	21.1	46.4	91.5	96.2	90.6	80.9	53.1
Specificity	90.5	88.9	89.0	90.2	90.0	89.9	92.2
Myoglobin							
Sensitivity	26.3	42.9	78.7	86.5	62.3	57.5	42.9
Specificity	87.3	89.4	89.4	90.2	88.3	88.8	91.3
Troponin T							
Sensitivity	10.5	35.7	61.7	86.5	84.9	78.7	85.7
Specificity	98.4	98.3	96.1	96.4	96.1	95.7	94.6
Troponin I							
Sensitivity	15.8	35.7	57.5	92.3	90.6	95.7	89.8
Specificity	96.8	94.2	94.3	94.6	92.2	93.4	94.2
Total CK-MB activity							
Sensitivity	21.1	40.7	74.5	96.2	98.1	97.9	89.8
Specificity	100.0	98.8	97.5	97.5	96.1	96.9	96.2
Total CK-MB mass							
Sensitivity	15.8	39.3	66.0	90.4	90.5	95.7	95.7
Specificity	99.2	98.8	100.0	99.6	98.9	99.6	99.1

Source: From Ref. 9.

finding is highly sensitive and specific for myocardial necrosis (8). Measurement of the subforms has the ability to detect myocardial necrosis as early as 3 hours after symptom onset and, important for emergency department use, has an excellent negative predictive value. In a recent study by Zimmerman and colleagues, CK-MB subforms was also the most sensitive (91%) and specific (89%) of all marker assays for the early diagnosis of myocardial infarction in emergency department patients with chest pain within 6 hours from onset of symptoms (9).

Cardiac Troponin T

The troponins comprise a group of three proteins (C, I, and T), which interact with tropomyosin to form the troponin-tropomyosin complex. This complex is part of the regulatory and structural backbone of the contractile apparatus of striated muscle (Fig. 3). Troponin T is the 33-kDa structural component of the troponin complex that binds it to tropomyosin. Troponin T exists in three isoforms—skeletal (slow- and fast-twitch) muscle, and cardiac muscle.

Table 3 Conditions with Elevated Creatine Kinase or Creatine Kinase-MB in the Absence of Acute Myocardial Infarction

Total creatine kinase
Muscular disorders
Surgery or trauma
Alcohol intoxication
Muscular injections
Convulsions (grand mal)
Vigorous exercise
Pulmonary emboli
Hypothyroidism
Collagen diseases
Malignant hypothermia
Creatine kinase-MB
Surgery of prostate or uterus
Surgery or trauma to small intestine, tongue, or diaphragm
Strenuous exercise (marathon running)
Cardiac surgery
Myocarditis
Chronic renal failure

Source: Ref. 7.

During fetal development, the cardiac and skeletal forms are coexpressed in both skeletal and cardiac tissues. In the adult, the cardiac isoform is expressed only in cardiac muscle and the skeletal form only in skeletal muscle (5). Although there is evidence in the stressed human heart and in animal models that the skeletal muscle isoform may be reexpressed (10,11), the current assay for cTnT does not appear to react with this isoform (12).

The majority of troponin T in the myocyte exists bound in the troponin-tropomyosin complex; however, there is a small cytoplasmic pool of about 6% of the total. Cardiac troponin T is detectable in the serum above the reference range as early as 4 to 6 hours after onset of symptoms of ischemia, probably reflecting early release of the cytoplasmic pool, and remains elevated for 10 days to 2 weeks as a result of slower and sustained release of troponin T bound in the troponin-tropomyosin complex.

With available monoclonal antibody techniques, cTnT is not detectable in serum from normal volunteers. Because of the sensitivity of the assay compared with CK-MB (the current gold standard for diagnosis of acute MI), the specificity of cTnT for acute MI is lower, although, as will be

MB Subforms

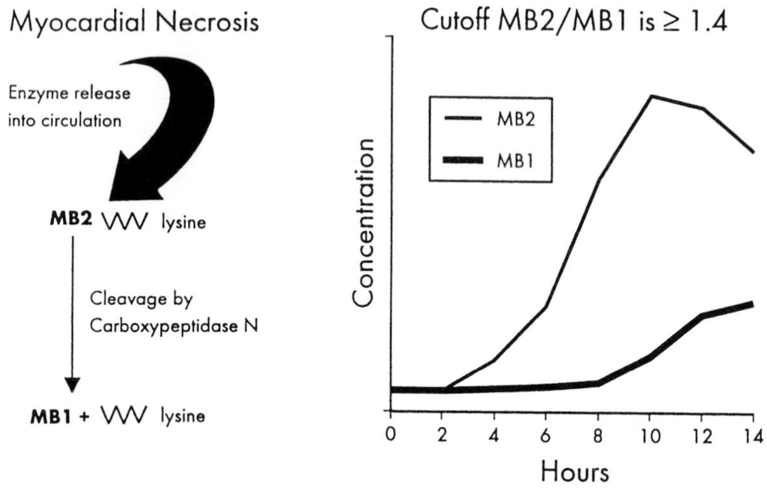

Figure 2 CK-MB isoform conversion.

The Troponins

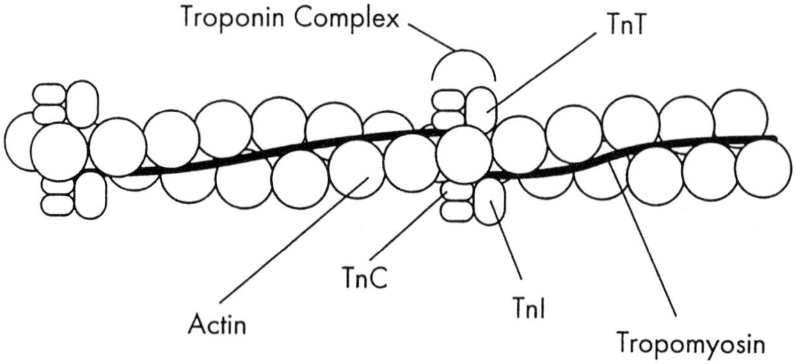

Figure 3 The troponin-tropomyosin complex. TnT = troponin T; TnC = troponin C; TnI = troponin I.

detailed later in the chapter, these "non-MI" elevations of cTnT in ACS patients appear to be prognostically important.

Cardiac Troponin I

Troponin I is a 23.5-kDa component of the troponin complex that inhibits the interaction of myosin cross-bridges with the actin/tropomyosin complex and thus regulates striated muscle contraction. Like troponin T, troponin I exists in three isoforms, cardiac and skeletal (slow- and fast-twitch), that are specific to the given tissue. Also similar to troponin T, troponin I exists predominantly bound within the troponin-tropomyosin complex, but it also has a small cytoplasmic pool of about 2.5% of the total. Unlike troponin T, the cardiac form of troponin I is never expressed in skeletal muscle, even during fetal development (5). Troponin I is detectable in the serum slightly later than cTnT, about 6 hours after the onset of ischemia, and remains elevated for 7 to 10 days. Because of their long serum half-lives, neither cTnT nor cTnI is suitable for detection of reinfarction using currently available assays. However, because they do remain elevated for days, they may be able to reveal an MI that occurred in days past (when presentation of the patient to medical attention is delayed, for example), when other markers of myocardial infarction have returned to normal.

Troponins in Renal Insufficiency

The utility of the troponins for diagnosis and risk stratification in patients with chronic renal insufficiency and end-stage renal disease has been questioned. Numerous reports have suggested that both troponin T and troponin I as well as CK-MB may be falsely elevated in patients with end-stage renal disease in the absence of characteristic diagnostic test abnormalities of coronary artery disease (13–24). In particular, concern about the use of troponin T in this group of patients has been raised.

Clinical considerations for elevation of cardiac troponin T and other markers in end-stage renal disease patients in the absence of documented myocardial injury have included subendocardial ischemia in the absence significant epicardial coronary atherosclerosis—not unlikely given the high prevalence of diabetes and hypertension in the end-stage renal disease population—and the presence of uremic myocardial injury (25). Another interesting finding proposed to explain many of the "false positives" in earlier reports was "interference" with the older ELISA assay for cTnT in patients with end-stage renal disease. The rate of positive cardiac troponin T using this assay has been reported to be as high as 71% to 75% (26,27). In part this may have been contributed to by the low-level crossreactivity of the labeling antibody in this assay with the skeletal isoform of troponin T

(28,29). One report comparing the older assay with a newer sandwich assay in a group of end-stage renal disease patients showed that only 17% of patients were positive with the newer assay, compared with 71% by the older assay (27). However, conflicting results have also been reported that show no difference in the incidence of positive results between the assays (26).

It has been shown in animals that in times of injury or stress there may be induction of expression of the cardiac isoform of troponin T in skeletal muscle (11). There has been speculation that in patients with end-stage renal disease on hemodialysis there is chronic skeletal muscle injury or inflammation with similar induced expression of the cardiac isoform of troponin T in human skeletal muscle. At least two groups have attempted to determine if this mechanism was active in end-stage renal disease patients. McLaurin and colleagues reported that by skeletal muscle biopsy and protein detection by Western blot technique, there was cardiac troponin T detected in the skeletal muscle of end-stage renal disease patients (27). However, Haller et al. demonstrated that there was no cardiac troponin T protein or RNA detectable by immunoblot and immunoflourescence or by reverse transcribed polymerase chain reaction, respectively, in biopsies of skeletal muscle from end-stage renal disease patients who were serum cardiac troponin T-positive (25). In addition, Ricchiuti and colleagues concluded from their work that several isoforms of cTnT are expressed in skeletal muscle, but that the second generation cTnT assay would not detect these isoforms if they were released into the circulation (12).

While uncertainty remains, several studies have attempted to address the clinical utility of the troponins in patients with renal insufficiency. Haller and colleagues have correlated serum cardiac troponin T level with presence or absence of known coronary artery disease or coronary artery disease risk factors (25). Further, Apple and colleagues showed that high levels of cardiac markers correlated with outcome, but were unable to show a clear relationship to outcome in the majority of patients with elevated marker levels and absence of other evidence of myocardial injury (26). More recently, McLaurin demonstrated that in 84 patients with a mean serum creatinine of 4.7 ± 3.3 mg/dL the sensitivities of CK-MB mass and cTnI were similar (68% and 77%, respectively) (30). Further, cTnI was more specific (92%) than CK-MB mass (80%). In addition, studies have shown that cTnT as well as cTnI may predict adverse outcomes in patients on chronic hemodialysis (26,31,32). However, the diagnostic and prognostic cutoffs applied to these patients may not be the same as for patients who are not renally impaired.

A recent study showed that cTnT and cTnI are important prognosticators in asymptomatic, otherwise "stable" patients on chronic renal dialysis (33). Also, in a case control study of 51 patients with renal insufficiency (mean creatinine 3.83 ± 2.68 mg/dL) and 102 control patients (mean creatinine 1.12 ± 0.59 mg/dL), Van Lente and colleagues compared the prognostic capabilities of cTnT and cTnI (34). For both cTnT and cTnI, the area under the receiver operator characteristics curve was significantly less for the renal group than for the nonrenal control group, leading to the conclusion that the ability of both cTnT and cTnI at the usual diagnostic thresholds to predict risk for subsequent adverse cardiac events is similarly reduced in patients with renal insufficiency. Further prospective study of the use of the troponins in renally impaired patients and standardization of assays will be needed to fully elucidate the best marker for detection of myocardial injury and prognosis in this group.

ROLE OF CARDIAC MARKERS

Diagnosis and Prognosis in ST-Segment Elevation Myocardial Infarction

When patients present with symptoms of acute myocardial ischemia and the electrocardiogram reveals ST-segment elevation, the diagnosis of acute MI is confirmed in >90% of cases by serial CK-MB sampling (35,36). The major decisions about acute treatment (thrombolytic therapy, direct angioplasty) and initial management (CCU-level care) in this group are made in response to the clinical and electrocardiographic diagnosis. Serum cardiac markers have played largely a confirmatory role or have been used to document the extent of the infarct or, as will be discussed in more detail, in the case of thrombolytic therapy, to assist in showing that reperfusion had occurred.

In the Global Use of Strategies to Open Occluded Arteries in Acute Coronary Syndromes (GUSTO-IIa) troponin T substudy, we showed that a single troponin T measurement at baseline was able to risk-stratify patients presenting with acute coronary ischemia into those at high or low risk of in-hospital complications. Further, it added significant information, despite the presence of ST-segment elevation, in predicting short-term mortality in these patients (37). Patients with ST-segment elevation who had cTnT ≥0.1 ng/mL had 13% mortality, compared with 4.7% in those with normal cTnT on admission. These findings have been confirmed by Stubbs and colleagues, who examined 240 patients with ST-segment elevation admitted to a general hospital (38). Mortality was significantly higher (32% vs. 13% at 3 years) in patients with cTnT >0.2 ng/mL.

The ability to risk-stratify patients with acute ST-segment elevation MI into high- and low-risk groups at admission could have important implications for both short- and long-term management decisions and for in-hospital resource use, length of stay, and costs. Lee and colleagues identified clinical characteristics at presentation that predicted mortality at 30 days in patients who underwent thrombolysis for ST-segment elevation MI (39). Conversely, several other groups have described clinical features at day 3 or 4 that identify a low-risk population that could be discharged earlier after MI (40–42). In the Global Use of Strategies to Open Occluded Coronary Arteries (GUSTO-III) troponin T substudy, Ohman and colleagues demonstrated in 12,666 patients with ST-segment elevation treated with either alteplase or reteplase, that a bedside whole-blood, qualitative troponin T result at presentation stratified risk for mortality and nonfatal postinfarction complications (43). Patients who were cTnT-positive had significantly higher 30-day mortality than cTnT-negative patients (15.7% vs. 6.2%, $P = .001$). Further, the troponin T result provided independent prognostic information (χ^2 46, $P = .001$) when added to the clinical risk model developed by Lee. Thus, the use of cardiac markers such as cTnT in this population might be used prospectively to improve triage decisions and management strategies, including timing of discharge.

Risk stratification by clinical variables alone can greatly reduce costs of hospitalization in the ST-segment elevation MI population, as shown by Eisenstein and colleagues in the Global Utilization of Streptokinase and TPA (alteplase) for Occluded Coronary Arteries (GUSTO-I) cohort and by Topol in a pilot study of clinical risk stratification to guide early discharge (42,44). Because the use of serum cardiac markers adds incrementally to short-term, clinical risk stratification, the potential economic impact of such a combined strategy should be evaluated.

Noninvasive Detection of Reperfusion After Thrombolytic Therapy

Animal models of acute coronary occlusion and more recent human studies of myocardial salvage after reperfusion with thallium imaging have shown that the duration of occlusion strongly correlates with the amount of infarcted tissue (45,46). Further, the GUSTO-I angiographic substudy has shown the critical relationship between TIMI flow grade after thrombolysis and improved left ventricular function and survival (47). Therefore, reperfusion status must be determined as early as possible, with intervention to complete the process if necessary. In this light, the ability to noninvasively assess reperfusion after thrombolysis should be considered an extension of baseline risk stratification in these patients.

Infarct-artery patency is generally reestablished (when it occurs) within 45 to 60 min after thrombolytic administration (48,49). To be practical for patient care, a noninvasive marker of reperfusion should be available during this window (ideally within 1 hour after the start of therapy), when definitive reestablishment of myocardial perfusion would have the greatest chance of myocardial salvage and the greatest effect on patient outcome.

Clinical indicators of reperfusion, such as partial or complete resolution of ST-segment elevation and relief of ischemic symptoms, have been of some use in predicting outcome. In 327 patients who underwent thrombolysis, Iparraguirre and colleagues showed that presence of a noninvasive clinical marker, *reperfusion clinical syndrome* (at least two of: significant relief of pain, ≥50% reduction in the sum of ST-segment elevation, or abrupt initial increase in CK level), was associated with significantly reduced mortality (odds ratio 0.20, $P < .0001$), but there was no assessment of coronary patency (50). In a Thrombolysis and Angioplasty in Myocardial Infarction (TAMI) cohort, 56% of patients with no ST-segment or symptom resolution had patent arteries at 90-min angiography. Only when ST-segment elevation had resolved completely was patency high (96%), yet this marker was present in only 6% of patients (51). For patients to benefit from early attempts at rescue therapy and to avoid unnecessary angiography, a noninvasive marker of perfusion status should be very sensitive and specific. To improve the diagnostic accuracy of noninvasive assessments of perfusion, investigators have studied the use of many serum cardiac markers, including myoglobin, CK and its subforms, CK-MB, CK-MB subforms, and most recently the troponins I and T.

Peak concentrations, time to peak concentrations, and rates of increase of markers can discriminate between patients with and without successful reperfusion. Unfortunately, in many cases the best discrimination occurs after the time window during which rescue reperfusion therapy would have the best chance of myocardial salvage or effect on survival (52–57). An estimation of the slope of the marker increase or relative increase in the marker over the first 90 min after thrombolysis has shown results equivalent to those for peak concentrations and time to peak concentrations and are available during the clinically useful time window.

Abe et al. (58) studied the ability of cTnT and CK-MB to predict patency in 38 patients undergoing reperfusion therapy with either angioplasty or thrombolytic therapy (alteplase, prourokinase, or intracoronary urokinase) within 7 hours of symptom onset. Reperfusion status was determined by comparing the angiogram taken before treatment with those taken every 5 to 8 min after treatment. Changes in cTnT of 0.5 ng/mL or in CK-MB of 25 mU/mL between baseline and 60 min after reperfusion therapy began had 100% sensitivity, specificity, and predictive accuracy for reperfusion in patients undergoing angioplasty as the means of reperfusion. For patients treated with thrombolytic therapy, the results were 83%, 100%, and 92%, respectively.

Laperche and colleagues evaluated the ability of the relative increase versus slope of increase of myoglobin, cTnT, CK, CK-MB, and CK-MM isoforms measured just before thrombolytic therapy and at 90 min to predict patency (TIMI grade 3 flow) of the infarct-related artery at angiography (59). Using receiver-operator curve (ROC) analysis, they found that the best diagnostic performance was shown for the relative increase in myoglobin, cTnT, and MM3/MM1 in patients treated beyond 3 hours after symptom onset (n = 49), with c-indices of 0.83, 0.84, and 0.85, respectively. For their entire cohort (n = 97), the relative increase in myoglobin appeared to have the best diagnostic performance, with c-indices of 0.72 for myoglobin, 0.66 for cTnT, 0.62 for CK-MB, 0.61 for CK, and 0.61 for MM3/MM1.

Christenson and colleagues also found myoglobin to be a good early marker for noninvasive detection of coronary patency after thrombolysis (60). Using the TAMI-7 population, they found that a single myoglobin measurement taken approximately 90 min after the start of thrombolysis performed better than measures of myoglobin ratio (90-min to baseline), slope, or change (90-min to baseline); χ^2 = 17.3, c-index 0.73 for TIMI grade 3 versus grade 0–2 flow. Further, they noted that this sampling strategy had the advantage of ease of use (only one blood draw) and lower cost than multiple samples required for the other variables.

Finally, in a prospective comparison of CK, CK-MB, myoglobin, and cTnT for early detection of reperfusion, Zabel and colleagues showed the difficulty with using "time to peak concentration" for noninvasive detection of reperfusion; all markers peaked too late to be clinically useful in guiding assessment of the need for rescue therapy (56). Myoglobin peaked earliest, at a mean 2.1 hours, followed by CK-MB (7.5 hours), CK (9.0 hours), and cTnT (11.6 hours). The time-activity relationship, expressed as a slope of each serum marker over the first 90 min after therapy, was an equally good indicator of successful reperfusion as time to peak for each marker. In comparing between the markers, the area under the ROC curve was 0.89 for myoglobin, 0.79 for CK, 0.79 for CK-MB, and 0.80 for cTnT. In univariable analysis, myoglobin slope (χ^2 = 36.7), followed by CK slope (χ^2 = 17.4), CK-MB (χ^2 = 15.5) slope, and cTnT slope (χ^2 = 9.7) were all predictors of coronary patency (TIMI grade 2 or 3 flow). When considered along with clinical indicators of reperfusion (ST-segment resolution, reperfusion arrhythmias, and relief of pain) in a logistic regression analysis, only myoglobin was an independent predictor of coronary artery patency.

Laperche and colleagues assessed the performance of published biochemical criteria for reperfusion when applied to a prospective cohort of thrombolytic-treated patients (Table 4) (59). For all methods tested, the actual sensitivities and specificities were lower than those in the original reports. This may have been related to the different marker assay techniques

Table 4 Sensitivity and Specificity of Biochemical Criteria of Reperfusion: Published versus Observed

Marker	Diagnostic threshold	Expected sensitivity	Observed sensitivity: TIMI grade 3 flow	Observed sensitivity: TIMI grade 2–3 flow	Expected specificity	Observed specificity: TIMI grade 3 flow	Observed specificity: TIMI grade 2–3 flow
Myoglobin	Slope >150 μg/L/h	94	84 (77–91)‡	82 (74–90)‡	88	40 (30–50)‡	48 (38–58)‡
	Slope >840 μg/L/h	54	47 (37–57)	48 (38–58)	83	71 (62–80)†	81 (73–89)
	90-min/baseline >3	95	81 (73–89)‡	78 (70–86)‡	100	51 (41–61)‡	61 (51–71)‡
Troponin T	Slope >0.2 μg/L/h	80	64 (54–74)‡	70 (60–80)*	65	53 (43–63)*	64 (54–74)
CK activity	Slope >60 U/L/h	87	74 (65–83)‡	77 (68–86)†	71	30 (20–40)‡	37 (27–47)‡
	90-min/baseline >1.9	70	45 (35–55)‡	39 (29–49)‡	82	77 (68–86)	80 (72–88)
CK-MB	Slope >17.5 μg/L/h	87	57 (47–67)‡	77 (68–86)†	71	54 (44–64)‡	61 (51–71)*
	2.2-fold increase, inferior MI	77	68 (59–77)*	68 (59–77)*	100	50 (40–60)‡	56 (46–66)‡
	2.5-fold increase, anterior MI	92	61 (51–71)‡	59 (49–69)‡	100	50 (40–60)‡	53 (43–63)‡
CK-MM3	Slope >0.18%/min	92	53 (42–64)‡	51 (40–62)‡	100	65 (54–76)‡	76 (66–86)‡
	Relative increase >0.83	40	42 (31–53)	40 (30–50)	75	62 (51–73)†	62 (51–73)†
CK-MM3/CK-MM1	Relative increase >3.5	30	47 (37–57)‡	44 (34–54)†	75	71 (61–81)	74 (65–83)

TIMI, Thrombolysis in Myocardial Infarction; CK, creatine kinase; MI, myocardial infarction.
Values are percentages (95% confidence intervals in parentheses).
*$P < .05$; †$P < .01$; ‡$P < .001$.
Source: Ref. 59.

and diagnostic criteria used. This analysis also highlights the lack of uniformity in the biochemical approach to assessment of perfusion.

The utility of combining cardiac markers with clinical variables has been shown by other investigators. Ohman and colleagues developed a predictive model containing CK-MB slope (CK-MB at 90- or 180-min angiography divided by the baseline value) and clinical variables (time from symptom onset to thrombolysis and chest pain at time of angiography), for which the area under the ROC curve was 0.85 (61). In an analysis by Christenson and colleagues, the myoglobin level 90 min after the start of therapy contributed significantly when combined with clinical variables and when assessed with the Ohman model (χ^2 for myoglobin contribution 4.04, P = .044, model c-index for detecting TIMI grade 3 flow 0.74) (60).

Apple and colleagues, in a study of cTnI, myoglobin, and CK-MB in 25 patients with acute MI treated with front-loaded alteplase, showed that cTnI also has potential use in predicting coronary patency at 90 min (62). In a pilot study of 24 patients, Tanasijevic and colleagues reported 100% sensitivity for detecting TIMI grade 2 or 3 flow with the ratio of 60-min to baseline cTnI, CK-MB, and myoglobin when the threshold values were 2.5, 3.0, and 5.7, respectively. The corresponding areas under the ROC curves were 0.96, 0.87, and 0.93 (63). These and other studies suggest that cardiac marker sampling early after beginning thrombolysis can provide useful insight into perfusion status, which might be helpful in directing care after thrombolytic therapy. Further prospective work in larger patient populations will be needed with all markers, however, to validate these early results and establish the most clinically useful tool for the noninvasive detection of reperfusion. With the evolution of new treatment strategies directed at microvascular, tissue-level perfusion, the cardiac markers may become even more important in the assessment of adequate reperfusion.

Assessment of Myocardial Damage

Since the early 1970s, investigators have used serum CK or CK-MB not only to confirm infarctions but also to estimate infarct size and prognosis (64–67). In the thrombolytic era, investigators have likewise described relationships between peak enzyme concentrations and infarct size and residual left ventricular function. Using a CK-MB mass assay, Christenson and colleagues studied the relationship between ventricular function, clinical outcomes, and CK-MB release in 145 patients who received accelerated alteplase for acute MI (Table 5) (68). This study showed significant inverse relationships between area under the CK-MB release curve and both ejection fraction (r = .21, P = .04) and infarct-zone function (r = .21, P = .04). There was also a trend toward more congestive heart failure and death in patients with larger CK-MB area (r = .12, P = .16).

Table 5 Relationship of Creatine Kinase-MB Release with Outcomes

	Data quintiles				
	0–20%	21–40%	41–60%	61–80%	81–100%
Median creatine kinase-MB area (ng/mL/min)	64,960	193,600	334,500	492,400	810,600
Congestive heart failure or death	17%	14%	21%	24%	31%

Source: Ref. 68.

Most recently, in the GUSTO-I enzyme substudy, Baardman and colleagues showed that the extent of the infarct measured by plasma α-hydroxybutyrate dehydrogenase activity correlated with infarct-artery patency and TIMI flow grade at 90-min angiography (69). Further, there was a relationship between smaller infarct size and treatment with accelerated alteplase or combined alteplase-streptokinase therapy versus streptokinase with either subcutaneous or intravenous heparin. Both findings mechanistically support the correlation between TIMI grade 3 flow and improved survival shown in the GUSTO-I angiographic substudy (47), the link between improved survival with accelerated alteplase relative to streptokinase monotherapies in the overall GUSTO-I trial, and the higher overall incidence of TIMI grade 3 flow seen with accelerated alteplase (70). These studies confirm the link between reduced infarct size and improved left ventricular function with improved patency and, most important, survival.

Diagnosis of Non-ST-Segment Elevation Myocardial Infarction

While the diagnosis of acute MI is relatively accurate in patients who present with ST-segment elevation, this group accounts for only a minority (about 5%) of the patients who ultimately are diagnosed with acute myocardial infarction (7,35,71). Beyond ST-segment elevation acute MI exists a diagnostic and risk continuum of acute coronary syndromes, including non-Q-wave or non-ST-segment elevation MI and unstable angina. The baseline electrocardiogram can help confirm a clinical suspicion of unstable angina but cannot differentiate non-ST-segment elevation MI from unstable angina (72–74). If a patient with a history of symptoms suggestive of unstable angina is symptom free upon examination, a baseline electrocardiogram with evidence of coronary artery disease (significant Q waves, deep symmetrical T-wave inversions, and resting ST-segment depression) supports the diagnosis. A normal electrocardiogram at baseline in the presence of symptoms does not exclude the diagnosis of unstable angina or non-ST-segment elevation MI, but it makes it less likely. Dynamic electrocardiographic changes with symptoms and symptom resolution strongly support the diagnosis, however.

Differentiation of non-ST-segment elevation MI from unstable angina is largely made in retrospect based on serial enzyme sampling over 24 hours. Even small amounts of myocardial necrosis, as measured by CK-MB enzyme sampling, portend a worse outcome (75), and because the best outcomes are likely obtained when specific therapy is started early, it is important to differentiate these two groups early and effectively. In addition, early risk assessment may improve triage decisions and facilitate development of diagnostic and management strategies. The use of very sensitive and "early" serum markers of myocardial necrosis may improve our diagnostic ability within this broad group of patients.

In general, sensitivities of all the commonly used serum cardiac markers are high. In the absence of skeletal muscle trauma, all are quite specific for myocardial injury except for myoglobin, for which no cardiac-specific isoform exists. Even for myoglobin, however, specificity is about 90% in patients with chest pain and no skeletal muscle injury. CK-MB is found to a small extent in skeletal muscle, which may produce false positive results for both the CK-MB mass assay and MB subform analysis in patients with muscle trauma. Collinson reported that cTnT was not elevated after strenuous exercise (76); therefore cTnT may be able to detect minor myocardial damage, even in trauma patients.

Of note is the lower reported specificity of cTnT for acute myocardial infarction in unstable angina populations. A number of studies have evaluated cTnT as a diagnostic tool for acute MI in acute coronary syndrome populations. In a meta-analysis, the cumulative sensitivities for cTnT (98.2%) and CK-MB (96.8%) were similar (77). The diagnostic specificity of cTnT compared with CK-MB was significantly lower, however (68.8% vs. 89.6%; $P < .001$). Because of the sensitivity of the assay and because cTnT is not found in the serum of control patients, minor myocardial damage may be detected. With CK-MB, a greater elevation above the detection limit is required to achieve high specificity for acute MI, because CK-MB may be detectable in control patients due to skeletal muscle release. Since CK-MB is the "gold standard" for the diagnosis of MI, cTnT may appear less specific because it picks up minor infarctions that are characterized by no elevation or only minor elevations of the CK-MB within the reference range. These patients would not traditionally be classified as having acute MI, but rather unstable angina. However, as will be discussed, the worse prognosis in patients who are cTnT positive but CK-MB negative suggests that the time has come to redefine the gold standard of MI by using cTnT.

Risk Stratification in Non-ST-Segment Elevation Acute Coronary Syndromes

Clinical Risk Stratification

Just as the diagnostic boundaries between non-ST-segment elevation MI and unstable angina are blurred, so too is there a gradation of risk within the acute coronary syndromes. Defining risk within the group is important for both patient management decisions and patient counseling. Clinical characteristics at presentation and diagnostic tools including the electrocardiogram and serum cardiac marker data can be used to help establish risk. The cardiac history and examination are often nonspecific, but prolonged pain at rest and the development of a transient S3 gallop, rales, or other signs of congestive heart failure, hypotension, or new or more severe mitral regurgitation during symptoms suggest left ventricular dysfunction with ischemia and a higher short- and long-term risk of mortality (72,74,78).

Other baseline characteristics may also be important in risk stratification. Calvin and colleagues identified previous infarction, lack of β-blocker or calcium-channel blocker treatment, baseline ST-segment depression, and diabetes mellitus as predictors of death or acute MI in 393 patients presenting with unstable angina (79). In a regression model developed in 1384 GUSTO-IIa patients with acute coronary ischemia, age, Killip class, systolic blood pressure, and previous hypertension were identified as significant predictors of 30-day mortality (80).

Electrocardiogram and Risk

Within the spectrum of non-ST-segment elevation acute coronary syndromes, the electrocardiogram remains an important prognostic tool. In particular, dynamic ST-segment elevation or depression and T-wave changes predict a higher risk of death or MI in unstable angina patients compared with normal tracings or nonspecific changes (71–74,81–83). In GUSTO-IIa, which included the spectrum of patients with acute coronary syndromes, the presenting electrocardiographic category (ST-segment elevation, ST-segment depression, T-wave inversion/normal, or confounding factors present) was an important predictor of short-term mortality in a multivariate survival model that also contained CK-MB and cTnT (37). In comparing the categories, patients with confounding electrocardiographic factors (such as left bundle branch block, left ventricular hypertrophy, or paced rhythms) had the highest short-term mortality (11.6%), followed by those with ST-segment depression (8.0%) and ST-segment elevation (7.4%). Short-term mortality was the lowest (1.2%) in the group with T-wave inversion or a normal tracing.

Risk Stratification with Cardiac Markers

Despite the potential criticism of the diagnostic specificity of cTnT, its measurement can provide important prognostic information in the unstable angina/non-Q-wave MI population (84–90). In a meta-analysis by Wu and colleagues, the odds ratio for death or infarction in cTnT-positive, unstable angina patients was 4.3 (95% confidence interval 2.8 to 6.8) (Table 6) (77,84–90). Recent larger clinical studies of cTnT for risk stratification have confirmed these early results, and a recent meta-analysis of both troponin T and troponin I studies has shown substantial increased risk in patients positive for either marker (cTnT: RR 2.7, 95% CI, 2.1 to 3.4; cTnI: RR 4.2, 95% CI, 2.7 to 6.4) (91).

In the Fragmin During Instability in Coronary Artery Disease (FRISC) trial, 976 patients with unstable angina were randomized to low-molecular-weight heparin or placebo. cTnT was measured within 12 hours of presentation, and patients were followed for cardiac death or MI for 5 months (92). The risk of events increased with increasing levels of cTnT (<0.06 ng/mL, 4.3%; 0.06 to 0.18 ng/mL, 10.5%; >0.18 ng/mL, 16.1%). In multivariable analysis, cTnT and the clinical variables age, hypertension, number of antianginal drugs, and electrocardiographic changes were identified as independent predictors of cardiac death or MI. Furthermore, Stubbs and colleagues have found similar results in a general unstable angina population (90).

A GUSTO-IIa substudy prospectively evaluated the prognostic significance of a single baseline measurement of cTnT in 855 patients across the spectrum of acute coronary syndromes (37). In all, 755 patients had complete cTnT, CK-MB, and electrocardiographic information; 36% were cTnT positive and 32% had elevated CK-MB. Mortality was highest in patients with electrocardiographic confounding factors (11.6%) and lowest in patients with normal tracings or only minor changes (1.2%). In cTnT-positive patients, 30-day mortality was 11.8% compared with 3.9% in cTnT-negative patients. As shown in Figure 4, mortality increased with increasing concentrations of cTnT. The same mortality relationship in cTnT-positive versus -negative patients held across all electrocardiographic categories (ST-segment elevation, ST-segment depression, confounders, and T-wave inversion/normal) (Table 7). In-hospital complications were likewise increased in the cTnT-positive patients. When the electrocardiographic category, CK-MB results, and cTnT value were considered in a mortality model, electrocardiographic findings followed by cTnT value and CK-MB were all predictors of 30-day mortality. The models were then adjusted for the presence of the other two

Table 6 Individual and Cumulative Odds Ratios of Cardiac Troponin T (cTnT) for the Development of Acute MI or Death

		Death/MI (n/total n)				
Study	Follow-up	High cTnT	Low cTnT	Odds ratio (95% CI)	χ^2	*P*
Hamm (63)	In-hospital	10/33	1/51	21.7 (2.6–180.5)	8.15	.0043
Ravkilde (64)	6 months	6/44	3/83	4.1 (1.0–17.7)	3.84	.0502
Seino (65)	In-hospital	2/14	0/8	—	—	—
Burlina (66)	In-hospital	5/16	0/12	—	—	—
Abbas (67)	3 weeks	8/27	3/104	14.2 (3.4–58.3)	13.50	.0002
Ravkilde (68)	28 months	6/25	5/99	5.9 (1.64–21.46)	7.38	.0066
Stubbs (69)	34 months	22/62	25/121	2.1 (1.1–4.2)	4.62	.0315
Cumulative		59/221	37/478	4.3 (2.8–6.8)	41.12	.0000

Source: Ref. 77.

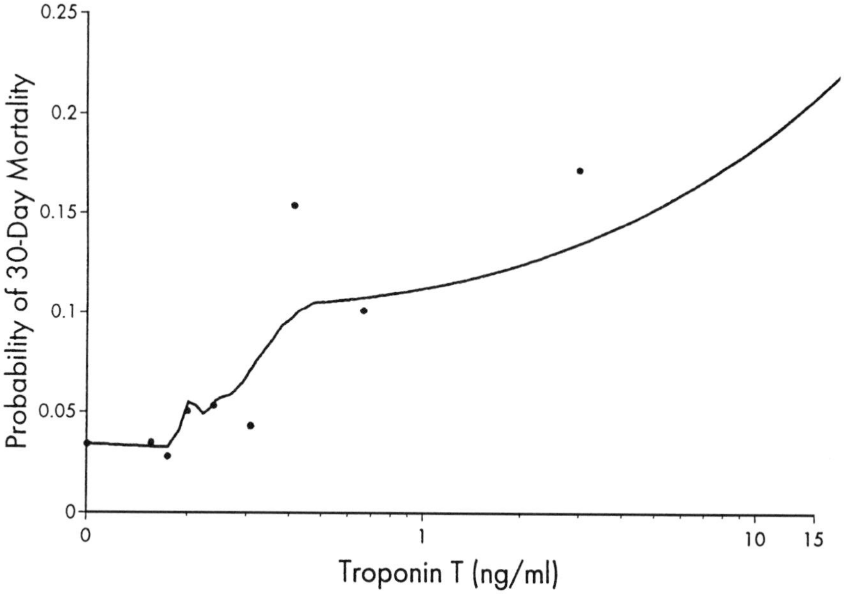

Figure 4 Nonparametric estimates of the probability of 30-day mortality versus admission troponin T level. Troponin T is plotted along a cube-root scale. Data density is shown at the top of the plot; each mark represents one patient. The solid circles represent simple mortality estimates from intervals of troponin T levels that were derived to contain at least 70 patients. (From Ref. 37. Copyright 1996 Massachusetts Medical Society.)

variables; once the electrocardiographic findings and cTnT value were known, CK-MB contributed no further prognostic information. Troponin T added significantly even after the other two variables were known.

Troponin I was a predictor of 42-day mortality in a retrospective analysis of 1404 patients with non-Q-wave MI or unstable angina randomized in the TIMI-3 trial (93). The cutoff value used in this analysis was 0.4 ng/mL using the Dade Stratus II assay, below the cutoff of 1.5 ng/mL for the diagnosis of acute MI with this test. Troponin I was positive in 41% of patients; 32% had elevated CK-MB. Mortality was 3.7% in cTnI-positive patients compared with 1.0% in cTnI-negative patients. The risk of morality increased with increasing concentration of cTnI. In multivariable analysis, ST-segment depression ($P < .001$), age >65 years ($P = .026$), and cTnI status on admission ($P = .03$) were independent predictors of 42-day mortality.

Evaluation of cTnT and cTnI (Sanofi assay) in 491 patients in a substudy of the TRIM trial showed that both identified similar groups of patients

Table 7 Complications and 30-Day Outcomes in the GUSTO-IIa Troponin T Substudy by Electrocardiographic Category and Troponin T and Creatine Kinase-MB

	ST-segment elevation				ST-segment depression			
30-day outcomes	cTnT (+)[a] (N = 138)	cTnT (−) (N = 297)	CK-MB (+) (N = 143)	CK-MB (−) (N = 292)	cTnT (+) (N = 43)	cTnT (−) (N = 45)	CK-MB (+) (N = 30)	CK-MB (−) (N = 58)
Death	18 (13.0)	14 (4.7)	15 (10.5)	17 (5.8)	5 (11.6)	2 (4.4)	4 (13.3)	3 (5.2)
Myocardial infarction	125 (90.6)	241 (81.1)	137 (95.8)	229 (78.4)	33 (76.8)	17 (37.8)	29 (96.7)	21 (36.2)
Bypass surgery	22 (15.9)	41 (13.8)	18 (12.6)	45 (15.4)	12 (27.9)	11 (24.4)	8 (26.7)	15 (25.9)
Angioplasty	35 (25.4)	107 (36.0)	43 (30.1)	99 (33.9)	9 (20.9)	11 (24.4)	8 (26.7)	12 (20.7)
	T-wave inversion, normal				Confounding electrocardiographic factors[b]			
30-day outcomes	cTnT (+) (n = 49)	cTnT (−) (n = 114)	CK-MB (+) (n = 44)	CK-MB (−) (n = 119)	cTnT (+) (n = 39)	cTnT (−) (n = 30)	CK-MB (+) (n = 28)	CK-MB (−) (n = 41)
Death	2 (4.1)	0	1 (2.3)	1 (0.8)	6 (15.4)	2 (6.7)	5 (17.9)	3 (7.3)
Myocardial infarction	43 (87.8)	40 (35.1)	43 (97.7)	40 (33.6)	31 (79.5)	15 (50.7)	27 (96.4)	19 (46.3)
Bypass surgery	10 (20.4)	22 (19.3)	8 (18.2)	24 (20.2)	3 (7.7)	4 (13.3)	0	7 (17.1)
Angioplasty	18 (36.7)	35 (30.7)	16 (36.4)	37 (31.1)	11 (28.2)	10 (33.3)	10 (35.7)	11 (26.9)

Values are medians (25th, 75th centiles) or frequencies (percentages).
[a]Troponin T (cTnT) (+) = >0.1 ng/mL, (−) = ≤0.1 ng/mL, by core laboratory determination.
[b]Left bundle branch block, left ventricular hypertrophy, or paced rhythms.
Source: Ref. 37.

at high risk for subsequent acute MI or death by 30 days (94). A comparison of cTnI (Dade Stratus II assay, cutoff 1.5 ng/mL) with cTnT within GUSTO-IIa showed that both predicted 30-day mortality (95), but in a mortality model that first considered ECG findings and troponin T results, cTnI did not add significantly to the prediction of 30-day mortality. Analytical characteristics such as minimum detection limit and measurement precision differ among various cTnI assays. These characteristics may translate into important differences in the ability to risk-stratify.

Because the baseline value of any cardiac marker may be affected by the time from symptom onset to sampling, the sensitivity of the assay, and the release and clearance kinetics of the marker after myocardial injury, a first measurement may be negative in patients who actually are at high risk. Because of this, serial sampling of CK-MB is routine for MI diagnosis. Newby and colleagues showed in a mortality model in 734 patients that even though the greatest prognostic information is conferred by the baseline cTnT measure, further measures at 8 or 16 hours add significant additional information, with the 16-hour sample carrying more additional information than the 8-hour sample, though not statistically significant (96). Because mortality was low in patients who were negative at 8 hours, an optimal sampling pattern with cTnT for risk stratification and that would maximize the ability to guide early therapy in patients with acute coronary syndromes might be at baseline and 8 hours. However, it should be emphasized that to be most effective for the individual patient, serial sampling must occur at a time that maximizes the likelihood of detection of the marker.

Cardiac Markers to Guide Treatment in Patients with Acute Coronary Syndromes

That the cardiac markers have diagnostic and prognostic utility across the spectrum of chest pain patients has now essentially been proven beyond doubt. The next step in the evolution of cardiac marker testing should take us one step further, using the information conveyed by the results of cardiac marker testing to most appropriately and cost-effectively apply the rapidly growing therapeutic options available for ACS patients. Studies are now beginning to show how knowledge of cardiac marker status in addition to clinical variables may be used to define high-risk populations who stand to gain the most from treatment with aggressive management strategies after an ACS or from the use of newer treatments such as the low-molecular-weight heparins or glycoprotein IIb/IIIa receptor antagonists.

Low-Molecular-Weight Heparins

The relationship of cardiac marker status with outcome by treatment strategy has been extensively studied in 976 patients in the FRISC study. Among cTnT-positive patients, the risk of death or myocardial infarction at 5 to 7 days was significantly reduced for patients receiving dalteparin compared with placebo (6.0% vs. 2.4%), such that the risk for troponin-positive dalteparin-treated patients approached that of cTnT-negative patients receiving standard therapy (2.4%) (97). Further, this treatment benefit was maintained for long-term follow-up. In contrast, among cTnT-negative patients at lower initial risk, the reduction in death or MI between treatment groups at 5 to 7 days was not statistically significant and was not present in long-term follow-up.

In a substudy of FRISC II, the relation of cTnT status with the effects of long-term (3 months) treatment with dalteparin versus placebo on the 3-month rate of death or myocardial infarction was assessed (98). In the overall cohort of 2266 patients, the rate of death or myocardial infarction was similar regardless of treatment strategy: 11.3% for placebo versus 9.9% for long-term treatment with dalteparin, $P = .16$. However, in the 1266 patients with cTnT >0.1 ng/mL there was a statistically significant reduction in death or myocardial infarction at 3 months for the dalteparin group compared with placebo (9.0% vs. 12.5%, $P < .05$). There was no difference in treatment effect among patients with cTnT <0.1 ng/mL.

Glyocoprotein IIb/IIIa Antagonists

Studies of platelet glycoprotein IIb/IIIa receptor antagonists administered intravenously in the settings of percutaneous coronary intervention and acute coronary syndromes have shown a consistent and durable reduction in death or myocardial infarction (99). As with low-molecular-weight heparin, data suggest that the results of cardiac marker testing along with clinical variables may identify subgroups of patients who benefit preferentially from the use of platelet glycoprotein IIb/IIIa antagonists.

Hahn and colleagues have shown that for the intravenous GP IIb/IIIa antagonist tirofiban in combination with heparin in patients with non-ST-segment elevation acute coronary syndromes, peak troponin I levels were significantly lower among patients who received tirofiban than in patients who received standard heparin therapy alone, suggesting a potential link between better outcomes in tirofiban-treated patients and troponin status (100). Further, in conjunction with the PRISM study, Heeschen and colleagues showed that among the 28% of patients with elevated troponin I (diagnostic threshold 1.0 μg/L) and the 29% of patients with elevated troponin T (diagnostic threshold 0.1 μg/L) measurements there was a significantly higher risk of 30-day rates of death or myocardial infarction (101). More importantly, they showed that troponin-positive status could be used to identify a subgroup of patients with acute coronary syndromes that benefited from the use of tirofiban. Among both the troponin I-positive patients who received tirofiban the hazard ratio for mortality (adjusted for other predictors) was 0.25 (95% CI 0.09 to 0.68). For myocardial infarction, the adjusted hazard ratio was 0.37 (95% CI 0.16 to 0.84). Table 8 reviews the event rates for these and other endpoints by troponin I status and treatment group in the PRISM study. Results were similar for troponin T. This marked reduction in 30-day death and myocardial infarction occurred regardless of the overall management strategy (medical or revascularization). There was no treatment benefit in the troponin-negative patients. Thus, troponin-positive status could be used to guide the use of tirofiban, reserving it for patients with the greatest benefit. This potential benefit of troponin testing to guide the appropriate use of therapy in acute coronary syndrome patients is also being explored with troponin T in a substudy of the PARAGON B trial of lamifiban.

These results are extended by the results of a troponin T substudy from the CAPTURE trial. In CAPTURE, patients with unstable angina were randomized to treatment with abciximab or placebo for 12 to 24 hours prior to, during, and 12 hours following percutaneous intervention (102). At all stages —before intervention, postprocedure, and in follow-up—rates of myocardial infarction were significantly lower in the abciximab-treated patients. The

Table 8 Event Rates for Three Periods of Time by Troponin I Status

	Troponin-I positive		Troponin-I negative	
	Heparin (n = 324)	Tirofiban (n = 305)	Heparin (n = 801)	Tirofiban (n = 792)
48 h				
Refractory ischemia	30 (9.3)	10 (3.3)	24 (3.05)	17 (2.1)
Death, MI	11 (3.4)	1 (0.3)	5 (0.6)	7 (0.9)
Death	2 (0.6)	0	0	3 (0.4)
MI	9 (2.8)	1 (0.3)	5 (0.6)	4 (0.5)
7 days				
Refractory ischemia	47 (14.5)	26 (8.5)	53 (6.6)	59 (7.4)
Death, MI	30 (9.3)	6 (2.0)	18 (2.2)	24 (3.0)
Death	12 (3.7)	2 (0.7)	3 (0.4)	7 (0.9)
MI	18 (5.6)	4 (1.3)	14 (1.8)	17 (2.1)
30 days				
Refractory ischemia	48 (14.8)	31 (10.2)	60 (7.5)	72 (9.1)
Death, MI	42 (13.0)	13 (4.3)	39 (4.9)	45 (5.7)
Death	20 (6.2)	5 (1.6)	18 (2.3)	18 (2.3)
MI	22 (6.8)	8 (2.6)	21 (2.6)	27 (3.6)

Percentages in parentheses. M = myocardial infarction.
Source: Reprinted from Ref. 101.

results of a troponin T substudy suggested that the observed treatment benefits were largely confined to patients who were troponin T-positive (103). The relative risk (RR) of death or myocardial infarction for abciximab treatment versus placebo in patients with cTnT >0.1 ng/mL was 0.32 (95% CI 0.12 to 0.49), but in patients with cTnT <0.1 ng/mL there was no significant difference for treatment with abciximab versus placebo, RR 1.26 (95% CI 0.74 to 2.31). In this study, in addition to showing that the most benefit was gained by treating troponin-positive patients, it was also demonstrated that the potential mechanism for this benefit related to the resolution of coronary thrombus (104). Among troponin T-positive patients, visible thrombus was present at baseline angiography in 14.6% of cases, compared with only 4.2% of troponin T-negative cases. Use of abciximab was highly associated with the resolution of thrombus and with greater improvement in TIMI flow among troponin T-positive patients (Table 9) suggesting the potential mechanism of the greater benefit of its use in troponin T-positive patients.

Aggressive Interventional Strategies

In the TIMI IIIb troponin I substudy, a retrospective analysis of outcome by cTnI status relative to treatment strategy (early invasive vs. conservative) showed that cTnI-positive patients who were treated with an early invasive strategy had significantly better outcome at 42 days than those treated conservatively (105). The 42-day outcome among patients who were cTnI positive and received the early invasive strategy was nearly equal to that of patients who were cTnI negative. In the cTnI-negative group, there was no significant difference in outcome by treatment strategy.

A more recent study (FRISC II) of early invasive evaluation and revascularization if indicated versus an early conservative strategy, reserving such evaluation and treatment for patients with recurrent symptoms or severe ischemia on treadmill testing showed a benefit favoring an early invasive strategy (106). In this study, however, the benefit on the endpoint of death or myocardial infarction for the early invasive strategy was present regardless of baseline cTnT status (overall comparison invasive vs. noninvasive: RR 0.77, 95% CI 0.61 to 0.97); cTnT <0.1: RR 0.80; 95% CI 0.54 to 1.19; cTnT >0.1: RR 0.75, 95% CI 0.56 to 1.01) (107).

Cardiac Markers in the Chest Pain Unit

Each year in the United States, about 6 million people arrive at emergency departments with complaints of chest pain or other symptoms of possible cardiac ischemia. As described in detail in Chapter 12, accurate diagnosis and triage of this diverse group of patients can be difficult but have important clinical, legal, and economic implications. Graff and colleagues have shown

Table 9 TIMI Flow After 18 to 24 Hours of Allocated Treatment According to TnT Status

TnT-positive (n = 263)				TnT-negative (n = 589)			
TIMI flow at baseline	Abciximab	Placebo	P	TIMI flow at baseline	Abciximab	Placebo	P
TIMI 0 n = 19	−1	+2	0.64	TIMI 0 n = 10	+1	−1	0.59
TIMI 1 n = 22	−5	+1	0.13	TIMI 1 n = 20	−1	Equal	0.87
TIMI 2 n = 65	−3	+1	0.16	TIMI 2 n = 119	+2	−1	0.43
TIMI 3 n = 157	+9	−4	<0.001	TIMI 3 n = 440	−2	+2	0.06

Source: Ref. 104.

that implementation of chest pain units can cut the historical "miss" rate of myocardial infarctions by 10-fold, from 4.3% to 0.4% (108).

Many strategies to improve diagnostic accuracy in these patients have been devised. Investigators have developed neural networks, diagnostic algorithms, and decision models to calculate the likelihood of acute MI (81,82,109–111), but the utility of these methods is generally limited by the available input. In part because they are cumbersome, the use of these algorithms has not become widespread despite testing and validation in multiple populations. Serial serum cardiac marker testing within short-stay observation units, sometimes called chest pain units, has become widespread to evaluate the diverse group of chest pain patients who are not at high risk for myocardial ischemia but in whom the diagnosis cannot be excluded.

Standard protocols for "ruling out" MI differ slightly from center to center, but generally involve serial sampling of CK-MB every 3 to 4 hours for 9 to 12 hours. Using a rule-out strategy such as this, Lee and colleagues showed that in the absence of recurrent chest pain and with negative CK-MB levels, 12 hours was sufficient to exclude the diagnosis of acute MI in 99.5% of low-risk patients (112). Using a similar strategy in a short-stay evaluation unit, Gaspoz showed that if serial CK-MB measurements were negative and there was no electrocardiographic evolution or recurrence of symptoms, the risk of MI was <1% (113). Gibler has shown that for the low-risk chest pain population, serial sampling of CK-MB over 9 hours is sufficient to rule out MI in nearly 100% of patients (114,115). The Rule Out Myocardial Infarction Observation Unit (ROMIO) study, in which 100 low-risk patients were randomized to a similar 9-hour CK-MB, short-stay, rule-out protocol or usual care, showed no difference in outcomes between the two groups (116).

The use of newer cardiac markers and testing strategies could change the diagnostic and management standards in this group of patients in many ways. The standard observation time of 9 to 12 hours for definitive rule-out of MI could probably be reduced using newer markers that are more sensitive and specific for myocardial necrosis and, in some cases, detectable above the reference limit in the serum earlier than CK-MB. The use of serum markers with high sensitivity and specificity for myocardial necrosis has the potential to greatly facilitate triage of these patients and the efficiency of the "rule-out" process for those who are sent to the chest pain unit for observation. In this light, for early diagnosis of myocardial necrosis in patients who present with varying duration of symptoms before presentation, the use of a panel that includes myoglobin or MB subforms as a very early marker, CK-MB mass (4 to 6 hours), and cTnT or cTnI (≥6 to 8 hours) could be ideal. The diagnostic accuracy and prognostic importance of such a strategy remain to be proved, but are currently being investigated in the

CHECKMATE study in which a multimarker strategy incorporating myoglobin, CK-MB, and cTnI is being studied in the chest pain unit setting.

Trahey and colleagues suggested that the use of serial sampling of MB isoforms could safely rule out acute MI in a chest pain unit population by 6 hours (117). If a later stress test was negative, 1.3% of patients eventually had an acute MI or documented acute coronary ischemia. Puleo and colleagues have also shown a high negative predictive value for MB isoform testing to rule out acute MI (8).

Troponin T testing has also shown promise for use in the low-risk chest pain unit population. In a meta-analysis of published reports of cTnT in chest pain patients, the odds ratio for coronary revascularization was 4.4 (95% confidence interval 3.0 to 6.5) with a positive cTnT result (Table 10) (77,86,88,90,118). Further, in an analysis of 383 consecutive patients in the Duke Chest Pain Unit, the rate of significant angiographic disease (>75% stenosis) in cTnT-positive (≥0.1 ng/mL) patients was 89% compared with 49% in the cTnT-negative group ($P = .002$); the rate of multivessel disease among the cTnT-positive patients was also significantly higher (67% vs. 29%, $p = .003$) (119). De Fillippi and colleagues have reported a similar association between troponin status and the presence of significant coronary artery disease at angiography in their chest pain cohort (120). Both of these studies point out the high prevalence of underlying coronary artery disease among even troponin-negative patients considered low to moderate risk by clinical features alone. Therefore, the importance of stress testing or other means of risk stratification in troponin-negative patients prior to release from chest pain units probably cannot be overemphasized. In support of this consideration, Lindahl and colleagues showed that in the FRISC study, among 963 patients at all levels of cTnT values, including those with negative values, the stress test provided prognostic information that was additive to the results of troponin testing (121).

The prognostic value of early serum cardiac markers in the chest pain unit setting is just being clearly defined. Sidman and colleagues showed that in 26 emergency department patients with a final diagnosis of unstable angina at hospital discharge, an elevated cTnT identified patients at higher risk for ischemic complications over the ensuing 2 months (122). In the longest follow-up of a chest pain unit population, the results from our study suggest that cTnT-positive status identifies a population at higher risk for total mortality (27% vs. 7%, $P = .0001$) and among those, a higher risk for cardiac mortality than cTnT-negative patients (119). As the clinical interpretation and application of such findings in the chest pain unit population evolves, management strategies for otherwise low-risk chest pain patients will likely change—perhaps more aggressive in the positive patients, both early and in secondary prevention.

Table 10 Individual and Cumulative Odds Ratios of Cardiac Troponin T (cTnT) for Predicting the Need for Cardiac Revascularization

Study	Follow-up	Death/MI (n/total n)		Odds ratio (95% CI)	χ^2	*P*
		High cTnT	Low cTnT			
Benjamin (84)	In-hospital	10/45	42/622	4.0 (1.8–8.5)	12.2	.0005
Seino (65)	In-hospital	8/14	0/8	—	—	—
Abbas (67)	3 weeks	17/27	38/104	3.0 (1.2–7.1)	5.9	.0156
Stubbs (69)	34 months	22/62	26/121	2.0 (1.0–4.0)	4.0	.0434
Cumulative		57/148	106/855	4.4 (3.0–6.5)	56.3	.000

Source: Ref. 77.

Table 11 Length of Stay and Financial Implications of Chest Pain Unit Rule-Out Protocols

	Reduction in length of stay (days)	Cost reduction[a] ($)
Gaspoz (112)		
CCU	4.0	7274 (76%)
Step-down	2.0	2104 (52%)
Wards	3.0	2785 (63%)
Gomez (115)	0.5	981 (47%)
DUMC chest pain program	2.3	1765 (47%)

[a]For hospital stay except Gaspoz, which reflects total costs through 6 months.
Source: Ref. 123.

Primarily through reduction in length of stay and use of less costly observation care, chest pain units significantly reduce the cost of chest pain evaluation. Table 11 summarizes the reductions in length of stay and cost through the use of chest pain unit "rule-out" protocols at different sites (116,123,124). Taking the situation at our institution as an example, if the use of MB subforms as described by Trahey were implemented (6-hour protocol), a further direct reduction in cost of 14.2% could result from the decrease in room charges alone (based on the hourly rate); if the rule-out period was shortened to 8 hours based on the results of cTnT testing, the reduction would be 9.5%. Thus, the use of sensitive and specific cardiac markers or panels of markers in an integrated chest pain unit program can provide rapid, early identification and better management of patients with acute MI or unstable coronary syndromes. This approach in low-risk patients assigned to a chest pain unit could also provide important prognostic information that can be used to guide short- and long-term care and counsel these patients.

BEDSIDE CARDIAC MARKER TESTING

Laboratory assays for most cardiac markers can now be done within 10 to 30 min of specimen receipt (Table 12). Lost time in specimen ordering, collection, and transport and result reporting add substantially to this time, however. In some institutions this process may take as long as 2 to 3 hours (125), greatly diminishing the value of a test for which there is a rapid laboratory assay. Point-of-care testing could circumvent many of these problems by putting not only the results but also the testing in the hands of the ordering physician. For example, real-time testing of blood glucose by a

Table 12 Laboratory Assay Times for Various Biochemical Markers of Myocardial Necrosis[a]

	Time (min)
Myoglobin	8–20
Creatine kinase, total	10–20
Creatine kinase-MB (mass assay)	8–30
Troponin T	45[b]
Troponin I	8–25
Creatine kinase-MB2/creatine kinase-MB1	25

[a]The times listed represent on-instrument duration only and do not take into account sample transport or specimen handling. Specimen handling routinely includes accessioning, labeling, centrifugation, and aliquoting, which typically requires about 15 minutes.
[b]12-min assay currently in final phase of FDA approval process.

bedside device allows rapid and precise adjustments to insulin regimens in diabetic patients, which could not be achieved with laboratory assessments. Further, rapid point-of-care testing of the activated partial thromboplastin time (aPTT) in GUSTO-I resulted in fewer bleeding complications compared with usual laboratory-based testing and had a substantially shorter turn-around time (126).

As suggested by the work of Downie and colleagues (127), bedside assessment of serum markers of myocardial necrosis in real time may offer physicians the greatest ability to make rapid decisions about diagnosis and patient management approaches. Particularly in a chest pain unit or to determine perfusion status after thrombolytic therapy, the availability of rapid bedside testing for cardiac markers would be important. This approach could offer not only the potential to improve the quality and effectiveness of critical management decisions but also the potential to advance the efficiency of patient care and reduce costs.

Rapid bedside assays for troponin T and I testing have now been developed and tested in clinical practice. In a GUSTO-III substudy, Ohman and colleagues demonstrated the ability of a rapid bedside assay for cTnT to risk-stratify patients rapidly at presentation with acute MI, alone and combined with known clinical predictors of risk (43). In addition, Hamm and colleagues showed that both cTnI and cTnT bedside qualitative assays were able to risk-stratify patients across the full spectrum of chest pain presentations in the emergency department (128). In their study the results for either marker sampled at presentation then 4 hours later was a strong independent predictor of 30-day mortality or myocardial infarction in this broad chest pain population.

As health care systems evolve to emphasize and reward more efficient patient care, and as rapid advances in technology provide improved early treatment options, it will be increasingly important to determine the benefits to patient care and costs of point-of-care testing and to establish what role, if any, this method of assessment should play for patients with acute coronary syndromes or in the evaluation of chest pain patients with less clear diagnoses. A concerted multidisciplinary effort involving basic researchers, clinicians, and clinical laboratory personnel will be required to develop and study new assays, devices, and testing strategies and to define the optimal approach.

CONCLUSIONS

The use of serum markers of myocardial necrosis will continue to play an important diagnostic role in patients with acute coronary syndromes. The use of newer, more sensitive, and more specific markers and innovative testing strategies could greatly facilitate the process of care across the spectrum of diagnostic indications. Certainly, the recently documented prognostic importance of the troponins (cTnI and cTnT) has the potential to change the way we think about acute coronary syndromes. In the unstable angina patient, conventionally diagnosed by negative serial testing of CK-MB, elevation of the troponins above control levels is associated with a prognosis similar to that of patients who "rule-in" for acute MI. It is not clear, however, whether this results from the process of micronecrosis (or infarctlet) or merely reflects a high-risk coronary disease state with active atherosclerotic lesions.

Perhaps even more interesting, the prognostic ability of a baseline cTnT measure extends across all electrocardiographic categories and is important even with positive CK-MB results. Although much work remains, these findings will likely change the way we define the acute coronary syndromes, in particular "acute myocardial infarction." The very important prognostic information provided by cTnT and cTnI suggests that we are entering an era in which we are redefining the "gold standard" for myocardial necrosis. Although such a change always induces a sense of uncertainty, there are many opportunities. By correctly identifying high- and low-risk patients, new treatment models can be applied. Future outcomes research will be essential to further our knowledge of the new markers of acute coronary syndromes. The application of these findings to patient care has the potential to revolutionize the way we manage and counsel patients with chest pain of suspected or conventionally documented coronary etiology.

REFERENCES

1. Lee KL, Pryor DB, Harrell FE Jr, Califf RM, Behar VS, Floyd WL, Morris JJ, Waugh RA, Whalen RE, Rosati RA. Predicting outcome in coronary disease. Statistical models versus expert clinicians. Am J Med 1986;80:553–560.
2. Kong DF, Lee KL, Harrell FE Jr, Boswick JM, Mark DB, Hlatky MA, Califf RM, Pryor DB. Clinical experience and predicting survival in coronary disease. Arch Intern Med 1989;149:1177–1181.
3. Roxin LE, Culled I, Groth T, Hallgren T, Venge P. The value of serum myoglobin determinations in the early diagnosis of acute myocardial infarction. Acta Med Scand 1984;215:417–425.
4. Bais R, Edwards JB. Creatine kinase. Crit Rev Clin Lab Sci 1982;16:291–335.
5. Adams JE, Abendschein DR, Jaffe AS. Biochemical markers of myocardial injury. Is MB creatine kinase the choice for the 1990s? Circulation 1993;88:750–763.
6. Ohman EM, Teo KK, Johnson AH, Collins PB, Dowsett DG, Ennis JT, Horgan JH. Abnormal cardiac enzyme responses after strenuous exercise: alternative diagnostic aids. Br Med J 1982;285:1523–1526.
7. Califf RM, Ohman EM. The diagnosis of acute myocardial infarction. Chest 1992;101:106S–115S.
8. Puleo PR, Meyer D, Wathen C, Tawa CB, Wheeler S, Hamburg RJ, Ali N, Obermueller SD, Triana JF, Zimmerman JL. Use of a rapid assay of subforms of creatine kinase MB to diagnose or rule out acute myocardial infarction. N Engl J Med 1994;331:561–566.
9. Zimmerman J, Fromm R, Meyer D, et al. Diagnostic Marker Cooperative Study for the diagnosis of myocardial infarction. Circulation 1999;99:1671–1677.
10. Anderson PAW, Malouf NN, Oakeley AE, Pagani ED, Allen PD. Troponin T isoform expression in humans. Circ Res 1991;69:1226–1233.
11. Saggin L, Gorza L, Ausoni S, Schiaffino S. Cardiac troponin T in developing, regenerating and denervated rat skeletal muscle. Development 1990;110:547–554.
12. Ricchiuti V, Voss EM, Ney A, Odland M, Anderson PAW, Apple FS. Cardiac troponin T isoforms expressed in renal diseased skeletal muscle will not cause false-positive results by the second generation cardiac troponin T assay by Boehringer Mannheim. Clin Chem 1998;44:1919–1924.
13. Keffer JH. Myocardial markers of injury: evolution and insights. Clin Chem 1996;105:305–320.
14. Bhayana V, Gougoulias T, Cohoe S, Henderson AR. Discordance between results for serum troponin T and troponin I in renal disease. Clin Chem 1995;41:312–317.
15. Li D, Keffer J, Corry K, Vazquez M, Jialal I. Nonspecific elevation of troponin T levels in patients with chronic renal failure. Clin Biochem 1995;28:474.

16. Wu AHB, Feng YJ, Contois JH, Pervaiz S. Comparison of myoglobin, creatine kinase-MB, and cardiac troponin I for diagnosis of acute myocardial infarction. J Clin Lab Sci 1996;26:291.
17. Frankel WL, Herold DA, Zeigler TW, Fitzgerald RL. Cardiac troponin T is elevated in asymptomatic patients with chronic renal failure. Am J Clin Pathol 1996;106:118.
18. Croitoru M, Taegtmeyer H. Spurious rises in troponin T in end-stage renal disease. Lancet 1995;346:974.
19. Hossein-Nia M, Nisbet J, Merton GK, Holt DW. Spurious rises of cardiac troponin T. Lancet 1995;346:1558.
20. Escalon JC, Wong SS. False-positive cardiac troponin T levels in chronic hemodialysis patients. Cardiology 1996;87:268.
21. Hafner G, Thome-Kromer B, Schaube J, et al. Cardiac troponins in serum in chronic renal failure. Clin Chem 1994;40:1790.
22. Katus HA, Haller C, Muller-Bardorff M, et al. Cardiac troponin T in end-stage renal disease patients undergoing chronic maintenance hemodialysis. Clin Chem 1995;41:1201.
23. Li D, Jailal I, Keffer J. Greater frequency of increased cardiac troponin T than cardiac troponin I in patients with chronic renal failure. Clin Chem 1996;42:114.
24. Braun SL, Baum H, Neumeier D, Vogt W. Troponin T and troponin I after coronary artery bypass grafting: discordant results in patients with renal failure. Clin Chem 1996;42:781.
25. Haller C, Zehelein J, Remppis A, Muller-Bardoff M, Katus HA. Cardiac troponin T in patients with end-stage renal disease: absence of expression in truncal skeletal muscle. Clin Chem 1998;44:930–938.
26. Apple FS, Sharkey SW, Hoeft P, et al. Prognostic value of serum cardiac troponin I and T in chronic dialysis patients: A 1-year outcomes analysis. Am J Kidney Dis 1997;29:399–403.
27. McLaurin MD, Apple FS, Voss EM, Herzog CA, Sharkey SW. Cardiac troponin I, cardiac troponin T, and creatine kinase MB in dialysis patients without ischemic heart disease: evidence of cardiac troponin T expression in skeletal muscle. Clin Chem 1997;43:976–982.
28. Wu AHB, Valdez R, Apple FS, et al. Cardiac troponin T immunoassay for diagnosis of acute myocardial infarction. Clin Chem 1994;40:900–907.
29. Katus HA, Looser S, Hallermayer K, et al. Development and in vitro characterization of a new immunoassay of cardiac troponin T. Clin Chem 1992;38:386–393.
30. McLaurin MD, Apple FS, Falahati A, Murakami MM, Miller EA, Sharkey SW. Cardiac troponin I and creatine kinase-MB mass to rule out myocardial injury in hospitalized patients with renal insufficiency. Am J Cardiol 1998;82:973–975.
31. Porter GA, Norton T, Bennett WB. Troponin T (TnT), a predictor of death in chronic haemodialysis patients. Eur Heart J 1998;19:N34–N37.
32. Martin GS, Becker BN, Schulman G. Cardiac troponin-I accurately predicts

myocardial injury in renal failure. Nephrol Dial Transplant 1998;13:1709–1712.

33. Roppolo LP, Fitzgerald R, Dillow J, Ziegler T, Rice M, Maisel A. A comparison of troponin T and troponin I as predictors of cardiac events in patients undergoing chronic dialysis at a Veteran's Hospital: a pilot study. J Am Coll Cardiol 1999;34:448–454.
34. Van Lente F, McErlean ES, DeLuca SA, Peacock WF, Rao JS, Nissen SE. Ability of troponins to predict adverse outcomes in patients with renal insufficiency and suspected acute coronary syndromes: a case-matched study. J Am Coll Cardiol 1999;33:471–478.
35. Rude RE, Poole WK, Muller JE, Turi Z, Rutherford J, Parker C, Roberts R, Raabe DS Jr, Gold HK, Stone PH. Electrocardiographic and clinical criteria for the recognition of acute myocardial infarction based on analysis of 3,697 patients. Am J Cardiol 1983;52:936–942.
36. Yusuf S, Pearson M, Sterry H, Parish S, Ramsdale D, Rossi P, Sleight P. The entry ECG in the early diagnosis and prognostic stratification of patients with suspected acute myocardial infarction. Eur Heart J 1984;5:690–696.
37. Ohman EM, Armstrong PW, Christenson RH, Granger CB, Katus HA, Hamm CW, O'Hanesian MA, Wagner GS, Kleiman NS, Harrell FE Jr, Califf RM, Topol EJ, for the GUSTO-IIa Investigators. Cardiac troponin T levels for risk stratification in acute myocardial ischemia. N Engl J Med 1996;335:1333–1341.
38. Stubbs P, Collinson P, Moseley D, Greenwood T, Noble M. Prognostic significance of admission troponin T concentrations in patients with myocardial infarction. Circulation 1996;94:1291–1297.
39. Lee KL, Woodlief LH, Topol EJ, Weaver WD, Betriu A, Col J, Simoons M, Aylward P, Van de Werf F, Califf RM, for the GUSTO-I Investigators. Predictors of 30-day mortality in the era of reperfusion for acute myocardial infarction. Results from an international trial of 14,021 patients. Circulation 1995;91:1659–1668.
40. Topol EJ, Burek K, O'Neill WW, Kewman DG, Kander NH, Shea MJ, Schork MA, Kirscht J, Juni JE, Pitt B. A randomized controlled trial of hospital discharge three days after myocardial infarction in the era of reperfusion. N Engl J Med 1988;318:1083–1088.
41. Mark DB, Sigmon K, Topol EJ, Kereiakes DJ, Pryor DB, Candela RJ, Califf RM. Identification of acute myocardial infarction patients suitable for early hospital discharge after aggressive interventional therapy: results from the Thrombolysis and Angioplasty in Acute Myocardial Infarction registry. Circulation 1991;83:1186–1191.
42. Newby LK, Califf RM, Guerci A, Weaver WD, Col J, Horgan JH, Mark DB, Stebbins A, Van de Werf F, Gore JM, Topol EJ, for the GUSTO-I Investigators. Early discharge in the thrombolytic era: an analysis of criteria for uncomplicated infarction from the Global Utilization of Streptokinase and t-PA for Occluded Coronary Arteries (GUSTO) Trial. J Am Coll Cardiol 1996;27:625–632.

43. Ohman EM, Armstrong PW, White HD, et al. Risk stratification with a point-of-care troponin T test in acute myocardial infarction. Am J Cardiol 1999;84:1281–1286.
44. Eisenstein EL, Newby LK, Knight JD, Shaw LJ, Mark DB. Cost avoidance through early discharge of the uncomplicated acute myocardial infarction patient. J Am Coll Cardiol 1996;27:244A–245A.
45. Reimer KA, Lowe JE, Rasmussen MM, Jennings RB. The wave-front phenomenon of ischemic cell death: myocardial infarct size versus duration of coronary occlusion in dogs. Circulation 1977;56:785–794.
46. Christian TF, Schwartz RS, Gibbons RJ. Determination of infarct size in reperfusion therapy for acute myocardial infarction. Circulation 1992;86:81–90.
47. GUSTO Angiographic Investigators. The effects of tissue plasminogen activator, streptokinase, or both on coronary-artery patency, ventricular function, and survival after acute myocardial infarction. N Engl J Med 1993;329:1615–1622.
48. TIMI Study Group. Thrombolysis in Myocardial Infarction (TIMI) trial. Phase I findings. N Engl J Med 1985;312:932–936.
49. Langer A, Krucoff MW, Klootwijk P, Veldkamp R, Simoons ML, Granger C, Califf RM, Armstrong PW, for the GUSTO Investigators. Noninvasive assessment of speed and stability of infarct-related artery reperfusion: results of the GUSTO ST segment monitoring study. J Am Coll Cardiol 1995;25:1552–1557.
50. Pomés Iparraguirre H, Tajer C, Sosa Liprandi A. Prognostic implications of early reperfusion coronary syndrome after thrombolysis in acute myocardial infarction. Fibrinolysis 1990;4:58.
51. Califf RM, O'Neill WW, Stack RS, Aronson L, Mark DB, Mantell S, George BS, Candela RJ, Kereiakes DJ, Abbottsmith C, and the TAMI Study Group. Failure of simple clinical measurements to predict perfusion status after intravenous thrombolysis. Ann Intern Med 1988;108:658–662.
52. Ohman EM, Christenson R, Clemmensen P, Wagner GS. Myocardial salvage after reperfusion. Observations from analysis of serial electrocardiographic and biochemical indices. J Electrocardiol 1992;25(suppl):10–14.
53. Kondo M, Yousuke Y, Arai M, Shimizu K, Morikawa M, Shimono Y. Comparison of early myocardial technetium-99m pyrophosphate uptake to early peaking of creatine kinase and creatine kinase-MB as indicators of early reperfusion in acute myocardial infarction. Am J Cardiol 1987;60:762–765.
54. Katus HA, Diederich KW, Scheffold T, Uellner M, Schwarz F, Kubler W. Non-invasive assessment of infarct reperfusion: the predictive power of the time to peak value of myoglobin. Eur Heart J 1988;9:619–624.
55. Katus HA, Scheffold T, Remppis A, Zehlein J. Proteins of the troponin complex. Lab Med 1992;23:311–317.
56. Zabel M, Hohnloser SH, Koster W, Prinz M, Kasper W, Just H. Analysis of creatine kinase, CK-MB, myoglobin, and troponin T time-activity curves for early assessment of coronary artery reperfusion after intravenous thrombolysis. Circulation 1993;87:1542–1550.

57. Grande P, Clemmensen P, Ohman EM, Wagner GS. Biochemical markers of early reperfusion. J Electrocardiol 1992;25(suppl):6–9.
58. Abe S, Arima S, Yamashita T, Miyata M, Okino H, Toda H, Nomoto K, Ueno M, Tahara M, Kiyonaga K. Early assessment of reperfusion therapy using cardiac troponin T. J Am Coll Cardiol 1994;23:1382–1389.
59. Laperche T, Steg G, Dehoux M, Benessiano J, Grollier G, Aliot E, Mossard JM, Aubry P, Coisne D, Hanssen M, for the PERM Study Group. A study of biochemical markers of reperfusion early after thrombolysis for acute myocardial infarction. Circulation 1995;92:2079–2086.
60. Christenson RH, Ohman EM, Topol EJ, Peck S, Newby LK, Duh S-H, Kereiakes DJ, Worley SJ, Alosozana GL, Wall TC, Califf RM, for the TAMI-7 Study Group. Assessment of coronary reperfusion after thrombolysis with a model containing myoglobin, creatine kinase-MB, and clinical variables. Circulation 1997;96:1776–1782.
61. Ohman EM, Christenson RH, Califf RM, George BS, Samaha JK, Kereiakes DJ, Worley SJ, Wall TC, Berrios E, Sigmon KN, and the TAMI-7 Study Group. Noninvasive detection of reperfusion after thrombolysis based on serum creatine kinase MB changes and clinical variables. Am Heart J 1993; 126:819–826.
62. Apple FS, Henry TD, Berger CR, Landt YA. Early monitoring of serum cardiac troponin I for assessment of coronary reperfusion following thrombolytic therapy. Am J Clin Pathol 1996;105:6–10.
63. Tanasijevsic MJ, Cannon CP, Wybenga DR, Fischer G, Grudzien C, McCabe CH. Cardiac troponin I, CK-MB, and myoglobin for early, noninvasive assessment of coronary reperfusion after thrombolysis for acute myocardial infarction. Results from TIMI 10 A. Circulation 1996;94(suppl I):I-322.
64. Sobel BE, Bresnahan GF, Shell WE, Yoder RD. Estimation of infarct size in man and its relation to prognosis. Circulation 1972;46:640–648.
65. Sobel BE, Roberts R, Larson KB. Estimation of infarct size from serum MB creatine phosphokinase activity: applications and limitations. Am J Cardiol 1976;37:474–485.
66. Thompson PL, Fletcher EE, Katavatis V. Enzymatic indices of myocardial necrosis, influence on short- and long-term prognosis after myocardial infarction. Circulation 1979;59:113–119.
67. Grande P, Hansen BF, Christianson C, Naestoft J. Estimation of acute myocardial infarct size in man by serum CK-MB measurements. Circulation 1982; 65:756–764.
68. Christenson RH, O'Hanesian MA, Newby LK, for the TAMI Study Group. Relation of area under the CK-MB release curve and clinical outcomes in myocardial infarction patients treated with thrombolytic therapy. Eur Heart J 1995;16(suppl):75.
69. Baardman T, Hermens WT, Lenderink T, Molhoek GP, Grollier G, Pfisterer M, Simoons ML. Differential effects of tissue plasminogen activator and streptokinase on infarct size and on rate of enzyme release: influence of early infarct related artery patency. The GUSTO enzyme substudy. Eur Heart J 1996; 17:237–246.

70. Simes RJ, Topol EJ, Holmes DR Jr, White HD, Rutsch WR, Vahanian A, Simoons ML, Morris D, Betriu A, Califf RM, for the GUSTO-I Investigators. Link between the angiographic substudy and mortality outcomes in a large randomized trial of myocardial reperfusion. Importance of early and complete infarct artery reperfusion. Circulation 1995;91:1923–1928.
71. Granger C, Moffie I, for the GUSTO Investigators. Under use of thrombolytic therapy in North America has been exaggerated: results of the GUSTO MI registry. Circulation 1994;90(suppl I):I-324.
72. Braunwald E, Mark DB, Jones RH, Cheitlin MD, Fuster V, McCauley KM, Edwards C, Green LA, Mushlin AI, Swain JA, Smith EE III, Cowan M, Rose GC, Concannon CA, Grines CL, Brown L, Lytle BW, Goldman L, Topol EJ, Willerson JT, Brown J, Archibald N. Unstable angina: diagnosis and management. Clinical Practice Guideline No. 10, AHCPR Publication 94-0602. Rockville, MD: Agency of Health Care Policy and Research and the National Heart, Lung and Blood Institute; 1994.
73. Karlson BW, Herlitz J, Pettersson P, Hallgren P, Strombom U, Hjalmarson A. One-year prognosis in patients hospitalized with a history of unstable angina pectoris. Clin Cardiol 1993;16:397–402.
74. Califf RM, Mark DB, Harrell FE Jr, Hlatky MA, Lee KL, Rosati RA, Pryor DB. Importance of clinical measures of ischemia in the prognosis of patients with documented coronary artery disease. J Am Coll Cardiol 1988;11:20–26.
75. Tardiff BE, Granger CB, Woodlief L, for the GUSTO-IIa Investigators. Prognostic significance of post-intervention isoenzyme elevations. Circulation 1995;92(suppl I):I-544.
76. Collinson PO, Chandler HA, Stubbs PJ, Moseley DS, Lewis D, Simmons MD. Measurement of serum troponin T, creatine kinase MB isoenzyme, and total creatine kinase following arduous physical training. Ann Clin Biochem 1995;32:450–453.
77. Wu AHB, Lane PL. Metaanalysis in clinical chemistry: validation of cardiac troponin T as a marker for ischemic heart diseases. Clin Chem 1995;41:1228–1233.
78. Betriu A, Heras M, Cohen M, Fuster V. Unstable angina: outcome according to clinical presentation. J Am Coll Cardiol 1992;19:1659–1663.
79. Calvin JE, Klein LW, Van den Berg BJ, Meyer P, Condon JV, Snell RJ, Ramirez-Morgen LM, Parrillo JE. Risk stratification in unstable angina: prospective validation of the Braunwald classification. JAMA 1995;273:136–141.
80. Woodlief LH, Lee KL, Califf RM, for the GUSTO IIa Investigators. Validation of a mortality model in 1384 patients with acute myocardial infarction. Circulation 1995;92(suppl I):I-776.
81. Selker HP, Griffith JL, D'Agostino RB. A tool for judging coronary care unit admission appropriateness, valid for both real-time and retrospective use. A time-insensitive predictive instrument (TIPI) for acute cardiac ischemia: a multicenter study. Med Care 1991;29:610–627.
82. Goldman L, Cook EF, Brand DA, Lee TH, Rouan GW, Weisberg MC, Acampora D, Stasiulewicz C, Walshon J, Terranova G. A computer protocol to

predict myocardial infarction in emergency department patients with chest pain. N Engl J Med 1988;318:797–803.

83. Rouan GW, Lee TH, Cook EF, Brand DA, Weisberg MC, Goldman L. Clinical characteristics and outcome of acute myocardial infarction in patients with initially normal or nonspecific electrocardiograms. A report from the Multicenter Chest Pain Study. Am J Cardiol 1989;64:1087–1092.
84. Hamm CW, Ravkilde J, Gerhardt W, Jorgensen P, Peheim E, Ljungdahl L, Goldmann B, Katus HA. The prognostic value of serum troponin T in unstable angina. N Engl J Med 1992;327:146–150.
85. Ravkilde J, Horder M, Gerhardt W, Ljungdahl L, Pettersson T, Tryding N, Moller BH, Hamfelt A, Graven T, Asberg A. Diagnostic performance and prognostic value of serum troponin T in suspected acute myocardial infarction. Scand J Clin Lab Invest 1993;53:677–685.
86. Seino Y, Tomita Y, Takano T, Hayakawa H. Early identification of cardiac events with serum troponin T in patients with unstable angina. Lancet 1993; 342:1236–1237.
87. Burlina A, Zaninotto M, Secchiero S, Rubin D, Accorsi F. Troponin T as a marker of ischemic myocardial injury. Clin Biochem 1994;27:113–121.
88. Wu AH, Abbas SA, Green S, Pearsall L, Dhakam S, Azar R, Onoroski M, Senaie A, Mckay RG, Waters D. Prognostic value of cardiac troponin T in unstable angina pectoris. Am J Cardiol 1995;76:970–972.
89. Ravkilde J, Nissen H, Horder M, Thygesen K. Independent prognostic value of serum creatine kinase isoenzyme MB mass, cardiac troponin T and myosin light chain levels in suspected acute myocardial infarction. Analysis of 28 months of follow-up in 196 patients. J Am Coll Cardiol 1995;25:574–581.
90. Stubbs P, Collinson P, Moseley D, Greenwood T, Noble M. Prospective study of the role of cardiac troponin T in patients admitted with unstable angina. Br Med J 1996;313:262–264.
91. Olatidoye AG, Wu AH, Feng YJ, Waters D. Prognostic role of troponin T versus troponin I in unstable angina pectoris for cardiac events with meta-analysis comparing published studies. Am J Cardiol 1998;81:1405–1410.
92. Lindahl B, Venge P, Wallentin L, for the FRISC Study Group. Relation between troponin T and the risk of subsequent cardiac events in unstable coronary artery disease. Circulation 1996;93:1651–1657.
93. Antman EM, Tanasijevic MJ, Thompson B, Schactman M, McCabe CH, Cannon CP, Fischer GA, Fung AY, Thompson C, Wybenga D, Braunwald E. Cardiac-specific troponin I levels to predict the risk of mortality in patients with acute coronary syndromes. N Engl J Med 1996;335:1342–1349.
94. Lüscher M, Ravkilde J, Thygesen K. Troponin T and troponin I in the detection of myocardial damage and subsequent events in 491 consecutive chest pain patients. A sub-study of the TRIM Trial. Circulation 1996;94(suppl I):I-323.
95. Christenson RH, Duh SH, Newby LK, et al., for the GUSTO-IIa Investigators. Cardiac troponin T and cardiac troponin I: relative values in short-term risk stratification of patients with acute coronary syndromes. Clin Chem 1998;44: 494–501.

96. Newby LK, Christenson RH, Ohman EM, et al., for the GUSTO-IIa Investigators. Value of serial troponin T measures for early and late risk stratification in patients with acute coronary syndromes. Circulation 1998;98:1853–1859.
97. Lindahl B, Venge P, Wallentin L, for the Fragmin in Unstable Coronary Artery Disease (FRISC) Study Group. Troponin T identifies patients with unstable coronary artery disease who benefit from long-term anti-thrombotic protection. J Am Coll Cardiol 1997;29:43–48.
98. Lindahl B, Diderholm E, Kontny F, et al. Long term treatment with low molecular weight heparin (dalteparin) reduces cardiac events in unstable coronary artery disease (UCAD) with troponin-T elevation: a FRISC II substudy. Circulation 1999;100:I-498. Abstract.
99. Kong DF, Califf RM, Miller DP, Moliterno DJ, White HD, Harrington RA, Tcheng JE, Lincoff AM, Hasselblad V, Topol EJ. Clinical outcomes of therapeutic agents that block the platelet glycoprotein IIb/IIIa integrin in ischemic heart disease. Circulation 1998;98:2829–2835.
100. Hahn SS, Chae C, Giugliano R, et al. Troponin I levels in unstable angina/non-Q wave myocardial infarction patients treated with tirofiban, a glycoprotein IIb/IIIa antagonist. J Am Coll Cardiol 1998;31:229A. Abstract.
101. Heeschen C, Hamm CW, Goldmann B, Deu A, Langenbrink L, White HD, for the PRISM Study Investigators. Troponin concentrations for stratification of patients with acute coronary syndromes in relation to therapeutic efficacy of tirofiban. Lancet 1999;354:1757–1762.
102. CAPTURE Investigators. Randomised placebo-controlled trial of abciximab before and during coronary intervention in refractory unstable angina: the CAPTURE study. Lancet 1997;349:1429–1435.
103. Hamm CW, Heeschen C, Goldmann B, et al. Benefit of abciximab in patients with refractory unstable angina in relation to serum troponin T levels. N Engl J Med 1999;340:1623–1629.
104. Heeschen C, van den Brand MJ, Hamm CW, Simoons ML, for the CAPTURE Investigators. Angiographic findings in patients with refractory unstable angina according to troponin T status. Circulation 1999;104:1509–1514.
105. Antman EM, Tanasijevic MJ, Cannon CP, et al. Cardiac troponin I on admission predicts death by 42 days in unstable angina and improved survival with an early invasive strategy: results from TIMI IIIB. Circulation 1995;92:I-663. Abstract.
106. Wallentin L, Kontny F, Lagerqvist B, Husted S, Stahle E, Swahn E. Early invasive versus early non-invasive strategy in the setting of long-term treatment with s.c. low-molecular-weight heparin in unstable coronary artery disease: a randomised trial with one year follow-up. Eur Heart J 1999;20:261. Abstract.
107. Lagerqvist B, Diderholm E, Lindahl B, et al. An early treatment strategy reduces cardiac events regardless of troponin levels in unstable coronary artery (UCAD) with and without troponin troponin-elevation: a FRISC II substudy. Circulation 1999;100:I-497. Abstract.

108. Graff LG, Dallara J, Ross MA, et al. Impact on the care of the emergency department chest pain patient from the Chest Pain Evaluation Registry (CHEPER) study. Am J Cardiol 1997;80:563–568.
109. Mair J, Smidt J, Lechleitner P, Deinstl F, Puschendorf B. A decision tree for the early diagnosis of acute myocardial infarction in nontraumatic chest pain patients at hospital admission. Chest 1995;108:1502–1509.
110. Selker HP, Griffith JL, Patil S, Long WJ, D'Agostino RB. A comparison of performance of mathematical predictive methods for medical diagnosis: identifying acute cardiac ischemia among emergency department patients. J Invest Med 1995;43:468–476.
111. Baxt WG, Skora J. Prospective validation of artificial neural network trained to identify acute myocardial infarction. Lancet 1996;347:12–15.
112. Lee TH, Juarez G, Cook EF, Weisberg MC, Rouan GW, Brand DA, Goldman, L. Ruling out acute myocardial infarction: a prospective multicenter validation of a 12-hour strategy for patients at low risk. N Engl J Med 1991;324:1239–1246.
113. Gaspoz JM, Lee TH, Cook EF, Weisberg MC, Goldman L. Outcome of patients who were admitted to a new short stay unit to "rule-out" myocardial infarction. Am J Cardiol 1991;68:145–149.
114. Gibler WB, Young GP, Hedges JR, Lewis LM, Smith MS, Carleton SC, Aghababian RV, Jorden RO, Allison EJ Jr, Otten EJ, for the Emergency Medicine Cardiac Research Group. Acute myocardial infarction in chest pain patients with nondiagnostic ECGs: serial CK-MB sampling in the emergency department. Ann Emerg Med 1992;21:504–512.
115. Gibler WB, Lewis LM, Erb RE, Makens PK, Kaplan BC, Vaughn RH, Biagini AV, Blanton JD, Campbell WB. Early detection of acute myocardial infarction in patients presenting with chest pain and nondiagnostic ECGs: serial CK-MB sampling in the emergency department. Ann Emerg Med 1990;19:1359–1366.
116. Gomez MA, Anderson JL, Karagounis LA, Muhlestein JB, Mooers FB, for the ROMIO Study Group. An emergency department-based protocol for rapidly ruling out myocardial ischemia reduces hospital time and expense: results of a randomized study (ROMIO). J Am Coll Cardiol 1996;28:25–33.
117. Trahey TF, Dunevant SL, Thompson AB, Hill DL, Fontana UG, Beard DC, Campbell PT. Early hospital discharge of chest pain patients using creatine kinase isoforms and stress testing—a community hospital experience. Circulation 1996;94(suppl I):I-569.
118. Benjamin RJ, Johnson P, Goldman L, Lee T, Sacks D. Cardiac troponin T as a diagnostic marker in patients with acute chest pain. Clin Chem 1994;40: 1041.
119. Newby LK, Kaplan AL, Granger BB, Sedor F, Califf RM, Ohman EM. Comparison of cardiac troponin T versus creatine kinase-MB for risk stratification in a chest pain evaluation unit. Am J Cardiol 2000;85:801–805.
120. de Fillippi CR, Parmar RJ, Potter MA, Tocchi M. Diagnostic accuracy, angiographic correlates and long-term risk stratification with the troponin T ultra

sensitive rapid assay in chest pain patients at low risk for acute myocardial infarction. Eur Heart J 1998;19:N42–N47.

121. Lindahl B, Andren B, Ohlsson J, Venge P, Wallentin L, for the FRISC Study Group. Risk stratification in unstable coronary artery disease. Additive value of troponin T determinations and pre-discharge exercise tests. Eur Heart J 1997;18:762–770.
122. Sidman RD, Sayre MR, Kaufmann K. Elevated serum troponin-T levels predict ischemic complications in patients with unstable angina. Acad Emerg Med 1994;1:A44.
123. Gaspoz JM, Lee TH, Weinstein MC, Cook EF, Goldman P, Komaroff AL, Goldman L. Cost effectiveness of a new short-stay unit to "rule-out" acute myocardial infarction in low risk patients. J Am Coll Cardiol 1994; 24:1249–1259.
124. Newby LK, Califf RM. Identifying patient risk: the basis for rational discharge planning after acute myocardial infarction. J Thromb Thrombol 1996; 3:107–115.
125. Zolaga GP. Evaluation of bedside testing options for the critical care unit. Chest 1990;97:185S–190S.
126. Zabel KM, Granger CB, Becker RC, Woodlief LH, Chesebro JH, Califf RM. Bedside aPTT monitoring is associated with less bleeding among GUSTO patients receiving IV heparin following thrombolytic administration. Circulation 1994;90(suppl I):I-553.
127. Downie AC, Frost PG, Fielden P, Joshi D, Dancy CM. Bedside measurement of creatine kinase to guide thrombolysis on the coronary care unit. Lancet 1993;341:452–454.
128. Hamm CW, Goldmann BU, Heeschen C, Kreymann G, Berger J, Meinertz T. Emergency room triage of patients with acute chest pain by means of rapid testing for cardiac troponin T or troponin I. N Engl J Med 1997;337:1648–1653.

14

Stenting in Acute Myocardial Infarction

Steven R. Steinhubl
Wilford Hall Medical Center
San Antonio, Texas

Eric J. Topol
The Cleveland Clinic Foundation
Cleveland, Ohio

INTRODUCTION

Percutaneous mechanical revascularization as primary therapy for restoring vessel patency during an acute myocardial infarction was first reported in 1983 (1). Since that time several randomized trials have confirmed that a mechanical intervention with balloon angioplasty can be as effective as, or superior to, pharmacologic therapy in the acute treatment of ST-segment elevation myocardial infarctions (2–4).

Stenting as a possible means of preventing reocclusion and restenosis following balloon angioplasty was first described in patients in 1987 (5). Initial experience with stents was hampered by unacceptably high rates of stent thrombosis and its associated frequent complications of Q-wave myocardial infarction or death (6). Due to early reports suggesting that thrombus-containing lesions were at especially high risk for stent thrombosis, stent placement in the setting of a recent myocardial infarction was considered contraindicated (7). Refinements in antithrombotic therapy and stent technique have subsequently led to a significant reduction in the incidence of stent thrombosis (8,9). This improvement in short-term outcomes, as well as the capacity for stents to decrease restenosis (10) have led to an exponential increase in the frequency of stent placement such that ~70% of patients in many interventional labs today are receiving stents.

The culprit lesions of an acute myocardial infarction are typically discrete and located proximally in a large caliber vessel, making them ideal candidates for stenting. However, just as the pathophysiology of a ruptured atherosclerotic plaque is distinct from that of a stable coronary lesion, the pathophysiologic response to stent placement is considerably different from that seen with balloon angioplasty alone (11,12). So while stenting following angioplasty provides mechanical support, it also alters the local hemostatic milieu. The interaction of these two processes with the inciting lesion will be what determines the short and long-term success of stenting as an adjunctive therapy. This chapter will explore what benefits and limitations of stenting compared with balloon angioplasty in the treatment of an acute myocardial infarction, as well as summarize the data currently available from clinical trials.

LIMITATIONS OF STANDARD ANGIOPLASTY

Angiographic Success and Abrupt Closure

Prospective randomized studies of primary balloon angioplasty in acute myocardial infarction have reported angiographic success rates (defined as residual stenosis of <50% and a Thrombolysis in Myocardial Infarction (TIMI) flow grade of 2 or 3) varying from as low as 80% to as high as 98% (3,4,13–15). However, in four of these five studies success was determined by the operator, and may therefore represent an overestimation. In the GUSTO IIb angioplasty substudy off-line quantitative angiographic analysis in a core laboratory found the percentage of lesions to have a residual stenosis of <50% to be 77.4%, compared with 91.4% as judged by the operators.

The distinction between successful and failed angioplasty in acute myocardial infarction is more than just a cosmetic one. Five observational studies of direct angioplasty have all shown more than a twofold, and up to a 10-fold greater mortality in patients with failed compared to successful angioplasty (16–20). Though the cause of this marked discrepancy in early mortality is uncertain, the rates in the failed group are significantly higher than pre-thrombolytic era historical controls with similar ejection fractions (21). This suggests that the unsuccessful intervention itself may have contributed to the increased mortality beyond the inability to restore patency. In further support of this tenet are the results of two studies evaluating rescue angioplasty (22,23). These trials not only demonstrated a similar six- to sevenfold increase in mortality in patients with failed compared with successful angioplasty, but they also showed that patients who did not undergo a percutaneous intervention despite angiographically proven occluded arteries had mortality rates comparable to the successful angioplasty group. These findings all suggest that by improving initial success rates stenting could potentially impact in-hospital mortality.

A role for stenting in improving acute procedural success is suggested by the results of a single-center study that retrospectively evaluated the mechanism for failure in 45 unsuccessful primary interventions preceding the stent era (24). In this series, nearly one-third of the failed interventions were due to acute closure. Another third of the patients failed secondary to suboptimal dilatation, with a substantial percentage of these patients having an angiographically discernable dissection. Another series of 34 patients evaluated with intravascular ultrasound following failed primary angioplasty, dissection was found to be the cause of failure in a majority of these patients (25). Similarly, angioscopy results have shown dissection to be the etiology behind acute closure following PTCA in 82% of patients studied (26). Interestingly, in these studies dissections were not recognized angiographically in one-third and two-thirds of the cases, respectively. The ability of stenting to successfully treat acute or threatened closure has been well documented in numerous observational studies in unselected patients, with the majority demonstrating 100% initial success (27). Randomized trials have also shown that the elective placement of a stent increases acute success when compared to balloon angioplasty alone. The Stent Restenosis Study (STRESS) showed a significantly higher angiographic success rate by core lab analysis of 99.5%, compared with 92.6% ($P < .001$) for angioplasty alone (28).

Recurrent Ischemia and Reocclusion

In-hospital recurrent ischemia occurs following primary angioplasty in 5% to 15% of patients—substantially higher than the ~4% seen with elective angioplasty (3,4,13–15). Evaluation of patients in the Primary Angioplasty in Myocardial Infarction (PAMI) II trial demonstrated that the angiographic appearance of a dissection or a >30% residual stenosis were markers for recurrent ischemia (29). When predischarge reocclusion was specifically addressed in this same group of patients, the presence of a dissection was again the strongest predictor of its occurrence (30). In one study of primary angioplasty with 3-week angiographic follow-up reocclusion had occurred in 12% of infarct-related arteries (31). In another series of 528 patients with angiographic follow-up 6 months after successful PTCA following a myocardial infarction, reocclusion had occurred in 17% (32). At long-term follow-up (mean 5.7 years), patients who had reoccluded had a significantly higher mortality than those who had a patent artery at 6 months (20% vs. 8%, $P = .002$). Stent placement in this patient population would be anticipated to decrease both recurrent ischemia and reocclussion.

Restenosis

Individual trials of primary angioplasty in acute myocardial infarction with angiographic follow-up have revealed restenosis rates between 32% and 52% with a pooled result of 43% (33). This high rate of restenosis considerably impacts the durability of the procedure and cost-effectiveness of primary angioplasty as a treatment strategy in acute myocardial infarction. This likely, at least in part, accounts for erosion of the early benefit conferred for PTCA over thrombolysis in the GUSTO IIb trial. The lack of durability was illustrated by results from the Myocardial Infarction Triage and Intervention (MITI) trial which demonstrated a significantly higher rate of repeat angiography (13.2% vs. 7.4%, $P < .001$) as well as angioplasty (9.0% vs. 6.6%, $P = .03$) at 1 year for patients treated with primary angioplasty compared with patients treated with thrombolytics (2).

The benefits of elective stenting for the prevention of restenosis have been consistently demonstrated in several randomized trials comparing balloon angioplasty with stenting in discrete, solitary lesions (10,28,34). In aggregate these trials have demonstrated a lower incidence of angiographic restenosis as well as a decreased need for repeat revascularizations with stenting.

CLINICAL TRIALS OF STENTING

Nonrandomized Trials

Due to the potential for stenting to overcome many of the limitations of primary angioplasty by improving acute success, preventing recurrent in-hospital ischemia, decreasing reocclusion, and limiting restenosis, there has been considerable interest in the role of stenting in the treatment of acute MI. However, with early studies showing such a dramatic increase in the risk of stent thrombosis with their use in acute coronary syndromes, most interventionalists did not even consider the use of stents in this setting. In the early 1990s, rare case reports of successful experiences in a very limited number of patients with acute myocardial infarction began appearing in the literature (35–38). Over the next several years, with increasing experience with stents in general, and improvements in poststenting antithrombotic regimens, an increasing number of observational studies were reported. By 1997 the results of nearly 30 nonrandomized studies involving ~2000 patients treated with stents in the setting of an acute MI had been published. Although the nature of these studies did not allow for the formation of specific conclusions regarding the role of stenting, the data were reassuring. Not only were stent thrombosis rates lower than initially feared, but also the results of these early trials consistently found that stenting could potentially minimize most of the limitations of primary angioplasty. A number of studies also evaluated that stenting in acute MI decreased restenosis. In 11 studies with angiographic follow-up, the combined binary restenosis rate in 580 patients was 23%. This compares quite favorably with the 32% to 52% restenosis rates published for primary angioplasty.

Another important observation from these early trials was that not all patients were amenable to stenting. In studies employing stenting as a primary therapy, only 54% to 77% of the eligible patients were able to receive stents (39,41). Interestingly, in studies where stents were reserved only for patients with a suboptimal angioplasty results, up to 48% of potential patients received stents (40,42,43).

Randomized Trials

To date, the results of nine randomized trials of stenting versus balloon angioplasty in the primary treatment of acute MI have been reported (44–52). In total these trials have randomized nearly 2500 patients, with individual studies ranging in size from 88 to 900 patients (Fig. 1). Importantly, all trials enrolled patients with angiographic characteristics allowing for optimal stent placement. In the Stent-PAMI (Primary Angioplasty in Myocardial Infarction) trial 38% of screened patients were not considered eligible, and in the Zwolle study nearly 50% of primary angioplasty candidates were excluded from randomization (48,51). With selective enrollment in these trials, successful stent placement was high—ranging from 86% (50) to 100% (45,52), with the majority achieving 97% to 98% success.

Whereas most of these trials randomized patients immediately after angiography demonstrated that they were stent-eligible, two trials, FRESCO (Florence Randomized Elective Stenting in Acute Coronary Occlusions) and PRISAM (Primary Stenting for Acute Myocardial Infarction) randomized patients to either stenting or no further treatment only after optimal balloon angioplasty (45,52). In both of these small studies, stenting compared to optimal angioplasty was associated with a significant decrease in the combined endpoint of death, re-MI and the need for urgent target vessel revascularization (TVR). In FRESCO, early recurrent ischemia was reduced from 15% in balloon-only treated patients compared with 3% in stented patients. Stenting compared with optimal balloon angioplasty also significantly decreased the cumulative incidence of restenosis or reocclusion at 6 months from 43% to 17% ($P = .001$) in the FRESCO trial.

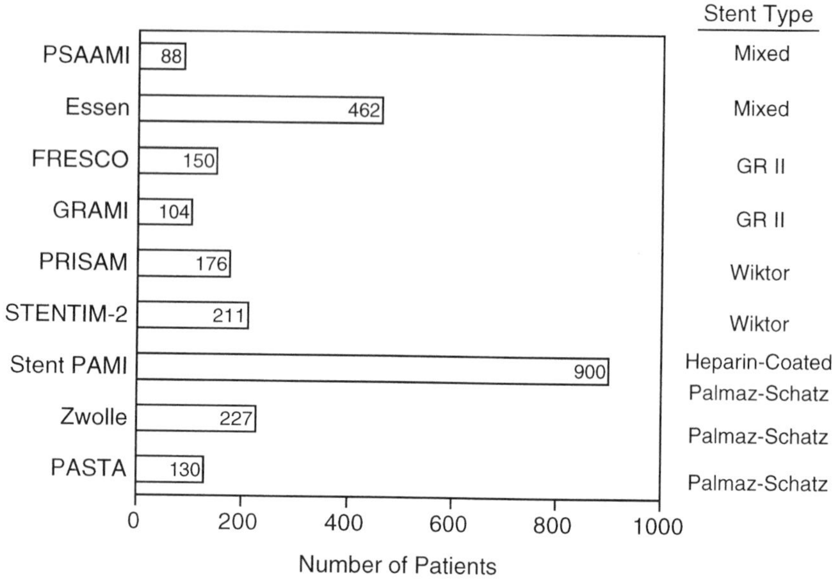

Figure 1 Randomized trials of stenting in acute myocardial infarction. Abbreviations: PSAAMI, Primary Stenting vs. Angioplasty in Acute Myocardial Infarction; FRESCO, Florence Randomized Elective Stenting in Acute Coronary Occlusions; GRAMI, Gianturco-Roubin in Acute Myocardial Infarction; PRISAM, Primary Stenting for Acute Myocardial Infarction; Stent PAMI, Primary Angioplasty in Myocardial Infarction; PASTA, Primary Angioplasty vs. Stent Implantation in AMI.

The remaining seven trials have reinforced the advantages of stenting over balloon angioplasty alone in terms of diminishing recurrent ischemia, and in particular improving restenosis (44,46–51) (Figs. 2, 3). In the trial from the Zwolle group (48), 217 patients with an acute MI presenting within 6 hours of symptom onset were randomized to Palmaz-Schatz stent placement or balloon angioplasty. Stenting led to a greater post-procedural minimal luminal diameter (2.57 ± 0.37 vs. 2.17 ± 0.45, $P < .0001$), and clinically was associated with a strong trend towards a decrease in death or re-MI (3% vs. 9%, $P = .08$) and a highly significant decrease in TVR at 6 months (4% vs. 17%, $P = .0016$). The largest randomized trial of stenting in acute MI is the Stent PAMI study, which evaluated a heparin-coated Palmaz-Schatz stent versus balloon angioplasty in 900 patients (51). In this trial patients were randomized only after blood flow had been established beyond the obstruction. Interestingly, core laboratory analysis of post procedure angiograms demonstrated that the balloon angioplasty cohort had a

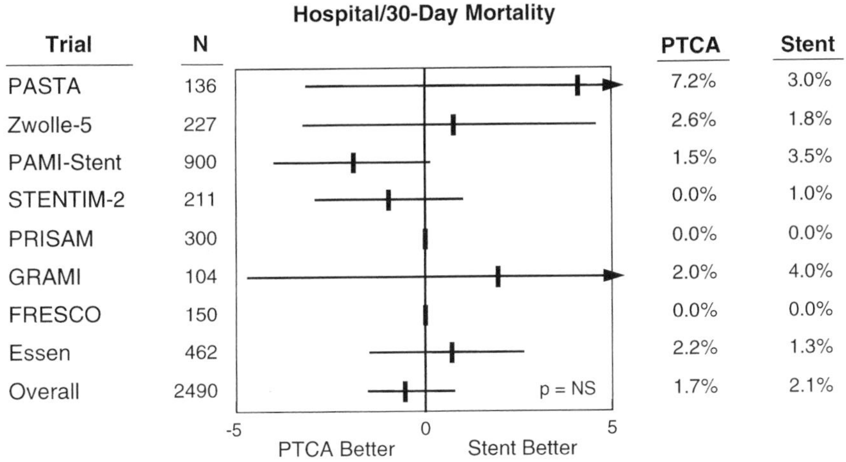

Figure 2 In-hospital or 30-day recurrent myocardial infarction in randomized trials of stenting in acute myocardial infarction. (Abbreviations as in Fig. 1.)

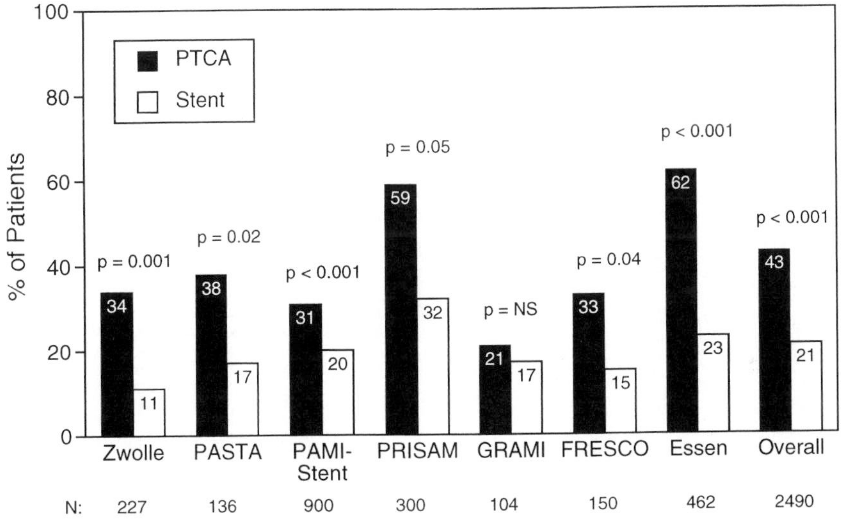

Figure 3 Restenosis in randomized trials of stenting in acute myocardial infarction. (Abbreviations as in Fig. 1.)

nonsignificant trend toward increased success (defined as TIMI grade 3 flow and <50% stenosis) compared to the stent group (91.6% and 89.4%, respectively; $P = .30$). This decrease in TIMI grade 3 flow in the stent arm occurred despite a significantly larger lumen being achieved in stented patients (2.56 ± 0.44 vs. 2.12 ± 0.45, $P < .001$). Also, unlike previous smaller trials, stenting did not have a significant impact on the incidence of in-hospital recurrent ischemia (2.9% stenting versus 4.0% angioplasty, $P = .37$). This trend towards diminished TIMI grade 3 flow and lack of a significant impact on recurrent ischemia likely contributed to the worrisome trend of increased mortality in the stent-treated patients compared with those receiving balloon angioplasty alone (3.5% vs. 1.8% at 1 month, $P = .15$; 4.2% vs. 2.7% at 6 months, $P = .27$). Like all previous trials, stenting did significantly decrease clinical restenosis compared with angioplasty (7.7% vs. 17.0%, $P < .001$).

Why Doesn't Stenting Decrease Mortality?

Although it is clear from the results of all trials to date that stenting of amendable infarct-related lesions does lead to a significant decrease in the incidence of clinical restenosis, its lack of affect on mortality has been disappointing (Fig. 4). One probable etiology for this is the decrease in TIMI grade 3 flow found in the stent arm of three of the four published randomized trials of stenting in acute MI (Table 1). The GUSTO-I (Global Utilization of Streptokinase and Tissue plasminogen activator for Occluded coronary ar-

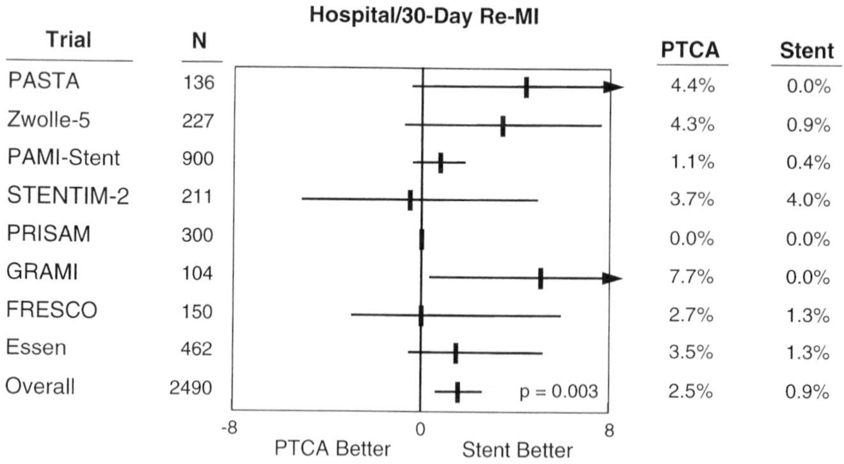
Hospital/30-Day Re-MI
Trial
N
PTCA
Stent
PASTA
136
4.4%
0.0%
Zwolle-5
227
4.3%
0.9%
PAMI-Stent
900
1.1%
0.4%
STENTIM-2
211
3.7%
4.0%
PRISAM
300
0.0%
0.0%
GRAMI
104
7.7%
0.0%
FRESCO
150
2.7%
1.3%
Essen
462
3.5%
1.3%
Overall
2490
p = 0.003
2.5%
0.9%
-8
0
8
PTCA Better
Stent Better

Figure 4 In-hospital or 30-day mortality in randomized trials of stenting in acute myocardial infarction. (Abbreviations as in Fig. 1.)

Table 1 Incidence of TIMI Grade 3 Flow in Published Randomized Trials of Stenting in Acute Myocardial Infarction

	N	% TIMI grade 3 flow		*P* value
		Angioplasty	Stent	
Stent PAMI (51)	884	92.7	89.4	0.10
Zwolle (66)	227	94	90	0.68
FRESCO (52)	150	100	98.7	1.0
GRAMI (47)	104	83	96	<0.02
Pooled Analysis	1365	93%	91%	0.222

PAMI = Primary Angioplasty in Myocardial Infarction; FRESCO = Florence Randomized Elective Stenting in Acute Coronary Occlusions; GRAMI = Gianturco-Roubin in Acute Myocardial Infarction.

teries) angiographic substudy was the first to demonstrate that complete reperfusion of the infarct-related artery with achievement of TIMI grade 3 flow was one of the strongest predictors of improved mortality over the long term (53). In the Stent PAMI trial, eight patients were identified who had TIMI grade 3 flow after initial angioplasty who developed TIMI grade 0 to 2 flow following stenting, with one of these patients dying (54). In a nonrandomized study of 361 patients with acute MI, <TIMI grade 3 flow was found in 17.4% of 109 stent-treated patients compared with 9.5% of 252 angioplasty-only patients ($P < .05$) (55). This decrease in TIMI grade flow was associated with poor recovery of left ventricular ejection fraction. In a final study, coronary blood flow was assessed by TIMI frame count after angioplasty and again after stenting in 75 patients with an acute MI (56). These investigators found that stenting caused a decrease in coronary blood flow in one-third of patients, no change in another third, and increased coronary blood flow in the final third, with no difference in minimal lumen diameter between groups. These results all clearly suggest that stenting can decrease coronary blood flow in a substantial number of patients.

Since all stent trials have consistently demonstrated an increase in luminal diameter with stenting compared with angioplasty alone, it appears likely that the diminished flow following stenting is related to microvascular injury or occlusion. In fact, the importance of achieving normal microvascular flow, even more so than normal epicardial flow, has recently been highlighted by several investigators. Ito and coworkers found that despite TIMI grade 3 epicardial flow in 126 patients following primary angioplasty, 37% had no microvascular flow as determined by myocardial contrast echocardiography (57). No reflow by myocardial contrast echocardiography was associated with a significant increase in left ventricular end-diastolic volume as well as less functional recovery. In a second study, microvascular obstruction post-MI as demonstrated by magnetic resonance imaging was found in 17% of 30 patients with TIMI grade 3 flow and 60% of 10 patients with TIMI grade 0 to 2 flow (58). These investigators found that microvascular obstruction was a more potent marker of postinfarction cardiovascular complications than epicardial flow. Two recent studies evaluating the filling and clearance of contrast in the myocardium during coronary angiography have confirmed that a large proportion of patients with TIMI grade 3 flow of the infarct-related epicardial artery do not achieve normal microvascular flow, and that diminished microvascular flow is more strongly associated with mortality than epicardial flow (59,60). The results of these trials suggest that protecting the microcirculation is crucial to optimizing coronary flow, and with it mortality, with stenting in the treatment of an acute MI.

The microvasculature of the myocardium can be compromised in the setting of an acute MI through various mechanisms including distal embolization of platelet microaggregates and atherosclerotic debris, the release of potent vasoconstrictors from activated platelets, and due to an inflammatory response to reperfusion injury. Since increased platelet activation has been demonstrated during an acute myocardial infarction as well as with stenting (11,61), the addition of a platelet glycoprotein IIb/IIIa receptor inhibitor could potentially decrease platelet-associated microvascular injury. In confirmation of this Neumann and colleagues compared coronary flow as measured by a Doppler wire in 200 patients undergoing stenting for an acute MI, half of whom were treated with abciximab and the other half with standard heparin (62). Although residual stenoses did not differ between the two groups, abciximab treatment was associated with a significant improvement of peak coronary flow velocity as well as improved wall motion index and recovery of global left ventricular function. This improved microvascular flow with abciximab translated into a significant decrease in the combined endpoint of death, re-MI, or urgent revascularization at 30 days, and a strong trend toward decreased mortality at 6 months (Fig. 6). These clinical benefits of abciximab in stenting for acute MI have been reinforced by the results of several randomized trials. In the ADMIRAL study, 300 patients with an acute MI were randomly assigned to either abciximab or placebo prior to PTCA and stenting (64). At 24 hours TIMI grade 3 flow was significantly improved in abciximab-treated patients compared to those receiving placebo from 82.5% to 92.0%. At 30 days the combined incidence of death, reinfarction and TVR was also significantly reduced from 14.7% in controls to 7.3% in abciximab-treated patients. The interim results of a second randomized trial, CADILLAC (Controlled Abciximab and Device In-

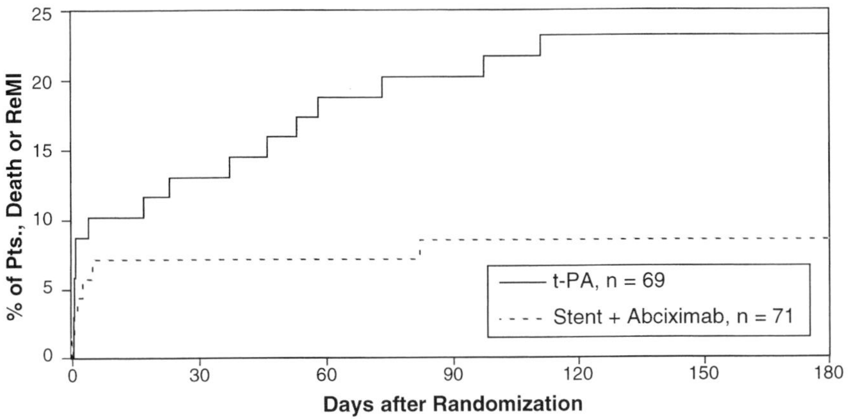

Figure 5 STOPMI trial demonstrating increased acute myocardial salvage with stenting + abciximab with an associated decrease in 6-month death and reinfarction.

vestigation to Lower Late Angioplasty Complications) were presented at the 1999 Scientific Sessions of the American Heart Association. In this trial 2081 patients were randomized to one of four treatment groups: abciximab + stent; placebo + stent; abciximab + balloon; or placebo + balloon. A report of the in-hospital outcomes demonstrated improved flow associated with abciximab treatment in acute MI patients treated with stents (96.7% vs. 92% TIMI 3 flow, respectively). A third trial, STOPMI, which compared fibrinolytic

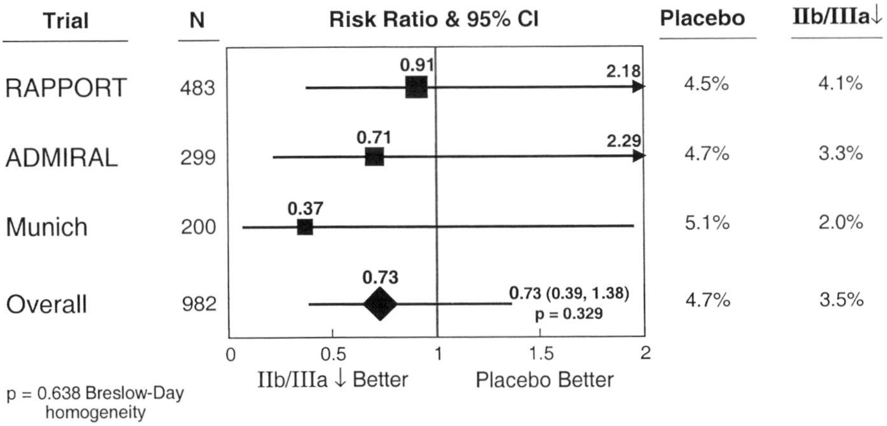

Figure 6 Mortality benefit in randomized trials of stenting ± abciximab in the treatment of acute myocardial infarction.

therapy with t-PA versus stent + abciximab in the treatment of acute MI, also demonstrated a consistent benefit of stenting plus GPIIb/IIIa inhibition. The combination of a stent plus abciximab led to increased myocardial salvage with an associated decrease in death and re-MI (Fig. 5).

When all of these trials are evaluated in aggregate, a clear benefit of abciximab is seen in patients treated with stents in acute MI (Fig. 6). Although the final data from these trials are needed before definitive recommendations can be made regarding adjunctive GPIIb/IIIa and stenting in acute MI, these results strongly support that a GPIIb/IIIa inhibitor plus stenting may offer additive benefit, similar to or even greater than that seen with abciximab and stenting in a nonacute setting (65).

CONCLUSION

While the vast majority of percutaneous coronary interventions performed in the United States today involve a stent, the culprit lesion associated with an acute myocardial infarction makes for an especially ideal target for stent placement. They are typically discrete, and proximally located in large caliber vessels. Since pathophysiologically they are initiated through plaque rupture, stenting can prevent the unprotected extension of this tear that occurs following balloon angioplasty. Unfortunately, the improvement in epicardial flow due to local scaffolding by the stent appears to be balanced by the potential for microcirculatory obstruction following stenting. The results of recently completed and ongoing studies will better define the promising role of the platelet GPIIb/IIIa receptor inhibitors as adjunctive therapy in stenting for an acute MI. With the addition of these agents it appears likely that stenting in the treatment of an acute MI can fulfill its promise as a means for improving initial success, preventing recurrent ischemia and decreasing restenosis.

REFERENCES

1. Hartzler GO, Rutherford BD, McConahay DR, Johnson WLJ, McCallister BD, Gura GMJ, Conn RC, Crockett JE. Percutaneous transluminal coronary angioplasty with and without thrombolytic therapy for treatment of acute myocardial infarction. Am Heart J 1983;106:965–973.
2. Every NR, Parsons LS, Hlatky M, Martin JS, Weaver WD, for the Myocardial Infarction Triage and Intervention Investigators. A comparison of thrombolytic therapy with primary coronary angioplasty for acute myocardial infarction. N Engl J Med 1996;335:1253–1260.
3. Grines CL, Browne KF, Marco J, Rothbaum D, Stone GW, O'Keefe J, Overlie P, Donohue B, Chelliah N, Timmis GC, Vlietstra RE, Strzelecki M, Puchrowicz-Ochocki S, O'Neill WW, for the Primary Angioplasty in Myocardial In-

farction Study Group. A comparison of immediate angioplasty with thrombolytic therapy for acute myocardial infarction. N Engl J Med 1993;328:673–679.

4. GUSTO IIb Angioplasty Substudy Investigators. An international randomized trial of 1138 patients comparing primary coronary angioplasty versus tissue plasminogen activator for acute myocardial infarction. N Engl J Med 1997; 336:1621–1628.
5. Sigwart U, Puel J, Mirkovitch V, Joffre F, Kappenberger L. Intravascular stents to prevent occlusion and restenosis after transluminal angioplasty. N Engl J Med 1987;316:701–706.
6. Serruys PW, Strauss BH, Beatt KJ, Bertrand ME, Puel J, Rickards AF, Meier B, Goy J-J, Vogt P, Kappenberger L, Sigwart U. Angiographic follow-up after placement of a self-expanding coronary-artery stent. N Engl J Med 1991;324: 13–17.
7. Nath CF, Muller DWM, Ellis SG, Rosenschein U, Chapkis A, Quain L, Zimmerman C, Topol EJ. Thrombosis of a flexible coil coronary stent: frequency, predictors and clinical outcome. J Am Coll Cardiol 1993;21:622–627.
8. Schomig A, Neumann F-J, Kastrati A, Schuhlen H, Blasini R, Hadamitzky M, Walter H, Zitzmann-Roth E-M, Richardt G, Alt E, Schmitt C, Ulm K. A randomized comparison of antiplatelet and anticoagulant therapy after the placement of coronary-artery stents. N Engl J Med 1996;334:1084–1089.
9. Colombo A, Hall P, Nakamura S, Almagor Y, Maiello L, Martini G, Gaglione A, Goldberg SL, Tobis JM. Intracoronary stenting without anticoagulation accomplished with intravascular ultrasound guidance. Circulation 1995;91:1676–1688.
10. Serruys PW, van Hout B, Bonnier H, Legrand V, Garcia E, Macaya C, Sousa E, Van der Giessen W, Colombo A, Seabra-Gomes R, Kiemeneij F, Ruygrok P, Ormiston J, Emanuelsson H, Fajadet J, Haude M, Klugmann S, Morel MA. Randomised comparison of implantation of heparin-coated stents with balloon angioplasty in selected patients with coronary artery disease (BENESTENT II). Lancet 1998;352:673–681.
11. Gawaz M, Neumann F-J, Ott I, May A, Rudiger S, Schomig A. Changes in membrane glycoproteins of circulating platelets after coronary stent implantation. Heart 1996;76:166–172.
12. Parsson H, Cwikiel W, Johansson K, Swartbol P, Norgren L. Deposition of platelets and neutrophils in porcine iliac arteries after angioplasty and Wallstent placement compared with angioplasty alone. Cardiovasc Intervent Radiol 1994; 17:190–196.
13. Gibbons RJ, Holmes DR, Reeder GS, Bailey KR, Hopfenspirger MR, Gersh BJ, for the Mayo Coronary Care Unit and Catheterization Laboratory Groups. Immediate angioplasty compared with the administration of a thrombolytic agent followed by conservative treatment for myocardial infarction. N Engl J Med 1993;328:685–691.
14. Ribeiro EE, Silva LA, Carneiro R, D'Oliveira LG, Gasquez A, Amino JG, Travares JR, Petrizzo A, Torossian S, Duprat R, Buffolo E, Ellis SG. Random-

ized trial of direct coronary angioplasty versus intravenous streptokinase in acute myocardial infarction. J Am Coll Cardiol 1993;22:376–380.
15. Zijlstra F, De Boer MJ, Hoorntje JCA, Reiffers S, Reiber JHC, Suryapranata H. A comparison of immediate coronary angioplasty with intravenous streptokinase in acute myocardial infarction. N Engl J Med 1993;328:680–684.
16. Ellis SG, Topol EJ, Gallison L, Grines CL, Langburd AB, Bates ER, Walton JAJ, O'Neill W. Predictors of success for coronary angioplasty performed for acute myocardial infarction. J Am Coll Cardiol 1988;12:1407–1415.
17. Miller PF, Brodie BR, Weintraub RA, LeBauer EJ, Katz JD, Stuckey TD, Hansen CJ. Emergency coronary angioplasty for acute myocardial infarction. Arch Intern Med 1987;147:1565–1570.
18. O'Keefe JH, Bailey WL, Rutherford BD, Hartzler GO. Primary angioplasty for acute myocardial infarction in 1,000 consecutive patients. Results in an unselected population and high-risk subgroups. Am J Cardiol 1993;72:107G–115G.
19. Rothbaum DA, Linnemeier TJ, Landin RJ, Steinmetz EF, Hillis JS, Hallam CC, Noble RJ, See MR. Emergency percutaneous transluminal coronary angioplasty in acute myocardial infarction: a 3 year experience. J Am Coll Cardiol 1987;10:264–272.
20. Weaver WD, Litwin PE, Martin JS, for the Myocardial Infarction Triage and Intervention Project Investigators. Use of direct angioplasty for treatment of patients with acute myocardial infarction in hospitals with and without on-site cardiac surgery. Circulation 1993;88:2067–2075.
21. Ellis SG, Van de Werf F, Ribeiro-daSilva E, Topol EJ. Present status of rescue coronary angioplasty: current polarization of opinion and randomized trials. J Am Coll Cardiol 1992;19:681–686.
22. Abbottsmith CW, Topol EJ, George BS, Stack RS, Kereiakes DJ, Candela RJ, Anderson LC, Harrelson-Woodlief SL, Califf RM. Fate of patients with acute myocardial infarction with patency of the infarct-related vessel achieved with successful thrombolysis versus rescue angioplasty. J Am Coll Cardiol 1990;16:770–778.
23. McKendall GR, Forman S, Sopko G, Braunwald E, Williams DO, and the Thrombolysis in Myocardial Infarction Investigators. Value of rescue percutaneous transluminal angioplasty following unsuccessful thrombolytic therapy in patients with acute myocardial infarction. Am J Cardiol 1995;76:1108–1111.
24. Bedotto JB, Kahn JK, Rutherford BD, McConahay DR, Giorgi LV, Johnson WL, O'Keefe JH, Shimshak TM, Ligon RW, Hartzler GO. Failed direct angioplasty for acute myocardial infarction: In-hospital outcome and predictors of death. J Am Coll Cardiol 1993;22:690–694.
25. Werner GS, Diedrich J, Kreuzer H. Causes of failed angioplasty for acute myocardial infarction assessed by intravascular ultrasound. Am Heart J 1997; 11337:517–525.
26. White CJ, Ramee SR, Collins TJ, Jain SP, Escobar A. Coronary angioscopy of abrupt occlusion after angioplasty. J Am Coll Cardiol 1995;25:1681–1684.
27. Eeckhout E, Kappenberger L, Goy J-J. Stents for intracoronary placement: current status and future directions. J Am Coll Cardiol 1996;27:757–765.

28. Fischman DL, Leon MB, Baim DS, Schatz RA, Savage MP, Penn I, Detre K, Veltri L, Ricci D, Nobuyoshi M, Cleman M, Heuser R, Almond D, Teirstein PS, Fish RD, Colombo A, Brinker J, Moses J, Shaknovich A, Hirshfeld J, Bailey S, Ellis S, Rake R, Goldberg S, for the Stent Restenosis Study Investigators. A randomized comparison of coronary-stent placement and balloon angioplasty in the treatment of coronary artery disease. N Engl J Med 1994; 331:496–501.
29. Grines C, Brodie B, Griffin J, Donohue B, Sampaolesi A, Constantini C, Sachs D, Wharton T, Esente P, Spain M, Stone G. Which primary PTCA patients may benefit from new technologies? Circulation 1995;92:I-146. Abstract.
30. Benzuly KH, O'Neill WW, Brodie B, Griffin J, Shimshak T, Jones DE, Graham M, Mitina L, Grines CL. Predictors of maintained infarct artery patency after primary angioplasty in high risk patients in PAMI-2. J Am Coll Cardiol 1996; 27:279A. Abstract.
31. Nakagawa Y, Iwasaki Y, Kimura T, Tamura T, Yokoi H, Yokoi H, Hamasaki N, Nosaka H, Nobuyoshi M. Serial angiographic follow-up after successful direct angioplasty for acute myocardial infarction. Am J Cardiol 1996;78:980–984.
32. Bauters C, Delomez M, Van Belle E, McFadden E, Lablanche J-M, Bertrand ME. Angiographically documented late reocclusion after successful coronary angioplasty of an infarct-related lesion is a powerful predictor of long-term mortality. Circulation 1999;99:2243–2250.
33. Horrigan MCG, Topol EJ. Direct angioplasty in acute myocardial infarction. State of the art and current controversies. Cardiol Clin 1995;13:321–338.
34. Serruys PW, De Jaegere P, Kiemeneij F, Magaya C, Rutsch W, Heyndrickx G, Emanuelsson H, Marco J, Legrand V, Materne P, Belardi J, Sigwart U, Colombo A, Goy JJ, van den Heuvel P, Delcan J, Morel M-A, for the Benestent Study Group. A comparison of balloon-expandable-stent implantation with balloon angioplasty in patients with coronary artery disease. N Engl J Med 1994; 331:489–495.
35. Cannon AD, Roubin GS, Macander PJ, Agrawal SK. Intracoronary stenting as an adjunct to angioplasty in acute myocardial infarction. J Invas Cardiol 1991; 3:255–258.
36. Tebbe U, Chemnitius JM, Brune S, Schmidt T, Scholz KH, Kreuzer H. Emergency stenting in acute myocardial infarction after failed thrombolysis and angioplasty. J Cardiovasc Technol 1991;10:49–53.
37. Wong SC, Franklin M, Teirstein PS, Yellayi SS, Morris N, De Remer VT, Schatz RA. Stenting in acute myocardial infarction secondary to delayed vessel closure following balloon angioplasty. J Invas Cardiol 1992;4:331–334.
38. Wong PH, Wong CM. Intracoronary stenting in acute myocardial infarction. Cathet Cardiovasc Diagn 1994;33:39–45.
39. Saito S, Hosokawa G, Kim K, Tanaka S, Miyake S. Primary stent implantation without coumadin in acute myocardial infarction. J Am Coll Cardiol 1996;28: 74–81.

40. Antoniucci D, Valenti R, Buanamici P, Santora GM, Leoncini M, Balognese L, Fazzini PF. Direct angioplasty and stenting of the infarct-related artery in acute myocardial infarction. Am J Cardiol 1996;78:568–571.
41. Stone GW, Brodie B, Griffin J, St. Gear FG, Morice M-C, Costantini C, Overlie PA, Jones D, O'Neill WW, Grines CL. Safety and feasibility of primary stenting in acute myocardial infarction—In hospital and 30 day results of the PAMI Stent Pilot Trial. J Am Coll Cardiol 1997;29:389A. Abstract.
42. Horstkotte D, Piper C, Andresen D, Linderer T, Schwimmbeck P, Oeff M, Schultheiss HP. Stent implantation for acute myocardial infarction: results of a pilot study with 80 consecutive patients. Eur Heart J 1996;17:297. Abstract.
43. Nakagawa Y, Yokoi H, Nosaka H, Yokoi H, Hamasaki N, Kimura T, Nobuyoshi M. Stent assisted direct balloon angioplasty for acute myocardial infarction, prospective trial. J Am Coll Cardiol 1996;27:249A. Abstract.
44. Scheller B, Hennen B, Severin-Kneib S, Markwirth T, Doerr T, Berg G, Schieffer H, Ozbek C. Follow-Up of the PSAAMI Study Population (Primary Stenting vs. Angioplasty in Acute Myocardial Infarction). J Am Coll Cardiol 1999;33: 29A. Abstract.
45. Kawashima A, Ueda K, Nishida Y, Inoue N, Uemura S, Miyazaki H, Tanaka N, Furukawa K, Okada T, Tanaka S, Kato O, Tamai H. Quantitative angiographic analysis of restenosis of primary stenting using Wiktor stent for acute myocardial infarction: results from a multicenter randomized PRISAM study. Circulation 1998;98:I-153.
46. Maillard L, Hamon M, Monassier J-P, Raynaud P, Investigators S. STENTIM 2. Six months angiographic results. Elective Wiktor stent implantation in acute myocardial infarction compared with balloon angioplasty. Circulation 1998;98: I-21.
47. Rodriguez A, Bernardi V, Fernandez M, Mauvecin C, Ayala F, Santaera O, Martinez J, Mele E, Roubin GS, Palacios I, Ambrosa JA, on behalf of the GRAMI Investigators. In-hospital and late results of coronary stents versus conventional balloon angioplasty in acute myocardial infarction (GRAMI trial). Am J Cardiol 1998;81:1286–1291.
48. Suryapranata H, van't Hof AWJ, Hoorntje JCA, de Boer M-J, Zijlstra F. Randomized comparison of coronary stenting with balloon angioplasty in selected patients with acute myocardial infarction. Circulation 1998;97:2502–2505.
49. Saito S, Hosokawa G. Primary Palmaz-Schatz stent implantation for acute myocardial infarction: the final results of the Japanese PASTA (Primary Angioplasty vs Stent Implantation in AMI in Japan) trial. Circulation 1997;96:I-595. Abstract.
50. Jacksch R, Niehues R, Knobloch W. PTCA versus stenting in acute myocardial infarction: single centre prospective randomized trial. Eur Heart J 1998;19:239. Abstract.
51. Grines CL, Cox DA, Stone GW, Garcia E, Mattos LA, Giambartolomei A, Brodie BR, Madonna O, Eijgelshoven M, Lansky AJ, O'Neill WW, Morice M-C, for the Stent Primary Angioplasty in Myocardial Infarction Study Group. Coronary angioplasty with or without stent implantation for acute myocardial infarction. N Engl J Med 1999;341:1949–1956.

52. Antoniucci D, Santoro GM, Bolognese L, Valenti R, Trapani M, Fazzini PF. A clinical trial comparing primary stenting of the infarct-related artery with optimal primary angioplasty for acute myocardial infarction. Results from the Florence Randomized Elective Stenting in Acute Coronary Occlusions (FRESCO) trial. J Am Coll Cardiol 1998;31:1234–1239.
53. Ross AM, Coyne KS, Moreyra E, Reiner JS, Greenhouse SW, Walker PL, Simoons ML, Draoui YC, Califf RM, Topol EJ, Van de Werf F, Lundergan CF, for the GUSTO-I Angiographic Investigators. Extended mortality benefit of early postinfarction reperfusion. Circulation 1998;97:1549–1556.
54. Stone GW, Garcia E, Maranon G, Griffin J, Grines L, Mattos L, Boura J, Cox D, Madonna O, Eijgelshoven M, Grines CL. Does stent implantation in acute myocardial infarction degrade TIMI flow and result in early higher mortality than PTCA? The PAMI stent randomized trial. Circulation 1998;98:I-151. Abstract.
55. Noma K, Tateisi H, Yumoto A, Nisioka K. No-reflow phenomenon during primary stenting in acute myocardial infarction: Comparison with primary PTCA. Circulation 1999;100:I-855. Abstract.
56. Escobar J, Marchant E, Fajuri A, Martinez A, Guarda E, Schnettler C. Stenting could decrease coronary blood flow during angioplasty in acute myocardial infarction. J Am Coll Cardiol 1999;33:361A. Abstract.
57. Ito H, Maruyama A, Iwakura K, Takiuchi S, Masuyama T, Hori M, Higashino Y, Fujii K, Minamino T. Clinical implications of the 'no reflow' phenomenon. A predictor of complications and left ventricular remodeling in reperfused anterior wall myocardial infarction. Circulation 1996;93:223–228. Abstract.
58. Wu KC, Zerhouni EA, Judd RM, Lugo-Olivieri CH, Barouch LA, Schulman SP, Blumenthal RS, Lima JAC. Prognostic significance of microvascular obstruction by magnetic resonance imaging in patients with acute myocardial infarction. Circulation 1998;97:765–772.
59. Gibson CM, Cannon CP, Murphy SA, Ryan KA, Mesley R, Marble SJ, McCabe CH, Van de Werf F, Braunwald E, of the TIMI (Thrombolysis in Myocardial Infarction) Study Group. Relationship of TIMI myocardial perfusion grade to mortality after administration of thrombolytic drugs. Circulation 2000;101:125–130.
60. Van't Hof AWJ, Liem A, Suryapranata H, Hoorntje JCA, de Boer M-J, Zijlstra F, on behalf of the Zwolle Myocardial Infarction Study Group. Angiographic assessment of myocardial reperfusion in patients treated with primary angioplasty for acute myocardial infarction. Myocardial blush grade. Circulation 1998;97:2302–2306.
61. Gawaz M, Neumann F-J, Ott I, Schiessler A, Schomig A. Platelet function in acute myocardial infarction treated with direct angioplasty. Circulation 1996; 93:229–237.
62. Neumann FJ, Blasini R, Schmitt C, Alt E, Dirschinger J, Gawaz M, Kastrati A, Schomig A. Effect of glycoprotein IIb/IIIa receptor blockade on recovery of coronary blood flow and left ventricular function after the placement of coronary artery stents in acute myocardial infarction. Circulation 1998;98: 2695–2701.

63. De Lemos JA, Antman EM, Gibson CM, McCabe CH, Giugliano RP, Murphy SA, Coulter SA, Anderson K, Scherer J, Frey MJ, Van der Wieken R, Van de Werf F, Braunwald E, for the TIMI 14 Investigators. Abciximab improves both epicardial flow and myocardial reperfusion in ST-elevation myocardial infarction. Observations from the TIMI 14 trial. Circulation 2000;101:239–243.
64. Montalescot G, Barragan P, Wittenberg O, Ecollan P, Elhadad S, Villain P, Boulenc J-M, Maillard L, Pinton P. Abciximab associated with promary angioplasty and stenting in acute myocardial infarction: the ADMIRAL study, 30-day final results. Circulation 1999;100:I-87. Abstract.
65. Topol EJ, Mark DB, Lincoff AM, Cohen E, Burton J, Kleiman N, Talley D, Sapp S, Booth J, Cabot CF, Anderson KM, Califf RM, for the EPISTENT Investigators. Outcomes at 1 year and economic implications of platelet glycoprotein IIb/IIIa blockade in patients undergoing coronary stenting: results from a multicentre randomised trial. Lancet 1999;354:2019–2024.
66. Van't Hof AWJ, Zijlstra F, Ottervanger JP, Hoorntje JCA, de Boer M-J, Suryapranata H. Primary stenting, compared with balloon angioplasty, in patients with acute MI does not improve reperfusion nor reduce infarct size. Circulation 1999;100:I-792. Abstract.

15

Early Invasive Versus Early Conservative Strategies for Acute Coronary Syndromes

Philippe L. L'Allier* **and A. Michael Lincoff**
The Cleveland Clinic Foundation
Cleveland, Ohio

Acute coronary syndromes (ACS) are a continuum of clinical entities that range from accelerated angina to acute myocardial infarction. The present chapter will use this term to designate unstable angina (UA) and non-Q-wave myocardial infarction (MI), excluding acute MI with ST-segment elevation and/or Q waves.

Acute coronary syndromes share a common pathophysiology, based on underlying atherosclerotic changes, plaque erosion or rupture, and initiation of the coagulation cascade and thrombus formation followed by infarction and disease progression. Understanding the basic processes involved is fundamental to design an optimal treatment strategy.

This optimal treatment strategy has been the subject of heated debate. Recent reports of more favorable outcomes with better anticoagulants (low-molecular-weight heparins, direct antithrombins) (1–6) and antiplatelet agents (platelet glycoprotein [GP] IIb/IIIa blockers) (7–9), have addressed some of the issues relating to the underlying thrombotic substrate. The present chapter will focus on the relative merits of early invasive versus early conservative strategies with regard to angiography and revascularization, and on the integration of new data to define an optimal approach to the treatment of ACS.

**Current affiliation*: McGill University and Montreal Heart Institute, Montreal, Quebec, Canada.

TREATMENT OPTIONS

When caring for patients with ACS, physicians are faced with conditions that may vary considerably with regard to disease severity and prognosis. Patients with mildly progressive anginal symptoms and minimal coronary disease have very favorable outcomes when compared with patients with rest pain, electrocardiographic changes, and evidence of myocardial necrosis (serum troponin, creatinine kinase) (10–16). Refining definitions and classifications for unstable angina has been one of many challenges in the evaluation of new therapies, partially explaining diverging results in clinical trials (17).

Opinions are polarized around two approaches to ACS: early conservative and early invasive strategies. This polarization arises from differing interpretations of the need for and timing of revascularization procedures following a course of optimal medical therapy. Most of the controversy relates to the delicate balance between the unacceptable event rates (death, reinfarction, revascularization, rehospitalization, etc.) associated with medical management alone, the documented excess in adverse events associated with revascularization procedures in the acute setting, and patient quality of life.

Early Conservative Strategy

This approach is based on the assumption that most patients can be stabilized with a short course of medical therapy, following which only patients with significant residual ischemia despite optimal medical therapy (failed medical therapy) are referred for catheterization and revascularization. This strategy relies heavily on the sensitivity and specificity of noninvasive stress testing (with or without imaging) to identify high-risk patients with significant residual ischemia. It has the advantages of avoiding the risks of revascularization in the acute setting and the costs of such procedures. On the other hand, length of stay may be considerably longer and patients with unrecognized high-risk anatomies may not receive attention and appropriate treatment. Furthermore, contemporary trials have confirmed incomplete plaque stabilization, at best, with medical therapy alone as death or reinfarction at 30 days occurs in 8% to 15% (depending on baseline characteristics and entry criteria), and refractory angina in approximately 25% (1–9,18). In fact, although the risk of adverse outcome is higher in the first days to weeks, events continue to occur at a significant rate months after the index hospitalization. Despite a 20% reduction in the composite endpoint of death or reinfarction at 30 days with new platelet GP IIb/IIIa receptor blockers (7,8,19) and a 20% reduction (1,3,20–23) with low-molecular-weight heparins, the absolute event rate is still unacceptably high, and other means of improving outcomes are needed.

Early Invasive Strategy

This approach is based on the assumption that patients with ACS cannot be adequately stabilized and symptomatically improved by medical therapy alone. Angiography with the intention to revascularize whenever possible is central to this strategy. After a short, intensive stabilization period, patients are brought to the angiographic suite and studied. Percutaneous coronary interventions (PCI) or coronary artery bypass grafting (CABG) are performed ad hoc or shortly thereafter if possible. This strategy relies on the safety and efficacy of coronary angiography and revascularization procedures in the acute setting. Proponents of this strategy believe that the "early procedural hazard" is largely offset by easier and faster initial patient management, better symptomatic relief, greater decrease in subacute events, and possibly better survival. Angiography plays a role in risk stratification, mainly by identifying patients with left main disease, severe three-vessel disease, or multivessel disease and decreased left ventricular function, all of whom benefit from aggressive myocardial revascularization. Angiography also reliably identifies patients with no or minimal disease who can be discharged early with a very good prognosis and who do not significantly benefit from extensive long-term medical therapy (24). This approach is becoming increasingly attractive due to recent developments in adjunctive pharmacotherapy with platelet GP IIb/IIIa inhibitors (which has been shown to provide long-term protection against ischemic complications following PCI) (25,26), and due to cost containment issues.

DEDICATED RANDOMIZED CONTROL TRIALS

Thrombolysis in Myocardial Infarction (TIMI) IIIB Study

This landmark multinational/multicenter study, published in 1994, was designed to determine the effect of a fibrinolytic agent added to conventional medical therapies and to compare an early invasive management strategy to a more conservative early strategy in patients with UA and non-Q-wave MI (18). Inclusion criteria for study entry were ischemic symptoms at rest, lasting 5 min or more but <6 hours. Furthermore, the discomfort must have occurred within 24 hours of study enrollment and been accompanied by objective evidence of ischemic heart disease. Patients who presented with pulmonary edema or had a myocardial infarction in the preceding 21 days, secondary unstable angina, a percutaneous intervention in the previous 6 months, or CABG at any time, or any of the usual contraindications to fibrinolytic therapy, were excluded.

Between October 1989 and June 1992, 1425 patients were randomly assigned by 2 × 2 factorial design to treatment with t-PA or placebo as well as to an early invasive or early conservative strategy. By protocol, baseline medical therapy consisted of bed rest, oxygen, metoprolol, diltiazem, and isosorbide dinitrate. Patients were to receive heparin as a 5000-U bolus followed by an infusion to maintain the activated partial thromboplastin time (aPTT) at 1.5 to 2.0 times the laboratory control value. Aspirin 325 mg daily was to be given on the second day and was administered daily for at least 1 year.

The early invasive strategy (n = 740) called for coronary angiography within 18 to 48 hours after randomization. Revascularization (as complete as possible) was to be performed at the time of catheterization or as soon as possible therafter (within 6 weeks for CABG).

The early conservative strategy (n = 733) called for medical management alone unless failure of such therapy had occurred. Failure was defined as: (1) a single anginal episode lasting at least 5 min and associated with ST-segment deviation greater or equal to 0.2 mV in two contiguous leads; (2) a single episode lasting more than 20 min or two or more anginal episodes lasting 5 min or more accompanied by electrocardiographic (ECG) criteria sufficient to satisfy inclusion criteria; (3) >20 min of ischemic ST deviation (>=0.1 mV) on 24-hour Holter monitoring; or (4) an unsatisfactory result (high-risk features) on the predischarge stress thallium test before the completion of stage II of a modified, low-level, Bruce protocol. After hospital discharge, angiography and revascularization were recommended only for patients who had to be rehospitalized for recurrent unstable angina at rest or who had moderate to severe stable angina despite optimal medical therapy (Canadian cardiovascular class III or IV) accompanied by a positive symptom-limited exercise treadmill test.

The primary endpoint of the study was the composite of death, reinfarction, or unsatisfactory exercise treadmill test at 6 weeks. Analyses for different subgroups were prespecified and included 6-week death or reinfarction for patients with unstable angina versus non-Q-wave myocardial infarction, age >65 years versus <65 years, and ST-T changes.

Of the patients assigned to the early invasive strategy, 98% underwent catheterization before 6 weeks (median of 1.5 days after randomization, 0.1% after discharge). Revascularization was performed in a total of 61% of cases (38% by PCI, 25% by CABG). Of the patients assigned to the early conservative strategy, 64% underwent unplanned cardiac catheterization (median of 7.1 days, 10% after discharge). Revascularization was performed in 49% (26% by PCI, 24% by CABG). Importantly, there was no difference in the procedural success or complication rates (death, infarction, emergency CABG, or abrupt closure) in the aggressive and conservative arms.

The primary endpoint of the study was reached in 16.2% of patients in the early invasive group, versus 18.1% in the early conservative group (P = .33). Specifically, death occurred in 2.4% versus 2.5%, and nonfatal myocardial infarction occurred in 5.1% versus 5.7%, respectively (P = ns), at 6 weeks. Importantly, length of initial hospital stay (10.2 days vs. 10.9 days, P = .01), percentage of patients requiring rehospitalization (7.8% vs. 14.1%, P < .001), and the number of days of rehospitalization (365 vs. 930, P < .001) at 6 weeks, were all significantly lower with the early invasive strategy. By 1 year (27), cumulative angiography and revascularization rates were higher in the early invasive arm (99% and 64% vs. 73% and 58%, P < .001), although angioplasty rates were only slighly different (39% vs. 32%, P < .001) and rates of bypass grafting by 1 year were identical (30% in each group, P = .50). The overall incidence of death and nonfatal infarction was substantial in this patient population by 1 year (4.3% mortality, 8.8% nonfatal infarction). Clinical outcomes (death/nonfatal MI) were not statistically different in the two groups (10.8% vs. 12.2%, in the invasive and conservative groups, respectively), but patients in the early invasive strategy were rehospitalized less frequently (26% vs. 33%, P < .001). It was concluded that the early invasive strategy provided more rapid relief of angina, without an excess in the risk of death or myocardial infarction.

The results of the TIMI IIIB trial may be largely inapplicable to contemporary practice due to a number of limitations. First, these results were obtained in the context of 50% of patients receiving fibrinolytic therapy shortly before revascularization procedures, and it has been established that such therapy activates platelets and provides an unfavorable milieu to perform PCI or CABG. Second, the difference in the rates of revascularization was small and therefore may have decreased the power of the study to detect a difference in outcome. Third, coronary stents and platelet GP IIb/IIIa receptor inhibitors, which have been shown to yield better and more durable acute results and decrease peri PCI and long-term ischemic complications, respectively, were not routinely used. Furthermore, CABG and anesthesiology techniques have also evolved to be safer and more appropriate for ACS patients (28).

Veterans Affairs Non-Q-Wave Infarction Strategies in Hospital (VANQWISH) Trial

This trial was designed to test the hypothesis that an early invasive strategy (characterized by routine angiography followed by revascularization, if feasible) is superior to an early conservative strategy (characterized by medical therapy, noninvasive testing, and referral for angiography and revascularization only if spontaneous or inducible ischemia is identified) in patients with acute non-Q-wave myocardial infarction. Patients were enrolled at 17 Veterans Administration hospitals between April 1993 and December 1995 (n = 920) (29).

Patients were randomly assigned to either strategy within 24 to 72 hours of onset of symptoms. To be eligible, patients had to have evolving myocardial infarction, a serum creatinine kinase MB isoenzyme level 1.5 or more times the local upper limit of normal, and no new pathologic Q-waves on serial electrocardiograms. Exclusion criteria were severe coexisting illness or high-risk clinical features (persistent or recurrent ischemia, refractory heart failure). Patients in both groups received aspirin 325 mg daily and diltiazem CD 180 to 300 mg daily. Patients could also receive any other standard medical therapy during hospitalization (including beta-blockers, ACE inhibitors, heparin, and nitrates).

The early invasive strategy (n = 462) specified coronary angiography soon after randomization. Importantly, however, the protocol did not require early myocardial revascularization.

Patients assigned to the early conservative strategy (n = 458) underwent radionuclide ventriculography as the initial noninvasive test, followed by predischarge exercise treadmill test (symptom-limited) with perfusion imaging. Failure of medical therapy, as an indication for angiogrphy, was defined by: (1) recurrent postinfarction angina with ischemic ECG changes; (2) ST-segment depression of at least 2 mm during peak exercise; or (3) redistribution deficits in two or more vascular territories on thallium scintigraphy or one redistribution defect with lung uptake.

A total of 96% of patients assigned to the early invasive strategy underwent angiography (median time from randomization 2 days, 98% predischarge), although revascularization was performed in only 44% of those patients (median time from randomization 8 days, 48% by PCI, 47% by CABG, and 5% by both). In patients assigned to the early conservative strategy, 48% underwent angiography (median time from randomization 14 days, 48% predischarge), and 33% received a revascularization procedure (median time from randomization 24.5 days, 36% by PCI, 57% by CABG, and 7% by both).

The primary endpoint of the study was the combination of death from any cause or recurrent nonfatal infarction during a minimum of 12 months of follow-up. This endpoint was reached in 26.9% versus 29.9% in the conservative and invasive groups, respectively (hazard ratio 0.87, 95% confidence interval 0.68 to 1.10, P = .35), during a mean follow-up of 23 months. There were 80 versus 59 deaths in the invasive versus conservative groups, respectively (hazard ratio 0.72, 95% confidence interval 0.51 to

1.01). There were no significant differences between groups in the incidence of reinfarction during follow-up. It was concluded that there was no evidence of improved clinical outcomes associated with a routine strategy of early angiography without revascularization in most patients with non-Q-wave MI.

Four important findings are noteworthy for the interpretation of the results of the VANQWISH study. First, procedural details were not presented for either PCI or CABG (angiographic success, abrupt or threatened closures, emergency CABG, number of grafts, completeness of revascularization, use of abciximab and stents, etc.). Second, 30-day mortality following CABG was reported to be 11.6%, an unexpectedly high rate in this group. Third, the extent of symptomatic relief, which is often regarded as an important endpoint in the evaluation of strategies to treat ACS, was not reported. Fourth, as might have been expected with a protocol that did not recommend revascularization per se, the absolute revascularization rate of 44% in the invasive arm is regarded by many as insufficient in light of contemporary standards and technical expertise. In effect, more than half of patients in this group were subjected to the risks of angiography without the benefits of revascularization. Furthermore, the differential between the two treatment arms in revascularization rates (44% vs. 33%) may also be insufficient to fully evaluate an invasive versus conservative strategy. As is the case with the TIMI IIIB study, the results of VANQWISH are difficult to incorporate into contemporary practice.

Fragmin and Fast Revascularization During Instability in Coronary Artery Disease (FRISC) II

The FRISC II trial was designed to compare an early invasive with a non-invasive strategy in patients with unstable coronary artery disease superimposed upon an intensive background antithrombotic medical regimen. Patients (n = 2457) were recruited between June 1996 and May 1998 (30).

Patients were eligible for randomization if they had increasing or rest symptoms of ischemia or if myocardial infarction was suspected, with the last anginal episode within 48 hours of hospitalization. Myocardial ischemia was to be accompanied by ECG changes (ST depression ≥0.1 mV or T-wave inversion ≥0.1 mV) or by elevated biochemical markers of myocardial damage (CK-MB >0.6 μg/L, troponin T >0.1 μg/L, or qualitative troponin T test positive). Patients were excluded on the basis increased risk of bleeding, anemia, indication for or treatment with a fibrinolytic agent in the past 24 hours, PCI within 6 months, being on a waiting list for revascularization, previous CABG, advanced age, or contraindications to treatment drugs.

Eligible patients were treated on admission with subcutaneous open-label dalteparin or intavenous unfractionnated heparin. As soon as possible after admission (up to 72 hours after start of open label treatment), patients were randomly assigned in a 2 × 2 factorial design to invasive versus noninvasive strategy and subcutaneous dalteparin versus placebo for 3 months. After randomization, patients received dalteparin for 5 days, until exercise testing or an invasive procedure. Aspirin was given to all patients on admission (300 to 600 mg initially, followed by a maintenance dose of 75 to 320 mg daily) and beta-blockers were used unless contraindicated. Other drugs were given at the discretion of the investigators. Use of abciximab (a platelet GP IIb/IIIa inhibitor) was encouraged during PCI and ticlopidine was recommended for 3 to 4 weeks following stenting.

In the invasive arms, the aim was to perform all revascularization procedures within 7 days of initiation of open-label treatment with dalteparin or unfractionated heparin (admission). Patients therefore underwent coronary angiography within a few days of randomization, and revascularization was recommended in all patients with a 70% stenosis or greater of any artery supplying a significant area of myocardium. Percutaneous procedures were recommended if there were one or two diseased vessels and CABG was recommended if there was left main or three-vessel disease.

In the noninvasive strategy, angiography was permitted for refractory or recurrent angina despite maximally tolerated medical therapy or severe ischemia on a symptom-limited exercise test before discharge. The exercise test criteria for referral for invasive management were: (1) ST depression ≥0.3 mV or T-wave inversion; (2) limiting anginal symptoms associated with a low maximum workload (<90 W in men and <70 W in women) or a decrease in blood pressure; or (3) ST elevation without preceding concomitant Q waves.

Of the patients assigned to the invasive strategy, 98% underwent angiography (median 4 days after initiation of open-label therapy, 96% within 7 days), and a total of 475 patients assigned to the noninvasive strategy underwent unplanned angiography (median 17 days after initiation of open-label therapy, 10% within 7 days). Seventy-eight percent of patients underwent a revascularization procedure as part of the invasive strategy (55% with PCI at a median of 4 days after initiation of treatment, 45% with CABG at a median of 7 days after initiation of treatment), versus 37% in the noninvasive strategy (49% with PCI at a median of 16.5 days after initiation of treatment, 51% with CABG at a median of 28 days after initiation of treatment).

Results of PCI were not different in the invasive versus noninvasive arms: mean number of treated segments 1.35 versus 1.34 and successfully treated segments 95% versus 91%, respectively. Procedural characteristics were also very similar, particularly with regard to rate of stenting (61% vs. 70%) and rate of abciximab use (10% vs. 10%).

This primary composite endpoint of death or MI by 6 months was reached in 9.4% of patients assigned to the invasive strategy and in 12.1% of patients assigned to the noninvasive strategy (risk ratio 0.78, 95% confidence interval 0.62 to 0.98, $P = .031$). Individual endpoints were also less frequent in the invasive group, with death rates of 1.9% versus 2.9% ($P = .10$) and reinfarction rates of 7.8% versus 10.1% ($P = .045$), respectively (Fig. 1). There was an approximately 50% relative reduction in anginal symptoms in the invasive compared with the noninvasive group, and a corresponding difference in the Canadian Cardiovascular Society score for angina. Furthermore, the need for readmission was halved in the invasive group due to the lower incidence of incapacitating angina or recurring unstable angina or myocardial infarction.

Summary

The TIMI IIIB trial confirmed that despite the use of fibrinolytic therapy in 50% of patients (31,32) and in the absence of stents or potent antiplatelet therapy, an early invasive strategy for ACS without ST-segment elevation was safe and provided more rapid and more effective symptomatic relief, lowering the need for rehospitalization. In addition, subgroup analysis revealed that the higher-risk patients (those with ECG changes, elevated cardiac enzymes, female gender, and age >65 years) tended to benefit the most for an early aggressive strategy (Fig. 2). Subsequently the VANQWISH trial reported that most patients with non-Q-wave MI did not benefit from routine angiography and that a more conservative strategy yielded equivalent results with regard to death/reinfarction during 23 months follow-up (despite very low revascularization rates and disturbingly high 30-day mortality following CABG).

The much more favorable results with an early invasive strategy in the FRISC II trial relative to TIMI IIIB and VANQWISH are likely explained by the greater absolute difference in revascularization rates in the invasive and noninvasive groups, the higher use of stents during PCI, the lower surgical mortality, and the use, although infrequent (10%), of abciximab during PCI (Table 1). As such, the early invasive strategy in FRISC II is much more representative of contemporary clinical practice than are those of either TIMI IIIB or VANQWISH. Furthermore, it is likely that these results can be at least reproduced and most likely improved upon with the increasing use of potent platelet inhibition (33–35).

DATA FROM NONRANDOMIZED REGISTRIES

In the Organization to Assess Strategies for Ischaemic Syndromes (OASIS) Registry, Yusuf and colleagues (36) studied the relation between different

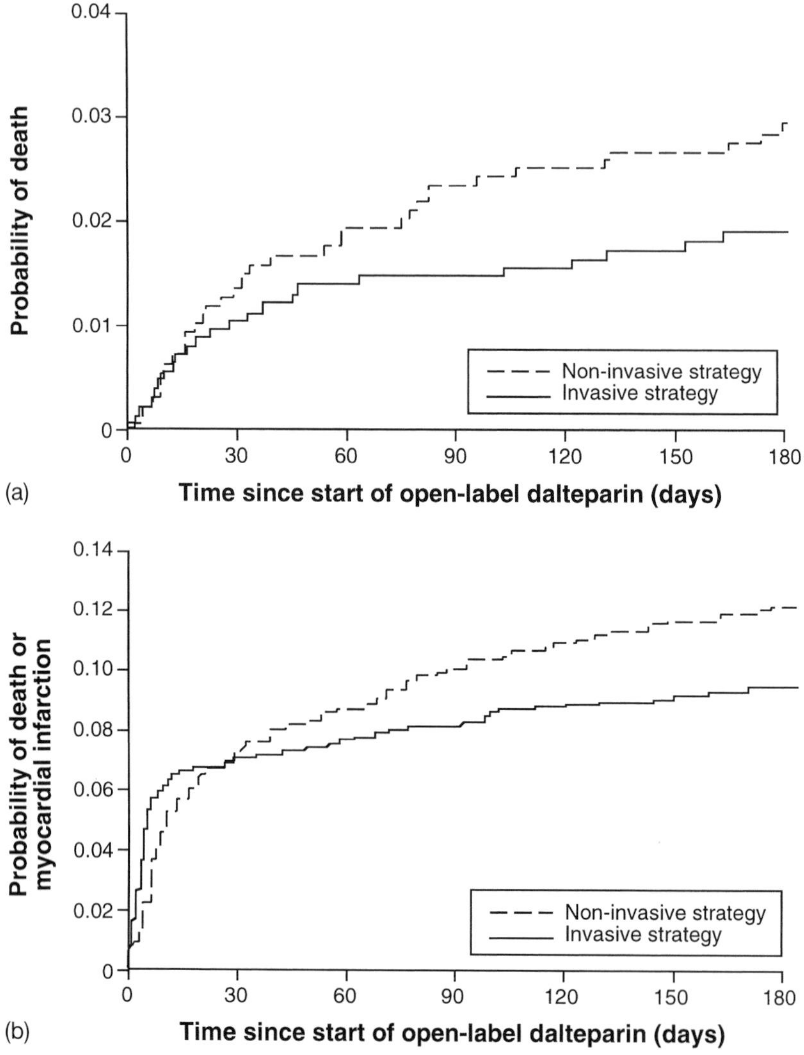

Figure 1 (Top) Probability of death and (bottom) of death or myocardial infarction in invasive and conservative groups. (From Ref. 30.)

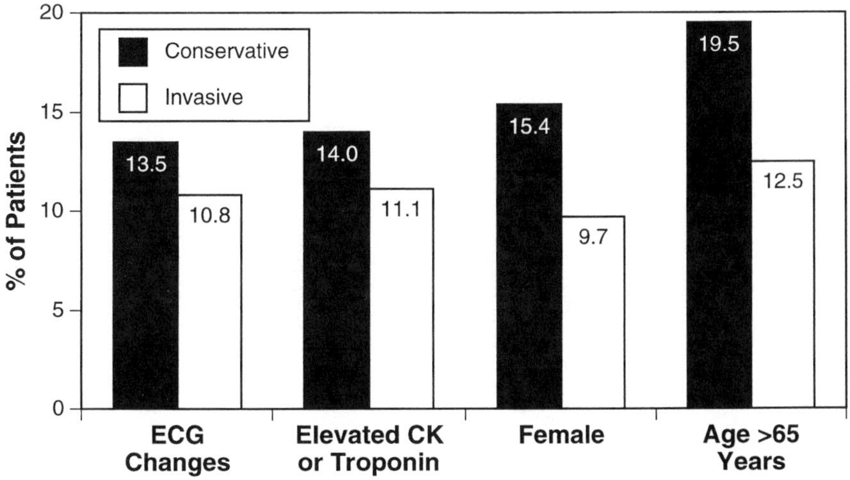

Figure 2 One-year death or myocardial infarction in selected high-risk subgroups from the TIMI IIIB trial. (From Ref. 18.)

rates of coronary angiography and revascularization procedures and the rates of cardiovascular death, myocardial infarction, stroke, refractory angina, and major bleeding in 7987 consecutive patients presenting with ACS without ST-segment elevation in six countries (95 hospitals in Australia, Brazil, Canada, Hungary, Poland, and the United States) with widely differing intervention rates. Eligibility criteria were admission to hospital with anginal symptoms within 48 hours of onset accompanied either by ECG changes or previously documented coronary artery disease. There were important variations in the use of angiography/revascularization procedures between countries (United States, 65% and 47%, respectively; Brazil, 72% and 47%; Canada, 57% and 38%; Australia, 41% and 28%; Hungary, 32% and 24%; Poland, 16% and 10%). They found no relation between the composite of death, myocardial infarction, or stroke and the use of invasive procedures in the various countries at 7 days and 6 months.

The adjusted odds ratios (OR) for death or myocardial infarction in the two countries with the highest revascularization rates (United States and Brazil) compared with the others was 0.88 (P = .27) at 7 days and 1.0 (P = .69) at 1 year. However, the rate of refractory angina or readmission for unstable angina at 6 months was lower in the two countries with the highest revascularization rates (13.9% vs. 20.1%, OR 0.63, P < .001). There was also a tradeoff in the form of an increased stroke rate (1.9% vs. 1.2%, OR 1.8, P = .004) and major bleeding complications (1.9% vs. 1.1%, OR 1.9,

Table 1 Randomized Trials of Early Invasive Versus Conservative Strategy in Acute Coronary Syndromes

Trial	Strategy	Revascularization rate (%)	Time to catheterization (days)	Time to revascularization (days)	Follow-up	Outcomes (%)	*P*
TIMI IIIB[a] (18)	Invasive	61	1.5	NA	6 weeks	16.2	ns
	Conservative	49	7.1	NA	6 weeks	18.1	
VANQWISH[b] (29)	Invasive	44	2	8	23 months	29.9	ns
	Conservative	33	14	24.5	23 months	26.9	
FRISC II[b] (30)	Invasive	78	4	4	6 months	9.4	.03
	Conservative	37	17	17	6 months	12.1	

[a]Death, myocardial infarction, or failed symptom-limited exercise treadmill test.
[b]Death or myocardial infarction.

P = .001) associated with a higher rate of catheterization. There are important limitations of this report that must be emphasized. First, there was no reported breakdown of the composite of death or myocardial infarction. Furthermore, the risk adjustment was limited to six clinical variables, and there are concerns regarding the completeness of such an adjustment. Also, the length of follow-up (6 months) may not allow assessment of the true benefit of a more aggressive strategy which is associated with an early hazard, and confounders associated with the decision to perform or not perform angiography and revascularization were not captured.

A different experience was reported from the GUSTO IIb trial (37) comparing hirudin versus heparin in patients with ACS. From this database, an analysis was performed to assess 30-day and 1-year mortality for invasive versus conservative strategies in patients with unstable angina and non-Q-wave myocardial infarction, defined by anginal symptoms within 12 hours associated with transient ST-segment elevation or depression of more than 0.5 mm, or with persistent T-wave inversion of more than 1 mm. Of the 7897 patients included, 57.4% and 42.6% underwent invasive and conservative therapy, respectively. The revascularization rate in the invasive group was 56% (58% of these with PCI, 42% with CABG). Of note, coronary angiography and revascularization were discouraged during the study drug infusion (3 to 5 days) unless there was evidence of refractory ischemia. In this study, mortality was 2.2% in the invasive group versus 3.1% in the conservative group at 30 days (relative reduction 28%, P = .02) and 5.4% versus 10.4% at 1 year (relative reduction 48%, $P < .0001$). Furthermore, the combination of death or myocardial infarction was significantly lower in the invasive group at 6 months (11.2% vs. 14.4%, relative reduction 22%, $P < .001$). The adjusted (multiple logistic regression) odds ratio for invasive therapy with regard to mortality was 0.46 (95% confidence interval 0.08 to 0.84). Rehospitalization at 6 months was 35.2% versus 39.9% for the invasive and conservative groups, respectively ($P < .001$). This analysis has important limitations that are noteworthy to ensure adequate interpretation, including lack of reported 1-year revascularization rates, procedural details, or time to revascularization.

ADJUNCTIVE PHARMACOTHERAPY

Following the demonstration that aspirin significantly improves outcomes in acute coronary syndromes, encouraging results have been obtained from research using platelet GP IIb/IIIa receptor inhibitors as an antithrombotic strategy in this setting (38). This surface integrin moderates platelet aggregation via binding of circulating fibrinogen or Von Willebrand factor. Therapeutic agents designed to block this receptor have been shown to improve ischemic complications associated with PCI and to improve outcomes in ACS (39).

Subgroup analyses of interventional trials have suggested that clinical benefit from GP IIb/IIIa antagonists is greatest among patients with ACS. In the EPIC trial (26), patients at high risk for periprocedural ischemic complications were randomized to abciximab (a GP IIb/IIIa inhibitor) or placebo. Of the 2099 patients enrolled, 489 had a diagnosis of unstable angina on entry and were the subject of a subanalysis (40). Unstable angina was defined by the presence of early (within 7 days) postinfarction angina or at least 2 episodes of angina occurring at rest or despite heparin and nitrate therapy. Accompanying ST-T changes were required to confirm the diagnosis of unstable angina. All patients received aspirin and heparin before and throughout the procedure in addition to abciximab. Administration of a bolus and 12-hour infusion of abciximab was associated with a 62% reduction in mortality (1.2% vs. 3.2%, $P = .16$) and an 80% reduction in myocardial infarction (1.8% vs. 9.0%, $P = .004$) at 30 days. These differences were amplified when only treated patients (n = 470) were considered: mortality in 0.0% versus 3.3% ($P = .004$) and infarction in 0.6% versus 9.2% ($P < .001$) of abciximab and placebo-treated patients respectively. This benefit was preserved throughout long-term follow-up. By 1 year, mortality among patients enrolled in EPIC with UA or acute MI was reduced by abciximab from 12.7% to 5.1% ($P = .01$). Subsets of patients with UA from EPILOG (41) and EPISTENT (25) also suggest an added benefit in this population (Table 2).

The CAPTURE trial (n = 1265) was specifically designed to evaluate whether abciximab, given during the 18 to 24 hours preceding PCI and continued 1 hour after PCI, could improve outcome (death, myocardial in-

Table 2 Analysis of 30-Day Endpoints for Patients with Unstable Angina at Entry in EPIC, EPILOG, and EPISTENT

Trial	Study therapy	n	Death/MI/ urgent TVR	% Change vs. placebo	*P*
EPIC (26)	Balloon + placebo	156	20 (13.1%)		
	Balloon + abciximab	165	6 (3.8%)	−71.0%	.004
EPILOG (41)	Balloon + placebo	474	44 (7.6%)		
	Balloon + abciximab	854	23 (5.9%)	−46.9%	.013
EPISTENT (25)	Stent + placebo	179	26 (14.8%)		
	Balloon + abciximab	152	11 (7.3%)	−50.4%	.033
	Stent + abciximab	156	7 (4.5%)	−69.6%	.002

farction, or urgent intervention) in patients with refractory unstable angina (42). All patients had undergone angiography for refractory angina (defined as chest pain at rest with concomitant ischemic electrocardiographic changes during therapy with intravenous heparin and glyceryl trinitrate, started at least 2 hours previously), and had significant coronary artery disease with a culprit lesion suitable for PCI. All patients received aspirin, and heparin was administered from before randomization to at least 1 hour after PCI. The trial was discontinued prematurely after interim analysis of 1050 patients (planned 1400 patients). By 30 days, the combined endpoint of death, myocardial infarction, or urgent revascularization had occurred in 11.3% versus 15.9% of patients receiving abciximab or placebo, respectively (P = .012). This trial demonstrated the potential for abciximab to stabilize patients with refractory ischemia prior to planned PCI.

Two large trials of platelet GP IIb/IIIa inhibitors (tirofiban and eptifibatide) in high-risk unstable angina have provided further insight into the optimal management of ACS with regard to the combination of potent platelet aggregation blockade and PCI. The PRISM-PLUS trial (7) investigated the clinical efficacy of tirofiban, an intravenously administered short-acting, nonpeptide inhibitor of platelet GP IIb/IIIa receptor, in the prevention of acute ischemic events in patients with unstable angina and non-Q-wave myocardial infarction. The composite primary endpoint of death, myocardial infarction, or refractory ischemia at 7 days was lower in patients who received tirofiban plus heparin versus heparin alone (12.9% vs. 17.9%, risk ratio 0.68, 95% confidence interval 0.53 to 0.88, P = .004), respectively. By study design, study drug was infused for 48 hours and revascularization procedures were postponed until after that period unless they were mandated by refractory ischemia or by new myocardial infarction. Investigators were encouraged to perform coronary angiography and revascularization of the culprit lesion, if indicated, between 48 and 96 hours after randomization while continuing study drug infusions. Death, myocardial infarction, refractory ischemia, or rehospitalization for unstable angina at 30 days was significantly lower in patients undergoing PCI in the tirofiban plus heparin group (n = 239) versus heparin alone group (n = 236) (8.8% vs. 15.3%, risk ratio 0.55, 95% confidence interval 0.32 to 0.94). In this trial, tirofiban was shown to reduce the occurence of death or MI both before PCI (during the 48-hour stabilization period: 2.6% vs. 0.9%, risk ratio 0.34) and after PCI (at 30 days: 5.9% vs. 10.2%, risk ratio 0.56) (Fig. 3).

The PURSUIT trial (19) assessed the clinical benefit of the platelet GP IIb/IIIa inhibitor eptifibatide, a short-acting cyclic heptapeptide, in patients with non-ST-segment elevation. Patients were enrolled if they presented within 24 hours of an episode of ischemic chest discomfort and had either ST depression, T-wave inversion, transient ST-segment elevation, or an in-

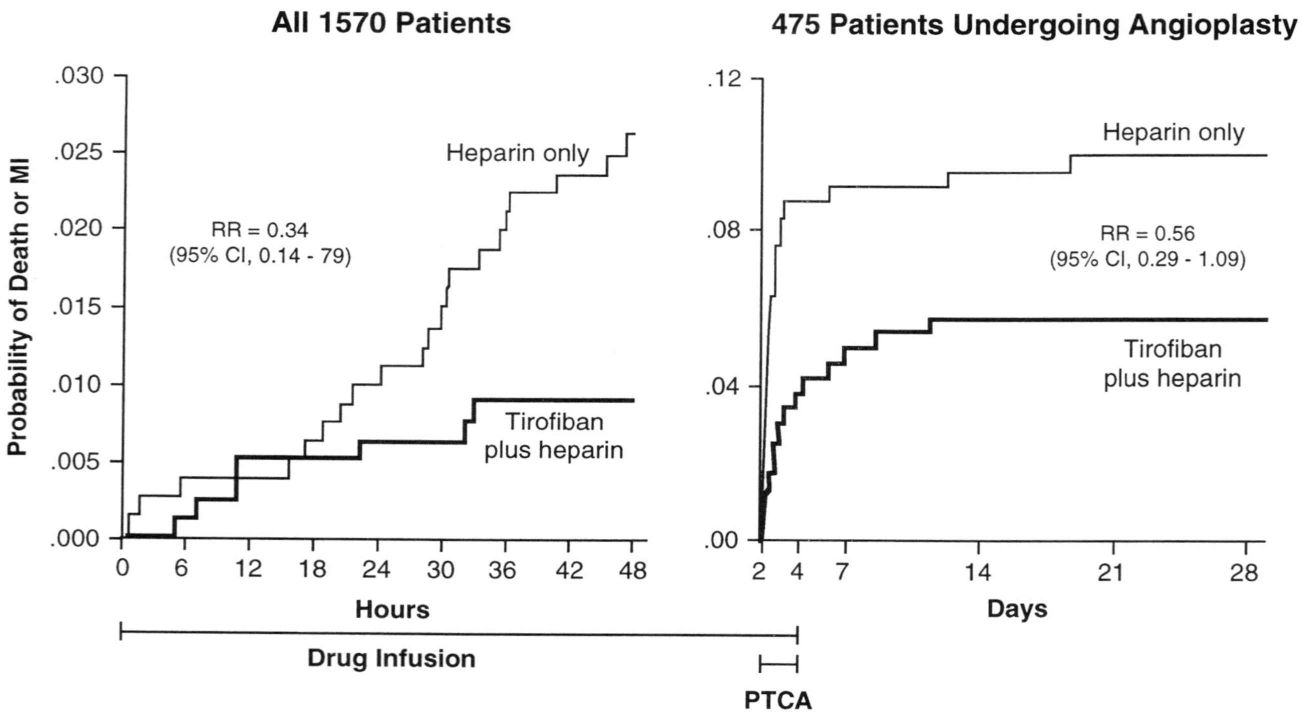

Figure 3 Kaplan-Meier curves showing the cumulative incidence of death or myocardial infarction among patients randomly assigned to heparin or to tirofiban plus heparin. The left-hand panel shows events during the initial 48 hours of medical treatment among all 1570 patients in the two groups, and the right-hand panel shows cumulative incidence of death or myocardial infarction from the time of procedure to 30 days after randomization among the 475 patients who underwent coronary intervention (angioplasty). RR, risk ratio; and CI, confidence interval. (From Ref. 7.)

crease in serum creatine kinase MB fraction. Patients were assigned to either eptifibatide or placebo for a maximum of 72 hours. When PCI was planned, investigators were encouraged (but not required) to perform it within 72 hours of randomization, with continuation of eptifibatide for 20 to 24 hours thereafter. Of the 9641 patients enrolled in the trial, 63% underwent coronary angiography, and 24% underwent PCI by 30 days (median time to index PCI: 67 hours, stents were used in approximately 50% of procedures). Eptifibatide-treated patients undergoing early (within 72 hours) PCI experienced a significant reduction in 30-day death or myocardial infarction (11.6% vs. 16.7%, odds ratio 0.65, 95% confidence interval 0.47 to 0.90, $P = .01$).

To assess the impact of early revascularization in the PURSUIT population, Kleiman and colleagues (43) developed a model to adjust for baseline characteristics (multiple logistic regression analysis) and selection bias for PCI (propensity analysis). After adjustment for randomized treatment and the propensity score, early PCI was not related to the composite endpoint of death or any myocardial infarction at 30 days (hazard ratio 1.239, $P = .075$). However, early PCI was associated with lower rates of the composite of death or Q-wave myocardial infarction at 30 days (3.3% vs. 4.8%, hazard ratio 0.68, $P = .055$). Of note, 42% of events in the PCI group occurred before the procedure. When excluding these events, there was a 17% relative reduction in death or myocardial infarction by eptifibatide at 30 days, while this reduction was 6% in patients who did not undergo early PCI. It was concluded that the benefits of eptifibatide appeared to be greater in patients undergoing PCI while receiving study drug, with an important suppression of events prior to the procedure. The results also suggest the possibility that early PCI was associated with early excess in periprocedural MIs (reduced by eptifibatide), but with a later reduction in more significant events (such as death and Q-wave MI).

Overall, platelet GP IIb/IIIa inhibitors improve outcomes in high-risk patients with ACS. They are efficacious in stabilizing patients during the initial phase of treatment and also suppress the early hazard associated with revascualrization procedures. With empiric therapy, there is a trend toward better treatment effect if PCI is performed. In addition, of patients undergoing PCI, those with a diagnosis of ACS tended to benefit more compared with more clinically stable patients (39) (Fig. 4). These agents are therefore expected to enhance any benefit associated with an early invasive strategy and become an integral part of such a strategy.

UNRESOLVED ISSUES

Although the weight of evidence generally favors an early invasive approach, there remain unresolved issues. The more pressing relate to: (1)

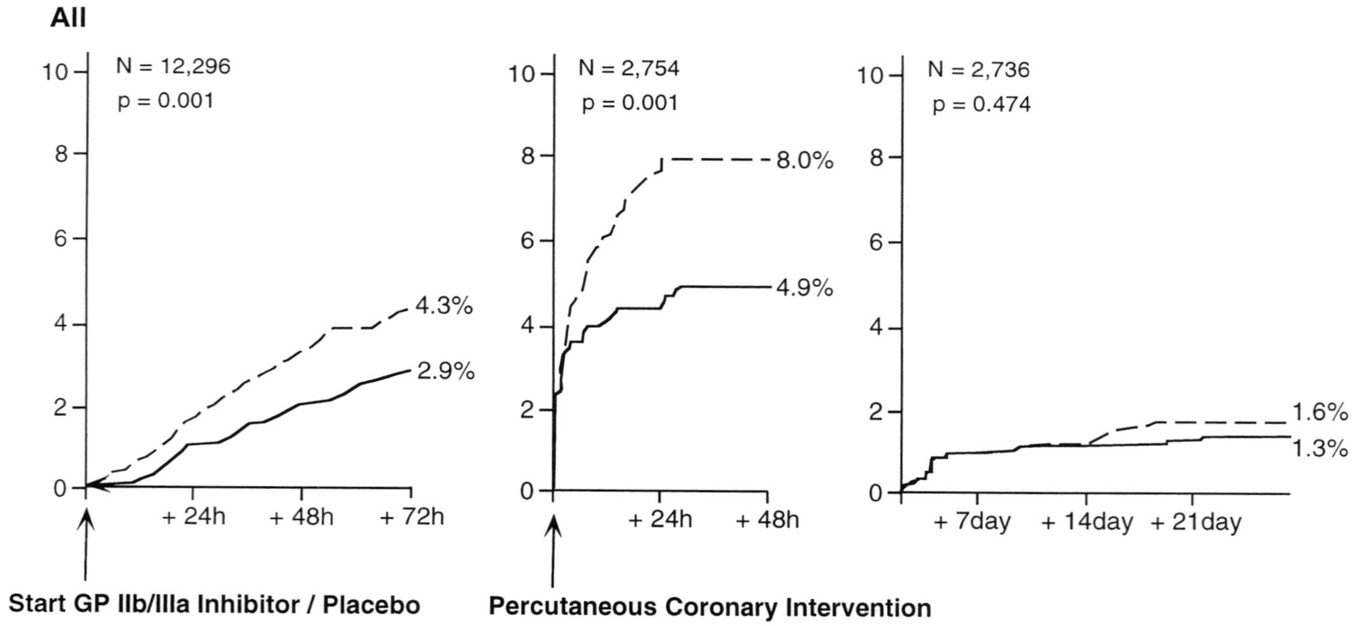

Figure 4 Kaplan-Meier curves showing cumulative incidence of death or myocardial infarction in patients randomly assigned to GP IIb/IIIa (bold lines) or placebo. Data were derived from CAPTURE (7), PURSUIT (19), and PRISM-PLUS (42).

stenting versus balloon angioplasty (with provisional stenting); (2) the optimal period (if any) of pretreatment or stabilization; (3) management of high versus low risk patients; and (4) culprit lesion versus complete revascularization.

Stenting has been shown to decrease restenosis and proportionally target vessel revascularization in early balloon versus stent trials (44,45). Since then, combination antiplatelet therapy with aspirin and thienopyridines has mutually improved the outcomes in stented patients, including those with acute myocardial infarction (46–48). These reports have set the stage for numerous trials of primary stenting versus balloon angioplasty for acute myocardial infarction. Collectively, preliminary results of these trials have shown a reduction in reinfarction and have confirmed the expected reduction in TVR rates. Although there are no dedicated trials of stenting versus balloon angioplasty in the context of ACS without ST-segment elevation, it is logical to extend the findings of the acute myocardial infarction trials to this population (48–54). Furthermore, in the EPISTENT trial (25,55), stenting plus placebo was compared with stenting plus abciximab and balloon angioplasty plus abciximab. In this trial, 487 patients had a diagnosis of unstable angina within 48 hours of randomization. The primary composite endpoint of death/myocardial infarction or urgent revascularization at 30 days was significantly reduced in the combined abciximab groups versus placebo (5.9% vs. 9.1%, $P < .001$). The combination of stenting plus abciximab was associated with a further 38% reduction in the same composite endpoint (4.5% vs. 7.3%) when compared with balloon angioplasty plus abciximab. Therefore, it appears that primary stenting plus abciximab is the best strategy in stent-eligible patients.

In early retrospective studies of angioplasty in ACS, patients pretreated with heparin for several days and patients who had their procedure >2 weeks after initiation of treatment had a lower rate of periprocedural complications. However, these studies were inherently flawed by an important selection bias in that only the more stable patients tolerated pretreatment. There is no evidence that a pretreatment period provides any clinical benefit prior to contemporary PCI, particularly with the use of GP IIb/IIIa. The Treat Angina with Aggrastat and Determine Cost of Therapy with an Invasive or Conservative Strategy (TACTICS-TIMI 18) was specifically designed to test whether an early invasive strategy (catheterization within 4 to 48 hours and revascularization if feasible) or a conservative strategy results in the best clinical outcomes (death, MI, or rehospitalization for ACS at 6 months) in the current era of platelet GP IIb/IIIa inhibition and contemporary intervention. The planned sample size of approximately 1720 moderate- to high-risk patients should have 80% power to detect a 25% difference between the two groups. This trial will also test the troponin hypothesis (secondary hypothesis), in which patients with elevated serum troponin levels benefit most from aggressive treatment.

Trials of platelet IIb/IIIa inhibitors and early invasive strategy in ACS have enrolled a spectrum of patients. To the extent that analyses have been performed, high-risk patients seem to benefit from more aggressive treatment (18,56–59) (Table 3). However, lower-risk patients may not derive as much benefit, particularly with regard to death and MI. Management of this group of patients has not been adequately studied, but it is possible that an early conservative strategy would be more appropriate.

Another important issue is the optimal revascularization strategy per se. There are two main strategies available in this regard: (1) treating the culprit lesion only in the acute setting, taking into consideration the patient's previous clinical status and factoring in the added risk of multivessel interventions; and (2) attempting complete revascularization with the expectation of providing optimal symptomatic relief and possibly improving survival in some subgroups of patients. No randomized data are available to address this issue. From nonrandomized studies, it appears that revascularization of the culprit lesion only provides adequate symptomatic relief in most of these patients while minimizing procedural risks. However, as procedural diminish over time with improved equipment and adjunctive therapy, this assessment may become outdated. Furthermore, certain subgroups of patients appear to particularly benefit from more complete revascularization (severe three-ves-

Table 3 Event Rates by Troponin Status and Treatment Strategy

Trial	Study therapy	Death or MI (%) (elevated troponin)	Death or MI (%) (normal troponin)
CAPTURE[a] (42)	Placebo (%)	19.6	4.9
	Abciximab (%)	5.8	5.2
	% Change	−70.4	+6.1
	P	<.001	ns
PRISM[a] (58)	Placebo (%)	13.0	4.9
	Tirofiban (%)	4.3	5.7
	% Change	−66.9	+16.3
	P	<.001	ns
FRISC II[b] (30)	Early invasive (%)	13.3	10.3
	Conservative (%)	10.1	8.3
	% Change	−24.1	−19.4
	P	NA	NA

[a]30-Day.
[b]6-Month.

sel disease, low ejection fraction, two-vessel disease including proximal left anterior descending artery, and diabetics).

INTEGRATED APPROACH

The ultimate goals of therapy in ACS are to improve survival, limit progression to myocardial infarction, and improve quality of life (anginal symptoms, anxiety, rehospitalization). A suggested management algorithm for these patients based on contemporary clinical data is as follows. Patients should be risk-stratified early after admission using recognized contemporary predictors of unfavorable outcome (physical examination, ECG, biochemical markers of disease severity such as CK-MB, troponin, CRP, etc.) (11–15,60–65). If moderate- to high-risk patients are candidates for revascularization, they should undergo early angiography within hours to days with the intent to perform revascularization if feasible (as clinical benefits are most likely related to revascularization, not angiography per se). The revascularization procedure of choice will depend on patient/physician preference and on coronary anatomy: complete revascularization seems an appropriate goal, but should be weighed against the inherent risks. For patients at low risk, the optimal strategy possibly involves a short stabilization period of medical therapy followed by noninvasive testing, leading to an ischemia-guided revascularization strategy, minimizing the early hazard of revascularization in patients without significant myocardium at risk and/or symptoms (66).

CONCLUSIONS AND FUTURE IMPLICATIONS

When assessing the best therapeutic strategy for patients with ACS, it is crucial to identify the true goals of therapy. These goals should predominantly relate to patient outcome, but also to practical management issues (resource utilization, length of stay, costs, etc.). In this context, the objective evidence favors the early invasive strategy for patients at moderate to high risk when considering residual symptoms and rehospitalization, and possibly for reduction of death and myocardial infarction. Furthermore, with the increasing use of the stents, platelet GP IIb/IIIa inhibitors, better anticoagulants (low-molecular-weight heparins, direct thrombin inhibitors), and potential emboli protection devices, the early invasive strategies will likely become the optimal therapy for moderate- to high-risk ACS patients.

REFERENCES

1. Fragmin during Instability in Coronary Artery Disease (FRISC). Low-molecular-weight heparin during instability in coronary artery disease Study Group. [see comments]. Lancet 1996;347(9001):561–568.

2. Long-term low-molecular-mass heparin in unstable coronary-artery disease: FRISC II prospective randomised multicentre study. Fragmin and Fast Revascularisation during Instability in Coronary artery disease Investigators. Lancet 1999;354(9180):701–707.
3. Swahn E, Wallentin L. Low-molecular-weight heparin (Fragmin) during instability in coronary artery disease (FRISC). FRISC Study Group. Am J Cardiol 1997;80(5A):25E–29E.
4. Wallentin L, Husted S, Kontny F, Swahn E. Long-term low-molecular-weight heparin (Fragmin) and/or early revascularization during instability in coronary artery disease (the FRISC II study). Am J Cardiol 1997;80(5A):61E–63E.
5. A comparison of recombinant hirudin with heparin for the treatment of acute coronary syndromes. The Global Use of Strategies to Open Occluded Coronary Arteries (GUSTO) IIb Investigators. N Engl J Med 1996;335(11):775–782.
6. OASIS-2 Investigators. Effects of recombinant hirudin (lepirudin) compared with heparin on death, myocardial infarction, refractory angina, and revascularisation procedures in patients with acute myocardial ischaemia without ST elevation: a randomised trial. Organisation to Assess Strategies for Ischemic Syndromes (OASIS-2) Investigators. Lancet 1999;353(9151):429–438.
7. PRISM-PLUS Investigators. Inhibition of the platelet glycoprotein IIb/IIIa receptor with tirofiban in unstable angina and non-Q-wave myocardial infarction. Platelet Receptor Inhibition in Ischemic Syndrome Management in Patients Limited by Unstable Signs and Symptoms (PRISM-PLUS) Study Investigators [published erratum appears in N Engl J Med 1998 Aug 6;339(6):415]. N Engl J Med 1998;338(21):1488–1497.
8. PRISM Investigators. A comparison of aspirin plus tirofiban with aspirin plus heparin for unstable angina. Platelet Receptor Inhibition in Ischemic Syndrome Management (PRISM) Study Investigators. N Engl J Med 1998;338(21):1498–1505.
9. PARAGON Investigators. International, randomized, controlled trial of lamifiban (a platelet glycoprotein IIb/IIIa inhibitor), heparin, or both in unstable angina. Platelet IIb/IIIa Antagonism for the Reduction of Acute coronary syndrome events in a Global Organization Network. Circulation 1998;97(24):2386–2395.
10. Antman EM, Tanasijevic MJ, Thompson B, Schactman M, McCabe CH, Cannon CP, et al. Cardiac-specific troponin I levels to predict the risk of mortality in patients with acute coronary syndromes. N Engl J Med 1996;335(18):1342–1349.
11. Hamm CW, Ravkilde J, Gerhardt W, Jorgensen P, Peheim E, Ljungdahl L, et al. The prognostic value of serum troponin T in unstable angina. N Engl J Med 1992;327(3):146–150.
12. Katus HA, Remppis A, Neumann FJ, Scheffold T, Diederich KW, Vinar G, et al. Diagnostic efficiency of troponin T measurements in acute myocardial infarction. Circulation 1991;83(3):902–912.
13. Lindahl B, Venge P, Wallentin L. Relation between troponin T and the risk of subsequent cardiac events in unstable coronary artery disease. The FRISC study group. Circulation 1996;93(9):1651–1657.

14. Lindahl B, Venge P, Wallentin L. Troponin T identifies patients with unstable coronary artery disease who benefit from long-term antithrombotic protection. Fragmin in Unstable Coronary Artery Disease (FRISC) Study Group. J Am Coll Cardiol 1997;29(1):43–48.
15. Lindahl B, Venge P, Wallentin L. The FRISC experience with troponin T. Use as decision tool and comparison with other prognostic markers. Eur Heart J 1998;19(suppl N):N51–N58.
16. Newby LK, Christenson RH, Ohman EM, Armstrong PW, Thompson TD, Lee KL, et al. Value of serial troponin T measures for early and late risk stratification in patients with acute coronary syndromes. The GUSTO-IIa Investigators. Circulation 1998;98(18):1853–1859.
17. Braunwald E. Unstable angina. A classification. Circulation 1989;80(2):410–414.
18. TIMI Investigators. Effects of tissue plasminogen activator and a comparison of early invasive and conservative strategies in unstable angina and non-Q-wave myocardial infarction. Results of the TIMI IIIB Trial. Thrombolysis in Myocardial Ischemia. Circulation 1994;89(4):1545–1556.
19. PURSUIT Trial Investigators. Inhibition of platelet glycoprotein IIb/IIIa with eptifibatide in patients with acute coronary syndromes. Platelet glycoprotein IIb/IIIa in unstable angina: receptor suppression using Integrelin therapy. N Engl J Med 1998;339(7):436–443.
20. Antman EM. TIMI 11B. Enoxaparin versus unfractionated heparin for unstable angina or non-Q-wave myocardial infarction: a double-blind, placebo-controlled, parallel-group, multicenter trial. Rationale, study design, and methods. Thrombolysis in Myocardial Infarction (TIMI) 11B Trial Investigators. Am Heart J 1998;135(6 Pt 3 Su):S353–S360.
21. Antman EM, Cohen M, Radley D, McCabe C, Rush J, Premmereur J, et al. Assessment of the treatment effect of enoxaparin for unstable angina/non-Q-wave myocardial infarction: TIMI 11B-ESSENCE meta-analysis. Circulation 1999;100(15):1602–1608.
22. Antman EM, McCabe CH, Gurfinkel EP, Turpie AG, Bernink PJ, Salein D, et al. Enoxaparin prevents death and cardiac ischemic events in unstable angina/non-Q-wave myocardial infarction: results of the Thrombolysis in Myocardial Infarction (TIMI) 11B Trial. Circulation 1999;100(15):1593–1601.
23. Gurfinkel E, Fareed J, Antman E, Cohen M, Mautner B. Rationale for the management of coronary syndromes with low-molecular-weight heparins. Am J Cardiol 1998;82(5B):15L–18L.
24. Diver DJ, Bier JD, Ferreira PE, Sharaf BL, McCabe C, Thompson B, et al. Clinical and arteriographic characterization of patients with unstable angina without critical coronary arterial narrowing (from the TIMI-IIIA Trial). Am J Cardiol 1994;74(6):531–537.
25. Randomised placebo-controlled and balloon-angioplasty-controlled trial to assess safety of coronary stenting with use of platelet glycoprotein-IIb/IIIa blockade. The EPISTENT Investigators. Evaluation of Platelet IIb/IIIa Inhibitor for Stenting. Lancet 1998;352(9122):87–92.

26. Use of a monoclonal antibody directed against the platelet glycoprotein IIb/IIIa receptor in high-risk coronary angioplasty. The EPIC Investigation. N Engl J Med 1994;330(14):956–961.
27. Anderson HV, Cannon CP, Stone PH, Williams DO, McCabe CH, Knatterud GL, et al. One-year results of the Thrombolysis in Myocardial Infarction (TIMI) IIIB clinical trial. A randomized comparison of tissue-type plasminogen activator versus placebo and early invasive versus early conservative strategies in unstable angina and non-Q wave myocardial infarction. J Am Coll Cardiol 1995;26(7):1643–1650.
28. Favaloro RG. Landmarks in the development of coronary artery bypass surgery. Circulation 1998;98(5):466–478.
29. Boden WE, O'Rourke RA, Crawford MH, Blaustein AS, Deedwania PC, Zoble RG, et al. Outcomes in patients with acute non-Q-wave myocardial infarction randomly assigned to an invasive as compared with a conservative management strategy. Veterans Affairs Non-Q-Wave Infarction Strategies in Hospital (VANQWISH) Trial Investigators [published erratum appears in N Engl J Med 1998 Oct 8;339(15):1091]. N Engl J Med 1998;338(25):1785–1792.
30. FRISC Investigators. Invasive compared with non-invasive treatment in unstable coronary-artery disease: FRISC II prospective randomised multicentre study. Fragmin and Fast Revascularisation during Instability in Coronary artery disease Investigators. Lancet 1999;354(9180):708–715.
31. Gurbel PA, Serebruany VL, Shustov AR, Bahr RD, Carpo C, Ohman EM, et al. Effects of reteplase and alteplase on platelet aggregation and major receptor expression during the first 24 hours of acute myocardial infarction treatment. GUSTO-III Investigators. Global Use of Strategies to Open Occluded Coronary Arteries. J Am Coll Cardiol 1998;31(7):1466–1473.
32. Moser M, Nordt T, Peter K, Ruef J, Kohler B, Schmittner M, et al. Platelet function during and after thrombolytic therapy for acute myocardial infarction with reteplase, alteplase, or streptokinase. Circulation 1999;100(18):1858–1864.
33. Abdelmeguid AE, Whitlow PL, Sapp SK, Ellis SG, Topol EJ. Long-term outcome of transient, uncomplicated in-laboratory coronary artery closure. Circulation 1995;91(11):2733–2741.
34. Califf RM, Abdelmeguid AE, Kuntz RE, Popma JJ, Davidson CJ, Cohen EA, et al. Myonecrosis after revascularization procedures. J Am Coll Cardiol 1998; 31(2):241–251.
35. Simoons ML, van den Brand M, Lincoff M, Harrington R, van der Wieken R, Vahanian A, et al. Minimal myocardial damage during coronary intervention is associated with impaired outcome. Eur Heart J 1999;20(15):1112–1119.
36. Yusuf S, Flather M, Pogue J, Hunt D, Varigos J, Piegas L, et al. Variations between countries in invasive cardiac procedures and outcomes in patients with suspected unstable angina or myocardial infarction without initial ST elevation. OASIS (Organisation to Assess Strategies for Ischaemic Syndromes) Registry Investigators. Lancet 1998;352(9127):507–514.
37. Cho L, Bhatt D, Marso S, Hsu C, Holmes D, Califf R, et al. An early invasive

strategy is associated with decreased mortality: GUSTO IIb trial. Circulation 1999;100(18):I-359.
38. Coller BS, Folts JD, Smith SR, Scudder LE, Jordan R. Abolition of in vivo platelet thrombus formation in primates with monoclonal antibodies to the platelet GPIIb/IIIa receptor. Correlation with bleeding time, platelet aggregation, and blockade of GPIIb/IIIa receptors. Circulation 1989;80(6):1766–1774.
39. Boersma E, Akkerhuis KM, Theroux P, Califf RM, Topol EJ, Simoons ML. Platelet glycoprotein IIb/IIIa receptor inhibition in non-ST-elevation acute coronary syndromes: early benefit during medical treatment only, with additional protection during percutaneous coronary intervention. Circulation 1999; 100(20):2045–2048.
40. Lincoff AM, Califf RM, Anderson KM, Weisman HF, Aguirre FV, Kleiman NS, et al. Evidence for prevention of death and myocardial infarction with platelet membrane glycoprotein IIb/IIIa receptor blockade by abciximab (c7E3 Fab) among patients with unstable angina undergoing percutaneous coronary revascularization. EPIC Investigators. Evaluation of 7E3 in Preventing Ischemic Complications. J Am Coll Cardiol 1997;30(1):149–156.
41. EPILOG Investigators. Platelet glycoprotein IIb/IIIa receptor blockade and low-dose heparin during percutaneous coronary revascularization. N Engl J Med 1997;336(24):1689–1696.
42. CAPTURE Study. Randomised placebo-controlled trial of abciximab before and during coronary intervention in refractory unstable angina [published erratum appears in Lancet 1997 Sep 6;350(9079):744]. Lancet 1997;349(9063):1429–1435.
43. Kleinman N, Lincoff A, Flaker G, Pieper K, Wilcox R, Berdan L, et al. Percutaneous coronary intervention, platelet inhibition with eptifibatide, and clinical outcomes in patients with acute coronary syndromes. Circulation 1999. In press.
44. Fischman DL, Leon MB, Baim DS, Schatz RA, Savage MP, Penn I, et al. A randomized comparison of coronary-stent placement and balloon angioplasty in the treatment of coronary artery disease. Stent Restenosis Study Investigators. N Engl J Med 1994;331(8):496–501.
45. Serruys PW, de Jaegere P, Kiemeneij F, Macaya C, Rutsch W, Heyndrickx G, et al. A comparison of balloon-expandable-stent implantation with balloon angioplasty in patients with coronary artery disease. Benestent Study Group. N Engl J Med 1994;331(8):489–495.
46. Schomig A, Neumann FJ, Kastrati A, Schuhlen H, Blasini R, Hadamitzky M, et al. A randomized comparison of antiplatelet and anticoagulant therapy after the placement of coronary-artery stents. N Engl J Med 1996;334(17):1084–1089.
47. Leon MB, Baim DS, Popma JJ, Gordon PC, Cutlip DE, Ho KK, et al. A clinical trial comparing three antithrombotic-drug regimens after coronary-artery stenting. Stent Anticoagulation Restenosis Study Investigators. N Engl J Med 1998; 339(23):1665–1671.

48. Schomig A, Neumann FJ, Walter H, Schuhlen H, Hadamitzky M, Zitzmann-Roth EM, et al. Coronary stent placement in patients with acute myocardial infarction: comparison of clinical and angiographic outcome after randomization to antiplatelet or anticoagulant therapy. J Am Coll Cardiol 1997;29(1):28–34.
49. Alfonso F, Rodriguez P, Phillips P, Goicolea J, Hernandez R, Perez-Vizcayno MJ, et al. Clinical and angiographic implications of coronary stenting in thrombus-containing lesions. J Am Coll Cardiol 1997;29(4):725–733.
50. Bauters C, Lablanche JM, Van Belle E, Niculescu R, Meurice T, Mc Fadden EP, et al. Effects of coronary stenting on restenosis and occlusion after angioplasty of the culprit vessel in patients with recent myocardial infarction. Circulation 1997;96(9):2854–2858.
51. Clarkson PB, Halim M, Ray KK, Doshi S, Been M, Singh H, et al. Coronary artery stenting in unstable angina pectoris: a comparison with stable angina pectoris. Heart 1999;81(4):393–397.
52. De Benedictis M, Scrocca I, Borrione M, Luceri S, Sala A, Baduini G. Coronary stenting in unstable angina: angiographic and clinical implications. G Ital Cardiol 1998;28(10):1099–1105.
53. Hamon M, Richardeau Y, Lecluse E, Saloux E, Sabatier R, Agostini D, et al. Direct coronary stenting without balloon predilation in acute coronary syndromes. Am Heart J 1999;138(1 Pt 1):55–59.
54. Walter H, Neumann FJ, Hadamitzky M, Elezi S, Muller A, Schomig A. Coronary artery stent placement with postprocedural antiplatelet therapy in acute myocardial infarction. Coron Artery Dis 1998;9(9):577–582.
55. Lincoff AM, Califf RM, Moliterno DJ, Ellis SG, Ducas J, Kramer JH, et al. Complementary clinical benefits of coronary-artery stenting and blockade of platelet glycoprotein IIb/IIIa receptors. Evaluation of Platelet IIb/IIIa Inhibition in Stenting Investigators. N Engl J Med 1999;341(5):319–327.
56. Diderholm E, Andren B, Frostfeldt G, Genberg M, Jernberg T, Lagerqvist B, et al. ST depression in ECG at entry identifies patients who benefit most from early revascularization in unstable coronary artery disease: a FRISC II substudy. Circulation 1999;100(18):I-497.
57. Hamm CW, Heeschen C, Goldmann B, Vahanian A, Adgey J, Miguel CM, et al. Benefit of abciximab in patients with refractory unstable angina in relation to serum troponin T levels. c7E3 Fab Antiplatelet Therapy in Unstable Refractory Angina (CAPTURE) Study Investigators. N Engl J Med 1999;340(21):1623–1629.
58. Heeschen C, Hamm CW, Goldmann B, Deu A, Langenbrink L, White HD. Troponin concentrations for stratification of patients with acute coronary syndromes in relation to therapeutic efficacy of tirofiban. PRISM Study Investigators. Platelet Receptor Inhibition in Ischemic Syndrome Management. Lancet 1999;354(9192):1757–1762.
59. Lagerqvist B, Diderholm E, Lindhal B, Husted S, Kontny F, Stahle E, et al. An early invasive treatment strategy reduces cardiac events regardless of troponin levels in unstable coronary with and without troponin-elevation: a FRISC II substudy. Circulation 1999;100(18):I-497.

60. Becker RC, Cannon CP, Bovill EG, Tracy RP, Thompson B, Knatterud GL, et al. Prognostic value of plasma fibrinogen concentration in patients with unstable angina and non-Q-wave myocardial infarction (TIMI IIIB Trial). Am J Cardiol 1996;78(2):142–147.
61. Ferreiros ER, Boissonnet CP, Pizarro R, Merletti PF, Corrado G, Cagide A, et al. Independent prognostic value of elevated C-reactive protein in unstable angina. Circulation 1999;100(19):1958–1963.
62. Garbarz E, Iung B, Lefevre G, Makita Y, Farah B, Michaud P, et al. Frequency and prognostic value of cardiac troponin I elevation after coronary stenting. Am J Cardiol 1999;84(5):515–518.
63. Lindahl B, Andren B, Ohlsson J, Venge P, Wallentin L. Noninvasive risk stratification in unstable coronary artery disease: exercise test and biochemical markers. FRISC Study Group. Am J Cardiol 1997;80(5A):40E–44E.
64. Liuzzo G, Biasucci LM, Gallimore JR, Grillo RL, Rebuzzi AG, Pepys MB, et al. The prognostic value of C-reactive protein and serum amyloid a protein in severe unstable angina. N Engl J Med 1994;331(7):417–424.
65. Toss H, Lindahl B, Siegbahn A, Wallentin L. Prognostic influence of increased fibrinogen and C-reactive protein levels in unstable coronary artery disease. FRISC Study Group. Fragmin during Instability in Coronary Artery Disease. Circulation 1997;96(12):4204–4210.
66. Madsen JK, Grande P, Saunamaki K, Thayssen P, Kassis E, Eriksen U, et al. Danish multicenter randomized study of invasive versus conservative treatment in patients with inducible ischemia after thrombolysis in acute myocardial infarction (DANAMI). Danish trial in Acute Myocardial Infarction. Circulation 1997;96(3):748–755.

16

Intravenous Glycoprotein IIb/IIIa Receptor Inhibitor Agents in Ischemic Heart Disease

Jeffrey Lefkovits
The Royal Melbourne Hospital
Melbourne, Australia

Eric J. Topol
The Cleveland Clinic Foundation
Cleveland, Ohio

INTRODUCTION

The important role of platelets in acute coronary syndromes has been increasingly recognized over recent years—both in terms of pathogenesis and as a target for treatment. With the platelet glycoprotein (GP) IIb/IIIa receptor being the key pathway leading to platelet aggregation, the proliferation of drugs that block the GP IIb/IIIa receptor has resulted in a large number of large-scale randomized, placebo-controlled drug trials in over 34,000 patients. There is now overwhelming evidence that these agents, particularly when administered in their intravenous form, reduce death and myocardial infarction in patients with acute coronary syndromes and those undergoing percutaneous intervention (Fig. 1). This chapter will review the background behind the applicability of GP IIb/IIIa receptor blockade in acute coronary disease, provide an up-to-date analysis of the evidence supporting intravenous GP IIb/IIIa receptor inhibition, and highlight some of the ongoing issues in their use in the context of acute coronary syndromes.

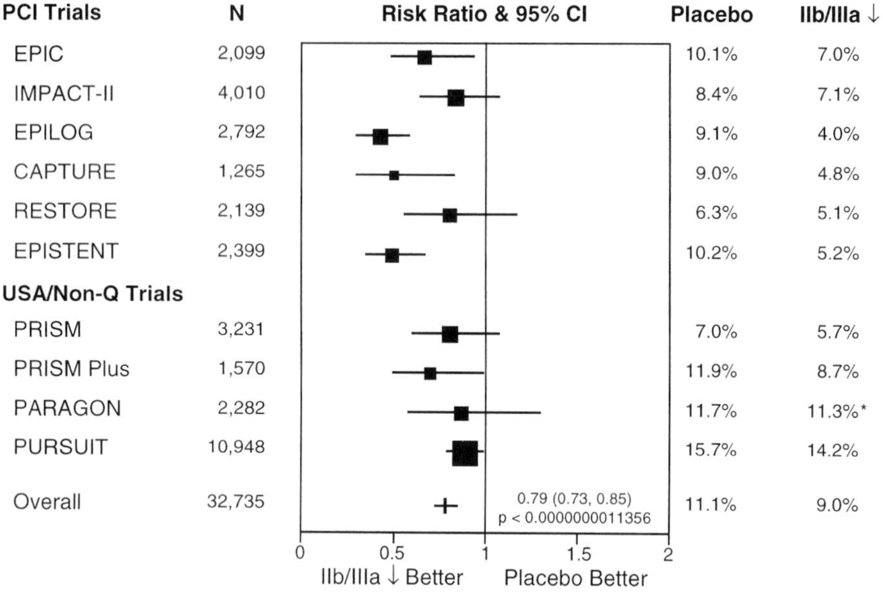

Figure 1 Risk ratios plots with 95% confidence intervals (CI) for the combined endpoint of death or nonfatal myocardial infarction for 10 large-scale randomized trials of GP IIb/IIIa receptor inhibition in percutaneous coronary intervention and unstable angina/non-ST-elevation myocardial infarction.

PLATELETS IN THE PATHOGENESIS OF ACUTE CORONARY SYNDROMES

The pathogenesis of acute coronary syndromes involves the fissuring or rupture of plaque and exposure of subendothelial collagen and the lipid-rich core (1). The syndrome of unstable angina differs from acute myocardial infarction with the formation of transient rather than more stable thrombotic arterial occlusion. Various factors influence the thrombotic response, including the character and extent of exposure of subendothelial plaque components (2–4), the degree of flow disturbance and resultant platelet activation that ensues (4,5), and the balance between endogenous thrombotic and thrombolytic processes (6–8). The formation of platelet-rich thrombus predominates in human coronary arteries.

Following platelet adhesion and activation, changes in platelet shape occur, thromboxane A2, plasminogen activator inhibitor-I (PAI-1), serotonin, and other pro-aggregatory substances are released and platelet aggregation follows. While adhesion of platelets to the damaged vessel site is dependent on the recognition of adhesive proteins by several platelet membrane glycoproteins, the GP IIb/IIIa receptor alone, is the principal receptor involved in platelet aggregation (9). Platelet activation triggers conformational changes in the unactivated GP IIb/IIIa receptor that transform it into its activated, ligand-competent state. This receptor then binds mainly fibrinogen, particularly at normal or low shear stress, and is the key event in the process of platelet aggregation. The fibrinogen molecules form cross-bridges between adjacent platelets, linking them together to form a scaffold for the advancing hemostatic plug (Fig. 2).

The GP IIb/IIIa (α_{IIb}/β_3) receptor (Fig. 3) belongs to the integrin family of heterodimeric adhesion molecules, which are formed by the noncovalent interaction of a series of α and β subunits (10–12). Integrins are found on virtually all cell types and mediate a diversity of physiological responses. Several other integrins are present on the platelet surface in addition to GP IIb/IIIa, many of which are involved in platelet adhesion. The GP IIb/IIIa

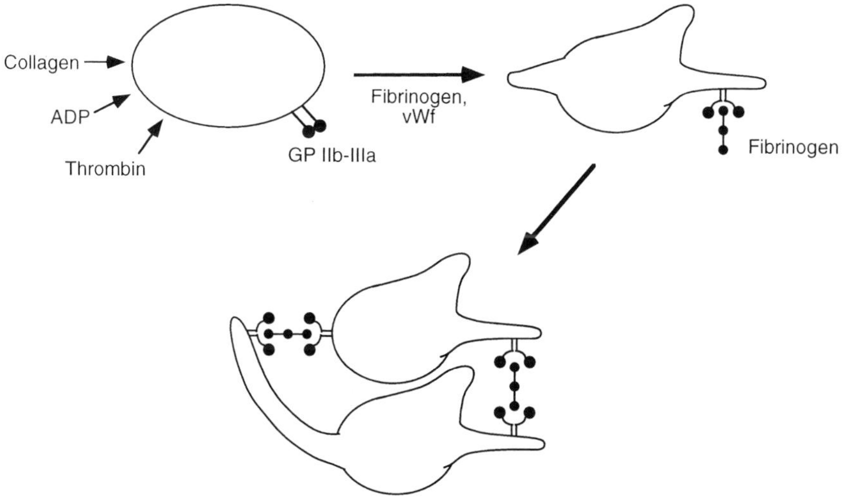

Figure 2 Illustration of key events that occur during the processes of platelet activation and aggregation. In the presence of agonists such as collagen, adenosine diphosphate (ADP), and thrombin, platelet activation leads to changes in platelet shape and activation of the GP IIb/IIIa receptor. Activated GP IIb/IIIa receptors bind mainly fibrinogen and this adhesive protein forms bridges between adjacent platelets —the principal mechanism resulting in platelet aggregation and formation of the advancing platelet plug. (From Phillips DR, et al. Am J Cardiol 1997;80:11B–20B.)

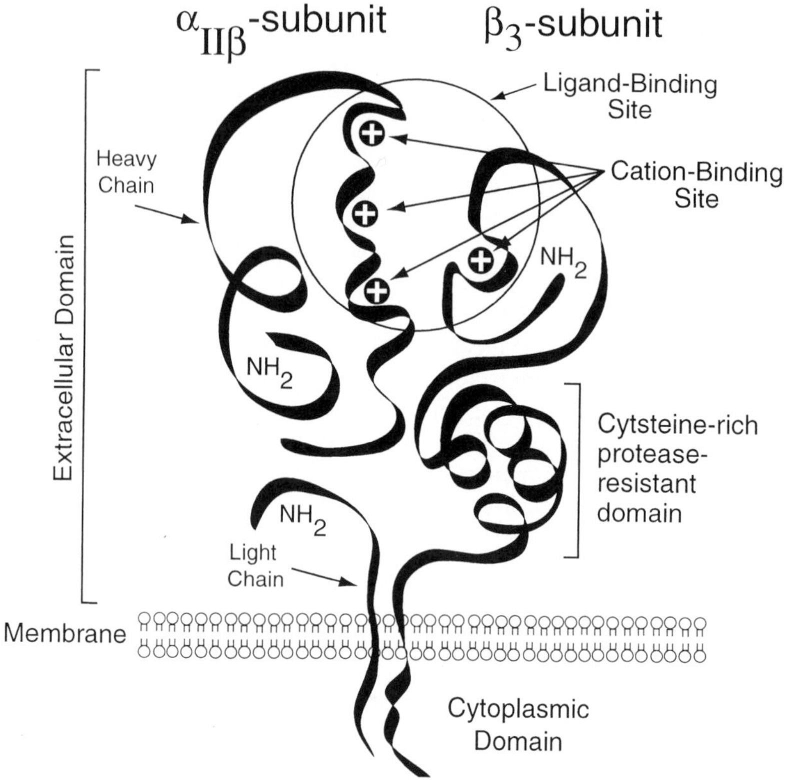

Figure 3 Schematic depiction of the $\alpha_{IIb}\beta_3$ (GP IIb/IIIa) integrin. (From Ref. 20.)

receptor is the most abundant on the platelet surface, with approximately 50,000 to 80,000 copies per platelet. Apart from its ability to bind fibrinogen, the receptor can bind other adhesive proteins such as fibronectin, vitronectin, and Von Willebrand factor (13–15). However, these proteins appear to have only minor roles in the process of aggregation (13). Two specific peptide sequences present in adhesive proteins are involved in binding to the GP IIb/IIIa receptor. The Arg-Gly-Asp (RGD) sequence was initially identified as the adhesive sequence in fibronectin (16), but is also present in fibrinogen, Von Willebrand factor, and vitronectin. The other major sequence involved is the Lys-Gln-Ala-Gly-Asp-Val (KQAGDV) sequence, located at the extreme carboxy terminus of the γ-chain of fibrinogen (17,18). Unlike the RGD sequence, this sequence is only found in fibrinogen.

PHARMACOLOGY OF THE INTRAVENOUS GP IIb/IIIa RECEPTOR INHIBITORS

Three parenteral agents—abciximab (ReoPro, Eli Lilly, Indianapolis, IN), eptifibatide (Integrilin, COR Therapeutics, South San Francisco, CA), and tirofiban (Aggrastat, MK-383, Merck White House Station, NJ)—are currently approved for clinical use by the U.S. Food and Drug Administration. The first to reach the clinical arena, abciximab, was developed from a murine monoclonal antibody directed against the GP IIb/IIIa integrin (19). Unlike the small-molecule agents, abciximab interacts with the GP IIb/IIIa receptor at sites distinct from the ligand-binding RGD sequence site, and probably exerts its inhibitory effect by steric hindrance (20). Abciximab also binds the $\alpha_v\beta_3$ integrin (a vitronectin receptor), suggesting that it is the β_3 (GP IIIa) subunit that contains conformational epitopes involved in ligand-receptor binding (21). The antibody has unique pharmacokinetics, with the majority of the drug cleared from plasma within 25 min, but much slower clearance from the body with a catabolic half-life up to 7 hours (22). Yet, platelet-associated abciximab can still be detected in the circulation for >14 days after cessation of infusion, in part related to its high affinity for the receptor (23). Throughout this time, the drug remains evenly distributed among the population of circulating platelets. With an average period of platelet circulation of about 7 days, it appears that abciximab molecules can freely dissociate and reassociate with GP IIb/IIIa as the turnover of platelets in the circulation continues, thus prolonging the "biological" half-life of the drug. Both preclinical studies and pharmacodynamic evaluation in patients have set the range of >80% inhibition of platelet aggregation as the target for effective antiplatelet activity (21). The appropriateness of this target has been validated by the clinical trials demonstrating both efficacy and safety with this level of platelet inhibition.

Synthetic peptides and small-molecule GP IIb/IIIa antagonists were developed because of concerns regarding potential immunogenicity, lack of reversibility, and cost of the monoclonal antibody agents. These contain the RGD sequence (or a variant of it) and occupy the RGD binding site of the GP IIb/IIIa receptor. The so-called KGD peptide GP IIb/IIIa receptor inhibitor, eptifibatide, has a lysine residue substituted for the arginine in the RGD sequence, while lamifiban (Hoffmann-La Roche, Basel, Switzerland) and tirofiban are small-molecule GP IIb/IIIa receptor antagonists based on the RGD motif. Unlike abciximab, these small-molecule agents are specific for GP IIb/IIIa without any appreciable binding to other integrins such as $\alpha_v\beta_3$ (20). Because of their small size, these drugs are also much less likely to induce an antibody response than abciximab. They have a high affinity for GP IIb/IIIa, but not as strong as abciximab, and are rapidly eliminated from the circulation once the infusion is stopped. Thus, they have the "biological" profile of short-acting agents whose effects on platelet aggregation rapidly dissipate (within 4 hours) once the drug infusion is terminated (21).

For eptifibatide, approximately 25% of the drug molecules in plasma are protein bound, leaving the remaining 75% to constitute the pool of pharmacologically active drug. The stoichiometry of both eptifibatide and tirofiban is >100 molecules of drug per GP IIb/IIIa receptor needed to achieve full platelet inhibition. This compares with a stoichiometry of 1.5 molecules of abciximab for each receptor. Eptifibatide has an elimination half-life of 2.5 hours, with the majority of the drug eliminated through renal mechanisms. Approximately 65% of tirofiban molecules end up bound to plasma proteins, with a half-life for that drug of around 2.0 hours. As with eptifibatide, the main route of excretion is through the renal tract. Plasma clearance of both eptifibatide and tirofiban is likely to be affected by significant renal impairment and the doses of these drugs should probably be adjusted where creatinine clearance is severely reduced.

THERAPEUTIC USE OF GLYCOPROTEIN IIb/IIIa RECEPTOR INHIBITORS IN ACUTE CORONARY SYNDROMES

Clinical Trials in Unstable Angina/Non-ST-Elevation Myocardial Infarction

The primary aims of any therapy for non ST-segment elevation acute coronary syndromes (ACS) are to relieve ischemia and prevent further coronary thrombosis. Four large-scale trials have now been completed with the GP IIb/IIIa receptor inhibitors in this clinical setting and have provided strong support for the inclusion if this class of agents in the medical treatment of non-ST-segment elevation ACS. These trials, listed in Table 1, have several important differences in their trial designs. Entry criteria were similar for Platelet IIb/IIIa in Unstable Angina Receptor Suppression Using Integrilin Therapy (PURSUIT) (24), Platelet Receptor Inhibition in Ischemic Syndrome Management in Patients Limited by Unstable Signs (PRISM PLUS) (25), and Platelet IIb/IIIa Antagonism for the Reduction of Acute Coronary Syndrome Events in the Global Organization Network (PARAGON) (26), but less rigorous for Platelet Receptor Inhibition in Ischemic Syndrome Management (PRISM) (27), with a lower-risk population included in this trial. The proportion of patients enrolled with a diagnosis of non-Q-wave myocardial infarction ranged from 25% in the lower-risk PRISM trial to 45% in PURSUIT and PRISM PLUS. The PARAGON and PRISM trials aimed for a conservative, medicine-based approach, with coronary angiography and revascularization allowed but discouraged. In contrast, the PRISM PLUS trial encouraged cath-

Table 1 Trial Design and Patient Population from Four Major Randomized Trials of GP IIb/IIIa Receptor Blockade in Unstable Angina or Non-ST-Elevation Myocardial Infarction

Trial	Agent	Number of patients	Entry criteria	Coadministration of heparin	Angiography and revascularization	Primary endpoint
PURSUIT	Eptifibatide	10,948	CP at rest within 24 h, and either ECG changes[a] or CK-MB rise	Heparin use encouraged, but not randomized	At discretion of attending physician	Death or MI at 30 days
PRISM PLUS	Tirofiban	1,915	CP at rest or minimal exertion within 12 h, and either ECG changes[a] or CK-MB rise	Yes	Deferred for 48 h then performed during study drug infusion	Death, MI, or refractory ischemia at 7 days
PRISM	Tirofiban	3,232	CP at rest or minimal exertion within 12 h, and either ECG changes[a] or CK-MB rise or history of coronary disease or positive stress test	No	Discouraged	Death, MI, or refractory ischemia at 48 h
PARAGON A	Lamifiban	2,282	CP at rest within 12 h, and ECG changes[a]	Randomized	Discouraged	Death or MI at 30 days

Abbreviations: CP, chest pain; CK-MB, creatine kinase MB isoenzyme fraction; MI, myocardial infarction.
[a]ECG changes include ST-segment depression, T-wave inversion, or transient ST-segment elevation.

eterization and revascularization after an initial 48-hour period of drug treatment. The PURSUIT trial did not stipulate guidelines for coronary angiography and revascularization but strongly encouraged the concomitant use of heparin.

Clinical Trial Outcomes

While the overall trend among the randomized trials was for a net clinical benefit with GP IIb/IIIa receptor blockade, individual studies varied in demonstrating statistically significant reductions in adverse outcomes (Table 2). It is also noteworthy that the magnitude of benefit of the GP IIb/IIIa receptor inhibitors in non-ST-segment elevation ACS has not been as great as observed in the trials of these same agents in the setting of percutaneous intervention. Nevertheless, there were significant reductions in the composite of death and myocardial infarction, particularly during the infusion period of the drug.

In PURSUIT, patients receiving eptifibatide had a 3.2% event rate after the scheduled 72 hours of study drug infusion versus 4.4% in the placebo arm ($P = .003$). The beneficial effects were maintained at 7 days and at 30 days. The PRISM trial demonstrated a reduction in events rates during the 48-hour period of study drug infusion (death, myocardial infarction, or refractory ischemia 3.8% tirofiban group vs 5.6% heparin group, $P = .001$). This reduction was largely a result of a lower rate of recurrent ischemia. Differences in outcomes between the two groups diminished by 30 days (27). The treatment benefit of tirofiban was more durable in the PRISM-PLUS trial (30-day rate of death, myocardial infarction, refractory ischemia, or rehospitalization for unstable angina—18.5% tirofiban plus heparin group vs. 22.3% heparin group, $P = .031$), although this treatment effect did not quite reach the prespecified requirement of statistical significance of $P < .025$ (25). The degree of benefit was clearly greater in those patients who proceeded to percutaneous intervention, with only a nonsignificant trend toward improved outcomes in medically treated patients (30-day composite endpoint rate of 14.8% in tirofiban plus heparin group vs. 16.8% heparin group, risk ratio 0.87 (95% CI 0.60 to 1.25).

The observation that most of the benefit of GP IIb/IIIa receptor inhibition in acute coronary syndromes occurs in patients who proceed to percutaneous revascularization is one of the more contentious issues relating to GP IIb/IIIa receptor blockade. However, in a recent meta-analysis of trials of GP IIb/IIIa inhibition in ACS, an overall 34% reduction in the rate of death or nonfatal myocardial infarction was found during the period of GP IIb/IIIa inhibitor therapy preceding the percutaneous intervention (2.5% vs. 3.8% in placebo group, odds ratio with 95% CI 0.66 [0.54 to 0.81]) (Fig. 4a). An additional 41% reduction in coronary intervention-related events was

Table 2 Short- and Medium-Term Clinical Outcomes from Four Major Randomized Trials of GP IIb/IIIa Receptor Blockade in Unstable Angina or Non-ST-Elevation Myocardial Infarction

	48–96 Hours			30 Days			6 Months		
	Death	MI	Death or MI	Death	MI	Death or MI	Death	MI	Death or MI
PURSUIT									
Placebo (n = 4739)	1.2	8.3	9.1	3.7	13.5	15.7	6.2	15.7	19.0
Eptifibatide (n = 4722)	0.9	7.1	7.6	3.5	12.6	14.2	6.4	14.7	17.8
PRISM PLUS									
Heparin (n = 797)	0.3	2.6	2.6	4.5	9.2	11.9	7.0	10.5	15.3
Tirofiban + heparin (n = 773)	0.1	0.9	0.9	3.6	6.6	8.7	6.9	8.3	12.3
PRISM									
Heparin (n = 1616)	0.4	1.4	1.4	3.6	4.3	7.1	—	—	—
Tirofiban (n = 1616)	0.2	0.9	0.9	2.3	4.1	5.8	—	—	—
PARAGON A									
Placebo (n = 758)	0.5	3.3	3.7	2.9	10.6	11.7	6.6	14.3	17.9
Lamifiban (low-dose) (n = 755)	0.3	3.5	3.5	3.0	9.4	10.6	5.2	10.8	13.7
Lamifiban (high-dose) (n = 769)	0.4	2.5	2.6	3.6	10.9	12.0	6.8	12.9	16.4

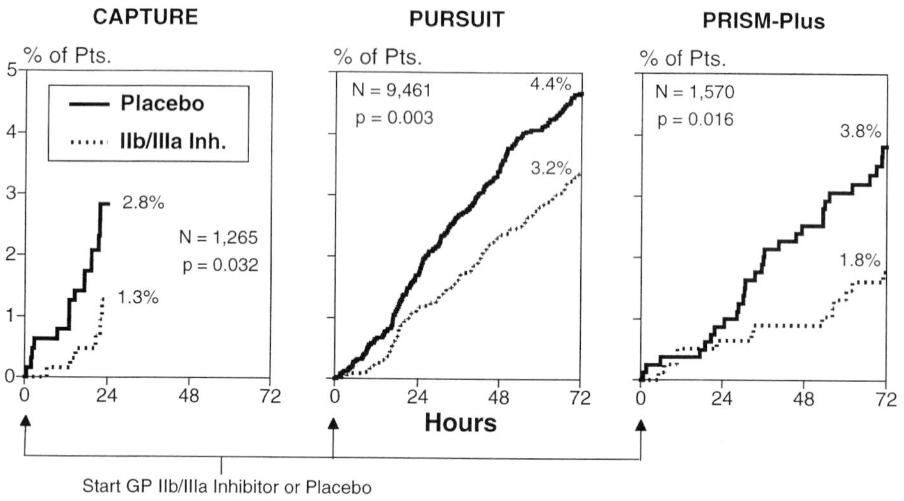

Figure 4a Kaplan-Meier curves showing the cumulative incidence of death or nonfatal myocardial infarction during the initial period of pharmacological therapy until time of percutaneous coronary intervention or coronary artery bypass surgery, if performed, from the CAPTURE, PURSUIT, and PRISM-PLUS trials.

also observed (4.9% vs. 8.0%, odds ratio 0.59 [0.44 to 0.81]) (Fig. 4b). Reductions in death rates were small but statistically significant with GP IIb/IIIa receptor inhibitor therapy both during the period of medical therapy and in the periprocedural period (28). Thus, the effect of glycoprotein IIb/IIIa receptor inhibition early in the management of acute coronary syndromes appears to be additive to its effects during percutaneous intervention.

From these data, significant clinical benefit can be anticipated from the early initiation of these drugs for the treatment of patients with non-ST-segment elevation acute coronary syndromes. Yet, the dilemma of whether patients should be taken to the catheterization laboratory early, or stabilized first with small-molecule GP IIb/IIIa receptor inhibitor treatment remains unresolved. The approach of early intervention with stenting and abciximab in patients presenting with acute coronary syndromes was highly effective in the EPISTENT trial, with a 47% reduction in death or large myocardial infarction at 6 months seen with the combination of stenting and abciximab compared with stenting alone (4.0% stent and abciximab vs. 9.5% stent and placebo) (29). In fact, combination therapies of GP IIb/IIIa receptor blockade and percutaneous revascularization may be the key to unravelling the apparent paradox that early invasive therapy after presentation with non-ST-segment elevation ACS is deleterious as suggested in the VANQWISH trial

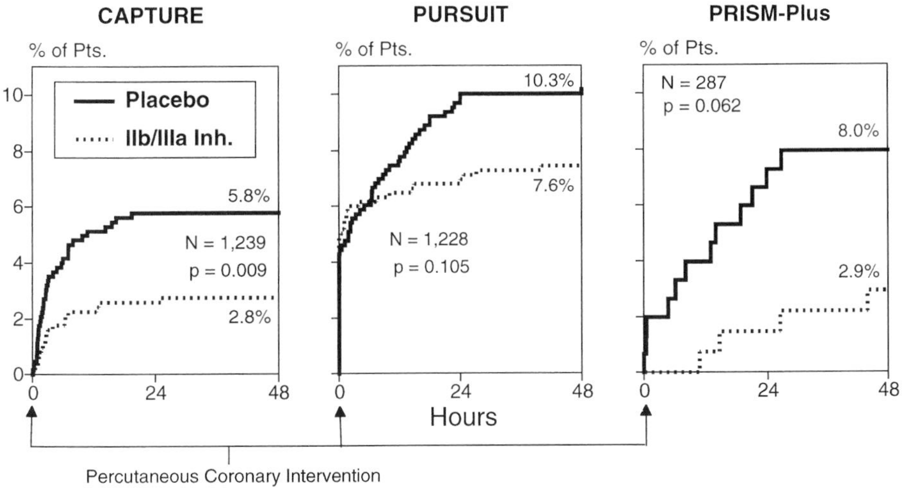

Figure 4b Kaplan-Meier curves showing the cumulative incidence of death or nonfatal myocardial infarction among patients undergoing percutaneous coronary intervention in the 48-hour period after the procedure. Patients received study medication during and for a short period after the procedure.

and other studies (30,31). These trials failed to reflect contemporaneous practices—particularly the widespread use of intravenous GP IIb/IIIa receptor blockade and coronary stents. In a recent trial of dalteparin therapy for unstable angina, stents were used in more than two-thirds of the study population, and an early invasive approach proved more beneficial in high-risk patients than a more conservative approach (32). The TACTICS trial was designed to further evaluate the use of tirofiban with either an early invasive or conservative approach to the treatment of unstable angina/non-ST-elevation myocardial infarction (33). Enrollment is complete and results of this trial will be available in late 2000.

The place of concomitant heparin therapy with GP IIb/IIIa receptor blockade in acute coronary syndromes has been difficult to determine from the results of the trials conducted to date. In the PRISM-PLUS trial, the arm of tirofiban without heparin was stopped prematurely because of an excess of early mortality. Therefore, a formal comparison of the heparin and no heparin arms was not possible. The PRISM trial directly compared tirofiban with a heparin control arm, but tirofiban combined with heparin was not tested. In PURSUIT, investigators were actively encouraged to use heparin with the study drug, eptifibatide, although this was not done in a systematic manner. The only truly randomized assessment of concomitant heparin usage

Table 3 Six-Month Efficacy Endpoints from the PARAGON Trial of High- or Low-Dose Lamifiban With or Without Heparin in Unstable Angina/Non-ST-Elevation Myocardial Infarction

Treatment arm	Death (%)	MI (%)	Death/MI (%)	Odds ratio death/MI (95% CI)
Heparin alone (control)	6.6	14.3	17.9	
Low-dose lamifiban + heparin	4.8	10.5	12.6	0.66 (0.46, 0.95)
Low-dose lamifiban + no heparin	5.6	11.1	14.7	0.79 (0.56, 1.12)
High-dose lamifiban + heparin	7.6	13.9	18.0	1.01 (0.73, 1.40)
High-dose lamifiban + no heparin	6.1	12.0	14.8	0.80 (0.57, 1.12)
All low-dose lamifiban ± heparin	5.2	10.8	13.7	0.73 (0.55, 0.97)
All high-dose lamifiban ± heparin	6.8	12.9	16.4	0.90 (0.69, 1.18)
All lamifiban + heparin	6.2	12.2	15.3	0.83 (0.63, 1.09)
All lamifiban + no heparin	5.9	11.6	14.8	0.80 (0.60, 1.05)

was conducted in the PARAGON A trial, and its results were inconclusive as shown in Table 3. However, the trial did show a late separation in ischemic event rates at 6 months between the lamifiban and placebo groups. The treatment effect was actually better in all lamifiban groups at 6 months compared with 30 days, with the benefit with low-dose lamifiban statistically significant (13.7% vs. 17.9% in the control group, $P = .027$) (26). Moreover, the mortality benefit in the low-dose lamifiban group was sustained to at least 1 year. These findings suggest a potential role for GP IIb/IIIa receptor inhibition prevention of complications in the longer term, possibly through vessel wall passivation. Results from the PARAGON B trial of lamifiban in unstable angina/non-ST-elevation myocardial infarction and the GUSTO-IV trial of abciximab in acute coronary syndromes, both due for release in late 2000, should help clarify these issues further.

Glycoprotein IIb/IIIa Receptor Inhibitors in Acute Myocardial Infarction

For over a decade, thrombolysis has set the standard for reperfusion therapy in evolving acute myocardial infarction. However, despite its ubiquity, failure to achieve complete and sustained reperfusion can be expected in up to

50% of treated patients (34). Thrombolytic therapy is still associated with rates of intracerebral hemorrhage of up to 1.0%, especially when its use is extended to elderly patients and those with a history of hypertension (35–37). Much lower rates of bleeding are seen with catheter-based reperfusion treatment, and although its comparative benefit with thrombolysis has been contentious (38,39), longer-term studies now point to percutaneous intervention as the more beneficial reperfusion treatment (40). The application of catheter-based reperfusion will never be as freely available as drug-based therapies, and both treatment options remain viable alternatives. Both techniques are strongly influenced by the effects of platelets and have become highly suitable targets for adjunctive potent platelet antagonism.

GP IIb/IIIa Receptor Inhibitors in Pharmacological Reperfusion Therapy

Platelets are at the core of coronary thrombosis, with their activation, adhesion to the exposed subendothelial matrix and resultant aggregation, and platelet plug formation forming the nidus for ongoing "red clot" formation with deposition of erythrocytes and fibrin. Platelet thrombus is resistant to thrombolytic therapy and paradoxically, further platelet aggregation can ensue in the presence of fibrinolytic agents due to exposure of thrombin within the clot, and the release of plasminogen activator inhibitor-I (PAI-1) from activated platelets (Fig. 5). Experimental studies have clearly demonstrated that more rapid, effective, and stable thrombolysis can be achieved with reduced doses of fibrinolytics in the presence of GP IIb/IIIa receptor blockade (41–44). Advantages of this approach include the avoidance of an overly prothrombotic environment seen with higher-dose fibrinolytics, reduced cost of thrombolytic and potential reduction in bleeding risk.

Three small pilot trials combined (full-dose) thrombolytic therapy with GP IIb/IIIa receptor blockade, with the resultant risk-benefit tradeoff favorable enough to trigger larger-scale evaluation of this therapeutic combination. Trends toward improvements in vessel patency and clinical outcomes were observed in the Eighth Thrombolysis and Myocardial Infarction (TAMI-8) project (45)—one of the earliest clinical trials with GP IIb/IIIa receptor inhibition as adjunctive therapy to thrombolysis—and the Integrilin to Minimize Platelet Aggregation and Prevent Coronary Thrombosis–Acute Myocardial Infarction (IMPACT-AMI) trial (46). Significant improvements in the speed and stability of reperfusion as measured by electrocardiographic monitoring were found in a dose-ranging Phase II trial with lamifiban (47). While encouraging trends were evident in this trial, there were no statistically significant differences in angiographic measures of reperfusion (TIMI grade 3 flow), assessed either early, at 60 to 90 min, or prior to discharge.

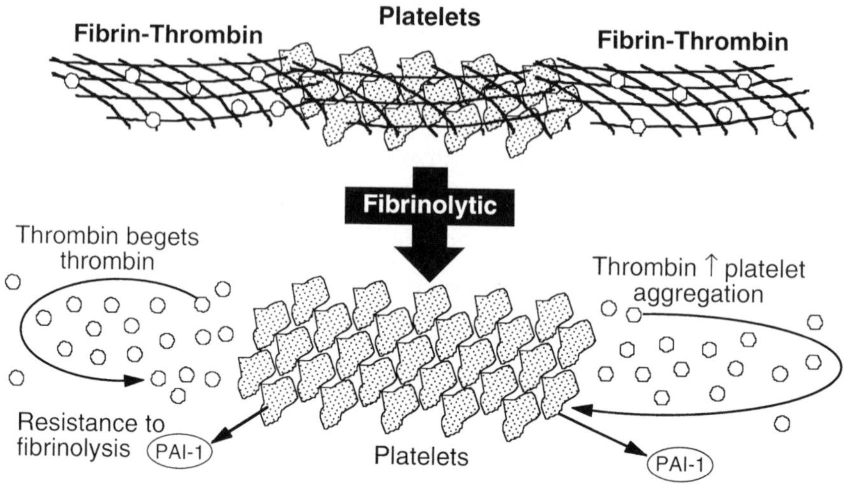

Figure 5 Schematic illustration of the prothrombotic effects of fibrinolytic therapy. With fibrinolysis, thrombin, previously bound to clot, is reexposed to the circulation. Thrombin is a potent platelet agonist and promotes further platelet aggregation. Platelets themselves are resistant to fibrinolytic therapy and secrete plasminogen activator inhibitor-1 (PAI-1) which antagonizes the action of the fibrinolytic agents. (From Topol EJ. Circulation 1998;97:211–218.)

Two Phase II trials significantly advanced the experience of combined reduced-dose thrombolytic and GP IIb/IIIa receptor blockade. In the Thrombolysis in Myocardial Infarction (TIMI)-14 dose escalation trial, patients with acute myocardial infarction were randomized to abciximab plus reduced dose t-PA or streptokinase or full-dose fibrinolytic therapy alone in an open-label design (48). Fourteen different reperfusion regimens were evaluated. The trial found that abciximab together with streptokinase regimens ranging in dose from 500,000 units to 1.25 million units resulted in modest improvements in restoration of normal (TIMI grade 3) flow at 90 min in the range of 34% to 46% of patients treated. The incidence of bleeding was related to the dose of streptokinase, ultimately producing an unacceptable bleeding risk with full-dose streptokinase and abciximab (even in the absence of heparin), and early termination of this arm of the trial. Greater therapeutic efficacy was achieved in the reduced-dose t-PA (alteplase) arms. With 50 mg of t-PA over 60 min, abciximab and low-dose, weight-adjusted heparin, 90-min TIMI 3 flow rates of 76% were achieved compared with TIMI-3 flow rates of 57% in the conventional accelerated full-dose t-PA arm ($P = .08$). Bleeding risk was no greater than with standard thrombolytic therapy. Both a low-dose and very low dose heparin regimen were tested in conjunction with alteplase and abciximab. The TIMI-3 flow rates were intermediate between the full-dose alteplase control arm and the most effective regimen of 50 mg alteplase and low-dose heparin (Fig. 6). The rate of major hemorrhage was 7% in the low-dose heparin group and 1% in the very low dose heparin arm (48).

The Strategies for Patency Enhancement in the Emergency Department (SPEED) trial restricted its thrombolytic use to reteplase only. Doses of reteplase ranging from 5 units to 10 units either as a single bolus or as a double bolus of 5 units and 5 units separated by 30 min were tested. Figure 7 provides a comparison of TIMI-3 flow rates at 60 min for various combinations of reteplase and abciximab. As seen in several other series, abciximab alone had only a modest effect on reperfusion. Overall, there appeared to be a dose relationship between reteplase and successful reperfusion, with the most successful strategy of a double bolus dose of 5 units and 5 units of reteplase and abciximab achieving complete reperfusion in 62% of patients. A very low dose heparin regimen was also tested against a low-dose

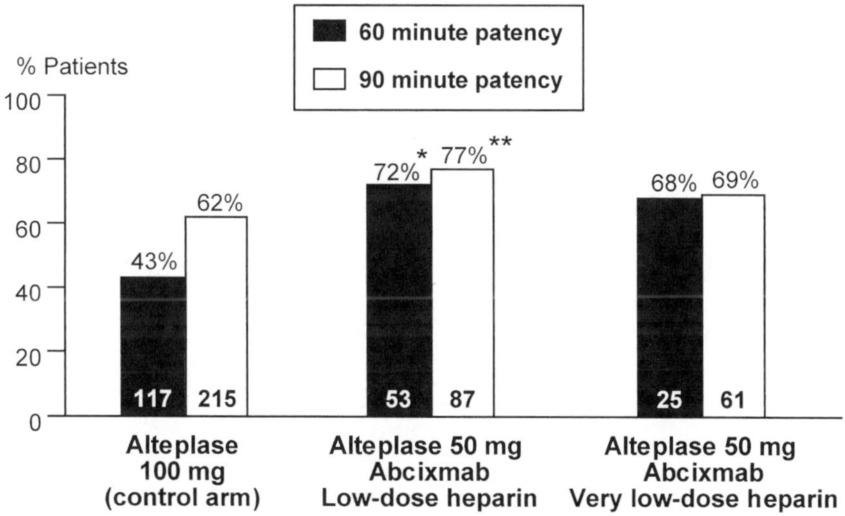

Figure 6 Percentage of patients with TIMI grade 3 flow at 60 min and 90 min in the TIMI-14 trial. The control group of alteplase 100 mg in accelerated dose regimen is compared with the regimens of alteplase 50 mg over 60 min, abciximab, and either low-dose heparin (60 U/kg bolus and infusion of 7 U/kg/h) or very low dose heparin (30 U/kg bolus and infusion of 4 U/kg/h). Significant increases in TIMI grade 3 flow rates were evident in the 50-mg alteplase, abciximab, and low-dose heparin regimen at 60 and 90 min, compared with the control arm.
**P* = .0009; ***P* = .01.

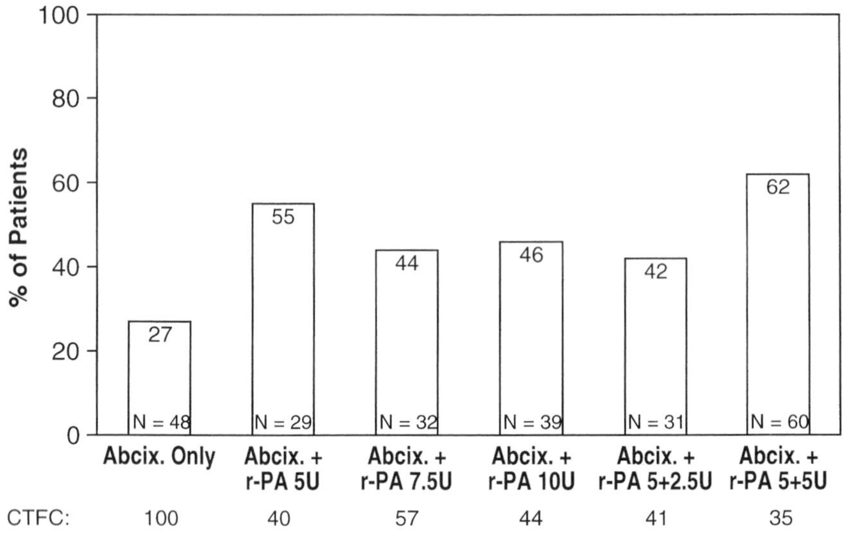

Figure 7 TIMI grade 3 flow rates at 60 min from in the GUSTO-IV pilot (SPEED) trial. CTFC—corrected TIMI frame count.

regimen with reteplase 5 + 5 units double bolus and abciximab. A trend toward better clinical outcomes was seen in the very low dose heparin arm, with no major differences in major bleeding event rates between the two groups (49).

While these trials collectively have ushered in an era of enhanced pharmacological reperfusion therapy, many therapeutic questions remain to be answered. The whole issue of appropriate heparin dosing in conjunction with combination GP IIb/IIIa receptor inhibition and thrombolysis is still uncertain, and to what extent very low dose heparin regimens will be both effective and safe will need further large-scale evaluation. Similarly, the interventional cardiological community is likely to demand randomized trials to establish the equivalence or superiority of enhanced pharmacological reperfusion therapy compared with emergent percutaneous intervention. Other trials will be needed to determine whether abciximab is the most effective GP IIb/IIIa inhibitor in combination with reduced dose thrombolysis, or whether there will be place for other GP IIb/IIIa receptor inhibitors as well. The combination of abciximab, a double bolus of 5 + 5 units reteplase, and low-dose, weight-adjusted heparin is currently being evaluated in the large-scale, clinical Phase III Global Use of Strategies to Open Occluded Arteries (GUSTO) IV trial (Fig. 8).

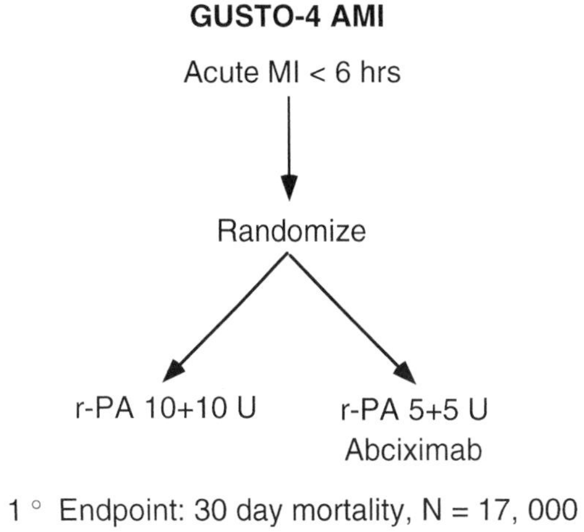

Figure 8 Schematic of the design of the large-scale, international, multicenter, randomized GUSTO-IV AMI trial.

GP IIb/IIIa Receptor Inhibitors as Adjuncts to Mechanical Reperfusion Therapy

Early indication of the potential benefit of GP IIb/IIIa receptor blockade in the setting of percutaneous intervention for acute myocardial infarction was evident in the Evaluation of c7E3 for Prevention of Ischemic Complications (EPIC) trial (50). Its use has subsequently been assessed both as a pretreatment and as conjunctive therapy during primary angioplasty. In small pilot studies, abciximab given as a pretreatment in the emergency room prior to primary angioplasty resulted in preprocedure TIMI-3 flow rates of around 20% (51,52). Similar reperfusion rates of between 20% and 40% were also seen among the control groups in TIMI-14 (48) and the GUSTO-IV pilot trials (49).

In the ReoPro and Primary PTCA Organization and Randomized Trial (RAPPORT) of adjunctive GP IIb/IIIa receptor inhibition during infarct angioplasty, a total of 483 patients with evolving myocardial infarction were assigned to either a bolus and 12-hour infusion of abciximab or matching placebo. A significant reduction in the composite of death, recurrent myocardial infarction, or need for urgent repeat revascularization was noted at 7 and 30 days (53) (Fig. 9). The results of RAPPORT were also notable for the excessive incidence of major bleeding—mainly owing to high conjunctive heparin dosing. The Abciximab before Direct Angioplasty and Stenting in Myocardial Infarction Regarding Acute and Long-Term Follow-Up (AD-

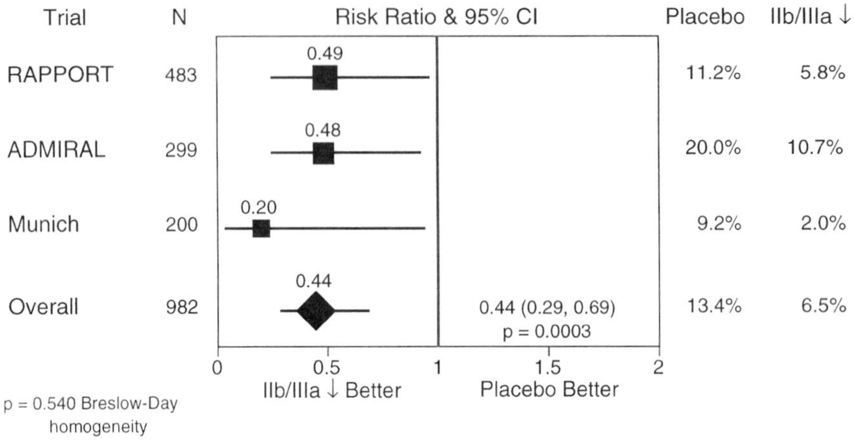

Figure 9 Risk ratios plots with 95% CI for the combined endpoint of death, (re)infarction, or urgent revascularization from the RAPPORT (53), ADMIRAL (54), and Munich (57) randomized trials of abciximab use during percutaneous intervention for acute myocardial infarction.

MIRAL) trial reflected a more contemporary approach to primary angioplasty (54). A much higher rate of stent usage was seen (85%), and low-dose, weight-adjusted heparin was administered to avoid the high incidence of bleeding complications as seen in RAPPORT. Once again, 30-day ischemic endpoints were significantly reduced by the use of abciximab, with a 46% reduction in the composite of death, nonfatal reinfarction, or need for urgent revascularization in the abciximab group ($P < .03$) (Fig. 9). Noncoronary artery bypass surgery major bleeding rates were similar in the two groups, although the incidence of minor bleeding events was approximately threefold greater in abciximab treated patients (6.7% abciximab group vs. 1.3% placebo group, $P = .02$).

The Controlled Abciximab and Device Investigation to Lower Late Angioplasty Complications (CADILLAC) trial (55) compared the effects of balloon angioplasty (with or without abciximab) and stenting (with or without abciximab) in acute myocardial infarction. Early results from this trial indicated that TIMI-3 flow rates are lower following stenting compared with balloon angioplasty alone (92.1% stent group vs. 94.8% PTCA group) and confirmed similar observations in other trials (56). The use of abciximab prevented this decline in TIMI-3 flow in stented patients, as well as reduced in-hospital recurrent ischemia and target lesion revascularization for recurrent ischemia. Further proof of benefit with abciximab use in stenting for acute myocardial infarction was seen at 14 days in a trial by Neumann and colleagues (57). Utilizing Doppler flow wire measurements and assessment of regional wall motion, they demonstrated significant improvements in microvascular perfusion and enhanced recovery of contractile function in the area at risk with the use of abciximab. Importantly, the coadministration of abciximab in all these trials of mechanical reperfusion in acute myocardial infarction did not increase the risk of intracerebral hemorrhage.

One of the strongest indications for concomitant GP IIb/IIIa receptor blockade is in the setting of urgent angioplasty for failed thrombolysis (rescue PTCA). While this particular clinical setting has not been subjected to a randomized comparison of GP IIb/IIIa receptor inhibition and placebo, a retrospective subgroup analysis of the GUSTO-III trial demonstrated markedly improved outcomes in patients undergoing rescue PTCA who also received abciximab (58). In a nonrandomized cohort of 392 patients requiring percutaneous intervention for failed thrombolysis, 83 (21%) received abciximab. There was a strong trend toward lower 30-day mortality in abciximab-treated patients (3.6% abciximab group vs. 9.7% no abciximab, $P = .076$), with the difference achieving statistical significance after adjustment for baseline differences ($P = .042$). Interestingly, the complications of death, reinfarction or stroke occurred less often when abciximab followed reteplase compared with alteplase (7% vs. 21%, $P = .08$). The numbers in each group were small (reteplase n = 55, alteplase n = 28), but this finding does raise the question of whether concomitant GP IIb/IIIa receptor inhibition may have differential effects when combined with various thrombolytic agents. Further studies are required to answer this question.

Percutaneous Coronary Intervention for Acute Coronary Syndromes

Extensive clinical trial experience has now been gained with the application of GP IIb/IIIa receptor blockade to percutaneous coronary intervention. Although the large-scale trials (59–65) were not primarily designed to evaluate patients with acute coronary syndromes, the EPIC and Randomized Efficacy Study of Tirofiban for Outcomes and Restenosis (RESTORE) trials limited enrollment to high-risk patients, with either an acute coronary syndrome or clinical and/or angiographic features indicating an increased risk of complications. The EPIC trial in particular showed a highly significant reduction in the composite event rate in the subgroup of patients with unstable angina (66). Follow-up in the EPIC trial extended to 3 years found a 60% reduction in long-term mortality with abciximab among the 555 patients enrolled with unstable angina or acute myocardial infarction (12.7% ACS group vs. 5.1% patients without ACS, $P = .01$) (67). In the more recent Evaluation of Platelet Inhibition in Stenting (EPISTENT) trial that evaluated the contemporary practice of stenting, the addition of abciximab to stenting resulted in significant reductions in the incidence of death or myocardial infarction at 6 months when abciximab was added to stenting or balloon angioplasty compared with stenting alone. This effect was particularly evident in patients presenting with unstable angina (63).

ONGOING CLINICAL ISSUES IN THE USE OF GLYCOPROTEIN IIb/IIIa RECEPTOR INHIBITORS

Effects of GP IIb/IIIa Receptor Blockade on the Microcirculation

There can now be little doubt about the prognostic importance of small elevations in markers of myocardial injury that would otherwise have been considered clinically insignificant (68). Several series have convincingly demonstrated worse long-term outcomes in patients with elevations in creatine kinase following percutaneous coronary intervention (69–72). Novel techniques with devices such as emboli containment guidewires have highlighted the frequency and extent of embolization that occur during percutaneous intervention (73). Release of creatine kinase, presumably by embolization of platelet thrombus, is suppressed with GP IIb/IIIa receptor blockade (63,74,75) with resultant reductions in virtually all of the major endpoints of death, emergency bypass surgery, and emergency repeat percutaneous coronary intervention.

In the setting of acute coronary syndromes, both troponin I and troponin T are identified as specific and highly sensitive markers of minor myocardial injury. Raised levels of these enzymes are strong predictors of cardiac risk (76–80). Recent analyses of both the PRISM (81) and CAPTURE (82) trials have indicated that as well as stratifying patients' cardiac risk, elevations in troponin I and troponin T may have important bearing on the responsiveness of these patients to GP IIb/IIIa receptor blockade. In the PRISM trial, the established relationship between elevation of these enzymes and worse outcomes was evident with a greater than twofold increase in 30-day death or myocardial infarction rates in patients with troponin I levels greater than the threshold of 0.1 μg/L (13.0% troponin I-positive patients vs. 4.9% troponin I-negative patients, $P < .001$). The interaction between elevations in troponins and benefit with tirofiban was striking, as shown in Figure 10. Tirofiban treatment resulted in significant reductions in the risk of both death and myocardial infarction in troponin I-positive patients, but no treatment effect was seen in troponin I-negative patients. This beneficial effect of tirofiban extended to both patients managed medically and to those who proceeded to percutaneous intervention (81) (Fig. 11).

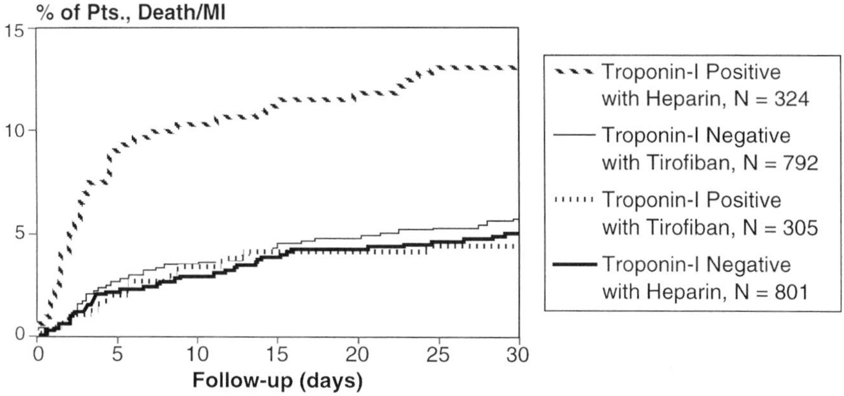

Figure 10 Event rate curves for death or nonfatal myocardial infarction for 30-day follow-up in patients with troponin I concentrations higher and lower than the threshold of 1.0 μg/L from the PRISM trial.

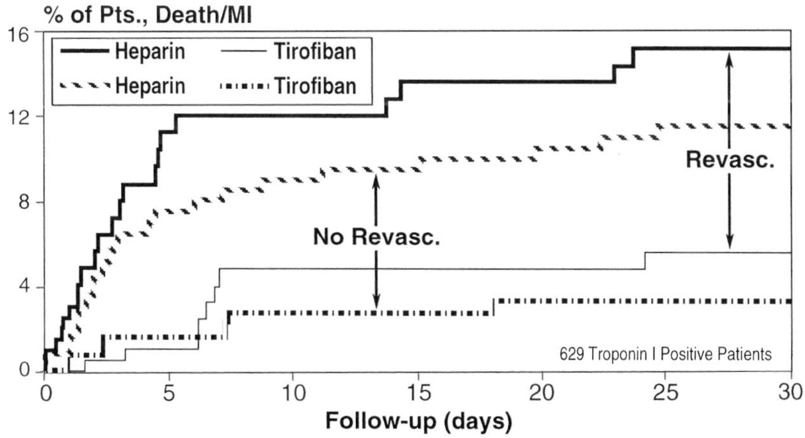

Figure 11 Event rate curves for death or nonfatal myocardial infarction for 30-day follow-up in patients with elevations in troponin I by treatment group after 48 hours of study medication in the PRISM trial. Patients treated medically are compared with those who underwent either surgical or percutaneous revascularization.

The interaction between GP IIb/IIIa receptor blockade and troponin elevations is not limited to the small-molecule GP IIb/IIIa antagonists. A similar effect was observed with abciximab in a posthoc analysis of the CAPTURE trial. Troponin T levels were elevated in 31% of 890 patients in the trial who had serum samples available for analysis. There was a relative risk of death or myocardial infarction of 0.32 (95% confidence interval 0.14 to 0.62) with abciximab therapy as compared with placebo in those patients with elevated troponin T, but no benefit of treatment with abciximab in troponin T-negative patients. The majority of the benefit of abciximab was in the reduction of myocardial infarction (82).

Elevations in troponin I and troponin T are associated with unstable coronary lesions and are considered surrogate markers for the presence of thrombus (83,84). In both coronary intervention and acute coronary syndromes, the prevention and treatment of intracoronary thrombus have key benefits on patient outcomes. The relationship of GP IIb/IIIa receptor blockade and troponin elevations is testament to the importance of treating platelet thrombus and protecting the microcirculation from platelet microthrombi embolization. It is intriguing that a similar relationship between GP IIb/IIIa inhibition and elevated creatine kinase MB fractions was not evident in either the PRISM or CAPTURE, and suggests that the troponin enzymes have specific characteristics as markers of disease extent and activity. These findings may serve as a basis for a more refined approach to the treatment of high-risk patients with unstable angina.

Comparative Efficacy of GP IIb/IIIa Receptor Inhibitors

Despite the consistency of effect of GP IIb/IIIa receptor blockade in the reduction of clinically important events of death and nonfatal myocardial infarction, disparate findings among individual trials raise the question of comparative efficacy among the various agents. No direct comparisons of the different intravenous agents have been made in a randomized clinical trial. However, in a comparison of ex vivo platelet function in a small cohort of patients randomized to abciximab, eptifibatide, or tirofiban, tirofiban had a delayed onset of maximal platelet inhibition and reduced intensity of platelet inhibition measured by platelet aggregometry compared to either of the other two agents (85). Yet, abciximab stands apart from the small molecule agents with its antithrombotic properties additional to its antiplatelet actions. By dampening and delaying thrombin generation, abciximab may affect the endothelium (86), cellular proliferation (87), and the release of platelet derived growth factor and other cytokines (88–90). Its equivalent blocking action on the vitronectin integrin receptor $\alpha_v\beta_3$ may also account for some of its beneficial effects in angioplasty, as the vitronectin receptor has been implicated in the processes of neointimal proliferation (91) and restenosis (92,93). Nevertheless, it remains uncertain whether any of these apparent differences among the various intravenous agents accounts for true differences in clinical outcomes.

Both the dose and duration of a particular GP IIb/IIIa inhibitor treatment may have a critical influence on the clinical efficacy of the agent. It is now clear that an inadequate dose of eptifibatide was used in the IMPACT II trial and may, at least in part, have been responsible for its less pronounced treatment effect. The use of citrate in the standard platelet aggregation assays employed in the pilot dose-ranging IMPACT I and the IMPACT II trials resulted in a gross overestimation of the platelet inhibitory capacity of doses of eptifibatide chosen (94). A more positive treatment effect was seen with eptifibatide when it was administered in higher doses in PURSUIT (24). On the other hand, patients undergoing coronary intervention with tirofiban in PRISM-PLUS had a more substantial treatment effect than was seen with the same drug in the RESTORE trial, even though the dose used in RESTORE was significantly higher. The longer minimum duration of tirofiban infusion in PRISM-PLUS of 48 hours may have played a role as compared with the 36 hours minimum in RESTORE. This would suggest that for the small-molecule agents, with their rapidly reversible pharmacokinetics, a more prolonged duration of treatment up to 72 hours or more may be more important than the actual dose of the drug used. However, it is important to highlight that differences in patient population, endpoints, and interventional procedures may also account for the variability in absolute or proportionate risk reduction.

GP IIb/IIIa Receptor Inhibition and Bleeding Risk

There is little doubt that the single greatest potential drawback of glycoprotein IIb/IIIa receptor blockade in any clinical setting is the risk of bleeding. The first ever major trial of a GP IIb/IIIa receptor inhibitor showed an unacceptable doubling of risk for major bleeds with bolus and infusion of abciximab (59). The hazards of an excessive bleeding risk go well beyond increasing the associated morbidity for treated patients. Length of stay, cost of treatment, and quality-of-life assessments can all be adversely affected. Major bleeding events are thought to have resulted in premature cessation of drug treatment in up to 3.5% of patients enrolled in the large clinical trials (95), further limiting the potential efficacy of this class of agent.

A relationship among patient weight, activated clotting time, and risk of bleeding with abciximab was seen in the EPIC trial of percutaneous intervention, and these findings suggested that dose weight adjustments and tight control of the degree of associated anticoagulation may result in a lower risk of bleeding (96). Similarly, the addition of intravenous heparin to GP IIb/IIIa receptor blockade for the treatment of acute coronary syndromes may also increase bleeding risk. In the pilot Canadian Lamifiban Study of patients with unstable angina (97) and the subsequent PARAGON trial, combination of high-dose lamifiban and heparin was associated with an approximately twofold increase in major bleeds compared with any of the other treatment arms (26). Nevertheless, the bleeding risk in this and other trials of acute coronary syndromes has generally been acceptably low (20). Importantly, the incidence of intracerebral hemorrhage remains very low, with no apparent increase across any of the placebo-controlled trials.

The lingering concern about the bleeding potential of GP IIb/IIIa receptor blockade relates to its use immediately prior to coronary artery bypass surgery. While emergency coronary artery bypass surgery following failed percutaneous intervention occurs rarely now, therapy with GP IIb/IIIa receptor blockade may frequently be encountered in patients with acute coronary syndromes who proceed to coronary artery bypass surgery. Data from the EPIC, IMPACT-II and EPILOG trials indicate that coronary artery bypass surgery accounted for 55% to 66% of all major bleeding complications in heparin-treated patients, and 41% to 53% of major bleeding episodes in patients treated with both heparin and a GP IIb/IIIa receptor inhibitor. This would suggest that GP IIb/IIIa receptor blockade itself is not a major factor in this bleeding risk. In the case of the small-molecule agents, the absence of an excessive perioperative bleeding risk (24,25) probably relates to their short duration of action and rapid reversibility of effect. However, even the longer-acting abciximab has been shown to actually be protective during coronary bypass, with less thrombocytopenia and better platelet function after cardiopulmonary bypass (98). Currently, there are no comparative data to indicate any differences in bleeding risk related to coronary artery bypass surgery among the various GP IIb/IIIa inhibitors. In cases of hemorrhagic complications, transfusion of mixed donor platelets prior to cardiac surgery can minimize the risk of bleeding associated with abciximab (99), while fresh-frozen plasma or cryoprecipitate provides additional fibrinogen to compete with the small-molecule antagonists for GP IIb/III receptor occupancy.

Economic Issues

In health environments with ever-increasing demands and limited resources, the clinical benefits of GP IIb/IIIa receptor blockade in both acute coronary syndromes and percutaneous intervention cannot be properly evaluated without regard to their associated costs and cost-effectiveness. An economic substudy from the EPIC trial was the first to prospectively collect cost data on glycoprotein IIb/IIIa receptor inhibitor use (100). Savings in medical costs due to reduced cardiac events at discharge and at 6-month follow-up partially offset the drug's procurements costs. The net incremental cost of abciximab treatment was approximately $1350 at hospital discharge and $300 at 6-month follow-up (100). Greater cost savings were expected in the EPILOG trial (61) because of the reduced rates of bleeding (and its associated costs) compared with EPIC. However, EPILOG did not demonstrate reductions in ischemic events at 6 months, as seen in the EPIC trial, and the incremental cost of abciximab in this trial was approximately $533 at hospital discharge, but $1180 at 6-month follow-up (101). Cost analysis from the RESTORE trial showed that the incremental cost of tirofiban use was similar to that of abciximab in the EPILOG trial (102).

To date, there have been no reports directly assessing costs of GP IIb/IIIa receptor inhibitor therapy for acute coronary syndromes. However, the incremental efficacy of the various GP IIb/IIIa receptor inhibitors (expressed as the number of patients needed to undergo treatment to prevent one adverse outcome) can be obtained from the various trials in ACS and used to calculate cost-effectiveness. From these data, Hillegass and colleagues performed a cost-effectiveness analysis of the GP IIb/IIIa receptor inhibitors, calculating the drug costs incurred to prevent one death or myocardial infarction at 30 days (103) (Table 4). As a group, GP IIb/IIIa receptor inhibitors appear to be more cost-effective when used in percutaneous intervention than in ACS. With angioplasty, the cost of preventing a death or

Table 4 Costs of GP IIb/IIIa Inhibitors to Prevent One Death or Myocardial Infarction at 30 Days

Drug	Mean duration of infusion (h)	Drug cost in 70-kg patient	Drug cost per death or MI prevented
Abciximab			
EPIC trial	12	$1407	$15,477
EPILOG trial	12	1407	22,512
EPISTENT trial	12	1407	13,648
Tirofiban			
PRISM trial	48	700	53,900
PRISM-PLUS trial	71	1050	32,550
RESTORE trial	36	700	37,100
Eptifibatide			
PURSUIT trial	72	1223	81,941
IMPACT trial	22	436	29,212

Source: Ref. 103.

myocardial infarction can range from $13,000 to $23,000 for abciximab and up to $57,000 for tirofiban. When used to treat acute coronary syndromes, the cost of tirofiban to prevent one death or myocardial infarction in medically treated patients in the PRISM trials was in the range of $40,000, while eptifibatide was associated with a cost of $80,000 for each death or myocardial infarction prevented in PURSUIT (103). While abciximab was more cost-effective than the small-molecule agents when used during percutaneous intervention, there are insufficient data to determine the relative cost-effectiveness of the various GP IIb/IIIa inhibitors in the treatment of ACS.

Several limitations exist with analyses like these, especially as they focus on drug procurement costs rather than the total cost of treatment which may also include other costs such as bed days. Known (and unknown) differences in the populations studied in these trials as well as different definitions of endpoints such as myocardial infarction may also affect the analyses. However, an economic analysis of the 1-year results of the EPISTENT trial of abciximab and stenting in percutaneous intervention demonstrated cost-effectiveness ratios for GP IIb/IIIa inhibitor usage that Western health care systems would consider affordable (29). Compared with the strategies of stenting alone or balloon angioplasty with abciximab, the combination of stenting with abciximab cover had an incremental cost effectiveness of $5300 to $6200 per added life-year. This compares quite favorably with other cardiac therapies such as CABG surgery for left main disease ($7000 per life-year saved), tissue plasminogen activator versus streptokinase ($32,000 per life-year saved), and cholesterol reduction as primary prevention therapy ($154,000 per life-year added). Drug procurement costs are much higher when used to treat acute coronary syndromes, and therefore from an economic standpoint it may be appropriate to focus the use of glycoprotein IIb/IIIa receptor inhibitors in this setting to patients at very high risk, in whom the potential clinical benefit is greatest. However, more data are needed in this important area to provide better estimates of the economic impact of these drugs in the setting of acute coronary syndromes.

CONCLUSION

The field of antiplatelet therapy for ischemic cardiovascular disease has rapidly advanced and continues to develop at an accelerated rate. The intravenously administered GP IIb/IIIa receptor inhibitors have proven potent and efficacious agents in the treatment of acute coronary syndromes. However, their role is still likely to evolve, as treating physicians gain more experience with these agents in a spectrum of disease states that is broader and more varied than those mandated by the various trials' inclusion criteria. New treatment modalities for acute ischemic heart disease continue to enter the clinical arena, and the relative place of agents as disparate as low-molecular-weight heparins, angiotensin-converting enzymes, and lipid-lowering agents will all need to be fitted in with platelet antagonists to tailor the most effective treatment strategy for an individual patient. The future promises other and novel approaches to control of platelet function, including inhibition of alternate platelet integrins and prevention of platelet adhesion. While much of this remains uncertain, it is now clear that we have moved into an era "beyond aspirin" in terms of antiplatelet therapeutics, and that control of the pivotal platelet thrombus will endure as a fundamental principle in the management of acute coronary disease.

REFERENCES

1. MacIsaac AI, Thomas JD, Topol EJ. Toward the quiescent plaque. J Am Coll Cardiol 1993;22:1228–1241.
2. Fuster V, Badimon L, Badimon JJ, Chesebro JH. The pathogenesis of coronary artery disease and the acute coronary syndromes (part 1). N Engl J Med 1992;326:242–250.
3. Fuster V, Badimon L, Badimon JJ, Chesebro JH. The pathogenesis of coronary artery disease and the acute coronary syndromes (part 2). N Engl J Med 1992;326:310–318.
4. Fernandez-Ortiz A, Badimon JJ, Falk E, et al. Characterization of the relative thrombogenicity of atherosclerotic plaque components: implications for plaque rupture. J Am Coll Cardiol 1994;23:1562–1569.
5. Badimon L, Badimon JJ. Mechanisms of arterial thrombosis in nonparallel streamlines: platelet thrombi grow on the apex of stenotic severely injured vessel wall. J Clin Invest 1989;84:1134–1144.
6. Trip MD, Cats VM, van Capelle FJL, Vreeken J. Platelet hyperreactivity and prognosis in survivors of myocardial infarction. N Engl J Med 1990;322:1549–1554.
7. Prins MH, Hirsh J. A critical review of the relationship between impaired fibrinolysis and myocardial infarction. Am Heart J 1991;122:545–551.
8. Lam J, Latour J, Lesperance J, Waters D. Platelet aggregation, coronary artery disease progression and future coronary events. Am J Cardiol 1994;73:333–338.
9. Lefkovits J, Plow EF, Topol EJ. Platelet glycoprotein IIb/IIIa receptors in cardiovascular medicine. N Engl J Med 1995;332:1553–1559.
10. Hynes RO. Integrins: a family of cell surface receptors. Cell 1987;48:549–554.
11. Ginsberg MH, Xiaoping D, O'Toole TE, et al. Platelet integrins. Thromb Haemost 1993;70:87–93.
12. Phillips DR, Charo IF, Scarborough RM. GPIIb-IIIa: the responsive integrin. Cell 1991;65:359–362.

13. Phillips DR, Charo IF, Parise LV, Fitzgerald LA. The platelet membrane glycoprotein IIb-IIIa complex. Blood 1988;71:831–843.
14. Ruggeri ZM, De Marco L, Gatti L, et al. Platelets have more than one binding site for von Willebrand factor. J Clin Invest 1983;72:1–12.
15. Pytela R, Pierschbacher MD, Ginsberg MH, et al. Platelet membrane glycoprotein IIb/IIIa: member of a family of RGD specific adhesion receptors. Science 1986;231:1559–1562.
16. Pierschbacher MD, Ruoslahti E. Cell attachment activity of fibronectin can be duplicated by small synthetic fragments of the molecule. Nature 1984;309: 30–33.
17. Kloczewiak M, Timmons S, Hawiger J. Recognition site for the platelet receptor is present on the 15-residue carboxy-terminal fragment of the gamma chain of human fibrinogen and is not involved in the fibrin polymerization reaction. Thromb Res 1983;29:249–255.
18. Kloczewiak M, Timmons S, Lukas TJ, Hawiger J. Platelet receptor recognition site on human fibrinogen. Synthesis and structure-function relationship of peptides corresponding to the carboxy-terminal segment of the gamma chain. Biochemistry 1984;23:1767–1774.
19. Coller B. A new murine monoclonal antibody reports on activation-dependent change in the conformation and/or microenvironment of the platelet glycoprotein IIb/IIIa complex. J Clin Invest 1985;76:101–108.
20. Topol EJ, Byzova TV, Plow EF. Platelet GPIIb-IIIa blockers. Lancet 1999; 353:227–231.
21. Kleiman NS. Pharmacokinetics and pharmacodynamics of glycoprotein IIb-IIIa inhibitors. Am Heart J 1999;138:S263-S275.
22. Kleiman NS, Raizner AE, Jordan R, et al. Differential inhibition of platelet aggregation induced by adenosine diphosphate or a thrombin receptor-activating peptide in patients treated with bolus chimeric 7E3 Fab: implications for inhibition of the internal pool of GPIIb/IIIa receptors. J Am Coll Cardiol 1995;26:1665–1671.
23. Mascelli MA, Lance ET, Damaraju L, et al. Pharmacodynamic profile of short-term abciximab treatment demonstrates prolonged platelet inhibition with gradual recovery from GP IIb/IIIa receptor blockade. Circulation 1998; 97:1680–1688.
24. PURSUIT Trial Investigators. Inhibition of platelet glycoprotein IIb/IIIa with eptifibatide in patients with acute coronary syndromes. N Engl J Med 1998; 339:436–443.
25. PRISM PLUS Study Investigators. Inhibition of the platelet glycoprotein IIb/IIIa receptor with tirofiban in unstable angina and non-Q-wave myocardial infarction. N Engl J Med 1998;338:1488–1497.
26. PARAGON Investigators. International, randomized controlled trial of lamifiban (a platelet glycoprotein IIb/IIIa inhibitor), heparin or both in unstable angina. Circulation 1998;97:2386–2395.
27. PRISM Study Investigators. A comparison of aspirin plus tirofiban with aspirin plus heparin for unstable angina. N Engl J Med 1998;338:1498–1505.

28. Boersma E, Akkerhuis KM, Theroux P, et al. Platelet glycoprotein IIb/IIIa receptor inhibition in non-ST-elevation acute coronary syndromes: early benefit during medical treatment only, with additional protection during percutaneous coronary intervention. Circulation 1999;100:2045–2048.
29. Topol EJ, Mark DB, Lincoff AM, et al. Outcomes at 1 year and economic implications of platelet glycoprotein IIb/IIIa blockade in patients undergoing coronary stenting: results from a multicentre randomised trial. Lancet 1999; 354:2019–2024.
30. Boden WE, O'Rourke RA, Crawford MH, et al. Outcomes in patients with acute non-Q-wave myocardial infarction randomly assigned to an invasive as compared with a conservative management strategy. Veterans Affairs Non-Q-Wave Infarction Strategies in Hospital (VANQWISH) Trial. N Engl J Med 1998; 338:1785–1792.
31. Yusuf S, Flather M, Pogue J, et al. Variations between countries in invasive cardiac procedures and outcomes in patients with suspected unstable angina or myocardial infarction without initial ST elevation. OASIS (Organisation to Assess Strategies for Ischaemic Syndromes) Registry. Lancet 1998;352:507–514.
32. FRISC II Investigators. Invasive compared with non-invasive treatment in unstable coronary artery disease: FRISC II prospective randomised multicentre study. Lancet 1999;354:708–715.
33. Cannon CP, Weintraub WS, Demopoulos LA, et al. Invasive versus conservative strategies in unstable angina and non Q-wave myocardial infarction following treatment with tirofiban: rationale and study design of the international TACTICS-TIMI 18 trial. Am J Cardiol 1998;82:731–736.
34. Lincoff AM, Topol EJ. Illusion of reperfusion: does anyone achieve optimal reperfusion during acute myocardial infarction? Circulation 1993;87:1792–1805.
35. GUSTO Investigators. An international randomized trial comparing four thrombolytic strategies for acute myocardial infarction. N Engl J Med 1993;329: 673–682.
36. The Global Use of Strategies to Open Occluded Coronary Arteries (GUSTO) IIb Investigators. A comparison of recombinant hirudin with heparin for the treatment of acute coronary syndromes. N Engl J Med 1996;335:775–782.
37. GUSTO-III Investigators. A comparison of reteplase with alteplase for acute myocardial infarction. The Global Use of Strategies to Open Occluded Coronary Arteries (GUSTO III). N Engl J Med 1997;337:1118–1123.
38. Every NR, Parsons LS, Hlatky M, et al. A comparison of thrombolytic therapy with primary coronary angioplasty for acute myocardial infarction. Myocardial Infarction Triage and Intervention Investigators. N Engl J Med 1996;335: 1253–1260.
39. GUSTO IIb Angioplasty Substudy Investigators. A clinical trial comparing primary coronary angioplasty with tissue plasminogen activator for acute myocardial infarction. N Engl J Med 1997;336:1621–1628.
40. Zijlstra F, Hoorntje JC, de Boer MJ, et al. Long-term benefit of primary

angioplasty as compared with thrombolytic therapy for acute myocardial infarction. N Engl J Med 1999;341:1413–1419.
41. Gold HK, Coller BS, Yasuda T, et al. Rapid and sustained coronary artery recanalization with combined bolus injection of recombinant tissue-type plasminogen activator and monoclonal antiplatelet GPIIb/IIIa antibody in a canine preparation. Circulation 1988;77:670–677.
42. Yasuda T, Gold HK, Leinbach RC, et al. Lysis of plasminogen activator-resistant platelet-rich coronary artery thrombus with combined bolus injection of recombinant tissue-type plasminogen activator and antiplatelet GPIIb/IIIa antibody. J Am Coll Cardiol 1990;16:1728–1735.
43. Coller B. Inhibitors of the platelet glycoprotein IIb/IIIa receptor as conjunctive therapy for coronary artery thrombolysis. Coron Artery Dis 1992;3:1016–1029.
44. Nicolini FA, Lee P, Rios G, et al. Combination of platelet fibrinogen receptor antagonist and direct thrombin inhibitor at low doses markedly improves thrombolysis. Circulation 1994;89:1802–1809.
45. Kleiman NS, Ohman ME, Califf RM, et al. Profound inhibition of platelet aggregation with monoclonal antibody 7E3 Fab following thrombolytic therapy: results of the TAMI 8 pilot study. J Am Coll Cardiol 1993;22:381–389.
46. Ohman EM, Kleiman NS, Gacioch G, et al. Combined accelerated tissue-plasminogen activator and platelet glycoprotein IIb/IIIa integrin receptor blockade with Integrilin in acute myocardial infarction: results of a randomized, placebo-controlled, dose-ranging trial. Circulation 1997;95:846–854.
47. PARADIGM Investigators. Combining thrombolysis with the platelet glycoprotein IIb/IIIa inhibitor lamifiban: results of the Platelet Aggregation Receptor Antagonist Dose Investigation and reperfusion Gain in Myocardial infarction (PARADIGM) trial. J Am Coll Cardiol 1998;32:2003–2010.
48. Antman EM, Giugliano RP, Gibson CM, et al. Abciximab facilitates the rate and extent of thrombolysis: results of the thrombolysis in myocardial infarction (TIMI) 14 trial. The TIMI 14 Investigators. Circulation 1999;99:2720–2732.
49. SPEED Group (Strategies for the Patency Enhancement in the Emergency Department). Randomized trial of abciximab with and without low-dose reteplase for acute myocardial infarction. Circulation 2000. In press.
50. Lefkovits J, Ivanhoe RJ, Califf RM, et al. Effects of platelet glycoprotein IIb/IIIa receptor blockade by a chimeric monoclonal antibody (abciximab) on acute and six-month outcomes after percutaneous transluminal coronary angioplasty for acute myocardial infarction. Am J Cardiol 1996;77:1045–1051.
51. Gold HK, Garabedian SM, Dinsmore RE, et al. Restoration of coronary flow in myocardial infarction by intravenous chimeric 7E3 antibody without exogenous plasminogen activators. Observations in animals and humans. Circulation 1997;95:1755–1759.
52. den Merkhof LF, Zijlstra F, Olsson H, et al. Abciximab in the treatment of acute myocardial infarction eligible for primary percutaneous transluminal coronary angioplasty. Results of the Glycoprotein Receptor Antagonist Patency Evaluation (GRAPE) pilot study. J Am Coll Cardiol 1999;33:1528–1532.

53. Brener SJ, Barr LA, Burchenai JEB, et al. A randomized, placebo-controlled trial of platelet glycoprotein IIb/IIIa blockade with primary angioplasty for acute myocardial infarction. Circulation 1998;98:734–741.
54. Montalescot G, Barragan P, Wittenberg O, et al. Abciximab associated with primary angioplasty and stenting in acute myocardial infarction: The ADMIRAL Study, 30-day final results. Circulation 1999;100:I-87. Abstract.
55. Stone GW. Controlled Abciximab an Device Investigation to Lower Late Angioplasty Complications (CADILLAC) trial. Paper presented at: 72nd Scientific Sessions of the American Heart Association; Atlanta, 1999.
56. Grines CL, Cox DA, Stone GW, et al. Coronary angioplasty with or without stent implantation for acute myocardial infarction. N Engl J Med 1999;341: 1949–1956.
57. Neumann F-J, Blasini R, Schmitt C, et al. Effect of glycoprotein IIb/IIIa receptor blockade on recovery of coronary flow and left ventricular function after the placement of coronary-artery stents in acute myocardial infarction. Circulation 1998;98:2695–2701.
58. Miller JM, Smalling R, Ohman EM, et al. Effectiveness of early coronary angioplasty and abciximab for failed thrombolysis (reteplase or alteplase) during acute myocardial infarction. Results from the GUSTO-III trial. Am J Cardiol 1999;84:779–784.
59. EPIC Investigators. Use of a monoclonal antibody directed against the platelet glycoprotein IIb/IIIa receptor in high-risk coronary angioplasty. N Engl J Med 1994;330:956–961.
60. Topol EJ, Califf RM, Weisman HF, et al. Randomised trial of coronary intervention with antibody against platelet IIb/IIIa integrin for reduction of clinical restenosis: results at six months. Lancet 1994;343:881–886.
61. EPILOG Investigators. Platelet glycoprotein IIb/IIIa receptor blockade and low-dose heparin during percutaneous coronary revascularization. N Engl J Med 1997;336:1689–1696.
62. CAPTURE Investigators. Randomized placebo-controlled trial of abciximab before and during coronary intervention in refractory unstable angina: The CAPTURE study. Lancet 1997;349:1429–1435.
63. EPISTENT Investigators. Randomised, placebo-controlled and balloon-angioplasty controlled trial to assess safety of coronary stenting with use of platelet glycoprotein IIb/IIIa blockade. Lancet 1998;352:87–92.
64. RESTORE Investigators. Effect of platelet glycoprotein IIb/IIIa blockade with tirofiban on adverse cardiac events in patients with unstable angina or acute myocardial infarction undergoing coronary angioplasty. Circulation 1997;96: 1445–1453.
65. IMPACT II Investigators. Randomised, placebo-controlled trial of effect of eptifibatide on complications of percutaneous coronary intervention: IMPACT II. Lancet 1997;349:1422–1428.
66. Lincoff AM, Califf RM, Anderson KM, et al. Evidence for prevention of death and myocardial infarction with platelet membrane glycoprotein IIb/IIIa receptor blockade by abciximab (c7E3 Fab) among patients with unstable angina undergoing percutaneous coronary revascularization. Evaluation of

7E3 in preventing ischemic complications. J Am Coll Cardiol 1997;30:149–156.

67. Topol EJ, Ferguson JJ, Weisman HF, et al. Long term protection from myocardial ischemic events after brief integrin β_3 blockade with percutaneous coronary intervention. JAMA 1997;278:479–484.
68. Califf RM, Abdelmeguid AE, Kuntz RE, et al. Myonecrosis after revascularization procedures. J Am Coll Cardiol 1998;31:241–251.
69. Abdelmeguid AE, Topol EJ, Whitlow PL, et al. Significance of mild transient release of creatine kinase-MB fraction after percutaneous coronary interventions. Circulation 1996;94:1528–1536.
70. Kugelmass AD, Cohen DJ, Moscucci M, et al. Elevation of the creatine kinase myocardial isoform following otherwise successful directional coronary atherectomy and stenting. Am J Cardiol 1994;74:748–754.
71. Kong TG, Davidson CJ, Meyers SN, et al. Prognostic implications of creatine kinase elevation following elective coronary artery interventions. JAMA 1997;277:461–466.
72. Simoons ML, van den Brand M, Lincoff AM, et al. Minimal myocardial damage during coronary intervention is associated with impaired outcome. Eur Heart J 1999;20:1112–1119.
73. Yadav J, Grube E, Rowold S, et al. Detection and characterization of emboli during coronary intervention. Circulation 1999;100:I-780. Abstract.
74. Lefkovits J, Blankenship JC, Anderson KM, et al. Increased risk of non-Q wave myocardial infarction after directional atherectomy is platelet dependent: evidence from the EPIC trial. Evaluation of c7E3 for the Prevention of Ischemic Complications. J Am Coll Cardiol 1996;28:849–855.
75. Ghaffari S, Kereiakes DJ, Lincoff AM, et al. Platelet glycoprotein IIb/IIIa receptor blockade with abciximab reduces ischemic complications in patients undergoing directional coronary atherectomy. Am J Cardiol 1998;82:7–12.
76. Antman EM, Tanasijevic MJ, Thompson B, et al. Cardiac-specific troponin I levels to predict the risk of mortality in patients with acute coronary syndromes. N Engl J Med 1996;335:1342–1349.
77. Hamm CW, Ravkilde J, Gerhardt W, et al. The prognostic value of serum troponin T in unstable angina. N Engl J Med 1992;327:146–150.
78. Ohman EM, Armstrong PW, Christenson RH, et al. Cardiac troponin T levels for risk stratification in acute myocardial ischemia. Circulation 1997;96:2578–2585.
79. Pettijohn TL, Doyle T, Spiekerman AM, et al. Usefulness of positive troponin-T and negative creatine kinase levels in identifying high-risk patients with unstable angina pectoris. Am J Cardiol 1997;80:510–511.
80. Stubbs P, Collinson P, Path MRC, et al. Prognostic significance of admission troponin T concentrations in patients with myocardial infarction. Circulation 1996;94:1291–1297.
81. Heeschen C, Hamm CW, Goldmann B, et al. Troponin concentrations for the stratification of patients with acute coronary syndromes in relation to therapeutic efficacy of tirofiban. Lancet 1999;354:1757–1762.

82. Hamm CW, Heeschen C, Goldmann B, et al. Benefit of abciximab in patients with refractory unstable angina in relation to serum troponin T levels. N Engl J Med 1999;340:1623–1629.
83. Heeschen C, van den Brand MJ, Hamm CW, et al. Angiographic findings in patients with refractory unstable angina according to troponin T status. Circulation 1999;100:1509–1514.
84. Benamer H, Steg PG, Benessiano J, et al. Elevated cardiac troponin I predicts a high-risk angiographic anatomy of the culprit lesion in unstable angina. Am Heart J 1999;137:815–820.
85. Kereiakes DJ, Broderck TM, Roth EM, et al. Time course, magnitude and consistency of platelet inhibition by abciximab, tirofiban or eptifibatide in patients with unstable angina pectoris undergoing percutaneous coronary intervention. Am J Cardiol 1999;84:391–395.
86. Theroux P, Lidon R. Anticoagulants and their use in acute ischemic syndromes. In: Topol EJ, ed. Textbook of Interventional Cardiology, 2nd ed., Vol. 1. Philadelphia: W.B. Saunders, 1993:23–45.
87. Graham DJ, Alexander JJ. The effect of thrombin on bovine aortic endothelial and smooth muscle cells. J Vasc Surg 1990;11:307–313.
88. Harlan JM, Thompson PJ, Ross RR, Bowen-Pope DF. Thrombin induces release of platelet-derived growth factor-like molecule(s) by cultured human endothelial cells. J Cell Biol 1986;103:1129–1133.
89. Bar-Shavit R, Hruska KA, Kahn AJ, Wilner GD. Hormone-like activity of human thrombin. In: Walz DA, Fenton JW, Shuman MA, eds. Bioregulatory Functions of Human Thrombin. New York: New York Academy of Sciences, 1986:335–348.
90. Jones A, Geczy CL. Thrombin and factor Xa enhance the production of interleukin-1. Immunology 1990;71:236–241.
91. Choi ET, Engel L, Callow AD, et al. Inhibition of neointimal hyperplasia by blocking $\alpha_v\beta_3$ integrin with a small peptide antagonist GpenGRGDSPCA. J Vasc Surg 1994;19:125–134.
92. Shattil SJ. Function and regulation of the beta 3 integrins in hemostasis and vascular biology. Thromb Haemost 1995;74:149–155.
93. Jones JI, Prevette T, Gockerman A, Clemmons DR. Ligand occupancy of the alphaV-beta3 integrin is necessary for smooth muscle cells to migrate in response to insulin-like growth factor. Proc Natl Acad Sci USA 1996;93:2482–2487.
94. Phillips DR, Teng W, Arfstent A, et al. Effect of Ca^{2+} on GP IIb/IIIa interactions with Integrilin. Enhanced GP IIb/IIIa binding and inhibition of platelet aggregation by reductions in the concentration of ionized calcium in patients anticoagulated with citrate. Circulation 1997;96:1488–1494.
95. Blankenship JC. Bleeding complications of glycoprotein IIb-IIIa receptor inhibitors. Am Heart J 1999;138:S287-S296.
96. Aguirre FV, Topol EJ, Ferguson JJ, et al. Bleeding complications with the chimeric antibody to platelet glycoprotein IIb/IIIa integrin in patients undergoing percutaneous coronary intervention. Circulation 1995;91:2882–2890.

97. Theroux P, Kouz S, Roy L, et al. Platelet membrane receptor glycoprotein IIb/IIIa antagonism in unstable angina. Canadian Lamifiban Study. Circulation 1996;94:899–905.
98. Boehrer JD, Keriakes DJ, Navetta FI, et al. Profound platelet inhibition with c7E3 prior to angioplasty does not increase emergency bypass surgery complications: experience from a randomized trial. Am J Cardiol 1994;74:1166–1170.
99. Juergens CP, Yeung AC, Oesterle SN. Routine platelet transfusion in patients undergoing emergency coronary bypass surgery after receiving abciximab. Am J Cardiol 1997;80:74–75.
100. Mark DB, Talley JD, Topol EJ, et al. Economic assessment of platelet glycoprotein IIb/IIIa inhibition for prevention of ischemic complications of high-risk coronary angioplasty. Circulation 1996;94:629–635.
101. Lincoff AM, Mark DB, Califf RM, et al. Economic assessment of platelet glycoprotein IIb/IIIa receptor blockade during coronary intervention in the EPILOG trial. J Am Coll Cardiol 1997;29:240A. Abstract.
102. Culler S, Boccuzzi S, Burnette J, et al. Costs after angioplasty: results from the RESTORE Trial. Am J Cardiol 1997;80:235. Abstract.
103. Hillegass WB, Newman AR, Raco DL. Economic issues in glycoprotein IIb/IIIa receptor therapy. Am Heart J 1999;138:S24–S32.

17

Oral Antiplatelet Agents

Aspirin, Ticlopidine, Clopidogrel, Cilostazol, and the Oral Glycoprotein IIb/IIIa Inhibitors

Peter B. Berger
Mayo Clinic
Rochester, Minnesota

INTRODUCTION

In most cases, myocardial infarction and stroke, and often sudden death, are caused by arterial thrombosis. Antiplatelet drugs may reduce the occurrence of arterial thrombosis, particularly among patients with vascular disease who are at increased risk for arterial thrombosis. Oral antiplatelet drugs, including aspirin; the thienopyridines, a class of drugs that currently includes only ticlopidine and clopidogrel; and cilostazol, a selective inhibitor of cyclic AMP phosphodiesterase, are used more and more frequently for the prevention of ischemic events in a wide variety of clinical settings. Several members of a relatively new class of drugs, the oral platelet glycoprotein IIb/IIIa inhibitors, have been studied in randomized trials involving tens of thousands of patients, although none are approved for use yet in the United States or elsewhere. The following is a review of these oral antiplatelet agents—aspirin, the thienopyridines, cilostazol, and the oral glycoprotein IIb/IIIa inhibitors—in the prevention and treatment of vascular events in patients with coronary artery disease.

ASPIRIN

Aspirin has now been around for more than 100 years, and was the only available oral antiplatelet agent for nearly all of that time. Aspirin inhibits platelet cyclooxygenase, and it does so irreversibly for the life of the platelet (5 to 10 days). This impairs the ability of platelets to produce thromboxane A_2, a potent vasoconstrictor and stimulant of platelet aggregation. Aspirin also inhibits endothelial cell production of prostacyclin, which counters the effects of thromboxane A_2. However, unlike platelets, which cannot synthesize new cyclo-oxygenase, endothelial cells can synthesize new cyclo-oxygenase. This enables endothelial cells to regain their capacity to synthesize prostacyclin within hours of aspirin administration. Aspirin has been studied in randomized controlled trials in which more than 100,000 patients were enrolled in a variety of clinical settings.

Secondary Prevention Trials

Aspirin has been studied for secondary prevention in placebo-controlled trials in which approximately 75,000 patients with vascular disease have been enrolled. In these studies, aspirin reduced the combined endpoint of vascular death, myocardial infarction, and stroke by 27% (Fig. 1) (1). Aspirin should be administered to all patients with vascular disease who do not have contraindications to its use, and be continued indefinitely.

Primary Prevention Trials

In a meta-analysis of aspirin of more than 28,000 patients without vascular disease enrolled in randomized controlled primary prevention trials, a sig-

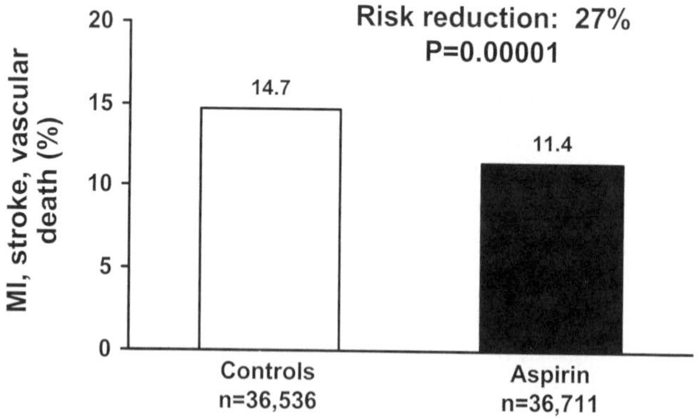

Figure 1 Meta-analysis of trials in which aspirin was used to reduce vascular events in patients with vascular disease.

nificant reduction in the frequency of nonfatal myocardial infarction of approximately 29% was seen, which represented five fewer nonfatal myocardial infarctions per 1000 patients treated ($P < .0005$) (1). This was partially offset, however, by a 21% increase in the frequency of stroke ($P = .05$). The overall benefit in terms of freedom from a vascular event over 5 years of follow-up was approximately four per thousand patients treated, which did not quite reach statistical significance ($P = .09$). The risk of vascular death was essentially unchanged by aspirin; a nonsignificant 5% odds reduction in death from any cause was seen among patients treated with aspirin.

Therefore, the benefits of aspirin for primary prevention are far less than that seen in the secondary prevention trials. Current recommendations are that aspirin be administered to patients with significant risk factors for vascular disease who are at low risk for stroke.

Catheterization Laboratory

The ability of aspirin to prevent ischemic complications among patients undergoing balloon angioplasty has been studied in two placebo-controlled randomized trials (2,3). (Although dipyridamole was used along with aspirin in both studies, the benefits of therapy were believed to be entirely due to aspirin, since other studies suggest that dipyridamole and aspirin are no more effective than aspirin alone.) Both studies revealed that the primary endpoint —Q-wave myocardial infarction in one trial, and acute vessel closure in the other—occurred less frequently among patients assigned to aspirin and dipyridamole. All patients undergoing balloon angioplasty, or percutaneous revascularization of any kind, should receive aspirin, unless contraindicated.

Aspirin Dose

The most appropriate dose of aspirin for chronic therapy has, until recently, been unclear. Even very low doses (20 to 40 mg/day) are able to irreversibly inhibit platelet cyclo-oxygenase; higher doses are required to impair endothelial cell production of postacycline, and higher doses cause more frequent gastrointestinal side effects as well. Therefore, there are theoretical reasons that low doses of aspirin might be preferable. In the randomized trials, different doses of aspirin have been examined (1). Meta-analysis of these trials in which different dosages of aspirin were compared with placebo failed to reveal greater benefit from doses ≤350 mg compared with higher doses (1).

However, the issue of the most appropriate dose of aspirin was directly examined in a recent trial in which 2849 patients undergoing carotid endarterectomy were assigned to receive either low doses of daily aspirin (81 or 325 mg) versus higher doses (650 or 1300 mg) (4). The results of the study indicated that the risk of death, myocardial infarction, or stroke was lower among patients receiving the two lower dosages of aspirin (5.4% vs. 7.0% at 30 days, $P = .07$) and at 3 months (6.2% vs. 8.4%, $P = .03$). The differences were even greater favoring the lower doses of aspirin when patients taking very high doses immediately prior to surgery were excluded (4.2% vs. 10.0% at 3 months, $P = .0002$). These are the first direct data to support the theoretical benefits of lower doses of aspirin. Comparison of the two lower doses of aspirin with one another has not yet been reported. It must be remembered that aspirin for stroke prophylaxis after carotid endarterectomy might not be generalizable to other clinical situations in which aspirin is used to prevent ischemic complications. Nonetheless, this study provides evidence that at least in this clinical situation, the theoretical advantages of low dose aspirin versus high dose aspirin were achieved.

For patients suffering acute myocardial infarction, however, the American College of Cardiology/American Heart Association guidelines for the treatment of acute myocardial infarction recommend an initial dose of 162 to 325 mg, rather than lower doses (5). This is in part because those doses were more frequently studied in the setting of acute myocardial infarction than other doses, and proven to be beneficial.

Aspirin Resistance

In recent years it has become clear that the remarkable efficacy of aspirin despite its relatively weak antiplatelet effect is all the more remarkable in view of data revealing that between 10% and 40% of patients appear to be resistant to its antiplatelet effects (6–10). In these studies, aspirin resistance has been variously defined as a failure by aspirin to prolong bleeding time; failure to reduce the production of 12-HETE (a metabolite of arachidonic acid); or failure to reduce platelet aggregation by >20% from baseline following a weak stimulus for aggregation, as determined by either whole-blood aggregometry or a rapid platelet function assay. All of these tests require comparison of platelet function both before and after the administration of aspirin, limiting the ease with which a diagnosis of aspirin resistance can be made. Failure to take aspirin should always be excluded as the cause of aspirin resistance when aspirin resistance is suspected. In several of these studies, compliance (that aspirin had actually been ingested) was confirmed by documenting that inhibition of platelet cyclooxygenase was present; in others, compliance was determined through interviews with the patient, their physician, or pill counts.

Significance of Aspirin Resistance

Regardless of how aspirin resistance is defined, it appears that more patients fail to respond to aspirin than was previously recognized. The question is,

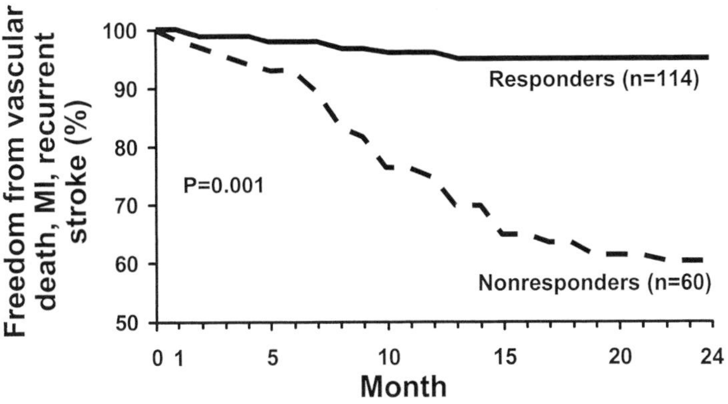

Figure 2 Frequency of adverse cardiovascular events among patients with a prior cerebrovascular event who were and were not resistant to aspirin. (Adapted from Ref. 9.)

however, whether failure to respond to aspirin, however determined, is clinically significant. The only two studies examining the issue indicate that resistance to aspirin is clinically significant, and that such patients are at increased risk of vascular events. In one study, patients who suffered a stroke were treated with large doses of aspirin, 500 mg three times daily; nearly 40% were found to be "nonresponders" based on the modified Wu and Hoak test of platelet function (9). All patients, both responders and nonresponders, were nonetheless maintained on the same daily dose of aspirin, 500 mg three times daily. After 2 years of follow-up, nonresponders had a nearly 40% rate of cardiovascular death, myocardial infarction, or recurrent stroke, compared with approximately 2% in aspirin responders (Fig. 2). In a second study examining the clinical significance of aspirin resistance, patients who did not respond or responded only partially to aspirin had a greater frequency of reocclusion after iliofemoral percutaneous transluminal angioplasty than patients who responded fully (or nearly so) to aspirin (11). Neither of these studies should be regarded as definitive, however, and additional studies are needed of the significance of aspirin resistance and the appropriate management of such patients, both in and out of the catheterization laboratory. Several such studies are under way.

THIENOPYRIDINES: TICLOPIDINE AND CLOPIDOGREL

Ticlopidine, approved for use in the United States in 1991, and clopidogrel, which was approved in March 1998, are the only two members of the thienopyridines class of drugs available for use. The chemical structure and function of the ticlopidine and clopidogrel are similar; clopidogrel has a carboxymethyl side group that ticlopidine does not. No common metabolites of the two drugs have yet been identified. Both ticlopidine and clopidogrel inhibit binding of adenosine 5′-diphosphate (ADP) to its receptors in platelets (12–14). This prevents up-regulation of the platelet glycoprotein IIb/IIIa receptor, reducing fibrinogen binding to these receptors. ADP-receptor blockade also reduces thrombosis due to sheer stress and abolishes cyclic flow variations, and prolongs the bleeding time by approximately twofold. These platelet functions are irreversibly inhibited for the life of the platelet. Both ticlopidine and clopidogrel inhibit vascular smooth muscle contraction in rabbits and rats in response to endothelin and serotonin, and inhibit platelet-induced expression of tissue factor in endothelial cells, although the clinical relevance of these latter actions in humans remains unclear (15). Neither ticlopidine nor clopidogrel influence heparin activity, or affect the partial thromboplastin time or activated clotting time. Despite the similarities between ticlopidine and clopidogrel, however, there are important differences between the two drugs.

Ticlopidine

Ticlopidine itself is not active, but it is metabolized to active metabolites by the liver (16). Although peak levels of ticlopidine's active metabolite are reached within 2 hours, it takes ticlopidine between 5 and 7 days to achieve maximal platelet inhibition (16). The reasons for the delay in antiplatelet effect have not been elucidated.

Secondary Prevention Trials

Ticlopidine has been studied in 39 randomized placebo-controlled trials in which a total of 6528 patients with vascular disease were enrolled for the prevention of vascular death, myocardial infarction, or stroke trials (Fig. 3) (1). Meta-analysis reveals that ticlopidine reduced the frequency of the combined endpoint of vascular death, infarction, and stroke in these trials by 33% (1). In one trial, enrollment was limited to patients with unstable angina (1). In that trial, ticlopidine with conventional therapy was compared with conventional therapy alone, but aspirin was not routinely administered to patients in either arm, by study design. Ticlopidine reduced the frequency of vascular death and nonfatal myocardial infarction by 46% in that trial (13.6% vs. 7.3%, $P = .009$).

Ticlopidine has been compared with aspirin in 3 randomized trials in which 3471 patients with either a stroke or a transient ischemic attack were enrolled (1). Meta-analysis revealed a 10% reduction in the frequency of the

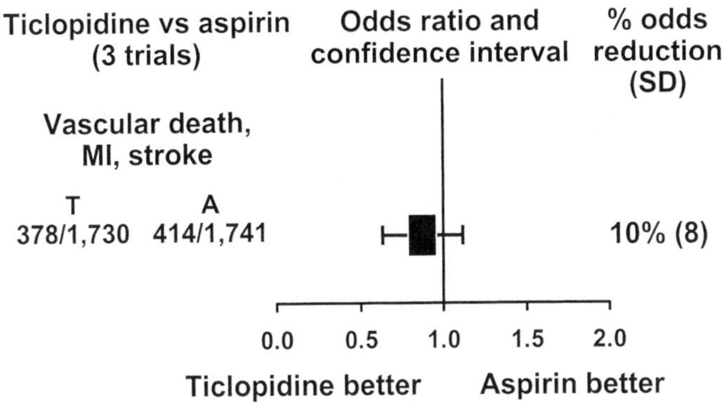

Figure 3 Meta-analysis of randomized trials comparing ticlopidine with aspirin in which patients with vascular disease were enrolled. (Adapted from Ref. 1.)

combined endpoint of vascular death, infarction, and stroke by ticlopidine (Fig. 4) (1).

Catheterization Laboratory

Two placebo-controlled randomized trials evaluated the efficacy of ticlopidine in patients undergoing balloon angioplasty who were not on aspirin (3,17). In both studies, ticlopidine significantly reduced the frequency of acute vessel closure (3,17).

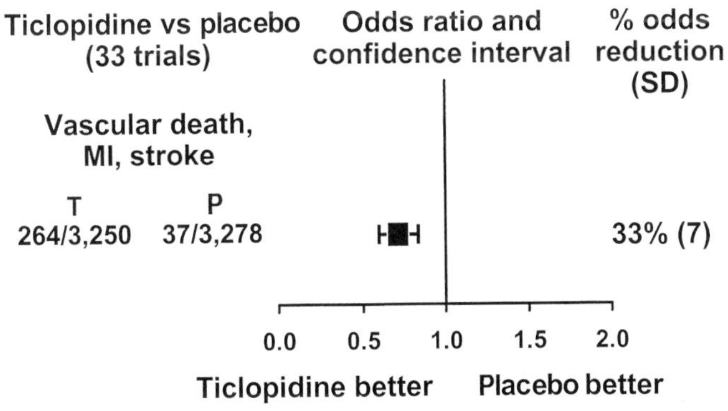

Figure 4 Meta-analysis of the reduction in adverse vascular events seen in randomized trials comparing ticlopidine with placebo in which patients with stroke or transient ischemic attacks were enrolled. (Adapted from Ref. 1.)

Little is known about whether aspirin combined with ticlopidine is more effective among patients undergoing balloon angioplasty than aspirin alone. Two retrospective studies addressing this issue have been performed (18,19). In the Total Occlusion Study of Canada (TOSCA) trial, 410 patients with a coronary occlusion were randomly assigned to receive one or more heparin-coated Palmaz-Schatz coronary stent or treatment with balloon angioplasty alone (19). Patients treated with balloon angioplasty alone received either aspirin and ticlopidine or aspirin alone, according to physician preference. The combination of aspirin and ticlopidine did not reduce the frequency of reocclusion or restenosis at six months, or adverse clinical events at one year. Although there were important differences in the baseline clinical, angiographic, and procedural characteristics among the two groups of patients, multivariate analysis used to adjust for these differences did not suggest benefit from adding ticlopidine to aspirin. An analysis of patients undergoing balloon angioplasty in the treatment of acute myocardial infarction in the STENT-PAMI trial revealed similar results (18). These two retrospective studies were not definitive; prospective randomized trials are needed to definitively determine whether combining ticlopidine with aspirin is more effective than aspirin alone among patients undergoing balloon angioplasty.

Coronary Stents

Five randomized trials have compared the combined use of aspirin and ticlopidine with aspirin alone, or aspirin with coumadin, in patients undergoing coronary stent placement (20–24). Aspirin and ticlopidine was the most effective regimen in all five trials (Fig. 5). Hemorrhagic complications were also less frequent with aspirin and ticlopidine than with aspirin and coumadin.

While aspirin and ticlopidine were both more efficacious and safe than aspirin and coumadin or aspirin alone among patients receiving coronary stents, the Full Anticoagulation versus Ticlopidine plus Aspirin after Stent Implantation (FANTASTIC) trial revealed an important limitation of therapy with ticlopidine (24). In FANTASTIC, the first dose of ticlopidine was administered on the day of stent implantation; pretreatment was not performed. The results of the trial reveal that stent thrombosis actually occurred more frequently in the 24 hours after stent placement among patients receiving ticlopidine than those receiving intravenous heparin while coumadin was being initiated (2.4% vs. 0.4%, respectively; $P = .06$). Subsequent to 24 hours, the frequency of stent thrombosis was reduced in the ticlopidine-treated patients, and the cumulative occurrence of stent thrombosis tended to be less in the ticlopidine patients (2.8% vs. 3.9%, P = NS). However, the trial indicates that when ticlopidine is first initiated the day of stent placement, as it frequently is in clinical practice, ticlopidine appears to provide

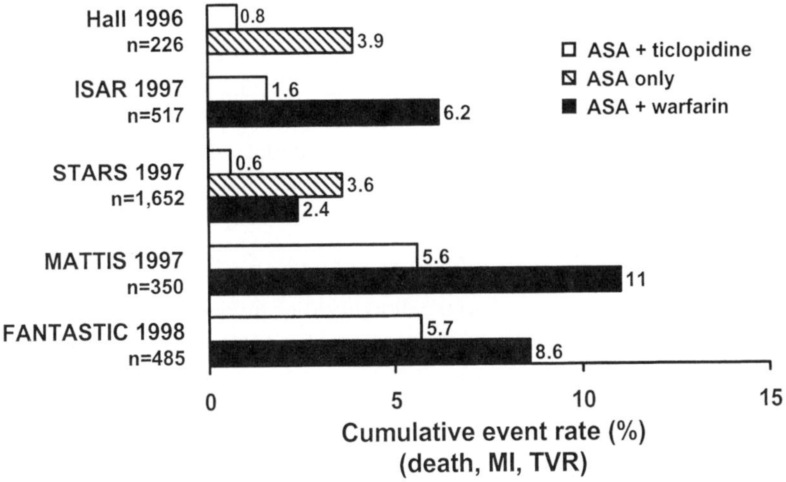

Figure 5 The five randomized trials in which aspirin and ticlopidine were compared with either aspirin alone, or aspirin and coumadin in patients following coronary stent placement. (Adapated from Ref. 83.)

insufficient antiplatelet inhibition for at least the first 24 hours after stent placement.

A hematological study of patients undergoing stent implantation randomly assigned to receive aspirin alone, ticlopidine alone, or aspirin and ticlopidine (with the first does of ticlopidine administered on the day of the procedure in both ticlopidine arms) confirms the inadequate platelet inhibition in the ticlopidine arm early after stent placement. In that study, platelet aggregation and fibrinogen binding to glycoprotein IIb/IIIa receptors were most inhibited on days 7 and 14 after stent placement in the group receiving aspirin and ticlopidine (25). However, in the 24 hours following stent implantation, platelet aggregation and fibrinogen binding were similar in the three groups, which may explain ticlopidine's inability to prevent stent thrombosis early after stent placement when pretreatment with ticlopidine has not been performed.

Side Effects

In many of the trials evaluating ticlopidine in patients with vascular disease, ticlopidine caused side effects, such as nausea, diarrhea, and rash, requiring discontinuation in as many as 20% of patients. The most serious side effects of ticlopidine, neutropenia and thrombotic thrombocytopenic purpura (TTP), are less frequent. Neutropenia occurs in approximately 1% to 3% of patients and can be life threatening; TTP which occurs much less frequently, perhaps in as few as 0.03% of patients, but is fatal in 25% to 50% of cases (26). Mortality from TTP is reduced if plasmapheresis is initiated rapidly. Because of these potentially lethal hematologic side effects and the need to make a diagnosis and begin treatment rapidly, blood counts should be examined serially in the first several months of ticlopidine use, the period during which these side effects are most likely to occur.

Duration of Therapy in Stent Patients

Based on the five randomized trials showing that ticlopidine, with aspirin, is the most efficacious therapy following stent placement to prevent stent thrombosis, and based on the increasing frequency with which stents are placed during percutaneous revascularization procedures, the frequency with which ticlopidine is prescribed has grown enormously. In an attempt to reduce not only the frequent minor side effects of ticlopidine but especially the risk of life-threatening neutropenia and TTP, studies have been performed of the safety and efficacy of administering ticlopidine for only 2 weeks after stent placement. Neutropenia is exceedingly rare during 2 weeks or less of therapy; TTP does occur with <2 weeks of ticlopidine therapy, although less frequently than after longer periods of therapy.

In a study of 827 consecutive patients at the Mayo Clinic in whom ticlopidine was discontinued 14 days after stent placement, 1.6% of patients suffered an adverse event (including death, myocardial infarction, or the need for a repeat angioplasty procedure or bypass surgery) in the first 14 days after stent placement, while ticlopidine was being administered (27). However, stent thrombosis did not occur in the days 15 through 30 after stent placement, after ticlopidine had been discontinued (27). The 95% confidence intervals for stent thrombosis, given no observed cases in 817 patients, range from 0 to 0.5%, suggesting that the risk of late stent thrombosis was less than the combined incidence of neutropenia and TTP when ticlopidine is given for 30 days. The investigators concluded that in patients undergoing stent implantation treated with ticlopidine, ticlopidine should be administered for only 14 days. In a subsequent substudy of the ATLAST (Antiplatelet Therapy Alone vs. Lovenox Plus Antiplatelet Therapy in Patients at Increased Risk of Stent Thrombosis) trial, 1102 patients at increased risk of stent thrombosis who did not receive a platelet glycoprotein IIb/IIIa inhibitor were randomized to receive either enoxaparin or placebo subcutaneously for 2 weeks; all patients received ticlopidine for only 2 weeks. In the third and fourth weeks after enrollment, after ticlopidine had been discontinued, there was one definite case of stent thrombosis and two possible cases, for a frequency of definite or possible stent thrombosis of 0.27% (95% confidence intervals 0.06–0.77). These data indicate that although longer periods of treatment with a thienopyridine (which are currently being studied) may well be helpful in terms of other reducing events other than stent thrombosis, they do not appear to be required to achieve a large reduction in the frequency of stent thrombosis in the 30 days after stent placement.

Consequences of the Slow Onset of Action of Ticlopidine

Stent Thrombosis Although limiting the duration of therapy of ticlopidine to 2 weeks after stent placement eliminates neutropenia and significantly reduces the frequency of TTP, there remain problems associated with ticlopidine not only due to its frequent nonlethal side effects, but related to the slow onset of action of ticlopidine, as described above. Most percutaneous revascularization procedures are not planned for days in advance of the procedure, precluding pretreament of patients with ticlopidine before a stent procedure. A study from the Mayo Clinic suggests that more complete platelet inhibition from a thienopyridine at the time of stent placement may decrease the risk of stent thrombosis (28). Wilson et al. (28) compared the frequency and timing of stent thrombosis rate in patients treated with aspirin and coumadin and in patients treated with aspirin and ticlopidine. In the aspirin and coumadin patients, the median time to stent thrombosis was 4 days. In contrast, in the aspirin and ticlopidine patients, the median time to stent thrombosis was 12 hours, during the time that maximal platelet inhibition with a thienopyridine has not yet occurred. Stent thrombosis was very rare after the first day. These data suggest that more complete platelet inhibition at the time of the stent procedure might reduce the risk of early stent thrombosis.

A study from Schomig et al. (29) also suggests that the slow onset of action of ticlopidine may well be important. These investigators examined their first 2833 patients who received coronary stents. Initially, patients were treated with aspirin and coumadin; subsequent patients were treated with aspirin and ticlopidine. Although the group who received aspirin and coumadin had a fivefold greater frequency of stent thrombosis, stent thrombosis was as likely to occur in the first day after stent placement in patients treated with heparin while coumadin was being initiated as it was in patients treated with ticlopidine. That stent thrombosis was most likely to occur in the first day of stent placement in the ticlopidine cohort, and less likely to occur subsequently when platelet aggregation was more inhibited by ticlopidine, also suggests that more complete platelet inhibition by a thienopyridine at the time of stent placement might reduce the risk of stent thrombosis.

Procedural Infarction Data from Steinhubl and others at Cleveland Clinic indicate that more complete platelet inhibition from ticlopidine at the time of stent placement procedure might reduce the frequency of procedural myocardial infarction (30). These investigators studied 175 patients undergoing elective stent placement and found that among patients who had received ticlopidine >3 days prior to the stent implantation procedure, the frequency of myocardial infarction (defined as any elevation of creatinine phosphokinase above normal with an elevation of CK-MB) was only 11%. If ticlopidine was administered for 1 to 2 days prior to stent placement, the frequency of myocardial infarction was 17%. If ticlopidine was first administered the day of the procedure, as is the practice at most hospitals where unplanned procedures are common, 29% of patients suffered a procedural myocardial infarction.

A second study by Steinhubl et al. also supports the theory that more complete platelet inhibition reduces procedural myocardial infarction (31). In the EPISTENT trial, 2399 patients requiring a percutaneous coronary intervention were randomly assigned to undergo coronary stent placement with aspirin and ticlopidine but without a platelet glycoprotein IIb/IIIa inhibitor; stent placement with aspirin, ticlopidine, and the glycoprotein IIb/IIIa inhibitor abciximab; or balloon angioplasty with aspirin and abciximab (32). Although the study protocol suggested that patients receive pretreatment with ticlopidine whenever possible, only about one-half of patients were pretreated with ticlopidine for >24 hours. A retrospective analysis indicated that the frequency of the combined endpoint of death, myocardial infarction, or urgent target vessel revascularization within 30 days after enrollment was significantly lower among stent patients who received pretreatment with ticlopidine (Fig. 6) (31). The reduction in the combined endpoint was driven by a reduction in procedural myocardial infarction. The addition of abciximab further reduced the frequency of adverse events among stent patients, even among those pretreated with ticlopidine, but the risk reduction from ticlopidine pretreatment was approximately equal to the reduction in risk seen with abciximab. These data indicate that pretreament with a thienopyridine may reduce procedural myocardial infarction, although they also indicate that the reduction in procedural myocardial infarction achieved with a thienopyridine is less than the reduction that can be achieved with abciximab.

These limitations of ticlopidine—its frequent side effects, the need to monitor blood counts during its administration, and its slow onset of action—stimulated interest in the more recently developed thienopyridine, clopidogrel.

Clopidogrel

Clopidogrel is a thienopyridine closely related to ticlopidine in chemical structure and function (14). Despite the similarities, no common metabolites of the two drugs have yet been identified. All known metabolites of clopi-

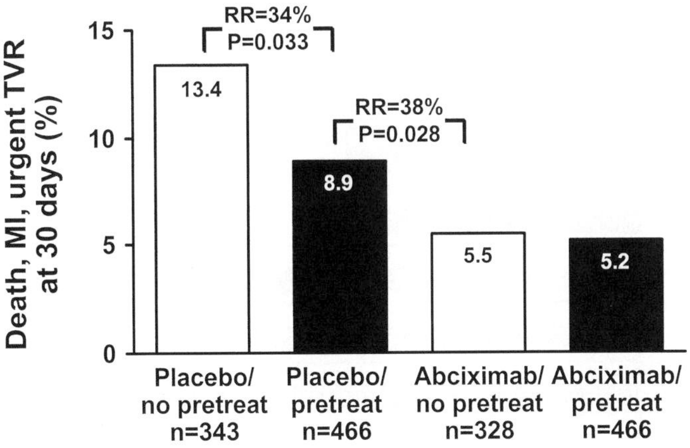

Figure 6 Data from the EPISTENT trial in which pretreatment with ticlopidine was associated with a risk reduction for procedural myocardial infarction and other adverse events of 34% in the 30 days following stent placement. The administration of abciximab further reduced adverse events 38%, even among patients pretreated with ticlopidine.

dogrel that have been identified contain a carboxymethyl side group that metabolites of ticlopidine lack.

Like ticlopidine, clopidogrel itself is not believed to be active; clopidogrel is metabolized by the liver to other compounds that account for its activity (14,33). Peak levels of the metabolite that account for its antiplatelet effect are reached in approximately 1 hour; however, like ticlopidine, it takes approximately 5 days to achieve maximal platelet inhibition from clopidogrel when no loading dose is administered.

Secondary Prevention

A dose-finding study of clopidogrel found that 75 mg/day achieved greater steady-state inhibition of platelets to 5 μM ADP than did lower doses; doses higher than 75 mg/day did not achieve greater platelet inhibition (Fig. 7) (34). A dose of 75 mg/day achieved the same degree of platelet inhibition as ticlopidine 250 mg twice daily.

On the basis of the dose-finding study, a daily dose of 75 mg of clopidogrel was used in the CAPRIE trial in which 19,185 patients, one-third of whom had peripheral vascular disease, one-third cerebrovascular disease, and one-third coronary artery disease, were enrolled (35). Patients were randomly assigned to receive clopidogrel 75 mg/day or aspirin 325 mg/day in addition to their other medications. After 3 years of follow-up, patients re-

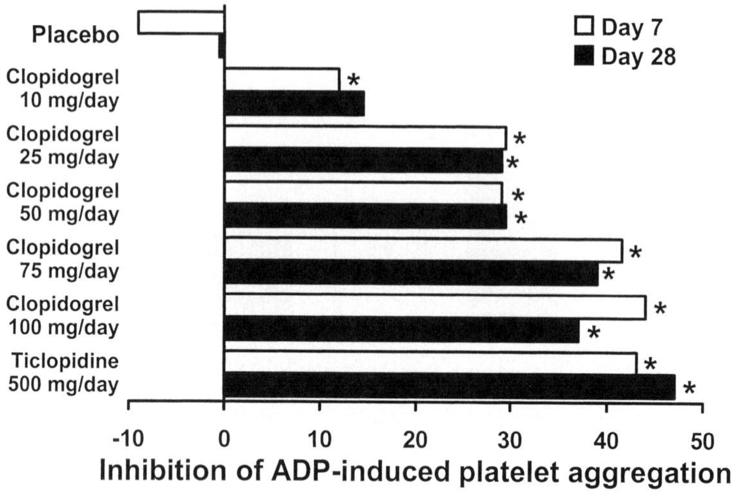

Figure 7 Results from a dose-ranging study in which clopidogrel 75 mg/day achieved greater steady-state inhibition of platelets than lower doses of clopidogrel, and the same degree of platelet inhibition as ticlopidine 250 mg twice daily. (Adapted from Ref. 34.)

ceiving clopidogrel had a slightly though statistically significant 8.7% lower rate of vascular death, myocardial infarction, or ischemic stroke (P = .043) (Fig. 8). The risk reduction of 8.7% was small in absolute terms, representing 0.5% fewer events per year. Perhaps the most impressive finding in CAPRI was the infrequency with which side effects required that the study drug be discontinued (Table 1). Clopidogrel was discontinued slightly less frequently than aspirin, even though only aspirin-tolerant patients were included in CAPRIE (35).

When the same endpoints are examined as were examined in the previously published meta-analysis of the three randomized trials comparing ticlopidine and aspirin—vascular death, nonfatal myocardial infarction, or any stroke—the risk reduction achieved with clopidogrel in CAPRIE was 10%, the same risk reduction seen with ticlopidine in the meta-analysis of trials comparing ticlopidine and aspirin (36). Therefore, not only is the amount of ex vivo inhibition of platelet aggregation with clopidogrel the same as is achieved with ticlopidine, but the reduction in adverse events with clopidogrel is also identical to the reduction with ticlopidine.

The benefits of clopidogrel in the CAPRIE trial are probably not sufficient to recommend that patients currently on aspirin be switched to clopidogrel. The results of CAPRIE do, however, indicate that in patients with

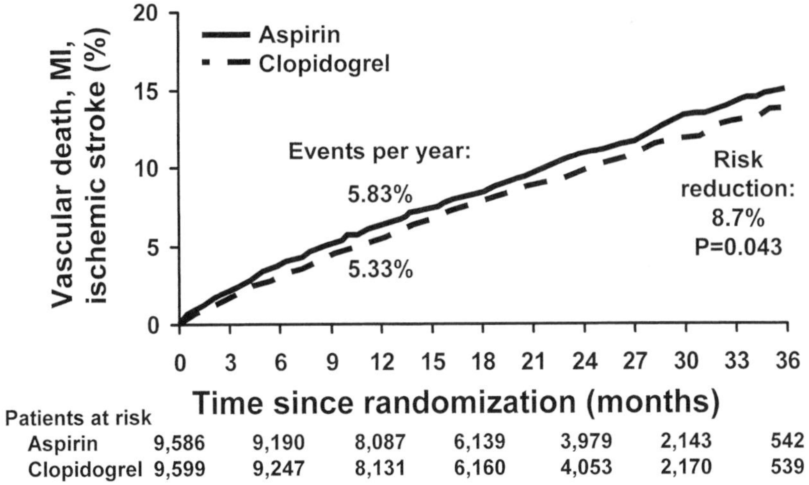

Figure 8 Results of the CAPRIE study. The 8.7% reduction in the risk of vascular death, hemorrhagic stroke, and nonfatal myocardial infarction with clopidogrel over aspirin during 3 years of follow-up corresponded to 0.5% fewer events per year. (Adapted from Ref. 35.)

Table 1 Frequency of Side Effects Requiring Permanent Discontinuation of Study Drug in CAPRIE (discontinuation of study drug among patients taking aspirin was more frequent than among those taking clopidogrel)

	Study drug permanently discontinued			
	Clopidogrel n = 9599		Aspirin n = 9586	
Adverse experience	No.	%	No.	%
Rash	86	0.90	39	0.41[a]
Diarrhea	40	0.42	26	0.27
Indigestion/nausea/vomiting	182	1.90	231	2.41[a]
Any bleeding disorder	115	1.20	131	1.27
Intracranial hemorrhage	20	0.21	32	0.33
Gastrointestinal hemorrhage	50	0.52	89	0.93[a]
Abnormal liver function	22	0.23	28	0.29
		5.3		6.0

[a]$p = 0.05$.
Source: Adapted from Ref. 35.

vascular disease intolerant of aspirin, clopidogrel is the antiplatelet treatment of choice, and it should be continued indefinitely (a position endorsed by the American Heart Association and American College of Cardiology) (37). The excellent safety profile of clopidogrel in CAPRIE also raises questions not addressed by the study, such as whether clopidogrel should be administered to patients who suffer a myocardial infarction or develop an acute coronary syndrome while on aspirin, or to patients at very high risk of myocardial infarction or death due to severe atherosclerosis, perhaps involving all three coronary arteries and perhaps the peripheral and cerebral circulations. It also raises the question whether clopidogrel should be administered to patients with biochemical evidence of aspirin resistance, as described above.

The Clopidogrel in Unstable Angina (CURE) study is examining some of these issues. In CURE, combination therapy with aspirin and clopidogrel is being compared with aspirin and placebo in 12,000 patients admitted to the hospital for treatment of an acute coronary syndrome. Only sites that generally pursue a noninvasive evaluation in such patients and infrequently perform coronary angiography are participating in the trial, so that the trial can determine the impact of aspirin and clopidogrel in patients managed medically rather than invasively.

Catheterization Laboratory

The available data suggest that clopidogrel and ticlopidine have similar efficacy among patients undergoing coronary revascularization procedures. However, there are reasons to believe that clopidogrel might be more effective than ticlopidine in such patients. Since maximal platelet inhibition is not achieved until after at least 5 days of treatment with ticlopidine, a 500-mg loading dose of ticlopidine is usually administered to speed the onset of platelet inhibition. Larger loading doses of ticlopidine frequently cause nausea and vomiting and are not recommended. Clopidogrel 75 mg, administered once daily, also takes many days to achieve maximal platelet inhibition but, in contrast to ticlopidine, large loading doses are well tolerated. A 375-mg dose of clopidogrel produced 60% platelet inhibition at 90 min in response to 5 μM ADP, and maximal platelet inhibition was achieved within 6 hours (38).

Patients Undergoing Stent Placement

Based on the data indicating that clopidogrel and ticlopidine produce equivalent ex vivo platelet inhibition, an equivalent reduction in adverse events among patients with vascular disease when compared with aspirin, and that both appeared to be very effective in animal models at reducing stent thrombosis, many laboratories changed their practice and began administering clopidogrel in place of ticlopidine to patients undergoing coronary stent procedures. In most cases, a 300-mg dose of clopidogrel has been administered immediately before or after the implantation procedure, when pretreatment was not possible, and 75 mg/day has been continued for 14 to 30 days. Data from several of these registries are now available (39,40,40A–40G). The frequency of stent thrombosis, and the frequency of any major ischemic event, has tended to be lower in the clopidogrel cohort than the comparator ticlopidine groups in nearly all of these retrospective studies (Fig. 9). Since newer-generation stents have become available which are generally superior in at least some way over the older stents, and operator experience has increased, it is difficult to be definitive about whether clopidogrel is truly superior to ticlopidine. However, taken together, the results of these registries suggest that clopidogrel is associated with a very low frequency of stent thrombosis and other ischemic events, and there is nothing to suggest

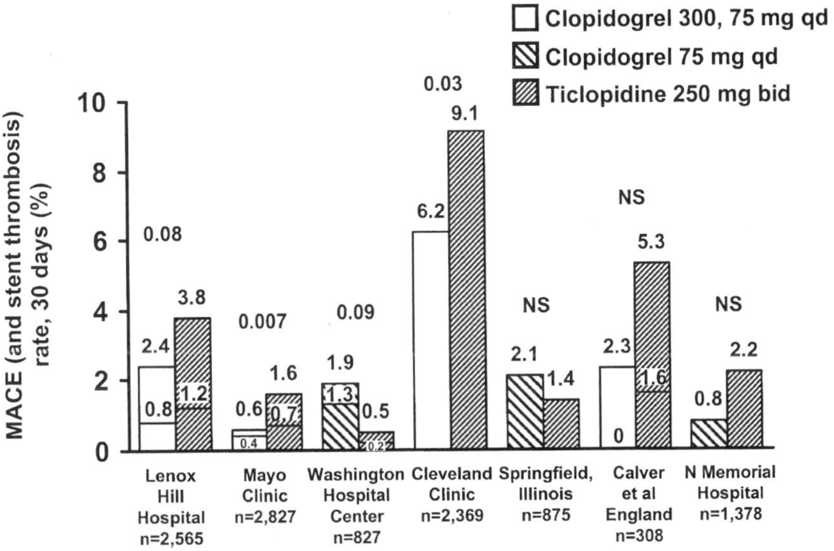

Figure 9 Data from registries in which patients treated with clopidogrel were compared with either a consecutive or matched series of patients who had received ticlopidine. In the registries from Washington Hospital Center and North Memorial Hospital, the initial dose of clopidogrel was either a 300-mg loading dose or 75 mg/day without a loading dose. In some series, patients were included even though stent thrombosis occurred before the first dose of thienopyridine was administered. Nonetheless, the data indicate a low rate of stent thrombosis and other major adverse events among stent patients treated with clopidogrel.

that the outcome of stent patients treated with clopidogrel is inferior to that of patients treated with ticlopidine.

Randomized Trials

Two randomized trials comparing ticlopidine and clopidogrel in stent patients have been performed (Fig. 10). In the Clopidogrel Aspirin Stent International Cooperative Study (CLASSICS) trial, performed in Europe, 1020 stent patients were randomly assigned to receive clopidogrel with a 300-mg loading dose followed by 75 mg/day for 28 days; clopidogrel 75 mg without a loading dose followed by 75 mg/day for 28 days; or ticlopidine 250 mg followed by 250 mg twice daily for 28 days (41). The initial dose of a thienopyridine was administered between 1 and 6 hours after stent placement, limiting the benefit one might hope to see from the most rapidly acting regimen, clopidogrel with a 300-mg loading dose. The results of the trial indicated that clopidogrel, with and without a loading dose, was better tolerated than ticlopidine (Fig. 11). Paradoxically, a 300-mg loading dose of clopidogrel was better tolerated than a 75-mg dose of clopidogrel with respect to side effects, which can only be attributed to chance. Although the study was sized to detect a difference in side effects and was too small to detect a difference in the frequency of stent thrombosis or other major ad-

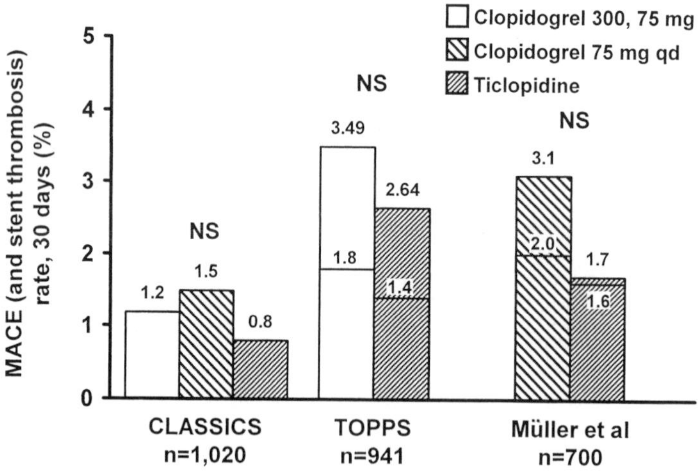

Figure 10 Data from randomized trials comparing ticlopidine with clopidogrel in patients receiving coronary stents. Although the trials suggest equivalence between the treatment arms, all the trials were underpowered to detect significant differences in stent thrombosis and other major adverse events between the treatment groups. (From Ref. 84.)

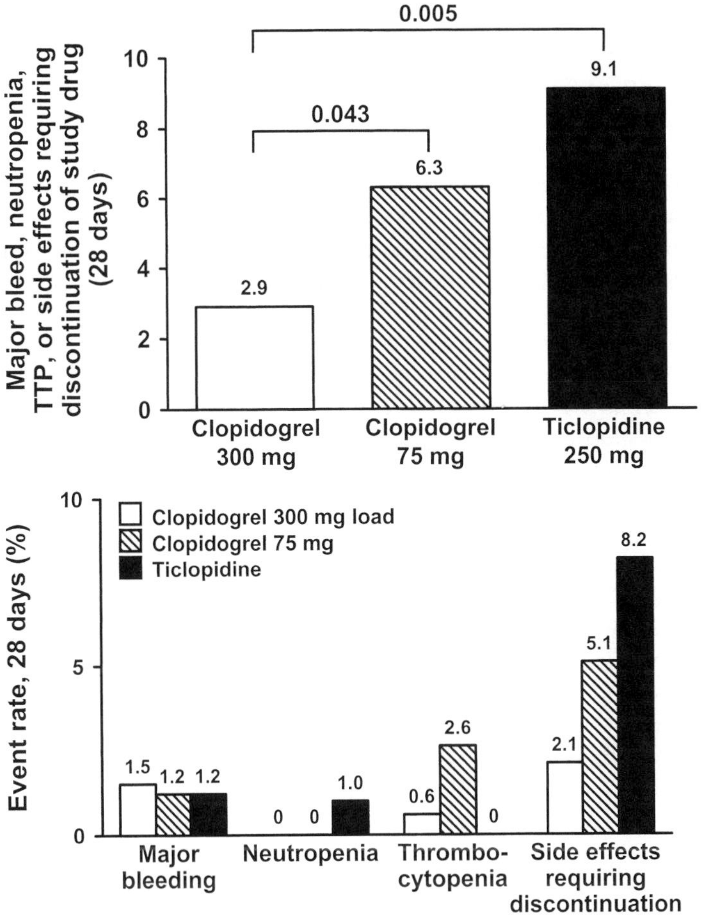

Figure 11 Results of the CLASSICS trial. (Top) Frequency with which the primary endpoint was reached in the three study groups. The finding that a 300-mg loading dose of clopidogrel was better tolerated than a 75-mg dose of clopidogrel can only be attributed to chance. (Bottom) Frequency with which each individual component of the primary endpoint was reached. (From Ref. 84.)

verse events, the frequency of such events was similar in all 3 arms—0.9% in the ticlopidine arm, 1.5% in the arm that received an initial dose of 75 mg of clopidogrel, and 1.2% in the group that received clopidogrel with a 300-mg loading dose (a difference of one event between each of the groups, P = NS for all comparisons) (Fig. 10).

In the second randomized trial comparing clopidogrel and ticlopidine, a single-center study from Barnes Hospital in St. Louis, Ticlid or Plavix Post-Stents (TOPPS), 1000 stent patients were randomly assigned to receive a 300-mg loading dose of clopidogrel followed by 75 mg/day for 14 days or 500-mg loading dose of ticlopidine followed by 250 mg twice daily for 14 days (42). The initial dose of study drug was administered within 2 hours after stent placement. An intravenous platelet glycoprotein IIb/IIIa inhibitor was administered to 48% of patients in the trial. The results of an interim analysis including the first 941 patients enrolled in the trial reveal that the frequency of stent thrombosis within 24 hours of stent placement was 0.62% in the ticlopidine arm versus 0.66% in the clopidogrel arm (P = .93). The frequency of stent thrombosis in the subsequent 29 days was 0.82% in the ticlopidine arm versus 1.10% in the clopidogrel arm (P = .66). The frequency of death, stent thrombosis, or need for a repeat target lesion revascularization procedure was 3.49% in the ticlopidine arm versus 2.64% in the clopidogrel arm (P = .45) (Fig. 10).

In the third randomized trial comparing clopidogrel and ticlopidine, this one from Germany, 700 stent patients were randomly assigned to receive a clopidogrel 75 mg/day without a loading dose, or a 500-mg loading dose of ticlopidine, followed by 250 mg twice daily, for 4 weeks (42A). The initial dose of study drug was administered within 1 hour after stent placement. The results of the study indicate that the frequency of a major adverse event (death, myocardial infarction, stent thrombosis, or need for a repeat target lesion revascularization procedure) was 1.7% in the ticlopidine arm versus 3.1% in the clopidogrel arm (P = .24). Stent thrombosis occurred in 0.6% of patients in the ticlopidine arm versus 2.0% in the clopidogrel arm (P = .10 (Fig. 10).

An ongoing randomized trial, the Clopidogrel for Reduction of Events During Extended Observation (CREDO) trial, is testing the hypothesis that more complete inhibition with a thienopyridine at the time of a percutaneous revascularization procedure. This trial will randomly assign 2000 patients undergoing percutaneous revascularization (with or without a stent) to a 300-mg loading dose of clopidogrel ≥3 hours before the procedure versus clopidogrel 75 mg/day beginning immediately before the procedure. Patients assigned to the clopidogrel 300-mg loading dose will receive clopidogrel 75 mg/day for one year (along with aspirin) whereas patients assigned to clopidogrel without a loading dose will receive clopidogrel for only 4 weeks, followed by placebo for 11 months, with aspirin.

The data, in aggregate, suggest that clopidogrel is at least equivalent to ticlopidine in preventing stent thrombosis and procedural infarction. Whether clopidogrel is superior to ticlopidine as one might hope, given it's more rapid onset of action, remains unproven. However, clopidogrel has nonetheless nearly completely replaced ticlopidine in the United States, both in and out of the catheterization laboratory, and is rapidly doing so around the world because frequent side effects such as nausea, vomiting, and diarrhea; and rare, potentially fatal side effects, such as neutropenia and TTP, are far fewer than with clopidogrel. With approximately 3 million patients treated with clopidogrel, TTP has been reported in 11 patients; several of these were on other drugs reported to be associated with the development of TTP. Therefore, the frequency of TTP in patients on clopidogrel appears to be very rare, and similar to the background frequency of TTP in the general population, reported to be 3.7 per million patients. Clopidogrel is also replacing ticlopidine because it is approximately 30% less expensive than ticlopidine (U.S. wholesale price), and the cost of clopidogrel is further reduced by not needing to monitor blood counts in patients receiving the drug, as is required every 2 weeks for the first 3 months of treatment with ticlopidine.

Unanswered Questions About Clopidogrel

Data from animal models of stent thrombosis (43,44), ex vivo platelet function data (34), data from clinical trials of secondary prevention (35,36,45), three randomized trials in stent patients (41,42), and seven observational studies of patients treated with coronary stents (39,40) suggest that clopidogrel is at least as effective as ticlopidine. However, there remain important unanswered questions about the thienopyridines: Is clopidogrel as effective as ticlopidine, or more effective as a result of clopidogrel's ability to administer a large loading dose and achieve platelet inhibition more rapidly in the setting of unplanned stent placement? Will the ability of clopidogrel to act more rapidly reduce stent thrombosis and procedural myocardial infarction? What is the optimal loading dose of clopidogrel? It remains unclear whether the thienopyridines are efficacious when combined with aspirin in patients undergoing balloon angioplasty and other interventions, as they clearly are in patients undergoing stent placement. Are aspirin and clopidogrel more effective than aspirin in patients with acute coronary syndromes not undergoing a revascularization procedure? Ongoing studies should provide the answer to all of these questions in the next few years.

CILOSTAZOL

Cilostazol (Otsuka Pharmaceutical Co, Ltd) is a selective inhibitor of cyclic AMP phosphodiesterase. Cilostazol both inhibits platelet aggregation and is a direct arterial vasodilator; these actions result from an increase in the intracellular concentration of cyclic AMP. Unlike aspirin, cilostazol does not inhibit prostacyclin synthesis, and its effect on platelets is reversible; the antiplatelet affect of cilostazol takes effect within 6 hours of ingestion, and platelet aggregation returns to normal within 48 hours of discontinuing the drug. Cilostazol is metabolized by the liver, and its metabolites are renally excreted; the standard dose of 100 mg twice daily need not be adjusted in mild liver disease or mild to moderate renal failure.

Cilostazol is approved for use in the United States for the treatment of claudication in patients with peripheral vascular disease; it has been shown, in randomized placebo-controlled trials in the United States, to improve exercise duration and the ankle:brachial index (46). However, among patients with coronary artery disease, cilostazol has been most extensively studied in Japan among patients undergoing balloon angioplasty, directional atherectomy, and stent placement for the prevention of both procedural complications and restenosis.

Percutaneous Coronary Revascularization

Among patients undergoing balloon angioplasty, cilostazol was added to aspirin in 71 patients undergoing stent implantation (47). One non-Q-wave infarction occurred due to occlusion of a branch vessel, but coronary thrombosis did not occur in any patient. Cilostazol alone was compared with other antiplatelet drugs (aspirin and/or ticlopidine) and coumadin in a nonrandomized trial in which 102 patients were enrolled (48). The results of this trial revealed a nonsignificant reduction in restenosis on follow-up angiography among patients treated with cilostazol (22% vs. 32%, $P = .24$), which led to many subsequent studies of cilostazol's ability to reduce restenosis.

Cilostazol was compared with aspirin alone in a trial that included 41 patients undergoing directional atherectomy (49). The primary endpoint, restenosis on follow-up angiography, was not reached by any patients treated with cilostazol versus 23.6% in the aspirin group ($P = .02$).

A subsequent study analyzed the frequency of restenosis in 211 patients who underwent balloon angioplasty of 273 lesions and were randomized to receive either cilostazol or aspirin (50). Both restenosis and target vessel revascularization occurred less frequently in the cilostazol group (17.9% vs. 39.5%, $P < .001$, and 11.4% vs. 28.7%, $P < .001$, respectively).

In a randomized trial in which cilostazol was compared with aspirin in 33 patients who underwent stent implantation with a Palmaz-Schatz stent, the late loss index was significantly lower in patients treated with cilostazol (51). In a study in which 63 patients underwent stent implantation with either a Palmaz-Schatz or Wiktor stent and were randomized to receive cilostazol or placebo, restenosis occurred less frequently in patients treated with cilostazol (12.7% vs. 31.7%, $P = .05$) (52). Among 70 patients who underwent implantation of a Palmaz-Schatz stent randomized to receive cilostazol or aspirin, restenosis was lower in patients treated with cilostazol (8.6% vs. 26.8%, $P = .05$) (53).

Cilostazol was compared with ticlopidine in a randomized trial in which 300 consecutive patients undergoing elective coronary stent placement were enrolled. In both groups, the study drug was begun 2 days before the procedure; both groups also received aspirin. The primary endpoint, a composite endpoint including stent thrombosis, death, myocardial infarction, or need for a repeat revascularization procedure within 30 days, occurred in 2.0% of the ticlopidine group versus 1.4% in the cilostazol group ($P = 1.0$) (54).

Potential to Reduce Restenosis

The mechanisms by which cilostazol might reduce restenosis may include reducing neointimal proliferation by inhibiting smooth muscle cell proliferation (55,56), and attenuating endothelial cell death and stimulating endothelial cell growth (57,58). It has also been hypothesized that cilostazol might reduce restenosis by reducing arterial remodeling through its vasodilatory properties (50). Cilostazol also reduces the induction of platelet-derived growth factors, which may be beneficial (50,59). However, the clinical trials in which cilostazol reduced restenosis were all small, making it all the more remarkable that a reduction in restenosis with cilostazol was found, but raising the possibility of a type 1 error due to the small sample sizes in all of these trials. Studies using other oral antiplatelet therapy in an attempt to prevent restenosis have been uniformly disappointing (2,17, 60–62).

Unanswered Questions

Whether patients taking cilostazol chronically should also be administered aspirin is unknown. A minority of patients in the placebo-controlled randomized trials who were taking cilostazol were also taking aspirin; in these patients, there was no short term increase in hemorrhagic complications. There is an approximately 30% increase in inhibition of ADP-induced aggregation when cilostazol is added to aspirin (63), but there are no data about the safety of long-term treatment with both cilostazol and clopidogrel.

Although cilostazol appeared to be well tolerated in the studies above, there are concerns about its safety among patients with significant (class 3 or 4) congestive heart failure, a group shown to have an increased mortality when treated with several other cyclic phosphodiesterase inhibitors. For that reason, cilostazol is contraindicated in patients with congestive heart failure of any severity.

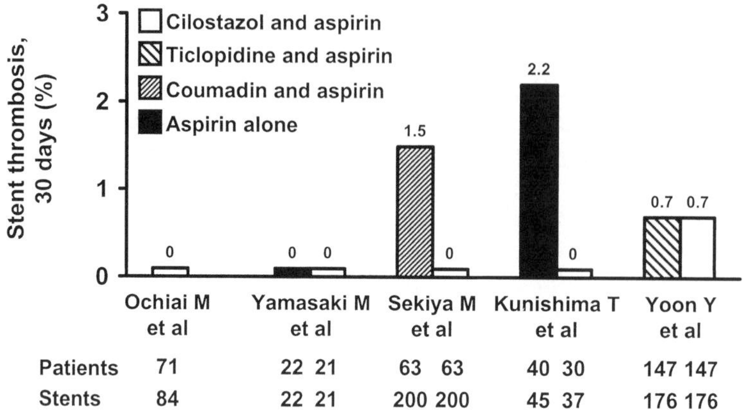

Figure 12 Studies reporting the frequency of stent thrombosis in patients treated with cilostazol. Cilostazol appeared to be more effective than aspirin alone and aspirin and coumadin, and equivalent to aspirin and ticlopidine, although all these studies were very undersized, enrolling far too few patients to provide strong evidence of the strength of therapeutic benefit.

Summary

Clearly, larger, properly designed trials will be required before the results of these studies lead to a change in clinical practice. The existing evidence suggests that cilostazol may have a role in the prevention of stent thrombosis, and based on the limited evidence available at present, it is probably reasonable to add cilostazol to aspirin among patients (without heart failure) undergoing stent placement intolerant of clopidogrel or ticlopidine (Fig. 12). More data are needed before cilostazol should be used in place of the clopidogrel or ticlopidine in patients tolerant of the thienopyridines, and before cilostazol should be used to prevent restenosis. There are no data yet suggesting a role for cilostazol in secondary or primary prevention. Further studies examining the ability of cilostazol to both prevent restenosis and stent thrombosis and other acute ischemic complications of percutaneous revascularization are planned.

ORAL PLATELET GLYCOPROTEIN IIb/IIIa RECEPTOR INHIBITORS

Platelet glycoprotein IIb/IIIa receptor inhibitors block the final common pathway of platelet aggregation. In view of the remarkable efficacy of intravenous platelet glycoprotein IIb/IIIa receptor inhibitors in the setting of percutaneous revascularization procedures (32,64,65), oral platelet glycoprotein IIb/IIIa receptor inhibitors have been developed to inhibit platelet aggregation for longer periods of time. Three oral platelet glycoprotein IIb/IIIa receptor inhibitors have been studied in very large clinical trials; others are being studied. Some of the trials have limited enrollment to patients undergoing percutaneous revascularization procedures; other trials have included patients with an acute coronary syndrome whether or not revascularization procedures were planned. The hope has been that orally active glycoprotein IIb/IIIa receptor blockers could provide the same benefits over the long term that the intravenous agents achieve over the short term, not only by reducing procedural complications during coronary revascularization but also by reducing adverse vascular events in the months and years following a revascularization procedure. There has also been the hope that the oral glycoprotein IIb/IIIa receptor blockers might reduce the frequency of restenosis.

Pharmacology

Several oral glycoprotein IIb/IIIa antagonists have been developed. The oral glycoprotein IIb/IIIa antagonists differ from one another in important ways. Orbofiban, xemilofiban, and sibrafiban, the best studied of the oral platelet glycoprotein IIb/IIIa receptor inhibitors, all are competitively bound to the platelet glycoprotein IIb/IIIa receptors, but differ in their kinetics. Twice or three times daily dosing is required for all three of these agents to maintain peak receptor blockade at levels approaching 70% to 80%, which corresponds to approximately 80% inhibition of platelet aggregation in response to a strong agonist for aggregation; 20 μM ADP has been used most frequently. The degree of inhibition at times of peak drug levels is much higher for all of the oral glycoprotein IIb/IIIa agents than at trough levels, which has generated safety concerns. It is possible that high peak levels account for high rates of bleeding (including the minor mucosal bleeding) that have been so frequent with these agents, and that low trough levels might expose the patient to insufficient levels of inhibition and fail to protect patients from platelet aggregation and ischemic events. Recent studies indicate that the oral platelet glycoprotein IIb/IIIa receptor inhibitors are associated with paradoxical activation of platelets during periods of trough drug levels, which might paradoxically increase the risk of arterial thrombosis and adverse clinical events (66,67). This might be even more clinically significant if aspirin were not simultaneously administered with the oral glycoprotein IIb/IIIa receptor inhibitor; aspirin was not administered to patients receiving an oral glycoprotein IIb/IIIa receptor in one of the large trials (the SYMPHONY trial; see below).

Potential Advantages and Disadvantages

A driving force behind the development of the oral glycoprotein IIb/IIIa inhibitors has been the recognition that aspirin as monotherapy, while effective, is far from optimal. It is a weak antiplatelet agent; many patients suffer ischemic events while on aspirin; aspirin is poorly tolerated in approximately 5% to 10% of patients; and between 10% and 40% of patients fail to respond to aspirin, depending on the platelet function test used to determine aspirin responsiveness and definition of response used (1,6–10). Although the addition of a thienopyridine to aspirin improves outcome in several clinical situations, it still does not inhibit platelet aggregation nearly as strongly as does an intravenous or oral platelet glycoprotein IIb/IIIa inhibitor (1,32,64,65,68).

The potential of both producing and administering an oral agent at a cost lower than that of the intravenous glycoprotein IIb/IIIa inhibitors has spurred the development of the oral glycoprotein IIb/IIIa inhibitors. It should be remembered, however, that since none of the oral agents have come to market, the cost of producing and price of the agents remains unknown.

The biggest concern surrounding the oral glycoprotein IIb/IIIa inhibitors IIb/IIIa antagonists has been the risk of bleeding. The more potent the agent, the greater the degree of platelet inhibition, the greater the risk of hemorrhagic complications. While the use of powerful intravenous glycoprotein IIb/IIIa antagonists for 12 to 24 hours after a revascularization procedure or during the early hospitalization for an acute coronary syndrome appears to be worth the bleeding risk in many patients, given the approximately 5% to 20% risk of an ischemic complication during this time period, the increased risk of bleeding from longer periods of treatment in lower risk individuals may not result in as favorable a risk:benefit ratio (32,64,65).

Fortunately, although thrombocytopenia has been reported for each of the oral glycoprotein IIb/IIIa antagonists, even the prolonged use of these agents causes thrombocytopenia less frequently than short-term therapy with the monoclonal antibody intravenous glycoprotein IIb/IIIa inhibitor (abciximab), and no more frequently than the small molecule intravenous glycoprotein IIb/IIIa inhibitors (tirofiban and eptifibatide) (32,64,65,69,70).

The belief that ≥80% of IIb/IIIa receptor blockade by an intravenous platelet glycoprotein IIb/IIIa inhibitor is necessary to prevent intraarterial thrombus formation in the presence of a strong thrombogenic stimulus largely results from a single study in a dog model of arterial thrombosis (71). This level of receptor blockade achieves levels of inhibition of platelet aggregation of ≤20% of baseline when 20 μM ADP, a strong stimulus of platelet aggregation, is used. The need for ≥80% of IIb/IIIa receptor blockade is indirectly supported by the results of the Evaluation of 7E3 for the

Prevention of Ischemic Complications (EPIC) trial (64). In that trial, patients receiving a bolus alone of abciximab were nearly completely protected from the need for urgent reintervention for the first 4 to 6 hours after the initial PTCA procedure, the time during which ≥80% receptor blockade is maintained. In patients treated with a bolus and 12-hour infusion of abciximab, protection from emergency repeat procedures extended almost throughout the infusion period, during which time receptor blockade was more likely to be ≥80%, with aggregation reduced to ≤20% of baseline. In contrast, patients treated with placebo required repeat procedures more frequently than the other two groups, and the period of risk in placebo-treated patients began immediately after the initial PTCA procedure. However, whether such a high level of inhibition needs to be maintained long-term following hospitalization for an acute coronary syndrome or following a coronary intervention, when the risk of arterial thrombosis is much lower, is unclear. Also, whether the "average level of inhibition" achieved with peak and trough levels of inhibition by the oral agents is efficacious is unknown. Efficacy has been conclusively demonstrated with the intravenous agents, but these maintain a relatively constant level of inhibition over the time course of the infusion.

Clinical Trials

Xemilofiban

Xemilofiban is a prodrug of a nonpeptide mimetic of the tetra-peptide RGDF. Xemilofiban is readily absorbed and metabolized to its active metabolite, SC-54701, which is a specific inhibitor of the platelet glycoprotein IIb/IIIa receptor. Elimination of xemilofiban is primarily renal.

The first study of xemilofiban was in patients undergoing a percutaneous coronary intervention; this was also the first study in which there was prolonged administration of an oral glycoprotein IIb/IIIa inhibitor (72) In this randomized, placebo-controlled, dose-ranging study in which 30 patients with an acute coronary syndrome undergoing percutaneous coronary revascularization were enrolled, 20 patients were randomized to receive a 35-mg loading dose of xemilofiban 1 to 3 hours prior to their revascularization procedure; 16 of these patients were subsequently treated with 25 mg TID, and four were treated with 20 mg TID. Ten patients received aspirin and placebo. All patients assigned to the xemilofiban arms also received aspirin. The study was terminated before completion due to an unacceptably high rate of severe bleeding. Of the 20 patients randomized to xemilofiban, four developed bleeding prior to hospital discharge sufficiently severe to require termination of the study drug. One patient developed gastric bleeding requiring 22 units of packed red blood cells, and a second died of bleeding complications following emergency bypass surgery requiring transfusion of 54 units of packed red blood cells. Only 10 xemilofiban patients completed their 30-day course of therapy, nine of whom reported minor bleeding. Pharmacodynamic analyses revealed that the majority of patients achieved peak levels of inhibition >80% in response to a 20-μM dose of ADP. However, there were large differences in platelet inhibition during peak and trough drug levels; 83% of patients had $\geq$80% inhibition during peak levels, but only 36% had $\geq$80% inhibition during trough levels.

Xemilofiban was next evaluated in a placebo-controlled study in which 170 patients receiving a coronary stent were randomized to receive either a lower dose of xemilofiban, 5 to 20 mg BID (n = 119) or ticlopidine (n = 51) (73). All patients received aspirin, and 30 patients also received the intravenous glycoprotein IIb/IIIa inhibitor abciximab during their procedure (for clinical indications at the discretion of the interventionalist). In this study, xemilofiban was not started until the morning after the interventional procedure. Only the 20-mg dose achieved $\geq$80% inhibition of aggregation. Hemorrhagic complications were infrequent; only 3 patients developed minor bleeding requiring discontinuation of xemilofiban. However, two patients developed stent thrombosis, both of whom had been treated with xemilofiban (without abciximab). Platelet inhibition was greater in patients treated with abciximab and xemilofiban than in those treated with xemilofiban alone. Among patients treated with xemilofiban alone, $\geq$80% inhibition of platelet aggregation was achieved after the initial dose of xemilofiban only in patients in whom 20 mg had been administered. No major hemorrhagic complications occurred among xemilofiban-treated patients in this study.

The Oral Glycoprotein IIb/IIIa Receptor Blockade to Inhibit Thrombosis (ORBIT) trial was a multicenter, randomized, placebo-controlled, dose-ranging trial of xemilofiban in 549 patients in whom a successful percutaneous coronary intervention had been performed (74). Four dosing strategies were evaluated in this trial, depending in part on whether abciximab was administered during the revascularization procedure. Patients receiving abciximab (29% of patients enrolled in the trial) were randomized to receive xemilofiban 10 mg three times daily for 2 weeks, followed by 15 or 20 mg twice daily for 2 weeks. Patients not receiving abciximab were randomized to receive either xemilofiban 15 mg three times daily for 2 weeks followed by 15 mg twice daily for 2 weeks, or 20 mg three times daily followed by 20 mg twice daily. Treatment with the study drug was initiated the day after the procedure and continued for 4 weeks; all patients received aspirin daily. Patients receiving placebo in whom a stent was placed (~50% of patients) received ticlopidine in addition to aspirin. Although not powered to detect a difference in clinical outcome, the primary endpoint of the study was the occurrence of death, myocardial infarction, urgent revascularization, and ischemic stroke at 90 days. Although the finding was emphasized that the composite endpoint was reached less frequently among patients who had received 20 mg xemilofiban than among those on placebo (3% vs. 12%, $P = .04$), close examination of the event curves is puzzling in that there was no suggestion of benefit from xemilofiban in the 2 weeks following the revascularization procedure, when most adverse events generally occur. Between days 30 and 90, placebo-treated patients had far more events than patients receiving xemilofiban, which is unusual in that adverse events in days 30 and 90 after a percutaneous revascularization procedure are rare except for restenosis, which is not believed to be reduced by xemilofiban. Among patients receiving abciximab, 26% patients treated with 20 mg xemilofiban had an event, compared with 15% in the placebo arm ($P = .36$). As in earlier studies, a correlation was noted between drug plasma concentrations and the degree of platelet inhibition, with a relatively steep dose response relationship. Bleeding complications were frequent, but generally mild. Analysis of patients not receiving abciximab revealed that "minor" bleeding in patients treated with placebo, 10 to 15 mg xemilofiban, or 10 to 20 mg xemilofiban was common (access site bleeding 6%, 6%, or 7%; gastrointestinal bleeding 1%, 5%, or 8%; genitourinary tract 2%, 8%, or 3%; oral/gingival 1%, 10%, 5%; or epistaxis 5%, 15%, 23%, respectively). Based on the suggestion of benefit in the xemilofiban patients not treated with abciximab, a large-scale Phase III trial was designed to further evaluate long-term glycoprotein IIb/IIIa inhibition with xemilofiban among patient s undergoing a percutaneous revascularization procedure.

The Evaluation of Oral Xemilofiban in Controlling Thrombotic Events (EXCITE) trial was a double-blind, placebo-controlled study of the efficacy and safety of xemilofiban when initiated prior to and continued for up to 6 months after a percutaneous coronary revascularization procedure (75). In EXCITE, 7233 patients were randomized to either placebo initiated 30 to 90 min prior to the revascularization procedure; xemilofiban 20 mg initiated 30 to 90 min prior to the procedure followed by either xemilofiban 10 mg TID for 6 months or xemilofiban 20 mg TID for 6 months. All patients also received aspirin. It was believed that xemilofiban 20 mg would inhibit ADP-induced platelet aggregation by ~40% at the time of the procedure, that 10 mg TID inhibit platelet aggregation by 30% to 60%, and that 20 mg TID would inhibit aggregation by 50% to 80%. In patients with minor bleeding, the dose of study drug could be adjusted in order to minimize the frequency of discontinuing the study drug.

The primary endpoint of the EXCITE trial was the occurrence of death, myocardial infarction, and urgent revascularization at 6 months. The results of the EXCITE revealed that the composite endpoint was reached in 13.6% of placebo-treated patients, 14.1% of patients treated with xemilofiban 10

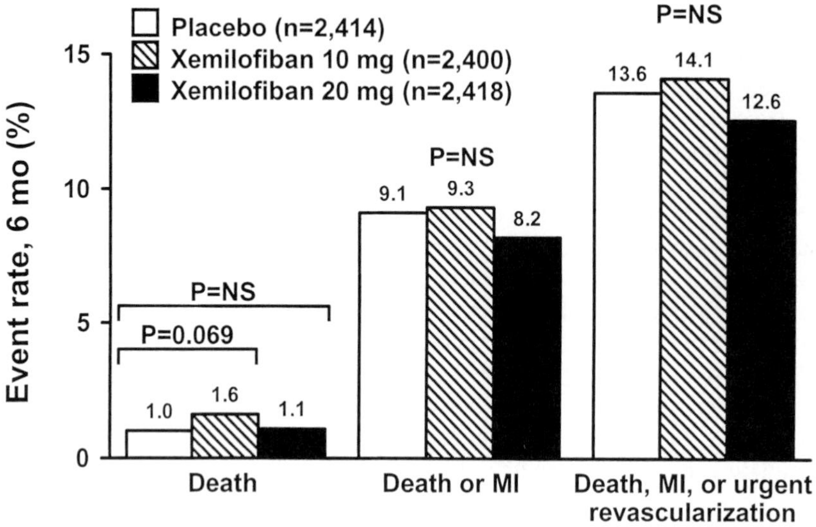

Figure 13 Results of the EXCITE trial in which xemilofiban was initiated prior to and continued for up to 6 months after a percutaneous coronary revascularization procedure.

mg, and 12.6% of patients receiving 20 mg xemilofiban (*P* = NS for all comparisons) (Fig. 13). Moderate or severe bleeding occurred in 0.9%, 3.8% (*P* = .001 vs. placebo group), and 5.1% (*P* = .001 vs. the placebo group, and *P* = .036 vs. the low-dose group) in the three groups, respectively. Minor bleeding occurred in 37.0%, 54.2%, and 66.0% of patients, respectively (*P* = .001 for all comparisons).

Based on these disappointing results, Searle, the manufacturer of xemilofiban, abandoned plans to further develop xemilofiban.

Orbofiban

Orbofiban is a synthetic peptide-mimetic glycoprotein IIb/IIIa inhibitor. Orbofiban's antiplatelet effect can be recognized 2 hours after administration; its peak effect occurs between at 4 and 6 hours. These kinetics are believed to be suitable for twice-daily dosing. Elimination of orbofiban is primarily renal.

The Safety of Orbofiban in Acute Coronary Research (SOAR) study was a dose-ranging study in which 520 patients hospitalized with an acute coronary syndrome were assigned to receive placebo or orbofiban 30, 40, or 50 mg twice daily or 50 mg once daily for up to 12 weeks; all patients also received aspirin 162 mg daily (76). Bleeding led to discontinuation of study drugs in 1%, 5%, 4%, 4% of the orbofiban groups, respectively. Severe bleeding, however, occurred in ≤1% of patients in each of the groups. These event rates were low enough to encourage further studies of orbofiban. A pharmacodynamic substudy of SOAR revealed a dose-related increase in inhibition of platelet aggregation in response to 20 mM ADP. Only the 50-mg twice-daily dose achieved both peak and trough levels of inhibition of platelet aggregation of 60% to 80% (77).

Subsequently, the Orbofiban in Patients with Unstable Coronary Syndromes–Thrombolysis in Myocardial Infarction-16 (OPUS-TIMI-16) study was performed in which patients hospitalized for treatment of an acute coronary syndrome within the prior 72 hours were randomly assigned to receive either 1) orbofiban 50 mg BID indefinitely; 2) orbofiban 50 mg twice daily for 30 days, which was then reduced to 30 mg twice daily thereafter; 3) placebo. All patients also received aspirin 150 to 162 mg (78). The primary endpoint of the study was a composite endpoint of death, myocardial infarction, urgent revascularization, rehospitalization for ischemia, or stroke.

The trial was halted by the Data Safety Monitoring Board after 10,302 patients had been enrolled due to safety concerns resulting from the first 30 days of treatment. The results of OPUS were unusual in that although therapy was identical in two of the three arms of the trial throughout the first 30 days, the results differed during this time period between these two arms (Fig. 14). Among patients taking placebo, the frequency in which the composite endpoint was reached within 30 days was 10.7%, versus 9.7% in the low-dose orbofiban arm and 9.3% in the high-dose orbofiban arm (*P* = .14 placebo vs. low-dose arm, and .05 placebo vs. high-dose arm). The finding that in the placebo, low-dose, and high-dose orbofiban arms, the frequency of death at 30 days was 1.4%, 2.3%, and 1.6%, respectively (*P* = .004 placebo vs. low-dose arm, and .53 placebo vs. high-dose arm) suggested that orbofiban increased early mortality. In the placebo, low-dose, and high-dose orbofiban arms, the frequency of myocardial infarction was 3.1%, 3.0%, and 2.6% (*P* = NS all comparisons); the frequency of urgent revascularization was 5.2%, 2.9%, and 3.3% (*P* = NS all comparisons); the frequency of urgent revascularization was 5.2%, 2.9%, and 3.3% (*P* = .001 all comparisons); the frequency of rehospitalization for recurrent ischemia was 4.1%, 4.0%, and 4.0% (*P* = NS all comparisons); and the frequency of stroke was 0.5%, 0.5%, and 0.6%, respectively (*P* = NS all comparisons). During follow-up through 300 days (median follow-up, 7 months), the composite endpoint was reached in 20.5% of patients in the placebo arm, 20.2% of patients in the low-dose orbofiban arm, and 19.5% of patients in the high-dose orbofiban arm (*P* = NS all comparisons). The mortality rates were 3.2%, 4.7%, and 4.0% for the placebo, low-dose, and high-dose arms, respectively (*P* =

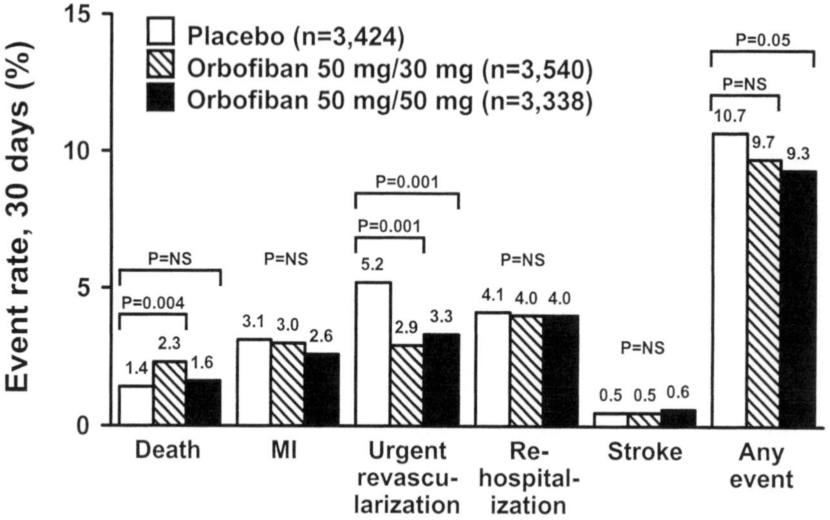

Figure 14 Results of the OPUS-TIMI 16 study in which patients with an acute coronary syndrome were randomly assigned to receive either orbofiban 50 mg BID indefinitely; orbofiban 50 mg twice daily for 30 days followed by 30 mg twice daily; or placebo.

.001 for the low-dose arm vs. placebo, and .06 for the high-dose arm vs. placebo); the rates of myocardial infarction were 4.8%, 4.9%, and 5.4% (P = NS all comparisons); the rates of urgent revascularization were 7.9%, 5.9%, and 5.8% (P = .002 favoring the low-dose arm over placebo, .004 favoring the high-dose arm versus placebo); the rates of rehospitalization for ischemia were 11.8%, 11.9%, and 10.9% (P = NS all comparisons), and the rates of stroke were 0.9%, 1.0%, and 1.1% (P = NS) in the placebo, low-dose, and high-dose arms, respectively. Severe bleeding occurred in 0.4% of placebo patients, 1.2% of high-dose patients (P = .0001), and 0.7% of high-dose patients (P = .04 vs. placebo).

In a pharmacodynamic substudy of OPUS, large variations between the peak and trough levels of orbofiban among patients taking 50 mg twice daily, and even larger differences among patients taking 30 mg twice daily, were found. These wide variations in drug levels may explain, in part, the increased frequency of both ischemic events (perhaps during trough levels of orbofiban) and bleeding (perhaps during peak levels of orbofiban) seen in the orbofiban arms of the trial (Fig. 15) (77).

Shortly after the OPUS trial was terminated by the Data and Safety Monitoring Committee, Searle, the manufacturer of orbofiban, announced

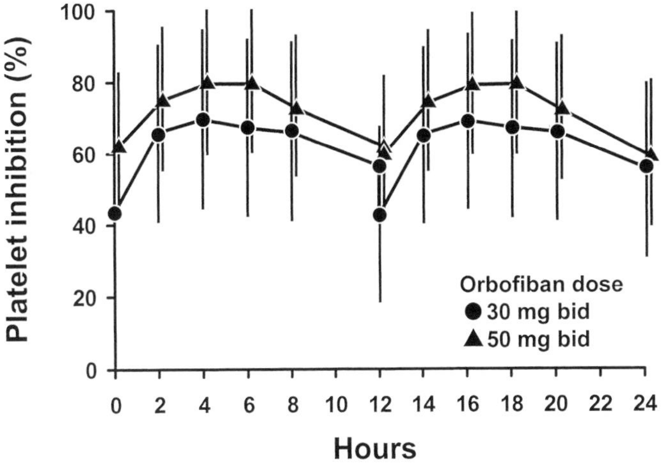

Figure 15 Degree of platelet inhibition in response to stimulation by 20 μM ADP in the OPUS-TIMI 16 study in patients receiving orbofiban 30 mg BID and 50 mg twice daily.

that the company was abandoning further development of orbofiban, as they had decided with xemilofiban.

Sibrafiban

Sibrafiban is a "doubly protected" prodrug in that it is first metabolized to a prodrug which is also inactive (Ro 48-3656), and then is further metabolized to its active metabolite (Ro 44-3888), a potent and highly selective reversible inhibitor of the platelet glycoprotein IIb/IIIa receptor.

In the TIMI 12 trial, a Phase II double-blind dose-ranging trial of sibrafiban, 329 patients with an acute coronary syndrome were enrolled in either a safety cohort, in which 223 patients were assigned to receive one of four dosages of sibrafiban ranging from 5 mg twice daily to 15 mg once daily, or aspirin, for 28 days; or they were enrolled into a pharmacokinetic cohort, in which 106 patients were randomly assigned to receive either one of seven dosages of sibrafiban ranging from 5 mg once daily to 10 mg twice daily for 28 days (79). In this trial, both the total daily dose of sibrafiban and peak plasma concentration of sibrafiban were associated with the risk of bleeding, and the peak concentration of sibrafiban and risk of bleeding were both affected by body weight and renal function (79). Minor hemorrhagic events occurred in >30% of patients, requiring discontinuation of sibrafiban in over half these patients. Discontinuation due to bleeding was required in 32% of patients in the group taking 15 mg once daily, versus only 13% of patients taking 10 mg twice daily. In the trial, twice daily dosing minimized differences between peak and trough levels and were associated with both greater sustained levels of platelet inhibition and lower rates of bleeding. Multivariate analysis indicated that the interpatient variability in peak drug concentrations was most influenced by renal function and body weight. Therefore, the dosages of sibrafiban utilized in subsequent studies (most notably the Sibrafiban Versus Aspirin to Yield Maximum Protection from Ischemic Heart Events Post Acute Coronary Syndromes [SYMPHONY] trial) were individually adjusted based on body weight and renal function. The goal was that peak plasma concentrations not exceed 40 ng/mL, since higher levels were associated with unacceptable levels of bleeding in TIMI-12, and that lower concentrations be at least approximately 7 ng/mL, a level that associated with approximately 25% inhibition of platelet aggregation in response to 20 μM ADP. This level of inhibition was modestly affective in the CAPRIE and IMPACT II trials in which drugs other than oral glycoprotein IIb/IIIa inhibitors (clopidogrel and eptifibatide, respectively) were studied.

In the SYMPHONY trial, a large Phase III trial of sibrafiban, 9233 patients with acute coronary syndrome were randomly assigned to receive either low-dose sibrafiban or high-dose sibrafiban (adjusted for renal function and weight), or placebo. The SYMPHONY trial differed from the other large Phase III trials of oral glycoprotein IIb/IIIa inhibitors in that only patients taking placebo were given aspirin; patients in the low-dose and high-dose sibrafiban arms did not receive aspirin. The primary endpoint of SYMPHONY was death, myocardial infarction, or severe recurrent ischemia within 90 days. After enrollment in SYMPHONY was completed, before the results of the trial were analyzed, investigators at participating sites began enrolling patients in the second SYMPHONY trial which was similar to the SYMPHONY trial except that patients in the low-dose sibrafiban arm also received aspirin.

The results of SYMPHONY were disappointing. The composite endpoint of death, myocardial infarction (or recurrent infarction, if an infarction had occurred prior to enrollment), or severe recurrent ischemia at 90 days was reached in 9.8% of aspirin patients, in 10.1% of patients in the low-dose sibrafiban arm, and in 10.1% of patients in the high-dose sibrafiban arm (P = NS for all comparisons) (Fig. 16) (80). Analysis of the frequency with which the individual components of the composite endpoint were reached (death 1.8%, 2.0%, and 2.0%; myocardial infarction 5.6%, 5.8%, and 6.5%; and severe recurrent ischemia 3.2%, 2.8%, and 2.5% in the placebo, low-dose sibrafiban, and high-dose sibrafiban arms, respectively) did not suggest benefit from sibrafiban.

Based on the disappointing results of SYMPHONY, enrollment was stopped in the second SYMPHONY trial after 6677 of a planned 8400 patients were enrolled. Now referred to by some as the "unfinished SYMPHONY,"

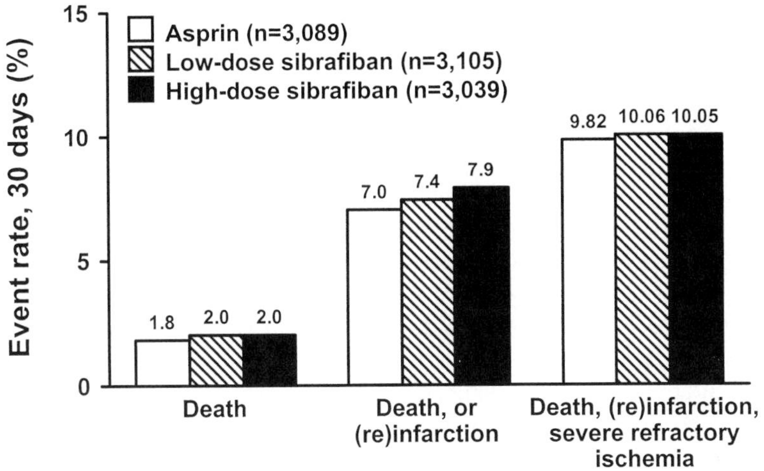

Figure 16 Results of the SYMPHONY trial in which patients with an acute coronary syndrome were randomly assigned in a double-blinded manner to receive either low- or high-dose sibrafiban (adjusted for renal function and body weight) or aspirin.

results from this trial have recently been reported. The primary endpoint of death, myocardial infarction (or recurrent infarction), or severe refractory ischemia occurred in 9.3% of patients treated with aspirin alone, in 9.2% of patients receiving low-dose sibrafiban and aspirin, and in 10.5% of patients receiving high-dose sibrafiban. Death or reinfarction occurred in 6.1%, 6.8%, and 8.6% of patients, respectively. Most troubling was the frequency of death, which was 1.3% among patients receiving aspirin alone, 1.7% among patients receiving low-dose sibrafiban and aspirin, and 2.4% in the high-dose sibrafiban arm ($P = .05$ vs. aspirin-alone arm).

Perhaps it was premature to perform these four large trials examining the safety and efficacy of the oral glycoprotein IIb/IIIa inhibitors in view of the fact that the optimal level of platelet inhibition with oral glycoprotein IIb/IIIa antagonists had not yet been established, nor had it been determined that that level could be maintained. Although plasma concentrations correlate well with the level of platelet inhibition achieved, the dose response is steep and a considerable amount of interpatient variability in plasma levels with identical doses of the oral glycoprotein IIb/IIIa inhibitors has been recognized. Also, it is unknown if the dose necessary to achieve a certain level of inhibition will change based on the clinical state. Studies have suggested that higher doses of an oral agent may be required in unstable coronary syndromes to achieve the same level of inhibition in patients with stable disease (81).

Overview of the Oral Glycoprotein IIb/IIIa Inhibitor Trials

The results of the four large trials of oral glycoprotein IIb/IIIa inhibitors, one of which (OPUS) suggested the study drug was harmful and the other two (EXCITE, SYMPHONY) suggested the study drug was of no benefit, have been disappointing. In fact, when the results of the four trials are analyzed together, a statistically significant increase in mortality associated with administration of an oral glycoprotein IIb/IIIa inhibitor can be seen (Fig. 17). The results of these studies have increased concerns that platelet-activating properties of these drugs may exist and be both clinically important and harmful. It has been reported that conformational changes in the glycoprotein IIb/IIIa receptor occur when binding to a IIb/IIIa inhibitor takes place (67). However, after these drugs dissociate from membrane receptors, the conformational changes persist, and platelets may actually be more likely to bind fibrinogen than before exposure to the IIb/IIIa receptor antagonist. Indeed, one study has indicated that oral glycoprotein IIb/IIIa inhibitors actually increase platelet activation, as assessed by P-selectin levels, compared with placebo (66). If true, the short half-life of these agents and large differences between peak and trough levels might not only increase the risk of

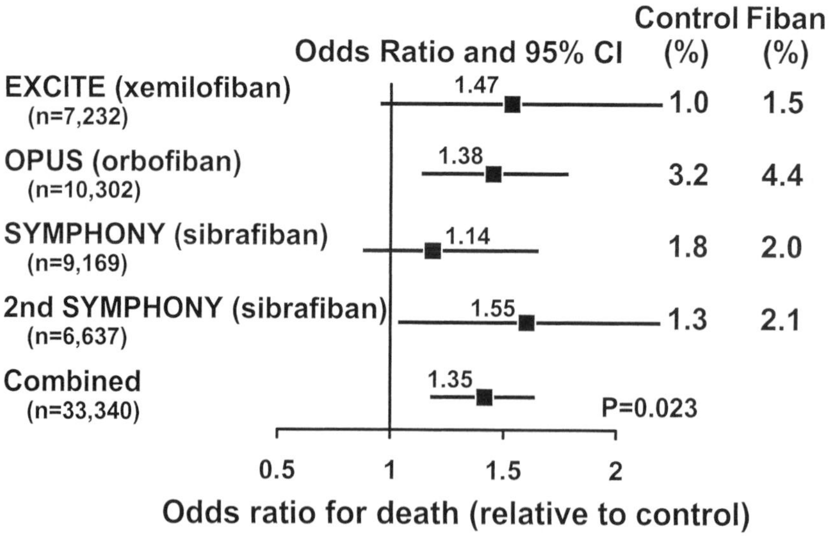

Figure 17 Analysis of the EXCITE, OPUS-TIMI 16, SYMPHONY, and second SYMPHONY trials. A statistically significant increase in mortality associated with administration of an oral glycoprotein IIb/IIIa inhibitor can be seen. (Courtesy of Dr. Kristin Newby.)

bleeding during peak levels, but might also paradoxically increase the risk of ischemic complications during periods of trough levels. Whether ischemic events in patients taking oral glycoprotein IIb/IIIa inhibitors do in fact cluster during periods of trough drug levels remains unproven.

Further development of many other oral glycoprotein IIb/IIIa inhibitors has been abandoned, in part because of disappointing results from preclinical and clinical trials, in part due to production costs believed to be too high for the drugs to ultimately be profitable, and in part due to the disappointing results of studies of these oral glycoprotein IIb/IIIa antagonists.

Ongoing Oral Glycoprotein IIb/IIIa Inhibitor Studies

There are two large ongoing trials of oral glycoprotein IIb/IIIa antagonists. In the Blockade of the Glycoprotein IIb/IIIa Receptor to Avoid Vascular Occlusion (BRAVO) trial, 9200 patients with an acute coronary syndrome will be randomized to receive the oral glycoprotein IIb/IIIa antagonist lotrafiban, either 30 mg or 50 mg depending on their body weight and renal function, and aspirin, or placebo and aspirin (82). The primary endpoint of the study is the occurrence of death, myocardial infarction, stroke, recurrent ischemia requiring hospitalization, or urgent revascularization. The existence of longer-acting oral glycoprotein IIb/IIIa receptor inhibitors like lotrafiban has encouraged investigators to investigate this drug further before abandoning the class of drugs based on the results of the EXCITE, OPUS-TIMI 16, and SYMPHONY.

Another trial, the ROCKET trial, had been planned in patients with an acute coronary syndrome who were to receive aspirin and be randomized to receive the oral glycoprotein IIb/IIIa antagonist roxifiban versus placebo. The manufacturers of roxifiban are weighing the disappointing results of the earlier four trials and deciding whether to proceed with the trial.

ANTIPLATELET DRUGS AND RESTENOSIS

Extended antiplatelet therapy with aspirin (with dipyridamole), ticlopidine, and thromboxane A_1-receptor inhibitors has been studied in randomized trials in an attempt to prevent restenosis after balloon angioplasty. None of the trials suggested that antiplatelet therapy with these drugs reduces restenosis (2,17,60–62). The studies of cilostazol have been promising, but the trials have been so small that a type 1 error may have been present (49–53). The positive results seen thus far must be duplicated in properly designed trials. The intravenous glycoprotein IIb/IIIa inhibitor abciximab has been associated with a reduced frequency of clinical restenosis in some trials, although the results have been inconsistent (32,64,65). Preliminary analyses of the trials in which oral glycoprotein IIb/IIIa antagonists were administered for prolonged periods of time do not suggest a reduction in clinical restenosis among patients who underwent percutaneous revascularization in those trials (2,17,60–62).

Despite the disappointing results of these trials, however, all patients undergoing percutaneous revascularization with any device should be maintained on aspirin indefinitely because of aspirin's ability to prevent ischemic events in patients with coronary disease (and vascular disease of any kind) (1). The duration of therapy that patients undergoing percutaneous revascularization should be treated with clopidogrel is being studied in the CREDO trial.

CONCLUSIONS

The large Phase III studies of the oral glycoprotein IIb/IIIa inhibitors have been extremely disappointing. Important lessons have been learned from these studies, and it is not yet appropriate to abandon hope for the entire class of agents. However, if the two large ongoing clinical trials are also negative (or reveal an increased risk associated with the use of the oral glycoprotein IIb/IIIa antagonists), it is unlikely that further investment in the development of this class of drugs will occur. This is particularly true if the CURE study examining combined therapy with aspirin and clopidogrel reveals these two drugs are both safe and efficacious when used in combination. This combination of inexpensive drugs would be formidable competition for the combination of an oral glycoprotein IIb/IIIa inhibitor and aspirin.

It is likely that future trials of oral antiplatelet drugs will include concomitant aspirin therapy. Studies such as CAPRIE, in which clopidogrel was found to be slightly more efficacious than aspirin, and SYMPHONY, in which the glycoprotein IIb/IIIa inhibitor sibrafiban was compared with aspirin, are less relevant to clinical practice because aspirin is so effective, well tolerated, and inexpensive. Even if the comparator drug is slightly more efficacious than aspirin and leads to approval of the drug, few patients will be treated with it in place of aspirin. Background aspirin might increase the efficacy of other antiplatelet drugs, such as the glycoprotein IIb/IIIa inhibitors, by inhibiting platelet aggregation during periods of trough levels of the glycoprotein IIb/IIIa inhibitor; the difference between platelet aggregation during peak and trough levels of aspirin is very small.

SUMMARY

For more than 100 years, aspirin was the only oral antiplatelet agent available for the primary and secondary prevention of myocardial infarction and for patients undergoing percutaneous coronary revascularization procedures. Then, ticlopidine became available and further improved clinical outcome, both in and out of the catheterization laboratory. Now, clopidogrel has become the thienopyridine of choice for most if not all indications. The role of cilostazol in the treatment of coronary disease and in patients undergoing percutaneous coronary revascularization procedures remains unclear. What role, if any, the oral platelet glycoprotein IIb/IIIa inhibitors will have in the treatment of patients with coronary disease is unknown; the future of this class of drugs is bleak. Ongoing studies of all of the newer oral antiplatelet drugs will further define their role in preventing adverse events in patients on aspirin, and in patients undergoing percutaneous revascularization procedures involving coronary stents and other interventions as well.

REFERENCES

1. Antiplatelet Trialists' Collaboration. Collaborative overview of randomised trials of antiplatelet therapy. I. Prevention of death, myocardial infarction, and stroke by prolonged antiplatelet therapy in various categories of patients. Antiplatelet Trialists' Collaboration. Br Med J 1994;308(6921):81–106.
2. Schwartz L, Bourassa MG, Lesperance J, et al. Aspirin and dipyridamole in the prevention of restenosis after percutaneous transluminal coronary angioplasty. N Engl J Med 1988;318(26):1714–1719.
3. White CW, Chaitman B, Knudson ML, Chisholm RJ, and the Ticlopidine Study Group. Antiplatelet agents are effective in reducing the acute ischemic complications of angioplasty but do not prevent restenosis: results from the ticlopidine trial. Coronary Artery Dis 1991;2:757–767.
4. Taylor DW, Barnett HJ, Haynes RB, et al. Low-dose and high-dose acetylsalicylic acid for patients undergoing carotid endarterectomy: a randomised controlled trial. ASA and Carotid Endarterectomy (ACE) Trial Collaborators. Lancet 1999;353:2179–2184.
5. Ryan TJ, Anderson JL, Antman EM, et al. ACC/AHA guidelines for the management of patients with acute myocardial infarction: a report of the American College of Cardiology/American Heart Association task force on practice guidelines (Committee of Management of Acute Myocardial Infarction). J Am Coll Cardiol 1996;28:1328–1428.
6. Helgason CM, Tortorice KL, Winkler SR, et al. Aspirin response and failure in cerebral infarction. Stroke 1993;24(3):345–350.
7. Helgason CM, Bolin KM, Hoff JA, et al. Development of aspirin resistance in persons with previous ischemic stroke. Stroke 1994;25(12):2331–2336.
8. Buchanan MR, Brister SJ. Individual variation in the effects of ASA on platelet function: implications for the use of ASA clinically. Can J Cardiol 1995;11(3):221–227.
9. Grotemeyer KH, Scharafinski HW, Husstedt IW. Two-year follow-up of aspirin responder and aspirin non responders. A pilot-study including 180 post-stroke patients. Thromb Res 1993;71(5):397–403.

10. Buchanan MR, Hirsh J. Effect of aspirin on hemostasis and thrombosis. N Engl Regional Allergy Proc 1986;7(1):26–31.
11. Mueller MR, Salat A, Stangl P, et al. Variable platelet response to low-dose ASA and the risk of limb deterioration in patients submitted to peripheral arterial angioplasty. Thromb Haemost 1997;78:1003–1007.
12. Savi P, Herbert JM. ADP receptors on platelets and ADP-selective antiaggregating agents. Med Res Rev 1996;16(2):159–179.
13. Mills DC, Puri R, Hu CJ, et al. Clopidogrel inhibits the binding of ADP analogues to the receptor mediating inhibition of platelet adenylate cyclase. Arterioscler Thromb 1992;12(4):430–436.
14. Coukell AJ, Markham A. Clopidogrel. Drugs 1997;54(5):745–750.
15. Yang LH, Fareed J. Vasomodulatory action of clopidogrel and ticlopidine. Thromb Res 1997;86(6):479–491.
16. Puri RN, Colman RW. ADP-induced platelet activation. Crit Rev Biochem Mol Biol 1997;3:437–502.
17. Bertrand ME, Allain H, LaBlanche JM, on behalf of the Investigators of the TACT study. Results of a randomized trial of ticlopidine versus placebo for prevention of acute closure and restenosis after coronary angioplasty (PTCA): the TACT study. Circulation 1990;82(suppl III):190.
18. Morice SP, Lefevre T, Grines C, Mattos L, den Heuvel PV, Nobuyoshi M, van der Giessen W, Brodie B, Katz S. Antiplatelet treatment with ticlopidine and aspirin does not prevent major adverse cardiac events in acute myocardial infarction patients treated with balloon alone: results from the Stent PAMI trial. Circulation 1998;98(suppl I):572. Abstract.
19. Berger PB, Dzavik V, Al-Rashdan I, et al. Does ticlopidine reduce reocclusion after successful balloon angioplasty of coronary occlusions? Insights from TOSCA. J Am Coll Cardiol 1999;33:40A. Abstract.
20. Hall P, Nakamura S, Maiello L, et al. A randomized comparison of combined ticlopidine and aspirin therapy versus aspirin therapy alone after successful intravascular ultrasound-guided stent implantation. Circulation 1996;93(2): 215–222.
21. Urban P, Macaya C, Rupprecht HJ, et al. Randomized evaluation of anticoagulation versus antiplatelet therapy after coronary stent implantation in high-risk patients: the multicenter aspirin and ticlopidine trial after intracoronary stenting (MATTIS). Circulation 1998;98(20):2126–2132.
22. Schomig A, Neumann FJ, Kastrati A, et al. A randomized comparison of antiplatelet and anticoagulant therapy after the placement of coronary-artery stents. N Engl J Med 1996;334(17):1084–1089.
23. Leon MB, Baim DS, Popma JJ, et al. A clinical trial comparing three antithrombotic-drug regimens after coronary-artery stenting. Stent Anticoagulation Restenosis Study Investigators. N Engl J Med 1998;339(23):1665–1671.
24. Bertrand ME, Legrand V, Boland J, et al. Randomized multicenter comparison of conventional anticoagulation versus antiplatelet therapy in unplanned and elective coronary stenting. The Full Anticoagulation Versus Aspirin and Ticlopidine (FANTASTIC) study. Circulation 1998;98(16):1597–1603.

25. Rupprecht HJ, Darius H, Borkowski U, et al. Comparison of antiplatelet effects of aspirin, ticlopidine, or their combination after stent implantation. Circulation 1998;97(11):1046–1052.
26. Steinhubl SR, Tan WA, Foody JM, Topol EJ, for the EPISTENT Investigators. Incidence and clinical course of thrombotic thrombocytopenic purpura due to ticlopidine following coronary stenting. JAMA 1999;281:806–810.
27. Berger PB, Bell MR, Grill DE, Melby S, Holmes DR Jr. Safety and efficacy of ticlopidine for only two weeks after successful intracoronary stent placement. Circulation 1999;99:248–253.
27A. Berger PB, Mahaffey KW, Buller CE, Meier SJ, Batchelor W, Zidar JP. Safety of only 2 weeks of ticlopidine therapy in patients at increased risk of coronary stent thrombosis: results from the ATLAST (Antiplatelet Therapy vs. Antiplatelet Therapy Alone in Patients at Increased Risk of Stent Thrombosis) trial. Circulation 1999;100(18):I-152.
28. Wilson S, Rihal CS, Bell MR, Holmes DRJ, Berger PB. Timing of coronary stent thrombosis in patients treated with ticlopidine and aspirin. Am J Cardiol 1999;83:1006–1011.
29. Schomig A, Kastrati A, Schuhlen H, et al. Risk factor analysis for stent occlusion within the first month after successful coronary stent placement. J Am Coll Cardiol 1998;31(suppl A):99A.
30. Steinhubl SR, Lauer MS, Mukherjee DP, et al. The duration of pretreatment with ticlopidine prior to stenting is associated with the risk of procedure-related non-Q-wave myocardial infarctions. J Am Coll Cardiol 1998;32(5): 1366–1370.
31. Steinhubl S, Balog C, Topol EJ. Pretreatment with ticlopidine prior to stenting is associated with a substantial decrease in complications: Data from the EPISTENT trial. Circulation 1998;98(suppl I):573. Abstract.
32. EPISTENT Investigators. Randomised placebo-controlled and balloon-angioplasty-controlled trial to assess safety of coronary stenting with use of platelet glycoprotein-IIb/IIIa blockade. Evaluation of Platelet IIb/IIIa Inhibitor for Stenting. Lancet 1998;352(9122):87–92.
33. Savi P, et al. Circulation 1999;100(suppl I):I-680.
34. Boneu B, Destelle G. Platelet anti-aggregating activity and tolerance of clopidogrel in atherosclerotic patients. Thromb Haemost 1996;76(6):939–943.
35. CAPRIE Steering Committee. A randomised, blinded, trial of clopidogrel versus aspirin in patients at risk of ischaemic events (CAPRIE). Lancet 1996; 348(9038):1329–1339.
36. Easton JD. Net benefit of clopidogrel over aspirin for the prevention of atherothrombotic events. Cerebrovasc Dis 1998;8(suppl 4):46.
37. Gibbons RJ, Chatterjee KD, Daley J, et al. ACC/AHA/ACP-ASIM guidelines for the management of patients with chronic stable angina: executive summary and recommendations: a report of the American College of Cardiology/American Heart Association Task Force on Practice Guidelines (Committee on Management of Patients With Chronic Stable Angina). Circulation 1999;99: 2829–2848.

38. Bachmann F, Savcic M, Hauert J, et al. Rapid onset of inhibition of ADP-induced platelet aggregation by a loading dose of clopidogrel. Eur Heart J 1996;suppl 263A.
39. Berger PB, Bell MR, Rihal CS, et al. Clopidogrel versus ticlopidine after intracoronary stent placement. J Am Coll Cardiol 1999;34:1891–1894.
40. Wang X, Oetgen M, Maida R, et al. The effectiveness of the combination of Plavix and aspirin versus Ticlid and aspirin after coronary stent implantation. J Am Coll Cardiol 1999;33:13A.
40A. Moussa I, Maida R, DeGregorio J, Chui M, Cohen N, Collins M. Prospective experience with clopidogrel use after coronary stent implantation in 1100 consecutive patients. Circulation 1999;100(suppl I):379. Abstract.
40B. Berger P. Clopidogrel versus ticlopidine after coronary stent placement. Presented at the Transcatheter Therapeutics conference, Washington, October 1999.
40C. Mehran R, Dangas G. Ticlopidine versus clopidogrel in patients receiving coronary stents. Presented at the Transcatheter Therapeutics Course, Washington, October 1999.
40D. L'Allier PL, Aronow HD, Cura FA, et al. Short term mortality lower with clopidogrel than ticlopidine following coronary artery stenting. J Am Coll Cardiol 2000;35(suppl A):66A.
40E. Mishkel GJ, Aguirre FV, Ligon RW, Rocha-Singh KJ, Lucore CL. Clopidogrel as adjunctive antiplatelet therapy during coronary stenting. J Am Coll Cardiol 1999;34:1884–1890.
40F. Calver AL, Blows LJ, Dawkins KD, Gray HH, Morgan JM, Simpson IA. The use of clopidogrel instead of ticlopidine after intra-coronary stent insertion: initial results in stents of ≤3 mm in diameter. Eur Heart J 1999;20:529. Abstract.
40G. Plucinski DA, Scheltema K, Krusmark J, Panchyshyn N. A comparison of clopidogrel to ticlopidine therapy for the prevention of major adverse cardiac events at thirty days and six months following coronary stent implantation. J Am Coll Cardiol 2000;35(suppl A):67A.
41. Bertrand ME, Rupprecht H-J, Urban P, Gershlick AJ. Comparative safety of ticlopidine and clopidogrel in coronary stent patients: data from CLASSICS. Circulation 1999;100(suppl 11):I-620.
42. Taniuchi M, Kurz HI, Smith SC, Lasala JM. Ticlid or Plavix Post-Stents (TOPPS). Circulation 1999;100(suppl I):379.
42A. Mueller C, Buttner HJ, Petersen J, Roskamm H. A randomized comparison of clopidogrel and aspirin versus ticlopidine and aspirin after the placement of coronary-artery stents. Circulation 2000;101:590–593.
43. Makkar RR, Eigler NL, Kaul S, et al. Effects of clopidogrel, aspirin and combined therapy in a porcine ex vivo model of high-shear induced stent thrombosis. Eur Heart J 1998;19:1538–1546.
44. Harker LA et al. Clopidogrel inhibition of stent, graft, and vascular thrombogenesis with antithrombotic enhancement by aspirin in nonhuman primates. Circulation 1998;1998:2461–2469.

45. Antiplatelet Trialists' Collaboration. Collaborative overview of randomised trials of antiplatelet therapy. II. Maintenance of vascular graft or arterial patency by antiplatelet therapy. Br Med J 1994;308(6922):159–168.
46. Money SR, et al. J Vasc Surg 1998;27:267–275.
47. Ochiai M, Isshiki T, Takeshita S, et al. Use of cilostazol, a novel antiplatelet agent, in a post-Palmaz-Schatz stenting regimen. Am J Cardiol 1997;79(11): 1471–1474.
48. Tsutsui M, Shimokawa H, Higuchi S, et al. Effect of cilostazol, a novel antiplatelet drug, on restenosis after percutaneous transluminal coronary angioplasty. Jpn Circ J 1996;60(4):207–215.
49. Tsuchikane E, Katoh O, Sumitsuji S, et al. Impact of cilostazol on intimal proliferation after directional coronary atherectomy. Am Heart J 1998;135(3): 495–502.
50. Tsuchikane E, Fukuhara A, Kobayashi T, et al. Impact of cilostazol on restenosis after percutaneous coronary balloon angioplasty. Circulation 1999; 100(1):21–26.
51. Yamasaki M, Hara K, Ikari Y, et al. Effects of cilostazol on late lumen loss after Palmaz-Schatz stent implantation. Cathet Cardiovasc Diagn 1998;44(4): 387–391.
52. Sekiya M, Funada J, Watanabe K, Miyagawa M, Akutsu H. Effects of probucol and cilostazol alone and in combination on frequency of poststenting restenosis. Am J Cardiol 1998;82(2):144–147.
53. Kunishima T, Musha H, Eto F, et al. A randomized trial of aspirin versus cilostazol therapy after successful coronary stent implantation. Clin Ther 1997;19(5):1058–1066.
54. Yoon-sup Y, Shim W-H, Lee D-H, et al. Usefulness of cilostazol versus ticlopidine in coronary artery stenting. Am J Cardiol 1999;84:1375–1380.
55. Matsumoto Y, Tani T, Watanabe K et al. Effects of cilostazol, an antiplatelet drug, on smooth muscle cell proliferation after endothelial denudation in rats. Jpn J Pharmacol 1992;58:284.
56. Kubota Y, Kichikawa K, Uchida H, et al. Pharmacologic treatment of intimal hyperplasia after metallic stent placement in the peripheral arteries. An experimental study. Invest Radiol 1995;30(9):532–537.
57. Morishita R, Nakamura S, Nakamura Y, et al. Potential role of an endothelium-specific growth factor, hepatocyte growth factor, on endothelial damage in diabetes. Diabetes 1997;1997:138–142.
58. Morishita R, Higaki J, Hayashi SI, et al. Role of hepatocyte growth factor in endothelial regulation: prevention of high D-glucose-induced endothelial cell death by prostaglandins and phosphodiesterase type 3 inhibitor. Diabetologia 1997;40(9):1053–1061.
59. Takahashi S, Oida K, Fujiwara R, et al. Effect of cilostazol, a cyclic AMP phosphodiesterase inhibitor, on the proliferation of rat aortic smooth muscle cells in culture. J Cardiovasc Pharmacol 1992;20(6):900–906.
60. Savage MP, Goldberg S, Bove AA, et al. Effect of thromboxane A_2 blockade on clinical outcome and restenosis after successful coronary angioplasty:

Multi-Hospital Eastern Atlantic Restenosis Trial (M-HEART II). Circulation 1995;92:3194–3200.

61. Serruys PW, Rutsch W, Heyndrickx GR, et al. Prevention of restenosis after percutaneous transluminal coronary angioplasty with thromboxane A_2-receptor blockade. A randomized, double-blind, placebo-controlled trial. Coronary Artery Restenosis Prevention on Repeated Thromboxane-Antagonism Study (CARPORT). Circulation 1991;84(4):1568–1580.
62. White CW, Chaitman B, Knudson ML, Chisholm RJ, and the Ticlopidine Study Group. Antiplatelet agents are effective in reducing the acute ischemic complications of angioplasty but do not prevent restenosis: results from the ticlopidine trial. Coron Artery Dis 1991;2:757–767.
63. Mallikaarjun S, et al. Clin Pharmacokinetics 1999;37(suppl 2):87–93.
64. EPIC Investigators. Use of a monoclonal antibody directed against the platelet glycoprotein IIb/IIIa receptor in high-risk coronary angioplasty. N Engl J Med 1994;330:956–961.
65. EPILOG Investigators. Platelet glycoprotein IIb/IIIa blockade and low-dose heparin during percutaneous coronary revascularization. N Engl J Med 1997; 336:1689–1696.
66. Casey M, Fornari C, Bozovich GE, Iglesias Varela ML, Mautner B, Cannon C. Increased expression of platelet p-selectin in patients treated with oral orbofiban in the OPUS-TIMI 16 study. Circulation 1999;100(suppl I):161. Abstract.
67. Peter K, Schwarz M, Ylanne J, et al. Induction of fibrinogen binding and platelet aggregation as a potential intrinsic property of various glycoprotein IIb/IIIa (aIIbb3) inhibitors. Blood 1998;92:3240–3249.
68. Bode L, Straub A, Kohler B, et al. Direct monitoring of c7E3 and fibrinogen binding to platelets allows differentiation of GP II/IIIa blockade and ticlopidine effects on platelet function. Circulation 1998;98(suppl I):250. Abstract.
69. PRISM-PLUS Study Investigators. Inhibition of the platelet glycoprotein IIb/IIIa receptor with tirofiban in unstable angina and non-Q-wave myocardial infarction. N Engl J Med 1998;338:1488–1497.
70. PURSUIT Study Investigators. Inhibition of platelet glycoprotein IIb/IIIa with eptifibatide in patients with acute coronary syndromes. N Engl J Med 1998; 339:436–443.
71. Coller BS, Scudder LE, Beer J, et al. Monoclonal antibodies to platelet GP IIb/IIIa as antithrombotic agents. Ann NY Acad Sci 1991;614:193–213.
72. Simpfendorfer C, Kottke-Marchant K, Lowrie M, et al. First chronic platelet glycoprotein IIb/IIIa integrin blockade. A randomized, placebo-controlled pilot study of xemilofiban in unstable angina with percutaneous coronary interventions. Circulation 1997;96(1):76–81.
73. Kereiakes DJ, Kleiman N, Ferguson JJ, et al. Sustained platelet glycoprotein IIb/IIIa blockade with oral xemilofiban in 170 patients after coronary stent deployment. Circulation 1997;96:1117–1121.
74. Kereiakes DJ, Kleiman NS, Ferguson JJ, et al. Pharmacodynamic efficacy, clinical safety, and outcomes after prolonged platelet glycoprotein IIb/IIIa

receptor blockade with oral xemilofiban: results of a multicenter, placebo-controlled, randomized trial. Circulation 1998;98(13):1268–1278.
75. O'Neill WW, et al. N. Engl J Med 2000;342:1316–1324.
76. Theroux P, Deedwania PC, Ferguson JJ, et al. Safety of orbofiban in acute coronary research (SOAR) study after three months of treatment. Circulation 1998;98:I-766.
77. Ferguson JJ, Deedwania PC, Kereiakes DJ, et al. Sustained platelet GP IIb/IIIa blockade with oral orbofiban: interim pharmacodynamic results of the SOAR study. J Am Coll Cardiol 1998;31:185A. Abstract.
78. Cannon CP, et al. Circulation 2000. In press.
79. Cannon CP, McCabe CH, Borzak S, et al. Randomized trial of an oral platelet glycoprotein IIb/IIIa antagonist, sibrafiban, in patients after an acute coronary syndrome. Results of the TIMI 12 trial. Circulation 1998;97:340–349.
80. SYMPHONY Investigators. Comparison of sibrafiban with aspirin for prevention of cardiovascular events after acute coronary syndromes: a randomised trial. Lancet 1999;355:337–345.
81. Catella-Lawson F, Kapoor S, Moretti DT, et al. Chronic oral glycoprotein IIb/IIIa antagonism in patients with unstable coronary syndromes: reduced antiplatelet effect in comparison to patients with stable coronary artery disease. Circulation 1998;98:I-251.
82. Topol EJ, et al. Am Heart J 2000. In press.
83. Berger PB. Aspirin, ticlopidine, and clopidogrel in and out of the catheterization laboratory. J Inves Cardiol 1999;11:20A–29A.
84. Berger PB. Clopidogrel instead of ticlopidine after coronary stent placement: is the switch justified? Am Heart J 2000:140. In press.

18

Aspirin Resistance

John H. Alexander
Duke University Medical Center
Durham, North Carolina

Steven R. Steinhubl
Wilford Hall Medical Center
San Antonio, Texas

INTRODUCTION

The central role of platelet activation and aggregation in the pathophysiology of acute coronary syndromes has been well documented through serological (1–3), angioscopic (4), and autopsy (5) studies. However, some of the strongest evidence supporting the importance of platelets in acute coronary syndromes has been the consistently beneficial results achieved with antiplatelet therapies in patients with unstable angina and acute myocardial infarction. Aspirin (acetylsalicylic acid), which has been commercially available for just over 100 years, even today remains the cornerstone of antiplatelet therapies in these patients.

The antipyretic and anti-inflammatory properties of salicylates were first described by Hippocrates 2400 years ago, and first published in the medical literature in 1763 (6). Acetylsalicylic acid was first synthesized in 1897 and was introduced commercially in 1899 as a powder and 1 year later became the first major drug sold in tablet form when 5 grains (~325 mg) of acetylsalicylic acid was mixed with starch and compressed. Although increased bleeding with salicylates was first described in 1891 (7), it wasn't until 1948 that it was first proposed that aspirin might be beneficial in the treatment of coronary thrombosis (8). This was rapidly followed by several nonrandomized observational reports of the benefit of aspirin in the prevention of acute coronary syndromes, but it wasn't until the 1970s and '80s that randomized, placebo-controlled, multicenter trials confirmed the valuable role of aspirin in this patient population. Early trials in unstable angina patients demonstrated that aspirin, compared to placebo, decreased the risk of death or myocardial infarction by 50% (9). The ISIS-2 trial in 1988 confirmed the critical role of aspirin in the treatment of acute myocardial infarction by showing a nearly 20% decrease in mortality with either aspirin or streptokinase alone, and a 40% reduction when used in combination (10).

PHARMACOLOGY OF ASPIRIN

In 1971 Smith and Willis described aspirin's inhibition of prostaglandin synthesis as the mechanism of its antiplatelet effect (11). Subsequent studies demonstrated that aspirin irreversibly acetylates prostaglandin H-synthase (PGHS), also referred to as cyclo-oxygenase (COX), and thereby prevents the conversion of arachadonic acid to PGH_2 and the eventual synthesis of thromboxane A_2. There are two isoforms of PGHS—PGHS-1 and PGHS-2, or COX-1 and COX-2. COX-1 is expressed in almost all cells, including platelets, whereas COX-2 is rapidly induced only after exposure to inflammatory cytokines. Aspirin is a relatively selective inhibitor of COX-1 and is 170-fold less potent in inhibiting COX-2 (12). Since the anucleated platelet lacks the biosynthetic capability to synthesize new COX-1, it remains inhibited throughout its 8- to 10-day life span.

Aspirin is rapidly absorbed in the stomach and small intestine with systemic bioavailability close to 50% over single dosages ranging from 20 to 1300 mg (13). When 325 mg of aspirin is given orally, either chewed or in solution, a significant decrease in thromboxane B_2 (a metabolite of thromboxane A_2) is detectable by 3 to 5 min, with near-maximal inhibition by 30 min (14). With chronic therapy, doses as low as 0.45 mg/kg/d have been shown to completely inhibit thromboxane B_2 production (15). However, it is unclear how generalizable the results of these ex vivo studies are to the entire aspirin-treated population as they were carried out in relatively small numbers of patients (5 to 46), and at least one study has demonstrated substantial inter- and intrapatient variability in the metabolism and subsequent platelet aggregation response to aspirin among healthy volunteers (16). The clinical significance of the variable pharmacokinetics of aspirin is unknown.

ASPIRIN RESISTANCE

Despite the clear benefit of aspirin in patients with coronary artery disease, there is growing evidence that a significant subset of patients may not benefit from therapy with standard doses of aspirin. This observation has raised the question of whether there are patients who are resistant to aspirin. Defining exactly what aspirin resistance is has been a challenge. There are no drugs that are 100% effective and one does not expect aspirin to prevent all recurrent thrombotic events; however, there may be an identifiable subset of patients in whom aspirin is less efficacious. These patients are aspirin resistant.

There are several possible explanations for the occurrence of recurrent thrombotic events in patients taking aspirin. Even if aspirin effectively inhibits thromboxane-mediated platelet activation, there are other factors in the physiologic milieu that may activate platelets despite a "therapeutic" aspirin effect. These factors, if present in sufficient strength, will overwhelm the platelet inhibitory effects of aspirin and result in platelet activation. In addition, because of fluctuations in their thrombotic milieu, patients may sometimes require higher doses of aspirin in order to obtain a "therapeutic effect." Finally, there may be yet unidentified patient characteristics that render some patients resistant to the effects of aspirin either all or some of the time.

Even if resistance to the beneficial effects of aspirin exists, the question remains how it should be identified and measured. Should it be identified pharmacodynamically by measuring aspirin's effect on platelet inhibition? This would ignore possible anti-inflammatory and other beneficial effects of aspirin. Alternatively, aspirin resistance can be "diagnosed" clinically in the subset of patients who have recurrent events despite aspirin. These "aspirin failures" can be considered resistant to the antithrombotic effects of aspirin, whether platelet mediated or not. In the following sections we will review the evidence that aspirin resistance exists, is measurable, both pharmcodynamically and clinically, and is of clinical consequence. We will also discuss some of the proposed mechanisms for resistance to aspirin. Finally, we will review the reported negative interaction between angiotensin-converting enzyme (ACE) inhibitors and aspirin.

Pharmacodynamic Evidence of Aspirin Resistance

The direct evidence that aspirin resistance exists comes from two major areas. The first is pharmacodynamic evidence that some patients have resistance to the antiplatelet effects of aspirin. Since the presumed primary mechanism of action of aspirin in patients with acute coronary syndromes is its effect on the platelet, a number of investigators, using different techniques, have attempted to demonstrate variability in the antiplatelet effects of aspirin across and within patients.

Variability in the effects of 80 and 325 mg/d aspirin has been demonstrated in healthy volunteers using assays which measure arachidonic acid induced platelet aggregation and adherence (16,17). A variable and even paradoxical response to 325 mg/d of aspirin has also been detected in normal subjects using flow cytometry for membrane glycoproteins expressed during platelet activation (18). Prior to receiving aspirin all subjects had >90% platelet activation. Following 325 mg/d of aspirin, 45% had <25% activation, 41% had 25% to 50% activation, and 14% even had >50% activation in response to arachidonic acid and epinephrine agonists. Aspirin resistance using bleeding time has also been demonstrated in both healthy subjects and patients undergoing coronary artery bypass surgery (19). A dose-related prolongation of bleeding time was found in between 30% and 90% of healthy subjects given between 80 and 1300 mg/d of aspirin and in 57% of patients undergoing coronary artery bypass grafting treated with 325 mg/d of aspirin (Fig. 1). Variability to the effects of aspirin has also been demonstrated in patients with atherosclerotic coronary artery disease, in patients following myocardial infarction, and in patients with peripheral vascular disease (20–22). Depending on the technique and criteria for aspirin resistance, between 8% and 26% of 113 patients with coronary artery disease were shown to have some resistance to the antiplatelet effects of 325 mg/d of aspirin (20). These data suggest that resistance to aspirin, as measured by bleeding time, platelet aggregation, or flow cytometry, occurs in a significant number of both normal volunteers and patients with atherosclerosis.

In addition to variability between patients, there is evidence that the effect of a given dose of aspirin may vary within a patient over time. The first study to document a variable response to aspirin within subjects over time was conducted in 306 patients following stroke (23). In this study, despite doses of aspirin ranging from 325 to 1300 mg/d, only 75% achieved complete inhibition of platelet aggregation. Importantly, of patients who did achieve complete inhibition of aggregation, over a third had only partial inhibition of aggregation when tested 6 months later. Overall, 8.4% (15.4% of those with partial and 5.0% of those with complete inhibition at hospital discharge) failed to achieve complete inhibition of platelet aggregation despite up to 1300 mg/d of aspirin. In another study of stroke patients, despite inhibition of platelet responsiveness at 2 hours after a 500-mg dose of aspirin, between 26% and 33% had the return of increased responsiveness at 12 hours (24). Similarly, data from the WARIS-II study investigating the effect of aspirin, warfarin, or combination aspirin and warfarin in a postinfarction population suggests that as many as 15% of patients treated with aspirin may be secondary nonresponders as assessed by platelet aggregate ratio 24 hours following aspirin ingestion (21). Finally, in patients with peripheral vascular disease treated with 100 mg/d of aspirin and classified as responders, nonresponders, or paradoxical responders, there was substantial movement of patients from one classification to another over the 52 weeks of

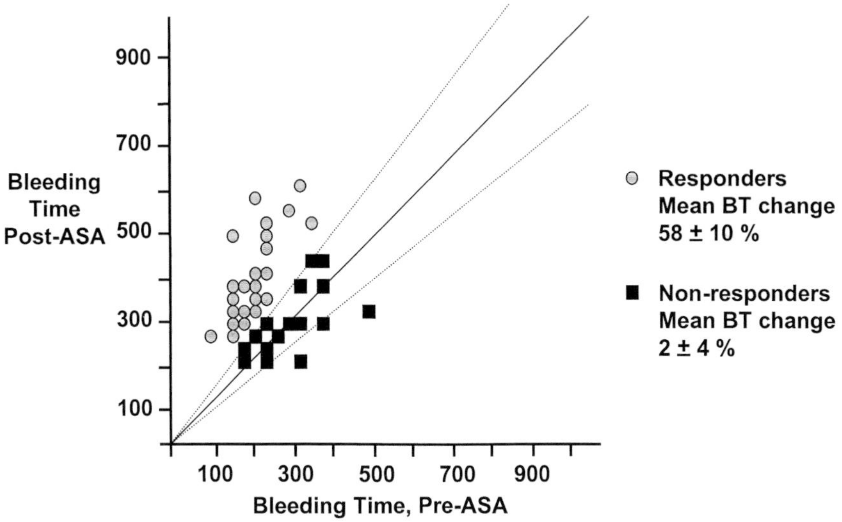

Figure 1 Effect of 325 mg/d aspirin on bleeding time in patients undergoing elective coronary artery bypass grafting. ASA, aspirin; BT, bleeding time. (Adapted from Ref. 19.)

follow-up (22). These data show that there is substantial intrapatient variability in the effects of aspirin as measured by any method studied. Aspirin resistance may be intermittently present either in all patients or in a poorly characterized subset of patients. More work is needed identifying an appropriate method of measuring a patient's response to aspirin that can be shown to correlate with the patient's long-term risk of a thrombotic event.

Not only are there patients who do not respond to aspirin and patients who respond differently over time, there is evidence that some patients respond paradoxically with an increase in platelet activity in response to aspirin. This paradoxical effect has been documented using flow cytometry to detect platelet activation and aggregometry to detect aggregation. In one study, patients were classified as responders (33%), nonresponders (45%), or paradoxical responders (22%). Responders had a reduction in activation with both 81 and 325 mg/d of aspirin, nonresponders demonstrated no significant reduction in activation with either dose, and paradoxical responders demonstrated a decrease in activation with 81 mg but an increase in activation with 325 mg/d (25). A paradoxical effect of aspirin on adenosine diphosphate and collagen-induced platelet aggregation was also seen in a subset of patients with peripheral vascular disease who had undergone percutaneous intervention treated with 100 mg/d of aspirin (22). Between 35%

and 41% were classified as responders (<80% of baseline aggregation), 41% to 55% as nonresponders (80% to 120% of baseline aggregation), and 6% to 18% as paradoxical responders (>120% of baseline aggregation). Not only do all patients not respond equally to aspirin, but also some patients may respond differently to different doses of aspirin having an increased platelet response to lower or even higher doses of aspirin.

Taken together, these studies demonstrate that between 8% and 50% of patients are likely to be resistant to the antiplatelet effects of aspirin and that this resistance may be dose related. Perhaps an even more important observation is that standard doses of aspirin are unlikely to provide consistent levels of protection over time. As the patient's thrombotic milieu changes, so may their response to aspirin and their need for the addition of alternative antiplatelet therapy.

Clinical Evidence of Aspirin Resistance

The second major body of evidence suggesting that aspirin resistance exists, and is of clinical consequence, comes from the clinical trial literature. Two studies have directly linked the presence of resistance to the antiplatelet effects of aspirin and adverse clinical outcomes. The first study to link aspirin resistance and worse outcomes was conducted in stroke patients. It demonstrated that a third of stroke patients, despite initial responsiveness to aspirin at 2 hours, developed resistance at 12 hours. These secondary aspirin nonresponders had a markedly higher rate of 2-year vascular mortality (25% vs. 3.5%) and a higher risk of the composite of vascular death, myocardial infarction, or recurrent stroke (44% vs. 4.4%) than aspirin responders (24)

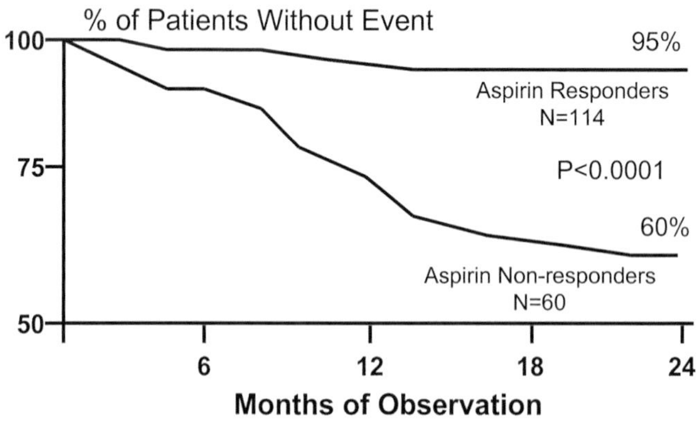

Figure 2 Worse outcomes in stroke patients not responsive to aspirin. Outcomes include stroke, myocardial infarction, and vascular death. (Adapted from Ref. 24.)

(Fig. 2). Similarly, in a study of patients with peripheral vascular disease, male nonresponders and paradoxical responders had an 87% higher risk of vessel reocclusion at 1 year compared to responders (22). These data demonstrate that not only does aspirin resistance exist but that patients who fail to respond to aspirin have markedly worse outcomes than those who respond.

A growing but indirect body of evidence in support of aspirin resistance comes from observations from recently conducted clinical trials in the acute coronary syndromes. Although it is well established that secondary prevention with aspirin results in an approximately 25% reduction in the incidence of death, nonfatal myocardial infarction, or stroke, a substantial number of patients continue to have recurrent thrombotic events despite aspirin (26). These patients are increasingly being considered resistant to the antithrombotic effects of aspirin. There is a growing body of evidence that patients who fail aspirin, that is, those who have recurrent clinical events despite therapy with aspirin, are at increased risk of long-term adverse outcomes.

Several studies have found that among patients presenting with acute coronary syndromes, prior aspirin users have less acute initial presentations. They have less non-Q-wave myocardial infarction compared to unstable angina (27–30), and even in those with myocardial infarction, prior aspirin users have smaller infarcts and more non-Q-wave infarcts than those not taking aspirin (30,31). Despite this lower incidence of myocardial infarction, an association between prior aspirin use and poorer longer-term outcomes has been demonstrated. In an analysis of over 10,000 non-ST-elevation acute coronary syndrome patients from the PURSUIT trial, prior aspirin users had a significantly higher incidence of 30-day death or myocardial infarction than patients not using aspirin prior to presentation (16.1% vs. 13.0%, odds ratio 1.3, 95% confidence interval 1.1 to 1.5) (28). Even after adjustment for differences in baseline characteristics, prior aspirin use remained significant, independent predictor of worse 30-day outcome (odds ratio 1.2, 95% confidence interval 1.0 to 1.3) (Fig. 3).

Similar findings have been demonstrated in a number of other databases. Two studies, including a total of 349 patients, found worse in-hospital and 14-day outcomes, but no difference at 3- and 6-month follow-up, in prior aspirin users versus nonusers (29,32). In data recently presented from the ESSENCE trial of the low-molecular-weight heparin enoxaparin the 3275 (84%) patients on aspirin prior to enrollment had worse outcomes with a higher incidence of death, myocardial infarction, or urgent revascularization at 43 days (19.7% vs. 8.3%, odds ratio 1.6, 95% confidence interval 1.3 to 2.1) even after adjustment for baseline characteristics (33) (Fig. 3). Similar findings with worse outcomes in prior aspirin users were observed in the PRISM-PLUS trial of the glycoprotein IIb/IIIa inhibitor tirofiban (27). Another

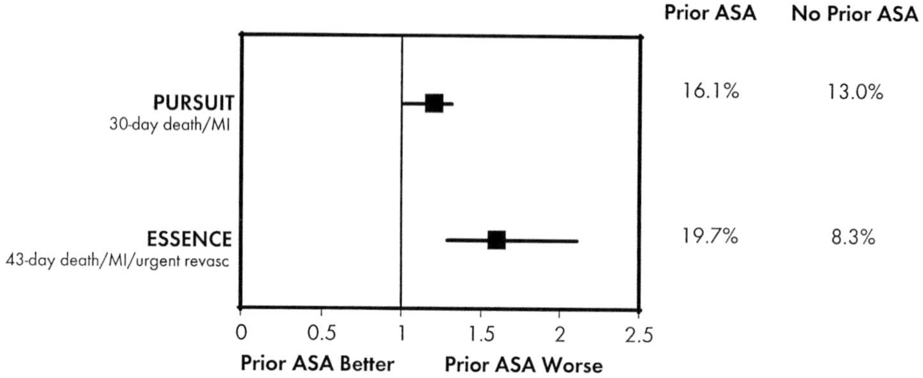

Figure 3 Worse outcomes in acute coronary syndrome patients who present despite chronic aspirin therapy after adjustment for baseline differences (28,33). Odds ratio and 95% confidence intervals for the occurrence of the primary endpoint in prior aspirin users versus non–prior aspirin users in the PURSUIT and ESSENCE trials.

small study of 410 patients with acute ischemic syndromes, however, found no difference in the incidence of death, nonfatal MI, or recurrent ischemia at 72 hours between prior aspirin users and nonusers (35).

Patients who have an acute coronary event while taking aspirin may be at higher risk for later events for several reasons. Prior aspirin use may simply be a surrogate marker for more extensive or aggressive cardiovascular disease. Alternatively, the worse outcomes observed in prior aspirin users may result from unmeasured hematological factors, endothelial dysfunction, or different atherosclerotic plaque characteristics, any of which may contribute to a more hostile local environment that overwhelms the relatively weak antiplatelet effects of aspirin. A third possibility is that patients who develop acute coronary syndromes while on aspirin may be aspirin resistant with relative or complete intrinsic resistance to the effects of aspirin.

If patients who have recurrent events despite aspirin are resistant to the antiplatelet effects of aspirin, they may derive particular benefit from the addition of other potent and effective antiplatelet or antithrombin therapies. A suggestion of such a preferential effect has been reported in three trials. In the PURSUIT trial, the 63% of patients who were prior aspirin users had a significant 16% reduction in 30-day death or nonfatal myocardial infarction with the glycoprotein IIb/IIIa inhibitor eptifibatide (17.3% vs. 14.9%, odds ratio 0.84, 95% confidence interval 0.73 to 0.96) (28) (Fig. 4). Nonprior aspirin users, on the other hand, did not have a significant reduction in death

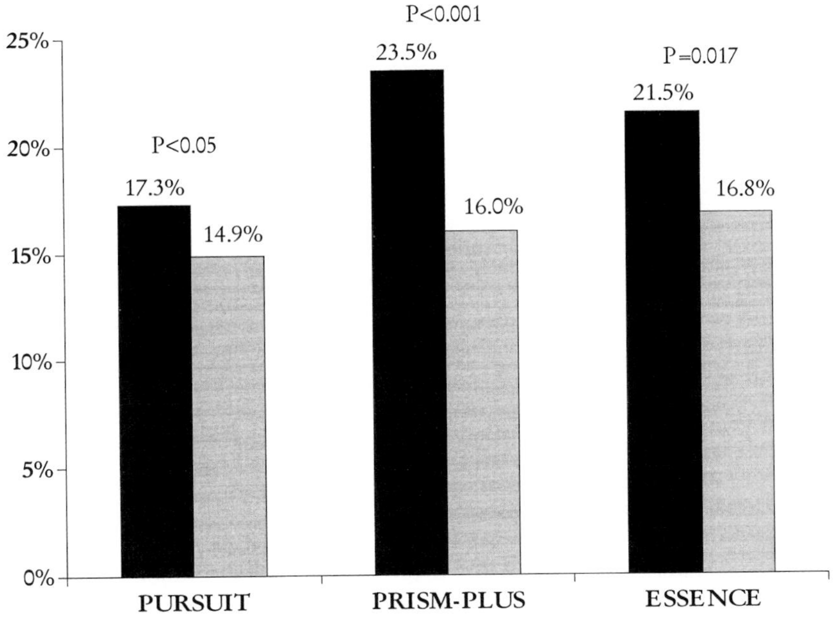

Figure 4 Beneficial effect of the antithrombotic therapies eptifibatide (PURSUIT), tirofiban (PRISM-PLUS), and enoxaparin (ESSENCE) in prior aspirin users. No effect was evidence in non–prior aspirin users (27,28).

or myocardial infarction with eptifibatide (12.9% vs. 13.0%, odds ratio 1.02, 95% confidence interval 0.84 to 1.25). When prior aspirin use was included in a multivariable model, however, the effect of eptifibatide was similar in prior aspirin users and nonprior aspirin users although the power to detect such an interaction was limited. Two other trials in patients with non-ST-elevation acute coronary syndromes, one with the low-molecular-weight heparin enoxaparin, (ESSENCE), and the other with the glycoprotein IIb/IIIa inhibitor, tirofiban (PRISM-PLUS) recently reported a treatment effect that was limited to prior aspirin users (27) (Fig. 4). In ESSENCE, prior aspirin users who received enoxaparin had a significant reduction in death, myocardial infarction, or urgent revascularization compared to those who received unfractionated heparin (16.8% vs. 21.5%, P = .009). Similarly, in PRISM-PLUS, prior aspirin users who received tirofiban had a significant reduction in death, myocardial infarction, and urgent revascularization (16.0% vs. 23.5%, P = .007). In both trials, patients who were not on prior aspirin at the time of enrollment had no apparent benefit with either enoxaparin in ESSENCE or tirofiban in PRISM-PLUS over unfractionated heparin. Whether prior aspirin users who have recurrent thrombotic events despite aspirin derive greater benefit from these potent antithrombotic medications after adjustment for differences in baseline characteristics remains to be seen.

Mechanisms of Aspirin Resistance

Several studies have proposed mechanisms for the resistance to the antiplatelet effects of aspirin observed in some patients. Importantly, however, none have explained why these mechanisms are active in some patients and not others. Buchanan observed that in both healthy subjects and in patients undergoing coronary artery bypass grafting, aspirin produced the expected complete inhibition of thromboxane A_2 synthesis. Patients who were aspirin resistant, with no prolongation of bleeding time, however, had increased levels of 12-hydroxyeicosatertraenoic acid (12-HETE), a compound known to increase platelet adhesivity (35) (Fig. 5). Like thromboxane A_2, 12-HETE is metabolized from arachidonic acid but via the enzyme lipoxygenase. When cyclo-oxygenase is inhibited by aspirin, 12-HETE production may be increased, resulting in increased platelet adhesivity in some patients.

Investigators from Germany have recently suggested another possible mechanism for aspirin resistance (36). The enzyme cyclo-oxygenase exists in two isoforms, COX-1 and COX-2. Aspirin effectively inhibits COX-1; however, aspirin is approximately 170-fold less potent in inhibiting COX-2. Recently presented data suggest that after cardiac bypass surgery-associated platelet turnover, the amount of COX-2 is increased 16-fold (37). This increase in COX-2 is paralleled by an increase in both collagen stimulated ex vivo thrombus formation and in platelet aggregation. Importantly, neither of these changes was inhibited by the addition of aspirin.

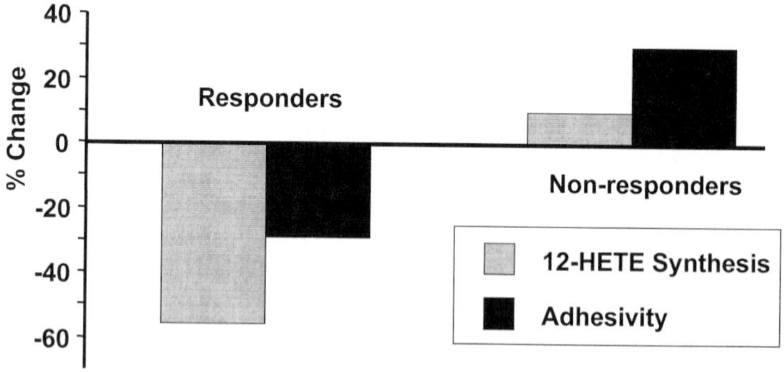

Figure 5 Relative effect of 325 mg/d aspirin on platelet 12-HETE synthesis and platelet adhesivity in coronary artery bypass patients classified as aspirin responders (n = 23) and aspirin nonresponders (n = 17). (Adapted from Ref. 19.)

It has also been proposed that the antiplatelet effects of aspirin can also be overcome by cyclo-oxygenase activity of a prostaglandin synthase produced by endothelial cells (38). Unlike platelet COX-1, which can not be regenerated after inhibition by aspirin, COX-2 can be rapidly regenerated by endothelial cells. Furthermore, prostaglandin synthase-2 production is upregulated in response to the inflammatory milieu of acute coronary syndromes. These investigators suggest that this increased endothelial production of COX-2 may be a potential extraplatelet source of thromboxane A_2 that is uninhibited by aspirin.

Patients with a certain genetic polymorphism of the platelet glycoprotein IIIa may be at increased risk for the complications of coronary artery disease. Patients with the polymorphism have less inhibition of thrombin generation from a bleeding time wound by aspirin than patients without the polymorphism (39). Interestingly, this polymorphism exists in approximately 25% of Caucasians. Whether these are the same patients who are aspirin resistant is unknown.

Finally, a number of investigators have demonstrated differential aspirin pharmacokinetics and pharmacodynamics in women (40–42), following exercise (43) or smoking (44), and in the presence of erythrocytes (45,46). Whether any of these play any role in clinical aspirin resistance has yet to be elucidated.

Angiotensin-Converting Enzyme (ACE) Inhibitors and Aspirin Interaction

Although not truly an "aspirin-resistant" population, the increasing number of patients treated with an ACE inhibitor represent an important subgroup of patients in which it has been postulated that aspirin may diminish the benefit (47). The clinical importance of this interaction has been suggested through the retrospective analysis of two large, placebo-controlled trials of ACE inhibitors. The Studies of Left Ventricular Dysfunction (SOLVD) investigators evaluated the impact of enalapril on mortality and morbidity in over 6797 patients with left ventricular systolic dysfunction with an ejection fraction of ≤0.35. At the time of randomization 46.3% of patients reported using antiplatelet therapy. Overall antiplatelet therapy at baseline was associated with a significant decrease in mortality compared to those not receiving it (RR 0.64, 95% CI 0.58 to 0.70, $P < .0001$) (48). However, patients receiving antiplatelet therapy at baseline who were randomized to enalapril experienced no survival benefit (adjusted HR 1.10, 95% CI 0.93 to 1.30), whereas those patients not receiving antiplatelet therapy had a significant decrease in mortality with enalapril (HR 0.77, 95% CI 0.67 to 0.87).

A similar interaction was noted between enalapril and aspirin in the Cooperative New Scandinavian Enalapril Survival Study II (CONSENSUS II).

This trial of 6090 patients assessed the impact of the early administration of enalapril in acute myocardial infarction (49). Results of CONSENSUS II demonstrated an overall 10% increase in the relative risk of death with early enalapril administration. When the results were reanalyzed by subgroups defined by the use of aspirin at baseline, a significant negative interaction was found between aspirin and enalapril on survival (50). In the ~24% of patients not receiving aspirin at baseline, enalapril actually decreased 30-day mortality (odds ratio 0.86, 95% CI 0.63 to 1.16, $P = .047$).

While it is possible that these findings could have occurred by chance, there is a physiologic basis for postulating that aspirin may negate some of the benefits of ACE inhibition. The production of vasodilating prostaglandins has been shown to play an important regulatory role in patients with heart failure (52), and several hemodynamic studies have consistently demonstrated that aspirin can substantially limit the vasodilator effects of ACE inhibitors (52–54). The WATCH (Warfarin-Antiplatelet Therapy in Chronic Heart Failure) is randomizing 4500 patients with congestive heart failure to either warfarin, aspirin, or clopidogrel and following them for 5 years to help determine the clinical significance of the ACE inhibitor/aspirin interaction.

CONCLUSION AND FUTURE DIRECTIONS

Despite aspirin's clear beneficial effects in the population of patients with coronary artery disease, it is becoming increasingly clear that not all patients benefit at all times from a standard dose of aspirin. Whether there are patients who are truly inherently resistant to the beneficial effects of aspirin is unclear. Another, equally plausible possibility is that patients become aspirin resistant when the antiplatelet effects of a fixed dose of aspirin are overcome by other prothrombotic stimuli. As it is likely that aspirin has beneficial mechanisms of actions other than its antiplatelet effect, more basic research is needed into multiple mechanisms of action of aspirin. A better understanding of how aspirin works may allow us to identify possible mechanisms of aspirin resistance and ultimately to identify patients who are not benefiting from aspirin.

As the thrombotic milieu within an individual patient changes over time, the antiplatelet effects of a fixed dose of aspirin may be overwhelmed by other stimulants to platelet activation and aggregation. In the future, bedside antiplatelet testing (Chap. 20) will allow us to measure aspirin's effect clinically and individualize antiplatelet therapy. Patients who are not achieving the desired level of antiplatelet effects from aspirin should either have their aspirin dose increased or be considered candidates for the substitution or addition of other antiplatelet agents. Currently only the adenosine diphosphate inhibitors ticlopidine and clopidogrel are available as alternatives; however, in the future other oral antiplatelet agents (Chap. 17) may also be available.

In the meantime, because routine clinical measurement of the antiplatelet effects of aspirin is not yet feasible, a more clinical approach should be taken. As has been discussed, patients who have recurrent acute coronary events despite therapy with standard doses of aspirin are at increased long-term risk, possibly owing to aspirin resistance. Until we can directly measure aspirin's effects, these high-risk patients with clinical aspirin failure should be considered candidates for the substitution or addition of other antiplatelet therapies.

REFERENCES

1. Mehta JL, Mehta P, Feldman RL, Horalek C. Thromboxane release in coronary artery disease: spontaneous versus pacing-induced angina. Am Heart J 1984; 107:859–869.
2. Fitzgerald DJ, Roy L, Catella F, Fitzgerald GA. Platelet activation in unstable coronary disease. N Engl J Med 1986;315:983–989.
3. Hirsh PD, Hillis D, Campbell WB, Firth BG, Willerson JT. Release of prostaglandins and thromboxane into the coronary circulation in patients with ischemic heart disease. N Engl J Med 1981;304:685–691.
4. Mizuno K, Satomura K, Miyamoto A, et al. Angioscopic evaluation of coronary-artery thrombi in acute coronary syndromes. N Engl J Med 1992;326: 287–291.
5. Davies MJ. Stability and instability: Two faces of coronary atherosclerosis. Circulation 1996;94:2013–2020.
6. Stone E. An account of the success of the bark of the willow in the cure of agues. Philos Trans R Soc Lond [Biol] 1763;53:195–200.
7. Mann CC, Plummer ML. The Aspirin Wars: Money, Medicine and 100 Years of Rampant Competition. New York: Alfred A. Knopf 1991.
8. Gibson PC. Salicylic acid for coronary thrombosis? Lancet 1948;1:965.
9. Lewis HDJ, Davis JW, Archibald DG, et al. Protective effects of aspirin against acute myocardial infarction and death in men with unstable angina. N Engl J Med 1983;309:396–403.
10. ISIS-2 Collaborative Group. Randomised trial of intravenous streptokinase, oral aspirin, both, or neither among 17,187 cases of suspected acute myocardial infarction: ISIS-2. Lancet 1988;2:349–360.
11. Smith JB, Willis AL. Aspirin selectively inhibits prostaglandin production in human platelets. Nature 1971;231:235–237.
12. Vane JR, Bakhle YS, Botting RM. Cyclooxygenases 1 and 2. Annu Rev Pharmacol Toxicol 1998;38:97–120.
13. Pedersen AK, FitzGerald GA. Dose-related kinetics of aspirin. Presystemic acetylation of platelet cyclooxygenase. N Engl J Med 1984;311:1206–1211.

14. Feldman M, Cryer B. Aspirin absorption rates and platelet inhibition times with 325-mg buffered aspirin tablets (chewed or swallowed intact) and with buffered aspirin solution. Am J Cardiol 1999;84:404–409.
15. Patrignani P, Filabozzi P, Patrono C. Selective cumulative inhibition of platelet thromboxane production by low-dose aspirin in healthy subjects. J Clin Invest 1982;69:1366–1372.
16. Benedek IH, Joshi AS, Pieniaszek HJ, King S-YP, Kornhauser DM. Variability in the pharmacokinetics and pharmicodynamics of low dose aspirin in healthy male volunteers. J Clin Pharmacol 1995;35:1181–1186.
17. Pappas JM, Westengard JC, Bull BS. Population variability in the effect of aspirin on platelet function. Implications for clinical trials and therapy. Arch Pathol Lab Med 1994;118:801–804.
18. Valettas N, Morgan CD, Reis M. Aspirin resistance using flow cytometry. Blood 1997;10:124b. Abstract.
19. Buchanan MR, Brister SJ. Individual variation in the effects of ASA on platelet function: implications for the use of ASA clinically. Can J Cardiol 1995;11:221–227.
20. Poggio ED, Kottke-Marchant K, Welsh PA, Brooks LM, Dela Rosa LR, Topol EJ. The prevalence of aspirin resistance in cardiac patients as measured by platelet aggregation and PFA-100. J Am Coll Cardiol 1999;33:254A. Abstract.
21. Hurlen M, Seljeflot I, Arnesen H. Platelet aggregability after myocardial infarction. Evidence of aspirin non-responsiveness in a subpopulation. Eur Heart J 1996;17:262. Abstract.
22. Mueller MR, Salat A, Stangl P, Murabito M, Pulaki S, Boehm D, Koppensteiner R, Ergun E, Mittlboeck M, Schreiner W, Losert U, Wolner E. Variable platelet response to low-dose ASA and the risk of limb deterioration in patients submitted to peripheral arterial angioplasty. Thromb Haemost 1997;78:1003–1007.
23. Helgason CM, Bolin KM, Hoff JA, Winkler SR, Mangat A, Tortorice KL, Brace LD. Development of aspirin resistance in persons with previous ischemic stroke. Stroke 1994;25:2331–2336.
24. Grotemeyer, KH, Scharafinski HW, Husstedt IW. Two-year follow-up of aspirin responders and aspirin non-responder. A pilot study including 180 post-stroke patients. Thromb Res 1993;71:397–403.
25. Farrell TP, Hayes KA, Tracy PB, Sobel BE, Schneider DJ. Unexpected, discordant effects of aspirin on platelet reactivity. J Am Coll Cardiol 1998;31:352A. Abstract.
26. Antiplatelet Trialists' Collaboration. Collaborative overview of randomised trials of antiplatelet therapy. I. Prevention of death, myocardial infarction, and stroke by prolonged antiplatelet therapy in various categories of patients. Br Med J 1994;308:81–106.
27. Lancaster GI, Lancaster CJ, Barr E, Radley D, Fromell GJ, Cohen M. Prior aspirin use in unstable coronary syndromes results in a lower incidence of non-Q-wave MI but a highter rate of medical therapy failure with unfractionated heparin: the aspirin paradox. Circulation 1999;100:I-620. Abstract.

28. Alexander JH, Harrington RA, Tuttle RH, Berdan LG, Lincoff AM, Deckers JW, Simoons ML, Guerci A, Hochman JS, Wilcox RG, Kitt MM, Eisenberg PR, Califf RM, Topol EJ, Karsh K, Ruzyllo W, Stepinska J, Widimsky P, Boland JB, Armstrong PW. Prior aspirin use predicts worse outcomes in patients with non-ST-elevation acute coronary syndromes. Am J Cardiol 1999; 83:1147–1151.
29. Cohen M, Adams PC, McBride R, Blanke H, Fuster V, and the Antithrombotic Therapy in Acute Coronary Syndromes Research Group. Prospective comparison of patient characteristics and outcome of non-prior aspirin users versus aspirin users with unstable angina or non-Q-wave myocardial infarction treated with combination antithrombotic therapy. J Thromb Thrombol 1997;4:275–280.
30. Garcia-Dorado D, Theroux P, Tornos P, Sambola A, Oliveras J, Santos M, Soler-Soler J. Previous aspirin use may attenuate the severity of the manifestation of acute ischemic syndromes. Circulation 1995;92:1743–1748.
31. Col NF, Yarzebski J, Gore JM, Alpert JS, Goldberg RJ. Does aspirin consumption affect the presentation or severity of acute myocardial infarction? Arch Intern Med 1995;155:1386–1389.
32. Haghani K, Shah PK, Cercek B. Unstable angina developing in patients on chronic aspirin therapy is associated with an increased risk of early adverse cardiac events. J Am Coll Cardiol 1993;21:270A. Abstract.
33. Santopinto J, Tajer C, Bozovich GE, Torres V, Gurfinkel EP, Marcos E, Antman EM. Prior aspirin users are at increased risk of cardiac events and should be treated with enoxaparin. Circulation 1999;100:I-620. Abstract.
34. Borzak S, Cannon CP, Kraft PL, Douthat L, Becker RC, Palmeri ST, Henry T, Hochman JS, Fuchs J, Antman EM, McCabe C, Braunwald E, for the TIMI 7 Investigators. Effects of prior aspirin and anti-ischemic therapy on outcome in patients with unstable angina. Am J Cardiol 1998;81:678–681.
35. Buchanan MR, Brister SJ. Individual variation in the effects of ASA on platelet function: implications for the use of ASA clinically. Can J Cardiol 1995;11: 221–227.
36. Weber A-A, Zimmermann KC, Meyer-Kirchrath J, Schror K. Cyclooxygenase-2 in human platelets as a possible factor in aspirin resistance. Lancet 1999; 353:900.
37. Zimmerman N, Kienzle P, Weber A, Gams E, Hohlfeld T, Schror K. Platelet aspirin resistance is associated with an increased platelet content of cyclooxygenase-2. Circulation 1999;100:I-327. Abstract.
38. Cipololone F, Patrignani P, Greco A, et al. Differential suppression of thromboxane biosynthesis by ibuprofen and aspirin in patients with unstable angina. Circulation 1997;96:1109–1116.
39. Undas A, Sanak M, Musial J, Szczeklik A. Platelet glycoprotein IIIa polymorphism, aspirin, and thrombin generation. Lancet 1999;353:982–983.
40. Canadian Cooperative Study Group. A randomized trial of aspirin and sulfinpyrazone in threatened stroke. N Engl J Med 1978;299:53–59.
41. Spranger M, Aspey BS, Harrison MJG. Sex difference in antithrombotic effect of aspirin. Stroke 1989;20:34–37.

42. Young VP, Giles AR, Pater J, Corbett WEN. Sex differences in bleeding time and blood loss in normal subjects following aspirin ingestion. Thromb Res 1980;20:705–709.
43. Li N, Wallen H, Hjemdahl P. Evidence for prothrombotic effects of exercise and limited protection by aspirin. Circulation 1999;100:1374–1379.
44. Davis JW, Hartman CR, Lewis HD Jr, Shelton L, Eigenberg DA, Hassanein KM, Hignite CE, Ruttinger HA. Cigarette smoking-induced enhancement of platelet function: lack of prevention by aspirin in men with coronary artery disease. J Lab Clin Med 1985;105:478–483.
45. Santos MT, Valles J, Aznar J, Marcus AJ, Broekman MJ, Safier LB. Prothrombotic effects of erythrocytes on platelet reactivity. Reduction by aspirin. Circulation 1997;95:63–68.
46. Valles J, Santos MT, Aznar J, Osa A, Lago A, Cosin J, Sanchez E, Broekman MJ, Marcus AJ. Erythrocyte promotion of platelet reactivity decreases the effectiveness of aspirin as an antithrombotic therapeutic modality. The effect of low-dose aspirin is less than optimal in patients with vascular disease due to prothrombotic effects of erythrocytes on platelet reactivity. Circulation 1998; 97:350–355.
47. Cleland JGF, Bulpitt CJ, Falk RH, et al. Is aspirin safe for patients with heart failure? Br Heart J 1995;74:215–219.
48. Al-Khadra A, Salem DN, Rand WM, Udelson JE, Smith JJ, Konstam MA. Antiplatelet agents and survival: a cohort analysis from the Studies of Left Ventricular Dysfunction (SOLVD) trial. J Am Coll Cardiol 1998;31:419–425.
49. Swedberg K, Held P, Kjekshus J, Rasmussen K, Ryden L, Wedel H. Effects of early administration of enalapril on mortality in patients in acute myocardial infarction: results of the Cooperative New Scandinavian Enalapril Survival Study II (CONSENSUS II). N Engl J Med 1992;327:678–684.
50. Nguyen KN, Aursnes I, Kjekshus J. Interaction between enalapril and aspirin on mortality after acute myocardial infarction: subgroup analysis of the Cooperative New Scandinavian Enalapril Survival Study II (CONSENSUS II). Am J Cardiol 1997;79:115–119.
51. Dzau VJ. Vascular wall renin-angiotensin pathway in control of the circulation. A hypothesis. Am J Med 1984;77:31–36.
52. Viecili PRN, Park M, Santos SR, Pamplona D, Ramires JAF, da Luz PL. Antagonism of captopril by aspirin in severe heart failure: haemodynamic and neurohormonal demonstration. Eur Heart J 1999;20:609. Abstract.
53. Spaulding C, Charbonnier B, Cohen-Solal A, et al. Acute hemodynamic interaction of aspirin and ticlopidine with enalapril. Results of a double-blind, randomized comparative trial. Circulation 1998;98:757–765.
54. Hall D, Zeitler H, Rudolph W. Counteraction of the vasodilator effects of enalapril by aspirin in severe heart failure. J Am Coll Cardiol 1992;20:1549–1555.

19

Antithrombin Therapy in Acute Coronary Syndromes

A. Vogt and K.-L. Neuhaus
Medizinische Klinik II
Klinikum Kassel
Kassel, Germany

INTRODUCTION

Thrombin plays a pivotal role in platelet-mediated thrombosis associated with atheromatous plaque rupture in patients with acute coronary syndromes. Thrombin inhibition is, therefore, a basic therapeutic goal in this setting together with thrombolysis and platelet inhibition.

HEPARIN

Heparin is a mixture of glycosaminglycans with an average molecular weight of 12,000 to 15,000. Heparin interacts with antithrombin III to inhibit the coagulation factors Xa and IXa, but especially thrombin. Inhibition of thrombin occurs via the formation of a ternary complex of heparin, antithrombin III, and thrombin. Low-molecular-weight (LMW) heparin is produced by depolymerization of standard heparin into polysaccharide fragments with a molecular weight of 4000 to 6500. The advantage of LMW heparin is a better bioavailability after subcutaneous injection, being close to 100% compared to 30% for standard heparin. The plasma half-life is two to four times that of standard heparin. The anticoagulant effect of LMW heparin is mostly due to inhibition of factor Xa (1).

Heparin in Unstable Angina and Non-Q-Wave Myocardial Infarction

Patients with unstable angina tend to have an activated coagulation system and especially heightened thrombin activity, which is associated with an early unfavorable outcome (2–5). Therefore, heparin has become a standard treatment for unstable angina and non-Q-wave myocardial infarction. Its efficacy has been well documented in terms of prevention of definite myocardial infarction and death, reducing the need for urgent revascularization, and reducing the incidence of recurrent ischemia (6–12) (Table 1). Most studies applied a dose regimen with an intravenous bolus of 5000 IU followed by an infusion of 1000 IU rh adjusted to a target aPTT around two times the control value. Dosing heparin by a weight-based nomogram instead of the standard doses results in a more reliable anticoagulation with respect to the target-aPTT (13). The clinical advantage of this technically more complicated regime has, however, not been demonstrated. Intermittent intravenous bolus injections of heparin were effective in one study (6) but did not prevent myocardial infarction of episodes of myocardial ischemia in two others (8,14). The Thrombolysis in Myocardial Infarction (TIMI) study group recommended a target aPTT of 45 to 60 sec according to the results of the TIMI-3 study (15). A more aggressive anticoagulation did not seem to result in further reduction of ischemic events.

Treatment with heparin is certainly superior to placebo and very probably better than aspirin alone (7,9,10,12). It seems reasonable to combine heparin with aspirin, since platelet inhibition is desirable in acute coronary syndromes and, moreover, heparin might enhance platelet function in unstable angina (16). The combination is widely used, but there is no proof evidence of a clinical benefit over heparin alone. While there was no significant difference in the incidence of ischemic events, the incidence of serious bleedings was 3.3% in patients treated with heparin and aspirin versus 1.7% in those on heparin only (7).

The vast majority of patients with unstable angina can be stabilized initially by maximal drug therapy including heparin and a combination of antianginal drugs; only 8.8% had truly refractory unstable angina in a cohort of 125 patients (17). Pretreatment of unstable angina patients with heparin over 3 days was reported to markedly reduce the incidence of major ischemic complications of a subsequent angioplasty procedure as compared to an immediate angioplasty (18).

Low-molecular weight heparin can be easily applied by SC injections and obviates the need of close monitoring of the aPTT. Dalteparin was shown to be more effective in unstable angina than aspirin alone to prevent ischemic events (21). Several studies have been performed to compare var-

Table 1 Heparin in Unstable Angina

Study	No. patients	Heparin	Controls	Endpoints/efficacy
Telford 1988 (6)	214	4 × 5000 IU IV	Placebo	MI 3% vs. 15%
Théroux 1988 (7)	479	a) IV (aPTT 1.5–2 × control) b) IV + 2 × 325 mg ASS	c) 2 × 325 mg ASS d) Placebo	Refractory angina/death/MI a) 9.3%; b) 11.5%; c) 16.5%; d) 26.3%
RISC 1990 (8)	796	a) 4 × 5000 IU bolus IV b) a + 1 × 75 mg ASS	c) 1 × 75 mg ASS d) Placebo	MI/death 5 days: a) 5.6%; b) 1.4%; c) 3.7%; d) 6.0%
Théroux 1993 (9)	484	IV (aPTT 1.5–2.5 × control)	2 × 325 mg ASS	MI 0.8% vs. 3.7%
Cohen 1994 (10)	214	IV (aPTT 2-fold) + ASS, contd. warfarin	1 × 162.5 mg ASS	Reischemia/MI/death 10.5% vs. 27%
Holdright 1994 (11)	285	IV (aPTT 1.5–2.5 × control) + ASS 1 × 150 mg	1 × 150 mg ASS	MI/death 27.3% vs. 30.5% Ischemia (Holter) no diff.
Serneri 1995 (12)	108	IV or SC + ASS (aPTT 1.5- to 2-fold)	1 × 325 mg ASS	Reischemia reduced by IV and SC heparin

ious preparations of LMW heparin given subcutaneously with IV standard heparin guided by aPTT values (Table 2). Dalteparin and nadroparin were equally effective as standard heparin, while enoxaparin 1 mg/kg BID proved to be superior in the ESSENCE and TIMI 11B studies (22,23). A meta-analysis of these two studies revealed about 20% reduction of definite myocardial infarction and death in patients with unstable angina or non-Q-wave infarction by this regimen of enoxaparin as compared to standard heparin (24). It is unclear yet why enoxaparin but not dalteparin or nadroparin was more effective than standard heparin. Enoxaparin has the smallest molecule size, the longest plasma half-life, and the most selective effect on factor Xa of these preparations (25). Whether these differences are clinically important could only be tested by head-to-head comparisons of enoxaparin with other LMW heparins.

Full-dose intravenous heparin as well as subcutaneous LMW heparin may both give rise to a rebound after cessation of treatment (21,29). The reason for this is unclear. It is probably not due to depletion of antithrombin III (30), but there is a transient rise in thrombin activity and activated protein C (31). It may well be that treatment with heparin over 2 to 7 days is too short to allow for healing of the underlying coronary plaque fissure. The rebound seems to be avoided when heparin is given in combination with aspirin. Fourteen of 107 patients given heparin alone had reactivation of unstable angina after discontinuation versus only 5 of 100 similar patients with concomitant aspirin treatment (29).

The necessary duration of therapy with heparin or LMW heparin has not been defined. Several trials tested prolonged treatment with LMW heparin after hospital discharge (21,22,26,32), but the results were mostly negative with respect to the prevention of clinical events. This is surprising, since the duration of initial treatment in these studies of only 2 to 8 days is probably not enough to passivate the underlying complicated coronary lesion. Only the FRISC-II study demonstrated a reduction of ischemic events by prolonged treatment with dalteparin in patients treated conservatively for approximately 2 months, but thereafter the benefit dissipated and was no more significant after 6 months (32,33).

Heparin as Adjunct to Thrombolysis in Acute MI

Streptokinase and other plasminogen activators cause a paradoxically increased local thrombin generation (34). This hypercoagulable state is associated with elevated plasma fibrinogen levels (35), an increase in thrombin-antithrombin III complexes and in prothrombin fragments (36), and a partial resistance to heparin (37). It seems reasonable, therefore, to combine thrombolytic treatment with adjunctive anticoagulation to improve early infarct

Table 2 Low-Molecular Weight Heparin SC in Unstable Angina

Study	No. patients	Heparin dose SC	Controls	Endpoints/efficacy
Correia 1995 (19)	314	160 or 320 IU/kg/day	Heparin IV by aPTT	Death/MI no difference
Gurfinkel 1995 (20)	219	a) 214 IU/kg BID + 1 × 200 mg ASS	b) 1 × 200 mg ASS c) Hep. IV (aPTT 2-fold) + ASS	MI/reischemia/urgent revasc. a) 22.1%; b) 58.9%; c) 60.0%
Frisc 1996 (21)	1506	120 IU/kg BID + ASS	ASS	Death/MI 1.8% vs. 4.8% Urgent revasc. 0.4% vs. 1.2%
Essence 1997 (23)	3171	1 mg/kg BID + ASS	Heparin IV aPTT 55–85 sec	Death/MI/rec. AP 19.8% vs. 23.3%
FRIC 1997 (26)	1482	120 IU/kg BID + ASS	Heparin IV aPTT 1.5-fold control	Death/MI/rec. AP 9.3% vs. 7.6%
TIMI 11B 1999 (22)	3910	1 mg/kg BID + ASS	Heparin IV aPTT 1.5- to 2.5-fold control	Death/MI/revasc. 12.4% vs. 14.5%
Fraxis (28)	3468	87 IU/kg BID (6 or 14 days)	Heparin IV aPTT 1.5–2.5 × control	Death/MI/rec. AP Heparin 18.1% LMW 6d 17.8%; LMW 14d 20.0%

vessel patency and prevent reocclusion. However, the available controlled clinical studies of adjunctive heparin in acute myocardial infarction treated with thrombolysis do not clearly support its routine use to improve the clinical outcome (38).

Most clearly the need of adjunctive heparin has been demonstrated when alteplase is given as thrombolytic agent (39–41). In one study, the patency of infarct vessels in subgroups with optimal, suboptimal, and inadequate anticoagulation was 90%, 80%, and 72%, respectively, at angiography 2 to 5 days after thrombolysis with alteplase (42). While the aPTT during heparin treatment correlated positively with infarct vessel patency at 18 hours after alteplase, there was no correlation with late reocclusion (43). Infarct vessel patency was also improved by an initial bolus of 5000 IU heparin before thrombolysis with saruplase. Angiography after 6 to 12 hours showed an open infarct vessel in 78.6% of the pretreated patients versus 56.5% of those receiving heparin only after thrombolysis (44).

The role of heparin as adjunct to other thrombolytic agents is less clear. The Duke University Clinical Cardiology (DUCCS) study group found no advantage of adjunctive heparin after thrombolysis with anistreplase; the only significant difference versus the control group was an increased bleeding risk (45). The Studio Sulla Calciparina nell'Angina e nella Trombosi Ventricolare nell'Infarto (SCATI) group randomized 733 patients with acute myocardial infarction to 12,500 IU SC heparin BID versus placebo; 433 of the patients received streptokinase when symptoms lasted <6 hours (46). Mortality was 5.8% versus 10.0% ($P = .03$), and in the subgroup of patients with streptokinase treatment it was 4.6% versus 8.8% ($P = .05$). These results, however, were in no way confirmed by the megatrials GISSI-2 and ISIS-3 (47,48). In both trials subcutaneous heparin was clinically ineffective in patients after thrombolysis with streptokinase, alteplase, or anistreplase (see Table 3). Furthermore, in GISSI-2, the 6-month survival rates as well as incidence of reinfarction were not different in patients with or without initial SC heparin treatment (49).

In the GUSTO-I trial the streptokinase-treated patients were randomly treated with SC heparin as in ISIS-3 or with full-dose IV heparin aiming at an aPTT of 60 to 85 sec (50). No differences were found between the clinical outcomes of the two groups, despite a slightly better early infarct vessel patency rate in the IV heparin group of 60% versus 54% (50,51). Some angiographic evidence has been presented that heparin might prevent late reocclusion of infarct vessels after thrombolysis with streptokinase (52). The much larger GUSTO angiographic substudy, however, could not confirm this; the rate of reocclusion at control angiograms on day 5 to 7 was 6.4% in patients on SC versus 5.5% of those on IV heparin (51). Prolonged treatment

Table 3 Megatrials of Heparin as Adjunct to Thrombolysis in AMI

Study	No. pts.	Heparin	Controls	Death (%)	Reinfarction (%)	Major bleeds (%)
GISSI-2 (47)	12,490	2 × 12,500 IU SC + ASS beginning after 12 h	No heparin, SK, or t-PA lysis	8.3 vs. 9.3	1.9 vs. 2.3	1.0 vs. 0.6
ISIS-3 (48)	41,299	2 × 12,500 IU SC + ASS beginning after 4 h	No heparin, SK, t-PA, or APSAC	10.3 vs. 10.6	3.2 vs. 3.5	Noncerebral 1.0 vs. 0.8; cerebral 0.6 vs. 0.4
GUSTO-I (50)	20,251	2 × 12,500 IU SC + ASS beginning after 4 h	Heparin IV, aPTT 60–85 s	7.2 vs. 7.4	3.4 vs. 4.0	Noncerebral 0.3 vs. 0.5; cerebral 0.5 vs. 0.5

with SC heparin after myocardinal infarction might prevent recurrent events when extended over 1 month (53).

GUSTO-I was the first trial to demonstrate a survival benefit of thrombolysis with alteplase versus streptokinase in acute myocardial infarction (50), which was not seen in the preceding megatrials GISSI-2 and ISIS-3 (47,48). The difference is very probably due to the front-loaded dosing of alteplase and to adjunctive full-dose heparin treatment in GUSTO but the relative importance of these cannot be estimated. The optimal intensity of anticoagulation is in the range of aPTT values 50 to 70 sec. Those patients had the lowest 30-day mortality, stroke, and bleeding rates in GUSTO-I (54). Interestingly, reinfarction was more common among patients with higher aPTT values, and there was a clustering of reinfarction in the first 10 hours after discontinuation of heparin (54). This may reflect a comparable rebound as seen in the treatment of unstable angina with heparin.

Left ventricular mural thrombi occur in about one-third of patients with anterior myocardial infarction (55–58). Subcutaneous heparin treatment with 2 × 12,500 IU was effective against left ventricular thrombus formation as compared to low-dose treatment with 2 × 5000 IU; in this randomized study left ventricular thrombi were observed in 11% versus 32% ($P = .0004$) (59). In a subgroup of GISSI-2, however, the incidence of echocardiographically detected left ventricular thrombi was similar in patients with and without 2 × 12,500 IU heparin (60). Full-dose heparin followed by oral anticoagulants was investigated in two small controlled studies in patients with first anterior myocardial infarction. Anticoagulants were effective against left ventricular thrombus formation in one study (61,62) but without any effect in the other (63).

When alteplase is given as thrombolytic agent in acute myocardial infarction, adjunctive heparin should be added aiming at an aPTT of 50 to 70 sec. No benefit has been convincingly demonstrated of IV heparin as adjunct to streptokinase or anistreplase, and adjunctive SC heparin seems not to be effective at all.

HIRUDIN

Hirudin is a most potent naturally occurring anticoagulant derived from the leech *Hirudo medicinalis*, and recently has become available in larger quantities as a result of production by recombinant techniques. It is a single polypeptide containing 65 amino acids which binds directly to thrombin forming an irreversible complex. In contrast to heparin hirudin does not need antithrombin III as cofactor, and it inhibits also clot-bound thrombin (for references see 64). Hirudin has been shown to be highly effective in preventing arterial thrombus formation in various experimental models (65–71).

Hirudin in Unstable Angina Pectoris

Hirudin has been compared to heparin treatment in a dose-escalating protocol with respect to its effect on the culprit lesion of 166 unstable angina patients as measured by paired quantitative coronary angiography (72). The doses of hirudin tested ranged from 0.05 mg/kg/h to 0.3 mg/kg/h in four sequential groups; the heparin dose was adjusted to an aPTT of 65 to 90 sec or 90 to 110 sec. The high-dose heparin group had similar aPTT values as the patients treated with ≥0.2 mg/kg/h hirudin, but there were wider fluctuations. Hirudin elicited a more stable prolongation of the aPTT, with 71% of the patients having sequential aPTT values within a 40-sec range versus only 16% of the heparin-treated patients. The effect of hirudin demonstrated a plateau at the 0.2 mg/kg/h level; further increase of the dose to 0.3 mg/kg/h caused no further prolongation of the aPTT. Hirudin tended to improve the angiographic parameters of the culprit lesion more than heparin leading to a greater stenosis diameter at the control angiogram after 72 to 120 hours ($P = .28$). The clinical outcome was not significantly different between the groups. Myocardial infarction occurred in 2.6% of the hirudin-treated patients versus 8% of those on heparin ($P = .11$).

The clinical relevance of these promising results was tested in the GUSTO-II study. In GUSTO-IIa, 2565 patients with acute coronary syndromes were randomized to treatment with hirudin (0.6 mg/kg bolus followed by 0.2 mg/kg/h infusion without aPTT adjustment), or heparin adjusted to an aPTT of 60 to 90 sec (73). Thrombolytic therapy was given to 1264 patients with ST elevation. The study was terminated early because of an excess of intracranial bleeding occurring in 1.3% and 0.7% of the hirudin- and heparin-treated groups, respectively. Most of the intracranial hemorrhages, however, occurred in patients receiving thrombolysis. Only 3 of 629 patients (0.5%) treated with hirudin without thrombolysis had an intracranial bleeding.

The study was reinitiated as GUSTO-IIb with reduced doses of both anticoagulants. Hirudin was given as a bolus of 0.1 mg/kg followed by an infusion with 0.1 mg/kg/h, and the aPTT was adjusted to 60 to 85 sec in both treatment groups (74). The study enrolled 12,142 patients of whom 8011 had unstable angina without ST elevation and did not receive thrombolysis. Confirming earlier results (72,75), the patients treated with hirudin had less fluctuation of the aPTT values than those on heparin. The incidence of severe bleeding was 1.3% and 0.9%, and the incidence of intracranial hemorrhage 0.2% and 0.02% of the patients treated with hirudin and heparin without additional thrombolysis. The combined incidence of death and myocardial infarction was 8.3% in the hirudin group and 9.1% in the heparin group. This small and statistically nonsignificant difference was mainly due to the prevention of myocardial infarction (5.6% vs. 6.4%), whereas the death rates were similar (3.7% vs. 3.9%).

A more favorable effect of higher doses of hirudin over heparin was reported from a pilot study of the Organization to Assess Strategies for Ischemic Syndromes (OASIS) in 909 patients with unstable angina. Of 267 patients treated with hirudin (0,4 mg/kg bolus followed by 0.15 mg/kg/h over 72 hours) 3.0% suffered cardiovascular death, myocardial infarction, or refractory angina until day 7, as opposed to 6.5% of 371 control patients treated with standard heparin (76). The subsequent OASIS-2 study in 10,141 patients with unstable angina or non-Q-wave MI demonstrated only a small advantage of hirudin over heparin with 3.6 versus 4.2% (P = .077) of the patients suffering death or MI within 7 days (77).

In the doses tested, hirudin seems to be marginally better than heparin with respect to the clinical outcome of patients with unstable angina. It causes a more reliable anticoagulation than heparin with less fluctuation of the aPTT values, however.

Hirudin as Adjunct to Thrombolysis in Acute MI

Hirudin was tested as adjunct to front-loaded alteplase in an open pilot study and subsequent dose-escalating study in 183 patients with acute myocardial infarction (78,79). In four dose groups hirudin was given as a bolus of 0.07 to 0.4 mg/kg followed by infusions of 0.05 to 0.15 mg/kg/h. Coronary angiography at 90 min after the initiation of treatment showed a completely perfused infarct-related artery (TIMI grade 3) in 67% to 76% of the patients. Of note, only 4.9% of the recanalized infarct vessels reoccluded. As compared to the earlier t-PA APSAC patency (TAPS) study (80) using the same protocol but heparin instead of hirudin, the initial patency rate was similar, but the reocclusion rate markedly lower (TAPS: 90-min TIMI grade 3 72%, reocclusion 12.3%). The incidence of reocclusion was slightly higher in patients with suboptimal anticoagulation as defined by the lowest aPTT <2 × baseline (8.8 vs. 3.1%, n.s.) (75).

The TIMI-5 study randomized 246 patients with acute myocardial infarction to heparin or one of four sequential hirudin dose groups as adjunct to front-loaded alteplase (81). The doses of hirudin ranged from 0.15 to 0.6 mg/kg bolus followed by infusions of 0.05 to 0.2 mg/kg/h. The 90-min patency rate (TIMI grade 3) was 64.8% in the hirudin-treated patients versus 57.1% in the heparin group. There were no significant differences in TIMI flow grade among the four dose groups of hirudin. As in the hirudin for the improvement of thrombolysis (HIT) studies (78,79), the reocclusion rate was markedly lower in the hirudin-treated patients (1.6% vs. 6.7%, $P = .07$). The combined incidence of death and reinfarction was 6.8% in the hirudin and 16.7% in the heparin group ($P = .02$), and there were more revascularization procedures in the heparin-treated patients (50% vs. 32%, $P = .006$).

Hirudin in comparable doses was also tested as adjunct to streptokinase in acute myocardial infarction. There is some evidence for improved early infarct vessel patency from the preliminary report of an angiographic study comparing hirudin with heparin (82). The TIMI-6 trial (83) randomized 193 patients treated with streptokinase for acute myocardial infarction to hirudin in three dose groups (0.15 to 0.6 mg/kg bolus, 0.05 to 0.2 mg/kg/h infusion). No differences were seen in the rate of major hemorrhage, and the hirudin-treated patients showed a nonsignificant trend to better clinical outcomes.

These preliminary data taken together demonstrate some advantages of hirudin over heparin as adjunct to thrombolysis in acute myocardial infarction: the rate of reocclusion after thrombolysis with alteplase seems to be markedly reduced compared to heparin, whereas the early-infarct vessel patency rate is similar. With streptokinase given as thrombolytic agent, the early patency might be improved by hirudin. The clinical relevance of these results was to be tested in large-scale trials. Three studies were simultaneously performed using the relatively high doses of hirudin as tested in the studies described above (73,84,85). In GUSTO-IIa patients with and without ST elevation were enrolled, 1264 of the total of 2564 received thrombolytic treatment (73). All three studies were terminated early because of an excess of intracranial hemorrhages (see Table 4). Of note, the high incidence of cerebral bleedings was not specific for hirudin, but the heparin-treated patients had also unexpectedly high bleeding rates. As compared to the earlier GUSTO-I study (50) using approximately 20% lower average doses of heparin, the bleeding risk was particularly high in patients treated with streptokinase irrespective of the anticoagulant given (Fig. 1).

The TIMI-9 and GUSTO-II studies were reinitiated with markedly lower doses of hirudin and the aPTT was targeted at lower values also in the heparin groups (Table 4). Both studies exhibited bleeding rates in the usually expected range for thrombolytic treatment of acute myocardial infarction, and the risk was similar for the hirudin- and heparin-treated groups (74,86). In GUSTO-IIb there was a small advantage of hirudin over heparin to prevent death and reinfarction, while TIMI-9b exhibited a trend in favor of heparin. Neither of those differences was statistically significant, and when the two studies are taken together the result is similar efficacy and safety of hirudin in the tested dose as compared to standard heparin. One reason for the generally disappointing clinical results with hirudin may be that thrombin is reliably inactivated, but thrombin generation is unaffected by hirudin (and

Table 4 Hirudin as Adjunct to Thrombolysis in AMI

Study	No. pts. thrombolytic	Target aPTT (s)	Hirudin (mg/kg) bolus/infusion	Cerebral bleeds (%) hirudin/heparin	Death/reinfarction (%) hirudin/heparin
GUSTO IIa (73)	1264[a]/SK or t-PA	60–90	0.6/0.2	2.2/1.5	
TIMI 9A (84)	757/SK or t-PA	60–90	0.6/0.2	1.8/2.0	
HIT-3 (85)	302/t-PA	2–3.5 × contr.	0.4/0.15	3.4/0	
GUSTO IIb (74)	4131[a]/SK or t-PA	55–85	0.1/0.1	0.5/0.4	9.9/11.3
TIMI 9B (86)	3.002/SK or t-PA	55–85	0.1/0.1	0.4/0.9	9.7/9.5
HIT-4 (90)	1.208/SK	2 × contr.	0.2/0.5 SC BID	0.2/0.3	10.4/11.0

[a]Only patients with ST elevation and thrombolytic treatment.

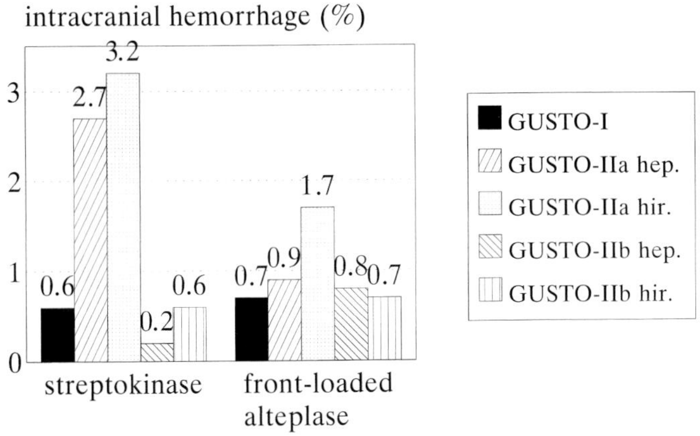

Figure 1 Cerebral bleeding in GUSTO studies. As compared to GUSTO-I (50) intercranial hemorrhages occurred markedly more often in GUSTO-IIa (73) not only in the hirudin-treated patients but also in the heparin group receiving about 20% higher average doses than GUSTO-I. This is particularly true for patients given streptokinase as thrombolytic agent. The cerebral bleeding risk is, therefore, not specifically increased by hirudin, but by more intense anticoagulant treatment in general. In GUSTO-IIb by reducing the dose of hirudin and only slightly reducing the target aPTT as compared to GUSTO-IIa the rates of intracranial hemorrhage were reduced to the usually expected range in thrombolytically treated patients.

heparin as well) (87,88). This may contribute to a rebound hypercoagulable state counteracting the initial benefit from hirudin treatment. Of note, in GUSTO-IIb the incidence of ischemic events was significantly reduced until 48 hours after randomization by hirudin, but the advantage dissipated over the following weeks.

A favorable treatment interaction was demonstrated of streptokinase, but not t-PA, with hirudin. The subgroup analysis of GUSTO-IIb patients treated with thrombolysis for AMI revealed a significant 36% reduction in the primary endpoint of death or reinfarction at 30 days in patients treated with streptokinase and hirudin versus those treated with streptokinase and heparin (see Fig. 2). In patients receiving front-loaded alteplase no significant reduction of events was noted by hirudin as compared to heparin (89). The mechanism of this specific interaction seems to be an improved early-infarct vessel patency achieved by adjunctive treatment with direct thrombin antagonists (82). In the HIT-IV study, adjunctive hirudin versus heparin with streptokinase in AMI coronary angiography at 90 min showed no significant difference in complete patency in a subgroup of 447 patients (90). However, complete ST resolution was observed in 28% versus 22% of the patients

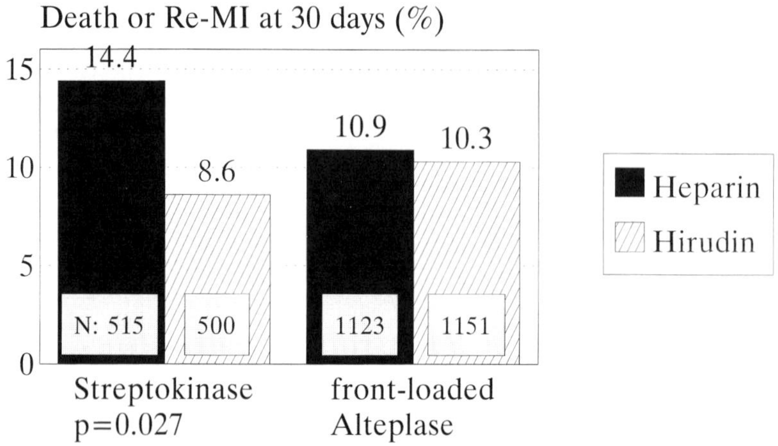

Figure 2 Treatment interaction of hirudin with streptokinase in GUSTO-IIb. Hirudin is more effective as adjunct to streptokinase than heparin, whereas thrombolysis with alteplase does not seem to be enhanced by hirudin more than by heparin. Rates of death or recurrent myocardial infarction are shown from the GUSTO-IIb study (89).

treated with hirudin (0.2 mg/kg IV bolus followed by 0.5 mg/kg SC BID) and heparin (P = .05).

HIRULOG

Hirulog is a dodecapeptide derived from hirudin. It binds to the active catalytic site of thrombin via a Phe-Pro-Arg linker molecule. Like hirudin, hirulog inhibits free as well as clot-bound thrombin (for references see 91).

Hirulog was investigated to treat unstable angina in 410 patients randomized to four dose groups of constant infusions over 72 hours with 0.02 to 1.0 mg/kg/h (92). All patients received 325 mg/d aspirin. The primary endpoint was unsatisfactory outcome by 72 hours defined as death, myocardial infarction, rapid clinical deterioration, or reischemia at rest occurred in 6.2% to 11.4% of the four dose groups without significant between-group differences. However, the secondary endpoint of in-hospital death or nonfatal myocardial infarction occurred in 10% of the patients of the lowest dose group versus 3.2 of those treated with the three higher doses (P = .008). Only two patients experienced a major hemorrhage attributed to hirulog.

Three studies compared hirulog to heparin as adjunct to thrombolysis with streptokinase in patients with acute myocardial infarction. In an angiographic pilot study of 45 patients hirulog yielded a higher 90-min patency rate of 77% versus 47% of the patients on heparin ($P < .05$). No reocclusions were seen at control angiography performed 4.7 days later (93). Théroux et al. (94) randomized 68 patients treated with streptokinase and aspirin for acute myocardial infarction to hirulog 0.5 mg/kg/h over 12 hours followed by 0.1 mg/kg/h (low dose), hirulog 1.0 mg/kg/h followed by placebo (high dose), or standard heparin treatment. At 90 min angiogram TIMI-grade 3 flow of the infarct vessel was found in 85%, 61%, and 31% of the low-dose, high-dose, and heparin groups, respectively ($P = .008$). Reocclusions during the following 4 days were more common in the patients without subsequent infusion after >12 hours. In the Hirulog Early Reperfusion Occlusion (HERO) trial of 412 patients treated with streptokinase for AMI, TIMI grade 3 flow in the infarct-related artery was achieved in 45% and 50% of patients treated with low- or high-dose hirulog, versus only 35% of patients treated with adjunctive heparin (95). Taking these results together, hirulog yields significantly better early patency rates of the infarct vessel than heparin when given as adjunct to streptokinase.

ARGATROBAN AND OTHER NOVEL SYNTHETIC THROMBIN ANTAGONISTS

Argatroban is a synthetic arginin derivative binding to a hydrophobic pocket near the active catalytic site of thrombin (96). Like other direct thrombin inhibitors, argatroban inhibits also clot-bound thrombin since it does not bind to the fibrin binding site of thrombin (97,98). In contrast to hirudin and hirulog, thrombin inhibition by argatroban is reversible (99). In experimental models of arterial thrombosis, argatroban was at least as effective as heparin in preventing thrombus formation (100–104). It was shown to inhibit the formation of thrombin-antithrombin III complexes as well as thrombus formation after coronary angioplasty (105,106). Thrombolysis by alteplase was enhanced by argatroban, and reocclusion after t-PA lysis was prevented in various experimental models of arterial thrombosis (107–110).

The clinical experience with argatroban is yet very limited. In a Phase I study argatroban was given to 43 patients with unstable angina as 0.5 to 5.0 μg/kg/min infusion over 4 hours (111). There was a dose-dependent increase of aPTT and a decrease of fibrinopeptide A, reflecting the thrombin inhibition. Surprisingly, 9 of the 43 patients experienced an episode of unstable angina 5.8 $\pm$ 2.6 hours after cessation of the infusion. This rebound was significantly correlated with higher argatroban doses. Argatroban was also investigated as adjunct to accelerated alteplase in 127 patients with acute myocardial infarction; the control group received heparin. The results were reported preliminary; the 90-min patency of the infarct-related arteries was 76% in the argatroban-treated patients versus 82% of those on heparin (TIMI grade 3 flow 57% vs. 67%) (112). Further clinical studies will be needed to define the future role of this novel thrombin antagonist in the management of acute coronary syndromes.

Another novel synthetic direct thrombin inhibitor, inogatran, was tested in 1209 patients with unstable angina in comparison to IV heparin (113). Inogatran was given in three dose groups increasing the aPTT values by 1.3- to 1.8-fold control. The rate of death or myocardial infarction was 7.6% to 9.0% in the inogatran-treated patients without evidence of a dose dependency, versus 5.9% in the heparin-treated control group. Interestingly, a later analysis of this study demonstrated ischemic clinical events to be associated with higher aPTT values in the inogatran-treated patients, while no such association was observed with heparin (114). This emphasizes the poorly defined optimal aPTT time range during treatment with direct thrombin inhibitors in acute coronary syndromes.

Efegatran is a tripeptide direct thrombin inhibitor inhibiting fibrin formation as well as thrombin-induced platelet aggregation. Efegatran markedly prolongs the thrombin time with only modest effects on the aPTT (115). In patients with unstable angina, efegatran elicited more stable prolongation of the aPTT than heparin, but the incidence of clinical events (death, myocardial infarction, or revascularization) was similar in patients treated with three different doses of efegatran and the control group on heparin (116).

SUMMARY

Antithrombin therapy is of utmost importance in all types of acute coronary syndromes. In unstable angina pectoris the standard treatment consists of intravenous heparin given as a bolus of 5000 IU followed by an infusion of 1000 IU/h adjusted to an aPTT around 2 × baseline. An alternative and at least equally effective treatment is subcutaneous application of LMW heparin. The combination with aspirin has not unequivocally been shown to be more effective than heparin alone, but it may prevent the rebound after cessation of heparin. The direct thrombin antagonists are at best marginally better than heparin in unstable angina.

In acute myocardial infarction treated with alteplase full-dose IV heparin should be given as adjunct to enhance thrombolysis and prevent early reocclusion. If streptokinase or anistreplase is given as thrombolytic agent, there is no proven benefit of adjunctive heparin therapy. Hirudin is very effective in preventing reocclusion after thrombolysis with alteplase without significantly affecting early-infarct vessel patency as compared to heparin. In contrast, direct thrombin inhibitors seem to accelerate thrombolysis by streptokinase, which may also improve the clinical outcome, whereas no clinical advantage of hirudin over heparin was demonstrated as adjunct to alteplase.

REFERENCES

1. Wallentin L. Low molecular weight heparins: a valuable tool in the treatment of acute coronary syndromes. Eur Heart J 1996;17:1470–1476.
2. Wilson JM, Dougherty KG, Ellis KO, Ferguson JJ, Blumenthal RS, Brinker JA. Activated clotting times in acute coronary syndromes and percutaneous transluminal coronary angioplasty. Cathet Cardiovasc Diagn 1995;34:1–7.
3. Fuchs J, Pinhas A, Davidson E, Rotenberg Z, Agmon J, Weinberger I. Plasma viscosity, fibrinogen and haematocrit in the course of unstable angina. Eur Heart J 1990;11:1029–1032.
4. Ardissino D, Merlini PA, Gamba G, Barberis P, Demicheli G, Testa S, Colombi E, Poli A, Fetiveau R, Montemartini C. Thrombin activity and early outcome in unstable angina pectoris. Circulation 1996;93:1634–1639.
5. Merlini PA, Ardissino D, Oltrona L, Broccolino M, Coppola R, Mannucci PM. Heightened thrombin formation but normal plasma levels of activated factor VII in patients with acute coronary syndromes. Arterioscler Thromb Vasc Biol 1995;15:1675–1679.
6. Telford AM, Wilson C. Trial of heparin versus atenolol in prevention of myocardial infarction in intermedicate coronary syndrome. Lancet 1981;I:1225–1228.
7. Théroux P, Quimet H, McCans J, Latour JG, Joly P, Lévy G, Pelletier E, Juneau M, Stasiak J, DeGuise P, Pelletier GB, Rinzler D, Waters DD. Aspirin, heparin, or both to treat acute unstable angina. N Engl J Med 1988;17:1105–1111.
8. Wallentin L. Risk of myocardial infarction and death during treatment with low dose aspirin and intravenous heparin in men with unstable coronary artery disease. Lancet 1990;336:827–830.
9. Théroux P, Waters D, Qiu S, McCans J, de Guise P, Juneau M. Aspirin versus heparin to prevent myocardinal infarction during the acute phase of unstable angina. Circulation 1993;88:2045–2048.
10. Cohen M, Adams PC, Parry C, Xiong J, Chamberlain D, Wieczorek I, Fox KAA, Chesebro JH, Strain J, Keller C, Kelly A, Lancaster G, Ali J, Kronmal F, Fuster V. Combination antithrombotic therapy in unstable rest angina and non-Q-wave infarction in nonprior aspirin users: primary end points analysis from the ATACS trial. Circulation 1994;89:81–88.
11. Holdright D, Patel D, Cunningham D, Thomas R, Hubbard W, Hendry G, Sutton G, Fox K. Comparison of the effect of heparin and aspirin versus aspirin alone on transient myocardial ischemia and in-hospital prognosis in patients with unstable angina. J Am Coll Cardiol 1994;24:39–45.
12. Serneri GGN, Modesti PA, Gensini GF, Branzi A, Melanari G, Poggesi L, Rostagno C, Tamburini C, Carnovali M, Magnani B. Randomised comparison of subcutaneous heparin, intravenous heparin, and aspirin in unstable angina. Lancet 1995;345:1201–1204.
13. Raschke RA, Reilly BM, Guidry JR, Fontana JR, Srinivas S. The weight-based heparin dosing nomogram compared with a ‘standard care’ nomogram: a randomized controlled trial. Ann Intern Med 1993;119:874–881.

14. Neri Serneri GG, Gensini GF, Poggesi L, Trotta F, Modesti PA, Boddi M, Ieri A, Margheri M, Casolo GC, Bini M, Rostagno C, Cranovali M, Abbate R. Effect of heparin, aspirin, or alteplase in reduction of myocardinal ischaemia in refractory unstable angina. Lancet 1990;335:615–618.
15. Becker RC, Cannon CP, Tracy RP, Thompson B, Bovill EG, Desvigne P, Randall AMY, Knatterud G, Braunwald E. Relation between systemic anticoagulation as determined by activated partial thromboplastin time and heparin measurements and in-hospital clinical events in unstable angina and non-Q wave myocardial infarction. Am Heart J. 1996;131:421–433.
16. Berglund U, Wallentin L. Influence on platelet function by heparin in men with unstable coronary artery disease. Thromb Haemost 1991;66:648–651.
17. Grambow DW, Topol EJ. Effect of maximal medical therapy on refractoriness of unstable angina pectoris. Am J Cardiol 1992;70:577–581.
18. Arai H, Saito S, Kim K, Aoki N, Hatano K, Hirashima O. Delayed catheter intervention for unstable angina pectoris. Jpn J Intervent Cardiol 1995;10: 157–162.
19. Correia LC, Neubauer C, Azevedo Jr A, Ribeiro F, Braga J, Passos LC, Teixeira M, Matos M, Aires V, Souza V, Rocha M, Camara E, Pericles Esteves J. The role of low molecular weight heparin in unstable angina, acute myocardial infarction and post-elective percutaneous transluminal coronary angioplasty. Arq Bras Cardiol 1995;65:475–478.
20. Gurfinkel EP, Manos EJ, Mejail RI, Cerda MA, Duronto EA, Garcia CN, Daroca AM, Mautner B. Low molecular weight heparin versus regular heparin or aspirin in the treatment of unstable angina and silent ischemia. J Am Coll Cardiol 1995;26:313–318.
21. Wallentin L, FRISC Study Group. Low-molecular-weight heparin during instability in coronary artery disease. Lancet 1996;347:561–568.
22. Antman EM, McCabe CH, Gurfinkel EP, Turpie AGG, Bernink PJLM, Salein D, Bayes de Luna A, Fox K, Lablanche J-M, Radley D, Premmereur J, Braunwald E, TIMI 11B Investigators. Enoxaparin prevents death and cardiac ischemic events in unstable angina/non-Q-wave myocardinal infarction. Results of the Thrombolysis in Myocardial Infarction (TIMI) 11B trial. Circulation 1999;100:1593–1601.
23. Cohen M, Demers C, Gurfinkel EP, Turpie AGG, Fromell G, Goodman S, Langer A, Califf RM, Fox KAA, Premmereur J, Bigonzi F. A comparison of low-molecular-weight heparin with unfractionated heparin for unstable coronary artery disease. N Engl J Med 1997;337:447–452.
24. Antman EM, Cohen M, Radley D, McCabe C, Rush J, Premmereur J, Braunwald E, for the TIMI 11B and ESSENCE Investigators. Assessment of the treatment effect of enoxaparin for unstable angina/non-Q-wave myocardinal infarction. TIMI 11B–ESSENCE meta-analysis. Circulation 1999;100:1602–1608.
25. Collignon F, Frydman A, Caplain H, Ozoux ML, Le Roux Y, Bouthier J, Thebault JJ. Comparison of the pharmacokinetic profiles of three low molecular mass heparins—dalteparin, enoxaparin and nadroparin—administered

subcutaneously in healthy volunteers (doses for prevention of thromboembolism). Thromb Haemost 1995;73:630–640.

26. Klein W, Buchwald A, Hillis SE, Monrad S, Sanz G, Turpie AGG, Van der Meer J, Olaisson E, Undeland S, Ludwig K, FRIC Investigators. Comparison of low-molecular-weight heparin with unfractionated heparin acutely and with placebo for 6 weeks in the management of unstable coronary artery disease. Fragmin in Unstable Coronary Artery Disease Study (FRIC). Circulation 1997;96:61–68.
27. Leizorovicz A. The FRAXIS Study. XXth Congress of the European Society of Cardiology 1998; Aug. 25, 1998.
28. FRAX.I.S. Study Group. Comparison of two treatment durations (6 days and 14 days) of a low molecular weight heparin with a 6-day treatment of unfractionated heparin in the initial management of unstable angina or non-Q wave myocardinal infarction: FRAX.I.S. (FRAXiparin in Ischaemic Syndrome). Eur Heart J 1999;20:1553–1562.
29. Theroux P, Waters D, Lam J, Juneau M, McCans J. Reactivation of unstable angina after the discontinuation of heparin. N Engl J Med 1992;327:141–145.
30. Lidon RM, Theroux P, Robitaille D. Antithrombin-III plasma activity during and after prolonged use of heparin in unstable angina. Thromb Res 1993;72: 23–32.
31. Granger CB, Miller JM, Bovill EG, Gruber A, Tracy RP, Krucoff MW, Green C, Berrios E, Harrington RA, Ohman EM, Califf RM. Rebound increase in thrombin generation and activity after cessation of intravenous heparin in patients with acute coronary syndromes. Circulation 1995;91:1929–1935.
32. FRISC II Investigators. Long-term low-molecular mass heparin in unstable coronary-artery disease: FRISC II prospective randomised multicentre study. Lancet 1999;354:701–707.
33. FRISC II Investigators. Invasive compared with non-invasive treatment in unstable coronary-artery disease: FRISC II prospective randomised multicentre study. Lancet 1999;354:708–715.
34. Aronson DL, Chang P, Kessler CM. Platelet-dependent thrombin generation after in vitro fibrinolytic treatment. Circulation 1992;85:1706–1712.
35. Vila V, Reganon E, Aznar J, Lacueva V, Ruano M, Laiz B. Hypercoagulable state after thrombolytic therapy in patients with acute myocardial infarction (AMI) treated with streptokinase. Thromb Res 1990;57:783–794.
36. Hoffman JJML, Michels HR, Windeler J, Gunzler WA. Plasma markers of thrombin activity coronary thrombolytic therapy with saruplase or urokinase: no prediction of reinfarction. Fibrinolysis 1993;7:330–334.
37. Zahger D, Maaravi Y, Matzner Y, Gilon D, Gotsman MS, Weiss AT. Partial resistance to anticoagulation after streptokinase treatment for acute myocardial infarction. Am J Cardiol 1990;66:28–30.
38. Mahaffey KW, Granger CB, Collins R, O'Connor CM. Overview of randomized trials of intravenous heparin in patients with acute myocardinal infarction treated with thrombolytic therapy. Am J Cardiol 1996;77:551–556.
39. Bleich SD, Nichols TC, Schumacher RR, Cooke DH, Tate DA, Teichman SL. Effect of heparin on coronary arterial patency after thrombolysis with tissue

plasminogen activator in acute myocardial infarction. Am J Cardiol 1990;66: 1412–1417.

40. De Bono DP, Simoons ML, Tijssen J, Arnold AER, Betriu A, Burgersdijk C, Lopez Bescos L, Mueller E, Pfisterer M, Van de Werf F, Zijlstra F, Verstraete M. Effect of early intravenous heparin on coronary patency, infarct size, and bleeding complications after alteplase thrombolysis: results of a randomised double blind European Cooperative Study Group trial. Br Heart J 1992;67: 122–128.
41. Hsia J, Hamilton WP, Kleiman N, Roberts R, Chaitman BR, Ross AM. A comparison between heparin and low-dose aspirin as adjunctive therapy with tissue plasminogen activator for acute myocardial infarction. N Engl J Med 1990;323:1433–1437.
42. Arnout J, Simoons M, De Bono D, Rapold HJ, Collen D, Verstraete M. Correlation between level of heparinization and patency of the infarct-related coronary artery after treatment of acute myocardial infarction with alteplase (rt-PA). J Am Coll Cardiol 1992;20:513–519.
43. Hsia J, Kleiman N, Aguirre F, Chaitman BR, Roberts R, Ross AM. Heparin-induced prolongation of partial thromboplastin time after thrombolysis: relation to coronary artery patency. J Am Coll Cardiol 1992;20:31–35.
44. Tebbe U, Windeler J, Boesl I, Hoffman H, Wojcik J, Ashmawy M, Schwarz ER, Von Loewis Of Menar P, Rosemeyer P, Hopkins G, Barth H. Thrombolysis with recombinant unglycosylated single-chain urokinase-type plasminogen activator (saruplase) in acute myocardial infarction: influence of heparin on early patency rate (LIMITS study). J Am Coll Cardiol 1995;26:365–373.
45. O'Connor CM, Meese R, Carney R, Smith J, Conn E, Burks J, Hartman C, Roark S, Shadoff N, Heard MIII, Mittler B, Collins G, Navetta F, Leimberger J, Lee K, Califf RM. A randomized trial of intravenous heparin in conjunction with anistreplase (anisoylated plasminogen streptokinase activator complex) in acute myocardial infarction: Duke University Clinical Cardiology Study (DUCCS) 1. J Am Coll Cardiol 1994;23:11–8.
46. SCATI Group. Randomised controlled trial of subcutaneous calcium-heparin in acute myocardial infarction. Lancet 1989;2:182–186.
47. Gruppo Italiano per lo Studio della Sopravvivenza nell'Infarto Miocardico (GISSI-2). A factorial randomised trial of alteplase versus streptokinase and heparin versus no heparin among 12,490 patients with acute myocardial infarction. Lancet 1990;336:65–71.
48. Third International Study of Infarct Survival Collaborative Group. ISIS-3: a randomised comparison of streptokinase vs tissue plasminogen activator vs anistreplase and of aspirin plus heparin vs aspirin alone among 41,299 cases of suspected acute myocardial infarction. Lancet 1992;339:753–770.
49. Gruppo Italiano per lo Studio della Sopravvivenza nell'Infarto Miocardico (GISSI-2) Six-month survival in 20,891 patients with acute myocardial infarction randomized between alteplase and streptokinase with or without heparin. Eur Heart J 1992;13:1692–1697.
50. GUSTO-1 Investigators. An international randomized trial comparing four

thrombolytic strategies for acute myocardial infarction. N Engl J Med 1993; 329:673–682.
51. GUSTO Angiographic Investigators. The effects of tissue plasminogen activator, streptokinase, or both on coronary-artery patency, ventricular function, and survival after acute myocardial infarction. N Engl J Med 1993;329:1615–1622.
52. Mahan EFII, Chandler JW, Rogers WJ, Nath HR, Smith LR, Whitlow PL, Hood WP, Reeves RC, Baxley WA. Heparin and infarct coronary artery patency after streptokinase in acute myocardial infarction. Am J Cardiol 1990; 65:967–972.
53. Glick A, Kornowski R, Michowich Y, Koifman B, Roth A, Laniado S, Keren G. Reduction of reinfarction and angina with use of low-molecular-weight heparin therapy after streptokinase (and heparin) in acute myocardial infarction. Am J Cardiol 1996;77:1145–1148.
54. Granger CB, Hish J, Califf RM, Col J, White HD, Betriu A, Woodlief LH, Lee KL, Bovill EG, Simes RJ, Topol EJ. Activated partial thromboplastin time and outcome after thrombolytic therapy for acute myocardial infarction: results from the GUSTO-I trial. Circulation 1996;93:870–878.
55. Funke Kupper AJ, Verheugt FWA, Peels CH, Galema TW, Roos JP. Left ventricular thrombus incidence and behavior studied by serial two-dimensional echocardiography in acute anterior myocardial infarction: left ventricular wall motion, systemic embolism and oral anticoagulation. J Am Coll Cardiol 1989;13:1514–1520.
56. Jugdutt BI, Sivaram CA, Wortman C, Trudell C, Penner P. Prospective two-dimensional echocardiographic evaluation of left ventricular thrombus and embolism after acute myocardial infarction. J Am Coll Cardiol 1989;13:554–564.
57. Keren A, Goldberg S, Gottlieb S, Klein J, Schuger C, Medina A, Tzivoni D, Stern S. Natural history of left ventricular thrombi: their appearance and resolution in the posthospitalization period of acute myocardial infarction. J Am Coll Cardiol 1990;15:790–800.
58. Nihoyannopoulos P, Smith GC, Maseri A, Foale RA. The natural history of left ventricular thrombus in myocardial infarction: a rationale in support of masterly inactivity. J Am Coll Cardiol 1989;14:903–911.
59. Turpie AGG, Robinson JG, Doyle DJ, Mulji AS, Mishkel GJ, Sealey BJ, Cairns JA, Skingley L, Hirsh J, Gent M. Comparison of high-dose with low-dose subcutaneous heparin to prevent left ventricular mural thrombosis in patients with acute transmural anterior myocardial infarction. N Engl J Med 1989;320:352–357.
60. Vecchio C, Chiarella F, Lupi G, Bellotti P, Domenicucci S. Left ventricular thrombus in anterior acute myocardial infarction after thrombolysis: a GISSI-2 connected study. Circulation 1991;84:512–519.
61. Johannessen KA, Nordrehaug JE, Von der Lippe G. Left ventricular thrombi after short-term high-dose anticoagulants in acute myocardial infarction. Eur Heart J 1987;8:975–980.

62. Nordrehaug JE, Johannessen KA, Von der Lippe G. Usefulness of high dose anticoagulants in preventing left ventricular thrombus in acute myocardial infarction. Am J Cardiol 1985;55:1491–1493.
63. Arvan S, Boscha K. Prophylactic anticoagulation for left ventricular thrombi after acute myocardial infarction: a prospective randomized trial. Am Heart J 1987;113:688–693.
64. Lefkovits J, Topol EJ. Direct thrombin inhibitors in cardiovascular medicine. Circulation 1994;90:1522–1536.
65. Haskel EJ, Prager NA, Sobel BE, Abendschein DR. Relative efficacy of antithrombin compared with antiplatelet agents in accelerating coronary thrombolysis and preventing early reocclusion. Circulation 1991;83:1048–1056.
66. Badimon L, Badimon JJ, Lassila R, Heras M, Chesebro JH, Fuster V. Thrombin regulation of platelet interaction with damaged vessel wall and isolated collagen type I at arterial flow conditions in a porcine model: effects of hirudins, heparin, and calcium chelation. Blood 1991;78:423–434.
67. Lam JYT, Chesebro JH, Steele PM, Heras M, Webster MWI, Badimon L, Fuster V. Antithrombotic therapy for deep arterial injury by angioplasty: efficacy of common platelet inhibition compared with thrombin inhibition in pigs. Circulation 1991;84:814–820.
68. Heras M, Chesebro JH, Webster MWI, Mruk JS, Grill DE, Penny WJ, Bowie EJW, Badimon L, Fuster V. Hirudin, heparin, and placebo during deep arterial injury in the pig. The in vivo role of thrombin in platelet-mediated thrombosis. Circulation 1990;82:1476–1484.
69. Agnelli G, Pascucci C, Cosmi B, Nenci GG. The comparative effects of recombinant hirudin (CGP 39393) and standard heparin on thrombus growth in rabbits. Thromb Haemost 1990;63:204–207.
70. Agnelli G, Pascucci C, Cosmi B, Nenci GG. Effects of hirudin and heparin on the binding of new fibrin to the thrombus in t-PA treated rabbits. Thromb Haemost 1991;66:592–597.
71. Heras M, Chesebro JH, Penny WJ, Bailey KR, Badimon L, Fuster V. Effects of thrombin inhibition on the development of acute platelet-thrombus deposition during angioplasty in pigs. Heparin versus recombinant hirudin, a specific thrombin inhibitor. Circulation 1989;79:657–665.
72. Topol EJ, Fuster V, Harrington RA, Califf RM, Kleiman NS, Kereiakes DJ, Cohen M, Chapekis A, Gold HK, Tannenbaum MA, Rao AK, Debowey D, Schwartz D, Henis M, Chesebro J. Recombinant hirudin for unstable angina pectoris: a multicenter, randomized angiographic trial. Circulation 1994;89:1557–1566.
73. GUSTO IIa Investigators. Randomized trial of intravenous heparin versus recombinant hirudin for acute coronary syndromes. Circulation 1994;90:1631–1637.
74. GUSTO IIb Investigators. A comparison of recombinant hirudin with heparin for the treatment of acute coronary syndromes. N Engl J Med 1996;335:775–782.
75. Zeymer U, von Essen R, Tebbe U, Niederer W, Mäurer W, Vogt A, Neuhaus KL. Frequency of "optimal anticoagulation" for acute myocardial infarction

after thrombolysis with front-loaded recombinant tissue-type plasminogen activator and conjunctive therapy with recombinant hirudin (HBW 023). Am J Cardiol 1995;76:997–1001.

76. OASIS Investigators. Comparison of the effects of two doses of recombinant hirudin compared with heparin in patients with acute myocardial ischemia without ST elevation: a pilot study. Circulation 1997;96:769–777.
77. OASIS-2 Investigators. Effects of recombinant hirudin (lepirudin) compared with heparin on death, myocardial infarction, refractory angina, and revascularisation procedures in patients with acute myocardial ischaemia without ST elevation: a randomised trial. Lancet 1999;353:429–438.
78. Zeymer U, von Essen R, Tebbe U, Michels HR, Jessel A, Vogt A, Roth M, Appel K-F, Neuhaus KL. Recombinant hirudin and front-loaded alteplase in acute myocardial infarction. Results of a pilot study: HIT-I (Hirudin for the Improvement of Thrombolysis). Eur Heart J 1995;16(suppl D):22–27.
79. Neuhaus KL, Niederer W, Wagner J, Mäurer W, Von Essen R, Tebbe U, von Leitner ER, Haerten K, Vogt A, Appel K-F, Mateblowski M, Zeymer U, ALKK study group. HIT (Hirudin for the Improvement of Thrombolysis): results of a dose escalation study. Circulation 1993;88(suppl I):I-292.
80. Neuhaus KL, Von Essen R, Tebbe U, Vogt A, Roth M, Riess M, Niederer W, Forycki F, Wirtzfeld A, Maeurer W, Limbourg P, Merx W, Haerten K. Improved thrombolysis in acute myocardial infarction with front-loaded administration of alteplase: results of the rt-PA-APSAC patency study (TAPS). J Am Coll Cardiol 1992;19:885–891.
81. Cannon CP, McCabe CH, Henry TD, Schweiger MJ, Gibson RS, Mueller HS, Becker RC, Kleiman NS, Haugland M, Anderson JL, Sharaf BL, Edwards SJ, Rogers WJ, Williams DO, Braunwald E, TIMI 5 Investigators. Pilot trial of recombinant desulfatohirudin compared with heparin in conjunction with tissue-type plasminogen activator and aspirin for acute myocardial infarction: results of the Thrombolysis in Myocardial Infarction (TIMI) 5 Trial. J Am Coll Cardiol 1994;23:993–1003.
82. Molhoek GP, Laarman GJ, Lok DJA, Luz M, Kingma JH, van den Bos AA, Bosma AH, den Heijer P. Effects of recombinant hirudin (HBW 023) on early and late coronary patency in acute myocardial infarction patients treated with streptokinase (the HIT-SK study). Eur Heart J 1995;16(abstract suppl):177.
83. Lee LV, TIMI 6 Investigators. Initial experience with hirudin and streptokinase in acute myocardial infarction: results of the thrombolysis in myocardial infarction (TIMI) 6 trial. Am J Cardiol 1995;75:7–13.
84. Antman EM, TIMI 9A. Investigators. Hirudin in acute myocardial infarction. Safety report from the thrombolysis and thrombin inhibition in myocardial infarction (TIMI) 9A trial. Circulation 1994;90:1624–1630.
85. Neuhaus KL, von Essen R, Tebbe U, Jessel A, Heinrichs H, Mäurer W, Döring W, Harmjanz D, Kötter V, Kalhammer E, Simon H, Horacek T. Safety observations from the pilot phase of the randomized r-hirudin for improvement of thrombolysis (HIT-III) study. Circulation 1994;90:1638–1642.
86. Antman EM, TIMI 9B Investigators. Hirudin in acute myocardial infarction.

Thrombolysis and Thrombin Inhibition in Myocardial Infarction (TIMI) 9B Trial. Circulation 1996;94:911–921.
87. Merlini PA, Bauer KA, Oltrona L, Ardissino D, Spinola A, Cattaneo M, Broccolino M, Mannucci PM, Rosenberg RD. Thrombin generation and activity during thrombolysis and concomitant heparin therapy in patients with acute myocardial infarction. J Am Coll Cardiol 1995;25:203–209.
88. Zoldhelyi P, Janssens S, Lefèvre G, Collen D, Van de Werf F. Effects of heparin and hirudin (GCP 39393) on thrombin generation during thrombolysis for acute myocardial infarction. Circulation 1995;92(suppl I):I-740. Abstract.
89. Metz BK, White HD, Granger CB, Simes RJ, Armstrong PW, Hirsh J, Fuster V, MacAulay CM, Califf RM, Topol EJ. Randomized comparison of direct thrombin inhibition versus heparin in conjunction with fibrinolytic therapy for acute myocardial infarction: results from the GUSTO-IIb Trial. J Am Coll Cardiol 1998;31:1493–1498.
90. Neuhaus KL, Molhoek GP, Zeymer U, Tebbe U, Wescheider K, Schröder R, Camez A, Laarman GJ, Grollier GM, Lok DJA, Kuckuck H, Lazarus P, HIT-4 Investigators. Recombinant hirudin (lepirudin) for the improvement of thrombolysis with streptokinase in patients with acute myocardial infarction. Results of the HIT-4 Trial. J Am Coll Cardiol 1999;34:966–973.
91. Topol EJ. Novel antithrombotic approaches to coronary artery disease. Am J Cardiol 1995;75:27B–33B.
92. Braunwald E, Fuchs J, Cannon CP, Antman EM, McCabe CH, DeFeo Fraulini T, Sollecito B, Wallman L, Tudor G, Williams DO, Sharaf B, Ferreira P, Miele N, Chaitman B, Stocke K, Hennekens C, Kelton J, Friesinger GC, Gersh B. Hirulog in the treatment of unstable angina: results of the Thrombin Inhibition in Myocardial Ischemia (TIMI) 7 Trial. Circulation 1995;92:727–733.
93. Lidón RM, Théroux P, Lespérance J, Adelman B, Bonan R, Duval D, Lévesque J. A pilot, early angiographic patency study using a direct thrombin inhibitor as adjunctive therapy to streptokinase in acute myocardial infarction. Circulation 1994;89:1567–1572.
94. Theroux P, Perez Villa F, Waters D, Lesperance J, Shabani F, Bonan R. Randomized double-blind comparison of two doses of Hirulog with heparin as adjunctive therapy to streptokinase to promote early patency of the infarct-related artery in acute myocardial infarction. Circulation 1995;91:2132–2139.
95. White HD. The hirulog early reperfusion occlusion (HERO) trial. American College of Cardiology 45th Annual Scientific Session, 1996. Abstract.
96. Okamoto S, Hijikata A. Potent inhibition of thrombin by the newly synthesized arginine derivative No. 805. The importance of stereostructure of its hydrophobic carboxamide portion. Biochem Biophys Res Commun 1981;101:440–445.
97. Hogg PJ, Jackson CM. Fibrin monomer protects thrombin from inactivation by heparin-antithrombin III: implications for heparin efficacy. Proc Natl Acad Sci USA 1989;86:3619–3623.
98. Lunven C, Gauffeny C, Lecoffre C, O'Brien DP, Roome NO, Berry CN. Inhibition by argatroban, a specific thrombin inhibitor, of platelet activation by fibrin clot-associated thrombin. Thromb Haemost 1996;75:154–160.

99. Callas DD, Hoppensteadt D, Fareed J. Comparative studies on the anticoagulant and protease generation inhibitory actions of newly developed site-directed thrombin inhibitor drugs. Efegatran registered, argatroban, hirulog, and hirudin. Semin Thromb Hemost 1995;21:177–183.
100. Kosugi T, Masuda Y, Kinjoh K, Yamashita S, Sungawa M, Nakamura M. Effects of argatroban on the formation of artificial thrombus on dogs. Int J Tissue React 1995;17:109–116.
101. Tomaru T, Nakamura F, Fujimori Y, Omata M, Kawai S. Okada R, Murata Y, Uchida Y. Local treatment with antithrombotic drugs can prevent thrombus formation: an angioscopic and angiographic study. J Am Coll Cardiol 1995; 26:1325–1332.
102. Jang IK, Gold HK, Ziskind AA, Leinbach RC, Fallon JT, Collen D. Prevention of platelet-rich arterial thrombosis by selective thrombin inhibition. Circulation 1990;81:219–225.
103. Jang IK, Gold HK, Leinbach RC, Rivera AG, Fallon JT, Bunging S, Collen D. Persistent inhibition of arterial thrombosis by a 1-hour intravenous infusion of argatroban, a selective thrombin inhibitor. Coron Artery Dis 1992;3:407–414.
104. Imura Y, Stassen JM, Vreys I, Lesaffre E, Gold HK, Collen D. Synergistic antithrombotic properties of G4120, a RGD-containing synthetic peptide, and argatroban, a synthetic thrombin inhibitor, in a hamster femoral vein platelet-rich thrombosis model. Thromb Haemost 1992;68:336–340.
105. Sakamoto S, Hirase T, Suzuki S, Tsukamoto T, Miki T, Yamada T, Matsuo T. Inhibitory effect of argatroban on thrombin-antithrombin III complex after percutaneous transluminal coronary angioplasty. Thromb Haemost 1995;74: 801–8-2.
106. Suzuki S, Sakamoto S, Adachi K, Mizutani K, Koide M, Ohga N, Miki T, Matsuo T. Effect of argatroban on thrombus formation during acute coronary occlusion after balloon angioplasty. Thromb Res 1995;77:369–373.
107. Fitzgerald DJ, Fitzgerald GA. Role of thrombin and thromboxane A-2 in reocclusion following coronary thrombolysis with tissue-type plasminogen activator. Proc Natl Acad Sci USA 1989;86:7585–7589.
108. Jang IK, Gold HK, Leinbach RC, Fallon JT, Collen D. In vivo thrombin inhibition enhances and sustains arterial recanalization with recombinant tissue-type plasminogen activator. Circ Res 1990;67:1552–1561.
109. Mellott MJ, Connolly TM, York SJ, Bush LR. Prevention of reocclusion by MCI-9038, a thrombin inhibitor, following t-PA-induced thrombolysis in a canine model of femoral arterial thrombosis. Thromb Haemost 1990;64:526–534.
110. Yasuda T, Gold HK, Yaoita H, Leinbach RC, Guerrero JL, Jang IK, Holt R, Fallon JT, Collen D. Comparative effects of aspirin, a synthetic thrombin inhibitor and a monoclonal antiplatelet glycoprotein IIb/IIIa antibody on coronary artery reperfusion, reocclusion and bleeding with recombinant tissue-type plasminogen activator in a canine preparation. J Am Coll Cardiol 1990; 16:714–722.

111. Gold HK, Torres FW, Garabedian HD, Werner W, Jang IK, Khan A, Hagstrom JN, Yasuda T, Leinbach RC, Newell JB, Bovill EG, Stump DC, Collen D. Evidence for a rebound coagulation phenomenon after cessation of a 4-hour infusion of a specific thrombin inhibitor in patients with unstable angina pectoris. J Am Coll Cardiol 1993;21:1039–1047.
112. Simoons ML, Vermeer F, van de Werf F, Radzik D, Vahanian A. Comparison of argatroban and heparin in patients treated for myocardial infarction with alteplase. 12th International Workshop George Washington University, New Orleans, Nov. 9, 1996.
113. Thrombin Inhibition in Myocardial Ischemia (TRIM) Study Group. A low molecular weight, selective thrombin inhibitor, inogatran, vs heparin, in unstable coronary artery disease in 1209 patients. Eur Heart J 1997;18:1416–1425.
114. Oldgren J, Linder R, Grip L, Siegbahn A, Wallentin L. Activated partial thromboplastin time and clinical outcome after thrombin inhibition in unstable coronary artery disease. Eur Heart J 1999;20:1657–1666.
115. Ohman EM, Slovak JP, Anderson RL, Grossman WJ, Barbeau GR, Butler JF, Frey MJ, Talley DJ, Leimberger JD, Scherer JC, Kleiman NS. PRIME Group. Potent inhibition of thrombin with efegatran in combination with tPA in acute myocardial infarction: results of a multicenter randomized dose ranging trial. Circulation 1996;94(suppl I):I-430.
116. Klootwijk P, Lenderink T, Meij S, Boersma E, Melkert R, Umans VAWM, Stibbe J, Müller EJ, Poortermans KJ, Deckers JW, Simoons ML. Anticoagulant properties, clinical efficacy and safety of efegatran, a direct thrombin inhibitor, in patients with unstable angina. Eur Heart J 1999;20:1101–1111.

20

Bedside Anticoagulant Testing

Christopher B. Granger
Duke University Medical Center
Durham, North Carolina

David J. Moliterno
Department of Cardiology
The Cleveland Clinic Foundation
Cleveland, Ohio

RATIONALE FOR ANTICOAGULANT MONITORING

Although some antithrombotic agents, such as aspirin, have efficacy without high bleeding risk over a wide range of doses, most others, such as thrombolytic agents and antithrombin agents, have a relatively narrow therapeutic window, making the appropriate dose of the agent critical for patient care. The need for anticoagulant monitoring is based on the premise that patient outcomes will be improved by the ability to adjust the anticoagulant to a range where the balance between preventing thrombosis and increasing bleeding risk is optimized.

The TIMI II pilot study provides one example of the importance of using the optimal dose of agents to treat thrombosis: the 150-mg dose of t-PA resulted in a 1.6% incidence of intracranial hemorrhage, while there was <0.5% incidence with 100 mg (1). A second example is the 90-min infusion of t-PA first studied by Neuhaus (2), which had substantially higher early coronary artery patency without more bleeding than the standard 3-hour infusion.

To optimize risk versus benefit of heparin by monitoring effect and adjusting dose, the optimal range must first be defined. Prior to the 1990s, even though standard practice was to avoid very high aPTTs due to concern about bleeding, data relating high levels of aPTT to higher bleeding risk were inconclusive, with some studies showing a relationship (3,4) and others not (5,6). In the early 1990s, the GUSTO-I trial showed that aPTTs >70 sec were found to have a linear relationship with increasing risk of hemorrhage, with each 10-sec increase in aPTT being associated with approximately a 1% absolute increase in moderate or severe hemorrhage and a 0.07% increase in risk of intracranial hemorrhage (7) (Fig. 1). There also appeared to be a higher risk of death with aPTTs below the 50-sec range and above the 75-sec range (Fig. 1). Although aPTT was associated with risk of both intracranial and other hemorrhage, patient-related factors are even more important (8,9), including both baseline features such as older age and lighter body weight, and performance of procedures such as angioplasty or bypass surgery. Patients known to be at high risk of hemorrhage should be managed even more carefully to avoid high levels of anticoagulation.

The relationship between greater heparin anticoagulant effect and higher risk of hemorrhage was further solidified in GUSTO IIa, where the 20% higher dose of heparin in GUSTO IIa (10) compared with GUSTO I, resulting in a 5- to 10-sec increase in aPTT, was associated with twice the risk of intracranial hemorrhage among patients treated with thrombolytic therapy. When the dose of heparin was lowered in GUSTO IIb, the median aPTT at 12 hours decreased from 85 to 65 sec among thrombolytic-treated patients, and the intracranial hemorrhage rate dropped in half to 0.6% (11). Likewise, a decrease in risk of intracranial hemorrhage was seen in the TIMI 9B trial with reduction of the anticoagulant doses (12).

Moreover, the median time to first symptoms of intracranial hemorrhage was approximately 12 hours after initiation of thrombolytic therapy, suggesting that if overanticoagulation is going to be recognized in time to make adjustments that will prevent intracranial hemorrhage, those changes must be made early following initiation of therapy. In GUSTO IIa, among patients treated with thrombolysis and heparin, the median aPTT at 6 hours was 150 sec for patients with intracranial hemorrhage versus 98 sec for patients without intracranial hemorrhage. The relationship of intracranial hemorrhage with high early aPTTs calls for careful monitoring of early aPTTs and rapid downtitration of heparin for markedly elevated aPTTs, for there to be any chance of reducing risk of intracranial hemorrhage. Halfway through the InTIME-2 trial comparing t-PA to lanoteplase, heparin monitoring was changed such that the first aPTT was 3 hours after starting heparin with downward adjustment in heparin dose for an aPTT >70 sec, and the intracranial hemorrhage rate dropped from 0.71% to 0.52% (13). The traditional initial heparin dosing of 5000-unit bolus followed by 1000 U/hr has been shown to result in a substantial portion of high early aPTTs both fol-

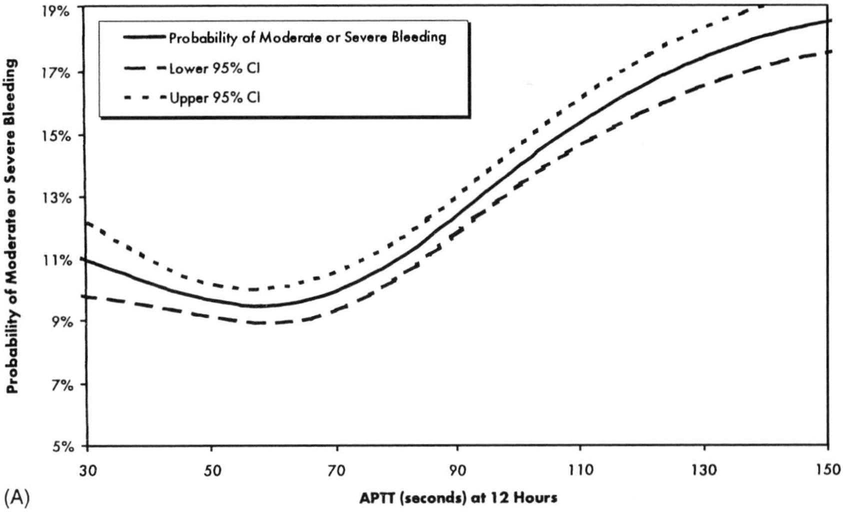

(A)

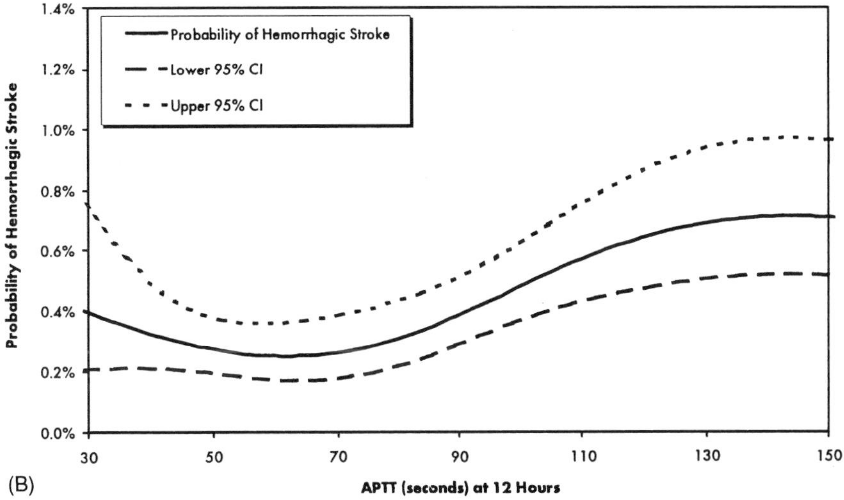

(B)

Figure 1 Probability of (A) moderate or severe bleeding, (B) intracranial hemorrhage, and (C) 30-day mortality according to aPTT at 12 hours after enrollment among patients on IV heparin in the GUSTO I trial. Dotted lines represent 95% confidence intervals. (Adapted from Ref. 7.)

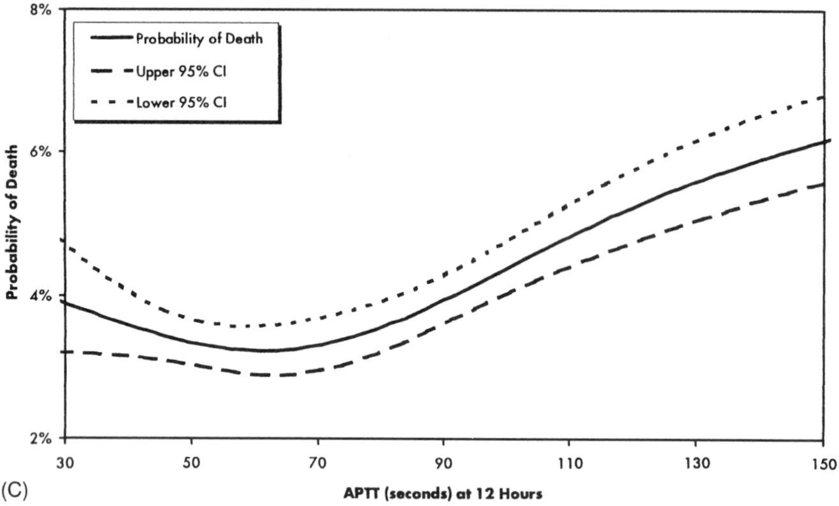

(C)

Figure 1 Continued

lowing thrombolytic therapy (7) and following acute coronary syndromes, compared to lower dose weight-adjusted therapy (14).

The concern over risk from high levels of heparin anticoagulation following thrombolytic therapy is reflected in the 1999 update of the ACC/AHA guidelines for the management of patients with acute myocardial infarction (15). These guidelines integrate data from observational studies, from the effect of varying heparin doses across trials, and from a small study testing a lower dose of heparin (14). The resulting recommendation is that heparin be administered at the lower weight-adjusted dose of 60 U/kg bolus followed by 12 U/kg/hr with a target aPTT of 50 to 70 sec (15).

Data relating aPTT to outcomes among patients with acute coronary syndromes other than acute myocardial infarction who are treated with thrombolytic therapy are less compelling. The randomized trials showing an advantage of heparin and aspirin over aspirin alone used a target aPTT in the 1.5 to 2.5 times control range (16). For standard aPTT reagents, this would correspond to a target range of 45 to 75 sec. In both the TIMI IIIb (17) and the GUSTO II trials (18), analyses have been performed assessing clinical outcomes according to degree of aPTT prolongation among patients with unstable angina or non-Q-wave myocardial infarction treated with intravenous heparin. Clinical outcomes were best with aPTTs in the 1.5 to 2 times control range, with no apparent advantage to aPTTs over the 70-to-75-sec range. These data suggest that the best aPTT range for patients with the entire spectrum of acute coronary syndromes is the 50-to-75-sec range.

The twofold higher dose of hirudin in GUSTO IIa than GUSTO IIb, which was associated with an 18-sec increase in the median aPTT at 12 hours, was also associated with three times the risk of intracranial hemorrhage. In the setting of coronary intervention in the EPILOG trial, a reduction in the dose of heparin from 100 U/kg to 70 U/kg with abciximab resulted in a reduction in major bleeding from 3.5% to 2.0% with no loss in benefit (19). These data in aggregate show that the dose of anticoagulants and the level of the anticoagulant effect are clinically important pieces of information that may be critical to optimize patient outcomes.

Three approaches can be considered to improve current dosing and monitoring of heparin therapy. First, dosing of intravenous heparin can be optimized by weight-adjusting the initial dose and using a nomogram to adjust the dose. Patient weight is the most important determinant of heparin dose requirement, with every additional 10 kg in patient weight being associated with a 6-sec lower aPTT with a given heparin dose (7). Several studies have shown better achievement and maintenance of a target aPTT range when a nomogram (20,21), and in particular a weight-adjusted nomogram (22–24), is used to guide heparin adjustment. A nomogram based on the aPTT target range of 50 to 75 sec is contained in the ACC/AHA Guidelines for the Management of Patients with Acute Myocardial Infarction (25) (Table 1).

Second, anticoagulants that require less monitoring to provide an adequate anticoagulant effect without high risk of bleeding may be used. Although it was hoped that direct thrombin inhibitors, due to the more predictable anticoagulant effect, might require less monitoring, the GUSTO IIa

Table 1 Heparin Adjustment Nomogram for Standard Laboratory Reagents with a Mean Control aPTT of 26 to 36 Sec

aPTT (sec)	Bolus dose (U)	Stop infusion (min)	Rate change (mL/h)	Repeat aPTT
<40	3000	0	+2	6 h
40–49	0	0	+1	6 h
50–75	0	0	0 (no change)	Next AM
76–85	0	0	−1	Next AM
86–100	0	30	−2	6 h
101–150	0	60	−3	6 h
>150	0	60	−6	6 h

Heparin infusion concentration = 50 U/mL. Target aPTT = 50–75 sec (for the CoaguChek Plus bedside monitor, target aPTT is 60–85 sec, and the nomogram should be modified accordingly). (From Ref. 25.)

(10), TIMI 9A (6), and HIT (26) trials demonstrated that there was a strong relationship between variation in anticoagulation effect and risk of bleeding, and therefore monitoring and adjusting the dose, albeit less frequently (11), is necessary. Low-molecular-weight heparins, on the other hand, which have a greater effect on inhibiting Factor Xa than thrombin, appear to have a similar bleeding risk compared with unfractionated heparin (27–29), and historically have not required anticoagulation monitoring. Contrary to popular belief, however, the variability of anticoagulant effect over time is substantial, due to the variation in drug level related to the twice-daily dosing (30).

Third, as long as unfractionated intravenous heparin continues to be the leading antithrombotic therapy, optimal monitoring techniques can be used which involve using methods that provide reliable and rapid measures of the anticoagulation effect. The extent to which bedside testing may assist in achieving that goal is discussed below.

PROBLEMS WITH TRADITIONAL METHODS

The standard method for monitoring heparin anticoagulation is the activated partial thromboplastin time (aPTT), a test that reflects the inhibitory effect of heparin on thrombin, Factor Xa, and Factor IXa. The therapeutic aPTT range was originally based on a rabbit jugular venous thrombosis model (31), in which aPTT of at least 1.5 times control (corresponding to an anti-Xa level of 0.2 U/mL) prevented thrombus extension.

Activiated PTT determination is usually made in a central laboratory on citrated plasma, using one of several commercially available instruments and one of many reagents, each with a different range of control values and a different aPTT-heparin level sensitivity relationship. Using a central laboratory involves a series of events, including venipuncture, transport to the lab, centrifugation, batching, testing, and communication of results back to the care provider. Not surprisingly, therefore, there is often a substantial delay in providing aPTT results to the care provider. In fact, this delay is typically approximately 2 hours. In 1992, data were collected on 60 aPTT samples ordered "STAT" that showed a 45-min delay from the time of blood draw to receipt of the sample in the laboratory and an additional 80 minutes until the results were available to the clinician (unpublished data) (Fig. 2). Data collected on 272 aPTT determinations in the cardiac care unit at the University of Massachusetts showed a mean time of 2 hours 6 min (32), with 36 min from sample acquisition until arrival in the laboratory. A survey of 79 hospitals that participated in the GUSTO I trial and collected data on timing on 387 aPTTs showed the mean time from blood draw until the aPTT was available to be 1 hour 46 min (33). Because patients with acute coronary

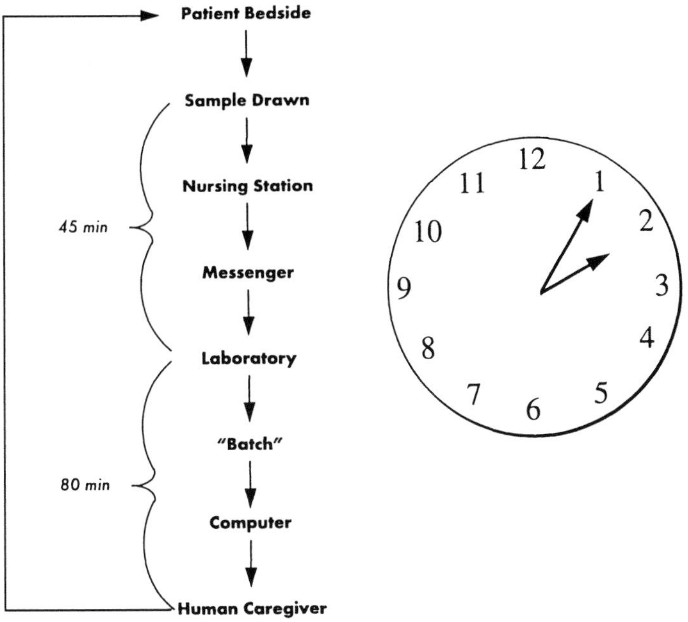

Figure 2 Delays in obtaining the aPTT by standard laboratory methods. Data are derived from 60 "STAT" samples from the Duke Cardiac Care Unit in 1992.

syndromes are at risk for both life-threatening thrombosis and serious hemorrhage, and the balance of the risk may change minute by minute, any unnecessary delay in obtaining a standard central laboratory aPTT could compromise optimal patient care.

In addition to the delay, aPTTs obtained from a central laboratory are subject to both artifact related to the sampling technique and handling, and considerable variability among different laboratory reagents and laboratories. Sources of sampling artifact include a difficult or poor venipuncture, collection of insufficient blood, delay between sampling and measurement of results, and incomplete centrifugation (34–36). Therefore, even in a laboratory with controlled conditions in which the aPTT is precise, accurate, and reproducible (low coefficient of variation), the aPTT may poorly reflect the level of anticoagulation in the patient due to variations related to events prior to the sample actually being tested (37). Moreover, there is substantial variability among different laboratories, related to differences between reagent-instrument combinations (38), different reagents (39), and even among different batches of the same reagent (40). In one study (39), seven commercially available reagents were tested, and the average amount of heparin required to double the baseline aPTT varied by twofold. In spite of efforts to do so, the hematology and laboratory societies have been unable to institute a standard aPTT measure (41), analogous to the International Normalized Ratio for the prothrombin time. Brill-Edwards and colleagues studied five different reagents and found that the aPTT ratio corresponding to a heparin level of 0.2 U/mL by protamine titration varied from 1.8 to 4.2 (42). Based on these results, many hospitals have established a target aPTT range based on a target heparin level of 0.2 to 0.4 U/mL by protamine titration or 0.3 to 0.7 U/mL by anti-Xa activity. Unfortunately, many hospitals have performed this range-finding by adding known amounts of heparin in vitro to a plasma pool, which can systematically underestimate the aPTT range needed in vivo (42).

The limitations to current standard methods of heparin monitoring are substantial. In addition to the typically long delay in obtaining the laboratory values, there is a substantial lack of consistency in the relationship of aPTT to heparin level between different labs and between different time periods in the same lab, and there is a lack of data to indicate whether aPTT, heparin level, or some other guide to adjusting dose is associated with the best patient outcomes. These issues are also present for assays of low-molecular-weight heparins which primarily assay the anti-Xa effect.

BEDSIDE "POINT OF CARE" TESTING

Technologies that enable rapid determination of laboratory values at the patient bedside—so called point-of-care testing—have required health care providers to decide when these methods provide an overall advantage in patient care and when they should therefore supplant traditional central laboratory testing. Typically, there is a trade-off when using point-of-care testing of less accuracy, less quality control, and higher cost per sample for more rapid and convenient determination of the result (Table 2). When time and convenience are more important than a high degree of accuracy—for example, with routine blood glucose monitoring in diabetics—point-of-care testing has been widely adopted. There has been a general trend towards the use of more point-of-care testing, although both regulatory requirements of the Clinical Laboratory Improvement Amendments of 1988 (43) and concern in the pathology community that loss of quality control may result in decreased quality of care (44) have limited the spread of bedside testing. Point-of-care testing raises logistic issues of training more individuals in the use of the chosen system, developing means of quality control, incorporating results into patient records and hospital information systems, and tracking use for billing purposes.

Table 2 Advantages and Disadvantages of Bedside "Point-of-Care" Testing

Advantages	Disadvantages
Rapid determination of results	Generally less accurate and reproducible
More convenient	Generally more costly per sample
Less nursing time in awaiting and retrieving results	More difficult to quality control
	More difficult to bill for
	Requires training more personnel
	More difficult to archive and integrate results into hospital information systems

Monitoring anticoagulation in patients with acute coronary syndromes has created controversy regarding point-of-care testing, with clinicians generally favoring institution of bedside testing (45) and laboratory-based physicians resisting (46). There is general consensus that studies evaluating outcome according to different approaches toward laboratory testing are needed, although few such data exist (44).

Activated Partial Thromboplastin Time (aPTT)

There are three commercially available bedside aPTT monitors in the United States designed for use in critical care settings (Table 3). Each has the advantage of rapid determination of the aPTT (typically within 3 min of application of the blood sample), use of small quantities of whole blood, and consistency in measurement among samples regardless of batch of reagent or institution of use. Each correlates reasonably well with standard laboratory testing, with correlation coefficients in the 0.80 range. Typical of whole-blood point-of-care testing, these devices have higher coefficients of variation than standard laboratory aPTT tests (5% to 10% vs. <2% to 3%, respectively). The incremental cost of a cartridge to perform a bedside test is generally \$3 to \$7, as opposed to <\$0.50 for the reagents to perform the traditional central laboratory test.

CoaguChek Plus

The CoaguChek Plus System (Roche Diagnostics and Boehringer-Mannheim Diagnostics) is a portable hand-held instrument that determines the aPTT based on the standard approach of using a phospholipid and an activator of the intrinsic system. It uses a single drop of whole blood (47) that can be obtained from a fingerstick puncture or venipuncture and is placed onto a disposable cartridge. The clotting time of blood is determined by sensing the cessation of blood flow through a capillary channel by detecting a change

Table 3 Devices Designed for Critical Care Use for Bedside Determination of aPTT

	Instrument		
	CoaguChek Plus	Hemochron Jr.	Thrombolytic assessment system
Manufacturer	Roche Diagnostics	International Technidyne Corp.	Cardiovascular Diagnostics, Inc.
Blood sample	Fresh whole blood	Whole blood or citrated plasma	Citrated whole blood or plasma
Sample volume	1 drop	1 drop	1 drop
Time to result	Minutes	Minutes	Minutes
Setting of clot formation	Capillary flow of unclotted blood	Forced movement of unclotted blood through a narrow channel	Chamber with magnetic particles with oscillating electric field
Clot detection method	Laser photometry	Optical light transmission	Optical light transmission
Correlation with standard lab	r = .78–.89 (42,49)	r = .87	r = .84 (46)
Therapeutic[a] aPTT range	60–85 sec (GUSTO III)	50–70 sec (PARAGON)	Customized to each hospital's standard aPTT range
Use in clinical trial of acute coronary syndromes	GUSTO-I, TIMI-5	PARAGON	None
Use associated with better achievement of target aPTT	Yes (GUSTO I, 23)	Unknown	Unknown
Use associated with improved clinical outcomes	Yes	Unknown	Unknown
Randomized evidence of clinical outcome advantage	No	No	No

[a]Corresponding to heparin level of 0.2–0.4 U/mL.

in light scatter from red blood cells measured by laser photometry. The time from reagent contact until clotting is approximately 3 min in anticoagulated patients and is mathematically converted to an aPTT, based on a conversion factor determined by studying a large number of normal and anticoagulated subjects.

Ansell reported that the correlation of the bedside monitor with a standard laboratory measurement was 0.79 to 0.83 in 319 subjects, similar to the correlation of 0.79 the investigators found when these patient samples were tested between two different standard laboratory reagents (47). The same group tested an additional 60 patients, including patients following thrombolytic therapy, and found similar results (32). Other groups have reported correlation coefficients of 0.89 in 100 patients undergoing coronary angioplasty (48) and 0.89 in a general population of heparinized patients (49). Data from the Duke University Cardiac Care Unit (unpublished data) demonstrate a correlation coefficient of 0.86 comparing the bedside monitor with the standard laboratory reagent in 66 patients, with the aPTT by the bedside monitor approximately 5 sec longer than the central laboratory for the same sample.

Hemochron Jr.

The Hemochron Jr. (International Technidyne Corporation) is similar to the CoaguChek Plus monitor in that it is a portable hand-held instrument that uses a disposable "cuvette" on which a drop of fresh whole blood is placed. Blood comes into contact with a kaolin and platelet factor substitute reagent to induce clotting. The unclotted blood is mechanically moved back and forth through a narrow channel, and clotting is detected as cessation of flow by a change in light transmission. An aPTT is calculated based on a conversion factor. The correlation coefficient between the Hemochron Jr. and standard laboratory aPTT measurement was 0.87 when simultaneous testing was performed on 492 samples at the Cleveland Clinic Foundation (unpublished data). In that series, the aPTT obtained with the Hemochron Jr. was 5 to 10 sec lower than the aPTT on the same patients from the central laboratory. Based on these data, a reasonable target range for aPTT with the Hemochron Jr. (and the one chosen for the PARAGON trial) is 50 to 70 sec.

Thrombolytic Assessment System

The Thrombolytic Assessment System (TAS) (Cardiovascular Diagnostics, Inc.) employs a technology which uses paramagnetic iron oxide particles that move in fluid uncoagulated blood in response to an oscillating magnetic field (50). Unlike the CoaguChek Plus and the Hemochron Jr., the TAS uses either citrated blood or plasma rather than fresh whole blood. Samples are typically run at a central location on a patient care unit and can be run several minutes after being obtained because the samples are citrated.

Studies of an earlier device using this technology showed a good correlation with standard laboratory methods, even in the hours following thrombolytic therapy (51), with a correlation coefficient in the 0.90 range. In a population of heparinized patients with acute coronary syndromes, correlation of the TAS with the standard lab using MDA Platelin L-Ca_2Cl reagent was 0.84 (46).

The aPTT target range can be customized to the hospital where the device is used by varying the conversion factor so that the target range for the TAS is identical to the target range for the hospital laboratory.

RATIONALE FOR USING ACT TO MEASURE HEPARIN EFFECT DURING CORONARY INTERVENTIONS

Since the early use of percutaneous coronary intervention (PCI), high-dose intravenous heparin has been used to prevent thrombosis related to both transient obstruction of coronary flow and endothelial disruption. Similar to cardiopulmonary bypass surgery, the doses and levels of heparin used during coronary intervention are above the level at which the heparin-aPTT response curve allows discrimination, and therefore the activated clotting time (ACT) has become the standard monitoring test. Because rapid turnaround time is essential to document the degree of anticoagulation and proceed expeditiously with the procedure, the ACT has evolved as a test used locally in the catheterization laboratory. Two common devices are used to measure ACT, the Hemochron and the HemoTec, both of which use whole blood and provide results within minutes. The two tests vary substantially, with the ACT from the Hemochron being approximately 50 sec longer than the HemoTec (52).

Although there are no randomized studies of different levels of heparin during PCI, a number of observational studies have found that the degree of heparin effect as measured by the ACT during the procedure is associated with risk of thrombotic complications (53–56), and all showed that lower ACTs are associated with greater risk of complications. One study compared 103 patients who died or had emergency bypass surgery with 400 uncomplicated patients, and found that the ACT, measured with the HemoTec device, was 60 to 80 sec lower among patients with complications (54). Another study compared 63 patients with abrupt closure to 124 controls matched for other predictors of abrupt closure. The median ACT, measured with the Hemochron device, was 30 to 40 sec shorter among patients with abrupt closure, and abrupt closure risk was twice as high with an ACT of 300 compared to 400 (55).

These two studies have led to the recommendation that heparin be titrated to an ACT of at least 300 (HemoTec) to 350 (Hemochron) sec before angioplasty (57). One study suggests that with the direct thrombin inhibitor bivalirudin, the relationship between ACT and abrupt vessel closure may be blunted, and ACT monitoring may not be necessary (56). When administered with abciximab, however, the reduction in bleeding without loss of efficacy in the EPILOG (19) compared to the EPIC trial (58) has led to the recommendation to use the less aggressive heparin regimen of ≤70 U/kg with an ACT of at least 200 sec (19,59). Moreover, in the presence of abciximab, the relationship of heparin dose and ACT is altered, such that after adjusting for patient weight, the ACT is prolonged by 35 sec on average by abciximab (60). As low-molecular-weight heparins have become utilized in hospitalized patients with acute coronary syndromes, more are presenting to the catheterization laboratory on such therapy. Several trials are assessing the safety, efficacy, and extent of anticoagulation patients undergoing PCI with low-molecular-weight heparins.

EXPERIENCE WITH BEDSIDE aPTT MONITORING IN CLINICAL TRIALS OF ACS

CoaguChek Plus

In the 41,000-patient GUSTO I trial evaluating thrombolytic strategies for acute myocardial infarction, a prospective observational study was planned to evaluate patient outcomes according to the method of monitoring anticoagulation. Each participating investigator was given the option of using the CoaguChek Plus bedside anticoagulation monitor. A nomogram was used to guide heparin adjustment for the trial, and a specialized nomogram was provided for use with the CoauguChek Plus monitor. This nomogram was developed using heparinized patients to generate a heparin-aPTT response curve, and the target range of 65 to 90 sec was chosen to correspond to a heparin level of 0.2 to 0.4 U/mL based on protamine titration. This target range corresponds to similar heparin levels as a range of approximately 60 to 85 sec for a standard aPTT reagent such as Dade Actin FS.

Of the 28,172 patients treated with intravenous heparin who had at least one aPTT determined, 1713 had all aPTT measurements by the CoaguChek Plus monitor (61). Patients having aPTTs monitored by the CoaguChek Plus (then called the Ciba-Corning M512 monitor) were enrolled in all 14 countries participating in the GUSTO I trial, with the greatest representation from Australia, Belgium, and the United States. Baseline characteristics were similar between the patients undergoing bedside monitoring versus central laboratory monitoring. The median aPTT at 24 hours was 11 sec higher among patients monitored with the bedside device, in spite of similar final heparin infusion. More patients were in the target aPTT range at 24 hours when the bedside monitor was used (26% vs. 22%). Taking into account the lower median body weight of patients being monitored with the bedside monitor, this suggests that in the 60-sec range, the same patient had a 5- to 10-sec higher aPTT using the CoaguChek Plus bedside monitor. This had been anticipated and adjusted for by having a higher aPTT range for the bedside monitor. Patients monitored with the bedside device had lower rates of bleeding, less of a drop from baseline to nadir hematocrit, less need for transfusion, and a tendency toward slightly higher reinfarction rate (Table 4). Mortality tended to be lower among the patients with bedside aPTT monitoring, both before and after adjustment for baseline differences in the populations. These data support the concept that bedside aPTT monitoring can provide a standardized, safe, and effective approach toward anticoagulation.

The CoaguChek Plus monitor was exclusively used to measure aPTTs in the 246-patient TIMI-5 pilot study, conducted at 16 United States hospitals, comparing heparin and hirudin in conjunction with accelerated t-PA (62). For the 84 patients randomized to heparin, the initial heparin dose was a 5000-unit bolus, with 1000 U/hr infusion, with a target aPTT range of 60 to 90 sec. At 24 hours, the median aPTT was 63 sec (25th to 75th percentile,

Table 4 Clinical Events by Monitoring Equipment in the GUSTO I Trial (61)

Event	CoaguChek aPTT (n = 1713)	Standard aPTT (n = 26,459)	*P*
Mortality			
30 Days (unadjusted)	4.3%	4.8%	.33
30 Days (adjusted[a])	4.3%	4.8%	.27
1 Year	7.1%	7.7%	.38
Reinfarction	4.9%	4.1%	.14
Bleeding			
Moderate	9.6%	11.8%	.01
Severe	0.7%	1.2%	.07
Moderate or severe	10.4%	13.0%	.001
RBC transfusion	7%	11%	<.001
Drop in hematocrit (%)	5.5 ± 5.2	6.7 ± 5.8	<.001
Stroke			
Hemorrhagic	0.7%	0.7%	.80
Overall	1.3%	1.4%	.71

[a]Adjusted for important baseline predictors of mortality following acute myocardial infarction.

48 to 75 sec), an achievement of target aPTTs at least as good as historical controls using standard methods (Table 5). Bleeding rates were high, although all patients underwent early angiography as part of the protocol. This study reinforces that the bedside monitor can be used in practice to effectively adjust heparin.

There has been one multicenter randomized trial testing different heparin dosing and monitoring strategies to determine effectiveness of achieving and maintaining target aPTT. A total of 113 patients with venous or arterial thrombotic disease were randomized in a factorial fashion to weight-adjusted versus non-weight-adjusted dose heparin and to point-of-care versus standard laboratory aPTT monitoring (23). Point-of-care testing with the CoaguChek Plus instrument reduced both the time from sample acquisition to adjustment of heparin dose (0.4 vs. 1.6 hours, $P < .0001$) and the time to reach therapeutic aPTT level (16.1 to 19.4 hours, $P = .24$). The mean proportion of time in the therapeutic range did not differ between the groups.

Hemochron Jr.

The PARAGON trial (63) randomized 2282 patients with unstable angina in 21countries in a blinded fashion to the intravenous glycoprotein IIb/IIIa receptor blocker lamifiban, with and without intravenous heparin, or placebo with intravenous heparin. APTT monitoring and heparin adjustment were achieved using both the Hemochron Jr. bedside aPTT monitor and a blinded, computerized system of using the aPTT results to determine heparin adjustment. Investigators ran the aPTT on the monitor, were given an encrypted code of the results, and entered the results into a computer via an automated telephone system, which in turn gave the investigator instructions on heparin (or placebo) adjustment. The target aPTT range was 50 to 70 sec. The median aPTT of the 758 patients randomized to the heparin control group was 62 sec (25th to 75th percentile, 48 to 78 sec) at 6 hours, and 50 sec (25th to 75th percentile, 40 to 63 sec) at 24 hours (64), ranges that compared favorably with standard care approaches of heparin adjustment (Table 5). Bleeding rates in the heparin control arm were likewise favorable compared with historical controls, at 5.5%.

The PARAGON experience shows that a bedside monitor, used with an automated blinded system of heparin adjustment, can achieve consistent therapeutic aPTT levels and low bleeding rates.

FUTURE OF BEDSIDE ANTICOAGULATION TESTING

It has been well established that antithrombotic therapy for the acute phase of coronary syndromes has potential for substantial benefit in preventing

Table 5 Target and Achieved aPTT Ranges According to Monitoring Method in Clinical Trials of ACS Among Patients Treated with IV Heparin

	GUSTO I, Central laboratory	GUSTO I, CoaguChek Plus	TIMI-5, CoaguChek Plus	GUSTO II, Central laboratory	PARAGON, Hemochron Jr.
n	25,766	1713	84	2868	758
Patient population	ST elevation, thrombolytic treated	ST elevation, thrombolytic treated	ST elevation, thrombolytic treated	Unstable angina/ non-Q-wave MI	Unstable angina/ non-Q-wave MI
Nomogram	Yes	Yes	Yes	Yes	Computer automated
Target aPTT	60–85 sec	65–90 sec	60–90 sec	60–85 sec	50–70 sec
Actual aPTT at 24 h	62 (47, 88)	71 (52, 103)	63 (48, 75)	61 (50, 75)	50 (40, 63)
Moderate or severe bleeding	13.0%	10.4%	23%[a]	8.4%	5.5%

[a]All patients underwent early angiography.

thrombotic complications while at the same time predisposing to serious hemorrhage. The concept that sophisticated, precise, and rapid monitoring of the effects of anticoagulants will be critical to optimize the benefit/risk ratio is the basis for the need for bedside anticoagulation testing. Although both observational and small randomized studies have suggested that bedside testing is associated with improved outcome, until more definitive outcome studies are performed to show that the additional cost, loss of precision, and challenge of quality control are warranted, it will be difficult to change practice so that bedside testing becomes the dominant strategy.

Beyond the relatively crude approach of using unfractionated heparin and even low-molecular-weight heparins to inhibit primarily thrombin and Factor Xa, development of specific inhibitors of the various factors in the coagulation cascade may provide the opportunity to use various combinations of inhibitors to achieve the optimal level of anticoagulation for a particular patient. Point-of-care systems are currently being developed to test both low-molecular-weight heparins and direct thrombin inhibitors. Beyond this advance, to develop and then to treat patients with combinations, however, insight will be needed into the effect of each agent on its target, and obtaining results rapidly would likely be important to be able to adjust doses to achieve optimal results during the acute phase. Data are beginning to emerge that link peptide markers of coagulation factor activity with patient outcomes (65–67), raising the possibility that monitoring of specific coagulation factor activity may be relevant. As new antithrombotic approaches are developed, establishing the optimal methods of dosing and monitoring, including at the patient's bedside, may be as important as which agents are used (68).

REFERENCES

1. Passamani E, Hodges M, Herman M, Grose R, Chaitman B, Rogers W, Forman S, Terrin M, Knatterud G, Robertson T, Braunwald E, for the TIMI Investigators. The Thrombolysis in Myocardial Infarction (TIMI) Phase II pilot study: tissue plasminogen activator followed by percutaneous transluminal coronary angioplasty. J Am Coll Cardiol 1987;10(suppl B):51B–64B.
2. Neuhaus KL, Feuerer W, Jeep-Tebbe S, Niederer W, Vogt A, Tebbe U. Improved thrombolysis with a modified dose regimen of recombinant tissue-type plasminogen activator. J Am Coll Cardiol 1989;14:1566–1569.
3. Arnout J, Simoons M, de Bono D, Rapold HJ, Collen D, Verstraete M. Correlation between level of heparinization and patency of the infarct-related coronary artery after treatment of acute myocardial infarction with alteplase (rt-PA). J Am Coll Cardiol 1992;20:513–519.
4. Bovill EG, Terrin ML, Stump DC, Berke AD, Frederick M, Collen D, Feit F, Gore JM, Hillis D, Lambrew CT, Leiboff R, Mann KG, Markis JE, Pratt CM,

Sharkey SW, Sopko G, Tracy RP, Chesebro JH, for the TIMI Investigators. Hemorrhagic events during therapy with recombinant tissue-type plasminogen activator, heparin, and aspirin for acute myocardial infarction. Results of the Thrombolysis in Myocardial Infarction (TIMI), Phase II trial. Ann Intern Med 1991;115:256–265.

5. Hsia J, Kleiman NS, Aguirre FV, Chaitman BR, Roberts R, Ross AM. Heparin-induced prolongation of partial thromboplastin time after thrombolysis: relation to coronary artery patency. J Am Coll Cardiol 1992;20:31–35.
6. Antman EM, for the TIMI 9A Investigators. Hirudin in acute myocardial infarction. Safety report from the thrombolysis and thrombin inhibition in myocardial infarction trial (TIMI) 9A trial. Circulation 1994;90:1624–1630.
7. Granger CB, Hirsh J, Califf RM, Woodlief LH, Bovill E, White HD, Topol EJ, for the GUSTO Trial Investigators. Activated partial thromboplastin time and outcome after thrombolytic therapy for acute myocardial infarction: results from the GUSTO Trial. Circulation 1996;93:870–888.
8. Gore JM, Granger CB, Sloan MA, Van de Werf F, Weaver WD, Califf RM, White HD, Barbash GI, Simoons ML, Aylward PE, Topol EJ, for the GUSTO Investigators. Stroke after thrombolysis: mortality and functional outcomes in the GUSTO-I Trial. Circulation 1995;92:2811–2818.
9. Berkowitz SD, Granger CB, Pieper KS, Lee KL, Gore JM, Simoons M, Armstrong PW, Topol EJ, Califf RM, for the GUSTO I Investigators. Incidence and predictors of bleeding following contemporary thrombolytic therapy for myocardial infarction. Circulation 1997;95(11):2508–2516.
10. GUSTO IIa Investigators. Randomized trial of intravenous heparin versus recombinant hirudin for acute coronary syndromes. Circulation 1994;90:1631–1637.
11. GUSTO IIb Investigators. A comparison of recombinant hirudin with heparin for the treatment of acute coronary syndromes. N Engl J Med 1996;335:775–782.
12. Antman EM. Hirudin in acute myocardial infarction. Thrombolysis and Thrombin Inhibition in Myocardial Infarction (TIMI) 9B trial. Circulation 1996;94:911–921.
13. Giugliano RP, Cutler SS, Llevodot J. Risk of intracranial hemorrhage with accelerated tPA: importance of the heparin dose. Circulation 1999;100:I-650. Abstract.
14. Hochman JS, Wali AU, Gavrila D, Sim MJ, Malhotra S, Palazzo AM, De La Fuente B. A new regimen for heparin use in acute coronary syndromes. Am Heart J 1999;138:313–318.
15. Ryan TJ, Antman EM, Brooks NH, Califf RM, Hillis LD, Hiratzka LF, Rapaport E, Riegel B, Russell RO, Smith EE, Weaver WD. 1999 update: ACC/AHA guidelines for the management of acute myocardial infarction: a report of the American College of Cardiology/American Heart Association Task Force on Practice Guidelines (Committee on Management of Acute Myocardial Infarction). J Am Coll Cardiol 1999;34:890–911.
16. Oler A, Whooley MA, Oler J, Grady D. Adding heparin to aspirin reduces the

incidence of myocardial infarction and death in patients with unstable angina. A meta-analysis. JAMA 1996;276:811–815.

17. Becker RC, Cannon CP, Tracy RP, Thompson B, Bovill EG, Desvigne-Nickens P, Randall AM, Knatternud G, Braunwald E. Relation between systemic anticoagulation as determined by activated partial thromboplastin time and heparin measurements and in-hospital clinical events in unstable angina and non-Q-wave myocardial infarction. Am Heart J 1996;131:421–423.
18. Granger CB, Califf RM, Van de Werf F, White HD, Topol EJ. Activated partial thromboplastin time and clinical outcome among patients with unstable angina or non-Q-wave MI treated with intravenous heparin. Circulation 1995;92 (suppl):I-416.
19. EPILOG Investigators. Platelet glycoprotein IIb/IIIa receptor blockade and low-dose heparin during percutaneous coronary revascularization. N Engl J Med 1997;336(24):1689–1696.
20. Cruickshank MK, Levine MN, Hirsh J, et al. A standard heparin nomogram for the management of heparin therapy. Arch Intern Med 1991;151:333–337.
21. Flaker G, Bartolozzi J, Davis V, McCabe C, Cannon C, for the TIMI 4 Investigators. Use of a standardized heparin nomogram to achieve therapeutic anticoagulation after thrombolytic therapy in myocardial infarction. Arch Intern Med 1994;154:1492–1496.
22. Raschke RA, Reilly BM, Guidry JR, Fontana JR, Srinivas S. The weight-based heparin dosing nomogram compared with a "standard care" nomogram. A randomized controlled trial. Ann Intern Med 1993;119:874–881.
23. Becker RC, Ball SP, Eisenberg P, Borzak S, Held AC, Spencer F, Voyce SJ, Jesse R, Hendel R, Ma Y, Hurley T, Hebert J. A randomized, multicenter trial of weight-adjusted intravenous heparin dose titration and point-of-care coagulation monitoring in hospitalized patients with active thromboembolic disease. Am Heart J 1999;137:59–71.
24. Patel VB, Moliterno DJ. Bedside activated partial thromboplastin time monitoring: just a matter of time? Am Heart J 1999;137:8–10. Editorial.
25. Ryan TJ. ACC/AHA guidelines for management of patients with acute myocardial infarction. J Am Coll Cardiol 1996;28:1328–1428.
26. Neuhaus KL, v. Essen R, Tebbe U, Jessel A, Heinrichs H, Maurer W, Doring W, Harmjanz D, Kotter V, Kalhammer E, Simon H, Horacek T. Safety observations from the pilot phase of the randomized r-Hirudin for Improvement of Thrombolysis (HIT-III) study. Circulation 1994;90:1638–1642.
27. Hirsh J, Raschke R, Warkentin TE, Dalen JE, Deykin D, Poller L. Heparin: mechanism of action, pharmacokinetics, dosing considerations, monitoring, efficacy, and safety. Fourth ACCP Consensus Conference on Antithrombotic Therapy. Chest 1995;108:258S–275S.
28. Cohen M, et al. A comparison of low-molecular-weight heparin with unfractionated heparin for unstable coronary artery disease. Efficacy and Safety of Subcutaneous Enoxaparin in Non-Q-Wave Coronary Events Study Group. N Engl J Med 1997;337:447–452.
29. Antman EM, McCabe CH, Gurfinkel EP, Turpie AG, Bernink PJ, Salein D, Bayes De Luna A, Fox K, Lablanche JM, Radley D, Premmereur J, Braunwald

E. Enoxaparin prevents death and cardiac ischemic events in unstable angina/non-Q-wave myocardial infarction. Results of the thrombolysis in myocardial infarction (TIMI) 11B trial. Circulation 1999;100:1593–1601.

30. Thrombolysis in Myocardial Infarction (TIMI) 11A Trial Investigators. Dose-ranging trial of enoxaparin for unstable angina: results of TIMI 11A. J Am Coll Cardiol 1997;29:1474–1482.
31. Chiu HM, Hirsh J, Yung WL, Regoeczi E, Gent M. Relationship between the anticoagulant and antithrombotic effects of heparin in experimental venous thrombosis. Blood 1977;49:171–184.
32. Becker RC, Cyr J, Corrao JM, Ball SP. Bedside coagulation monitoring in heparin-treated patients with active thromboembolic disease: a coronary care unit experience. Am Heart J 1994;128:719–723.
33. GUSTO Gazette, July/August, 1992, p. 2.
34. Peterson P, Gottfried EL. The effects of inaccurate blood sample volume on prothrombin (PT) and activated partial thromboplastin time (APTT). Thromb Haemost 1982;47:101–103.
35. Thomson JM. Pre-test variables in blood coagulation testing. In: Thomson JM, ed. Blood Coagulation and Hemostasis, A Practical Guide. New York, NY: Churchill Livingstone; 1985:340–369.
36. Brandt JT, Triplett DA. Laboratory monitoring of heparin. Effects of reagents and instruments on the activated partial thromboplastin time. Am J Clin Pathol 1981;76:530–537.
37. Watts N. Reproducibility (precision) in alternate site testing. A clinician's perspective. Arch Pathol Lab Med 1995;119:914–917.
38. D'Angelo A, Seveso MP, D'Angelo SV, et al. Effect of clot-detection methods and reagents on activated partial thromboplastin time (APTT): implications in heparin monitoring by APTT. Am J Clin Pathol 1990;94:297–306.
39. Bjornsson TD, Nash PV. Variability in heparin sensitivity of aPTT reagents. Am J Clin Pathol 1986;86:199–204.
40. Shojania AM, Tetreault J, Turnbull G. The variations between heparin sensitivity of different lots of activated partial thromboplastin time reagent produced by the same manufacturer. Am J Clin Pathol 1988;89:19–23.
41. Poller L, Thomson JM, Taberner DA. Use of the activated partial thromboplastin time for monitoring heparin therapy: problems and possible solutions. Res Clin Lab 1989;19:363–370.
42. Brill-Edwards P, Ginsberg JS, Johnston M, Hirsh J. Establishing a therapeutic range for heparin therapy. Ann Intern Med 1993;119:104–109.
43. Ehrmeyer SS. Laessig RH. Regulatory requirements (CLIA '88, JCAHO, CAP) for decentralized testing. Am J Clin Pathol 1995;104(4 suppl 1):S40–S49.
44. Howanitz PJ. College of American Pathologists Conference XXVIII on alternate site testing. What must we now do? Arch Pathol Lab Med 1995;119:979–983.
45. Becker RC. Exploring the medical need for alternate site testing. A clinician's perspective. Arch Pathol Lab Med 1995;119:894–897.
46. Macik BG. Designing a point-of-care program for coagulation testing. Arch Pathol Lab Med 1995;119:929–938.

47. Ansell J, Tiarks C, Hirsh J, McGehee W, Adler D, Weibert R. Measurement of the activated partial thromboplastin time from a capillary (fingerstick) sample of whole blood. A new method for monitoring heparin therapy. Am J Clin Pathol 1991;95:222–227.
48. Reiner JS, Coyne KS, Lundergan CF, Ross AM. Bedside monitoring of heparin therapy: comparison of activated clotting time to activated partial thromboplastin time. Cathet Cardiovasc Diagn 1994;32:49–52
49. Ruzicka K, Kapiotis S, Quehenberger P, Handler S, Hornykewycz S, Michitsch A, Huber K, Clemens D, Susan M, Pabinger I, Eichinger S, Jilma B, Speiser W. Evaluation of bedside prothrombin time and activated partial thromboplastin time measurement by coagulation analyzer CoaguCheck plus in various clinical settings. Thromb Res 1997;87:431–440.
50. Oberhardt BJ, Drmott SC, Taylor M, Alkadi ZY, Abruzzini AF, Gresalfi NJ. Dry reagent technology for rapid, convenient measurements of blood coagulation and fibrinolysis. Clin Chem 1991;37:520–526.
51. Sane DC, Gresalfi NJ, Enney-O'Mara LA, Califf RM, Greenberg CS, Bovill EG, Oberhardt BJ. Exploration of rapid bedside monitoring of coagulation and fibrinolysis parameters during thrombolytic therapy. Blood Coagul Fibrinolysis 1992;3:47–54.
52. Avendano A, Ferguson JJ. Comparison of Hemochron and HemoTec activated coagulation time target values during percutaneous transluminal coronary angioplasty. J Am Coll Cardiol 1994;23:907–910.
53. McGarry TF Jr, Gottlieb RS, Morganroth J, Zelenkofske SL, Kasparian H, Duca PR, Lester RM, Kreulen TH. The relationship of anticoagulation level and complications after successful percutaneous transluminal coronary angioplasty. Am Heart J 1992;23:1445–1451.
54. Ferguson JJ, Dougherty KG, Gaos CM, Bush HS, Marsh KC, Leachman DR. Relation between procedural activated coagulation time and outcome after percutaneous transluminal coronary angioplasty. J Am Coll Caridol 1994;23: 1061–1065.
55. Narins CR, Hillegass WB Jr, Nelson CL, Tcheng JE, Harrington RA, Phillips HR, Stack RS, Califf RM. Relation between activated clotting time during angioplasty and abrupt closure. Circulation 1996;93:667–671.
56. Bittl JA, Ahmed WH. Relation between abrupt vessel closure and the anticoagulant response to heparin or bivalirudin during coronary angioplasty. Am J Cardiol 1998;82:50P–56P.
57. Popma JJ, Coller BS, Ohman EM, Bittle JA, Weitz J, Kuntz RE, Leon MB. Antithrombotic therapy in patients undergoing coronary angioplasty. Chest 1995;108(suppl):486S–501S.
58. EPIC Investigators. Use of a monoclonal antibody directed against the platelet glycoprotein IIb/IIIa receptor in high-risk coronary angioplasty. N Engl J Med 1994;330:956–961.
59. Lincoff AM, Tcheng JE, Califf RM, Bass T, Popma JJ, Teirstein PS, Kleiman NS, Hattel LJ, Anderson HV, Ferguson JJ, Cabot CF, Anderson KM, Berdan LG, Musco MH, Weisman HF, Topol EJ. Standard versus low-dose weight-adjusted heparin in patients treated with the platelet glycoprotein IIb/IIIa re-

ceptor antibody fragment abciximab (c7E3 Fab) during percutaneous coronary revascularization. Am J Cardiol 1997;79:286–291.
60. Moliterno DJ, Califf RM, Aguirre FV, Anderson K, Sigmon KN, Weisman HF, Topol EJ. Effect of platelet glycoprotein IIb/IIIa integrin blockade on activated clotting time during percutaneous transluminal coronary angioplasty or directional atherectomy (the EPIC trial). Evaluation of c7E3 Fab in the Prevention of Ischemic Complications trial. Am J Cardiol 1995;75:559–562.
61. Zabel KM, Granger CB, Bovill R, Hirsh J, Topol EJ, Califf RM, for the GUSTO Investigators. The use of a bedside activated partial thromboplastin time (aPTT) monitor to adjust level of anticoagulation following thrombolysis in a large, multinational trial of acute myocardial infarction. Am Heart J 1998;136:868–876.
62. Cannon CP, McCabe CH, Henry TD, Schweiger MJ, Gibson RS, Mueller HS, Becker RC, Kleiman NS, Haugland JM, Anderson JL, Sharaf BL, Edwards SJ, Rogers WJ, Williams DO, Braunwald E, for the TIMI 5 Investigators. A pilot trial of recombinant desulfatohirudin compared with heparin in conjunction with tissue-type plasminogen activator and aspirin for acute myocardial infarction: results of the Thrombolysis in Myocardial Infarction (TIMI) 5 trial. J Am Coll Cardiol 1994;23:993–1003.
63. PARAGON Investigators. A randomized trial of potent platelet IIb/IIIa antagonism, heparin, or both in patients with unstable angina: the PARAGON study. Circulation 1996;94(suppl I):I-553.
64. Newby KL, Harrington RA, Bhapkar M, Granger CB, van de Werf F, Keech A, Rames A, Moliterno D. Tight control of aPTT in acute coronary syndrome patients using an automated strategy for bedside heparin adjustment: results for the PARAGON A trial. Circulation 1997;96(suppl):I-748.
65. Scharfstein JS, Abendschein DR, Eisenberg PR, George D, Cannon CP, Becker RC, Sobel B, Cupples LA, Braunwald E, Loscalzo J. Usefulness of fibrinogenolytic and procoagulant markers during thrombolytic therapy in predicting clinical outcomes in acute myocardial infarction. TIMI-5 Investigators. Thrombolysis in Myocardial Infarction. Am J Cardiol 1996;78:503–510.
66. Granger CB, Becker R, Tracy RP, Califf RM, Topol EJ, Pieper K, Ross AM, Roth S, Lambrew C, Bovill EG, for the GUSTO-I Hemostasis Substudy Group. Thrombin generation, inhibition and clinical outcomes in patients with acute myocardial infarction treated with thrombolytic therapy and heparin: results from the GUSTO-I trial. J Am Coll Cardiol 1998;31:497–505.
67. Ardissino D, Merlini PA, Eisenberg PR, Kottke-Marchant K, Crenshaw BS, Granger CB. Coagulation markers and outcomes in acute coronary syndromes. Am Heart J 1998;136(4)(suppl part 2):S7–S18.
68. Patel VB, Moliterno DJ. Bedside activated partial thromboplastin time monitoring: just a matter of time? Am Heart J 1999;137:8–11.

21

Bedside Platelet Monitoring

Debabrata Mukherjee and David J. Moliterno
The Cleveland Clinic Foundation
Cleveland, Ohio

INTRODUCTION

Platelet function tests measure the capacity of platelets to adhere, activate, aggregate, and secrete. The goal of platelet function testing is to provide information about the platelet contributions to the risk of thrombotic or hemorrhagic events. Important clinical questions in acute coronary syndromes are whether an antiplatelet agent is having the desired effect on platelet inhibition (efficacy) and whether the patient has sufficient residual platelet function to avoid bleeding (safety). The role of aspirin and thienopyridines is well established in management of coronary artery disease and in the setting of coronary interventions. The last several years have demonstrated the unequivocal efficacy of intravenously administered platelet GPIIb/IIIa antagonists in the management of acute coronary syndromes (ACS) and in the setting of percutaneous interventions.

PLATELET GPIIb/IIIa INHIBITORS

Twenty-five years ago, an important insight into the molecular basis for platelet aggregation was provided by the discovery that two major membrane glycoprotein bands, GPII and GPIII, were missing from the surface of thrombasthenic platelets (1). To date, more than 60,000 patients with ischemic heart disease have been treated in clinical trials with a new class of potent and highly effective antiplatelet agents, specifically targeting this IIb/

IIIa receptor (2). Three such drugs have been licensed by the U.S. Food and Drug Administration, and many more GPIIb/IIIa antagonists are in Phase II and III trials for a potentially expanding series of clinical indications. Four parenterally administered GPIIb/IIIa antagonists (abciximab, eptifibatide, tirofiban, and lamifiban) have been tested for two different clinical indications, percutaneous coronary interventions and acute coronary syndromes. The trials show a drug class effect, with all agents reducing ischemic events.

Efficacy

The abciximab trials, most of which have been done in the setting of percutaneous coronary intervention, showed a drug-specific effect (i.e., there was a more pronounced reduction in the 30-day composite endpoint of death, nonfatal myocardial infarction, or urgent revascularization than that seen with the other GPIIb/IIIa antagonists). Three-year follow-up of the patients who entered the first trial (EPIC) with an acute coronary syndrome demonstrated a 60% decrease in mortality with an overall mortality reduction of 35% at the latest point of follow-up in abciximab trials (3). The most impressive effect of mortality reduction was reported in EPISTENT with a 58% reduction in 1-year mortality among stented patients treated with abciximab (4). Empiric treatment (i.e., not necessarily associated with PCI) with eptifibatide or tirofiban for unstable angina or non-Q-wave MI has been shown to reduce death or myocardial infarction by 10% to 35%, and the effects are persistent at 6 months (5,6). It remains unclear how much of the apparent difference in efficacy among the agents is related to the clinical setting or trial design or drug itself or the extent and duration of antiplatelet effect. It has been postulated that the protracted inhibition afforded by the antibody fragment or its binding to other integrins may explain the interagent differences in clinical outcome.

Safety

In the early trials, GPIIb/IIIa blockade was associated with a higher rate of bleeding complications (7,8). This was subsequently learned to be due to excessive and prolonged concurrent heparin administration and delayed sheath removal. Thus, later trials, which incorporated reduced weight-adjusted heparin regimens and earlier sheath removal, demonstrated no excess in major bleeding as compared with placebo (4–6,9,10). However, there remains an increase in minor bleeding with these agents, and it is conceivable that "optimal dosing" of the GPIIb/IIIa antagonist would further reduce bleeding complications. Previous studies have suggested that >80% of GPIIb/IIIa receptors must be occupied for the antagonist to block thrombus formation, and that receptor blockade >90% increases the risk of bleeding

(11). Likewise, the frequency of thrombocytopenia ($\leq$100,000 platelets/μL) is low with the intravenously used GPIIb/IIIa agents (~1%), but better titration of the dosage used may minimize this side effect.

In addition to abciximab (Reopro, c7E3), a number of low-molecular-weight GPIIb/IIIa antagonists patterned on the arginine-glycine-asparatic acid (RGD) recognition sequence have also shown benefit in the prevention and treatment of ischemic thrombotic coronary artery disease (12–15). Correlative studies of the antithrombotic effects of 7E3 compared with its effects on bleeding time, platelet aggregation, and GPIIb/IIIa receptor blockade were performed prior to clinical studies with abciximab (16–19). These studies provided information for dosing for the first Phase III study (EPIC) (7).

Similar preclinical studies have been reported with the other GPIIb/IIIa antagonists (20,21). The rapid off rates of the low-molecular-weight compounds as compared with abciximab made it technically more difficult to directly and accurately assess GPIIb/IIIa receptor blockade with these agents, but binding studies have been reported with fluorescent and radiolabeled compounds (22–25). The pharmacokinetics for the synthetic peptide and the nonpeptide GPIIb/IIIa antagonists differ from that of the monoclonal antibody. These small-molecule compounds are cleared renally, and dosage likely needs to be adjusted in patients with renal insufficiency.

Current Questions

The introduction of GPIIb/IIIa antagonists as therapeutic agents raises several important questions:

1. What is the interindividual variability in dose response (blockade of platelet aggregation) with the current weight-adjusted GPIIb/IIIa bolus?
2. Is variability in dose response associated with clinical (ischemic or bleeding) events?
3. Could patient-specific bolus dosing (beyond weight adjustment) improve efficacy or safety of therapy?
4. Is there inter- or intrapatient variability in platelet blockade over time (i.e., during the drug infusion period)?
5. Could monitoring and adjustment of the drug infusion improve outcome?
6. Are there differences among drugs in this class (antibody, peptides, nonpeptides) regarding predictability of response?
7. What is the optimal target to measure: plasma drug levels, number of IIb/IIIa receptors occupied, percentage of IIb/IIIa receptors blocked, or extent of aggregation inhibition?

8. What is the best agonist (collagen, ADP, TRAP) and at what concentration (1 μM, 10 μM, 20 μM) for the assay?
9. Would a functional assay (e.g., clot formation in whole blood) be more clinically relevant than a platelet-specific (platelet-rich plasma) assay?
10. Can an ideal assay be developed that is rapid, simple, accurate, and inexpensive?

PLATELET RECEPTOR AGONISTS

Platelet activation can be induced by a variety of chemical and mechanical methods that work through several distinct intracellular pathways (Fig. 1). Recognition of these pathways and the receptors and ligands is important in assessing platelet aggregation. Agonists are classified as weak or strong agonists with the strong agonists leading to platelet degranulation, exteriorization of GPIIb/IIIa receptors, and release of fibrinogen stored within the alpha granules. Several agonists are shown in Figure 1. Historically, adenosine diphosphate (ADP) has been the agonist most commonly used for turbidimetric aggregation studies. The aggregation response to ADP is concentration dependent. Aggregation in response to low concentrations of ADP (1 to 5 μM) is spontaneously reversible, whereas aggregation induced by higher concentration (10 to 20 μM) is not (26). Most physiological studies of congenital platelet defects have been performed using concentrations of

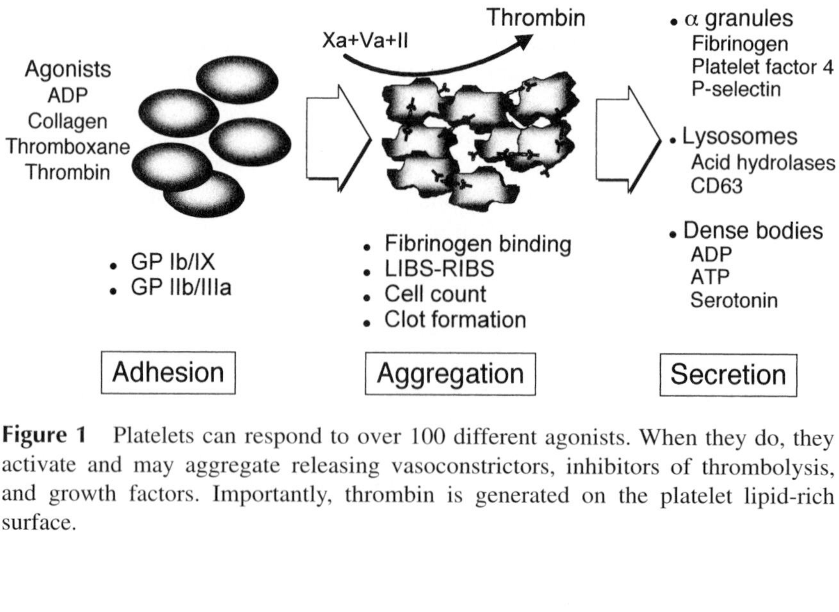

Figure 1 Platelets can respond to over 100 different agonists. When they do, they activate and may aggregate releasing vasoconstrictors, inhibitors of thrombolysis, and growth factors. Importantly, thrombin is generated on the platelet lipid-rich surface.

1 to 5 μM ADP or less (27–29). Studies of GPIIb/IIIa antagonists have required more intense stimulation of the platelets in order to discriminate among doses and have been conducted using concentrations of 10 to 20 μM (21,30–34).

The strength of collagen as an agonist also depends on the concentration used. The relevance of collagen as an agonist stems from the abundance of collagen in the subendothelium exposed at the time of arterial injury. Unlike ADP-induced aggregation, aggregation in response to collagen is sensitive to the effects of aspirin. The use of collagen as an agonist is limited by variability between production lots that occurs at the time of harvest. Arachidonic acid and thromboxane A_2 are weak platelet agonists that are completely inhibited by aspirin. Arachidonic acid-induced platelet aggregation is sometimes used to assess compliance with aspirin regimens.

Thrombin is the most potent platelet agonist and in addition to stimulating aggregation, it also stimulates platelet degranulation. The use of α-thrombin as a platelet agonist has been well accepted. However, thrombin-induced platelet aggregation has several limitations including lot-to-lot variability, storage requirements, and thrombin's ability to activate the clotting cascade and thus interfere with the assay. Recently, a thrombin receptor agonist peptide (TRAP) has been used in place of thrombin to allow activation of platelets through the thrombin receptor without activating the clotting cascade. Thus, they do not suffer from the limitations affecting the use of thrombin and can be produced inexpensively. The substitution of isoserine for serine has led to the development of iso-TRAP, which is more resistant than TRAP to degradation by the plasma enzyme aminopeptidase and is thus likely to yield more reproducible results (35). When aggregation to ADP or collagen is blocked, stimulation with TRAP is able to recruit more activated receptors to the platelet surface and may still produce aggregation (36,37). Increasing the plasma concentration of GPIIb/IIIa antagonist can further block this aggregation (36). TRAP is thus useful for discriminating effects of higher doses of GPIIb/IIIa antagonists when ADP-induced aggregation appears to be inhibited maximally. It is usually used in concentration ranging from 5 to 10 μM.

GP IIb/IIIa Antagonist Pharmacodynamics

The dose response curves of GPIIb/IIIa antagonists are generally considered steep. Figure 2 shows receptor blockade and platelet aggregation response to 5 μmol of ADP in subjects who received 0.25 mg/kg bolus and 12-hour infusion of abciximab. There is little inhibition of platelet aggregation initiated by ADP and similar antagonists until ≥50% of the receptors are blocked (17,38). At ≥80% GPIIb/IIIa receptor blockade, platelet aggregation

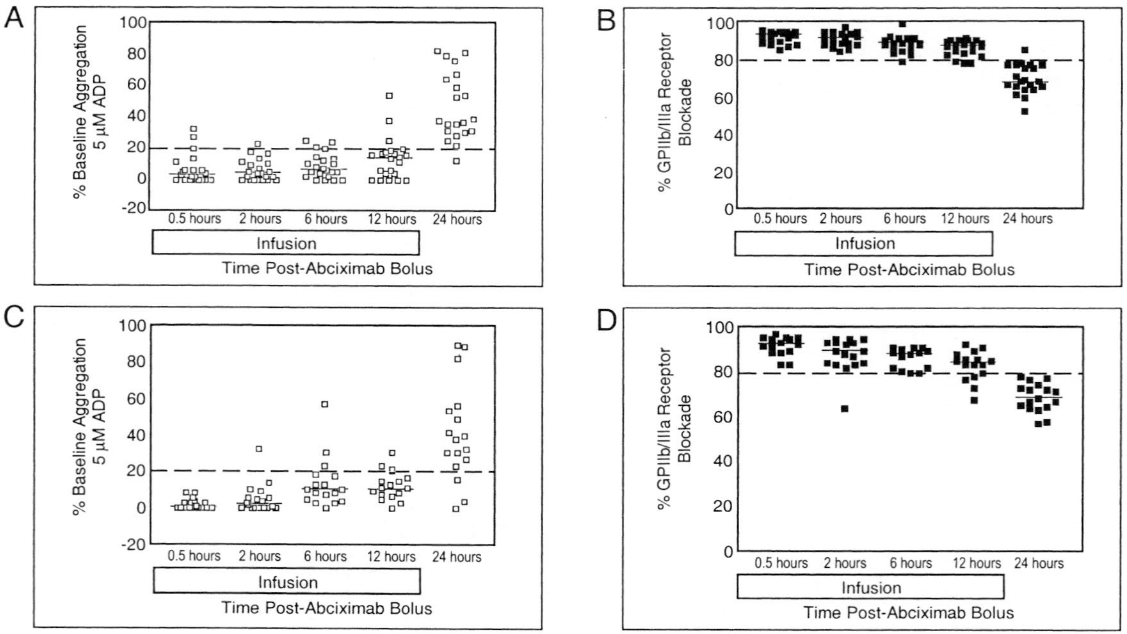

Figure 2 GP IIb/IIIa receptor blockade (B and D) and platelet aggregation response to 5 μmol/L ADP (A and C) of subjects who received 0.25-mg/kg bolus and 12-hour infusion of abciximab. Degrees of GP IIb/IIIa receptor blockade and platelet aggregation are expressed as percent of baseline values. Symbols represent individual subject values; solid lines, median values; and dashed line, 80% blockade of both GP IIb/IIIa receptors and aggregation. (A and B) Test subjects who received 10 μg/min (non-weight-adjusted; n = 24) infusion regimen. (C and D) Individuals who received 0.125 μg/kg/min (weight-adjusted; n = 17) infusion regimen. (Adapted from Ref. 17.)

with conventional agonists is nearly abolished (17,38). However, giving an additional dose of either antibody 10E5 or 7E3 (both of which block IIb/IIIa) to animals which already have complete inhibition of platelet aggregation, further prolongation of bleeding time results, demonstrating that the additional antibody has functional consequences that are not detected by turbidimetric aggregometry (18).

For acute GPIIb/IIIa blockade during coronary interventions, monitoring may not be necessary if a dosing regimen consistently achieves receptor blockade in all patients and if there is no increase in clinical hemorrhage in patients having the greatest receptor blockade. Previous studies of the pharmacokinetics of abciximab support the hypothesis that most, but not all, patients achieve and sustain ≥80% threshold level with the current dose of 0.25 mg/kg bolus and infusion of either 10 μg/min or 0.125 μg/kg/min (31,39,40). However, some individual variation in receptor blockade has been observed (31,40,41), and as demonstrated by Mascelli et al. (39), mean GPIIb/IIIa receptor blockade was ≈80% at 6 and 12 hours after therapy was initiated, so some patients were below this level. The theoretical peak whole-blood level of abciximab exceeds the amount of antibody required to fully saturate the GPIIb/IIIa receptors on a normal number of circulating platelets by approximately twofold. Despite this, it is plausible that patients with thrombocytosis or more activated receptors per platelet will not achieve as high a degree of receptor blockade as patients with normal platelet counts. A systematic assessment of the effects of elevated platelet counts on the efficacy of abciximab would be desirable, and dose adjustments have the potential to improve efficacy. Assessment of receptor blockade after discontinuation of GPIIb/IIIa will also be important in determining the return of platelet function toward normal. This information will help physicians decide whether platelet transfusion or more time for renal clearance is necessary before surgery or other invasive procedures. In general, there is little hemostasis compromise at receptor blockade levels <50%.

GPIIb/IIIa Antagonist Monitoring

An important question which needs to be answered is the optimum way to monitor GPIIb/IIIa dose to impact clinical outcome. Table 1 lists some scenarios in which platelet monitoring would be clinically useful. Drug levels are usually used as surrogate for drug effect, but in the case of GPIIb/IIIa antagonists, interindividual variations in platelet count, density of GPIIb/IIIa receptors, intrinsic platelet functional competence, or levels of platelet cofactors may affect the response to a given plasma level of a GPIIb/IIIa antagonist. It is not clear whether the best parameter is the percentage of GPIIb/IIIa receptors blocked or the effect of GPIIb/IIIa antagonism on plate-

Table 1 Scenarios in Which Platelet Monitoring Would Be Clinically Useful

Patient
Confirm ≥80% aggregation inhibition
Prior to PCI
In patients with refractory ischemia on IIb/IIIa inhibitors
Interruption of intravenous therapy
Abnormal platelet count
Renal insufficiency
High or low body weight
Clinical
Bleeding
Confirm excess inhibition
Guidance during reversal of therapy
Emergent Surgery
Confirm ≤50% aggregation inhibition
Guidance to reverse therapy if needed
Other
Drug-specific
Switching among intravenous agents
Transition from intravenous to oral agents
Combination with other antiplatelet/anticoagulants

let function. Expressing GPIIb/IIIa antagonism as percentage of receptors blocked avoids some variables that affect platelet function such as anticoagulant use, platelet preparation, agonist use, endpoint measured, and equipment used.

However, a monitoring system based on receptor blockade has several drawbacks. These include the potential need for different reagents and assay techniques for each individual drug, concerns about the impact of variability in drug uptake by platelets on the result of binding studies, the need for expensive equipment and technical expertise with the current assays used, and the difficulty in performing and interpreting receptor blockade studies during transition periods when two different GPIIb/IIIa antagonists are present simultaneously as when switching from an intravenous to an oral agent or vice versa (32). The original correlation between receptor blockade and inhibition of platelet function was based on studies of apparently normal individuals; extrapolation of these data to a wider population of patients with chronic illnesses that may affect platelet function, and more intercurrent medications may not be justified.

Using a "functional" platelet assay to monitor GPIIb/IIIa therapy has the advantage of directly assessing the goal of therapy as well as integrating the effects of nearly all of the variables listed above. For example, standard doses of a GPIIb/IIIa antagonist may be excessive in patients with low platelet counts, on other medications which affect platelet function, or with illnesses that may affect platelet function. Another major advantage of a "functional assay" is that a single assay may be applicable to monitor all of the available GPIIb/IIIa antagonists.

Conventional turbidimetric platelet aggregometry using citrated platelet-rich plasma is the most accepted and most widely used method of testing platelet function but involves sample preparation, extensive quality control, operator experience, and expensive equipment. Also, the calcium chelation caused by citrate anticoagulation may artifactually enhance the inhibition observed with some GPIIb/IIIa antagonists such as eptifibatide (42). Citrate chelation reduces the Ca^{2+} concentration of PRP to 40 to 50 μmol/L, partially removing Ca^{2+} from the divalent cation binding sites on GP IIb-IIIa. Although the reduced Ca^{2+} lowers the affinity of fibrinogen for GP IIb/IIIa on the surface of activated platelets, sufficient binding persists to allow for platelet aggregation. Reduced Ca^{2+} simultaneously increases the binding of eptifibatide, possibly because eptifibatide and Ca^{2+} occupy overlapping sites on GP IIb-IIIa. The increased binding of eptifibatide to GP IIb/IIIa and the decreased binding of fibrinogen together serve to increase the inhibitory activity of eptifibatide.

The characteristics of an ideal platelet function assay include the requirement of small amount of whole blood, the requirement of minimal processing or pipetting, and the availability of accurate results within a few minutes. Table 2 shows the desired characteristics of an ideal test. For obvious reasons, undiluted whole blood is preferable for bedside testing rather than PRP as it involves an extra processing step. Tests that involve dilution of whole blood may not accurately measure inhibition due to low-molecular-weight agents with rapid GP IIb/IIIa off rates. There is currently no test which fulfills all the criteria for an ideal test. There is also no gold standard against which other tests can be compared, and there are few data on clinical outcomes using the currently available tests.

PLATELET FUNCTION TESTS

Table 3 lists the currently available platelet function tests, their substrates and principles of assessment.

Table 2 Characteristics of an Ideal Platelet Assay

Whole blood
No pipetting or exposure
No reagent preparation
Small sample
Small device (POCT)
Ease of use
Automated
Quick
Inexpensive
Easily interpretable
Accurate
Reliable
Reproducible

Table 3 Currently Available Platelet Function Assays, Their Substrate, and Principles of Assessment

	Whole blood	Platelet-rich plasma (PRP)	Point-of-care test	Principle
Ivy bleeding time	√		√	Primary hemostasis
Photo-optical aggregometer		√		Aggregation
Impedance aggregometer	√	√		Aggregation
Flow cytometry	√			Activation
Receptor blockade		√		Receptor blockade
Thromboelastograph	√			Clot strength
Sonoclot analyzer	√			Clot strength
PFA-100	√		√	Primary hemostasis
PACT assay	√			Activation
Hemostasis analyzer	√			Clot retraction
Clot signature analyzer	√		√	Adhesion, aggregation
Platelet count ratio	√			Aggregation
Rapid platelet function assay	√		√	Aggregation
Cone and plate viscometer	√			Aggregation, clot strength

Ivy Bleeding Time

Bleeding time evaluates primary hemostasis (platelet adhesion, release reaction, aggregation, and primary plug formation) and assesses the overall ability of platelets to form a thrombus.

Clinical Utility

This is a rapid, noninvasive test that can assess overall platelet function. However, the test requires a dedicated technologist and can take up to 30 min to perform. Also the accuracy, validity, and predictability of this test are not proven. A number of other patient- and technique-related factors may affect bleeding time. The normal range of bleeding time is 7 to 10 min.

Photo-Optical (Turbidometric) Platelet Aggregometry

This is the most commonly practiced assay of platelet function. Instruments used with this technique include the Chrono-Log (Havertown, PA), Bio-Data (Hatboro, PA), Payton-Scientific (Buffalo, NY), and Helena Laboratories (Beaumont, TX). For this assay platelet-rich plasma (PRP) and platelet-poor plasma (PPP) are prepared from citrated blood, pipetted into matched cuvettes, placed in the appropriate positions in the instrument, and equilibrated at 37°C. The instrument is calibrated so that the amount of light transmitted through the PPP is defined as 100% aggregation and light transmitted through unstimulated PRP is defined as 0% aggregation. In some laboratories, platelet count in the PRP is adjusted by the addition of PPP to achieve a standardized count between 250,000 and 350,000/μL (43). Aggregation is initiated by adding a measured aliquot of platelet agonist such as ADP, collagen, or epinephrine; stirring is achieved by means of a magnetic stirbar, and the change in light transmitted through the PRP is monitored. As aggregation proceeds, large platelet aggregates form, turbidity decreases, and light transmitted through the sample is increased. The light received through the sample is converted into electrical signals, amplified, and recorded. Results are expressed as percentage of aggregation. Figure 3 illustrates the principles of this assay.

Clinical Utility

This widely available method has been used for more than 30 years. This method can be standardized, is well accepted, and has been most widely used for clinical correlation. However, the process is laborious, time-consuming, and limited by the optical quality of the PRP. The centrifugation step involved in the procedure may also modulate platelet behavior as a subpopulation of platelets may be lost during centrifugation. Hospitals may standardize their tests differently, and it is often somewhat difficult to com-

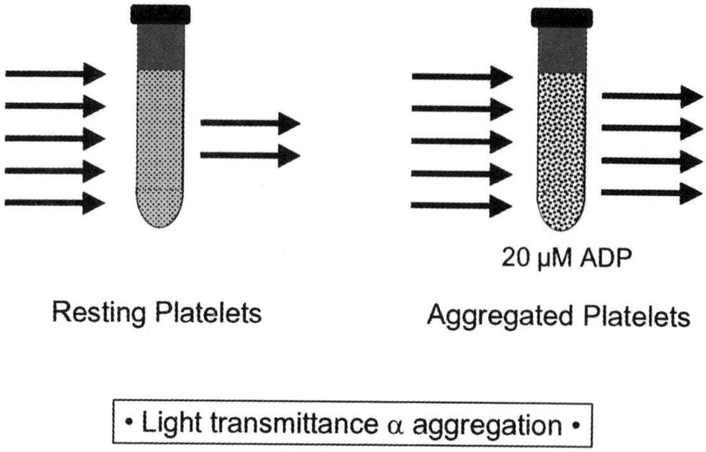

Figure 3 In photo-optical turbidimetric aggregometry, as platelets aggregate more light is able to pass through the sample and this light is converted into an electrical signal.

pare results from one clinical site with those of another using this test. Clinical areas of variation in procedure include PRP (preparation, centrifugation), use of adjusted or unadjusted platelet count, cuvette size, stirbar speed, choice of agonist or agonist concentration, paper speed, and use of aggregation versus slope of aggregation as the primary endpoint. This method is useful in detecting platelet function defects in patients with congenital or acquired bleeding disorders. This assay has been used for Phase II studies for drug development of GP IIb/IIIa inhibitors and can be used clinically though it is time-consuming. A rapid assay using this principle yet limiting pitfalls of variability, would be ideal.

Impedence Aggregometry

Cardinal et al. (26) introduced this method as an alternative to photo-optical aggregometry, and it can be used with whole blood or PRP. Instruments using this method are made by Chrono-Log (Havertown, PA) and Bio-Data (Hatboro, PA). When whole blood is used, it is diluted with normal saline 1:1, placed in a plastic cuvette at 37°C, and stirred. A probe composed of two closely spaced platinum wires is inserted, and the resistance between them is measured. On addition of a platelet agonist, platelet aggregates accumulate between the wires and the resistance increases. Results are reported as the maximal change in resistance in ohms or the change in resistance at a specified time after addition of agonist. Figure 4 illustrates the principle used in this method.

Clinical Utility

The advantages of this method include use of whole blood, a smaller quantity of blood, and the rapidity of the assay. The disadvantages are a significantly higher variability than PRP aggregometry, and poor correlation between the turbidimetric and impedence methods when ADP is used as the agonist. Disadvantages of this technique also include that it requires relatively expensive equipment, the need to prepare and pipette reagents, delicate care of the electrodes, and detailed quality control procedures. This method appears to be suitable for use in catheterization laboratories with a high volume of patients, but it is less likely to be useful in monitoring long-term therapy in large number of patients. Also, the whole-blood dilution step may limit its utility in monitoring low-molecular-weight agents with rapid receptor off rates since even modest dilutions of blood for brief periods of time may falsely lower the extent of inhibition.

Flow Cytometry

Flow cytometry can rapidly measure specific characteristics of a large number of individual platelets. In response to agonists such as thrombin, collagen, or ADP, a spectrum of specific activation-dependent modifications of

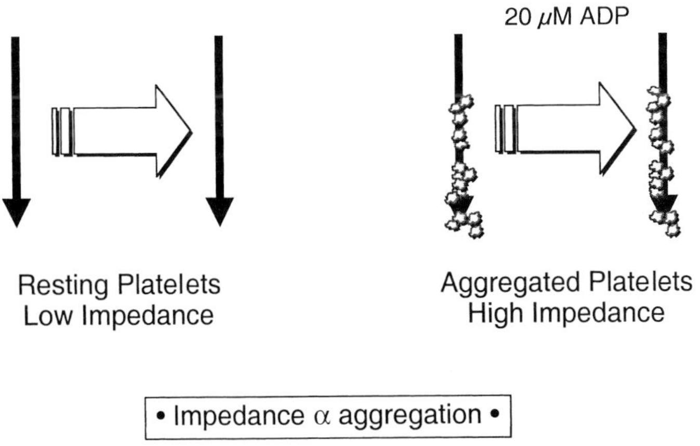

Figure 4 In whole-blood impedance aggregometry on addition of a platelet agonist, platelet aggregates accumulate between the wires and the resistance increases. Results are reported as the maximal change in resistance in ohms or the change in resistance at a specified time after addition of agonist.

platelet surface antigens can be detected. This process leads to an intracellular signal transduction cascade involving ion fluxes and activation of the cytoskeleton. The end result is secretion of endosomes, which causes reorganization and conformational changes of surface receptor expression through inside-out signaling. Platelet activation also leads to an altered expression of already constitutively expressed surface glycoproteins. Increased numbers of GPIIb/IIIa complexes and reduced numbers of GPIb-IX complexes result from bidirectional trafficking of these glycoproteins among the cell surface, the surface-connected canalicular system, and intracellular storage. Inside-out signaling leads to conformational changes of GPIIb-IIIa complexes, exposing conformation-dependent activation epitopes with high affinity for their ligands. The release reaction of platelets is associated with the neoexpression of α-granule glycoproteins such as CD62P or CD63. Thus, measuring the expression of these antigens on circulating platelets reflects not only the activation state of the platelets but also the extent to which secretion has occurred.

Flow cytometry is a sensitive and rapid research tool for the study of both inherited and acquired platelet disorders. By quantitation of the surface expression of the principal adhesion and aggregation receptors (GPIb-IX, GPIIb-IIIa) and of secreted platelet proteins (CD62P, CD63, thrombospondin, fibrinogen), conformational changes in platelet glycoproteins, especially GPIIb-IIIa, can be measured using monoclonal antibodies recognizing receptor-induced binding sites (RIBS) on the ligand, or ligand-induced binding sites (LIBS) on the receptor. Increased amount of platelet-bound ligands such as fibrinogen, Von Willebrand factor, P-selectin, or thrombospondin can be quantified using ligand-directed antibodies.

To perform cytometry platelets are labeled with a fluorescent-conjugated monoclonal antibody and placed in the flow chamber. The cells are passed at a rate of 1000 to 10,000 cells/min through the focused light beam of a laser. Exposure of labeled cells to light at the excitation wavelength results in emitted fluorescence, which is detected and processed along with the forward and side light scattering properties of the cell. Activation state of circulating platelets is assessed with an activation-dependent monoclonal antibody. Such antibodies bind strongly to activated platelets and weakly or undetectably to unstimulated platelets. The number of fluorescent platelets is directly related to the activation of the pathway being assessed.

Clinical Utility

In addition to the benefits of whole-blood analysis and the small amount of blood required, the minimal handling of samples needed prevents artifactual in vitro platelet activation. Also, with this assay both the activation state and the reactivity of platelets can be assessed. The disadvantages include the need for expensive equipment and a dedicated technologist. Flow cytometry is helpful in assessing specific platelet functions, activity, and hyperreactivity. Thus, this test can be used to monitor the inhibition of the GPIIb/IIIa receptor by specific antagonists, but its use is mainly limited to use as a research tool.

Receptor Blockade

Direct measurement of receptor blockade has been shown to correlate with the antithrombotic efficacy of derivatives of the IIb/IIIa monoclonal antibody 7E3 in animal studies (18). To measure receptor blockade by 7E3, platelets with and without the inhibitor are incubated with a saturating concentration of radiolabeled 7E3. Bound radioactivity is separated from free by spinning the platelets through a layer of sucrose. The difference in the amount of radioactivity bound to platelets with versus without the inhibitor represents the amount of receptors that are blocked. Clinical dosing with abciximab is targeted to approximately 80% receptor blockade. This method, however, is not accurate for small-peptide or nonpeptide inhibitors, which do not compete with 7E3 for binding to GPIIb/IIIa receptors.

A new assay called DART (D3 Assay for Receptor Targeting) has been developed to calculate the percentage of total GPIIb/IIIa receptors that have bound drug by measuring the D3 binding on platelets compared with the total number of receptors measured by D3 after in vitro addition of excess drug (Fig. 5) (44). This assay evaluates the extent of receptor blockade without requiring a predrug or baseline sample. DART can be used in conjunction with GPIIb/IIIa inhibitors that do not express the D3 LIB site. Peptides are added to the sample, and percentage of receptors blocked by the target drug can be determined by measuring the remaining available receptors that bind D3 compared with the total number of surface receptors.

Clinical Utility

Unlike aggregation studies, the DART assay is not affected by antiplatelet agents such as aspirin, ticlopidine, or clopidogrel. The samples can be analyzed up to 72 hours after blood collection. However, this method remains a surrogate for platelet inhibition as it does not measure the functional extent of inhibition directly.

Thromboelastography

Thromboelastograph measures clot strength (45). A clot is allowed to form between a cup and a sensing device (pin suspended from a torsion wire). Platelet participation in clot retraction results in increased fibrin rigidity. In this device, Figure 6a (Thromboelastograph coagulation analyzer, Haemo-

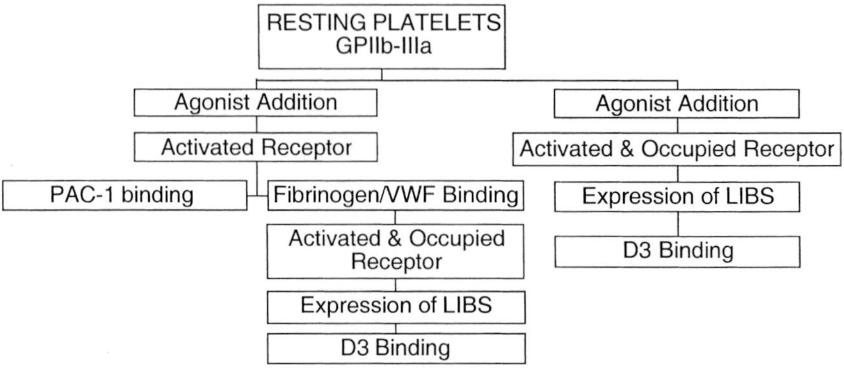

Figure 5a Events leading to activation and binding of GPIIb/IIIa ligands. Resting platelets are activated by agonists that lead to expression of activated GPIIb/IIIa. This activated receptor may be recognized by murine monoclonal antibody PAC-1. However, if large ligand binds to activated receptor or antagonist binds to GPIIb/IIIa complex, receptor converts to high affinity state and expresses neoepitopes called LIBS. (Adapted from Ref. 44.)

scope, Morton Grove, IL) (Fig. 6a), the cup is oscillated and the transduction of the oscillatory movement to the torsion wire is measured and represented graphically. The measurement is most directly related to the physical properties of the clot. Several parameters, reflecting different stages of clot development are measured as shown in Figure 6b. The strength of a clot is graphically represented over time as a characteristic cigar-shaped curve. The five parameters of the Thromboelastograph tracing—R, K, alpha angle, MA, and MA60—measure different stages of a clot development. R is the time from initiation of the test to the initial fibrin formation. K is a measure of the time from the beginning of clot formation until the amplitude of thromboelastogram reaches 20 mm, and represents the dynamics of clot formation. Alpha angle is the angle between the line in the middle of the tracing and the line tangential to the developing body of the tracing. Alpha angle represents the kinetcs of fibrin buildup and cross-linking. MA is the maximum amplitude of movement and reflects the strength of the clot, which is dependent on the number and function of platelets and its interaction with fibrin. MA60 measures the rate of amplitude reduction 60 min after MA and represents the stability of the clot. Platelet function is evaluated at physiologic calcium concentrations and under maximal thrombin generation. The test is allowed to run until clot lysis or retraction occurs, which can take up to 1 hour.

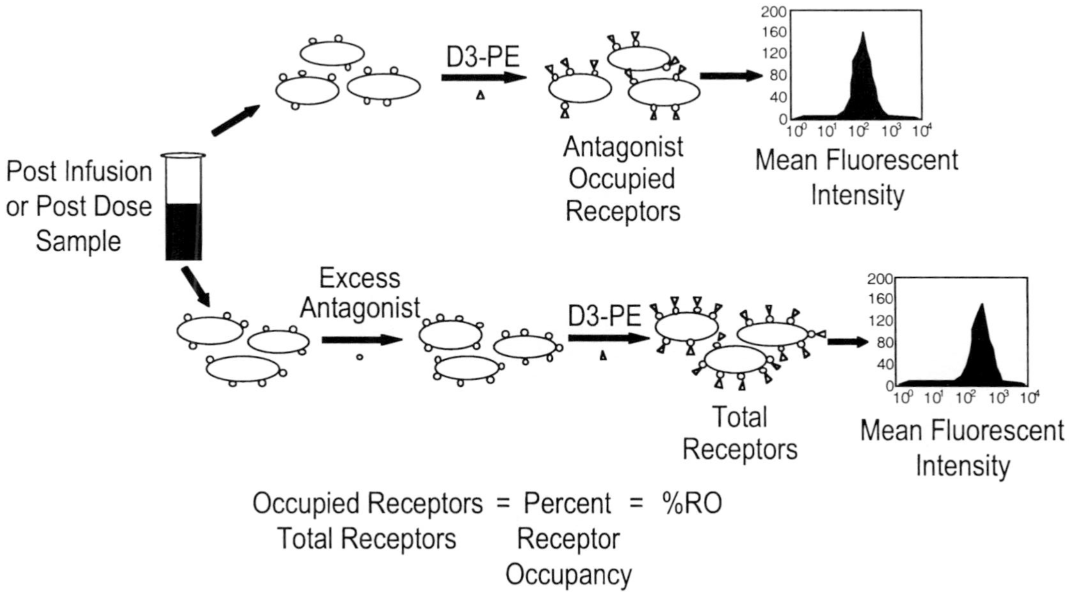

Figure 5b DART assay. Samples are analyzed for receptor occupancy. Postinfusion sample or postdose sample from administration of either intravenous or oral antagonist formulation, respectively, is divided into two aliquots for measurement of receptors blocked and total platelet surface receptors. Measured mean fluorescent intensity is converted to number of molecules bound and percent receptor occupancy is determined. (Adapted from Ref. 44.)

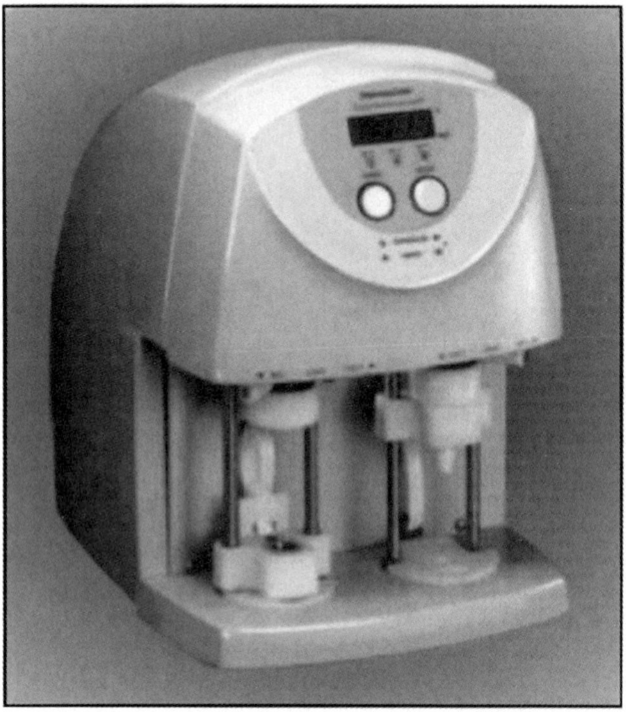

Figure 6a The Thromboelastograph.

Clinical Utility

This method uses whole blood and assesses multiple components of thrombosis. However, the method requires a long time, is cumbersome, and requires pipetting. Recently a modified thromboelastographic method was described for monitoring heparinized patients receiving abciximab (46). Addition of abciximab in vitro resulted in a linearly dose-dependent reduction in clot strength and platelet force. The currently available method is unlikely to be applicable to rapid point-of-care testing.

Sonoclot Analyzer

The Sonoclot analyzer (Sienco, Morrisson, CO), like the thromboelastograph, assesses clot strength by vibrating the clot and recording its response to agitation. The patient sample is contained in a glass cuvette into which a plastic probe is inserted. The amount of power required to maintain probe oscillation is measured and increases with increasing clot viscosity.

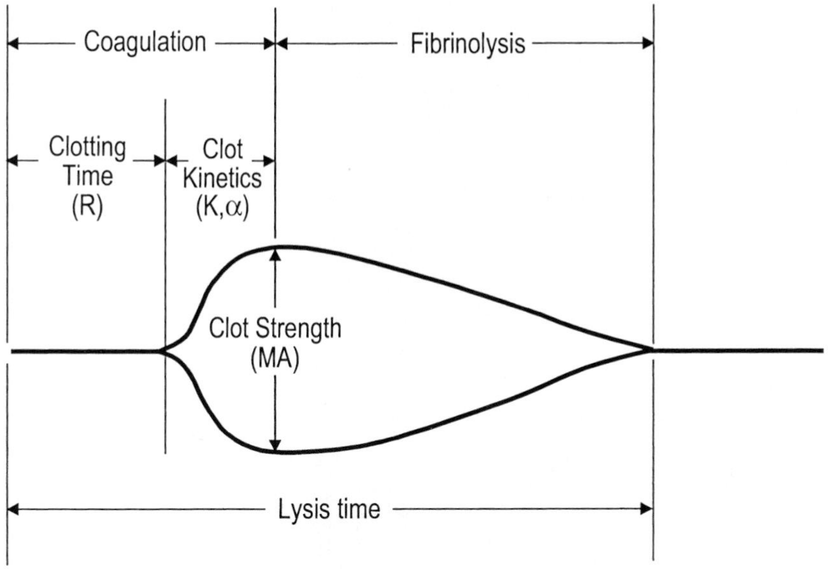

Figure 6b The five parameters of the Thromboelastograph tracing: R, K, alpha-angle, MA and MA60, which measures different stages of clot development.

Clinical Utility

The absence of correlation with physiologic events and the curve characteristics of the assay and lack of objective parameters at present make this assay of limited use.

PFA-100 Analyzer

The Dade Behring (Miami, FL) Platelet Function Analyzer (PFA-100) evaluates primary hemostasis through platelet-platelet interaction as whole blood flows under shear stress conditions through an aperture (47). The instrument (Fig. 7) uses citrated whole blood which is drawn by means of a vacuum through a capillary tube producing high shear forces and then through a precisely defined aperture in a membrane that has been coated with either collagen and epinephrine or collagen and ADP. The platelets adhere and aggregate at the aperture until it is occluded, and the results are reported as a closure time. The testing process takes about 10 min. Occlusion is blocked by antibodies directed at GP Ib, vWF, GP IIb/IIIa, and RGD-containing peptides, which suggests a critical role for these molecules. A polyclonal antifibrinogen antibody did not permit occlusion, presumably because of the

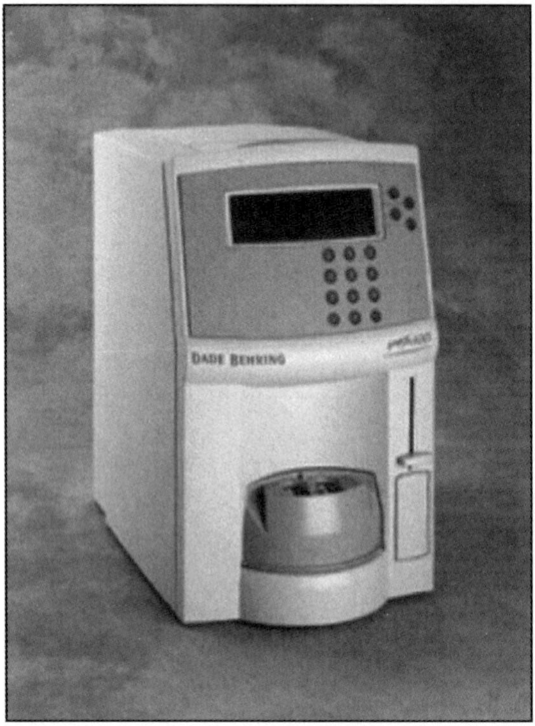

Figure 7a The Platelet Function Analyzer (PFA-100).

high shear rate involved. The proposed molecular mechanism evaluated in this system—initial binding of vWF by GP Ib followed by GP IIb/IIIa-dependent binding of vWF and possibly collagen—is distinct from that of fibrinogen-mediated platelet aggregation. This distinction may have clinical relevance because different GP IIb/IIIa inhibitors may preferentially block binding of vWF over fibrinogen, or vice versa. Blood can be collected in routine vacutainer tubes, and can be kept in room temperature for up to 4 hours. The instrument can run two tests in sequence. With the two test cartridges, the dysfunction of platelets caused by aspirin can be detected as a prolonged closure time with collagen/epinephrine cartridge but normal with collagen/ADP cartridge. This is a high shear system generating capillary shear rates on the order of 4000 to 5000 reciprocal seconds. A constant vacuum of 40 mBar is maintained in the system that mimics the pressure in a microcapillary in the human body.

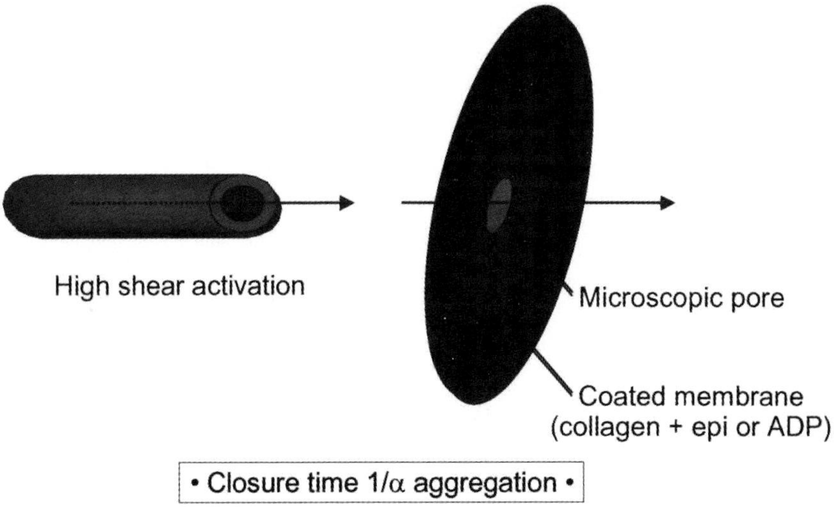

Figure 7b The PFA-100 analyzer uses citrated whole blood which is drawn by means of a vacuum through a capillary tube producing high shear forces and then through a precisely defined aperture in a membrane that has been coated with either collagen and epinephrine or collagen and ADP. The platelets adhere and aggregate at the aperture until it is occluded, and the results reported as a closure time.

Clinical Utility

This assay evaluates multiple factors involved in primary hemostasis similar to the template bleeding time without the incisional variability. It uses whole blood, is simple to perform, and is quick and automatic. The normal closure time is 100 sec and the instrument can detect a closure time of up to 300 sec, so this assay has a limited range. Its usefulness in monitoring GPIIb/IIIa therapy requires further study, but in general the closure times are increased beyond 300 sec with GP IIb/IIIa antagonists. The PFA-100 with the collagen-ADP cartridge correlates well with optical aggregometry at lower levels of aggregation inhibition (Fig. 8).

PACT Assay

Platelet-activated clotting test (PACT) is a modified activated clotting time (ACT) test of platelet function, based on the ability of activated platelets to contribute a surface on which contact-activated platelet factors can be generated (48). The assay requires a modified Hepcon HMS device (Medtronic Hemotec, Englewood, CO) with software adjustments to preset plunger lift and drop rates. Platelet-activating factor (PAF)-accelerated coagulation is

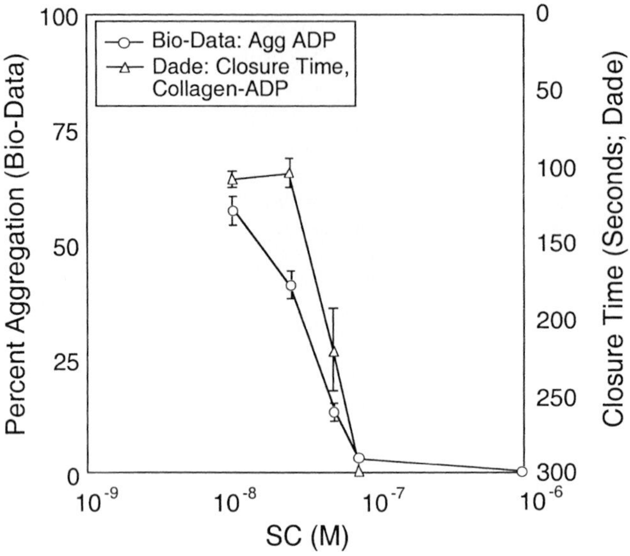

Figure 8 Closure time (collagen-ADP membrane) and ADP-induced aggregation in PRP. Concentrations of SC ranging from 10.8 to 10.6 mol/L were added to citrated blood samples and added to test cartridge. Sample was through capillary under high shear flow conditions. Sample then passed through aperture in membrane coated with collagen and ADP. Instrument determined time required for occlusion of aperture (closure time). PRP was prepared from same samples by differential centrifugation and ADP-induced aggregation measured the PFA-100 with the collagen-ADP cartridge correlates well with optical aggregometry at lower levels of aggregation. (Adapted from Ref. 49.)

measured in a six-channel cartridge in which platelet activation and clotting of heparinized blood are initiated by the combination of kaolin and varied concentration of PAF within the multiwell cartridge. For patients with normal platelet function, higher concentration of PAF yield shorter clotting time. The assay is sensitive to inhibition of platelet responsiveness, exposure to platelet factor 3, and indirectly to the extent that GPIIb/IIIa receptors contribute to this process.

Clinical Utility

This is a rapid assay requiring <3 min. However, the sensitivity and specificity of this test are less than that seen with the thromboelastograph technique. The instrument used is large and cumbersome for routine use. ACT measurements were not closely related to PRP aggregation across the range of in vitro saline control (SC) levels (49). As tested, the assay is highly variable and not suitable for monitoring the effects of GPIIb/IIIa inhibitors.

Hemostasis Analyzer

The Hemostasis Analyzer (Hemodyne, Richmond, VA) measures the strength of clot retraction as a means of assessing platelet function (Fig. 9) (50). The sample chamber consists of a thermostated cup and a parallel upper plate, which is attached to a displacement transducer. Citrated whole blood or PRP is introduced into the sample chamber, and clotting is initiated by addition of thrombin and calcium. Fibrin strands adhere to the cup and transducer, and platelets bind to and contract the fibrin strands resulting in movement of the transducer. A downward force is produced on the probe when the platelets within the clot contract it. The downward force generates a voltage signal that is converted to force and reported in dynes.

Clinical Utility

Limitations of this assay include a long test time ($\approx$20 min) and multiple pipetting steps. Carr et al. (51) reported suppression of force development

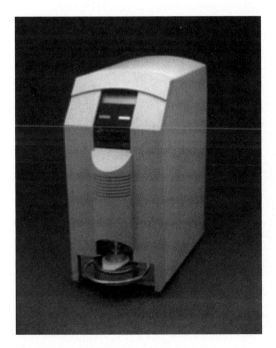

Figure 9 The Hemostasis Analyzer.

with RGD peptide. However, sufficient data are not yet available to assess reproducibility for clinical use.

Clot Signature Analyzer

This assay measures several aspects of platelet function and clotting properties. The instrument Clot Signature Analyzer (Xylum Corporation, Scarsdale, NY) (Fig. 10a) has a collagen channel to simulate the exposure of blood to thrombogenic subendothelial tissue. Blood is perfused over the collagen fiber at a high shear rate (approximately 6200 s^{-1}). Platelets activated by collagen adhere and aggregate to form a thrombus. The clot signature analyzer (CSA) has a punch channel that provides information on platelet function (Fig. 10b). While blood flows through the channel, the channel is punched by a 0.15-mm needle, resulting in two fine holes. A high shear rate at the punch point promotes platelet adhesion to the injury site and recruitment of activated platelets and resultant aggregation at the site.

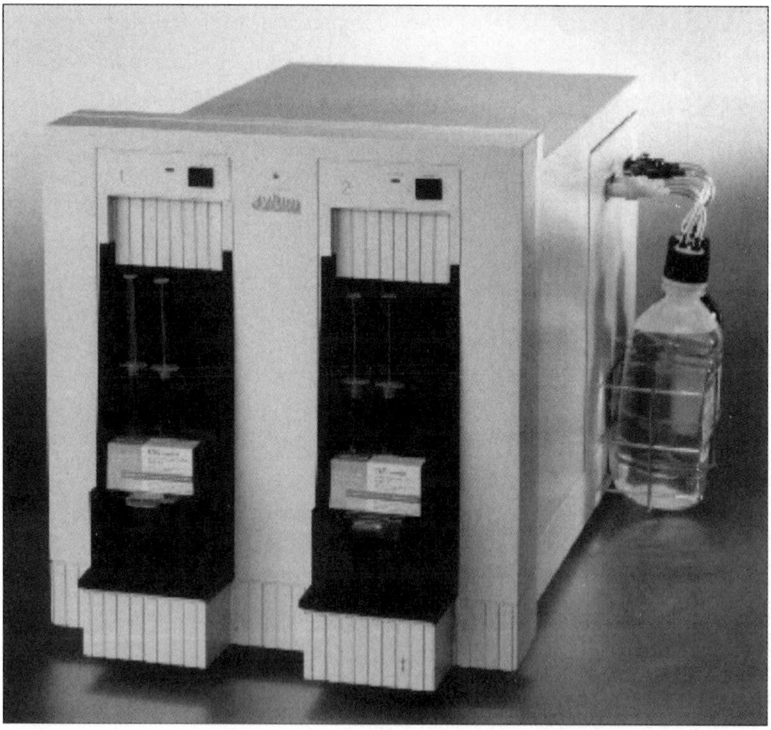

Figure 10a The Clot Signature Analyzer.

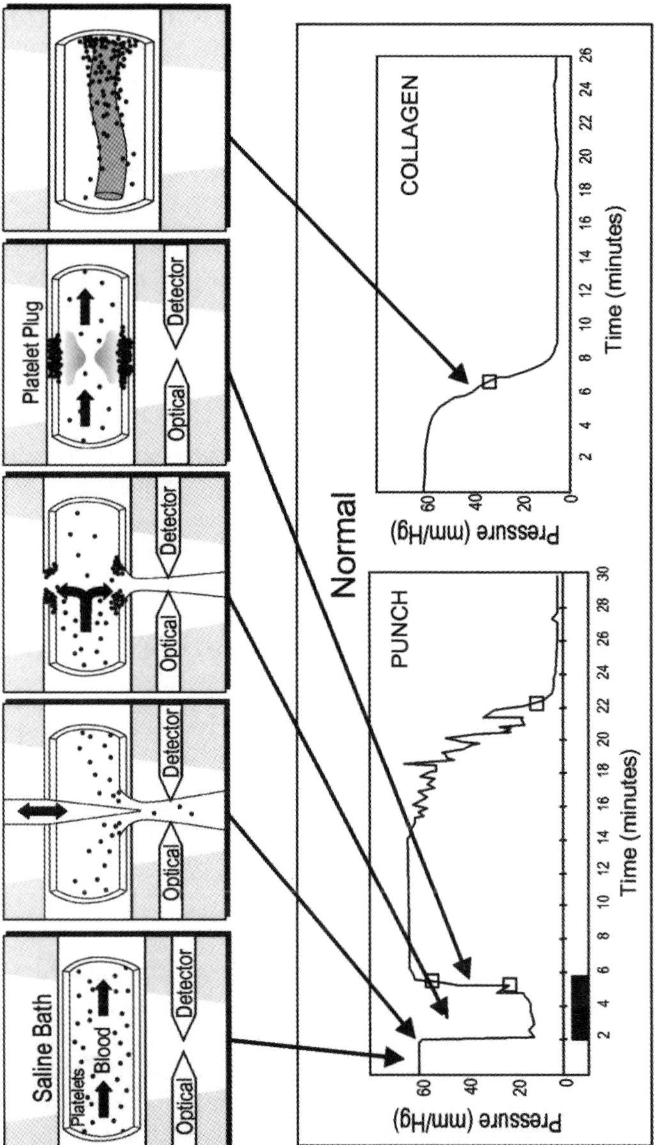

Figure 10b Principle of the Clot Signature Analyzer, which has a punch channel that provides information on platelet function.

A growing fibrin clot gradually occludes the pathway, resulting in reduction of the flow as evidenced by decrease in the pressure. Pressure in millimeters of mercury is plotted against time for both channels to produce a clot signature.

Clinical Utility

This is an automated assay that uses whole nonanticoagulated blood under conditions of physiologic flow and temperature. It evaluates both platelet activation and aggregation. These ideal features are somewhat offset since the current instrument is rather large for routine use and interpretation of the results is complex.

Platelet Count Ratio

Platelets in whole blood respond to agonists by forming aggregates, thereby decreasing the number of free platelets. This assay measures the number of free platelets in an ADP-stimulated blood sample compared with the same sample in which aggregation has been prevented by addition of EDTA (49).

Clinical Utility

The assay uses counting equipment available in most hospitals, and the time for analysis is flexible (up to 4 hours). The count ratio assay is a good predictor of PRP aggregation but is not a bedside assay.

Cone and Plate Viscometer

This is an in vitro assay of platelet thrombus formation after adhesion (52), not suited for rapid clinical testing.

Rapid Platelet Function Assay

The Ultegra-RPFA (Accumetrics, San Diego, CA) is an automated, whole-blood, cartridge-based, point-of care device that allows for the rapid and reproducible evaluation of platelet function in patients treated with GPIIb/IIIa inhibitors (Fig. 11). It is designed to assess platelet function utilizing the ability of activated platelets to bind fibrinogen (14). Fibrinogen-coated polystyrene microparticles agglutinate in whole blood in proportion to the number of unblocked platelet GPIIb/IIIa receptors. Pharmacologic blockade of GPIIb/IIIa receptors prevents this interaction and therefore diminishes agglutination in proportion to the degree of receptor blockade achieved. Because the speed of bead agglutination is more rapid and reproducible if platelets are activated, the thrombin receptor-activating peptide iso-TRAP [(iso-S)FLLRN] is incorporated into the assay.

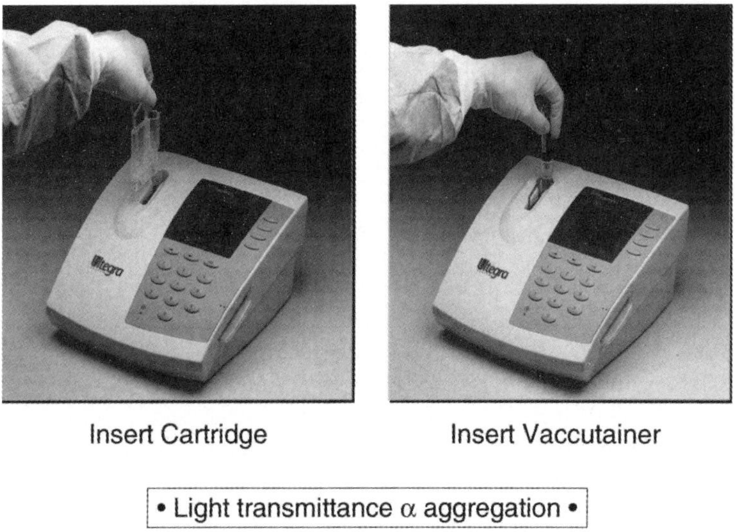

Figure 11 The Rapid Platelet Function Analyzer (Ultegra™) device.

Blood samples are obtained in either a standard citrate blood tube or, if eptifibatide is the agent being used, PPACK (Phe-Pro-Arg chloromethyl ketone) for the anticoagulant instead of citrate. The tube is inserted into a disposable plastic cartridge and the blood is automatically drawn into two sample channels containing lyophilized iso-TRAP and fibrinogen-coated beads. The sample is then mixed for 70 sec by the movement of a steel ball driven by a microprocessor. The light absorbance of the sample is measured 16 times/sec by an automated detector. As the platelets interact with the fibrinogen-coated beads, resulting in agglutination, there is a progressive increase in light transmission. The rate of agglutination is quantified as the slope of the change of absorbance over a fixed time interval and reported as millivolts per 10 sec (mV/10 sec). An individual patient's pre-GPIIb/IIIa inhibitor baseline slope is retained in memory, and all additional specimens are reported as the raw slope as well as a percentage of the baseline slope.

The Ultegra-RPFA has several advantages over turbidimetric aggregometry, including: 1) use of whole blood, thus avoiding the need for sample preparation and eliminating variables in sample preparation; 2) semiautomated format, which avoids operator errors and subjective endpoint assessments; 3) rapid test completion; 4) digital readout; 5) duplicate analysis to minimize random errors. Studies involving simultaneous measurement of platelet function measured by RPFA and turbidimetric platelet aggregometry induced by 20 μM ADP of samples treated in vivo with increasing doses of abciximab demonstrated a close correlation between the results (r^2 = .95), as well as between the RPFA results and the percentage of unblocked GPIIb/IIIa receptors assessed directly by radiolabeled monoclonal antibody binding (r^2 = .96). Similarly, the mean difference in measurements between RPFA and aggregometry was only −4% (±4% SD) and the mean difference in measurements between RPFA and free GPIIb/IIIa receptors was −2% (±6% SD) (53).

Comparison of RPFA and Turbidimetric Aggregometry

Figure 12 shows data from the SOAR study with close correlation between RPFA and aggregometry using orofiban as a GPIIb/IIIa antagonist (54). A functional assay such as RPFA provides information on the total effect of the agents on platelet function, independent of the agent, and so provides a measure that is likely to be biologically relevant. To further increase the automation of the RPFA, work is under way on a system that does not require an interface with a personal computer and that will require only the insertion of the vacutainer tube cartridge. When normalized to baseline control values, the percentage inhibition of the RPFA correlated well with both the percentage inhibition of turbidimetric platelet aggregometry and GPIIb/IIIa receptor blockade. In blood obtained from four separate donors, the correlation between RPFA and turbidimetric aggregometry was r^2 = .98, and that between RPFA and unblocked GPIIb/IIIa receptors was r^2 = .96. The

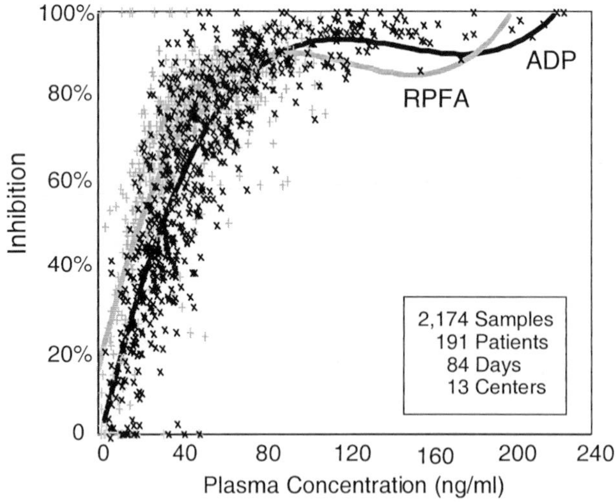

Figure 12 Orbofiban—correlation between the Rapid Platelet Function Analyzer and traditional aggregometry. (Adapted from SOAR study.)

disadvantages of RPFA is that it requires a baseline sample comparison, a specific agonist and there are little outcome data currently available using this technique.

CLINICAL STUDIES

There are several clinical studies under way to assess platelet function assays to evaluate optimum GPIIb/IIIa blockade. These include the GOLD (55) and the PARADISE (41) studies. The PARADISE study involved 100 patients, and demonstrated substantial interpatient variability in response to standard, weight-adjusted abciximab (41). Almost all patients achieved ≥80% of platelet inhibition following an abciximab bolus, but ~13% of patients did not maintain this level of inhibition during the infusion (Fig. 13). Even a wider range of variability was noted following the termination of the infusion. Although this study was not designed to evaluate clinical outcomes, routine monitoring of in-hospital adverse events, with systematic monitoring of postprocedural myocardial enzymes, was carried out. Interestingly, of the 13 patients with platelet function inhibited by <80% at 8 hours, six (46%) experienced an adverse cardiac event. This is in comparison to only five events among 75 (7%) patients with >80% inhibition at 8 hours ($P < .001$). Although not a predefined objective of the study, these results are consistent with the hypothesis that a specific level of platelet inhibition needs to be

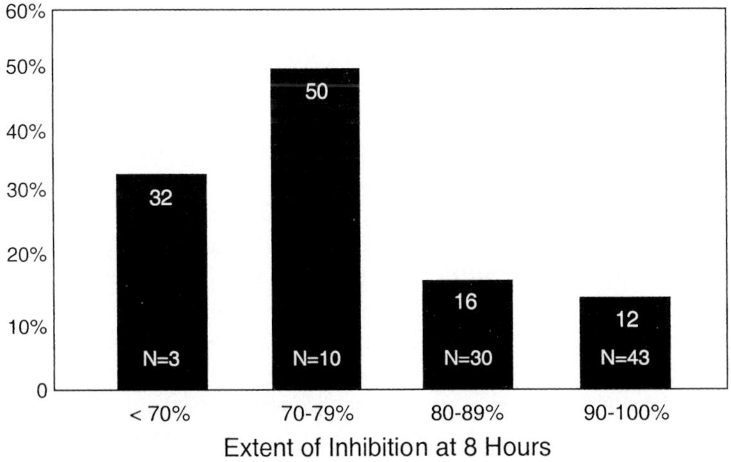

Figure 13 Data from PARADISE study showing incidence of major adverse cardiac events (MACE) and percent GPIIb/IIIa inhibition. (Adapted from Ref. 41.)

maintained in order to prevent thrombotic complications associated with a PCI.

The GOLD study (55) will prospectively evaluate the association between the level of platelet inhibition achieved at various time points as determined by the Ultegra-RPFA and the occurrence of major adverse cardiac events in a population of 500 patients undergoing a PCI treated with any of the three currently approved GPIIb/IIIa inhibitors—abciximab, eptifibatide, and tirofiban. Platelet function will be determined at five time points: baseline (just prior to receiving bolus); 10 min postbolus; 1 hour following the bolus or completion of the procedure; 8 hours following the bolus; and 24 hours following the bolus or at discharge. Patients will be monitored while hospitalized for the occurrence of any major adverse cardiac events defined as death, need for urgent revascularization, or myocardial infarction. All pertinent clinical, laboratory, and procedural characteristics will be evaluated in terms of their association with response to GPIIb/IIIa inhibitor therapy and the risk of adverse events. Major hemorrhagic complications will also be tracked.

Based on the results of earlier studies, it is hypothesized that by being able to monitor the response to treatment with GPIIb/IIIa antagonists in a large population of patients, a lower limit of effective platelet inhibition will be able to be identified. However, recent data from the PARAGON study (56) suggest that there may also be an upper limit of optimal platelet inhibition. Of the 2282 patients enrolled in the study, 810 had their plasma concentration measured. The plasma level was directly related to the patient's renal function, and correlated with the level of GPIIb/IIIa receptor occupancy and platelet inhibition. Interestingly, it was only patients with a plasma concentration in the middle range (18 to 42 ng/mL), corresponding to 80% to 90% GPIIb/IIIa receptor occupancy, that experienced a significant reduction in death and MI at 30 days and 6 months.

Patients with <80% or >90% receptor blockade as determined by plasma concentration experienced no clinical benefit compared with patients receiving placebo. The etiology of this upper limit of benefit of platelet inhibition is unclear, but in light of a number of small studies suggesting an intrinsic ability of various GPIIb/IIIa inhibitors to induce platelet activation, further evaluation and optimum dosing is warranted (57–60).

Use of parenteral platelet GPIIb/IIIa antagonists have been consistently shown to reduce the risk of thrombotic complications in the setting of acute coronary syndrome and PCI. However, many important issues remain unresolved regarding these agents. The ability to rapidly and reproducibly monitor the effects of these agents in individual patients is likely important to optimizing their use. For example, if via monitoring a similarly well-controlled and maintained therapeutic level of IIb/IIIa blockade was obtained using several different agents (antibody vs. small-molecule peptidomimetics), a more similar clinical outcome may be obtained. If long-term GPIIb/IIIa receptor blockade for primary or secondary prophylaxis of ischemic vascular disease becomes clinically useful, it will likely require a monitoring strategy more important than that considered for short-term therapy. Minor bleeding such as excess bruising, epistaxis, and gingival bleeding is likely to be unacceptable to patients treated with GPIIb/IIIa antagonists for prophylaxis. Therefore, a targeted upper limit of GPIIb/IIIa receptor blockade may be necessary. Also, a lower limit of receptor blockade will be required to achieve efficacy and avoid rebound.

Thus a therapeutic window will need to be defined as has been done for other antithrombotic drugs. Maintaining patients within a therapeutic window by use of a single dosing regimen is very unlikely, because the pharmacokinetics of the low-molecular-weight agents are likely too dependent upon individual renal and hepatic function. At the same time, as intravenous GPIIb/IIIa antagonists become incorporated as standard therapy during percutaneous revascularization procedures, monitoring will also become integral.

REFERENCES

1. Nurden AT, Caen JP. An abnormal platelet glycoprotein pattern in three cases of Glanzmann's thrombasthenia. Br J Haematol 1974;28:253–260.
2. Topol EJ, Byzova TV, Plow EF. Platelet GPIIb-IIIa blockers. Lancet 1999;353: 227–231.
3. Topol EJ, Ferguson JJ, Weisman HF, et al. Long-term protection from myocardial ischemic events in a randomized trial of brief integrin beta$_3$ blockade with percutaneous coronary intervention. EPIC investigator group. Evaluation of platelet IIb/IIIa inhibition for prevention of ischemic complication. JAMA 1997;278:479–484.
4. EPISTENT Investigators. Randomised placebo-controlled and balloon-angioplasty-controlled trial to assess safety of coronary stenting with use of platelet glycoprotein-IIb/IIIa blockade. Evaluation of platelet IIb/IIIa inhibitor for stenting. Lancet 1998;352:87–92.
5. Platelet Receptor Inhibition in Ischemic Syndrome Management (PRISM) Study Investigators. A comparison of aspirin plus tirofiban with aspirin plus heparin for unstable angina. N Engl J Med 1998;338:1498–1505.
6. PRISM-PLUS Study Investigators. Inhibition of the platelet glycoprotein IIb/IIIa receptor with tirofiban in unstable angina and non-Q-wave myocardial infarction. N Engl J Med 1998;338:1488–1497.
7. EPIC Investigation. Use of a monoclonal antibody directed against the platelet glycoprotein IIb/IIIa receptor in high-risk coronary angioplasty. N Engl J Med 1994;330:956–961.
8. CAPTURE Study. Randomised placebo-controlled trial of abciximab before and

during coronary intervention in refractory unstable angina. Lancet 1997;349: 1429–1435.

9. IMPACT-II. Randomised placebo-controlled trial of effect of eptifibatide on complications of percutaneous coronary intervention. Lancet 1997;349:1422–1428.
10. EPILOG Investigators. Platelet glycoprotein IIb/IIIa receptor blockade and low-dose heparin during percutaneous coronary revascularization. N Engl J Med 1997;336:1689–1696.
11. Chong PH. Glycoprotein IIb/IIIa receptor antagonists in the management of cardiovascular diseases. Am J Health Syst Pharm 1998;55:2363–2386.
12. Coller BS. Platelet GPIIb/IIIa antagonists: the first anti-integrin receptor therapeutics. J Clin Invest 1997;100:S57–S60.
13. Coller BS. Platelet GPIIb/IIIa antagonists: the first anti-integrin receptor therapeutics. J Clin Invest 1997;99:1467–1471.
14. Coller BS, Lang D, Scudder LE. Rapid and simple platelet function assay to assess glycoprotein IIb/IIIa receptor blockade. Circulation 1997;95:860–867.
15. Ammar T, Scudder LE, Coller BS. In vitro effects of the platelet glycoprotein IIb/IIIa receptor antagonist c7E3 Fab on the activated clotting time. Circulation 1997;95:614–617.
16. Gold HK, Gimple LW, Yasuda T, et al. Pharmacodynamic study of F(ab′)2 fragments of murine monoclonal antibody 7E3 directed against human platelet glycoprotein IIb/IIIa in patients with unstable angina pectoris. J Clin Invest 1990;86:651–659.
17. Coller BS, Scudder LE, Beer J, et al. Monoclonal antibodies to platelet glycoprotein IIb/IIIa as antithrombotic agents. Ann NY Acad Sci 1991;614:193–213.
18. Coller BS, Folts JD, Smith SR, Scudder LE, Jordan R. Abolition of in vivo platelet thrombus formation in primates with monoclonal antibodies to the platelet GPIIb/IIIa receptor. Correlation with bleeding time, platelet aggregation, and blockade of GPIIb/IIIa receptors. Circulation 1989;80:1766–1774.
19. Wagner CL, Mascelli MA, Neblock DS, Weisman HF, Coller BS, Jordan RE. Analysis of GPIIb/IIIa receptor number by quantification of 7E3 binding to human platelets. Blood 1996;88:907–914.
20. Barrett JS, Murphy G, Peerlinck K, et al. Pharmacokinetics and pharmacodynamics of MK-383, a selective non-peptide platelet glycoprotein-IIb/IIIa receptor antagonist, in healthy men. Clin Pharmacol Ther 1994;56:377–388.
21. Harrington RA, Kleiman NS, Kottke-Marchant K, et al. Immediate and reversible platelet inhibition after intravenous administration of a peptide glycoprotein IIb/IIIa inhibitor during percutaneous coronary intervention. Am J Cardiol 1995;76:1222–1227.
22. Askew BC, Bednar RA, Bednar B, et al. Non-peptide glycoprotein IIb/IIIa inhibitors. 17. Design and synthesis of orally active, long-acting non-peptide fibrinogen receptor antagonists. J Med Chem 1997;40:1779–1788.
23. Kouns WC, Kirchhofer D, Hadvary P, et al. Reversible conformational changes induced in glycoprotein IIb-IIIa by a potent and selective peptidomimetic inhibitor. Blood 1992;80:2539–2547.

24. Tsao PW, Bozarth JM, Jackson SA, Forsythe MS, Flint SK, Mousa SA. Platelet GPIIb/IIIa receptor occupancy studies using a novel fluoresceinated cyclic Arg-Gly-Asp peptide. Thromb Res 1995;77:543–556.
25. Bednar B, Cunningham ME, McQueney PA, et al. Flow cytometric measurement of kinetic and equilibrium binding parameters of arginine-glycine-aspartic acid ligands in binding to glycoprotein IIb/IIIa on platelets. Cytometry 1997; 28:58–65.
26. Cardinal DC, Flower RJ. The electronic aggregometer: a novel device for assessing platelet behavior in blood. J Pharmacol Methods 1980;3:135–158.
27. Di Minno G, Cerbone AM, Mattioli PL, Turco S, Iovine C, Mancini M. Functionally thrombasthenic state in normal platelets following the administration of ticlopidine. J Clin Invest 1985;75:328–338.
28. Herbert JM, Bernat A, Samama M, Maffrand JP. The antiaggregating and antithrombotic activity of ticlopidine is potentiated by aspirin in the rat. Thromb Haemost 1996;76:94–98.
29. Kuzniar J, Splawinska B, Malinga K, Mazurek AP, Splawinski J. Pharmacodynamics of ticlopidine: relation between dose and time of administration to platelet inhibition. Int J Clin Pharmacol Ther 1996;34:357–361.
30. Kleiman NS, Ohman EM, Califf RM, et al. Profound inhibition of platelet aggregation with monoclonal antibody 7E3 Fab after thrombolytic therapy. Results of the Thrombolysis and Angioplasty in Myocardial Infarction (TAMI) 8 pilot study. J Am Coll Cardiol 1993;22:381–389.
31. Tcheng JE, Ellis SG, George BS, et al. Pharmacodynamics of chimeric glycoprotein IIb/IIIa integrin antiplatelet antibody Fab 7E3 in high-risk coronary angioplasty. Circulation 1994;90:1757–1764.
32. Kereiakes DJ, Runyon JP, Kleiman NS, et al. Differential dose-response to oral xemilofiban after antecedent intravenous abciximab. Administration for complex coronary intervention. Circulation 1996;94:906–910.
33. Cannon CP, McCabe CH, Borzak S, et al. Randomized trial of an oral platelet glycoprotein IIb/IIIa antagonist, sibrafiban, in patients after an acute coronary syndrome: results of the TIMI 12 trial. Circulation 1998;97:340–349.
34. Kereiakes DJ, Kleiman N, Ferguson JJ, et al. Sustained platelet glycoprotein IIb/IIIa blockade with oral xemilofiban in 170 patients after coronary stent deployment. Circulation 1997;96:1117–1121.
35. Coller BS, Springer KT, Scudder LE, Kutok JL, Ceruso M, Prestwich GD. Substituting isoserine for serine in the thrombin receptor activation peptide SFLLRN confers resistance to aminopeptidase M-induced cleavage and inactivation. J Biol Chem 1993;268:20741–20743.
36. Kleiman NS, Raizner AE, Jordan R, et al. Differential inhibition of platelet aggregation induced by adenosine diphosphate or a thrombin receptor-activating peptide in patients treated with bolus chimeric 7E3 Fab: implications for inhibition of the internal pool of GPIIb/IIIa receptors. J Am Coll Cardiol 1995; 26:1665–1671.
37. Theroux P, Kouz S, Roy L, et al. Platelet membrane receptor glycoprotein IIb/IIIa antagonism in unstable angina. The Canadian Lamifiban Study. Circulation 1996;94:899–905.

38. Coller BS, Peerschke EI, Scudder LE, Sullivan CA. A murine monoclonal antibody that completely blocks the binding of fibrinogen to platelets produces a thrombasthenic-like state in normal platelets and binds to glycoproteins IIb and/or IIIa. J Clin Invest 1983;72:325–338.
39. Mascelli MA, Worley S, Veriabo NJ, et al. Rapid assessment of platelet function with a modified whole-blood aggregometer in percutaneous transluminal coronary angioplasty patients receiving anti-GP IIb/IIIa therapy. Circulation 1997;96:3860–3866.
40. Simoons ML, de Boer MJ, van den Brand MJ, et al. Randomized trial of a GPIIb/IIIa platelet receptor blocker in refractory unstable angina. European Cooperative Study Group. Circulation 1994;89:596–603.
41. Steinhubl SR, Kottke-Marchant K, Moliterno DJ, et al. Attainment and maintenance of platelet inhibition through standard dosing of abciximab in diabetic and nondiabetic patients undergoing percutaneous coronary intervention. Circulation 1999;100:1977–1982.
42. Phillips DR, Teng W, Arfsten A, et al. Effect of Ca^{2+} on GP IIb-IIIa interactions with integrilin: enhanced GP IIb-IIIa binding and inhibition of platelet aggregation by reductions in the concentration of ionized calcium in plasma anticoagulated with citrate. Circulation 1997;96:1488–1494.
43. Berkowitz SD, Frelinger AL 3rd, Hillman RS. Progress in point-of-care laboratory testing for assessing platelet function. Am Heart J 1998;136:S51–S65.
44. Jennings LK, White MM. Expression of ligand-induced binding sites on glycoprotein IIb/IIIa complexes and the effect of various inhibitors. Am Heart J 1998;135:S179–S183.
45. Mallett SV, Cox DJ. Thrombelastography. Br J Anaesth 1992;69:307–313.
46. Greilich PE, Alving BM, O'Neill KL, Chang AS, Reid TJ. A modified thromboelastographic method for monitoring c7E3 Fab in heparinized patients. Anesth Analg 1997;84:31–38.
47. Mammen EF, Comp PC, Gosselin R, et al. PFA-100 system: a new method for assessment of platelet dysfunction. Semin Thromb Hemost 1998;24:195–202.
48. Despotis GJ, Levine V, Filos KS, et al. Evaluation of a new point-of-care test that measures PAF-mediated acceleration of coagulation in cardiac surgical patients. Anesthesiology 1996;85:1311–1323.
49. Nicholson NS, Panzer-Knodle SG, Haas NF, et al. Assessment of platelet function assays. Am Heart J 1998;135:S170–S178.
50. Greilich PE, Carr ME Jr, Carr SL, Chang AS. Reductions in platelet force development by cardiopulmonary bypass are associated with hemorrhage. Anesth Analg 1995;80:459–465.
51. Carr ME Jr, Carr SL, Hantgan RR, Braaten J. Glycoprotein IIb/IIIa blockade inhibits platelet-mediated force development and reduces gel elastic modulus. Thromb Haemost 1995;73:499–505.
52. Varon D, Dardik R, Shenkman B, et al. A new method for quantitative analysis of whole blood platelet interaction with extracellular matrix under flow conditions. Thromb Res 1997;85:283–294.
53. Smith JW, Steinhubl SR, Lincoff AM, et al. Rapid platelet-function assay: an

automated and quantitative cartridge-based method. Circulation 1999;99:620–625.

54. Theroux P, Gosselin G, Nasmith J, et al. The accumetrics rapid platelet function analyzer (RPFA) to monitor platelet aggregation during oral administration of a gpIIb/IIIa antagonist. J Am Coll Cardiol 1999;33(2):330A.
55. Steinhubl S. Assessing the optimal level of platelet inhibition with GP IIb/IIIa inhibitors in patients undergoing coronary intervention. Rationale and design of GOLD study. J Thromb Thrombol 2000. In press.
56. PARAGON Investigators. International, randomized, controlled trial of lamifiban (a platelet glycoprotein IIb/IIIa inhibitor), heparin, or both in unstable angina. Circulation 1998;97:2386–2395.
57. Peter K, Schwarz M, Ylanne J, et al. Induction of fibrinogen binding and platelet aggregation as a potential intrinsic property of various glycoprotein IIb/IIIa (alphaIIbbeta3) inhibitors [see comments]. Blood 1998;92:3240–3249.
58. Hezard N, Metz D, Nazeyrollas P, et al. Free and total platelet glycoprotein IIb/IIIa measurement in whole blood by quantitative flow cytometry during and after infusion of c7E3 Fab in patients undergoing PTCA. Thromb Haemost 1999;81:869–873.
59. Du XP, Plow EF, Frelinger AL, O'Toole TE, Loftus JC, Ginsberg MH. Ligands "activate" integrin alpha IIb beta 3 (platelet GPIIb-IIIa). Cell 1991;65:409–416.
60. Gawaz M, Ruf A, Neumann FJ, et al. Effect of glycoprotein IIb-IIIa receptor antagonism on platelet membrane glycoproteins after coronary stent placement. Thromb Haemost 1998;80:994–1001.

22

Hypolipidemic Intervention and Plaque Stabilization

Robert A. Vogel
University of Maryland School of Medicine
Baltimore, Maryland

INTRODUCTION

Hypercholesterolemia contributes substantially to the development and clinical expression of atherosclerosis, especially in the coronary circulation (1–9). Considerable evidence suggests that cholesterol lowering stabilizes atherosclerotic plaques and reduces cardiovascular events, including all-cause mortality (10–36). Of all patients, those with established coronary heart disease benefit the most from cholesterol lowering (15–20). Twenty-two of 23 angiographic or ultrasound trials of hypolipidemic therapy have shown a reduction in disease progression and a 24th study has shown an anatomic advantage for aggressive over moderate treatment (37–92). Six large primary and secondary prevention event trials, completed between 1994 and 1999, have demonstrated significant reductions in cardiovascular events in patients with a wide range of cholesterol levels (93–118). These findings suggest that aggressive lipid management can accomplish the same treatment goals as traditional antianginal and interventional therapy, namely, reductions in anginal frequency, exercise intolerance, cardiovascular events, and mortality (13,117). This chapter reviews the pathophysiology and impact of hypolipidemic therapy on atherosclerosis (119–140) and vascular biology (141–200) and outlines the lipid management for coronary artery disease patients (201–251), including those undergoing interventional procedures.

PATHOPHYSIOLOGY OF ATHEROSCLEROSIS

In broad terms, coronary atherosclerosis is an initially slow process of endothelial dysfunction, intimal lipid, monocyte, and T lymphocyte accumulation with inflammation leading to the migration and proliferation of smooth muscle cells and elaboration of collagen and matrix (119–140). In its more advanced stages, this process is punctuated by acute episodes of plaque disruption, thrombosis, and vessel reorganization, which underlie the clinical syndromes of unstable angina and acute myocardial infarction (122–124,127,130,131,134,137). The disease, beginning in the first few decades of life (6), remains asymptomatic until significant luminal compromise develops or sudden occlusion occurs. In the former circumstance, stable exertional angina may be the presenting symptom, although this occurs in only 12% to 26% of men and 47% of women (5,7). Unstable angina, urgent need for coronary revascularization, acute myocardial infarction, and sudden death together make up the majority of the initial presenting symptoms of coronary heart disease. Important early pathophysiological processes include endothelial dysfunction (141–181) caused by coronary risk factors, mechanical trauma, and infections (possibly chlamydia, CMV, and herpes viruses), and the progressive modification of LDL, predominantly by oxidation (121,126). Once atherosclerotic plaques develop, the combined factors of local plaque inflammation (130,140), dissolution of internal plaque collagen, and vasomotion lead to plaque disruption, with ensuing partial or complete vessel thrombosis (119,122–125). Cholesterol lowering has been shown to slow the progression of coronary atherosclerosis and reduce plaque rupture (37–67,71,72,75). It may also decrease thrombogenicity and platelet adhesion to the denuded or ruptured vessel wall (24,25,32–34). Beyond its effects on the atherosclerotic process, improvements in endothelial function are thought to decrease the ischemic manifestations of coronary artery disease by increasing flow-mediated vasodilation at both the conduit and arteriolar vessel level (21,26,27,29,30,35,36).

Endothelial Pathway

Two processes play key roles in the initiation of atherosclerosis: endothelial dysfunction and lipid accumulation and modification (18,121,125,126,142,160,167,169,170,173,175) (Fig. 1). The endothelium is a major regulator of vasodilatation, vasoconstriction, vessel growth, aggregation of platelets, adhesion of monocytes, inflammation, immune responses, plaque remodeling, and fibrinolysis (18,141,145,147,150,173,175). Endothelium-derived relaxing factors in conduit and resistance vessels include nitric oxide (NO) or an NO adduct, prostacyclin, and hyperpolarizing factor which operate through the intermediate signaling mechanisms of cyclic-GMP, cyclic-AMP, and K^+

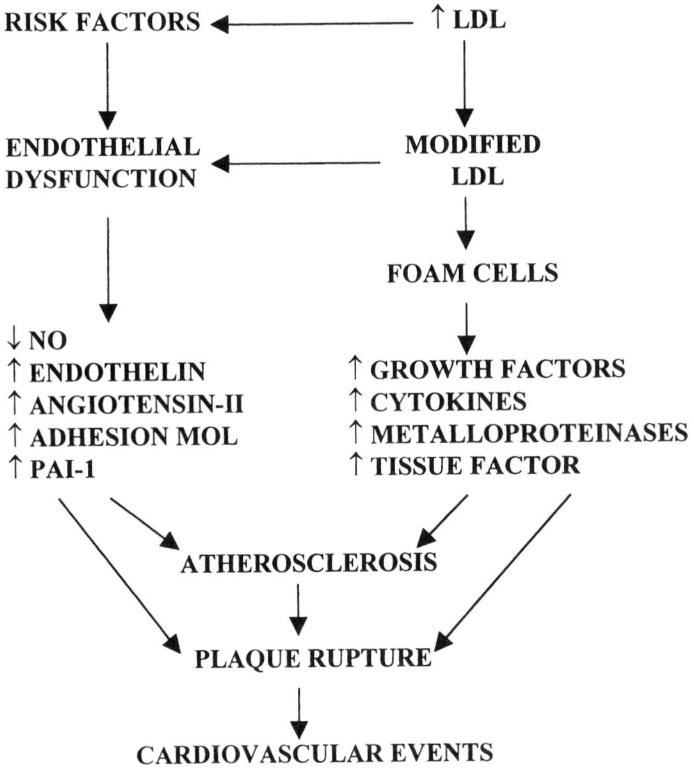

Figure 1 Pathogenesis of atherosclerosis demonstrating two important pathways, endothelial dysfunction and LDL accumulation and modification.

channels, respectively) (151,154). Endothelium-mediated or activated vasocontrictors include endothelin-1, angiotensin II, thromboxane, prostacyclin-H_2 and oxygen free radicals. Endothelin-1 also potentiates renin and catecholamines. The endothelium also expresses several monocyte adhesion molecules and coagulation altering factors (18,147). These factors are released in response to endothelium-dependent stimuli, such as acetylcholine, serotonin, thrombin, and blood flow shear. Normal endothelium prevents the development of atherosclerosis by promoting vasodilatation (NO) and thrombolysis (increased tPA:PAI-1) and inhibiting platelet aggregation (NO) and monocyte adhesion (decreased adhesion molecule expression). Experimental studies have demonstrated that NO synthesis inhibition (L-NAME) accelerates the development of atherosclerosis, whereas increasing NO availability (L-arginine) retards its development, at least for a period of several weeks (162,163). Preliminary reports suggest that clinical events occur more frequently in patients with the least endothelial-dependent vasodilation, even in individuals with similar extent of coronary artery stenosis (176).

All major coronary risk factors (both modifiable and immutable) are associated with endothelial dysfunction (146,149,152,157,161,169,173,175). Several mechanisms have been postulated for the decrease in NO availability with hypercholesterolemia, including increased production of oxygen free radicals (predominantly superoxide anion) which combine with and deactivate nitric oxide, abnormal intermediate signaling, and decreased NO production, possibly through reduced NO synthase expression caused by oxidized LDL (158,173,175). Other postulated mechanisms include reduced microdomain availability of the substrate L-arginine, increased asymmetric dimethyl arginine (ADMA), and increased activity of caveolin, a membrane inhibitor of NO synthase. Nitric oxide deactivation and endothelial dysfunction result in increased vasocontriction, smooth muscle cell proliferation, platelet aggregation, monocyte adhesion, inflammation, metalloproteinase and tissue factor production, and decreased fibrinolysis, all of which are important factors in the development of atherosclerosis, plaque rupture, and vessel thrombosis. The vasoregulatory aspect of endothelial function can be assessed in the coronary circulation using intracoronary infusions of acetylcholine, serotonin, or substance P and in the brachial circulation using a postocclusion hyperemic vasodilatation (flow-mediated) or forearm plethysmographic assessment of blood flow following cholinergic stimulation. Normal responses to these stimuli are manifest as vasodilation, whereas endothelial dysfunction is associated with reduced vasodilatation or vasoconstriction (142,144,145,148,150,152,155,168,173,175). Vasoregulation is, however, spatially variable, distal and smaller vessels generally being more reactive (153,164–166). Endothelial dysfunction is thought to be an important component in the pathophysiology of coronary ischemia. In the presence of endothelial dysfunction, clinical stimuli such as exercise-induced hyperemia, cold exposure, and emotional stress have been shown to result in vasoconstriction in the stenotic regions (167). Resistance vessel endothelial dysfunction also contributes to ischemia (21,27,30,35,36).

To date, 17 of 19 clinical studies have reported significant or borderline improvements in coronary or brachial artery endothelial function with cholesterol lowering in subjects both with and without coronary heart disease (Table 1) (182–200). Initial subject cholesterol has ranged from 195 to 373 mg/dL. Endothelium-dependent vasodilation improves with cholesterol lowering to about 150 mg/dL. Certain high-fat meals, hypertriglyceridemia, and elevated remnant particle levels have also been demonstrated to impair en-

Table 1 Effect of Cholesterol Lowering on Endothelial Function

Study	Pts.	Chol	Circ	Interv	Months	Result
Egashira (183)	CAD	272	CA	PRAVA	6	(+)
Treasure (184)	CAD	226	CA	LOVA	6	(+)
Anderson (185)	CAD	209	CA	LO/CH	12	(±)
				LO/PROB	12	(+)
Seiler (189)	CAD	300	CA	BEZAFIB	7	(+)
Yeung (190)	CAD	230	CA	SIMVA	6	(−)
CARE (191)	CAD	209	FMV	PRAVA	54	(+)
Tamai (192)	CAD	195	FVR	APHER	1 Hour	(+)
O'Driscol (193)	CAD	254	FVR	SIMVA	1	(+)
Andrews (194)	CAD	202	FMV	GEM/NIA/CH	30	(−)
Dupuis (199)	CAD	246	FMV	PRAVA	1.5	(+)
Herrington (200)	CAD	200	FMV	LOVA	1.5	(+)
Leung (182)	NL	239	CA	CH	6	(+)
Stroes (186)	NL	354	FVR	SIM/CO	3	(+)
Goode (187)	NL	373	EVR	UNSPEC	10	(+)
Vogel (188)	NL	200	FMV	SIMVA	0.5–3	(+)
De Man (195)	NL	1065 (TG)	FVR	ATORVA	1.5	(+)
Simons (196)	NL	320	FMV	SIMVA/CH	7	(+)
				ATORVA	7	(+)
Vogel (197)	NL	198	FMV	PRAVA	1 Day	(−)
					1	(+)
John (198)	NL	278	FVR	FLUVA	6	(+)

APHER = apheresis, ATORVA = atorvastatin, BEZA = bezafibrate, CA = coronary artery, CAD = coronary artery disease, CH = cholestyramine, CHOL = mean cholesterol (mg/dL), CIRC = circulation studied, CO = colestipol, EVR = excised vascular ring, FLUVA = fluvastatin, GEM = gemfibrozil, INTERV = study intervention, LO = lovastatin, NIA = niacin, NL = normal, PET = positron emission tomography, PRAVA = pravastatin, PROB = probucol, SIMVA = simvastatin, TG = triglycerides, UNSPEC = unspecified, (+) = improvement, (±) = borderline, (−) = no improvement.

dothelial function, a phenomenon which appears to be caused by free radical release and can be reversed by antioxidant vitamins and ACE inhibitors (172,174,178–181). Improvements in endothelium-dependent vasodilatation have been demonstrated with antioxidant vitamins (consistently with vitamin C, inconsistently with vitamin E or combinations), B-complex vitamins, and estrogen and ACE inhibitor administration (169,173,175). Antioxidant vitamin administration has also been shown to reduce the endothelial expression of monocyte adhesion molecules in smokers (171).

Cholesterol Pathway

Cholesterol deposition (predominantly from LDL) and modification is the second major process initiating atherosclerosis (121,122,125,126). Initially, LDL passes through the endothelial barrier by a process termed transcytosis. This process is accelerated by increased serum LDL and endothelial injury. HDL accomplishes reverse cholesterol transport, and exerts an antioxidant effect (129). With time, intimal LDL undergoes progressive modification through oxidation, glycosylation, and acetylation. Macrocytes, endothelial cells, and smooth muscle cells are the likely sources of LDL oxidation. Minimally modified LDL is a potent inhibitor of endothelial function. Maximally modified LDL is recognized as foreign material by macrophages and taken up by the unregulated scavenger receptors, creating metabolically active foam cells. These express a number of growth factors and cytokines which induce smooth muscle cell migration, proliferation, and matrix generation, leading to the formation of complex atheroma. Remodeling of the vessel wall in the form of abluminal dilation occurs in the majority of plaques during the development of early atherosclerosis, reducing luminal compromise. The adaptive mechanism is reduced in patients with diabetes and possibly in those with hypertension or reduced HDL. Eventually, expansion of the atheroma exceeds this locally variable compensatory mechanism, leading to luminal narrowing (120,133).

Plaque Disruption

Cardiovascular events usually occur as a consequence of disruption or ulceration of "vulnerable" atheromas (122,123,125,130,131). Hypercholesterolemia and cigarette smoking have been shown to be directly associated with plaque disruption and ulceration, respectively (134,137). Plaque disruption is associated with variable degrees of intramural hemorrhage and luminal thrombosis. Incomplete luminal thrombosis may produce accelerated or unstable angina. Complete thrombosis may produce myocardial infarction if inadequate collaterals are present. Intramural hemorrhage and luminal thrombosis are important mechanisms for rapid progression of stenosis severity (124). Vulnerable plaques tend to be eccentric and have large, soft (cholesterol ester), coalescent lipid pools, thin fibrous caps, and reduced internal plaque collagen (130,131). High concentrations of T-lymphocytes, foam and mast cells, and cytokines have been identified in the region of plaque rupture, suggesting an inflammatory mechanism (140). This process is often localized to the "shoulder" region of the plaque at the intersection of the atheroma and normal vessel wall. Through the elaboration of interferon-gamma, T-lymphocytes may suppress smooth muscle cell proliferation and induce foam cells to digest internal plaque collagen through the secretion of metalloproteinases (130). These factors are predominantly responsible for plaque instability. The effectiveness of aspirin in secondary prevention may be, in part, due to its anti-inflammatory properties (139). In contrast to plaque morphology (histologic and angiographic "complexity"), stenosis severity correlates poorly with vulnerability to plaque disruption (68–70,78,134). The most severe stenosis is often not the site of plaque rupture, which usually occurs in intermediate-grade stenoses. High-grade stenoses are often associated with collaterals and progress to total occlusion without accompanying myocardial infarction. Angiographic "complex" stenoses demonstrate more progression and are associated with acute ischemic events more commonly than smooth lesions (78).

Plaque Stabilization

In addition to improving endothelial function, cholesterol lowering stabilizes plaques by decreasing plaque inflammation and foam cell number and activity and by increasing plaque collagen matrix (71,75,130). Normalization of diet in cholesterol-fed monkeys reduces macrophage number, increases collagen, and depletes and hardens plaque lipids, resulting in a smaller, stiffer atheroma and larger lumen. These changes theoretically reduce plaque vulnerability to disruption. In contrast to experimental studies, only modest degrees of regression have been observed with clinical cholesterol lowering (Table 2), although the rate of disease progression is considerably reduced (71,72,75). It is likely that this reduced disease progression is associated with plaque stabilization because of the associated marked reduction in the incidence of cardiovascular events (73,78,82,83).

Disruption of lipid-rich plaques with ensuing intramural hemorrhage and luminal thrombosis accounts for 55% to 85% of acute ischemic events (119,122–124,131,137). A second mechanism is thrombosis on superficial erosions of proteoglycan-rich and smooth muscle cell-rich plaques lacking a lipid core (134,137). These lesions are more often seen in younger individuals, smokers, and women, and are associated with less luminal narrowing, calcification, macrophages, and T lymphocytes. For both plaque disruption and superficial erosions, the extent of luminal thrombosis depends on intramural concentrations of tissue factor and systemic factors, including Lp(a), platelet aggregability, fibrinogen, and other procoagulants. Cholesterol lowering has been shown to decrease thrombogenicity and platelet adhesion to denuded endothelium (24,25,32–34).

CLINICAL STUDIES

The landmark Framingham Heart (3,5), Seven Countries (2,8), and MRFIT (12) studies firmly established that hypercholesterolemia was a major risk

Table 2 Angiographic Changes and Clinical Cardiovascular Event Reductions in the Randomized Placebo-Controlled Cholesterol-Lowering Studies

Trial	Angiographic change		% Event reduction
	Treated pts.	Control pts.	
NHLBI (37,38)	32%/7%[a]	49%/7%[a]	33
CLAS I (40)	+0.35%DS	+2.65%DS	25
FATS (41)	−0.8%DS[b]	+2.1%DS	75
SCOR (42)	−1.5%DS	+0.8%DS	(0/1)
LHT (43,66)	−3.1%DS	+5.4%DS	44
POSCH (44)	55/6[a]	85/4[b]	35
Heidelberg (45)	28%/39%[a]	33%/6%[a]	27
STARS (46)	−1.5%DS[b]	+5.8%DS	75
CLAS II (47)	−0.05 mm IMT	+0.05 mm IMT	43
MARS (48)	+1.6%DS	+2.2%DS	24
HARP (49)	−0.14 mm	−0.15	33
MAAS (50)	+0.9%DS	+3.6%DS	22
SCRIP (51,57)	+0.3%DS	+0.9%DS	50
CCAIT (52)	+1.66%DS	+2.89%DS	25
PLAC I (54)	+0.67%DS	+1.11%DS	38
PLAC II (55)	+0.059 mm/yr IMT	+0.068 mm/yr IMT	60
ACAPS (56)	−0.009 mm IMT	+0.006 mm IMT	64
KAPS (58)	+0.017 mm/yr IMT	+0.031 mm/yr IMT	40
REGRESS (59)	+1.10%DS	+3.26%DS	42
BECAIT (60)	+1.70%DS	+4.25%DS	77
CIS (63)	−0.20 mm MLD	−0.58 mm MLD	21
LCAS (64)	−0.028 mm MLD	−0.100 mm MLD	24
LOCAT (65)	−0.04 mm MLD	−0.09 mm MLD	0

%DS = percent diameter stenosis, IMT = intima-media thickness, MLD = minimal lumen diameter.

[a]Patients with progression/patients with regression.

[b]Mean of two treatment groups.

factor for cardiovascular morbidity and mortality. The Lipid Research Clinics Coronary Primary Prevention (93,94) and Helsinki Heart (95) trials demonstrated significant reductions in cardiac events with cholesterol lowering in healthy subjects. Initially in 1987, and revised in 1993, the Adult Treatment Panel of the National Cholesterol Education Program (NCEP) (211,212) published guidelines on testing and treating hypercholesterolemic patients which outlined a more aggressive approach to cholesterol lowering than was then in practice (203). During the late 1980s and early 1990s, several angiographic trials demonstrated reduced progression of coronary artery disease using lifestyle, drug, and surgical means for reducing cholesterol (37–67). The later trials commonly employed HMG-CoA reductase inhibitors ("statins") reflecting their increasing clinical usage. Although these trials demonstrated statistically significant but modest anatomical benefit associated with cholesterol lowering, on average 48% reductions in major cardiovascular event rates were observed (Table 2) (15–21,71,75,107, 108,114,115). Since 1994, six large cardiovascular event trials (Scandinavian Simvastatin Survival Study [97–102], West of Scotland Coronary Prevention Study [103], Cholesterol and Recurrent Events Trial [104,105,110,111,116], Long-Term Intervention with Pravastatin in Ischemic Disease [113], Air Force Coronary Atherosclerosis Prevention Study/Texas Coronary Atherosclerosis Prevention Study [109], and Veterans Affairs HDL Intervention Trial [118]), a large aggressive versus moderate cholesterol lowering angiographic trial (Post-CABG Trial [62]), and a small aggressive versus usual cholesterol lowering event trial (Atorvastatin vs. Revascularization Trial [117]) have reported that aggressive cholesterol lowering reduces both cardiovascular morbidity and mortality, largely substantiating the NCEP guidelines.

Primary Prevention Trials

The strongest evidence that cholesterol is causally related to the development of coronary heart disease is derived from randomized, controlled primary and secondary prevention clinical trials. The Lipid Research Clinics Coronary Primary Prevention Trial (LRC-CPPT) (92,93) studied 3806 middle-aged men (35 to 59 years) without symptomatic coronary heart disease but with total cholesterol >265 mg/dL. During the 7-year trial, cholestyramine 24 g daily decreased total cholesterol 13% and LDL cholesterol 20%. Definite coronary heart disease death occurred in 155 treated men and 187 control men (19% difference). Significant reductions were observed in angina (20%), positive exercise tests (25%), surgical revascularization (21%), and congestive heart failure (28%). The study found that cardiovascular events are reduced about 2% for every 1% reduction in cholesterol.

The Helsinki Heart Study (94), randomized 4081 middle-aged (40 to 55 years) men with non-HDL cholesterol >200 mg/dL. Gemfibrozil 600 mg twice daily resulted in decreases in total cholesterol (8%), LDL cholesterol (8%), and triglycerides (35%) and an increase in HDL cholesterol (10%). The treated population experienced 34% fewer cardiovascular events in this 5-year trial. In both the LRC-CPPT and the Helsinki Heart Study, no differences were observed in all-cause mortality.

More recently, two primary prevention trials employed HMG-CoA reductase inhibitors. The West of Scotland Coronary Prevention Study (103) randomized 6695 men between the ages of 45 and 64 years with LDL-cholesterol >155 mg/dL to either pravastatin 40 mg daily or placebo. Associated with the reductions in total cholesterol (20%) and LDL cholesterol (26%), the primary endpoint, coronary heart disease mortality and nonfatal myocardial infarction, was reduced 31%. All-cause mortality, which fell 22% (P = .51), became statistically significant (P = .39) after adjustment for baseline risk factors.

Most recently, the Air Force Coronary Atherosclerosis Prevention Study/Texas Coronary Atherosclerosis Prevention Study (109) randomized 6605 healthy, middle-aged men and women with HDL cholesterol <50 mg/dL, LDL cholesterol 130 to 190 mg/dL, and an increased LDL cholesterol to HDL cholesterol level to lovastatin in stepwise dose to achieve LDL cholesterol <110 mg/dL versus placebo. This 5-year study demonstrated a 36% reduction in death, myocardial infarction, or hospital admission for unstable angina (162 vs. 105, $P < .001$), which was evident by the end of the first year of the trial. Subsequent analysis has shown 45% and 44% risk reductions in those with HDL cholesterol <35 mg/dL and 35 to 39 mg/dL, respectively, suggesting that healthy individuals with HDL cholesterol <40 mg/dL and LDL cholesterol >130 mg/dL benefit from treatment with an HMG-CoA reductase inhibitor. The majority of such individuals would not require treatment under the 1993 NCEP guidelines, and the vast majority are not currently receiving treatment.

Angiographic Trials

During the past two decades, 23 randomized, controlled trials have investigated whether cholesterol lowering was associated with reduced rates of angiographic or ultrasonic progression of coronary or carotid atherosclerosis, respectively (Table 2) (37–67). Cholesterol reduction in these trials was achieved by widely differing regimens including low-fat diet (LHT [43,66], STARS [46]), exercise (Heidelberg [45]), single drug (NHLBI type II [37,38], MARS [48], STARS [46], MAAS [50], CCAIT [52], PLAC I [54], PLAC II [55], ACAPS [56], KAPS [58], REGRESS [59], BECAIT [60], CIS [63], LCAS [64], LOCAT [65]), multiple drugs (CLAS I [40], FATS [41], SCOR [42], CLAS II [47], HARP [49], SCRIP [51,57], LCAS [64]), and partial ileal bypass surgery (POSCH [44]). Later trials consistently employed quantitative coronary arteriography and more commonly employed HMG-CoA reductase inhibitors reflecting their widespread clinical use (MARS, MAAS, CCAIT, PLAC I, PLAC II, REGRESS, CAPS, ACAPS, CIS, LCAS). Trials ranged from 1 to 10 years in duration and enrolled from 43 to 838 patients. All but one of the trials (HARP), undertaken in patients with the lowest cholesterol, demonstrated angiographic improvement in those randomized to lipid lowering in the form of less disease progression, more stability of existing lesions, fewer new lesions, fewer progressions to total occlusion, and/or more disease regression than in the control group. Although absolute differences in coronary luminal dimensions between the treatment and control groups were found to be significant but small, on average this represented a 50% to 75% relative reduction in disease progression. The reduction in disease progression was associated with substantial decreases in cardiovascular events. Seven trials (LHT, FATS, STARS, SCOR, Heidelberg, CLAS II, ACAPS) demonstrated an average minimal reduction in percent diameter stenosis or intima-media thickness. Although this finding suggests disease regression, the angiographic trials provided data only on luminal dimensions and were unable to provide data on changes in plaque volume. Preliminary intravascular ultrasound data suggest that cholesterol lowering reduces atherosclerosis plaque area, even if luminal diameter is not increased. A large angiographic trial (REVERSAL) using intravascular ultrasound is under way to test this observation.

The angiographic trials have provided important information on which patients benefit from cholesterol lowering. There was a trend for more angiographic benefit from cholesterol lowering in those studies with higher initial cholesterol levels (79,112), although this correlation was primarily driven by the results of the very positive STARS trial (46) and the negative HARP trial (19). In contrast, three retrospectively evaluated studies (CLAS [40], FATS [41], MARS [48]) failed to show differences between those subjects with higher or lower initial total or LDL-cholesterol levels, although all three studied very hypercholesterolemic individuals. Similar results were obtained in the Scandinavian Simvastatin Survival Study (97–102), but the Cholesterol and Recurrent Events Study (104,105,110,111,116) found no risk reduction in those subjects with LDL cholesterol levels initially <125 mg/dL. Overall, the angiographic trials demonstrated less disease progression with lower on-treatment LDL cholesterol levels (Fig. 2) (112). This finding is strongly supported by the results of the Post-CABG trial, which compared on-treatment LDL cholesterol of 95 and 135 mg/dL (see below). The angiographic trials generally that found disease progression correlated more closely with high initial levels of triglyceride-rich particles (elevated triglycerides, IDL, apo C-III, and/or decreased HDL) than with initial LDL levels (72,74,82,83,91). These patients tend to have small, dense LDL particles which is associated with insulin resistance, truncal obesity, and hypertension (236,237,240). More treatment-induced reduction in disease progression was also observed in patients with small, dense LDL and/or low HDL cholesterol (91). The Scandinavian Simvastatin Survival Study also found greater event reductions in initially hypertriglyceridemic patients, but the Cholesterol and Recurrent Events Trial did not. In contrast to most other

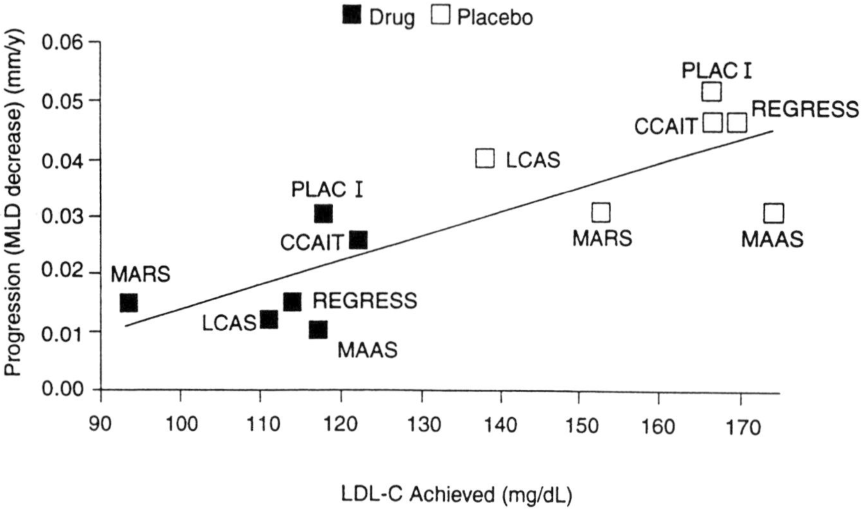

Figure 2 Association between on-treatment LDL cholesterol and progression of coronary artery disease in angiographic trials. (From Ref. 112.)

trials, the latter study found greater event risk in subjects with large, buoyant LDL, perhaps reflecting a somewhat different etiology of the atherosclerosis in these borderline hypercholesterolemic individuals. Importantly, disease progression tended to predict cardiovascular events, reinforcing the concept that events are associated with plaque disruption and that cholesterol lowering stabilizes plaques (73,78,82,83).

Secondary Prevention Trials

Scandinavian Simvastatin Survival Study (4S)

Although earlier event and angiographic secondary prevention trials had demonstrated reductions in cardiovascular events, cholesterol lowering had not been clearly shown to reduce all-cause mortality. This question was addressed in the 4S study (97–102). The 4S study enrolled 4444 men (81%) and women, aged 35 to 70 years with prior myocardial infarction (79%) and/or angina, initial cholesterol levels 213 to 310 mg/dL, and triglycerides <200 mg/dL. Simvastatin was administered at 20 or 40 mg/day with the intent to lower cholesterol below 200 mg/dL. Over the 5.4-year mean follow-up period, simvastatin lowered mean cholesterol from 260 to 189 mg/dL (−25%). A 30% reduction in all-cause mortality was observed (182 vs. 256 deaths, $P = .0003$). Significant reductions were also observed in myocardial infarction, need for coronary angioplasty or bypass surgery, stroke or transient ischemic attack, and hospitalizations. Benefit was generally demonstrated in all subgroups. Although all-cause mortality was not reduced in women, probably due to the smaller subgroup size, total cardiovascular events were reduced to the same extent in both sexes. Of all the subgroups studied, diabetic patients received the greatest relative and absolute benefit (55% risk reduction). The risk of major cardiovascular events was reduced to the same extent at all initial cholesterol levels. Patients with either higher triglyceride and/or lower HDL cholesterol levels appeared to derive more benefit. Both the magnitude of LDL cholesterol decrease and on treatment LDL cholesterol levels correlated with decrease in mortality.

Hospitalizations for acute cardiovascular events or coronary revascularization were reduced from 1905 (average duration 7.9 days) in the placebo group to 1403 (average duration 7.1 days) in the simvastatin group (100,101). The corresponding number of hospital days was 15,089 and 9951, respectively (−34%). Cost-benefit analysis suggested a $3000 to $10,000 cost per year of life saved (100,101,105,106). In comparison, primary prevention is less cost-effective, with substantial variations dependent on whether individuals are high or low risk (106).

Cholesterol and Recurrent Events (CARE) Study

The majority of coronary heart disease patients in the United States have "borderline" elevated cholesterol levels (mean 225 mg/dL), leading to the incorrect impression that they would not benefit from cholesterol lowering. The CARE study (104,105,110,111,116) was designed to determine the value of cholesterol lowering (pravastatin 40 mg/day) in 4159 men (86%) and women with a prior myocardial infarction and "average" cholesterol, i.e., <240 mg/dL. Mean lipid values for the patients studied were total cholesterol 209 mg/dL, LDL cholesterol 139 mg/dL, HDL cholesterol 39 mg/dL, and triglycerides 155 mg/dL. This mean cholesterol is almost equal to the American average (208 mg/dL). Pravastatin reduced total and LDL cholesterol by 20% and 32%, respectively. Over the 5 years of the trial, the primary endpoint, coronary heart disease mortality and nonfatal myocardial infarction, was reduced from 274 in the control group to 212 in the pravastatin group (−24%, $P = .003$). As in the 4S study, the need for coronary angioplasty or bypass surgery, episodes of unstable angina, and stroke were also reduced (13% to 31%).

Benefit from cholesterol lowering was observed in all subgroups except those with initial LDL cholesterol <125 mg/dL (851 patients). There was, however, equal benefit in the groups with initial cholesterol above and below the mean (209 mg/dL). These contrasting observations combined with the small number of patients at the lowest LDL cholesterol level leave in doubt whether patients with established disease and LDL cholesterol <125 mg/dL might benefit from HMG-CoA reductase inhibitor therapy. Almost statistically significant ($P = .06$), more reduction in the primary endpoint was observed in women (−46%) compared with men (−20%). Unlike the results of the 4S study, less reduction in cardiovascular endpoints was observed in those with higher initial triglycerides and event risk was increased in subjects with large, buoyant LDL. The CARE trial results extend the important observations of the 4S study to the majority of coronary heart disease patients in the United States, including women.

Long-Term Intervention with Pravastatin in Ischemic Disease (LIPID) Trial

The third large secondary prevention trial, LIPID (113), conducted in Australia and New Zealand, enrolled 9014 men and women with cholesterol 155 to 271 mg/dL. Treatment with pravastatin 40 mg/day reduced the primary endpoint coronary heart disease mortality 24%, $P < .001$. As observed in the other secondary prevention trials, stroke risk was reduced 19% (28,115). In the LIPID trial, risk reduction was determined in prespecified tertiles of initial cholesterol. Although the lowest tertile trended to less risk reduction, the trend did not reach statistical significance, and a similar reduction in progression of carotid intima-media thickness was observed in all initial cholesterol tertiles. The three secondary prevention trials demonstrate a continuous reduction in cardiovascular events with cholesterol lowering to <100 mg/dL (Fig. 3).

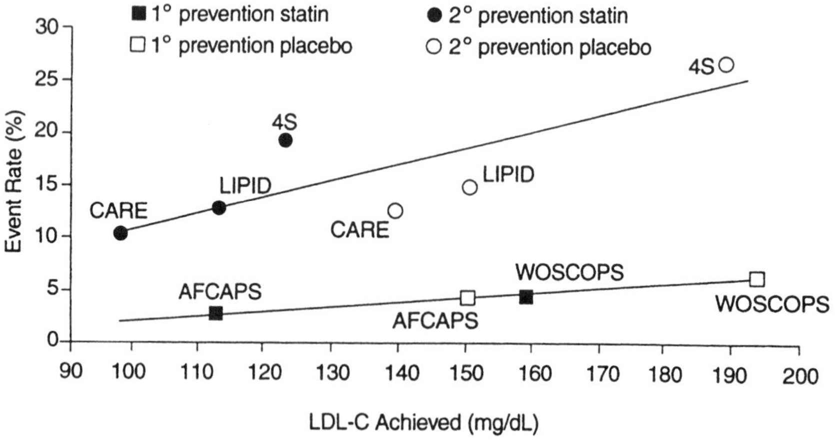

Figure 3 Association between on-treatment LDL cholesterol and cardiovascular events in the recent primary and secondary prevention trials. (From Ref. 112.)

Post-CABG Trial

Although the 4S and CARE trials demonstrated clear benefits in secondary-prevention populations over a wide range of initial cholesterol levels, they were not intended to assess the benefit afforded by different degrees of cholesterol lowering. The Post-CABG trial (62,67) was designed to address this issue. Predominantly an angiographic trial, it compared disease progression in 1351 men (92%) and women who had undergone prior bypass surgery in a 2×2 factorial design trial of moderate versus aggressive cholesterol lowering and low-dose warfarin versus placebo administration. The moderate cholesterol lowering group received a mean of 4 mg lovastatin daily resulting in a mean LDL cholesterol of 135 mg/dL and the aggressive cholesterol lowering group received a mean of 76 mg of lovastatin daily (30% also took cholestyramine 8 g/day) resulting in a mean LDL cholesterol of 95 mg/dL. By a composite angiographic index, the aggressive cholesterol lowering group had less bypass graft disease progression than the moderate treatment group over 4 years. No benefit was observed in the low-dose warfarin group. Preliminary long-term data suggest that cardiovascular event risk was reduced 25% ($P < .01$). This was the first trial to document an additional benefit for an aggressive treatment program designed to meet the National Cholesterol Education Program's (NCEP) (211,212) recommendations for lowering LDL cholesterol to <100 mg/dL in patients with coronary heart disease.

Atorvastatin Versus Revascularization Trial (AVERT)

The findings of the Post-CABG trial were substantiated by the AVERT trial (117) which compared aggressive cholesterol reduction (atorvastatin 80 mg/day) to usual cholesterol reduction and angioplasty in 341 coronary heart disease subjects with stable mild angina. Atorvastatin reduced LDL cholesterol from 144 to 77 mg/dL and the usual cholesterol lowering regimen from 147 to 119 mg/dL (higher than NCEP recommendations). The primary composite clinical endpoint was reduced 36% in the aggressive treatment group, mostly due to reduced hospitalizations for unstable angina, $P = .048$ (prespecified trial significance 0.045 because of two interim analyses). Time to first event was significantly reduced ($P < .03$). Although the AVERT trial supports the findings of the other secondary prevention studies regarding aggressive cholesterol lowering, a possible adverse effect of elective angioplasty in the usual cholesterol lowering group complicates the interpretation of this study.

Veterans Affairs HDL Intervention Trial (VA-HIT)

In distinction to the HMG-CoA reductase inhibitor secondary prevention trials, the VA-HIT trial (118) investigated coronary heart disease patients with

HDL cholesterol <40 mg/dL (mean 32 mg/dL), but with LDL cholesterol <140 mg/dL (mean 111 mg/dL). The mean total cholesterol of the 2531 male, <75-year-old cohort was 175 mg/dL, the lowest of any trial to date. Gemfibrozil 600 mg twice daily increased HDL cholesterol 8%, reduced triglycerides 25%, but did not change LDL cholesterol. The latter is unique among the secondary prevention trials. The primary endpoint coronary heart disease mortality and nonfatal myocardial infarction was reduced 22% (P = .006). Stroke and carotid endarterectomy were also reduced significantly. Risk reduction correlated with increase in HDL cholesterol, but not with triglyceride reduction (mean initial triglycerides 161 mg/dL). The VA-HIT trial underscores the value of increasing HDL cholesterol in coronary heart disease patients with isolated low HDL cholesterol.

TREATMENT GOALS

The NCEP Adult Treatment Panel recomendations (211,212) are based on measurements of LDL and HDL cholesterol and triglycerides which require fasting conditions. Patient management is divided into three categories based on the presence of coronary risk factors and established cardiovascular disease. The highest treatment priority is given to those patients with established disease for whom LDL cholesterol should be reduced to <100 mg/dL. The American Diabetic Association now includes diabetic patients in this highest risk group. Those individuals without cardiovascular disease but with multiple risk factors (men >45 years, women >55 years, smoking, hypertension, diabetes mellitus, HDL cholesterol <35 mg/dL, family history of premature cardiovascular disease) should have LDL cholesterol reduced to <130 mg/dL (intermediate risk). An HDL cholesterol >60 mg/dL is considered a negative risk factor. Those individuals without established cardiovascular disease or multiple risk factors (low risk) should maintain an LDL cholesterol <160 mg/dL. The 1993 Adult Treatment Panel also recommends achieving an HDL cholesterol >35 mg/dL, especially if LDL cholesterol and/or triglycerides are elevated. Triglycerides >200 mg/dL is considered borderline, and >400 mg/dL considered high. Based on the recent trials, desirable lipoproteins can be considered <100 and <115 mg/dL for LDL cholesterol in coronary heart disease and high-risk healthy individuals, and >40 mg/dL for HDL cholesterol (Table 3).

Dietary Treatment

Before patient management is undertaken, secondary causes of hypercholesterolemia should be excluded (hypothyroidism, diabetes mellitus, pregnancy, nephrotic syndrome, obstructive hepatic disease, dysproteinemias, an-

Table 3 1993 National Cholesterol Education Program Recommendations vs. 1999 Evidence-Based Desirable Lipoprotein Levels

	1993 NCEP (211)	1999 Evidence-based (62,109,117,118)
LDL-C, CAD, CVD, DM	<100 mg/dL	<100 mg/dL
≥2 risk factors:	<130 mg/dL	<115 mg/dL
HDL-C	>35 mg/dL	>40 mg/dL

CAD = coronary artery disease, CVD = cardiovascular disease, DM = diabetes mellitus, HDL-C = high-density cholesterol, LDL-C = low-density cholesterol.

orexia, porphyria, and use of progestins, anabolic steroids, corticosteroids, diuretics, and beta-blockers) (9,211,212). Most Westernized individuals have elevated cholesterol levels because of excess saturated fat and calorie intake, and inadequate physical activity levels. Some Westernized societies, however, have particularly low rates of coronary heart disease. Examples include the Pacific Rim which consumes a low-fat diet and the Mediterranean region which consumes a high monounsaturated fat, fruit, and vegetable diet. Low total fat, low saturated fat, and Mediterranean diets have been shown to reduce the progression of coronary disease and cardiovascular events (8,43,45,46,202,205,209,215,222–225,228,234,238,239). Dietary saturated fat reduces the activity of hepatic LDL receptors, dietary cholesterol reduces their production, and obesity leads to an overproduction of lipoproteins. Dietary therapy remains the cornerstone of cholesterol reduction in primary prevention (especially for low-risk individuals [211,212]) and is an important addition to drug therapy in secondary prevention. In addition to improving cholesterol levels, appropriate diet can achieve weight loss and improve blood pressure, hyperglycemia, and insulin resistance.

Replacing saturated fat with monounsaturated and polyunsaturated fats reduces serum total and LDL cholesterol, and the latter may also decrease HDL cholesterol. In general, reductions in dietary saturated fat and calories are more effective in lowering cholesterol than is reducing dietary cholesterol. Although effective in reducing cholesterol, a high-carbohydrate diet may actually increase triglycerides. In addition to increases in cholesterol, some high-fat foods also directly impair endothelial function through an oxidative stress mechanism in a manner similar to hypercholesterolemia and smoking (172,174,178–180). This may explain the benefit of high dietary intake of antioxidants in the form of flavanoid-rich fruits and vegetables observed in the Seven Countries study (8).

The physician plays a pivotal role in suggesting and reinforcing dietary modification, but implementation is greatly assisted by dietitians and/or nurses (203,205,210–213,214,219,221,226). The most important change from the average American diet, consisting of 37% of calories derived from fat, 15% from saturated fat, and 450 mg of cholesterol intake daily, are reductions in saturated fat and total calories (Table 4). Importantly, 30% of American are currently >20% overweight (9). Reduction in saturated fat can be achieved by eating less meat, whole-milk products, tropical oils (palm, coconut), and hydrogenated vegetable oils. Omega-3 fatty acids found in fish and vegetable oils, such as canola oil, have several vascular benefits, including improvements in endothelial function, membrane stabilization, reduction in platelet aggregability, and reductions in triglycerides (177,202, 222–225,228,238,242). One of two angiographic trials has demonstrated a reduction in disease progression with administration of fish oil (80,89). The GISSI study group recently reported a 20% decrease in all-cause mortality with addition of omega-3 fatty acid (1 g/day) in postmyocardial infarction patients (177). Low-glycemic-index, complex carbohydrate intake is strongly encouraged in a heart-healthy diet. Moderate alcohol intake (1 to 2 oz/day) is associated with reduced cardiovascular risk and total mortality compared with either abstinence or heavier intake. Overall mortality is increased with more alcohol consumption, however, because of other alcohol-related diseases, as well as increased hypertension and myocardial dysfunction (9). Regular physical activity decreases weight, LDL cholesterol, triglycerides, and the risk of myocardial infarction and sudden death, and increases HDL cholesterol, cardiovascular conditioning, and a sense of well-being.

In contrast to the generally prudent recommendations of the NCEP, which produce approximately 5% reductions in cholesterol, the Mediterranean diet rich in fruits, vegetables, fish, pasta, and wine appears to offer a substantial advantage in reducing cardiovascular risk (222–225,228,238). The Lyon Diet Heart Trial demonstrated a 70% reduction in cardiovascular events and mortality with the following dietary advice: more bread, fruits, vegetables, and beans; less meat and whole-milk dairy products; and use of

Table 4 Drug Effects on Lipoproteins

	Total C	LDL C	HDL C	Triglycerides
HMG-CoA RI	↓20–50%	↓25–60%	↑5–15%	↓10–30%
Bile acid sequestrants	↓10–20%	↓15–30%	↑3–5%	↑5–15%
Fibric acid derivatives	↓0–10%	↓0–15%	↑5–15%	↓20–35%
Nicotinic acid	↓10–20%	↓15–25%	↑10–30%	↓15–30%

C = cholesterol, HDL-C = high-density cholesterol, LDL-C = low-density cholesterol, HMG-CoA RI = 3-hydroxy-3-methylglutaryl-coenzyme A reductase inhibitor.

omega-3-enriched canola oil. An alternative approach is the very low fat diet (Pritikin, Ornish) (43,66) containing approximately 10% of calories from fat. Fewer long-term data is available of these diets, but small angiographic trials have reported angiographic disease regression. Although scientifically sound, few patients and physicians are willing and/or able to implement these diets.

Drug Treatment

Drug treatment of hypercholesterolemia is generally more effective than dietary treatment (9,209,230). Drug therapy may be postponed in low-risk primary prevention patients for at least 6 months to allow patients to modify their diet. In contrast, secondary prevention and high-risk primary prevention patients should be begun on both drug and dietary therapy as soon as hypercholesterolemia is identified (244). Cholesterol-modifying drugs can generally be divided into two classes—those which predominantly lower LDL cholesterol (HMG-CoA reductase inhibitors or "statins," and bile acid sequestrants), and those which predominantly lower triglycerides and increase HDL cholesterol (nicotinic acid and fibric acid derivatives) (9,208,220,235, 248,251). HMG-CoA reductase inhibitors secondarily increase HDL cholesterol and lower triglycerides (Table 4). Higher doses of HMG-CoA reductase inhibitors are more effective in lowering triglycerides in hypertriglyceridemic subjects and in increasing HDL cholesterol in low-HDL cholesterol subjects. In contrast, bile acid sequestrants may increase triglycerides, as can a high-carbohydrate diet, alcohol, and estrogen. In addition to their triglyceride-lowering, HDL cholesterol-raising effects, nicotinic acid and fibric acid derivatives lower LDL cholesterol (especially nicotinic acid in higher doses).

LDL Cholesterol

A general approach to drug therapy is shown in Table 5. In determining drug therapy, the physician should first set goals for LDL and HDL cholesterol and triglycerides depending on patient risk as recommended by the NCEP (211,212,220,251). Drug therapy should not be initiated until the lipid abnormality is verified on repeat determination. Determinations of LDL cholesterol require a fasting blood sample, and transient reductions occur with myocardial infarctions, acute illnesses, and hospitalizations (231). The majority of coronary artery disease patients will have an elevated LDL cholesterol (91% in a prospective study). HMG-CoA reductase inhibitors are the agents of first choice for elevated LDL cholesterol because of their high effectiveness (25% to 60% LDL cholesterol lowering) and infrequent side effects (208,220,235,251). This drug class inhibits the hepatic synthesis of cholesterol, which increases the expression of hepatic LDL receptors. At

Table 5 Suggested Drug Treatment for Dyslipidemias

High LDL-C	1. HMG-CoA RI
	2. HMG-CoARI + BAS
Low HDL-C	
With lower LDL-C	1. Fibric acid derivative
	2. Nicotinic acid
With higher LDL-C	1. HMG-CoA RI
	2. Nicotinic acid
High triglycerides	1. Fibric acid derivative
	2. Nicotinic acid
	3. HMG-CoA RI
Mixed dyslipidemia	1. HMG-CoA R + fibric acid derivative
	2. HMG-CoA RI + nicotinic acid

BAS = bile acid sequestrant, HMG-CoA RI = 3-hydroxy-3-methylglutaryl-coenzyme A reductase inhibitor.

present, six HMG-CoA reductase inhibitors are available in the United States: atorvastatin, cerivastatin, fluvastatin, lovastatin, pravastatin, and simvastatin. In general, doubling a dose of an HMG-CoA reductase inhibitor will lower LDL cholesterol an additional 6% to 7%. HMG-CoA reductase inhibitors are usually given once a day in the evening, since most cholesterol is synthesized at night. Dividing the HMG-CoA reductase inhibitors into twice-a-day doses adds 2% to 4% cholesterol lowering (atorvastatin should be given only once a day at any time). After initiating an HMG-CoA reductase inhibitor, a lipid panel should be repeated in about 6 weeks and diet modification should again be emphasized at this time. If the LDL cholesterol goal is not reached, a more effective drug and/or higher dose should be instituted. After reaching a high dose of an effective HMG-CoA reductase inhibitor, a bile acid sequestrant may be added to the regimen if the goal is not reached. Up to 70% reductions in LDL cholesterol are expected with current drug therapy except in those patients with absent or defective LDL receptors (familial hypercholesterolemia).

HMG-CoA reductase inhibitors are generally well-tolerated drugs. Infrequently, hepatocellular injury or myositis occurs. HMG-CoA reductase inhibitors commonly produce minimal elevations in liver function tests and should not be discontinued unless values exceed three times normal upper limit. Increased alcohol intake should also be considered if abnormal liver function tests are observed. Hepatic dysfunction is reversible after drug discontinuation, and a lesser dose or another agent may be tried. Myositis (diffuse muscle pain and weakness) with markedly elevated CPKs (>10 times upper normal limit) rarely occurs with HMG-CoA reductase inhibitors, although the frequency rises with concomitant use of gemfibrozil, nicotinic acid, immunosuppressives, erythromycin, and antifungals. In the extreme, rhabdomyolysis associated with renal failure rarely occurs. Some patients report myalgias without elevated CPK while on HMG-CoA reductase inhibitors, which probably does not warrant drug discontinuation.

Bile acid sequestrants (cholestyramine, colestipol) increase cholesterol excretion by binding bile acids in the intestine during enterohepatic recirculation (9,220,251). These agents lower LDL cholesterol about 25% when used in maximum dose (24 to 30 g/d). Gastrointestinal side effects are common, including constipation, bloating, and flatulence. Lower doses (8 to 12 g divided daily) are better tolerated. These agents may also interfere with the absorption of other drugs, including coumadin and other cholesterol-lowering agents. Patients should be advised to take other drugs >1 hour before or 4 to 5 hours after taking sequestrants.

HDL Cholesterol

The second most frequent lipid abnormality, a low HDL cholesterol (<35 to 40 mg/dL), is present in at least 56% of coronary disease patients. HDL cholesterol is primarily responsible for reverse cholesterol transport, and its level generally varies inversely with triglycerides (9). The ratio of LDL to HDL cholesterol correlates well with coronary heart disease risk for total cholesterol levels above 150 mg/dL (201,207,218). Larger HDL particles with predominately apo AI are most antiatherogeic (87,88). Non-Westernized societies usually have both low LDL and low HDL cholesterol. HDL cholesterol is increased by exercise, alcohol, smoking cessation, estrogen, and weight loss (9). A low-fat diet and anabolic steroids lower HDL cholesterol, although the former is useful for LDL cholesterol reduction.

Drugs are generally not as effective in increasing HDL cholesterol as they are in lowering LDL cholesterol (9,220,251). Increasing a low HDL cholesterol is easier to achieve in those with concomitant elevated triglycerides. Nicotinic acid is the most effective HDL cholesterol-raising agent (up to 25%). A delayed (15-year) reduction in all-cause mortality (11%) was observed with nicotinic acid in the Coronary Drug Project (10). The side effects of flushing, headache, dyspepsia, and dry skin are common, especially when initiating the drug or increasing a dose. The use of aspirin reduces flushing. Nicotinic acid toxicity includes gout (elevated uric acid), worsening of diabetes, peptic ulcer disease, and hepatic dysfunction. Patients should be started on a nicotinic acid at a low dose (50 mg BID) and increased slowly to 1.0 to 1.5 g BID. Alternatively, slow-release nicotinic acid preparations can be used, especially using nighttime administration. These are associated with fewer side effects, but are more expensive and may have greater hepatic toxicity.

Fibric acid derivatives (gemfibrozil, fenofibrate) are also useful in increasing HDL cholesterol (~10%) (251) and have been shown to reduce the progression of coronary artery disease and cardiovascular events (BECAIT [60], LOCAT [65], Helsinki Heart Study [95], VA-HIT [118]). The fibric acid derivative clofibrate is still occasionally used to lower triglycerides, but is associated with cholelithiasis and adenocarcinoma. Fibric acid derivatives are generally well-tolerated drugs, but the concomitant use of an HMG-CoA reductase inhibitor and gemfibrozil increases the risk of myositis. Fibric acid derivatives are recommended for coronary heart disease patients with low HDL cholesterol (<40 mg/dL) and low LDL cholesterol (<130 mg/dL) (118,248). Coronary heart disease patients with low HDL cholesterol and elevated LDL cholesterol (>130 mg/dL) should probably be begun on an HMG-CoA reductase inhibitor. Simvastatin has been reported to elevate a low HDL cholesterol up to 17% in such patients.

Triglycerides

Elevated triglycerides are a risk factor for coronary heart disease, especially in women, but the correlation is weakened by adjustment for HDL cholesterol (9). Hypertriglyceridemia, however, strongly predicts cardiovascular events in those with established cardiovascular disease, and hypertriglyceridemic patients derive greater benefit from LDL cholesterol lowering (4S study [97–102]) and HDL cholesterol raising (Helsinki Heart Study [95]). Postprandial rather than fasting hypertriglyceridemia may be more predictive of coronary disease risk (9), and increases in postprandial triglycerides have been shown to correlate with the transient endothelial dysfunction observed after a fatty meal (172,174). The NCEP Adult Treatment Panel considers a fasting triglyceride >200 mg/dL as borderline high, and >400 mg/dL as definitely elevated (211,212). Hypertriglyceridemia is commonly observed in diabetic patients in whom it should be considered a sign of poor control.

Hypertriglyceridemia should be initially managed by exclusion of secondary causes followed by lifestyle modification, including weight reduction, decreased dietary fat and alcohol intake, exercise, and smoking cessation. Estrogen, bile acid sequestrants, and very high carbohydrate diets increase triglycerides (9). Fish oil is effective in reducing triglycerides (20% to 40%) and reduces cardiovascular events (177,202,222–225,228,238,242). Fibric acid derivatives and secondarily nicotinic acid are the most effective drugs in lowering triglycerides (35%) (9,251). HMG-CoA reductase inhibitors also lower elevated triglycerides up to 30% when used in high doses.

Mixed Dyslipidemia

A reduced HDL cholesterol combined with elevated triglycerides is frequently associated with small, dense LDL particles which are particularly atherogenic (87,88,92,236,237,240). Coronary heart disease patients with small, dense LDL appear to derive the greatest benefit from lipid management. Fibric acid derivatives and nicotinic acid are the most effective agents in changing the LDL pattern to larger, buoyant LDL, but HMG-CoA reductase inhibitors decrease the number of both types of LDL particles. Elevated LDL cholesterol associated with low HDL cholesterol and/or elevated triglycerides is most often managed with a combination of an HMG-CoA reductase inhibitor and either nicotinic acid or a fibric acid derivative (208,251). The risk of myositis with combined therapy should be considered, but this is relatively uncommon especially if the HMG-CoA reducatse inhibitor dose is kept low.

TREATMENT GAP

Despite the widespread lay and physician education programs stressing the importance of cholesterol management over the past decade, many patients potentially benefiting from cholesterol lowering remain untreated (9,203, 210,213,219,226,227). Recent surveys of hypercholesterolemic coronary heart disease patients demonstrate that drug treatment is provided to only 14% of those with cholesterol 200 to 240 mg/dL, 41% of those with cholesterol 241 to 300 mg/dL, and 78% of those with cholesterol >300 mg/dL. In essence the first two groups represent the CARE (104) and 4S (97) study populations in which 25% to 40% reductions in cardiovascular event rates were observed. Moreover, a recent survey of community practice (ARIC Study [227]) found that only 4% of coronary disease patients were managed sufficiently to meet the NCEP criterion. Several explanations for this treatment gap have been proposed (9,203,210,219,227), including: lack of belief in the cholesterol hypothesis; confusion regarding guidelines; routine nature of cholesterol treatment; lack of knowledge of lifestyle and drug management; extended reliance on diet treatment; missed communication between generalists and specialists; concerns over adverse effects and/or expense of drug treatment; and poor reimbursement for cholesterol management. Reducing the treatment gap in cholesterol reduction remains one of the most important therapeutic opportunities to improve patient care today.

REFERENCES

1. Anitschkow N. Experimental atherosclerosis in animals. In Cowdry EV (ed): Arteriosclerosis: A Survey of the Problem. New York: Macmillan, 1933;271–322.
2. Keys A, Araranis C, Blackburn H, et al. Epidemiologic studies related to coronary heart disease: characteristics of men aged 40–59 in seven countries. Acta Med Scand 1967;180(suppl 460):1-392.

3. Gordon T, Kannel WB. Premature mortality from coronary heart disease. Framinghan Heart Study. JAMA 1971;215:1617–1625.
4. AHA Committee Report. Risk factors and coronary heart disease. A statement for physicians. Circulation 1980;62:449A–455A.
5. Anderson M, Castelli WP, Levy D. Cholesterol and mortality: 30 years of follow-up from the Framingham Study. JAMA 1987;257:2176–2180.
6. Joseph A, Ackerman D, Talley D, et al. Manifestations of coronary atherosclerosis in young trauma victims: an autopsy study. J Am Coll Cardiol 1993; 22:459–469.
7. Thaulow E, Erikssen J, Sansvik L, et al. Initial presentation of cardiac disease in asymptomatic men with silent myocardial ischemia and angiographically documented coronary artery disease (the Oslo Ischemia Study). Am J Cardiol 1993;72:629–633.
8. Verschuren WMM, Jacobs DR, Bloemberg BPM, et al. Serum total cholesterol and long-term coronary heart disease mortality in different cultures. Twenty-five year follow-up of the Seven Countries Study. JAMA 1995;274:131–136.
9. Miller M, Vogel R. The Practice of Coronary Disease Prevention. Baltimore: Williams and Wilkins, 1996.
10. Holme I. An analysis of randomized trials evaluating the effect of cholesterol reduction on total mortality and coronary heart disease incidence. Circulation 1990;82:1916–1924.
11. Rossouw J, Lewis B, Rifkind BM. The value of lowering cholesterol after myocardial infarction. N Engl J Med 1990;323:1112–1119.
12. Multiple Risk Factor Intervention Trial Research Group. Mortality rates after 10.5 years for participants in the Multiple Risk Factor Intervention Trial. Findings related to a priori hypothesis of the trial. JAMA 1990;263:1795–1801.
13. Vogel RA. Comparative clinical consequences of aggressive lipid management, coronary angioplasty and bypass surgery in coronary disease. Am J Cardiol 1992;69:1229–1233.
14. Manson JE, Tosteson H, Ridker PM, et al. Medical progress: the primary prevention of myocardial infarction. N Engl J Med 1992;326:1406–1416.
15. LaRosa JC, Cleeman JI. Cholesterol lowering as a treatment for established coronary heart disease. Circulation 1992;85:1229–1235.
16. LaRosa JC. Cholesterol lowering, low cholesterol, and mortality. Am J Cardiol 1993;72:776–786.
17. Stamler J, Stamler R, Brown WV, et al. Serum cholesterol. Doing the right thing. Circulation 1993;88:1954–1960.
18. Levine GN, Keaney JF Jr, Vita JA. Medical progress: cholesterol reduction in cardiovascular disease. N Engl J Med 1995;332:512–521.
19. Gotto AM. Lipid lowering, regression and coronary events. A review of the Interdisciplinary Council on Lipids and Cardiovascular Risk Intervention, seventh council meeting. Circulation 1995;92:646–656.
20. Gould AL, Rossouw JE, Santanello NC, et al. Cholesterol reduction yields clinical benefit. A new look at old data. Circulation 1995;91:2274–2282.

21. Gould KL, Ornish D, Scherwitz L, et al. Changes in myocardial perfusion abnormalities by positron emission tomography after long-term, intense risk factor modification. JAMA 1995;274:894–901.
22. Lacoste L, Lam JYT, Hung J, et al. Hyperlipidemia and coronary disease. Correction of the increased thrombogenic potential with cholesterol reduction. Circulation 1995;92:3172–3177.
23. Ganz P, Creager MA, Fang JC, et al. Pathogenic mechanisms of atherosclerosis: effect of lipid lowering on the biology of atherosclerosis. Am J Med 1996;101(suppl 4A):10S–16S.
24. Nofer J-R, Tepel M, Kehrel B, et al. Low-density lipoproteins inhibit the Na^+/H^+ antiport in human platelets. A novel mechanism enhancing platelet activity in hypercholesterolemia. Circulation 1997;95:1370–1377.
25. Rosenson RS, Tangney CC. Antiatherothromboic properties of statins. Implications for cardiovascular event reduction. JAMA 1998;279:1643–1650.
26. Andrews TC, Raby K, Barry J, et al. Effect of cholesterol reduction on myocardial ischemia in patients with coronary disease. Circulation 1997;95:324–328.
27. van Boven AJ, Jukema JW, Zwinderman AH, et al. Reduction of transient myocardial ischemia with pravastatin in addition to the conventional treatment in patients with angina pectoris. Circulation 1996;94:1503–1505.
28. Crouse JR, Byington PB, Hoen HM, et al. Reductase inhibitor monotherapy and stroke prevention. Arch Intern Med 1997;157:1305–1310.
29. Pedersen TR, Kjekshus J, Pyorala K, et al. Effect of simvastatin on ischemic signs and symptoms in the Scandinavian Simvastatin Survival Study (4S). Am J Cardiol 1998;81:333–335.
30. Huggins GS, Pasternak RC, Alpert NM, et al. Effects of short-term treatment of hyperlipidemia on coronary vasodilator function and myocardial perfusion in regions having substantial impairment of baseline vasodilator reserve. Circulation 1998;98:1291–1296.
31. Bustos C, Hernandez-Presa MA, Ortego M, et al. HMG-CoA reductase inhibition by atorvastatin reduces neointimal inflammation in a rabbit model of atherosclerosis. J Am Coll Cardiol 1998;32:2057–2064.
32. Szczeklik A, Musial J, Undas A, et al. Inhibition of thrombin generation by simvastatin and lack of additive effects of aspirin in patients with marked hypercholesterolemia. J Am Coll Cardiol 1999;33:1286–1293.
33. Dangas G, Badimon JJ, Smith DA, et al. Pravastatin therapy in hyperlipidemia: effects on thrombus formation and the systemic hemostatic profile. J Am Coll Cardiol 1999;33:1294–1304.
34. Kearney D, Fitsgerald D. The anti-thrombotic effects of statins. J Am Coll Cardiol 1999;33:1305–1307.
35. Yokoyama I, Momomura S, Ohtake T, et al. Improvement of impaired myocardial vasodilatation due to diffuse coronary atherosclerosis in hypercholesterolemics after lipid-lowering therapy. Circulation 1999;100:117–122.
36. Baller D, Notomamiprodjo G, Gleichmann U, et al. Improvement in coronary reserve determined by positron emission tomography after 6 months of cho-

lesterol-lowering therapy in patients with early stages of coronary atherosclerosis. Circulation 1999;99:2871–2875.
37. Brensike JF, Levy RL, Kelsey SF, et al. Effects of therapy with cholestyramine on progression coronary arteriosclerosis: results of the NHLBI Type II Coronary Intervention Study. Circulation 1984;69:313–324.
38. Levy RI, Brensike JF, Epstein SE, et al. The influence of changes in lipid values induced by cholestyramine and diet on progression of coronary artery disease: results of the NHLBI Type II Coronary Intervention Study. Circulation 1984;69:325–337.
39. Arntzenius AC, Kromhout D, Barth JD, et al. Diet, lipoproteins, and the progression of coronary atherosclerosis. The Leiden Intervention Trial. N Engl J Med 1985;312:805–811.
40. Cashin-Hemphill L, Mack WJ, Pogoda JM, et al. Beneficial effects of colestipol-niacin on coronary atherosclerosis. A 4-year follow-up. JAMA 1990;264: 3013–3017.
41. Brown G, Albers JJ, Fisher LD, et al. Regression of coronary artery disease as a result of intensive lipid-lowering therapy in men with high levels of apolipoprotein B. N Engl J Med 1990;323:1289–1298.
42. Kane JP, Malloy MJ, Ports TA, et al. Regression of coronary atherosclerosis during treatment of familial hypercholesterolemia with combined drug regimen. JAMA 1990;264:3007–3012.
43. Ornish D, Brown SE, Scherwitz, et al. Can lifestyle changes reverse coronary heart disease? The Lifestyle Heart Trial. Lancet 1990;336:129–133.
44. Buchwald H, Varco RL, Matts JP, et al. Effect of partial ileal bypass surgery on mortality and morbidity from coronary heart disease in patients with hypercholesterolemia. Report of the Program on the Surgical Control of the Hyperlipidemias (POSCH). N Engl J Med 1990;323:946–955.
45. Schuler G, Hambrecht R, Schlierf G, et al. Myocardial perfusion and regression of coronary artery disease in patients on a regimen of intensive physical exercise and low fat diet. J Am Coll Cardiol 1992;19:34–42.
46. Watts GF, Lewis B, Brunt JNH, et al. Effects on coronary artery disease of lipid-lowering diet, or diet plus cholestyramine, in the St Thomas Atherosclerosis Regression Study (STARS). Lancet 1992;339:563–569.
47. Blankenhorn DH, Selzer RH, Crawford DW, et al. Beneficial effects of colestipol-niacin therapy on the common carotid artery. Two- and four-year reduction of intima-media thickness measured by ultrasound. Circulation 1993;88:20–28.
48. Blankenhorn DH, Azen SP, Kramsch DM, et al. Coronary and angiographic changes with lovastatin therapy: the Monitored Atherosclerosis Regression study (MARS). Ann Intern Med 1993;119:969–976.
49. Sachs FM, Parternak RC, Gibson CM, et al. Effect on coronary atherosclerosis of decrease in plasma cholesterol concentration in normocholesterolemic patients. Lancet 1994;344:1182–1186.
50. MAAS Investigators. Effect of simvastatin on coronary atheroma: the Multicentre Anti-Atheroma Study. Lancet 1994;344;633–638.

51. Haskell WL, Alderman EL, Fair JM, et al. Effects of intensive risk factor reduction on coronary atherosclerosis and clinical events in men and women with coronary artery disease. The Stanford Coronary Risk Intervention Project (SCRIP). Circulation 1994;89:975–990.
52. Waters D, Higginson L, Gladstone P, et al. Effects of monotherapy with an HMG-CoA reductase inhibitor on the progression of coronary atherosclerosis as assessed by serial quantitative arteriography. The Canadian Coronary Atherosclerosis Trial. Circulation 1994;89:959–968.
53. Walldius G, Erikson U, Olsson AG, et al. The effect of probucol on femoral atherosclerosis: the Probucol Quantitative Regression Swedish Trial (PQRST). Am J Cardiol 1994;74:875–883.
54. Pitt B, Mancini GBJ, Ellis SG, et al. Pravastatin limitation of atherosclerosis in the coronary arteries (PLAC-I): reduction in atherosclerosis progression and clinical events. J Am Coll Cardiol 1995;26:1133–1139.
55. Crouse JR III, Byington RP, Bond MG, et al. Pravastatin, lipids, and atherosclerosis in the carotid arteries (PLAC-II). Am J Cardiol 1995;75:455–459.
56. Furberg CD, Adams HP, Applegate WB, et al. Effect of lovastatin and warfarin on early carotid atherosclerosis and cardiovascular events. Circulation 1994:90:1679–1687.
57. Haskell WL, Alderman EL, Fair JM, et al. Effects of intensive multiple risk factor reduction on coronary atherosclerosis and clinical events in men and women with coronary artery disease: the Stanford Coronary Risk Intervention Project (SCRIP). Circulation 1994;89:975–990.
58. Salonen R, Nyyssonen K, Porkkala E, at al. Kuopio Atherosclerosis Prevention Study (KAPS). A population-based primary prevention trial of the effect of LDL lowering on atherosclerosis progression of the carotid and femoral arteries. Circulation 1995;92:1758–1764.
59. Jukema JW, Bruschke AVG, van Boven AJ, et al. Effects of lipid lowering by symptomatic men with normal to moderately elevated serum cholesterol levels. The Regression Grown Evaluation Study (REGRESS). Circulation 1995; 91:2528–2540.
60. Ericsson C-G, Hamsten A, Nilsson, et al. Angiographic assessment of effects of bezafibrate on progression of coronary artery disease in young male postinfarction patients. Lancet 1996;347:849–853.
61. Kroon AA, Aengevaeren WRM, van der Werf T, et al. LDL-Apheresis Atherosclerosis Regression Study (LAARS). Effect of aggressive versus conventional lipid lowering treatment on coronary atherosclerosis. Circulation 1996; 93:1826–1835.
62. Post Coronary Artery Bypass Graft Trial Investigators. The effect of aggressive lowering of low-density lipoprotein cholesterol levels and low-dose anticoagulation on obstructive changes in saphenous-vein coronary-artery bypass grafts. N Engl J Med 1997;336:153–162.
63. Bestehorn HP, Rensing UFE, Roskamm H, et al. The effect of simvastatin on progression of coronary artery disease. The multicenter coronary intervention study (CIS). Eur Heart J 1997;18:226–234.

64. Herd JA, Ballantyne CM, Farmer JA, et al. Effects of fluvastatin on coronary atherosclerosis in patients with mild to moderate cholesterol elevations (lipoprotein and coronary atherosclerosis study [LCAS]). Am J Cardiol 1997;80: 278–286.
65. Frick MH, Syvanne M, Nieminen MS, et al. Prevention of the angiographic progression of coronary and vein-graft atherosclerosis by gemfibrozil after coronary bypass surgery in men with low levels of HDL cholesterol. Circulation 1997;96:2137–2143.
66. Ornish D, Schweritz LW, Billings JH, et al. Intensive lifestyle changes for reversal of coronary heart disease. JAMA 1998;280:2001–2007.
67. Campeau L, Hunninghake DB, Knatterud GL, et al. Aggressive cholesterol lowering delays saphenous vein graft atherosclerosis in women, the elderly, and patients with associated risk factors. Circulation 1999;99:3241–3247.
68. Little WC, Constantinescu M, Applegate RJ, et al. Can coronary arteriography predict the site of a subsequent myocardial infarction in patients with mild-to-moderate coronary artery disease. Circulation 1988;78:1157–1166.
69. Ellis S, Alderman E, Cain K, et al. Prediction of risk on anterior myocardial infarction by lesion severity and measurement method of stenoses in the left anterior descending coronary distribution: a CASS Registry Study. J Am Coll Cardiol 1988;11:908–916.
70. Giroud D, Li JM, Urban P, et al. Relationship of the site of acute myocardial infarction to the most severe coronary arterial stenosis at prior angiography. Am J Cardiol 1992;69:729–731.
71. Brown BG, Zhao X-Q, Sacco DE, Albers JJ. Lipid lowering and plaque regression. New insights into prevention of plaque disruption and clinical events in coronary disease. Circulation 1993;87:1781–1789.
72. Phillips NR, Waters D, Havel RJ. Plasma lipoproteins and progression of coronary artery disease evaluated by angiography and clinical events. Circulation 1993:88:2762–2770.
73. Waters D, Craven TE, Lesperance J. Prognostic significance of coronary atherosclerosis. Circulation 1993;87:1067–1075.
74. Hodis HN, Mack WJ, Azen SP, et al. Triglyceride- and cholesterol-rich lipoproteins have a differential effect on mild/moderate and severe lesion progression as assessed by quantitative coronary angiography in a controlled trial of lovastatin. Circulation 1994;90:42–49.
75. Brown BG, Maher VMG. Reversal of coronary heart disease by lipid-lowering therapy. Observations and pathological mechanisms. Circulation 1994; 89:2928–2933.
76. Maher VMG, Clinics Program. The Lipid Research Clinics Coronary Primary Prevention Trial Result. I. Reduction in incidence of coronary heart disease. JAMA 1984;251:351–364.
77. Stewart BF, Brown BG, Zhao X-Q, et al. Benefits of lipid lowering therapy in men with elevated apolipoprotein B are not confined to those with very high low density lipoprotein cholesterol. Circulation 1994;23:899–906.
78. Kaski JC, Chester MR, Chen L, Katritsis D. Rapid angiographic progression

of coronary artery disease in patients with angina pectoris. The role of complex stenosis morphology. Circulation 1995;92:2058–2065.
79. Sachs FM, Gibson M, Rosner B, et al. The influence of pretreatment low density lipoprotein cholesterol concentrations on the effect of hypocholesterolemic therapy on coronary atherosclerosis in angiographic trials. Am J Cardiol 1995;76:78C–85C.
80. Sacks FM, Stone PH, Gibson CM, et al. Controlled trial of fish oil for regression of human coronary atherosclerosis. J Am Coll Cardiol 1995;25: 1492–1498.
81. Thompson GR, Hollyer J, Waters DD. Percentage change rather than plasma level of LDL-cholesterol determines therapeutic response in coronary heart disease. Curr Opin Lipidiol 1995;6:386–388.
82. Phillips NR, Waters D, Havel RJ. Plasma lipoproteins and progression of coronary artery disease evaluated by angiography and clinical events. Circulation 1993:88:2762–2770.
83. Azen SP, Mack WJ, Cashin-Hemphill L, et al. Progression of coronary artery disease predicts clinical coronary events. Long-term follow-up from the Cholesterol Lowering Atherosclerosis Study. Circulation 1996;93:34–41.
84. Lamarche B, Tchernof A, Cantin B, et al. Small, dense low-density lipoprotein particles as a predictor of the risk of ischemic heart disease in men. Prospective results from the Quebec Cardiovascular Study. Circulation 1997;95:69–75.
85. Syvanne M, Nieminen MS, Frick H, et al. Associations between lipoproteins and the progression of coronary and vein-graft atherosclerosis in a controlled trial with gemfibrozil in men with low baseline levels of HDL cholesterol. Circulation 1998;98:1993–1999.
86. Ruotolo G, Ericsson C-G, Tetamanti C, et al. Treatment effects of serum lipoprotein lipids, apolipoproteins and low density lipoprotein particle size and relationships of lipoprotein variables to progression of coronary artery disease in the bezafibrate coronary atherosclerosis intervention trial (BECAIT). J Am Coll Cardiol 1998;32:1648–1656.
87. Freedman DS, Otvos JD, Jeyarajah EJ, et al. Relation of lipoprotein subclasses as measured by proton nuclear magnetic resonance spectroscopy to coronary artery disease. Arterioscler Thromb Vasc Biol 1998;18:1046–1053.
88. Otvos J. Measurement of triglyceride-rich lipoproteins by nuclear magnetic resonance spectroscopy. Clin Cardiol 1999;22(suppl II):21–27.
89. von Schacky C, Angerer P, Kothny W, Theisen K, Mudra H. The effect of dietary ω-3 fatty acids on coronary atherosclerosis. A randomized, double-blind, placebo-controlled trial. Ann Intern Med 1999;130:554–562.
91. Ballantyne CM, Her JA, Ferlic LL, et al. Influence of low HDL on progression of coronary artery disease and response to fluvastatin therapy. Circulation 1999;99:736–743.
92. Lamarche B, Tchernof A, Moorani S, et al. Small, dense low-density lipoprotein particles as a predictor of the risk of ischemic heart disease in men. Prospective results from the Quebec Cardiovascular Study. Circulation 1997; 95:69–75.

93. Lipid Research Clinics Program. The Lipid Research Clinics Coronary Primary Prevention Trial Result. I. Reduction in incidence of coronary heart disease. JAMA 1984;251:351–364.
94. Lipid Research Clinics Program. The Lipid Research Clinics Coronary Primary Prevention Trial Results. II. The relationship of reduction in incidence of coronary heart disease to cholesterol lowering. JAMA 1984;251:365–374.
95. Frick MH, Elo O, Haapa K, et al. Helsinki Heart Study: primary-prevention trial with gemfibrozil in middle-aged men with dyslipidemia. Safety of treatment, changes in risk factors, and incidence of coronary heart disease. N Engl J Med 1987;317:1237–1245.
96. Byington RP, Jukema JW, Salonen JT, et al. Reduction in cardiovascular events during pravastatin therapy. Pooled analysis of clinical events of the Pravastatin Atherosclerosis Intervention Program. Circulation 1995;92:2419–2425.
97. Scandinavian Simvastatin Survival Study Group. Randomised trial of cholesterol lowering in 4444 patients with coronary heart disease. Lancet 1994;344:1383–1389.
98. Kjekshus J, Pedersen TR. Reducing the risk of coronary events: evidence from the Scandinavian Simvastatin Survival Study (4S). Am J Cardiol 1995;76:64C–68C.
99. Scandinavian Simvastatin Survival Study Group. Baseline serum cholesterol and treatment effect in the Scandinavian Simvastatin Survival Study (4S). Lancet 1995;345:1274–1275.
100. Pedersen TR, Kjekshus J, Olsson AG, et al. Cholesterol lowering and the use of healthcare resources. Results of the Scandinavian Simvastatin Survival Study. Circulation 1996;93:1796–1802.
101. Johannesson M, Jonsson B, Kjekshus J, et al. Cost effectiveness of simvastatin to lower cholesterol levels in patients with coronary heart disease. N Engl J Med 1997;336:332–336.
102. Pyorala K, Olsson AG, Pedersen TR, et al. Cholesterol lowering with simvastatin improves prognosis of diabetic patients with coronary heart disease. A subgroup analysis of the Scandinavian Simvastatin Survival Study. Diabetes Care 1997;20:614–620.
103. Shepherd J, Cobbe SM, Ford I, et al. Prevention of coronary heart disease with pravastatin in men with hypercholesterolemia. N Engl J Med 1995;333:1301–1307.
104. Sachs FM, Pfeffer MA, Moye LA, et al. The effect of pravastatin on coronary events after myocardial infarction in patients with average cholesterol. N Engl J Med 1996;335:1001–1009.
105. Ashraf T, Hay JW, Pitt B, et al. Cost-effectiveness of pravastatin on coronary events after myocardial infarction in patients with average cholesterol. N Engl J Med 1996;335:1001–1009.
106. Hay JW, Wittels EH, Gotto AM Jr. An economic evaluation of lovastatin for cholesterol lowering and coronary disease reduction. Am J Cardiol 1991;67:789–796.

107. Gotto AM Jr. Results of recent large cholesterol-lowering trials and their implications for clinical management. Am J Cardiol 1997;79:1663–1669.
108. Vogel RA. Clinical implications of recent cholesterol lowering trials for the secondary prevention of coronary heart disease. Am J Managed Care 1997; 3:S83–S92.
109. Downs JR, Clearfield M, Weiss S, et al. Primary prevention of acute coronary events with lovastatin in men and women with average cholesterol levels. Results of the AFCAPS/TexCAPS. JAMA 1998;279:1615–1622.
110. Sacks FM, Moye LA, Davis BR, et al. Relationship between plasma LDL concentrations during treatment with pravastatin and recurrent coronary events in the cholesterol and recurrent events trial. Circulation 1998;97:1446–1452.
111. Goldberg RB, Mellies MJ, Sacks FM, et al. Cardiovascular events and their reduction with pravastatin in diabetic and glucose-intolerant myocardial infarction survivors with average cholesterol levels. Subgroup analyses in the Cholesterol and Recurrent Events (CARE) trial. Circulation 1998;98:2513–2519.
112. Ballantyne CM. Low-density lipoproteins and risk for coronary artery disease. Am J Cardiol 1998;82:3Q–12Q.
113. Long-Term Intervention with Pravastatin in Ischemic Disease (LIPID) Study Group. Prevention of cardiovascular events and death with pravastatin in patients with coronary heart disease and a broad range of initial cholesterol levels. N Engl J Med 1998;339:1349–1357.
114. Gould AL, Rossouw JE, Santanello NC, et al. Cholesterol reduction yields clinical benefit. Impact of statin trials. Circulation 1998;97:946–952.
115. Plehn JF, Davis BR, Sacks FM, et al. Reduction of stroke incidence after myocardial infarction with pravastatin. The Cholesterol and Recurrent Events (CARE) study. Circulation 1999;99:216–223.
116. Pfeffer MC, Sacks FM, Moye LA, et al. Influence of baseline lipids on effectiveness of pravastatin in the CARE trial. J Am Coll Cardiol 1999;33:125–130.
117. Pitt B, Watrs D, Brown WV, et al. Aggressive lipid-lowering therapy compared with angioplasty in stable coronary artery disease. N Engl J Med 1999; 341:70–76.
118. Rubins HB, Robind SJ, Collins D, et al. Gemfibrozil for the secondary prevention of coronary heart disease in men with low levels of high-density lipoprotein cholesterol. N Engl J Med 1999;341:410–418.
119. Fuster V, Steele PM, Chesebro JH. Role of platelets and thrombosis in coronary atherosclerotic disease and sudden death. J Am Coll Cardiol 1986;5: 175B–184B.
120. Glagov S, Weisenberg E, Zarins CK, et al. Compensatory enlargement of human atherosclerotic coronary arteries. N Engl J Med 1987;316:1371–1375.
121. Steinberg D, Parthasarathy S, Carew TE, Khoo JC, Witztum JL. Beyond cholesterol. Modifications of low-density lipoprotein that increase its atherogenicity. N Engl J Med 1989;320:915–924.

122. Davies MJ. A macro and micro view of coronary vascular insult in ischemic heart disease. Circulation 1990;82(suppl II):38–46.
123. Fuster V, Stein B, Ambrose JA, et al. Atherosclerotic plaque rupture and thrombosis-evolving concepts. Circulation 1990;82(suppl II):47–59.
124. Ip JH, Fuster V, Badimon L, et al. Syndromes of accelerated atherosclerosis: role of vascular injury and smooth muscle cell proliferation. J Am Coll Cardiol 1990;15:1667–1687.
125. Fuster V, Badimon L, Badimon JJ, Chesebro JH. The pathogenesis of coronary artery disease. N Engl J Med 1992;326:242–250, 310–318.
126. Witstum JL. Role of oxidized low density lipoprotein in atherosclerosis. Br Heart J 1993:69(suppl):S12–S18.
127. Stary HC, Chandler AB, Glagov JR, et al. A definition of initial, fatty streak, and intermediate lesions of atherosclerosis. A report from the Committee on Vascular Lesions of the Council on Arteriosclerosis, American Heart Association. Circulation 1994;89:2462–2478.
128. Clarkson TB, Pritchard RW, Morgan TM. Remodeling of coronary arteries in human and nonhuman primates. JAMA 1994;271:289–294.
129. Segrest JP, Anantharamaiah GM. Pathogenesis of atherosclerosis. Curr Opinion Cardiol 1994;9:404–410.
130. Libby P. Molecular basis of the acute coronary syndromes. Circulation 1995; 91:2844–2850.
131. Falk E, Shah PK, Fuster V. Coronary plaque disruption. Circulation 1995;92: 657–671.
132. Grayston JT, Kuo C, Coulson AS, et al. *Chlamydia pneumoniae* (TWAR) in atherosclerosis of the carotid artery. Circulation 1995;92:3397–3400.
133. Nishioka T, Luo H, Eigler NL, et al. Contribution of inadequate compensatory enlargement to development of human coronary artery stenosis: an in vitro intravascular ultrasound study. J Am Coll Cardiol 1996;27:1571–1576.
134. Farb A, Burke AP, Tang AL, et al. Coronary plaque erosion without rupture into a lipid core. A frequent cause of coronary thrombosis in sudden coronary death. Circulation 1996;93:1354–1363.
135. Zhou YF, Leon MB, Waclawiw MA, et al. Association between prior cytomegalovirus infection and the risk of restenosis after coronary atherectomy. N Engl J Med 1996;335:624–630.
136. Mann JM, Davies MJ. Vulnerable plaque. Relation of characteristics to degree of stenosis in human coronary arteries. Circulation 1996;94:928–931.
137. Burke AP, Farb A, Malcom GT, et al. Coronary risk factors and plaque morphology in men with coronary disease who die suddenly. N Engl J Med 1997; 336:1276–1282.
138. Ridker PM, Cushman M, Stampfer MJ, et al. Inflamation, aspirin, and the risk of cardiovascular disease in apparently healthy men. N Engl J Med 1997; 336:973–979.
139. Ridker PM, Rifai N, Pfeffer MA, et al. Inflammation, pravastatin, and the risk of coronary events after myocardial infarction in patients with average cholesterol levels. Circulation 1998;98:839–844.

140. Ross R. Atherosclerosis—an inflammatory disease. N Engl J Med 1999;340: 115–126.
141. Furchgott RF, Zawadski JV. The obligatory role of endothelial cells in the relaxation of arterial smooth muscle by acetylcholine. Nature 1980;288:373–376.
142. Ludmer PL, Selwyn AP, Shook TL, et al. Paradoxical vasoconstriction induced by acetylcholine in atherosclerotic coronary arteries. N Engl J Med 1986;315:1046–1051.
143. Osborne JA, Siegman MJ, Sedar AW, et al. Lack of endothelium-dependent relaxation in coronary resistance arteries of cholesterol-fed rabbits. Am J Physiol 1989;256:C591–C597.
144. Drexler H, Zeiher AM, Wollschlager H, et al. Flow-dependent coronary artery dilatation in humans. Circulation 1989;80:466–474.
145. Harrison DG. From isolated vessels to the catheterization laboratory. Studies of endothelial function in the coronary circulation of humans. Circulation 1989;80:703–706.
146. Vita JA, Treasure CB, Nabel EG, et al. Coronary vasomotor responses to acetylcholine relates to risk factors for coronary artery disease. Circulation1990;81:491–497.
147. Vane JR, Anggard EE, Botting RM. Regulatory functions of the vascular endothelium. N Engl J Med 1990;323:27–36.
148. Creager MA, Cooke JP, Mendelsohn ME, et al. Impaired vasodilation of forearm resistance vessels in hypercholesterolemic humans. J Clin Invest 1990; 86:228–234.
149. Kuhn FE, Mohler ER, Reagan K, et al. Effects of high-density lipoprotein on acetylcholine-induced coronary vasoreactivity. Am J Cardiol 1991;1425–1430.
150. Lerman A, Burnett JC Jr. Intact and altered endothelium in regulation of vasomotion. Circulation 1992;86(suppl III):12–19.
151. Flavahan NA. Atherosclerosis or lipoprotein-induced endothelial dysfunction. Potential mechanisms underlying reduction in EDRF/nitric oxide activity. Circulation 1992;85:1927–1938.
152. Celermajer DS, Sorensen KE, Gooch VM, et al. Non-invasive detection of endothelial dysfunction in children and adults at risk of atherosclerosis. Lancet 1992;340:1111–1115.
153. Vogel RA. Endothelium-dependent vasoregulation of coronary artery diameter and blood flow. Circulation 1993;88:325–327.
154. Mocada S, Higgs A. The L-arginine-nitric oxide pathway. N Engl J Med 1993; 329:2002–2012.
155. Lefroy DC, Crake T, Uren NG, et al. Effect of inhibition of nitric oxide synthesis on epicardial coronary artery caliber and coronary blood flow in humans. Circulation 1993;88:43–54.
156. Matsuda Y, Hirata K, Inoue N, et al. High density lipoprotein reverses inhibitory effect of oxidized low density lipoprotein on endothelium-dependent arterial relaxation. Circ Res 1993;72:1103–1109.

157. Seiler C, Hess M, Buechi M, et al. Influence of serum cholesterol and other coronary risk factors on vasomotion of angiographically normal coronary arteries. Circulation 1993;88(part 1):2139–2148.
158. Ohara Y, Pederson TE, Harrison DG. Hypercholesterolemia increases endothelial superoxide production. J Clin Invest 1993;91:2546–2551.
159. Reddy KG, Nair RN, Sheehan HM, et al. Evidence that selective endothelial dysfunction may occur in the absence of angiographic or ultrasound atherosclerosis in patients with risk factors for atherosclerosis. J Am Coll Cardiol 1994;23:833–843.
160. Benzuly KH, Padgett RC, Kaul S, et al. Functional improvement precedes structural regression of atherosclerosis. Circulation 1994;89:1810–1818.
161. Celermajer DS, Sorensen KE, Bull C, et al. Endothelium-dependent dilation in the systemic arteries of asymptomatic subjects relates to coronary risk factors and their interaction. J Am Coll Cardiol 1994;24:1468–1474.
162. Cayette AJ, Palacino JJ, Cohen RA. Chronic inhibition of nitric oxide production accelerates neointimal formation and impairs endothelial function in hypercholesterolemic rabbits. Arterioscler Thromb 1994;14:753–759.
163. Hamon M, Vallet B, Bauters C, et al. Long-term administration of L-arginine reduces intimal thickening and enhances neoendothelium-dependent acetylcholine relaxation after arterial injury. Circulation 1994;90:1357–1362.
164. El-Tamimi H, Mansour M, Wargovich TJ, et al. Constrictor and dilator responses to intracoronary acetylcholine in adjacent segments of the same coronary artery in patients with coronary artery disease. Circulation 1994;89:45–51.
165. Penny WF, Rockman H, Long J, et al. Heterogeneity of vasomotor response to acetylcholine along the human coronary artery. J Am Coll Cardiol 1995;25:1046–1055.
166. Kuo L, Davis MJ, Chilian WM. Longitudinal gradients for endothelium-dependent and -independent vascular responses in the coronary microcirculation. Circulation 1995;92:518–525.
167. Zeiher AM, Krause T, Schachinger V, et al. Impaired endothelium-dependent vasodilation of coronary resistance vessels is associated with exercise-induced myocardial ischemia. Circulation 1995;91:2345–2352.
168. Shiode N, Nakayama K, Morishima N, et al. Nitric oxide production by coronary conductance vessels in hypercholesterolemic patients. Am Heart J 1996;131:1051–1057.
169. Glasser SP, Selwyn AP, Ganz P. Atherosclerosis: risk factors and the vascular endothelium. Am Heart J 1996;131:379–384.
170. Anderson TJ, Meredith IT, Charbonneau F, et al. Endothelium-dependent coronary vasomotion relates to the susceptibility of LDL to oxidation in humans. Circulation 1996;93:1647–1650.
171. Weber C, Erl W, Weber K, et al. Increased adhesiveness of isolated monocytes to endothelium is prevented by vitamin C intake in smokers. Circulation 1996;93:1488–1492.
172. Vogel RA, Corretti MC, Plotnick GD. Effect of a single high-fat meal on endothelial function in healthy subjects. Am J Cardiol 1997;79:350–354.

173. Vogel RA. Coronary risk factors, endothelial function, and atherosclerosis: a review. Clin Cardiol 1997;20:426–432.
174. Plotnick GD, Corretti MC, Vogel RA. Antioxidant vitamins blunt the transient impairment of endothelium-dependent brachial artery vasoactivity following a fatty meal. JAMA 1997;278:1682–1686.
175. Vogel RA, Corretti MC, Gellman J. Cholesterol, cholesterol lowering, and endothelial function. Progr Cardiovasc Dis 1998;41:117–136.
176. Murakami T, Mizuno S, Kaku B. Clinical morbidities in subjects with Doppler-evaluated endothelial dysfunction of coronary artery. J Am Coll Cardiol 1998;31:419A.
177. GISSI Investigators. Dietary supplementation with n-3 polyunsaturated fatty acids and vitamin E after myocardial infarction: results of the GISSI-Prevenzione trial. Lancet 1999;354:447–455.
178. Djousse L, Ellison RC, McLennan CE, et al. Acute effects of a high-fat meal with and without red wine on endothelial function in healthy subjects. Am J Cardiol 1999;84:660–664.
179. Williams MJA, Sutherland WHF, McCormick MP, et al. Impaired endothelial function following a meal rich in used cooking oil. J Am Coll Cardiol 1999; 33:1050–1055.
180. Wilmink HW, Banga JD, Hijmering M, et al. Effect of angiotensin-converting enzyme inhibition and angiotensin II type 1 receptor anatagonism on postprandial endothelial function. J Am Coll Cardiol 1999;34:140–145.
181. Lewis TV, Dart AM, Chin-Dusting JPF. Endothelium-dependent relaxation by acetylcholine is impaired in hypertriglyceridemic humans with normal levels of plasma LDL cholesterol. J Am Coll Cardiol 1999;33:805–812.
182. Leung W-H, Lau C-P, Wong C-K. Beneficial effect of cholesterol-lowering therapy on coronary endothelium-dependent relaxation in hypercholesterolaemic patients. Lancet 1993;341:1496–1500.
183. Egashira K, Hirooka Y, Kai H, et al. Reduction in serum cholesterol with pravastatin improves endothelium-dependent coronary vasomotion in patients with hypercholesterolemia. Circulation 1994;89:2519–2524.
184. Treasure CB, Klein JL, Weintraub WS, et al. Beneficial effects of cholesterol-lowering therapy on the coronary endothelium in patients with coronary artery disease. N Engl J Med 1995;332:481–487.
185. Anderson TJ, Meredith IT, Yeung AC, et al. The effect of cholesterol-lowering and antioxidant therapy on endothelium-dependent coronary vasomotion. N Engl J Med 1995;332:488–493.
186. Stroes ESG, Koomans HA, de Bruin TWA, et al. Vascular function in the forearm in hypercholesterolaemic patients off and on lipid-lowering medication. Lancet 1995;346:467–471.
187. Goode GK, Heagerty AM. In vitro responses of human peripheral small arteries in hypercholesterolemia and effects of therapy. Circulation 1995;91: 2898–2903.
188. Vogel RA, Corretti MC, Plotnick GP. Changes in flow-mediated brachial artery vasoactivity with lowering of desirable cholesterol levels in healthy middle-aged men. Am J Cardiol 1996;77:37–40.

189. Seiler C, Suter TM, Hess OM. Exercise-induced vasomotion of angiographically normal and stenotic coronary arteries improves after cholesterol-lowering drug therapy with bezafibrate. J Am Coll Cardiol 1995;26:1615–1622.
190. Yeung A, Hodgson JMcB, Winniford M, et al. Assessment of coronary vascular reactivity after cholesterol lowering. Circulation 1996;94(suppl I):I-402. Abstract.
191. Drury J, Cohen JD, Veerendrababu B, et al. Brachial artery endothelium-dependent vasodilation in patients enrolled in the Cholesterol and Recurrent Events (CARE) study. Circulation 1996;94(suppl I):I-402. Abstract.
192. Tamai O, Matsuoka H, Itabe H, et al. Single LDL apheresis improves endothelium-dependent vasodilatation in hypercholesterolemic humans. Circulation 1997;95:76–82.
193. O'Driscoll G, Green D, Taylor RR. Simvastatin, an HMG-CoA reductase inhibitor, improves endothelial function within 1 month. Circulation 1997;95:1126–1131.
194. Andrews TC, Whitney EJ, Green G, et al. Effect of gemfibrozil ± niacin ± cholestyramine on endothelial function in patients with serum low-density lipoprotein cholesterol levels <160 mg/dL and high-density lipoprotein cholesterol levels <40 mg/dL. Am J Cardiol 1997;80:831–835.
195. de Man FH, Weverling AW, Smelt AH, et al. Impaired endothelium-dependent vaodilation in the forearm of patients with endogenous hypertriglyceridemia: reversal upon lipid-lowering therapy by atorvastatin. Circulation 1998;98:I-243.
196. Simons A, Sullivan D, Simons J, et al. Effects of atorvastatin monotherapy and simvastatin plus cholestyramine on arterial endothelial function in patients with severe primary hypercholesterolemia. Atherosclerosis 1998;137:197–203.
197. Vogel RA, Corretti MC, Plotnick GD. The mechanism of improvement in endothelial function by pravastatin: direct effect or through cholesterol lowering. J Am Coll Cardiol 1998;31:60A.
198. John S, Schlaich M, Langenfeld M, et al. Increased bioavailability of nitric oxide after lipid-lowering therapy in hypercholesterolemic patients. A randomized, place-controlled, double-blind study. Circulation 1998;98:211–216.
199. Dupuis J, Tardif J-C, Cernacek P, et al. Cholesterol reduction rapidly improves endothelial function after acute coronary syndromes. The RECIFE (Reduction of Cholesterol in Ischemia and Function of the Endothelium) trial. Circulation 1999;99:3227–3233.
200. Herrington DM, Werbel BL, Riley WA, et al. Individual and combined effects of estrogen/progestin therapy and lovastatin on lipids and flow-mediated vasodilation in postmenopausal women with coronary artery disease. J Am Coll Cardiol 1999;33:2030–2037.
201. Abbott RD, Wilson PWF, Kannel WB, et al. High density lipoprotein cholesterol, total cholesterol screening, and myocardial infarction—the Framingham experience. Arteriosclerosis 1988;8:207–211.

202. Burr ML, Fehily AM, Gilbert JF, et al. Effects of changes in fat, fish, and fibre intakes on death and myocardial reinfarction: Diet and Reinfarction Trial (DART). Lancet 1989:757–761.
203. Cohen MV, Byrne M-J, Levine B, et al. Low rate of treatment of hypercholesterolemia by cardiologists in patients with suspected and proven coronary artery disease. Circulation 1991;83:1294–1304.
204. Vogel RA. The case for aggressive lipid lowering in CAD patients. J Myo Ischemic 1991;3:30–44.
205. Wood, Stefanick ML, Williams PT, et al. The effects on plasma lipoproteins of a prudent weight-reducing diet, with or without exercise in overweight men and women. N Engl J Med 1991;325:461–466.
206. Manninen V, Tenkanen L, Koskinen P, et al. Joint effects of serum triglyceride and LDL cholesterol and HDL concentrations on coronary heart disease risk in the Helsinki Heart Study. Implications for treatment. Circulation 1992;85: 37–45.
207. Assmann G, Schulte H. Relation of high-density lipoprotein cholesterol and triglycerides to incidence of atherosclerotic coronary artery disease (the PROCAM experience). Am J Cardiol 1992;70:733–737.
208. Levy RI, Troendle AJ, Fattu JM. A quarter century of drug treatment of dyslipoproteinemia, with a focus on the new HMG-CoA reductase inhibitor fluvastatin. Circulation 1993(suppl III):45–53.
209. Huninghake DB, Stein EA, Dujoune CA, et al. The efficacy of intensive dietary therapy alone or in combination with lovastatin in outpatients with hypercholesterolemia. N Engl J Med 1993;328:1213–1219.
210. Roberts WC. Getting cardiologists interested in lipids. Am J Cardiol 1993; 72:744–745.
211. Expert Panel on Detection, Evaluation, and Treatment of High Blood Cholesterol in Adults. Summary of the second report of the National Cholesterol Education Program (NCEP) Expert Panel on Detection, Evaluation and Treatment of High Blood Cholesterol in Adults (Adult Treatment Panel II). JAMA 1993;269:3015–3023.
212. Grundy SM, Bilheimer D, Chait A, et al. National cholesterol education program expert panel on detection, evaluation, and treatment of high blood cholesterol in adults (Adult Treatment Panel II). NIH Publication 93-3095, 1993: O-1-R-32; and Circulation 1994;89:1329–1448.
213. DeBusk RF, Miller NH, Superko HR, et al. A case-management system for coronary risk factor modification after acute myocardial infarction. Ann Intern Med 1994;120:721–729.
214. Cupples ME, McKnight A. Randomized trial of health promotion in general practice for patients at high cardiovascular risk. Br Med J 1994;309:993–996.
215. Watts GF, Jackson P, Mandalia S, et al. Nutrient intake and progression of coronary artery disease. Am J Cardiol 1994;73:328–332.
216. Krumholtz HM, Seeman TE, Merrill SS, et al. Lack of association between cholesterol and coronary heart disease mortality and morbidity and the all-cause mortality in persons older than 70 years. JAMA 1994;272:1335–1340.

217. Tervahaura M, Pekkanen J, Nissinen A. Risk factors of coronary heart disease and total mortality among elderly men with and without preexisting coronary heart disease. Finnish cohorts of the Seven Countries Study. J Am Coll Cardiol 1995;26:1623–1629.
218. Burchfiel CM, Laws A, Benafante R, et al. Combined effects of HDL cholesterol, triglyceride, and total cholesterol concentrations on 18-year risk of atherosclerotic disease. Circulation 1995;92:1430–1436.
219. Miller M. Maximizing secondary prevention of CAD: a model program. J Myocard Ischemia 1995;7:166–169.
220. Havel RJ, Rapoport E. Drug therapy: management of primary hyperlipidemia. N Engl J Med 1995;332:1491–1498.
221. Vogel RA. Risk factor intervention and coronary heart disease: clinical strategies. Coron Art Dis 1995;6:466–471.
222. Renaud S, de Longeril M, Delaye J, Guidollet J, Jacquard F, Mamelle N, Martin J-L, Monjaud I, Salen P, Toubol P. Cretan Mediterranean diet for prevention of coronary heart disease. Am J Clin Nutr 1995;61(suppl):1360S–1367S.
223. de Longeril M, Salen P, Martin J-L, Mamelle N, Monjaud I, Touboul P, Delaye J. Effect of a Mediterranean type of diet on the rate of cardiovascular complications in patients with coronary artery disease. Insights into the cardioprotective effect of certain nutrients. J Am Coll Cardiol 1996;28:1103–1108.
224. de Longeril M, Salem P, Martin J-L, Monjaud I, Boucher P, Mamelle N. Mediterranean dietary pattern in a randomized trial. Prolonged survival and possibly reduced cancer rate. Arch Intern Med 1998;158:1181–1187.
225. de Longeril M, Salem P, Martin J-L, Monjaud I, Delaye J, Mamelle N. Mediterranean diet, traditional risk factors, and the rate of cardiovascular complications after myocardial infarction. Final report of the Lyon Diet Heart Study. Circulation 1999;99:779–785.
226. Clinical Quality Improvement Network (CQUIN) Investigators. Low incidence of assessment and modification of risk factors in acute care patients with high risk for cardiovascular events, particularly among females and the elderly. Am J Cardiol 1995;76:570–573.
227. Nieto FJ, Alonso J, Chambless LE, et al. Population awareness and control of hypertension and hypercholesterolemia. The Atherosclerosis Risk in Communities Study. Arch Intern Med 1995;155:677–684.
228. Renaud S, de Longeril M, Guidollet J, et al. Cretan Mediterranean diet for prevention of coronary heart disease. Am J Clin Nutr 1995;61(suppl):1360S–1367S.
229. Iribarren C, Reed DM, Chen R, et al. Low serum cholesterol and mortality. Which is the cause and which is the effect? Circulation 1995;92:2396–2403.
230. Nawrocki JW, Weiss SR, Davidson MH, et al. Reduction of LDL cholesterol by 25% to 60% in patients with primary hypercholesterolemia by atorvastatin, a new HMG-CoA reductase inhibitor. Arterioscler Thromb Vasc Biol 1995; 15:678–682.

231. Van Dis F, Keilson LM, Rundell CA, et al. Direct measurement of serum low-density lipoprotein cholesterol in patients with acute myocardial infarction on admission to the emergency room. Am J Cardiol 1996;77:1232–1234.
232. Smith SC Jr, Blair SN, Criqui MH, et al. Preventing heart attack and stroke in patients with coronary disease. Circulation 1995;92:2–4.
233. Smith SC Jr. Risk-reduction therapy: the challenge to change. Circulation 1996;93:2205–2211.
234. Rimm EB, Ascherio A, Giovannucci E, et al. Vegetable, fruit, and cereal fiber intake and risk of coronary heart disease among men. JAMA 996;275:447–451.
235. Rackley CE. Monotherapy with HMG-CoA reductase inhibitors and secondary prevention in coronary artery disease. Clin Cardiol 1996;19:683–689.
236. Gardner CD, Fortman SP, Krauss RM. Association of small low-dense lipoprotein particles with the incidence of coronary artery disease in men and women. JAMA 1996;276:875–881.
237. Stampfer MJ, Krauss RM, Ma J, et al. A prospective study of triglyceride level, low-density lipoprotein particle diameter, and risk of myocardial infarction. JAMA 1996;276:882–888.
238. de Lorgeril M, Salen P, Martin J-L, et al. Effect of a Mediterranean type of diet on the rate of cardiovascular complications in patients with coronary artery disease. Insights into the cardioprotective effects of certain nutrients. J Am Coll Cardiol 1996;28:1103–1108.
239. Rodriguez BL, Sharp DS, Abbott RD, et al. Fish intake may limit the increase in risk of coronary heart disease morbidity and mortality among heavy smokers. The Honolulu Heart Program. Circulation 1996;94:952–956.
240. Superko HR. Beyond LDL cholesterol reduction. Circulation 1996;94:2351–2354.
241. Fortmann SP, Marcovina SM. Lipoprotein(a), a clinically elusive lipoprotein particle. Circulation 1997;95:295–296.
242. Daviglus ML, Stamler J, Orencia AJ, et al. Fish consumption and the 30-year risk of fatal myocardial infarction. N Engl J Med 1997;336:1046–1053.
243. Tosteson ANA, Weinstein MC, Hunink MGM, et al. Cost-effectiveness of population wide educational approaches to reduce serum cholesterol levels. Circulation 1997;95:24–30.
244. Grundy SM, Balady GJ, Criqui MH, et al. When to start cholesterol-lowering therapy in patients with coronary heart disease. A statement for healthcare professionals from the Task Force on Risk Reduction. Circulation 1997;95:1683–1685.
245. Grundy SM, Balady GJ, Criqui MH, et al. Guide to primary prevention of cardiovascular diseases. A statement for healthcare professionals from the Task Force on Risk Reduction. Circulation 1997;95:2329–2331.
246. Gotto AM Jr. Cholesterol management in theory and practice. Circulation 1997;96:4424–4430.
247. Grundy SM. Statin trials and goals of cholesterol-lowering therapy. Circulation 1998;97:1436–1439.

248. Fruchart JC, Brewer HB, Leitersdorf E. Consensus for the use of fibrates in the treatment of dyslipidemia and coronary heart disease. Am J Cardiol 1998: 81:912–917.
249. Sposito AC, Mansur AP, Coelho OR, et al. Additional reduction in blood pressure after cholesterol-lowering treatment by statins (lovastatin or pravastatin) in hypercholesterolemic patients using angiotensin-converting enzyme inhibitors (enalapril or lisinopril). Am J Cardiol 1999;83:1497–1499.
250. Brunzell JD, Hohanson JE. Low-density and high-density lipoprotein subspecies and risk for premature coronary artery disease. Am J Med 1999;107: 16S–18S.
251. Knopf RH. Drug treatment of lipid disorders. N Engl J Med 1999;341:498–511.

23

Myocardial Rupture

Pathobiology, Diagnosis, Medical Management, and Surgical Intervention

Richard C. Becker and A. Thomas Pezzella
University of Massachusetts Medical School
Worcester, Massachusetts

INTRODUCTION

Myocardial rupture is a well-recognized complication of myocardial infarction that is responsible for 10% to 15% of all in-hospital deaths. Written descriptions of this feared entity, which most often involves the left ventricular free wall and less frequently the interventricular septum, papillary muscle, right ventricular free wall, and atrium, have appeared in the medical and surgical literature for centuries. William Harvey (1647) is credited with the initial report (1), followed some years later by a detailed account of myocardial rupture found within the autopsy notes from King George II (1727).

The anatomist Morgani collected 10 cases of myocardial rupture in 1765 (2). In 1859 Malmsten reported a case of myocardial rupture and for the first time described "softening of the myocardium" within the involved area due to occlusive coronary artery thrombosis (3,4). By 1925, Krumbhaar and Crowell (5) had collected 632 cases of rupture from the literature and added 22 cases of their own, emphasizing its association with coronary artery disease and acute myocardial infarction. Despite enjoying considerable notoriety, there are many unanswered questions regarding the pathobiology, prevention, premorbid diagnosis, medical management, and surgical intervention of myocardial rupture.

The reperfusion era has heightened an existing interest in myocardial rupture, and has raised additional questions about the potential contribution of reperfusion injury, fibrinolytic therapy, and adjunctive antithrombotic treatment that includes anticoagulants and potent platelet antagonists.

ACUTE MYOCARDIAL INFARCTION

General Pathologic Features

Necrosis is defined as an irreversible change or death of an individual cell or group of cells. Acute myocardial infarction is characterized by ischemic coagulative necrosis with a surrounding neutrophilic response. The gross pathologic changes do not appear in the myocardium for 6 hours after the onset of cellular damage. Initially, the involved region is soft, swollen, and pale. Over the ensuing 18 to 36 hours, the myocardium becomes tan or reddish-purple and the epicardium (visceral pericardium) develops a fibrinous exudate. In nontransmural infarction, the epicardial surface remains relatively unchanged. By 48 hours, the zone of infarction appears gray, and yellow lines representing areas of neutrophilic infiltration extend to the periphery. Eight to 10 days after the onset of infarction, the myocardium (within the involved zone) thins as necrotic muscle is removed by mononuclear cells. At this point in time, the infarction appears yellow but is surrounded by a reddish-purple band referred to as the hyperemic zone. Granulation tissue appears approximately 7 days later and extends throughout the infarcted area by 3 to 4 weeks. Within 1 month of the initial event, and continuing over the ensuing 2 to 3 months, the infarction becomes gray in color and gelatinous in appearance. In time (typically within 3 to 4 months) the zone of infarction shrinks to become a white, thin, and firm scar (Fig. 1) (6–9).

Histology

On light microscopy, severe ischemia produces cell swelling and hydropic degeneration. Cells that are irreversibly damaged (by definition necrotic) exhibit cytoplasmic hypereosinophilia and nuclear pyknosis. Myocardial cells typically develop a wavy appearance. Accordingly, the combination of myocyte waviness and cellular hypereosinophilia bordering on a zone of hydropic cell swelling and contraction bands is considered diagnostic of myocardial infarction.

Approximately 8 hours later interstitial edema is present and intracellular fatty deposits can be seen. Neutrophilic infiltration can also be observed at this point (Fig. 2). Small and well-localized areas of hemorrhage appear in the interstitial spaces from small, disrupted/necrotic blood vessels. In the

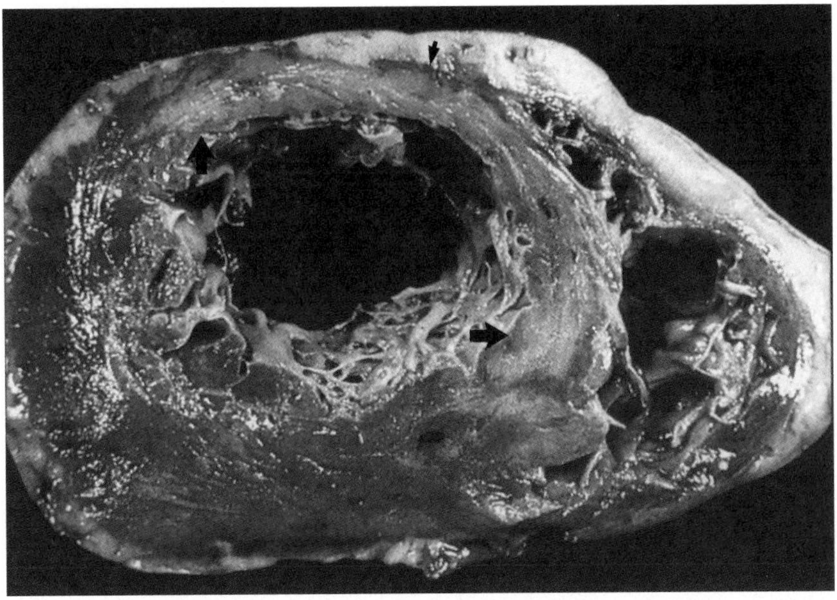

Figure 1 Gross pathology (cross section). The anterior wall of the left ventricle is thin and light in appearance, representing scar tissue that extends to the mid and superior aspects of the interventricular septum (arrows).

absence of reperfusion, the interstitial extravasation of erythrocytes is mild and visualized only on histologic examination. Thus most infarctions are classified as *anemic*.

Approximately 24 hours after the onset of infarction, the cytoplasm becomes clumped, cross-striations are lost, and focal hyalinization appears. Nonnecrotic capillaries within both the involved and surrounding areas dilate, allowing further neutrophil accumulation. Typically, the leukocyte response begins at the periphery of the infarct zone and moves centrally over time.

Within 96 hours of infarction, removal of necrotic fibers begins, first in the peripheral zones followed later within the central region.

Cellular Characteristics of Wound Healing

The infiltration of inflammatory cells is an early component of tissue repair following myocardial infarction. The process is mediated by neutrophils, lymphocytes, macrophages, and fibroblasts (Fig. 3). Collagen degradation is also an early response to myocardial necrosis. Matrix metallopro-

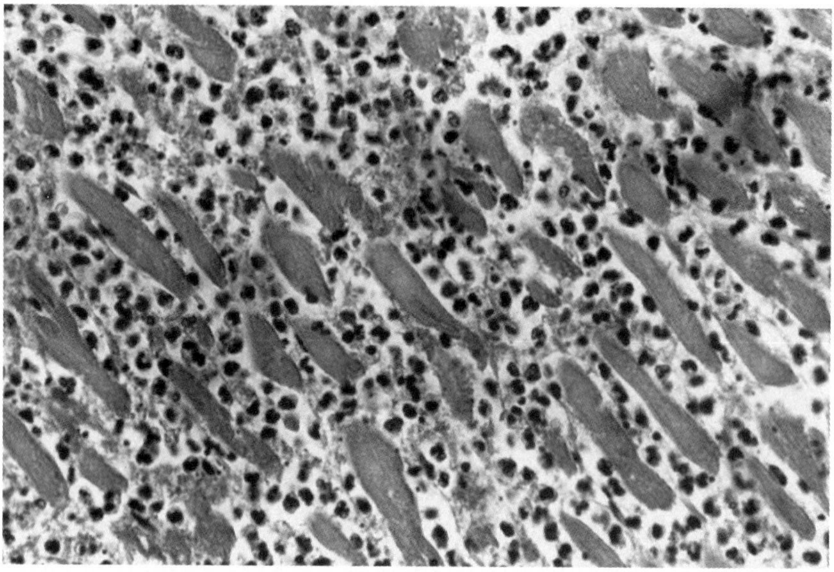

Figure 2 Neutrophic infiltration within an area of myocardial necrosis. Interstitial edema and myocyte atrophy are also present.

teinases (MMPs) reside in the myocardium as latent forms and, upon activation, degrade fibrillar collagen. A transient increase in collagenase activity appears within the infarcted myocardium by day 2, peaking at day 7. Increased collagenase activity does *not* occur in sites remote from the infarction (10–13).

The fibrous stage of wound healing follows the initial inflammatory stage. Increased synthesis of fibrillar type III collagen and later type I collagen is preceded by a heightened expression of their respective messenger RNA transcripts. Collagen fibers are evident by day 7 after infarction with an organized assembly (early component of scar development) evident by day 14. Interestingly, proliferation of fibroblasts and fibroblastlike cells is also evident at sites remote from the infarction.

A fibrillar fibronectin scaffolding represents an important precursor to the attachment of myofibroblasts and to the subsequent deposition of type III followed by type I collagen. Myofibroblasts synthesize and metabolize a number of substances involved in the regulation of collagen turnover. Over the subsequent weeks, blood vessels and fibroblasts continue to increase and proliferate, respectively, with removal of necrotic cells and deposition of collagen. By 4 to 6 weeks, most of the necrotic myocardium has been removed and replaced by fibrous scar tissue.

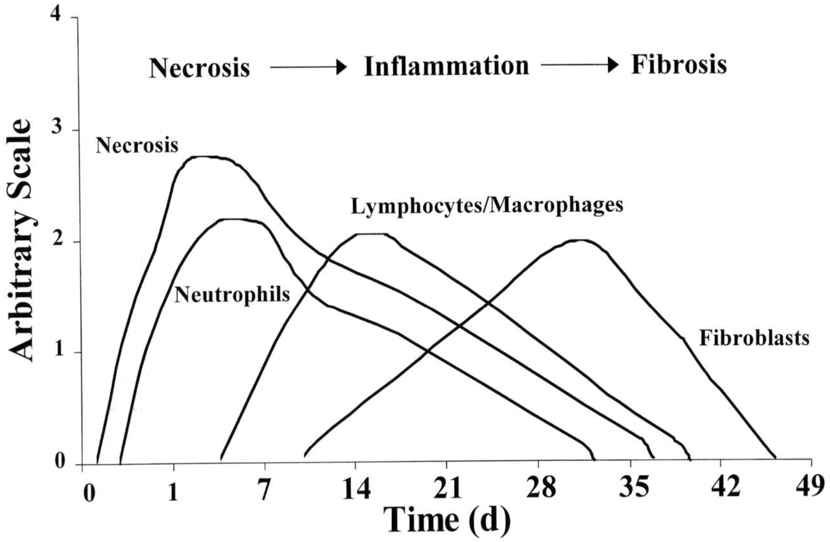

Figure 3 Histologic "time line" characteristic of acute myocardial infarction. Tissue necrosis is followed rapidly by an acute inflammatory response predominated by neutrophil infiltration. Removal of necrotic fibers begins within 4 days and granulation tissue first appears by day 12 (see text for discussion). (Adapted from Ref. 8.)

Patterns of Myocardial Necrosis

Three distinct pathologic patterns of myocardial necrosis have been described—coagulation necrosis, contract band necrosis, and myocytolysis (14). Each pattern is briefly described.

Coagulation Necrosis

Coagulation necrosis is the end-product of severe, persistent ischemia and is found within the central portion of the infarct zone. The gross and microscopic findings have already been reviewed.

Contraction Band Necrosis

Contraction band necrosis, also referred to as reperfusion necrosis and myofibrillar degeneration, is caused by severe ischemia and increased calcium ion flux into dying cells within a contracted state. It is typically observed at the border of large infarctions and constitutes the major pathologic substrate following reperfusion. Grossly, areas of contraction band necrosis are dark red. The appearance is caused by distension of capillary beds within the damaged zone, and extravasation of red blood cells from disrupted capillary vessels, leading to focal interstial hemorrhage.

Myocytolysis

Myocytolysis, also referred to as colliquative necrosis, is caused by prolonged moderate ischemia and is most often observed in surrounding areas (border zones) of the infarction. Histologically, myocytolysis is characterized by cell swelling, early lysis of myofibrils, late lysis of cell nuclei, and an absence of neutrophilic infiltration (6,14).

Hemorrhagic Infarction

Hemorrhagic infarction, defined grossly as visible blood within the myocardium, is a phenomenon that coexists with extensive coagulative necrosis. Although hemorrhagic infarction has been recognized by pathologists for decades, it was not a common occurrence prior to the advent of reperfusion therapy (Fig. 4). An autopsy study of 119 patients with fatal myocardial

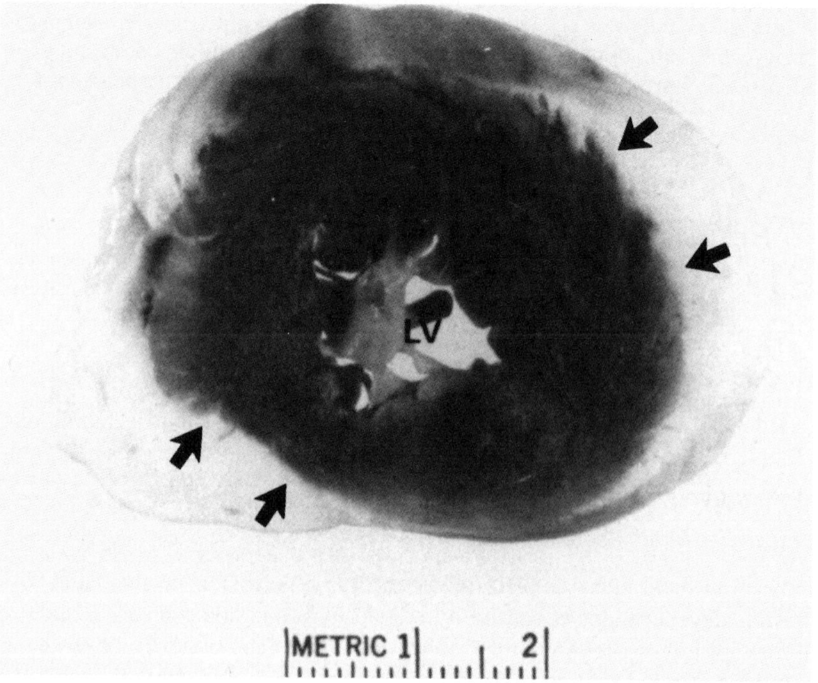

Figure 4 Transmural hemorrhagic infarction in a patient who received fibrinolytic therapy in the setting of an acute inferolateral myocardial infarction.

infarction (15) performed in the prereperfusion era revealed hemorrhagic infarction in only 2% of hearts. A separate study of 200 patients (16) did not observe hemorrhagic infarction in any of the autopsy specimens. In distinct contrast, Waller and colleagues (17) reported a 74% incidence of hemorrhagic infarction in patients who had received reperfusion therapy (fibrinolysis alone or combined fibrinolysis and coronary angioplasty).

The debate continues whether hemorrhagic infarction is detrimental to the overall wound healing process. In at least one study (16) an area of hemorrhagic infarction (following reperfusion therapy) failed to exhibit histologic evidence of repair after 8 days.

MYOCARDIAL RUPTURE

Epidemiology

Autopsy series serve as the basis for determining the overall incidence of rupture associated with myocardial infarction (Table 1) (18–52). Several large series are commonly cited. Malmo General Hospital (Sweden) reported a total of 2477 myocardial infarctions between 1935 and 1959. One-third of the events were fatal, and autopsies performed in 95% of cases revealed myocardial rupture with pericardial tamponade in 12.5% of patients (53). An overview of 1326 patients suffering either in-hospital or out-of-hospital death in Rochester, MN (1947–1959), cited a 24% rupture rate (from 691 patients autopsied), among persons ≥20 years of age (54). The most common cause of myocardial rupture is acute myocardial infarction; other, less common causes include infective endocarditis, myocardial abscesses, aortic dissection, myocarditis, tuberculosis, ecchinococcal cysts, trauma (blunt or penetrating) (with or without pericardial rupture), and malignancy (primary or metastatic).

Site of Involvement

Rupture associated with acute myocardial infarction can involve the ventricular free wall, ventricular septum, papillary muscles, and rarely the atrium (Fig. 5).

Ventricular Free Wall Rupture

Rupture of the ventricular free wall is the most common variety of rupture. According to descriptions offered in the prereperfusion era, left ventricular free wall rupture can occur at any time between 1 day and 3 weeks after infarction, but most develop between days 3 and 5 (Fig. 6). Overall, left ventricular rupture is seven times more frequent than right ventricular rupture, and typically involves the anterior and lateral walls. The myocardial tear is commonly identified near the junction of infarcted tissue and adjacent

Table 1 Myocardial Rupture in Acute Fatal Myocardial Infarction: Historic Time Line of Necropsy-Based Series

Author(s)	Year	Cases of fatal myocardial infarction	Cases of cardiac rupture	
			Total	%
Parkinson and Bedford	1928	51	5	9.8
Levine	1929	46	9	19.6
Bean	1938	114	17	14.9
Mallory	1939	72	8	11.0
Edmondson and Hoxie	1942	865	72	8.3
Friedman and White	1944	105	10	9.5
Mintz and Katz	1947	46	5	10.4
Wartman and Hellerstein	1948	111	6	5.5
Selzer	1948	95	8	8.4
Diaz-Rivera and Miller	1948	53	5	9.4
Foord	1948	264	33	12.5
Wang	1948	267	23	8.6
Howell and Turnbull	1950	111	8	7.2
Zinn and Cosby	1950	430	34	7.9
Oblath	1952	1,026	91	8.9
Wessler	1952	256	14	6.0
Waldron	1954	545	40	7.5
Goetz and Gropper	1954	145	14	9.6
McDonnieal	1955	144	12	8.0
Lee	1956	500	25	5.0
Maher	1956	183	21	11.5
Aarseth	1958	1,229	89	7.3
Zeman and Rodstein	1960	81	16	19.7
Griffith	1961	3,103	215	6.9
Spiekerman	1962	87	21	24.0
Ross and Young	1963	606	43	7.0
Sievers	1964	811	104	12.8
London and London	1965	1,001	47	5.0
Lautsh	1967	585	43	7.3
Sugiura	1968	129	17	15.0
Sahebjamin	1969	933	37	3.8
Lewis	1969	1,228	106	8.6
Beutler	1970	250	20	8.0
Meurs	1970	34	8	23.5
Gjol	1972	440	51	12.0
Naeim	1972	989	44	4.0
Hammer	1972	47	7	15.0
Havig	1973	122	14	11.5
Total		17,109	1,342	7.8

Source: Ref. 152.

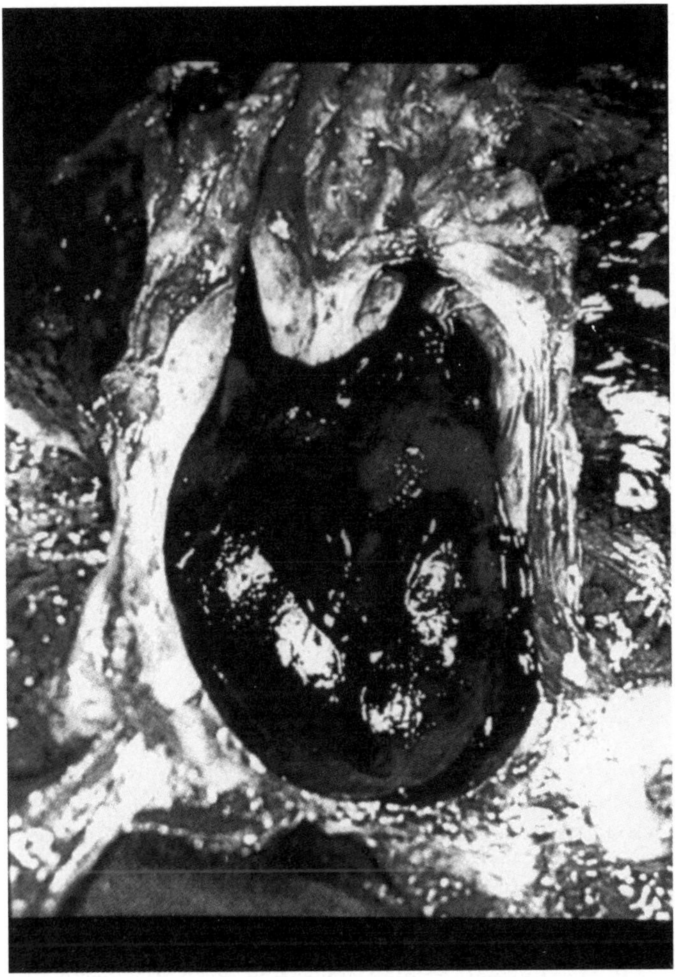

Figure 5 Gross specimen of the heart in situ with a layer of fresh blood on its surface and within the pericardial space resulting from acute myocardial rupture.

healthy muscle. A classification of rupture has been proposed by Becker and Van Mantgem (55):

Type I Rupture Type I rupture is characterized by an abrupt tear in the left ventricular wall. In most cases, there is no appreciable decrease in wall thickness, suggesting that type I rupture occurs early after infarction and is an *acute* process (Fig. 7). Single-vessel disease is present in a majority of cases.

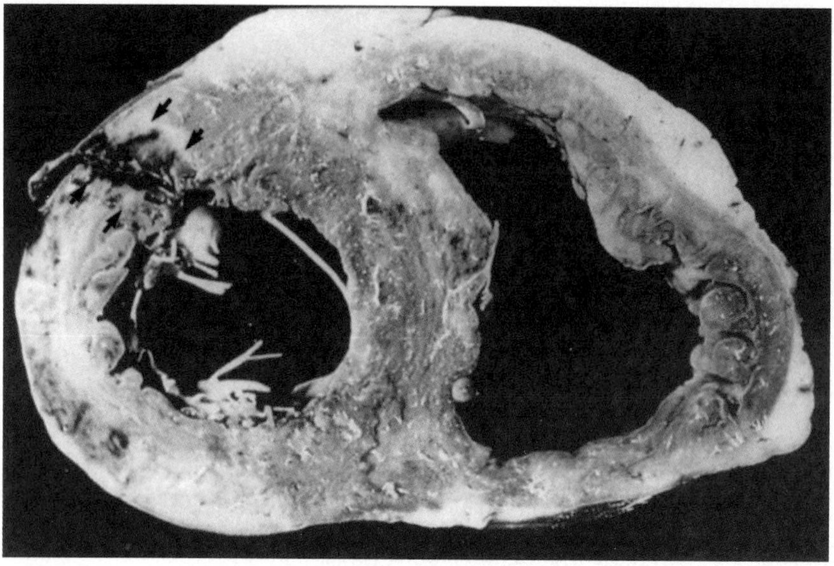

Figure 6 Acute left ventricular free wall rupture (arrows) causing cardiac tamponade and death. A serpiginous path from the endocardium to the epicardial surface is evident.

Type II Rupture Type II rupture is characterized by an advanced but well-localized loss of myocardium and an area of erosion blended with thrombus and necrotic tissue. These features suggest that type II rupture is a *subacute* process where overt rupture is preceded by myocardial erosion (Fig. 8). Multivessel disease is present in a majority of cases.

Type III Rupture Type III rupture occurs in areas of extensive myocardial thinning and aneurysmal bulging consistent with a subacute *or* chronic process (Fig. 9). Rupture is almost always localized to aneurysm's central portion. The extent of coronary artery disease varies.

The age of infarction, determined histologically, differs considerably among the three types of myocardial rupture. In general, hearts with type I rupture exhibit the most recent infarcts with nearly 50% being <24 hours old. In contrast, type II and III ruptures show a much wider age range, averaging 8 and 21 days, respectively.

Ventricular Septal Rupture

Rupture of the ventricular septum occurs in 1.0% to 3.0% of individuals with acute myocardial infarction (one-tenth the incidence of ventricular free

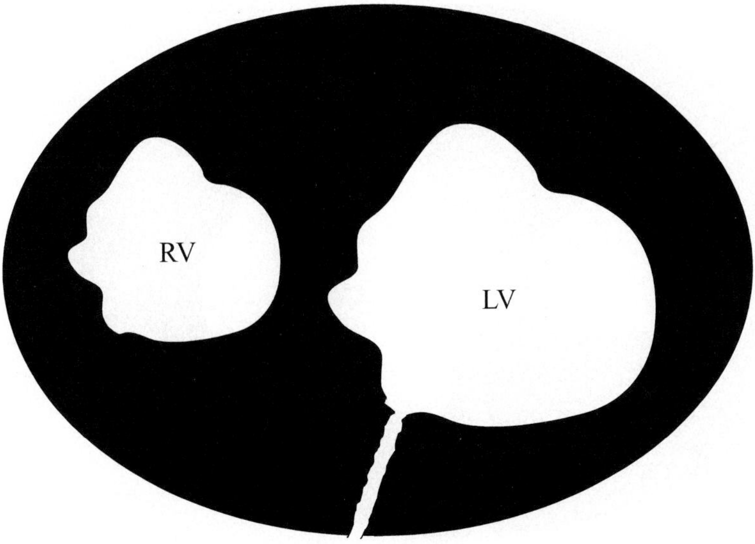

Figure 7 Type I cardiac rupture is an acute process characterized by a "slitlike" tear in the myocardium.

wall rupture) (Fig. 10) (43,56,57). It is reported to be more common in the elderly and among women, and typically occurs within 7 days of infarction. An anterior site of infarction is most common.

Papillary Muscle Rupture

Complete rupture of the papillary muscle causing sudden and torrential mitral insufficiency is a rare but often fatal complication of acute myocardial infarction. It occurs in <1% of all patients; however, papillary muscle rupture carries an 80% mortality (Fig. 11). Rupture of the posteromedial papillary muscle is five to 10 times more common than rupture of the anterolateral papillary muscle owing to its single-vessel blood supply. Rupture of the right ventricular papillary muscle is rare but can cause tricuspid insufficiency and right-sided heart failure.

Partial papillary muscle rupture is more common than complete rupture and can often be addressed surgically. Like ventricular free wall and septal ruptures, papillary muscle rupture typically occurs within the first week of an acute myocardial infarction.

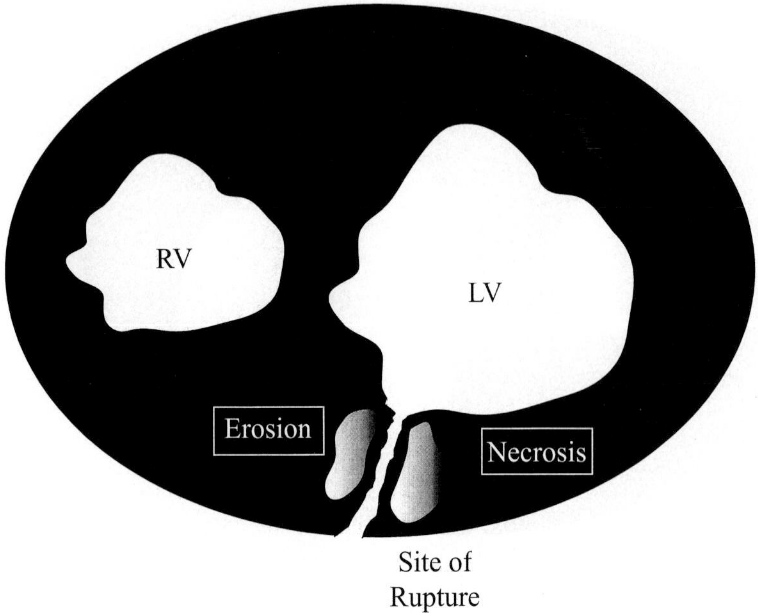

Figure 8 Type II cardiac rupture is a subacute process preceded by myocardial erosion.

Section Summary

Although a majority of ruptures occur within the first 5 days of myocardial infarction, nearly one-quarter take place within the first 24 hours. The proportion of early rupture events may increase with reperfusion therapy (discussed in a section to follow). Rupture after 2 weeks typically involves a site of aneurysm formation or may be a complication of recurrent infarction. In a majority of instances, rupture does *not* represent a myocardial "blowout," but a process that progresses from a small endocardial tear through a zone of extensive transmural necrosis.

PATHOBIOLOGY OF MYOCARDIAL RUPTURE

Between 1936 and 1950 a total of 1641 autopsies were performed at the Beth Israel Hospital in Boston (33). Overall there were 19 cases (1.2%) of spontaneous myocardial rupture (7.0% of all myocardial infarction cases). In each instance there was evidence of a recent infarction. A group of 104 hearts with a fresh infarction but *without* myocardial rupture was examined for comparison. All ruptures were limited to the left ventricle and septum;

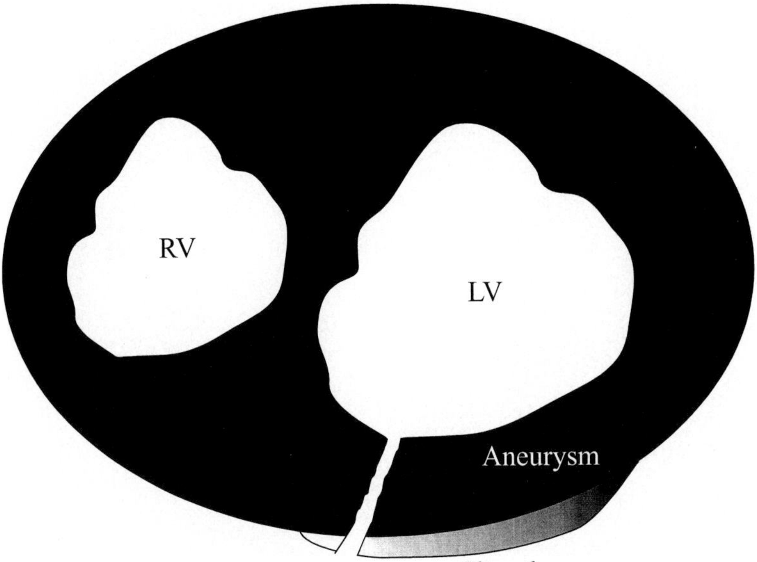

Figure 9 Type III cardiac rupture is a chronic process that occurs in an area of myocardial thinning and aneurysmal bulging.

six involved the anterior and nine the posterior walls, and there was considerable variability in size and shape. Some were described as ragged with gaping holes, while others were linear slits. Tears on the epicardial surface were easily found and varied in length from 3.0 to 30.0 mm. In contrast, the endocardial rents were often small and hidden behind ventricular trabeculae. Old coronary occlusions antedating the acute infarction were present in one-third of hearts with rupture, compared to three-fourths in nonruptured hearts. There was a high incidence of fresh coronary artery occlusions (100%) in hearts with rupture; however, a well-developed collateral circulation was uncommon. There was minimal myocardial fibrosis within the infarct zone and site of rupture. The overall size of the infarct zone did not differ significantly between hearts with rupture and those without; however, transmural infarction was *always* present in hearts with myocardial rupture. In most instances, the path of rupture traversed an area of recent infarction that was free of fibrosis. These observations suggest that the major pathologic findings among hearts with myocardial rupture are 1) fresh coronary artery occlusion, 2) recent infarction, 3) transmural necrosis, 4) a poorly

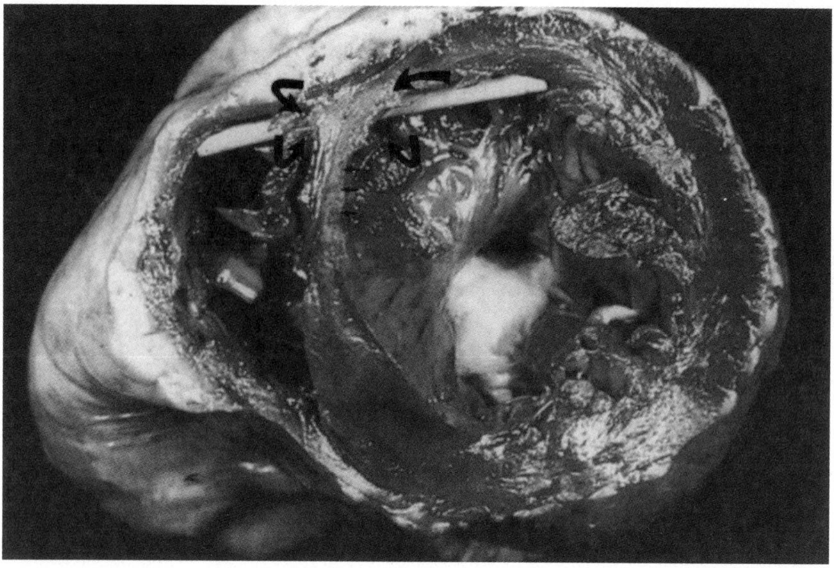

Figure 10 Acute rupture of the interventricular septum (large arrows, marker). A zone of infarction extends from the anterior wall to the septum (small arrows).

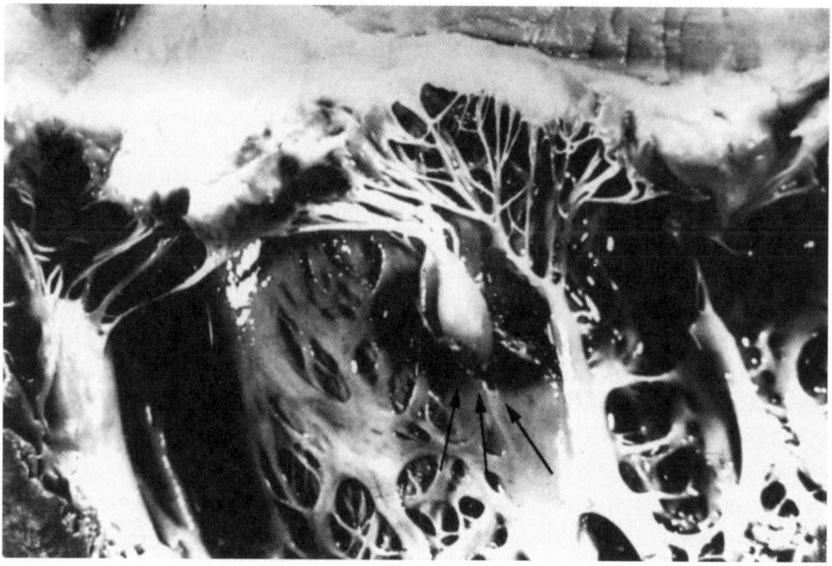

Figure 11 Acute rupture of the posteromedial papillary muscle (arrows) causing torential mitral insufficiency.

developed collateral circulation, and 5) minimal or absent myocardial fibrosis.

One of the largest published series (58) consisting of 9109 autopsies performed at Temple University between 1945 and 1963 reported a 6.4% incidence of rupture in men and 9.1% in women. Several pathologic characteristics of the hearts contained rupture were notable: 1) There was extensive necrosis and neutrophil infiltration; 2) intramural hemorrhage was not marked nor was there evidence of intramural hematoma; and 3) the plane of rupture was invariably through the most necrotic zone. With regard to the tears themselves, 65% contained thrombus, suggesting progression rather than a sudden event. Ruptures were not observed in areas with completed (healed) infarction.

A total of 3416 consecutive autopsies performed at the Miami Heart Institute and Mt. Sinai Hospital contained 1001 cases of acute myocardial infarction, including 47 cases of rupture (59). The average age of the patients with fatal rupture was 69 years, supporting the association between advanced age and mechanical complications of myocardial infarction. A majority of deaths (rupture, nonrupture) occurred within the first 3 days.

Mechanisms: Mechanical and Cellular

While a model for studying myocardial rupture has not yet been developed, hypotheses based on pathologic descriptions have been proposed.

Pressure Theory

The development of an endocardial tear may result either from increased or sustained intracavitary pressure or from forces generated by the contracting heart directed toward the infarct zone. The "pull" of contracting healthy muscle on an adjacent zone of softened necrotic muscle could produce the initial tear, widening with subsequent systolic contractions. In addition to the pulling action, healthy muscle could conceivably produce paradoxical pulsations within the infarcted area (because of differences in elasticity). These actions, coupled with a sustained increase in diastolic pressure at the endocardial surface commonly observed in myocardial ischemia and infarction, could create the "pressure substrate" for rupture, particularly at the junction of normal and abnormal (necrotic) tissue (Fig. 12).

The pressure theory has been extended further to include a transient, acquired dynamic outflow tract obstruction with systolic anterior motion of the mitral valve leaflets in the setting of acute anterior wall myocardial infarction. The focal increase in end-systolic wall stress could facilitate rupture in areas of "vulnerable" myocardium (Fig. 13) (60). Lastly, the impor-

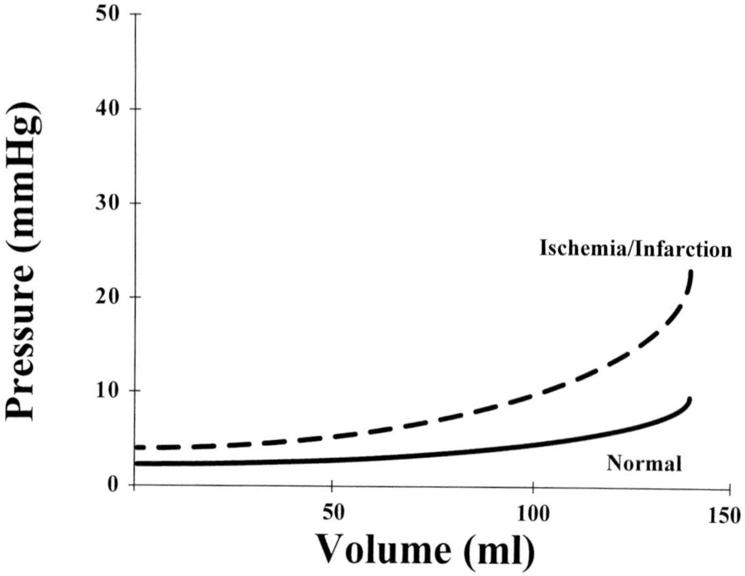

Figure 12 In the setting of myocardial ischemia and infarction a greater increase in left ventricular end-diastolic pressure is generated (steep pressure-volume relationship) in response to a given ventricular volume when compared to a healthy (compliant) heart.

tant contribution of wall stress "surges" to myocardial rupture is supported by reported events during dobutamine stress testing (61).

Collagen Matrix Theory

Although increased intracavitary pressure may play an important role in myocardial rupture, the event itself in all likelihood requires a "vulnerable" myocardium. In other words, the myocardium must be weakened, even if only in a small, well-localized region, for the effects of increased pressure

Figure 13 (Top) Schematic representation of a two-dimensional longitudinal plane through the left ventricle during systole in a patient with an anterior myocardial infarction. (Ao = aorta; LA = left atrium; LV = left ventricle; LVOT = left ventricular outflow tract; RV = right ventricle; Ø = diameter; SAM = systolic anterior movement of the mitral valve). (Bottom) Cascade of events potentially contributing to the development of a left ventricular outflow tract gradient and to myocardial rupture in patients with an anterior myocardial infarction. (From Ref. 60.)

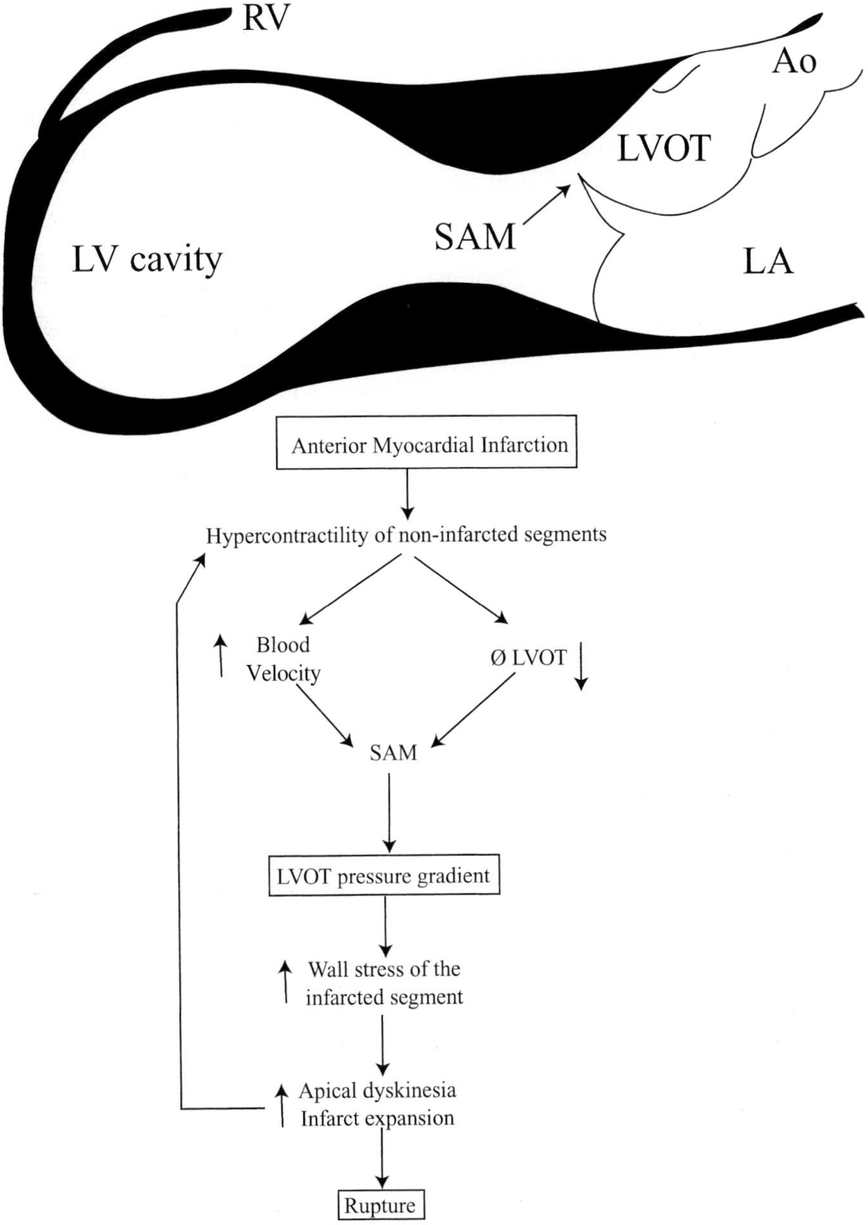
RV
Ao
LVOT
SAM
LV cavity
LA
Anterior Myocardial Infarction
Hypercontractility of non-infarcted segments
↑ Blood Velocity
Ø LVOT ↓
SAM
LVOT pressure gradient
↑ Wall stress of the infarcted segment
↑ Apical dyskinesia Infarct expansion
Rupture

to have important pathologic consequences. Indeed, areas of rupture are often heavily infiltrated by neutrophils, proteolytic enzymes, and a poorly developed supporting collagen framework (Fig. 14). The importance of a strong matrix scaffold for infarct healing is highlighted by the protection from myocardial rupture observed in mice given a plasminogen-activator inhibitor or matrix metalloproteinase inhibitor after coronary artery ligation (62).

Risk Factors for Myocardial Rupture

The major demographic and clinical features associated with myocardial rupture, as determined by necropsy series performed in the prereperfusion era, include advanced age (60 years or older), female sex, first infarction, and hypertension (in the acute phase of infarction).

Section Summary

Myocardial rupture occurs in upward of 10% of individuals following acute myocardial infarction and is most commonly experienced by older individuals within the first 5 days. In a majority of cases, there is extensive necrosis and neutrophilic infiltration caused by sudden coronary occlusion in the absence of a well-developed collateral circulation. Early weakening of a poorly developed collagen framework and increased intracavitary pressure are potentially important contributing factors.

REPERFUSION ERA

Pathologic Features

Animal Models

Coronary ligation experiments designed to investigate the pathologic and histologic features of myocardial infarction following reperfusion have been conducted in animals and nonhuman primates. NcNamara and colleagues (63) documented hemorrhagic infarction in all hearts (nonhuman primates) with coronary occlusion followed by reperfusion (releasing an occlusive clamp). Hemorrhage within the infarct zone was greatest with reperfusion after 4 or more hours of occlusion. Similar observations were made by Vandersalm (64) and Higginson (65), who also found that hemorrhage after reperfusion occurred predominantly in zones of severe myocardial necrosis. The impact of fibrinolytic agents on myocardial hemorrhage has been investigated by Kloner and colleagues (66), who randomly assigned anesthetized, open-chest dogs to reperfusion alone (release of an occlusive clamp) or reperfusion plus intracoronary streptokinase. All animals had 3 hours of

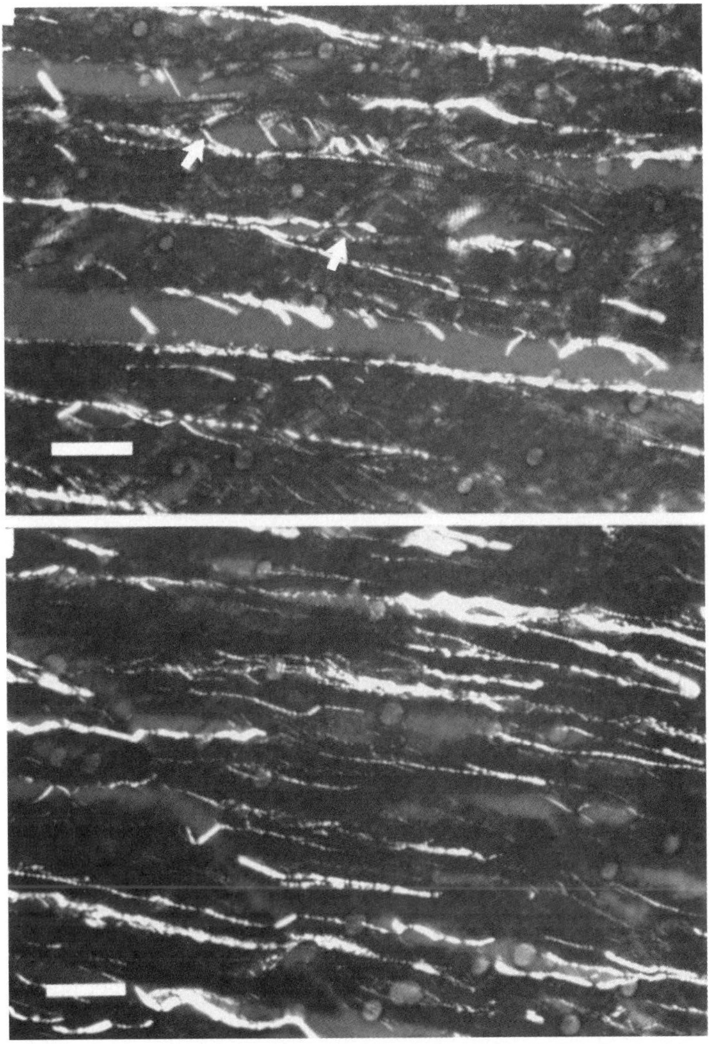

Figure 14 (Top) Micrograph of noninfarcted myocardium revealing normal collagen fibers. (Bottom) Micrograph of infarcted myocardium 3 days after coronary artery occlusion. Fewer collagen fibers are present and their internal structure has been altered. (From Ref. 64.)

occlusion followed by 3 hours of reperfusion. There were no differences in the extent of gross hemorrhage or the calculated intramyocardial hemoglobin concentrations between the two experimental groups.

Stunned myocardium (ischemia followed by reperfusion) exhibits increased collagenase activity and procollagenase activation. Following permanent coronary occlusion (with or without reperfusion), collagen degradation can be observed within 24 hours of infarction. The fewer the number of collagen fibers, the greater the degree of subsequent infarct expansion (67). Coronary ligation followed by reperfusion leads to myocardial necrosis with a hemorrhagic component and a loss of the collagen supporting framework.

Necropsy-Based Experience in Humans with Acute Myocardial Infarction

Myocardial hemorrhage has been observed in humans following coronary reperfusion. In a report by Mathey (68), 6 of 101 patients with myocardial infarction whose coronary arteries were initially recanalized using intracoronary streptokinase (average time to recanalization 2.9 hours) subsequently died in the ensuing weeks (range 1 to 18 days). Hemorrhagic infarction was identified in three patients and was confined to areas of necrosis. Similar observations were made by Fugiwara based on an autopsy study of 30 patients who had received intracoronary urokinase (69). In five patients, myocardial hemorrhage was observed in the absence of reperfusion. Marked focal hemorrhage was *not* identified in patients dying within 4 hours of receiving fibrinolytic therapy.

A necropsy-based series by Waller and colleagues (70), including 19 patients who underwent either pharmacologic (fibrinolytic) or mechanical (predominantly balloon coronary angioplasty) reperfusion, reported a 74% rate of hemorrhagic infarction. Each of the patients with hemorrhagic infarction had received fibrinolytic therapy (or a combination of lytics and angioplasty). In contrast, anemic infarctions were found in patients undergoing mechanical reperfusion.

A study of 23 patients with suspected myocardial infarction, 17 of whom received fibrinolytic therapy, was carried out to determine the effects of plasmin generation on collagen breakdown (71). Amino terminal propeptide of type III procollagen and carboxy terminal propeptide of type I procollagen were assayed. During a streptokinase infusion, serum concentrations of both type I and type III procollagen increased rapidly by 50%, suggesting that fibrinolytics, by generating the nonspecific protease plasmin from its inactive precursor plasminogen, stimulate collagen breakdown.

The hearts of 52 patients (age 67 ± 11 years) participating in the TIMI II study who died between 5 hours and 260 days (medium 2.7 days) after myocardial infarction were examined (72). A total of 38 patients received tissue plasminogen activator (without coronary angioplasty or bypass surgery). A comparison of 23 patients with hemorrhagic infarction and 20 patients with nonhemorrhagic infarction revealed 1) similar frequencies of myocardial rupture—26% of patients with rupture had hemorrhagic infarction while 25% did not; 2) similar infarct size; and 3) similar extent of coronary artery disease.

Observations from necropsy studies suggest that myocardial hemorrhage and collagen breakdown are hallmarks of reperfusion therapy in humans.

Proposed Mechanisms For Myocardial Rupture

There is evidence that transmural infarction is a prerequisite for myocardial rupture. Although hemorrhagic infarction could conceivably weaken the supporting framework, few studies have shown that hemorrhage extends beyond the zone of myocardial necrosis. Thus, based on the available information the critical factor in rupture appears to be disruption of the myocardial connective tissue matrix (73).

Areas of infarction have diminished collagen density (75), and hearts with rupture have a virtual absence of collagen at the involved site (75). Fibrinolytic therapy, by generating plasmin, activates latent tissue collagenases, thereby contributing to early collagen breakdown (71). The added feature of increased endocardial pressure within ischemic/infarcted regions is likely an important contributor.

Section Summary

Observations derived from necropsy studies suggest that myocardial hemorrhage and collagen breakdown are common following reperfusion. Beyond the loss of collagen expected in the early phase of infarction, the nonspecific protease plasmin generated following fibrinolytic administration may initially augment collagen breakdown. The contribution of myocardial hemorrhage to rupture is not clear. In most instances, myocardial salvage achieved through successful reperfusion will prevent transmural injury and minimize the depth and overall extent of necrosis.

CLINICAL EXPERIENCE: RANDOMIZED CLINICAL TRIALS AND LARGE-SCALE REGISTRIES

Prereperfusion Era

The incidence of myocardial rupture was determined among 849 patients enrolled in the MILIS (Multicenter Investigation of Limitation of Infarct Size) study (76). Although there were only 14 cases (1.7%) of rupture, it accounted for 14% of all in-hospital deaths. The following characteristics were associated with a near 10-fold increase of myocardial rupture events: 1) no prior history of angina or myocardial infarction; 2) electrocardiographic ST-segment elevation or the development of Q-waves; and 3) a peak creatine kinase >150 IU/L (Table 2).

Reperfusion Era

A total of 9720 patients participating in the GISSI-2 study (77) who had experienced their first myocardial infarction were analyzed. The in-hospital

Table 2 Infarct-Related Features Among Patients With Subsequent Rupture: Prereperfusion Era

Characterization	Free wall rupture (N = 8)	Ventricular septal rupture (N = 8)	No rupture (N = 831)	*P* value
Location of MI				
Anterior	5	3	389	.79[a]
Inferior	3	3	376	
Lateral or other	0	0	65	
Peak MB-CK (IU/L)				
Sample size	8	6	830	
Mean	312	210	145	.01[b]
Infarct size index by MB-CK (CK-g-eq/m^2)				
Sample size	4	5	713	
Mean	56	21	17	.01[b]
% Dyskinetic segments on admission RVG				
Sample size	7	4	731	
Mean	20	4.5	3.9	.01[b]
LVEF on admission RVG				
Sample size	7	4	718	
Mean	26	42	46	.01[b]

MI = myocardial infarction; RVG = radionuclide ventriculogram; LVEF = left ventricular ejection fraction.
P values reported are from chi-square test of homogeneity or analysis of variance.
[a]Chi-square test may be invalid because of the limited size of the sample in certain groups.
[b]$P < .05$ when the three groups were tested with one another.
Source: Ref. 76.

mortality was 1.9% for patients <40 years of age, but increased to 31.9% among those >80 years. Autopsies were performed in 20% of 772 patients dying in-hospital. The frequency of myocardial rupture was 19% in patients <60 years of age, increasing to 86% (72 of a total of 84 patients) for those >70 years. Approximately half of all deaths occurred within the initial 48 hours of infarction. The findings suggest that myocardial rupture is a particularly common cause of early death in older patients.

The TIMI II study included a total of 3534 patients with suspected myocardial infarction. From the overall cohort, 23 patients had myocardial rupture verified at either autopsy or surgery, and an additional 10 patients died following an episode of EMD (electromechanical dissociation) (without preceding pump heart failure, ventricular tachycardia, or ventricular fibrillation). The incidence of myocardial rupture was 0.95. In a subset of patients undergoing protocol-directed coronary angiography, complete occlusion of the infarct-related coronary artery was more common among patients with rupture compared with the overall study population (40% vs. 11%, $P = .03$). Advanced age and female sex were independent predictors of myocardial rupture (Currier JW: personal communication).

Among 350,755 patients enrolled in the National Registry of Myocardial Infarction (Phase 1) (*NRMI*), 122,243 received fibrinolytic therapy (78). In-hospital mortality rates for the overall patient population, those not treated with fibrinolytics (n = 228,512) and those given fibrinolytics, were 10.4%, 12.9%, and 5.9%, respectively. Cardiogenic shock from primary pump failure was the most common cause of death in each patient group. The overall incidence of myocardial rupture was low (<1.0%), but was responsible for an increasing proportion of hospital deaths among patients given fibrinolytics (7.3%, 6.1%, and 12.1%, respectively) (Table 3). Death from rupture also occurred earlier with fibrinolytic treatment (Table 4). Despite the early occurrence of rupture among fibrinolytic-treated patients, death rates were lower for this group during each of the first 30 postinfarction days (Figs. 15, 16). By multivariable analysis, older age, female sex, and fibrinolytic therapy were associated with early myocardial rupture.

The GISSI-1 trial (79), in which patients were enrolled up to 12 hours from symptom onset, reported an increased incidence of myocardial rupture among late-entry patients treated with fibrinolytics. An overview of four clinical trials that included a total of 1638 patients (58 cases of myocardial rupture) (80) identified a correlation between increasing time to treatment and rupture. However, these data are not conclusive. A prospectively designed ancillary study including a total of 5711 patients randomized to fibrinolytic therapy or placebo 6 to 24 hours from symptom onset (81) revealed no evidence of increased rupture events with treatment beyond 12 hours.

Table 3 National Registry of Myocardial Infarction: Patient Population with In-Hospital Mortality

	All MI patients (%, n)	No fibrinolytic therapy (%, n)	Fibrinolytic therapy (%, n)	*P* value[a]
Number of patients (n)	36,581	29,408	7,173	
Cause of death				
Cardiogenic shock	33.5% (12,262)	32.1% (9,437)	39.4% (2,054)	<.001
Sudden cardiac arrest	27.9% (10,251)	28.7% (8,435)	24.8% (2,282)	<.001
Arrhythmias	14.7% (5,385)	14.6% (4,279)	15.4% (794)	.068
Recurrent MI	6.9% (2,511)	6.8% (1,993)	7.2% (384)	.153
EMD/rupture	7.3% (2,671)	6.1% (1,801)	12.1% (631)	<.001
Other cardiac	11.5% (4,221)	12.1% (3,556)	9.3% (468)	<.001

[a]Pearson chi-square test, patients with versus those without fibrinolytic therapy.
EMD = electromechanical dissociation; MI = myocardial infarction.
Source: Ref. 78.

Table 4 National Registry of Myocardial Infarction: Timing of In-Hospital Death

Hospital	All MI patients	No fibrinolytic therapy	Fibrinolytic therapy	*P* value[a]
Time from presentation to death, mean ± SEM (n)	6.1 ± 0.0 days (35,442)	6.3 ± 0.1 days (28,488)	4.9 ± 0.1 days (6,954)	<.001
Subanalysis				
Rupture/EMD: yes mean ± SEM (n)	3.4 ± 0.1 days (2,621)	3.7 ± 0.1 days (1,762)	2.7 ± 0.1 days (859)	<.001
Rupture/EMD: no mean ± SEM (n)	6.3 ± 0.0 days (32,821)	6.5 ± 0.1 days (26,726)	5.2 ± 0.1 days (6,095)	<.001
P value[b]	<.001	<.001	<.001	

[a]Patients with versus those without fibrinolytic therapy.
[b]Patients with versus those without myocardial rupture/electromechanical dissociation (EMD).
The Wilcoxon test was used to compare time intervals.
MI = myocardial infarction.
Source: Ref. 78.

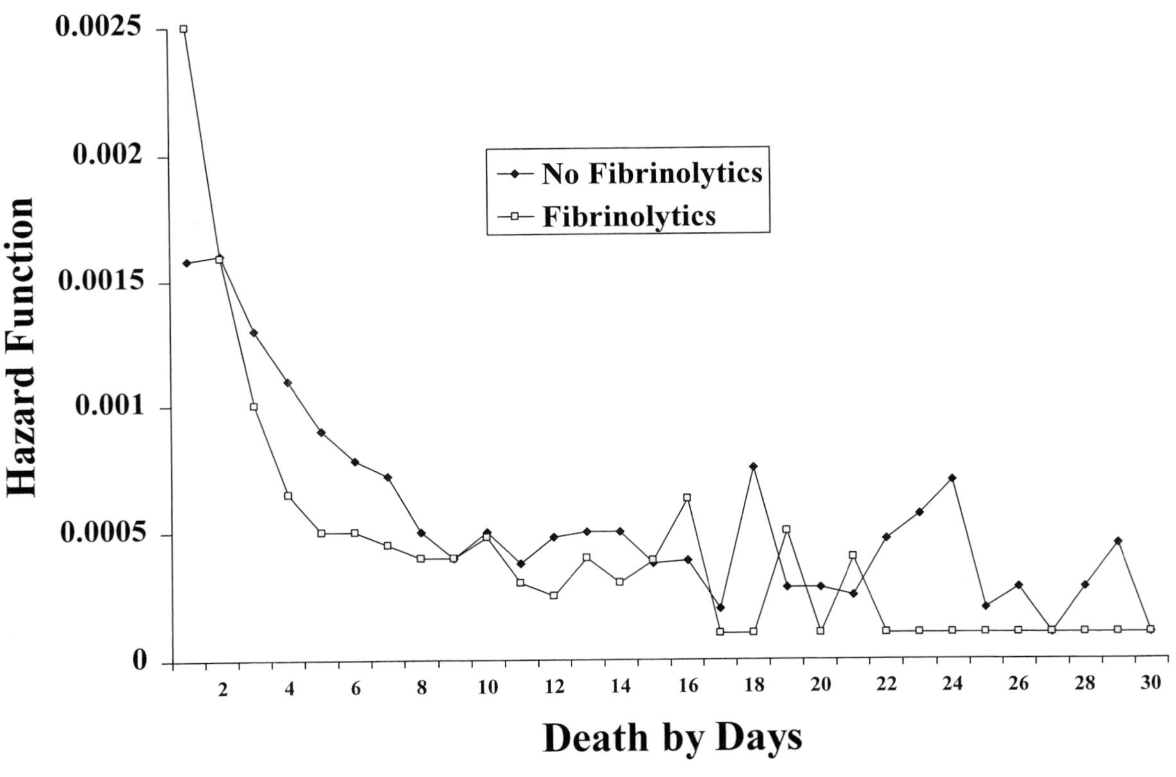

Figure 15 Hazard function for myocardial rupture death in patients enrolled in the National Registry of Myocardial Infarction (Phase 1). Rupture was a more common cause of early death among fibrinolytic-treated patients. (From Ref. 75).

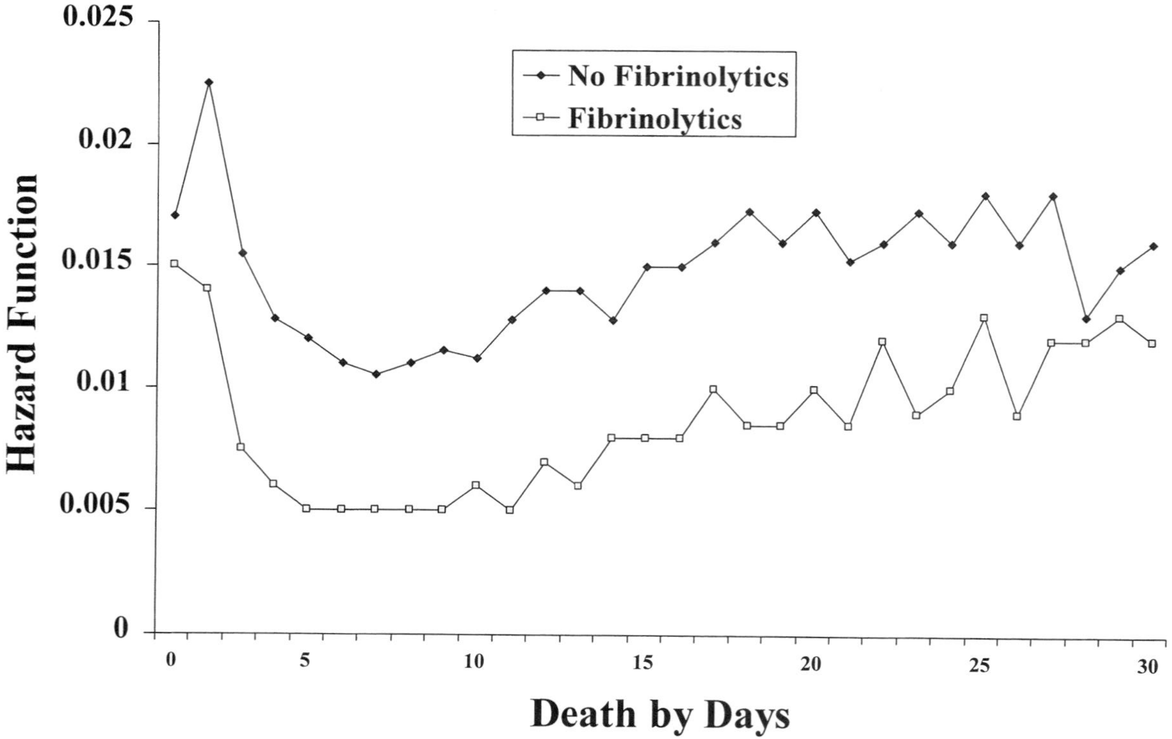

Figure 16 Hazard function for deaths (all cause) among patients enrolled in the National Registry of Myocardial Infarction (Phase 1). Despite having an increased number of early myocardial rupture-related events, patients treated with fibrinolytics experienced a lower overall mortality than those not treated with fibrinolytics. (From Ref. 78.)

Does Fibrinolytic Therapy Increase the Risk of Myocardial Rupture?

Although fibrinolytic therapy represents an established means to reduce mortality in the setting of myocardial infarction, some clinicians remain concerned that its use is accompanied by an "early hazard" attributable to myocardial rupture. A comparison with studies carried out in the prereperfusion era does *not* reveal a major increase in events, mitigating against reperfusion itself as a potential cause for a myocardial rupture. In addition, the incidence of rupture has also not differed between groups in placebo-controlled fibrinolytic therapy trials. There is clear evidence that reperfusion reduces the extent of transmural injury and necrosis (82), still considered a prerequisite for rupture. Accordingly, successful thrombolysis should reduce the overall occurrence of mechanical events that are themselves the end result of extensive myocardial necrosis (83). The low incidence of ventricular septal defects in GUSTO-1 coupled with the observation that a majority of patients with this mechanical event had an occluded infarct-related coronary artery support the "closed artery hypothesis" for myocardial rupture (83a).

The most common cause of death among patients dying within 18 hours of enrollment in TIMI II was pump failure (84). In a separate report by the GUSTO investigators (85), early death (within the first 4 hours) was *not* influenced by coronary arterial patency status. This observation has several important implications. First, it suggests that very early death may not be preventable even with the restoration of coronary blood flow (at least with current treatment strategies). Second, deaths occurring between 6 and 24 hours may, because of a predominant ischemic component, be preventable by means of reestablishing coronary blood flow. Lastly, the available evidence does not support the contention that myocardial rupture is a manifestation or form of "reperfusion injury."

The very low incidence of mechanical complications following primary angioplasty suggests strongly that reperfusion (or reperfusion injury) is not a cause of rupture (86). A recent overview of the *PAMI I* and *PAMI II* trials (1295 patients undergoing primary angioplasty) reported a 0.31% combined incidence of acute mitral insufficiency and ventricular septal defects.

Does the Choice of Fibrinolytic Agent Influence the Risk of Myocardial Rupture?

There is limited clinical and pathologic information that permits a direct comparison of fibrinolytic agents. However, based on the proposed mechanistic algorithm for rupture, one would anticipate a higher incidence of mechanical defects with agents (strategies) that yield relatively low patency rates (reduced myocardial salvage) and higher circulatory concentrations of plasmin. In the GUSTO-1 study, the incidence of rupture (mitral insufficiency/VSD) correlated inversely with early TIMI grade 3 flow.

Does Fibrinolytic Therapy Accelerate Myocardial Rupture?

The beneficial impact of reperfusion therapy on overall patient outcome must never be overlooked when investigating specific causes of death. Indeed, as the mortality from early pump failure and malignant ventricular arrhythmias declines with more effective reperfusion and adjunctive therapies, the contribution attributable to early rupture could potentially increase. This "shift" may also be influenced by a reduced number of late ruptures—a direct reflection of myocardial preservation, reduced infarct expansion, and limited substrate for aneurysm development.

An acceleration of myocardial rupture, typically to within the initial 24 to 48 hours, was appreciated in the TIMI II study, the LATE study (81), GUSTO 1 (83a), and in the NRMI-1 (78). Although there is limited information on the subject, it is conceivable that fibrinolytic therapy, through plasmin generation, accelerates type I and possibly type II ruptures.

Does Antithrombotic Therapy Increase the Risk of Myocardial Rupture?

Anticoagulant therapy, either as a primary form of treatment or used adjunctively with fibrinolytics or primary angioplasty, is commonly utilized in the management of myocardial infarction. The association between anticoagulation and myocardial rupture has been examined; however, data from randomized trials are not available.

From a series of 47 cases with myocardial rupture (43), 45% of patients had received either intravenous unfractionated heparin or oral anticoagulants. A comparative group of patients with fatal myocardial infarction (nonrupture) had a similar proportion of anticoagulant use. Among anticoagulated patients with rupture, a majority had subtherapeutic levels (determined by the prothrombin time or Lee White clotting time). The investigators concluded that anticoagulant therapy did not affect the likelihood of myocardial rupture. Similar observations were made by Maher (87); however, somewhat differing conclusions have been drawn by other investigators (88–90), who found a threefold increase in myocardial rupture and/or hemopericardium (with or without rupture) with anticoagulant use, particularly when the level of systemic anticoagulation was excessive. Considering all of the available information (964 patients in five moderate-size case series), the likelihood of myocardial rupture with and without anticoagulation was 4.2% and 3.7%, respectively.

The discrepant findings are difficult to explain; however, methodologic limitations within existing studies must be considered. First, anticoagulant therapy was not administered in a randomized fashion. Second, it is likely that heparin (and warfarin) was given to inherently sicker patients (larger infarctions). Lastly, several studies reporting an association between anticoagulant use and rupture compared patients from different time periods, introducing potentially important confounding variables.

Anticoagulant therapy is not known to have an adverse effect on myocardial healing following infarction, nor does it increase the extent of hemorrhage within the necrotic zone (91). In the TIMI 9 study (92), hirudin, a potent and direct thrombin antagonist, when given adjunctively with either streptokinase or tPA did not increase the likelihood of rupture compared to heparin (Table 5). Hirudin also did not accelerate rupture events. Although there was a clear relationship between the intensity of anticoagulation (as determined by the activated partial thromboplastin time) and the incidence of major hemorrhage, no correlation was found with myocardial rupture (Fig. 17).

Do Platelet GPIIb/IIIa Antagonists Influence the Risk for Myocardial Rupture?

The available evidence derived from clinical trials of medically treated patients with acute coronary syndromes, those undergoing percutaneous cor-

Table 5 Independent Predictors of Myocardial Rupture: TIMI 9B Trial

Variable	Odds ratio	*P* value
Age >70 yrs	4.96	.0001
Female sex	3.59	.0005
Streptokinase	1.69	.10
Hypertension	1.32	.42
Q-wave MI	1.28	.52
Smoker	1.19	.64
Prior MI	1.06	.90
Systolic BP >160 mm Hg	0.94	.01
Hirudin	0.79	.48
Diabetes	0.65	.38
Fibrinolytic therapy >6 hr from symptom onset	1.00	.98

Source: Ref. 92.

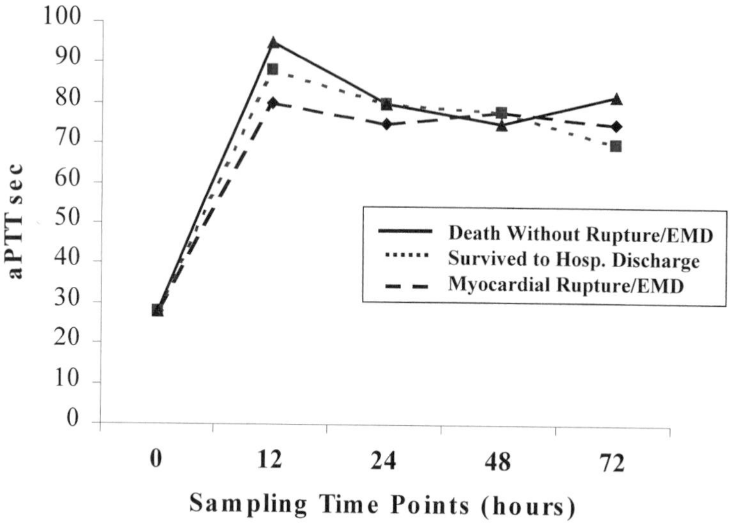

Figure 17 Serial coagulation measurements (activated partial thromboplastin times; aPTT) for patients with and without cardiac rupture-related death and those surviving to hospital discharge. There were no differences in the intensity of anticoagulation at the 12-, 24-, 48- and 72-hr sampling time points. (From Ref. 92.)

onary interventions, and combination low-dose fibrinolytic/anticoagulant therapy Phase II studies has not uncovered an increased occurrence of myocardial rupture. Phase III studies (GUSTO IV acute MI) will provide a large enough experience to examine the question in greater detail.

Are Age and Gender Important Contributing Factors for Myocardial Rupture?

In the TIMI 9 study (92) age >70 years, female gender, and prior angina were associated independently with myocardial rupture (Fig. 18a). Non-rupture-related death was associated with age >70 years, initial pulse >100 beats per minute, and prior MI (Fig. 18b). Thus, myocardial rupture-related death may be responsible for the high early-mortality rates experienced by older women.

Section Summary

The overall incidence of myocardial rupture has not increased substantially in the reperfusion era; however, rupture is observed earlier "accelerated" by fibrinolytic therapy. The available evidence suggests that coronary arterial

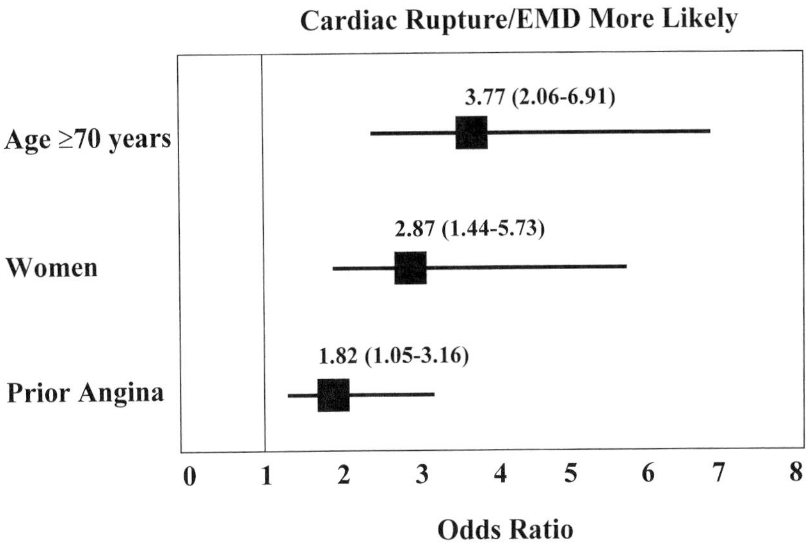

Figure 18a Multivariable analysis of patients experiencing myocardial rupture or electromechanical dissociation (EMD). Age ≥70 years, female gender, and prior angina were independent predictors of an in-hospital event.

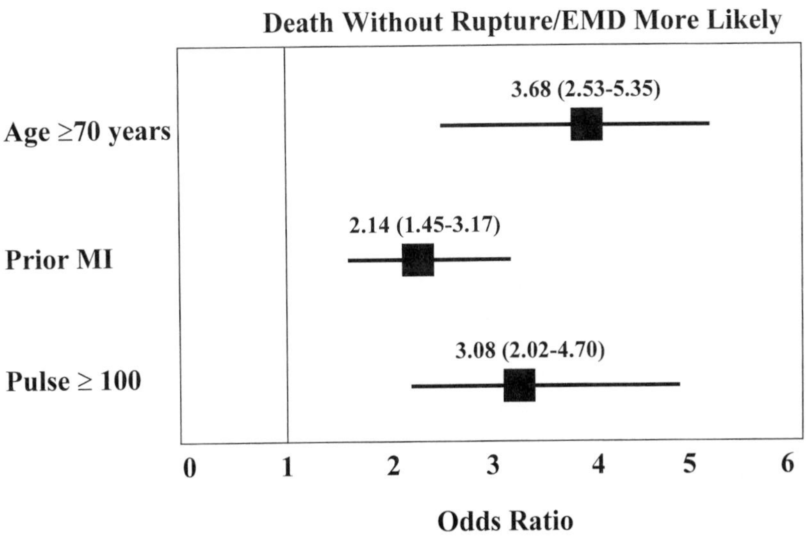

Figure 18b Multivariable analysis of patients with non-rupture-related death. Female gender was *not* independently associated with non-cardiac rupture death.

patency, by limiting myocardial injury, reduces the overall likelihood of mechanical complications, including rupture. The potential impact of treatment strategies utilizing lower doses of fibrinolytics in combination with GPIIb/IIIa antagonists will be determined by ongoing clinical trials. The increased occurrence of myocardial rupture among elderly women must be investigated to determine the causative mechanism, prevention, and preferred treatment of acute myocardial infarction.

DIAGNOSING MYOCARDIAL RUPTURE

Acute Free Wall Rupture

The primary obstacle to preventing death following acute free wall rupture is the limited time available to secure a diagnosis and rapidly proceed to the operating room for definitive treatment. Although free wall rupture most often causes progressive clinical deterioration, characterized by hypotension, electromechanical dissociation (93), and ultimately death, there are several preceding clinical features that may herald its occurrence. The clinical course and evolutionary electrocardiographic changes in 70 consecutive patients with myocardial rupture were described by Oliva and colleagues (94). Patients experiencing rupture had an increased incidence of pericarditis, repetitive emesis, restlessness, and agitation compared to patients without rupture. A deviation from the normal ST and T-wave evolutionary pattern (persistent ST elevation or upright T waves) following infarction was observed in a majority of patients. An abrupt but transient period of hypotension and bradycardia was experienced by nearly one-quarter of patients within 24 hours of rupture. Free wall rupture may be the presenting manifestation of acute myocardial infarction in diabetic patients (95).

Subacute Free Wall Rupture

In some cases, free wall rupture can progress over a 24- to 48-hour period —starting as a small endocardial tear followed by an intramyocardial hematoma that subsequently dissects to the myocardial surface. The sensitivity and specificity of clinical, hemodynamic, and electrocardiographic variables in diagnosing subacute free wall rupture were prospectively studied in 1247 consecutive patients with acute myocardial infarction, including 33 patients with rupture diagnosed at the time of surgery. The incidence of syncope, recurrent chest pain, hypotension, EMD, cardiac tamponade, pericardial effusion, echocardiographic right atrial or right ventricular wall collapse, and hemopericardium (demonstrated by pericardiocentesis) was significantly higher among patients with rupture than among those without (96).

Ventricular Septal Rupture

Rupture of the ventricular septum causes less abrupt hemodynamic deterioration than free wall rupture and should be suspected in patients with unexplained hemodynamic deterioration, particularly in the presence of a new holosystolic murmur. The diagnosis can be strengthened by echocardiographic findings and confirmed by the presence of an oxygen "step up" at the level of the right ventricle. Progressive hemodynamic deterioration represents the combined effects of decreased left ventricular stroke volume and right ventricular failure. Accordingly, fluid resuscitation, inotropic support, and balloon counterpulsation represent the therapeutic mainstays that are designed to provide initial stabilization followed by definitive surgical intervention (97). The use of intrapulmonary balloon counterpulsation should be considered a perioperative management option for patients undergoing surgical repair.

Section Summary

A high index of suspicion is an absolute prerequisite for the early diagnosis of myocardial rupture. Clinical deterioration with sustained hypotension and EMD are diagnostic features of acute free wall rupture. While subacute rupture is characterized by transient periods of agitation, restlessness, bradycardia, and hypotension, myocardial rupture may be a presenting feature of acute myocardial infarction.

SURGICAL ASPECTS OF MYOCARDIAL RUPTURE

The surgical approach to myocardial rupture has historically been individualized and approached on a case-by-case basis. In the acute setting death is inevitable unless prompt relief of pericardial tamponade can be followed by expedient surgical repair. Since the natural history of subacute or "delayed" rupture is largely unknown, emergent or urgent surgery is warranted if the patient is deemed an operative candidate. Attempts to optimize comorbid conditions must be factored against progressive hemodynamic deterioration or sudden death. The goals of surgery are 1) relief of tamponade, 2) cardiac resuscitation, 3) repair or containment of the defect, and 4) concomitant myocardial revascularization.

Repair of the infarcted area ranges from wide debridement of infarcted myocardial muscle and linear buttressed closure or patch closure around a pledgeted base. The current technique, which includes placing a prosthetic or bovine pericardial patch over the unresected area, is expedient and technologically appealing; however, long-term follow-up of this technique is incomplete. A case study from our institution underscores the potential hazard of pseudoaneurysm formation within infarcted regions. Long-term follow-up and echocardiographic surveillance are recommended in all cases.

Case Presentation

A 68-year-old man with a past medical history of hypertension and diabetes experienced progressive angina of 3 weeks' duration culminating in an acute inferior wall myocardial infarction. He was treated with fibrinolytic therapy (tissue plasmogen activator [TPA]). Transthoracic echocardiography identified a moderate-size pericardial effusion with right ventricular wall compression. Cardiac catheterization was recommended and revealed an ejection fraction of 35%, severe three vessel coronary artery disease and moderate pulmonary hypertension. There was inferior wall hypokinesis and a left ventricular subacute rupture with intramyocardial dissection (Fig. 19).

The patient was taken to the operating room where a large pericardial effusion containing old defibrinated blood was confirmed. There was gross evidence of fibrinous pericarditis. Although no discrete perforation was detected, there was a "weakened" (2 cm in diameter) area of recent infarction

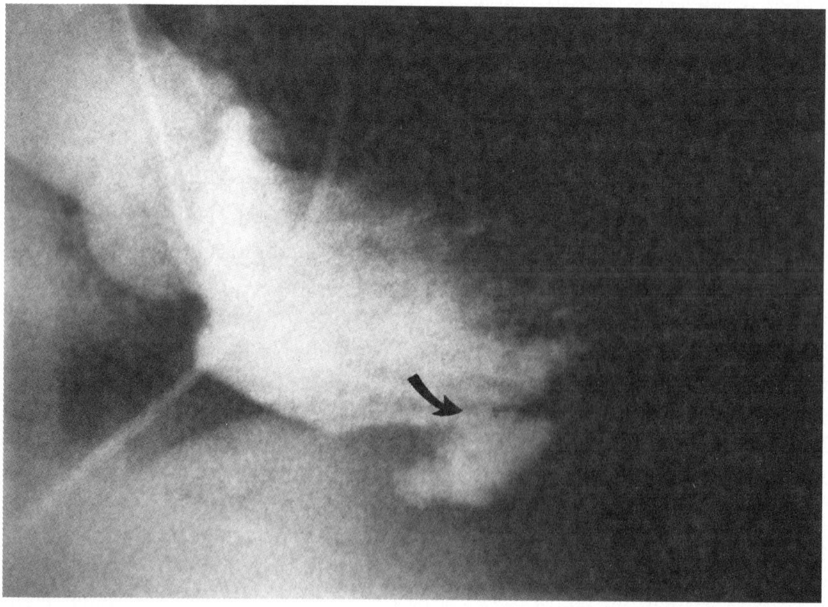

Figure 19 Left ventriculogram revealing posterior extravasation of blood or intramyocardial dissection within an area of infarction (arrow).

involving the left inferior ventricular wall and evidence of subepicardial hemorrhage.

Coronary artery bypass surgery was performed with reversed saphenous vein grafts to the left anterior descending, first obtuse marginal branch of the left circumflex, and right coronary arteries. A bovine pericardial patch was applied to the weakened, infarcted left ventricular inferior wall over a resorcinol glue base. This was sewn circumferentially to the healthy myocardium using 4-0 polypropylene prolene. A femoral intra-aortic balloon pump was placed and removed 2 days after surgery. The patient's postoperative course was complicated by atrial flutter and a pulmonary embolism for which he was anticoagulated initially with intravenous heparin followed by oral warfarin.

An elective left ventriculogram performed 5 months later revealed a large left ventricular pseudoaneurysm (Fig. 20) and patent vein grafts. On reoperation, the left ventricular inferior wall contained a discrete rupture with a fibrous rim contained by the bovine pericardium. This was repaired by closing the fibrous defect using 3-0 pledgeted polypropylene sutures reinforced with adjacent bovine pericardium and the patient's own pericardium

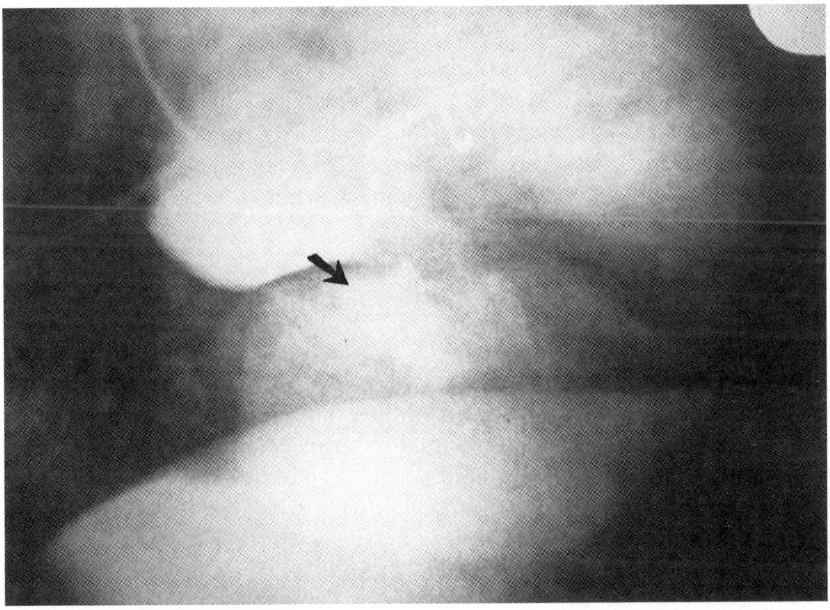

Figure 20 Postoperative left ventriculogram at 5 months revealing a posterior pseudoaneurysm in area of previous repair (arrow).

as a second, "reinforcing" layer. The patient's recovery was uneventful and he was discharged to home on the fourth postoperative day. At 24 months he remains physically active and is clinically well.

The operative approach to myocardial rupture has several important features. In the presence of tamponade physiology the operative field should be prepared prior to full anesthetic delivery. This may prevent sudden hemodynamic collapse when compensatory tachycardia is suppressed. Femoral arterial and venous cannulation should be considered. At the very least exposure of the femoral vessels is recommended. Manipulation of the ventricle should be avoided until the patient has been placed on cardiopulmonary bypass. Full cardiopulmonary bypass coupled with antegrade cardioplegia and hypothermia (25 to 28°C) allows complete evacuation of the pericardial space, assessment and repair of the defect, and concomitant coronary artery bypass grafting. With rupture involving the posterior myocardium, retrograde cardioplegia may be technically difficult and hazardous.

There are several other technical points of importance. Wide excision and debridement of the infarcted area with subsequent patch reconstruction has been performed successfully, as has linear closure over bolstered sutures or strips with minimal debridement. Purse-string closure of myocardial rupture has also been reported (98).

Historically the surgical approach to myocardial rupture has evolved through three phases. The first phase includes anecdotal case reports of dramatic attempts to resuscitate and repair the life-threatening defect. The second phase introduced a variety of surgical techniques for closure. The third (current) phase emphasizes early diagnosis and aggressive surgical management. This exciting phase involves intermediate and long-term results of less aggressive methods of surgical management, namely, biological glues and patching techniques (99).

Surgical History of Myocardial Rupture Repair

Lillehei in 1969 (100) is credited with the first attempt at surgical repair of myocardial rupture. In March 1968 a 50-year-old man underwent repair 10 days following an acute myocardial infarction. He died 37 days postoperatively. In 1971 Friedman reported an unsuccessful attempt to repair a posterior rupture without cardiopulmonary bypass. FitzGibbon (101) successfully repaired a cardiac rupture developing 21 days after a large anteroseptal myocardial infarction.

The early cases, while considered anecdotal by current standards, were nonetheless vital to the development of surgical techniques (98,100–127,153–154). The majority of patients were male and had either anterior or posterior sites of infarction, surgical infarctectomy, debridement, and buttressed repair. Few patients underwent concomitant myocardial revascularization; however, cardiopulmonary bypass did play a pivotal role in the initial resuscitation of patients (35 of 49; 70%) who survived the operation. The reports, however, focused solely on short-term outcome with little diagnostic or investigative follow-up.

There are several case studies that have included complex ruptures and at least two published reports of cardiac rupture following myocardial revascularization. Charnvechai (128) reported seven patients with rupture of the left ventricular free wall following internal mammary artery implantation (Vineberg procedure). Few details were provided, yet false passage to the subepicardial area is a potential explanation. Fortunately, this procedure is rarely performed today. Bojar (129) reported successful left ventricular free wall rupture repair in a patient 5 days following bypass surgery.

Myocardial cardiac rupture does occur in association with left ventricular true or false aneurysms. Abel in 1976 (109) observed a rupture at the junction of a left ventricular aneurysm and normal myocardium. This observation is in conflict with the findings of Vlodaver (130), who reported that fibrous left ventricular aneurysms rarely rupture. There is little question, however, that false aneurysms do rupture. Yaku in 1995 (131) reported the successful repair of an early false aneurysm (<10 days).

Recent advances in surgery have focused on an aggressive approach to patients with subacute myocardial rupture, including patients with dissection, hematoma, or "concealed" ruptures. Pliam reviewed 12 cases from 1944 to 1991 (132,141–151). All five surgical cases survived while only one of seven patients receiving medical management did so. The appealing features of the surgery are omission of cardiopulmonary bypass and avoidance of resection/debridement. Instead, biological glues buttressed with pericardial or synthetic patches are used. Although the short-term results are dramatic, long-term data regarding survival or pseudoaneurysm formation are incomplete. The role of concomitant myocardial revascularization is also unknown. We recommend preoperative coronary angiography if the clinical status of the patient permits.

Advances in the surgical approach to myocardial rupture were highlighted by Padró in 1989 (133). A 62-year-old woman underwent emergency operation 7 days following an acute myocardial infarction. A large anterolateral transmural infarction was found with several epicardial bleeding points and a large volume of blood in the pericardium. Without the institution of cardiopulmonary bypass, the bleeding points were controlled with butyl-2-cyanoacrylate glue. A large Teflon patch was then placed over the entire area. She was alive at 15-month follow-up. Zogno (134) applied the same technique successfully. Utilizing cardiopulmonary bypass a 2-cm linear anterolateral tear was coated with fibrin glue. A glutaraldehyde stiffened patch of autologous pericardium was then placed over the area and sewn to surrounding normal myocardium with a running 5-0 polypropylene suture. Padró (135) summarized his own surgical experience with myocardial rupture in 1993. Thirteen patients underwent repair with cyanoacrylate and Teflon patch. Only one patient (with a posterior wall rupture) required cardiopulmonary bypass. All patients survived surgery. At follow-up (26 months) there was a 100% survival. Five patients had transthoracic echocardiography performed at 3 to 7 months without evidence of psuedoaneurysms development. A similar result was reported by Almdahl (136).

Coletti and Torracca (137) reported three cases of myocardial rupture repaired with fibrin glue (two) and GRF biological glue (one) covered by an autologous glutaraldehyde-stiffened pericardial patch and fixed with running sutures on the adjacent healthy myocardium. Echocardiography performed serially to 3 months did not reveal evidence of pseudoaneurysm formation.

Current Considerations for Surgical Repair

The natural history of cardiac rupture that includes a 50% mortality within 5 days and 87% within 2 weeks of infarction justifies the urgency of surgical repair. Traditional methods of repair including infarctectomy, debridement, and buttressed linear or patch closure has been challenged in recent years. The employment of biological glues with patch reinforcement has provided encouraging short-term results. It should be stressed that preoperative use of intraaortic balloon counterpulsation and pericardiocentesis are temporizing modalities. Although the use of cardiopulmonary bypass is not universally accepted, supporters point out that a more precise repair, concomitant myocardial revascularization, and optimization of resuscitative efforts are more successfully accomplished while the patient is on bypass.

In emergent or urgent situations the presence of cardiac tamponade following acute myocardial infarction represents left ventricular free wall rupture until proven otherwise. Immediate echocardiography followed by surgery is the best chance for survival. Lopez-Sendon (96) in a series of 33 operative cases 25 (76%) survived with an aggressive approach. Six additional patients undergoing emergent surgery did not have rupture. Five survived, with the remaining patient dying of cardiogenic shock. A recent series by Cheriex (138) showed 9 of 12 (75%) surviving myocardial rupture with aggressive treatment. The trend toward rapid diagnosis and aggressive surgical intervention has yielded a >70% chance of survival.

Percutaneous Strategies for Myocardial Rupture

Although surgical intervention represents the standard of care for patients with free wall myocardial rupture in whom aggressive intervention is deemed appropriate, percutaneous strategies have been investigated as a means to achieve rapid stabilization. A recent report outlined the potential use of intrapericardial fibrin glue administration following a pericardial drainage as a therapeutic option (155).

Section Summary

Once a diagnosis of acute myocardial rupture is seriously entertained immediate surgery is required for patient survival. Temporizing pericardiocentesis and intrapericardial administration of fibrin glue represent "bridging" therapies en route to the operating room. In the subacute setting coronary angiography should be performed because the high incidence of concomitant multivessel disease.

The surgical literature can be divided historically into two eras. The first included isolated case reports of cardiac rupture. The second has highlighted the importance of subacute rupture associated with intramyocardial dissection and/or hematomas. These patients also benefit from early diagnosis and aggressive treatment. Long-term objective data are needed to determine whether less aggressive surgical techniques utilizing a biological glue and patching will prevent subsequent rupture or pseudoaneurysm development.

CHAPTER SUMMARY

Myocardial rupture is an infrequent but well-recognized and typically fatal complication of acute myocardial infarction that can involve the left ventricular free wall, ventricular septum, papillary muscle, right ventricular free wall, and atrium. Although typically occurring between 4 and 7 days from the time of infarction, myocardial rupture can manifest within the first 24 to 48 hours, particularly among patients receiving fibrinolytic therapy. For reasons that are not entirely clear, older women are at increased risk for myocardial rupture, possibly due to unique features of reparative processes, collagen matrix, proteolytic enzymes, and wall stress. Early β-blockade and ACE inhibitor therapy do offer protective effects.

The diagnosis of myocardial rupture begins with a high index of suspicion and must be considered strongly in the setting of sudden or rapidly progressive hemodynamic compromise. Prompt diagnosis and stabilization achieved with pericardiocentesis, intravenous fluid administration, and hemodynamic support followed by definitive surgical intervention are the keys to a favorable clinical outcome.

REFERENCES

1. Harvey W. Complete Works. London: Syndenham Society, 1847.
2. Morgagni JB. The Seats and Causes of Disease Investigated by Anatomy: In Five Books, Containing a Great Variety of Dissections with Remarks. Translated by B. Alexander. London: A. Millar & T. Cadell, 1769 Letter 27, Vol. 1 (Book 2), p. 830.
3. Malmsten. Cited by Benson et al. (Ref. 4).
4. Benson RL, Hunter WC, Manlove CH. Spontaneous rupture of heart: report of 40 cases in Portland, Oregon. Am J Pathol 1933;9:295–328.
5. Krumbhaar EB, Crowell C. Spontaneous rupture of heart: clinicopathologic study based on 22 unpublished cases and 632 from literature. Am J Med Sci 1925;170:828–856.
6. Braunwald E. Heart Disease: A Textbook of Cardiovascular Medicine, Vol. 2. Philadelphia: W.B. Saunders, 1984:1262–1300.
7. Buja LM, Willerson JT. Clinicopathological correlates of acute ischemic heart disease syndromes. Am J Cardiol 1981;47:343–356.
8. Fishbein MC, Maclean D, Maroko PR. The histopathological evolution of myocardial infarction. Chest 1978;73:843–849.
9. Henson DE, Najafi H, Callaghan R, Coogan P, Julian OC, Eisenstein R. Myocardial lesions following open heart surgery. Arch Pathol 1969;88:423–430.
10. Tyagi SC, Ratajska A, Weber KT. Myocardial matrix metalloproteinase(s): localization and activation. Mol Cell Biochem 1993;126:49–59.
11. Cleutjens JPM, Kandala JC, Guarda E, Guntaka RV, Weber KT. Regulation of collagen degradation in the rat myocardium after infarction. J Mol Cell Cardiol 1995;27:1281–1292.
12. McCormick RJ, Musch TI, Bergman BC, Thomas DP. Regional differences in LV collagen accumulation and mature cross-linking after myocardial infarction in rats. Am J Physiol 1994;266:H354-H359.
13. Finesmith TH, Broadley KN, Davidson JM. Fibroblasts from wounds of different stages of repair vary in their ability to contract a collagen gel in response to growth factors. J Cell Physiol 1990;144:97–107.
14. Hutchins GM. Time course of infarct and healing. In: Wagner GS, ed. Myocardial Infarction: Measurement and Intervention. The Hague: Martinus Nijhoff, 1982:3–20.
15. Waller BF. Pathology of new interventions used in the treatment of coronary heart disease. Curr Probl Cardiol 1986;11:665–740.
16. Mathey DG, Schofer J, Kuck KH, Beil U, Kloppel G. Transmural hemorrhagic myocardial infarction after intracoronary streptokinase. Clinical, angiographic and necropsy finding. Br Heart J 1982;48:546–551.
17. Waller BF, Rothbaum DA, Pinkerton CA, Cowley MJ, Linnemeier TJ, Orr C, Irons M, Helmuth RA, Wills ER, Aust C. Status of the myocardium and infarct-related coronary artery in 19 necropsy patients with acute recanalization using pharmacologic (streptokinase, r-tissue plasminogen activator), mechanical (percutaneous transluminal coronary angioplasty) or combined types of reperfusion therapy. J Am Coll Cardiol 1987;9:785–801.

18. Parkinson J, Bedford DE. Cardiac infarction and coronary thrombosis. Lancet 1928;1:4–11.
19. Levine SA. Coronary thrombosis: its various clinical features. Medicine 1929; 8:245–418.
20. Bean WB. Infarction of heart. III. Clinical course and morphological findings. Ann Intern Med 1938;12:71–94.
21. Mallory GK, White PD, Sahedo-Salgar J. The speed of healing of myocardial infarction. Am Heart J 1939;18:647–671.
22. Edmondson HA, Hoxie HJ. Hypertension and cardiac rupture. Am Heart J 1942;24:719–733.
23. Friedman S, White PD. Rupture of the heart in myocardial infarction. Ann Intern Med 1944;21:778–782.
24. Mintz SS, Katz LN. Recent myocardial infarction: Analysis of 572 cases. Arch Intern Med 1947;80:205–236.
25. Wartman WB, Hellerstein HK. Incidence of heart disease in 2,000 consecutive autopsies. Ann Intern Med 1948;28:41–65.
26. Selzer A. Immediate sequelae of myocardial infarction: their relation to prognosis. Am J Med Sci 1948;216:172–178.
27. Diaz-Rivera RS, Miller AJ. Rupture of heart following acute myocardial infarction: incidence in public hospital, with five illustrative cases including one of perforation of interventricular septum diagnosed antemortem. Am Heart J 1948;35:126–133.
28. Foord AG. Embolism and thrombosis in coronary artery disease. JAMA 1948; 138:1009.
29. Wang CH, Bland EF, White PD. Note on coronary occlusion and myocardial infarction found postmortem at Massachusetts General Hospital during twenty year period from 1926 to 1945 inclusive. Ann Intern Med 1948;29:601–606.
30. Howell DA, Tumbell GC. Hypertension and effort in cardiac rupture following acute myocardial infarction. Q Bull NWU Med School 1950;24:100–103.
31. Zinn WJ, Cosby RS. Myocardial infarction. I. Statistical analysis of 679 autopsy proven cases. Am J Med 1950;8:169–176.
32. Oblath RW, Levenson DC, Griffith GC. Factors influencing rupture of the heart after myocardial infarction. JAMA 1952;149:1276–1281.
33. Wessler S, Zoll PM, Schlesinger MI. The pathogenesis of spontaneous cardiac rupture. Circulation 1952;6:334–351.
34. Waldron BR, Fennel RH, Castelman B, Bland EF. Myocardial rupture and hemopericardium associated with anticoagulant therapy. A postmortem study. N Engl J Med 1954;251:892–894.
35. Goetz AA, Gropper AN. Perforation of interventricular septum. Am Heart J 1954;48:130–140.
36. Mcdonniael SH, Humbrecht M, Voorhies NW. Cardiac rupture. J Louisiana Med Soc 1955;107:171–177.
37. Maher JF, Mallory GK, Laurenz GA. Rupture of the heart after myocardial infarction. N Engl J Med 1956;255:1–10.
38. Zeman F, Rodstein M. Cardiac rupture complicating myocardial infarction in the aged. Arch Intern Med 1960;105:431–433.

39. Griffith GC, Hedge B, Oblath RW. Factors in myocardial rupture. An analysis of 204 cases at Los Angeles County Hospital between 1924–1959. Am J Cardiol 1961;8:792–798.
40. Friedberg CK. General treatment of acute myocardial infarction. Circulation 1969;39:40(suppl IV):252–260.
41. Ross RM, Young JA. Clinical and necropsy findings in rupture of the myocardium. A review of 43 cases. Scott Med J 1963;8:222–226.
42. Sievers J. Cardiac rupture in acute myocardial infarction. Geriatrics 1966;21: 125–130.
43. London RE, London SB. Rupture of the heart. A critical analysis of 47 consecutive autopsy cases. Circulation 1965;31:202–208.
44. Sugiura M, Okada R, Morii T, Hiraoka K, Shimada H, Nakanishi A. A clinicopathological study on the cardiac rupture following myocardial infarction in the aged. Jpn Heart J 1968;9:265–280.
45. Sahebjaml H. Myocardial infarction and cardiac rupture. Analysis of 37 cases and a brief review of the literature. South Med J 1969;62:1058–1063.
46. Lewis JL, Burchell HB, Titus JL. Clinical and pathologic features of postinfarction cardiac rupture. Am J Cardiol 1969;23:43–53.
47. Beutler SM, Toscano M. Cardiac rupture in the University of Chicago. Personal observations. Am Heart J 1942;23:455–467.
48. Meurs AAH, Vos AK, Verhey JB, Gerbrandy J. Electrocardiogram during cardiac rupture by myocardial infarction. Br Heart J 1970;32:232–235.
49. Gjol N. Cardiac rupture and acute myocardial infarction. Geriatrics 1972;26: 126–137.
50. Naeim F, de al Maza, LM, Robbins SL. Cardiac rupture during myocardial infarction: a review of 44 cases. Circulation 1972;45:1231–1239.
51. Hammer J, Fabian J, Pavlovic J, Smid J. Myocardial rupture in acute myocardial infarction. Cor Vasa 1972;14:180–187.
52. Havig O. Cardiac rupture in recent myocardial infarction. Acta Pathol Microbiol Scand [A] 1973;81:501–506.
53. Sievers J. Cardiac rupture in acute myocardial infarction: Geriatrics 1996;21: 125–130.
54. Spiekerman RE, Brandenburg JT, Achor RWP. The spectrum of coronary artery disease in a community of 30000. A clinicopathologic study. Circulation 1962;25:57–65.
55. Becker AE, van Mantgem J-P. Cardiac tamponade. A study of 50 hearts. Eur J Cardiol 1974;3/4:349–358.
56. Kassis E, Vogelsang M, Lyngborg K. Cardiac rupture complicating myocardial infarction. A study concerning early diagnosis and possible management. Dan Med Bull 1981;48:164–167.
57. Matsui K, Kay JH, Mendez M. Ventricular septal rupture secondary to myocardial infarction. Clinical approach and surgical results. JAMA 1981;245: 1537–1539.
58. Lautsch EV, Lanks KW. Pathogenesis of cardiac rupture. Arch Pathol 1967; 84:264–271.

59. London RE, London SB. The electrocardiographic signs of acute hemopericardium. Circulation 1962;25:780–786.
60. Bartunek J, Vanderheyden M, De Bruyne B. Dynamic left ventricular outflow obstruction after anterior myocardial infarction. Eur Heart J 1995;16:1439–1442.
61. Reisenhofer B, Squarcini G, Picano E. Cardiac rupture during dobutamine stress test. Ann Intern Med 1998;128:605.
62. Heymens S, Lutten A, Nuyens D, et al. Inhibition of plasminogen activators or matrix metalloproteinases prevents cardiac rupture but impairs therapeutic angiogenesis and causes cardiac failure. Nature Med 1999;5:1135–1142.
63. McNamara JJ, Lacro RV, Yee M, Smith GT. Hemorrhagic infarction and coronary reperfusion. J Thorac Cardiovasc Surg 1981;81:498–501.
64. Vander Salm TJ, Pape LA, Price J, Burke M. Hemorrhage from myocardial revascularization. J Thorac Cardiovasc Surg 1981;82:768–772.
65. Higginson LAJ, White F, Heggtveit HA, Sanders TM, Bloor CM, Covell JW. Determinants of myocardial hemorrhage after coronary reperfusion in the anesthetized dog. Circulation 1982;65:62–69.
66. Kloner RA, Alker KJ. The effect of streptokinase on intramyocardial hemorrhage, infarct size, and the no-reflow phenomenon during coronary reperfusion. Circulation 1984;70:513–521.
67. Whittaker P, Boughner DR, Kloner RA. Role of collagen in acute myocardial infarct expansion. Circulation 1991;84:2123–2134.
68. Mathey DG, Schofer J, Kuck K-H, Beil U, Klöppel G. Transmural, haemorrhagic myocardial infarction after intracoronary streptokinase. Clinical, angiographic, and necropsy findings. Br Heart J 1982;48:546–551.
69. Fujiwara H, Onodera T, Tanaka M, Fujiwara T, Wu D-J, Kawai C, Hamashima Y. A clinicopathologic study of patients with hemorrhagic myocardial infarction treated with selective coronary thrombolysis with urokinase. Circulation 1986;73:749–757.
70. Waller BF. The pathology of acute myocardial infarction: definition, location, pathogenesis, effects of reperfusion, complications and sequelae. Cardiol Clin 1988;6:1–28.
71. Peuhkurinen KJ, Risteli L, Melkko JT, Med C, Linnaluoto M, Jounela A, Risteli J. Thrombolytic therapy with streptokinase stimulates collagen breakdown. Circulation 1991;83:1969–1975.
72. Gertz SD, Kalan JM, Kragel AH, Roberts WC, Braunwald E, and the TIMI Investigators. Cardiac morphologic findings in patients with acute myocardial infarction treated with recombinant tissue plasminogen activator. Am J Cardiol 1990;65:953–961.
73. Whittaker P. Unravelling the mysteries of collagen and cilatrix after myocardial infarction. Cardiovasc Res 1996;31:19–26.
74. Charney RH, Takahashi S, Zhao M, Sonnenblick EH, Eng C. Collagen loss in the stunned myocardium. Circulation 1992;85:1483–1490.
75. Factor SM, Robinson TF, Dominitz R, Cho S. Alterations of the myocardial skeletal framework in acute myocardial infarction with and without ventricular rupture. A preliminary report. Am J Cardiovasc Pathol 1986;1:91–97.

76. Pohjola-Sintonen S, Muller JE, Stone PH, Willich SN, Antman EM, Davis VG, Parker CB, Braunwald E, and the MILIS study group. Ventricular septal and free wall rupture complicating acute myocardial infarction: experience in the multicenter investigation of limitation of infarct size. Am Heart J 1989; 117:809–816.
77. Maggioni AP, Maseri A, Fresco C, Franzosi MG, Mauri F, Santoro E, Tognoni G on behalf of the Investigators of the Gruppo Italiano per lo Studio della Sopravvivenza nell'Infarto Miocardico (GISSI-2). Age-related increase in mortality among patients with first myocardial infarctions treated with thrombolysis. N Engl J Med 1993;11:1442–1448.
78. Becker RC, Gore JM, Lambrew C, Weaver WD, Rubison RM, French WJ, Tiefenbrunn AJ, Bowlby LJ, Rogers WJ. A composite view of cardiac rupture in the United States National Registry of Myocardial Infarction. J Am Coll Cardiol 1996;27:1321–1326.
79. Mauri F, DeBiase AM, Franzosi MD, Pampallona S, Foresti A, Gasparini M. GISSI analisis cause di morte intraspedaliera. G Ital Cardiol 1987;17:37–44.
80. Honan MB, Harrell FE, Reimer KA, Califf RM, Mark DB, Pryor DB, Hlatky MA. Cardiac rupture, mortality and the timing of thrombolytic therapy: a meta-analysis. J Am Coll Cardiol 1990;16:359–367.
81. Becker RC, Charlesworth A, Wilcox RG, Hampton J, Skene A, Gore JM, Topol EJ. Cardiac rupture associated with thrombolytic therapy: impact of time to treatment in the Late Assessment of Thrombolytic Efficacy (LATE) study. J Am Coll Cardiol 1995;25:1063–1068.
82. Correale E, Maggioni AP, Romano S, Ricciardiello V, Battista R, Salvarola G, Santoro E, Tognoni G on behalf of the Gruppo Italiano per lo Studio della Sopravvivenza nell'Infarto Miocardico (GISSI). Am J Cardiol 1993;71:1377–1381.
83. Nakamura F, Minamino T, Higashino Y, Ito H, Fujii K, Fujita T, Nagano M, Higaki J, Ogihara T. Cardiac free wall rupture in acute myocardial infarction: ameliorative effect of coronary reperfusion. Clin Cardiol 1992;15:244–250.
83a. Crenshaw BS, Granger CB, Birnbaum T, et al. for the GUSTO-1 trial investigators. Risk factors, angiographic patterns and outcomes in patients with ventricular septal defect complicating acute myocardial infarction. Circulation 2000. In press.
84. Kleimen NS, Terrin M, Mueller H, and the TIMI Investigators. Mechanisms of early death despite thrombolytic therapy: experience from the TIMI II study. J Am Coll Cardiol 1992;19:1129–1135.
85. Kleimen NS, White HD, Ohman EM for the GUSTO Investigators. Mortality within 24 hours of thrombolysis from myocardial infarction: the importance of early reperfusion. Circulation 1994;20:2658–2665.
86. Brodie B, et al. Timing and mechanism of death determined clinically after primary angioplasty for acute myocardial infarction. Am J Cardiol 1997;79: 1586–1591.
87. Maher JF, Mallory GK, Laurenz GA. Rupture of the heart after myocardial infarction. N Engl J Med 1956;255:1–10.

88. Aarseth S, Lange HF. The influence of anticoagulant therapy on the occurrence of cardiac rupture and hemopericardium following heart infarction. I. A study of 89 cases of hemopericardium (81 of them cardiac ruptures). Am Heart J 1958;56:250–256.
89. Lee KT, O'Neal RM. Anticoagulant therapy of acute myocardial infarction. An evaluation from autopsy data with special reference to myocardial rupture and thromboembolic complications. Am J Med 1956;21:555–559.
90. Capeci NE, Levy RL. The influence of anticoagulant therapy on the incidence of thromboembolism, hemorrhage and cardiac rupture in acute myocardial infarction. Am J Med 1959;26:76–80.
91. Blumgart HL, Freedberg AS, Zoll PM, Lewis HB, Wessler S. Effect of Dicumarol on heart in experimental acute coronary occlusion. Am Heart J 1948; 36:13–27.
92. Becker RC, Hochman JS, Cannon CP, et al. for the TIMI 9 Investigators. Fatal cardiac rupture among patients treated with thrombolytic agents and adjunctive thrombin antagonists. Observations from the TIMI 9 study. J Am Coll Cardiol 1999;33:479–487.
93. Figueras J, Curós A, Cortadellas J, Soler-Soler J. Reliability of electromechanical dissociation in the diagnosis of left ventricular free wall rupture in acute myocardial infarction. Am Heart J 1996;131:861–864.
94. Oliva PB, Hammill SC, Edwards WD. Cardiac rupture, a clinically predictable complication of acute myocardial infarction: report of 70 cases with clinicopathologic correlations. J Am Coll Cardiol 1993;22:720–726.
95. Zahger D, Milgalter E, Pollak A, Hasin Y, Merin G, Beeri R, Gotsman MS. Left ventricular free wall rupture as the presenting manifestation of acute myocardial infarction in diabetic patients. Am J Cardiol 1996;78:681–682.
96. López-Sendón J, González A, López de Sá E, Coma-Canella I, Roldán I, Domínguez F, Maqueda I, Jadraque LM. Diagnosis of subacute ventricular wall rupture after acute myocardial infarction: sensitivity and specificity of clinical, hemodynamic and echocardiographic criteria. J Am Coll Cardiol 1992;19:1145–1153.
97. Radford MJ, Johnson RA, Daggett WM, Fallon JT, Buckley MJ, Gold HK, Leinbach RC. Ventricular septal rupture: a review of clinical and physiologic features and an analysis of survival. Circulation 1981;64:545–553.
98. John LC, O'Riordan JB. Peri-infarct pursestring for repair of subacute cardiac rupture. Ann Thorac Surg 1996;61:728–730.
99. Basu S, Marini CP, Bauman FG, Shirazian D, Damiani P, Robertazzi R, Jacobowitz IJ, Acinapura A, Cunningham JN. Comparative study of biological glues: cryoprecipitate glue, two-component fibrin sealant, and "French" glue. Ann Thorac Surg 1995;60:1255–1262.
100. Lillehei CW, Lande AJ, Rassman WR, Tanaka S, Bloch JH. Surgical management of myocardial infarction. Circulation 1969;39(suppl IV):315–333.
101. FitzGibbon GM, Hooper GD, Heggtveit HA. Successful surgical treatment of postinfarction external cardiac rupture. J Thorac Cardiovasc Surg 1972;63: 622–630.

102. Hatcher CR, Mansour K, Logan WD, Symbas PN, Abbott OA. Surgical complications of myocardial infarction. Am Surg 1970;36:163–170.
103. Friedman HS, Kuhn LA, Katz AM. Clinical and electrocardiographic features of cardiac rupture following acute myocardial infarction. Am J Med 1971;50: 709–720.
104. Löfström B, Mogensen L, Nyquist O, Orinius E, Sjögren A, Werner B. Attempts at emergency surgical treatment. Chest 1972;61:10–13.
105. Montegut FJ. Left ventricular rupture secondary to myocardial infarction. Ann Thorac Surg 1972;14:75–78.
106. Cobbs BW, Hatcher CR, Robinson PH. Cardiac rupture. JAMA 1973;223: 532–535.
107. O'Rourke MF. Subacute heart rupture following myocardial infarction. Lancet 1973;2:124–126.
108. Calick A, Kerth W, Barbour D, Cohn K. Successful surgical therapy of ruptured myocardium. Chest 1974;66:188.
109. Abel RM, Buckley MJ, Friedlich AL, Austen WG. Survival following free rupture of left ventricular aneurysm: report of a case. Ann Thorac Surg 1976; 21:175–179.
110. Anagnostoupoulos E, Beutler S, Levett JM, Lawrence JM, Lin CY, Replogle RL. Myocardial rupture: major left ventricular infarct rupture treated by infarctectomy. JAMA 1977;238:2715–2716.
111. Eisenmann B, Bareiss P, Pacifico AD, Jeanblanc B, Kretz JG, Baehrel B, Warter J, Kieny R. Anatomic, clinical, and therapeutic features of acute cardiac rupture. J Thorac Cardiovasc Surg 1978;76:78–82.
112. Kendall RW, DeWood MA. Postinfarction cardiac rupture: surgical success and review of the literature. Ann Thorac Surg 1978;25:311–315.
113. Parr GV, Pae WE, Pierce WS, Zellis R. Cardiogenic shock due to ventricular rupture. J Thorac Cariovasc Surg 1981;82:889–891.
114. Windsor HM, Chang VP, Shanahan MX. Postinfarction cardiac rupture. J Thorac Cardiovasc Surg 1982;84:755–761.
115. Bashour T, Kabbani SS, Ellertson DG, Crew J, Hanna ES. Surgical salvage of heart rupture: report of two cases and review of the literature. Ann Thorac Surg 1983;36:209–213.
116. Feneley MP, Chang VP, O'Rourke MF. Myocardial rupture after acute myocardial infarction. Br Heart J 1983;49:550–556.
117. Nunez L, de la Llana R, López-Sendon J, Coma I, Gil-Aguado M, Larrea JL. Diagnosis and treatment of subacute free wall ventricular rupture after infarction. Ann Thorac Surg 1983;35:525–529.
118. Pifarré R, Sullivan HJ, Grieco J, Montoya A, Bakhos M, Scanlon PJ, Gunnar RM. Management of left ventricular rupture complicating myocardial infarction. J Thorac Cardiovasc Surg 1983;86:441–443.
119. Hochreiter C, Goldstein J, Borer JS, Tyberg T, Goldberg HL, Subramanian V, Rosenfeld I. Myocardial free-wall rupture after acute infarction. Circulation 1982;65:1279–1284.
120. Choo MH, Chia BL, Chia F. Cardiac tamponade from ventricular rupture:

value of two-dimensional echocardiography in guiding acute surgical management. Crit Care Med 1985;13:446–447.
121. McMullan MH, Kilgore TL, Dear HD, Hindman SH. Sudden blowout rupture of the myocardium after infarction: urgent management. J Thorac Cardiovasc Surg 1985;89:259–263.
122. Stiegel M, Zimmern SH, Robicsek F. Left ventricular rupture following coronary occlusion treated by streptokinase infusion: successful surgical repair. Ann Thorac Surg 1987;44:413–415.
123. Pierli C, Lisi G, Mezzacapo B. Subacute left ventricular free wall rupture. Chest 1991;100:1174–1176.
124. Luciani GB, Tappainer E, Pessotto R, Fabbri A, Mazzucco A. Mechanical support for decompression of the left ventricle in repair of ischemic cardiac rupture. J Card Surg 1993;8:638–640.
125. Komeda M, Mickleborough LL. Concealed rupture of the left ventricle: successful surgical repair. Ann Thorac Surg 1994;57:1333–1335.
126. Sakakibana T, Matsuwaka R, Shintani H, Yagura A, Yamaguchi T, Nirayama A, Kodama K. Successful repair of postinfarction left ventricular free wall rupture: new strategy with hypothermic percutaneous cardiopulmonary bypasss. J Thorac Cardiovasc Surg 1996;111:276–276.
127. Sutherland FW, Guell FJ, Pathi VL, Naik SK. Postinfarction ventricular free wall rupture: strategies for diagnosis and treatment. Ann Thorac Surg 1996; 61:1281–1285.
128. Charnvechai C, Effler DB. Postoperative myocardial rupture. Ann Thorac Surg 1972;13:458–463.
129. Bojar RM, Overton JW, Madoff IM. Successful management of left ventricular rupture following myocardial revascularization. Ann Thorac Surg 1987; 44:312–314.
130. Vlodaver Z, Coe JI, Edwards JE. True and false left ventricular aneurysms. Propensity for the latter to rupture. Circulation 1975;51:567–572.
131. Yaku H, Fermanis G, Horton DA, Guy D, Lvoff R. Successful repair of a ruptured postinfarct pseudoaneurysm of the left ventricle. Ann Rhorac Surg 1995;60:1097–1098.
132. Pliam MB, Sternlieb JJ. Intramyocardial dissecting hematoma: an unusual form of subacute cardiac rupture. J Card Surg 1993;8:628–637.
133. Padró JM, Caralps JM, Montoya JD, Cámara ML, Garcia-Picart JG, Arís A. Sutureless repair of postinfarction cardiac rupture. J Card Surg 1988;3:491–493.
134. Zogno M, Lacanna GC, Ceconi C, Ferrari M, Latini L, Lorusso R, Sandrelli L, Alfieri O. Postinfarction left ventricular free wall rupture: original management and surgical technique. J Card Surg 1991;6:396–399.
135. Padró JM, Mesa JM, Silvesre J, Larrea JL, Caralps JM, Cerrón F, Aris A. Subacute cardiac rupture: repair with a sutureless technique. Ann Thorac Surg 1993;55:20–24.
136. Almdahl SM, Hotvedt R, Larsen U, Srlie DG. Postinfarction rupture of left ventricular free wall repaired with a glued-on pericardial patch. Scan J Thorac Cardiovasc Surg 1993;27:105–107.

137. Coletti G, Torracca L, Zogno M, LaCanna G, Lorusso R, Pardini A, Alfieri O. Surgical management of left ventricular free wall rupture after acute myocardial infarction. Cardiovasc Surg 1995;3:181–186.
138. Cheriex EC, deSwart H, Dijkman LW, Havenith MG, Maessen JG, Engelen DJ, Wellens HJ. Myocardial rupture after myocardial infarction is related to the perfusion status of the infarct-related coronary artery. Am Heart J 1995; 129:644–649.
139. Pliam MB, Sternlieb JJ. Intramyocardial dissecting hematoma: an unusual form of subacute cardiac rupture. J Card Surg 1993;8:628–637.
140. Wright IS, et al. Myocardial Infarction: Its Clinical Manifestations and Treatment with Anticoagulants—a Study of 1031 Cases. New York: Grune & Stratton, 1954:392–455.
141. Wood A. Perforation of the interventricular septum due to cardiac infarction. Br Heart J 1944;6:191–193.
142. Peel AAF. Dissecting aneurysm of the interventricular septum. Br Heart J 1948;10:239–243.
143. Lewis AJ, Burchell HB, Titus JL, et al. Clinical and pathologic features of postinfarction cardiac rupture. Am J Cardiol 1969;23:43–53.
144. Awan NA, Ikeda R, Olson H, Hata J, DeMaria AN, et al. Intraventricular free wall dissection causing acute interventricular communication with intact septum in myocardial infarction. Chest 1976;69:782–785.
145. Daubert J, Mattheyses M, Fourdilis M, Pony JC, Gouffault J, et al. L'infarctus du ventricule droit. 2. Incidences pronostiques et therapeutiques. Arch Mal Coeur 1977;70:257–264.
146. Stewart S, Huddle R, Stuard I, Schreiner BF, De Weese JA, et al. False aneurysm and pseudo-false aneurysm of the left ventricle: etiology, pathology, diagnosis, and operative management. Ann Thorac Surg 1981;31:259–265.
147. Hodsden J, Nanda NC. Dissecting aneurysm of the ventricular septum following acute myocardial infarction: diagnosis by real time two-dimensional echocardiography. Am Heart J 1981;101:671–672.
148. Tanimoto M, Iwasaki T, Yamamoto T, Makihata S, Konisiike A, Mihata S, Matsumori Y, Yasutomi N, Koide T, Kawai Y. Two-dimensional echocardiography in ventricular septal rupture after acute myocardial infarction. J Cardiogr 1985;15:625–637.
149. Scanu P, Lamy E, Commeau P, Grollier G, Charbonneau P, et al. Myocardial dissection in right ventricular infarction: two-dimensional echocardiographic recognition and pathologic study. Am Heart J 1986;111:422–425.
150. Kanemoto N, Hirose S, Goto Y, Matsuyama S, et al. Disappearing false aneurysm of the ventricular septum without rupture: a complication of acute inferior myocardial infarction—a case report. Angiology 1988;39:263–271.
151. Savage MP, Hopkins JT, Templeton JY, Goldburgh WP, Goldberg S, et al. Left ventricular pseudopseudoaneurysm: angiographic features and surgical treatment of impending cardiac rupture. Am Heart J 1988;116:864–866.
152. Bates RJ, Beutler S, Resnekov L, Anagnostopoulos CE, et al. Cardiac rupture —challenge in diagnosis and management. Am J Cardiol 1977;3:429–437.

153. Reardon MJ, Carr CL, Diamond A, Letsou GV, Safi HJ, Espada R, Baldwin JC. Ischemic left ventricular free wall rupture: prediction, diagnosis, and treatment. Ann Thorac Surg 1997;64:1509–1513.
154. Zeebregts CJ, Noyez L, Hensens AG, Skotnicki SH, Lacquet LK. Surgical repair of subacute left ventricular free wall rupture. J Card Surg 1997;12: 416–419.
155. Kyo S, Ogiwara M, Miyamoto N, et al. Clinical effect of percutaneous intrapericardial fibrin flue infusion therapy for the treatment of rupture of left ventricular free wall following acute myocardial infarction. Circulation 1999; 100:I-867.

24

Reperfusion Injury

Mitchell J. Silver and John P. Gassler
The Cleveland Clinic Foundation
Cleveland, Ohio

HISTORICAL BACKGROUND AND INTRODUCTION

Both clinicians and experimentalists have long been concerned that reperfusion of ischemic myocardium may precipitate a series of unanticipated events that limit the benefit expected of restoring blood flow and oxygen to the heart. This limitation of benefit has been vaguely defined as "reperfusion injury," and embraces a variety of functional, metabolic, and ionic disturbances, some of which may be transitory and only of temporary concern, whereas others could cause permanent damage. Probably the most fundamental, and controversial, question is whether the process of reperfusion actually contributes to the destruction of myocytes that are not yet necrotic at the time of reperfusion and that might be anticipated to recover normal function. Alternatively, reperfusion might simply accelerate the death of cells that are irreversibly injured at the time of reperfusion and destined to die from the ischemic injury alone. Certainly the resolution of this controversy is paramount in this era of thrombolytic therapy, primary angioplasty, and surgical revascularization, since if reperfusion injury occurs, then there certainly is an opportunity to improve further on the benefits derived from these procedures (1–3).

Reperfusion injury has been applied to several categories of pathophysiological changes that occur when ischemic myocardium is reperfused with arterial blood. The first major category is the most deleterious response to reperfusion—lethal reperfusion injury (Fig. 1). Lethal reperfusion injury

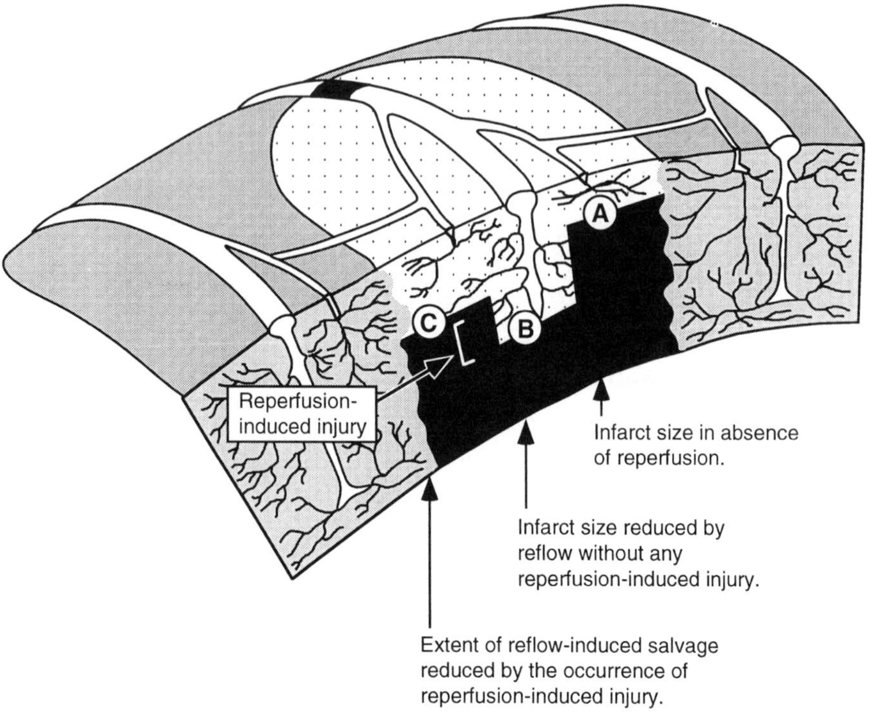
A
B
C
Reperfusion-
induced injury
Infarct size in absence
of reperfusion.
Infarct size reduced by
reflow without any
reperfusion-induced injury.
Extent of reflow-induced salvage
reduced by the occurrence of
reperfusion-induced injury.

Figure 1 Lethal reperfusion injury. A transmural section through an area of regional ischemia in which a zone of lethal injury (dark shading) is initiated in the endocardium and extends, with time, toward the epicardial surface. In the absence of reperfusion but in the presence of sufficient collateral flow, the infarct may eventually stabilize in the midmyocardial region (A). Early reperfusion would be expected to salvage tissue and reduce the extent of necrosis such that the infarct interface stabilized near the endocardium (B). However, if lethal reperfusion induced injury exists, it might attenuate the extent of salvage achieved by reperfusion (C). (From Hearse DJ, Yellon DM. Why are we still in doubt about infarct size limitation? The experimentalists viewpoint. In: Hearse DJ, Yellon DM, eds. Therapeutic Approaches to Infarct Size Limitation. New York: Raven Press, 1984:17–41.)

is defined as the death of myocytes, alive at the time of reperfusion, as a direct result of some aspect of the process of reperfusion (4,5). Even though reperfusion with arterial blood is the only means known that will salvage the myocytes destined to die in a zone of sustained ischemia, a body of evidence has been produced that suggests that lethal reperfusion injury occurs when such areas of ischemia are reperfused with arterial blood (5–12). The second category of reperfusion injury is termed myocardial "stunning"

(13,14), and refers to the fact that reversibly injured living myocardium contracts less efficiently after reperfusion than it did in the control state. The duration of the dysfunction greatly exceeds that of the antecedent ischemia (15), for example, after 15 min of ischemia in dogs, myocardial function remains depressed for 24 hours (16). The third category of reperfusion injury was described by Kloner and colleagues (17), who popularized the concept of the "no-reflow" phenomenon. No-reflow is defined as the inability to perfuse previously ischemic myocardium, even when blood flow has been restored to the large epicardial arteries supplying the tissue. Recent research efforts have focused on the microcirculation whereby distal embolization of platelet aggregates following either mechanical or pharmacological reperfusion is likely a key component of the no-reflow phenomenon. Lastly, arrhythmogenesis as a manifestation of reperfusion injury was first noted in animal models whereby brief (5 to 15 min) periods of coronary artery occlusion followed by reperfusion were associated at the time of reflow with dramatic arrhythmias, including ventricular fibrillation and ventricular tachycardia (18–20). Since these arrhythmias develop promptly upon reflow, this has been considered to be a form of reperfusion injury.

ROLE OF OXYGEN FREE RADICALS

In keeping with the concept of reperfusion injury is the notion that certain harmful substances formed following ischemia reperfusion may cause cell damage. Oxygen free radicals have been implicated in the pathogenesis of tissue injury in a variety of organ systems. Several lines of evidence suggest that oxygen free radicals may play an important role in the pathogenesis of reperfusion injury (Fig. 2). It is well documented by several techniques that tissue oxygen free radical levels increase markedly upon reperfusion of ischemic heart tissue. Also, in the absence of ischemia reperfusion, exposure of hearts to oxygen free radical generating systems causes irreversible cardiac injury similar to that caused by ischemia reperfusion and precipitates nonreentrant arrhythmias similar to reperfusion arrhythmias. Finally, many interventions designed to scavenge or rapidly metabolize free radicals have been shown to decrease reperfusion injury (21–23).

The cytotoxic effects of oxygen free radicals are thought to be due to the peroxidation of cellular lipids and proteins (24). There is evidence in humans that ischemia reperfusion can result in detectable levels of lipid peroxidation products. Roberts and colleagues (25) performed balloon angioplasty on 10 patients with stable angina pectoris. They observed a significant increase in malondialdehyde venous blood concentration in the great cardiac vein immediately after a first 60-sec balloon inflation in the left anterior descending coronary artery.

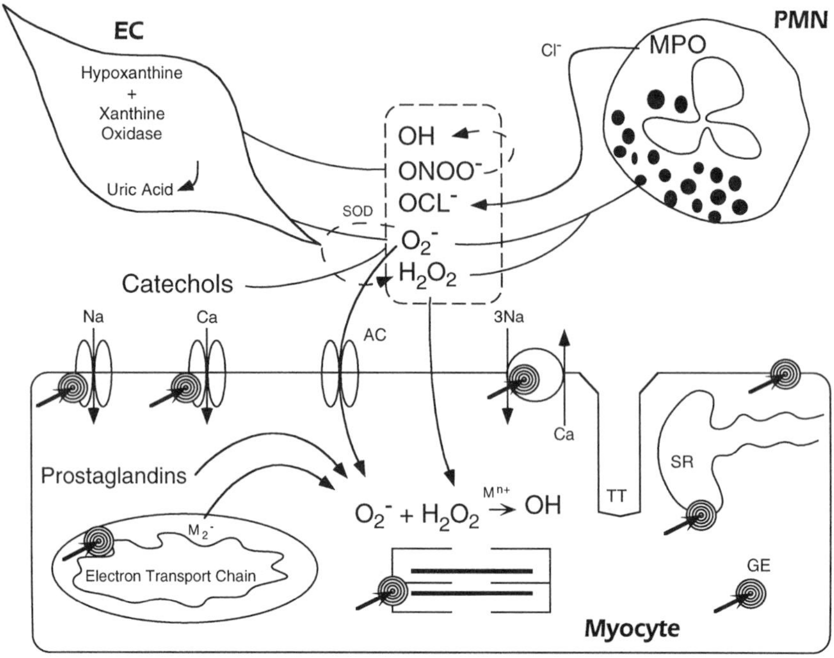

Figure 2 Schematic drawing shows sources and cellular targets of oxygen free radicals during myocardial ischemia/reperfusion. EC, endothelial cell; NO, nitric oxide; OH, hydroxyl radical; ONOO, peroxide anion; OCL, Hypochlorous anion; O_2, superoxide anion; H_2O_2, hydrogen peroxide; SOD, superoxide dismutase; PMN, polymorphonuclear leukocyte. MPO, myeloperoxidase; Cl, chloride anion; AC, anion channel; TT, T tubule; SR, sarcoplasmic reticulum; GE, glycolytic enzymes; M, transition metal. Arrows and bull's-eyes represent specific targets of oxygen free radical toxicity. (From Goldhaber JI, Weiss JN. Oxygen free radicals and cardiac reperfusion abnormalities. Hypertension 1992;20:118–127.)

A clinical role for the use of oxygen free radical scavengers or inhibitors in ischemic heart disease is still evolving. At the present time, oxygen free radical scavengers and inhibitors have been successfully tested for use in cardioplegic solutions designed to promote the preservation of transplanted organs (26) and to protect the myocardium during circulatory arrest during open heart surgery (27). The first moderate-size clinical trial specifically designed to assess therapy targeted to oxygen free radical mediated reperfusion injury was performed using superoxide dismutase (SOD) (28) (Table 1). The design of the study called for the administration of intrave-

Table 1 Summary of Clinical Trials Targeted at Reducing Myocardial Infarct Size by Reducing Reperfusion Injury

Trial	Agent studied	Proposed mechanism	Effect on animal model infarct size	n	Primary endpoint	Trial result
TIMI-II	IV metoprolol	Lowers O_2 demand	143% (reperfusion, canine)	1,390	LVEF	Negative (50.5% vs. 50.0%)
TAMI-4	Prostacyclin	Inhibits neutrophils	147% (reperfusion, canine)	50	Patency, EF	Negative (both lower)
TAMI-9	Fluosol	Improves O_2 delivery	67% better LV function	430	Infarct size	Negative (22% vs. 17%)
ISIS-4	Magnesium	Stabilizes membranes	160% (reperfusion, canine)	58,050	35-day survival	Negative (7.6% vs. 7.2%)
CORE	RheothRx	Improves O_2 delivery	42% better EF (canine)	2,607	Death, shock, re-MI	Negative (14.0% vs. 12.6%)
EMIP-FR	Trimetazidine	Inhibits neutrophils	Significant reduction (rabbit)	19,665	35-day mortality	Negative (12.2% vs. 12.3%)
Calypso	Cylexin	Inhibits p-selectin	169% (reperfusion, canine)	153	Infarct size	Negative (larger)
HALT MI	Hu23F2G	Inhibits neutrophil-endothelial interaction	Reduction (several models)	374	Infarct size	Negative (19% vs. 16% vs. 17%)
AMISTAD	Adenosine	Reduces free radical generation and platelet aggregation	Reduction (several models)	236	Infarct size	Negative for non-AWMI; positive for AWMI (15% vs. 45.5%)
GUARDIAN	Cariporide	Na/H exchange inhibitor	Significant reduction (rabbit and rat models)	11,500	Death, (re-)MI	Negative (except decreased MI in CABG patients)

nous SOD to patients undergoing direct coronary angioplasty or "rescue" coronary angioplasty so that certainty would exist that the drug was present at the time of reperfusion. Unfortunately, clinical outcomes were not different between placebo and SOD. Another agent, Fluosol, a fluorohydrocarbon emulsion that is capable of carrying much higher concentrations of oxygen than blood, has been able to ameliorate the effects of reperfusion on the elaboration of toxic substances thought to be free radicals in previous animal studies (29). TAMI-9 was designed specifically to determine whether these initially promising results with Fluosol could be replicated in the setting of thrombolytic agent administration (30) (Table 1). No difference in outcome measured by thallium infarct size, ejection fraction, or regional wall motion results was found. It is a sobering thought to realize that not one of the antioxidants, when used in a clinical trial of ischemia reperfusion, has made any impact on reduction of myocardial infarct size.

NEUTROPHIL ACTIVATION

The rapid accumulation of polymorphonuclear leukocytes (PMNs) in reperfused areas of the myocardium was first described by Sommers and Jennings (2) in 1964 using a canine model of 40-min coronary occlusion followed by reperfusion. This accelerated PMN accumulation has been since validated using histological (12), enzymatic (31), and radiolabeled techniques (32). Recent studies (32) have demonstrated that the rate of PMN accumulation is greatest within the first hour of reperfusion, where it can increase six- to sevenfold, and declines there after, although cumulatively the influx of PMNs proceeds probably for 18 to 24 hours. The most direct evidence for PMNs participating in the process of reperfusion injury is provided by four independent studies that used different methods to deplete PMNs, and demonstrated that cell depletion was associated with a reduction in infarct size, even when the depletion was affected only at reperfusion (33–36).

The adhesion of PMNs to the vascular endothelium is a prerequisite for their recruitment and accumulation in damaged tissue. Adherence of PMNs to coronary vascular endothelium involves the interaction of specific molecules belonging to one of three major families: the selectins, the immunoglobulin superfamily, and the integrins (Table 2). The selectin family has three major adhesion glycoproteins; two are localized on endothelial cells (P- and E-selectin), and one is localized on neutrophils (L-selectin). Intercellular adhesion molecule 1 (ICAM-1) is a member of the immunoglobulin superfamily located on endothelial cells. The third major player in the adhesion process is the CD11/CD18 complex, which is a β-2-integrin.

Once PMNs adhere to the vascular endothelium, they can induce vascular dysfunction and tissue injury by a variety of mechanisms. First, they

Table 2 Adhesion Molecules Involved in Neutrophil-Coronary Endothelial Cell Interactions

Type	Location	Expression	Time course	Ligand
Selectins				
P	Platelet, endothelium	Stimulated: thrombin, histamine, H_2O_2	10–20 min	Sle^x on PMN, Sle^a on PMN
E	Endothelium	Stimulated: cytokines, LPS	4–6 hr	Sle^x on PMN, Sle^a on PMN
L	Leukocyte	Constitutive	Shed on activation	Sle^x on PMN
Immunoglobulins				
ICAM-1	Endothelium, monocyte, lymphocyte	Constitutive, low concentrations	Constitutive, increases slowly over 6–12 hr	CD11a/CD18, CD11b/CD18
β_2 integrins				
CD11a/CD18	Neutrophils	Stimulated by chemotactic stimuli	Activated in minutes	ICAM-1, ICAM-2
CD11b/CD18	Neutrophils	Stimulated by chemotactic stimuli	Activated in minutes	ICAM-1

Source: Lefer AM. Role of selectins in myocardial ischemia reperfusion injury. Ann Thorac Surg 1995;60:773–777.

can attract other PMNs and platelets by releasing chemotactic humoral mediators (leukotriene B_4, thromboxane A_2, and platelet activating factor). The adherence of these circulating blood elements can lead to plugging of the microvasculature, a finding that has been observed in reperfusion injury (37) and one that could contribute to the no-reflow phenomenon following ischemia reperfusion. Secondly, most of the PMNs that remain intravascular are adherent to the microvasculature, particularly the coronary capillaries and venules (38). Due to this location, the PMNs are positioned one endothelial cell thickness away from the cardiac myocytes, and could release injurious mediators (elastase, collagenase, cytokines, eicosanoids, free radicals) which could diffuse this short distance to the cardiac myocytes and injure them. The third explanation has to do with the fact that 15% to 25% of the marginated pool of PMNs at 4 to 5 hours postreperfusion undergo transendothelial migration (39). These extravascular PMNs could migrate to the cardiac myocyte and, since cardiac myocytes have been shown to express ICAM-1 on their cell surface, these PMNs could adhere to the myocytes (39), where they would be able to exacerbate cell injury and death.

CORONARY MICROVASCULATURE AND MACROVASCULATURE

In 1974, Kloner and colleagues (17) reported that myocardial blood flow in dogs was reduced after release of coronary artery occlusion, an event they referred to as the "no-reflow" phenomenon. As a result of intensive experimentation, several investigators have observed abnormalities involving both the microvasculature and the epicardial macrovasculature to explain this manifestation of reperfusion injury. More recently, it has become apparent that the microvascular damage following ischemia reperfusion can be explained by two broad categories (Fig. 3). The first category, or earlier phase, that causes microvascular obstruction is likely due to platelet microembolism and de novo thrombosis. The second category, or later phase, represents reperfusion injury and involves tissue edema, neutrophil aggregation, and oxygen free radical release.

Regarding the epicardial macrovasculature, several theories have been put forth in an effort to explain no-reflow following ischemia reperfusion. First, interstitial edema, intracellular edema, or both could cause extravascular compression of the coronary arteries and arterioles, thereby preventing normal blood flow (40). Second, the decrease in epicardial flow could be the result of impaired autoregulatory responses, or alternatively, this might represent "appropriate autoregulation" caused by decreased demands of the postischemic heart (41). Third, agonist-stimulated endothelial nitric oxide release in coronary conduit arteries and coronary resistance vessels has been

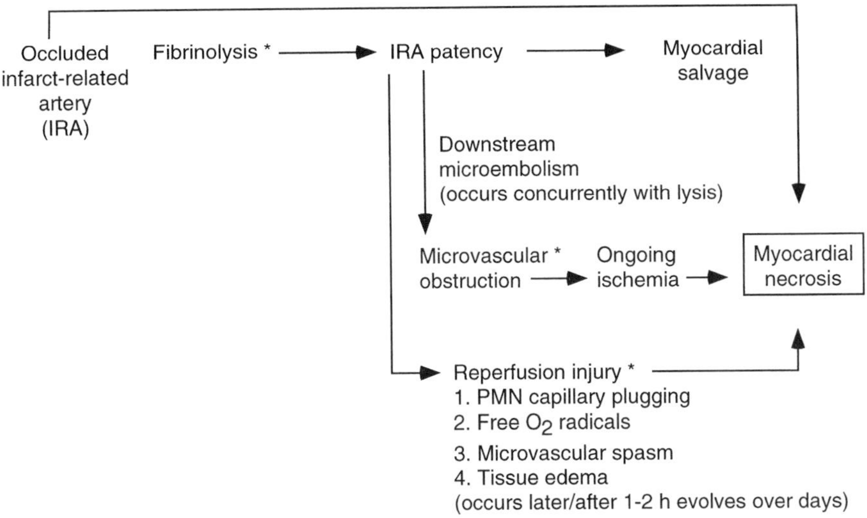

Figure 3 Schematic demonstrating potential outcomes at the microvascular and myocardial level after fibrinolysis. *Potential target for therapeutic intervention to increase myocardial salvage. PMN, polymorphonuclear monocyte. (From Ref. 51.)

demonstrated to be diminished following ischemia reperfusion, with consequent reduced dilator activity (42). Finally, coronary artery smooth muscle damage might augment vascular tone and impair the ability of the vascular smooth muscle to relax in response to normal mechanisms.

Microvascular damage following ischemia reperfusion has been documented by electron microscopic examination, which reveals a loss of pinocytotic vesicles to the endothelium, endothelial blisters or blebs, and gaps within the endothelium (17,37,43). This expression of reperfusion injury leads to abnormalities in myocardial microvascular transport of fluid and solutes. An increase in myocardial tissue water content and capillary permeability has been observed following reperfusion after even brief (i.e., 5 min.) periods of experimental myocardial ischemia (44–46), and these effects can be attenuated by antioxidants (47,48). Perhaps the one potential etiology for microvascular-related no-reflow that received much attention in earlier studies was "neutrophil plugging." Engler and colleagues (37,49) have shown that neutrophils can be identified in capillaries of the no-reflow area with red cells lodged or "stacked up" behind, suggesting that the leukocytes are causing the obstruction. Mehta (50) also described neutrophil infiltration and capillary plugging in dogs subjected to 1 hour of coronary occlusion and 1 hour of reperfusion. More recent evidence has become available that describes a combination of red (fibrin- and red blood cell-rich) and white (platelet-rich) clots being responsible for microembolization resulting in coronary obstruction after plaque rupture in patients with acute coronary syndromes (51). Current myocardial infarction therapy does not affect the platelet component, such that as fibrinolysis occurs (and fibrin is lysed), and fragments consisting of platelet aggregates may be dislodged and become microemboli which then can cause abnormalities in the microcirculation via obstruction to flow at that level. Indeed, the most promising advance in the treatment of myocardial reperfusion abnormalities affecting the microvasculature, the glycoprotein IIb/IIIa antagonists, are directed against platelet microembolism formation causing early microvascular obstruction. A more detailed discussion on embolization can be found in the accompanying chapter in this text.

"Microvascular stunning," the last manifestation of microvascular reperfusion injury, refers to an abnormality in function of viable microvessels after ischemia reperfusion. Nicklas and Gips (52) measured reactive hyperemia in dogs after brief 30-sec coronary occlusions or after an intracoronary bolus of adenosine. Maximum flow during reactive hyperemia and intracoronary adenosine decreased by 20% and 24%, respectively, after ischemia, and these parameters remained depressed for at least 1 hour into reperfusion. Human data also exist that support the notion of no-reflow following coronary ischemia reperfusion. Utilizing myocardial contrast echocardiography, Ito demonstrated that patients with significant no-reflow zones immediately after thrombolysis had poorer functional recovery of the left ventricle than that of patients without such zones (53). A summary of three studies correlating microvascular malperfusion and clinical outcomes can be found in Table 3.

Schofer and colleagues (54) injected intracoronary thallium and intracoronary technetium-99m-labeled albumin microspheres into patients with acute myocardial infarction after thrombolytic therapy. Perfusion defects of both tracers were observed both immediately and late (2 to 4 weeks) after reperfusion. Utilizing intracoronary Doppler flow velocity measurements obtained during primary or rescue angioplasty for acute myocardial infarction, Kern (55) demonstrated markedly impaired coronary flow reserve (coronary flow reserve 1.67 ± 0.88 for TIMI ≤ 2 and 1.49 ± 0.49 for TIMI 3), which suggests a variable degree of microvascular injury following reperfusion. Finally, regarding the role of the macrovasculature in reperfusion injury, it is of interest that the GUSTO-1 angiographic substudy demonstrated mortality at 24 hours to be higher in patients with TIMI grade 2 flow, than those patients with TIMI grade 0 or 1 flow (Table 4) (56).

Table 3 Summary of Clinical Outcomes on the Basis of Myocardial Malperfusion

Study	Patients (n)	Diagnostic modality	Follow-up	Results
Sakuma et al. (155)	50	MCE	22 months (median)	Compared with patients with <45% risk area and minimal defect Major cardiac events of death, MI, CHF, admission with relative risk of 10.7 Major cardiac events and target lesion revascularization with relative risk of 3.69
Ito et al. (53)	126	MCE	Hospital stay	Comparison with patients with MCE-defined reflow Reperfusion arrhythmia 19% vs. 14% Any arrhythmia except reperfusion 10% vs. 6% Early CHF 21% vs. 12% Late CHF (after 3 days) 6% vs. 1%
Wu et al. (156)	44	MRI	16 months (median)	Cardiac death, reinfarction, CHF, stroke Comparison of patients with vs. without MRI defect (45% vs. 9%)

MCE, myocardial contrast echocardiography; MI, myocardial infarction; CHF, congestive heart failure; MRI, magnetic resonance imaging.
Source: Ref. 51.

Table 4 24-Hour Mortality Versus TIMI Flow Grade Taken from the GUSTO 1 Angiographic Substudy

TIMI flow	24-hr mortality (%)
0	2.8
1	1.0
2	3.0
3	0.9

Note that patients with TIMI grade 2 flow had a higher 24-hour mortality than those with either TIMI grade 0 or 1 flow.
Source: GUSTO Angiographic Investigators. The effects of tissue plasminogen activator, streptokinase, or both on coronary artery patency, ventricular function, and survival after acute myocardial infarction. N Engl J Med 1993;329:1615–1622.

MYOCARDIAL STUNNING

Experimental studies have demonstrated that although early reperfusion limits or even prevents necrosis, this beneficial effect does not lead to immediate functional improvement; rather, the return of contractility in tissue salvaged by reperfusion is delayed for hours, days, or even weeks (13,57–60). This phenomenon has been termed "myocardial stunning" (61). The essential element from these experimental and clinical observations is that postischemic dysfunction, no matter how severe or prolonged, is a fully reversible abnormality. It follows that the diagnosis of myocardial stunning should not be made unless reasonable assurance can be provided that the tissue in question is still entirely viable.

One of the earliest explanations for the mechanism of myocardial stunning was that resynthesis of adenosine triphosphate (ATP) was delayed because the precursors were washed out during the reperfusion period. In fact, it was demonstrated that ATP levels in stunning were depressed and recovered slowly with a time course similar to that of contractile function (59,62). Additional experimentation by others found that there is no correlation between the myocardial ATP level and recovery of contractility. The content of phosphocreatine in the stunned myocardium is normal or supernormal; and the stunned myocardium responds to inotropic stimuli without a further decrease in ATP, indicating that energy production is not impaired (63–65).

Others have proposed that alterations in calcium homeostasis and free radical formation might be involved in the genesis of stunning, the two mechanisms being not necessarily mutually exclusive (14). The ability of oxygen metabolites to depress myocardial function has been demonstrated in vitro and in vivo (66,67). The results of studies that have measured free radicals in the stunned myocardium provide evidence that these toxic metabolites are produced in excess (15,68,69).

There is an emerging body of literature on cardioprotection utilizing a new group of compounds that inhibit the cardiac sodium/hydrogen exchanger. The sodium/hydrogen exchanger is a cell membrane protein that is activated primarily in response to intracellular acidosis. Many endogenous mediators such as catecholamines, thrombin, and endothelin (70,71) play a role in the expression of this cell membrane protein (Fig. 4). Animal studies have suggested that inhibition of the sodium/hydrogen exchanger with selective and potent inhibitors (cariporide and its structurally related congener) reduces the susceptibility of cardiac tissue to severe ventricular arrhythmias (72–74), attenuates contractile dysfunction (75–77), and limits myocardial infarct size following ischemia and reperfusion (78–84). Given the mechanism of action of the sodium/hydrogen exchange inhibitors, this observed benefit is likely to result from the attenuation of calcium overload, which has been documented to occur with all of these conditions. Based on these animal studies, sodium/hydrogen exchange inhibitors may provide meaningful adjunctive therapy to reperfusion agents by limiting myocardial infarct size, reducing the incidence of reperfusion arrhythmias, and potentially slowing the process of irreversible myocyte injury which could extend the time period for reperfusion therapy. Finally, other theories regarding the cause of postischemic myocardial stunning have included impairment of sympathetic neural responsiveness (85), impairment of myocardial perfusion (86), and damage of the extracellular collagen matrix (87).

A considerable amount of clinical evidence has accumulated which suggests stunned myocardium occurs in humans (Table 5). Fournier reported a case of variant angina in which marked anteroapical hypokinesis (noted during pain free intervals) persisted for days and then gradually disappeared (88). Thrombolytic trials (89–91) have shown that functional recovery of ischemic myocardium salvaged by reperfusion may require several days to perhaps months. Some patients with coronary artery disease who undergo exercise treadmill tests demonstrate regional wall motion abnormalities that persist for at least 30 to 60 min after termination of exercise (92–94). Reversible myocardial postischemic dysfunction has also been shown to occur following cardiopulmonary bypass and cardiac transplantation (95,96). Patients with unstable angina pectoris have been found to have prolonged regional wall motion abnormalities on transthoracic echocardiography,

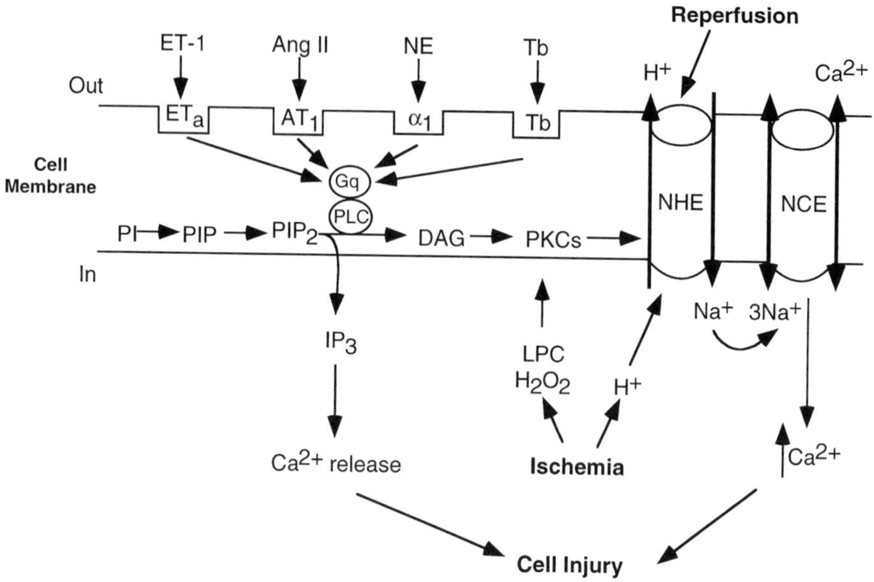

Figure 4 Factors that activate Na-H exchange (NHE) and the likely mechanisms for NHE involvement in mediating injury in the ischemic and reperfused myocardium. Stimulation of NHE occurs as a consequence of receptor activation by various hormones or autocrine and paracrine factors, including endothelin-1 (ET-1), angiotensin II (Ang II), norepinephrine (NE), and thrombin (Tb), through a common signal transduction mechanism involving a G-protein (Gq)-dependent activation of phospholipase C (PLC), which catalyzes the breakdown of phosphatidylinositol bisphosphate (PIP2) to diacylglycerol (DAG), which in turn activates various protein kinase Cs (PKCs). Phosphatidylinositol (PI) breakdown also results in the production of inositol trisphosphate (IP3), which causes the release of calcium from intracellular stores. NHE is also activated by various ischemic metabolites, including hydrogen peroxide (H_2O_2) and lysophosphatidylcholine (LPC), most likely by a PKC-dependent mechanism, as well as by protons (H^+) generated during ischemia. Reperfusion of the ischemic myocardium and the concomitant establishment of a transmembrane pH gradient also activates NHE. NHE activation during ischemia results in the influx of sodium ions, which cannot be effectively removed because of the inhibited sodium-potassium pump (not shown). The increased intracellular sodium will therefore increase intracellular calcium levels through the sodium-calcium exchanger (NCE). The increased calcium from this process, as well as a consequence of IP3-induced release, will produce cell injury from calcium overloading. (From Karmazyn M. Mechanisms of protection of the ischemic and reperfused myocardium by sodium-hydrogen exchange inhibition. J Thromb Thrombol 1999;8:33–38.)

Table 5 Clinical Settings Potentially Associated with Myocardial Stunning and Their Experimental Equivalents

Experimental setting	Clinical setting
Regional ischemia	
Completely reversible ischemic episode (coronary occlusion <20 min)	Percutaneous transluminal coronary angioplasty, unstable angina, variant angina
Partially irreversible ischemic episode (subendocardial infarction) (coronary occlusion >20 min)	Acute myocardial infarction with early reperfusion
Exercise-induced ischemia	Exercise-induced ischemia
Global ischemia	
Cardioplegic arrest	Cardiac surgery, cardiac transplant

Source: Bolli R. Myocardial "stunning" in man. Circulation 1992;86:1674.

which improves after stabilization (97). Finally, transient periods of total coronary artery occlusion induced by percutaneous transluminal coronary angioplasty have been demonstrated to cause a relatively prolonged increase in diastolic stiffness, present for at least 12 to 15 min after balloon deflation (98).

REPERFUSION ARRHYTHMIAS

One potentially catastrophic consequence of reperfusion, particularly following regional ischemia, is the phenomenon of reperfusion-induced arrhythmias. These may include ventricular premature beats, ventricular tachycardia, ventricular fibrillation, and idioventricular rhythm. Many possible mechanisms have been identified (18), including the stimulation of adrenergic receptors and the elevation of cyclic adenosine monophosphate (99), disturbances of lipid metabolism and the formation of lysophosphatides (100), and disturbances of ionic homeostasis, particularly of calcium and potassium (101,102). Most recently, attention has been focused on the possibility that oxygen free radicals, produced during early reperfusion, may cause oxidant stress to membrane lipids or proteins (18,103) that, in turn, may lead to arrhythmogenic events such as loss of potassium and redistribution of calcium. Experimental evidence also demonstrates the high frequency of ventricular fibrillation that follows abrupt reperfusion after relatively short periods of ischemia (15 to 20 min) in anesthetized animals with previously normal coronary arteries (104). However, the frequency of ventricular fibrillation drops substantially with more prolonged ischemia and with staged, as distinct from abrupt, reflow (105) (Fig. 5).

In general, trials of intravenous thrombolytic agents have not demonstrated any increase in life-threatening ventricular arrhythmias that could be attributed to reperfusion (106,107). In fact, arrhythmias do not appear to be a valid marker of successful reperfusion in patients with acute myocardial infarction receiving thrombolysis (108). Although reperfusion arrhythmias are consistently observed in experimental models, the occurrence of true reperfusion related ventricular arrhythmias in patients receiving thrombolytic therapy is probably low (109,113). There are several potential reasons for this experimental-clinical dissociation including: 1) atherosclerotic coronary disease is absent in animal models; 2) gradual reperfusion by thrombolytic treatment bears little resemblance to abrupt mechanical reopening of the coronary vessel in most animal studies (110); 3) previous episodes of symptomatic or silent myocardial ischemia may protect the heart from subsequent reperfusion arrhythmias (a preconditioning phenomenon) (111); and 4) myocardial collateral flow during ischemia is higher in humans than in many animal species (112).

MYOCARDIAL PRECONDITIONING

Ischemic preconditioning is a process by which a brief ischemic episode confers a state of myocardial protection against subsequent sustained periods of ischemia (114–116). This increased tolerance is manifest by slower ischemic metabolism and by a delayed onset of irreversible cell injury, which translates into limitation of infarct size if the test episode of ischemia is terminated by timely reperfusion (114). It is well established that ischemic preconditioning affords an immediate protection against infarction, which lasts approximately 1 hour (101,116). Recent data, however, suggest the existence of a second, more prolonged window of protection. Marber and coworkers (117) reported that preconditioning with four 5-min occlusions significantly reduced infarct size after a 30-min occlusion performed 24 hours after the preconditioning protocol; this effect was associated with an increase in myocardial heat shock protein 70 and 60. Similarly, Sun and others (118) found that a brief ischemic stress triggers a powerful, long-lasting (at least 48 hours), adaptive response that renders the heart partially resistant to the same ischemic stress applied 24 hours later. Indeed, the clinical counterpart as described by Ottani and colleagues (119) suggests that despite a similar area at risk, patients with new-onset prodromal angina showed a significantly smaller infarct size than patients without prodromal symptoms.

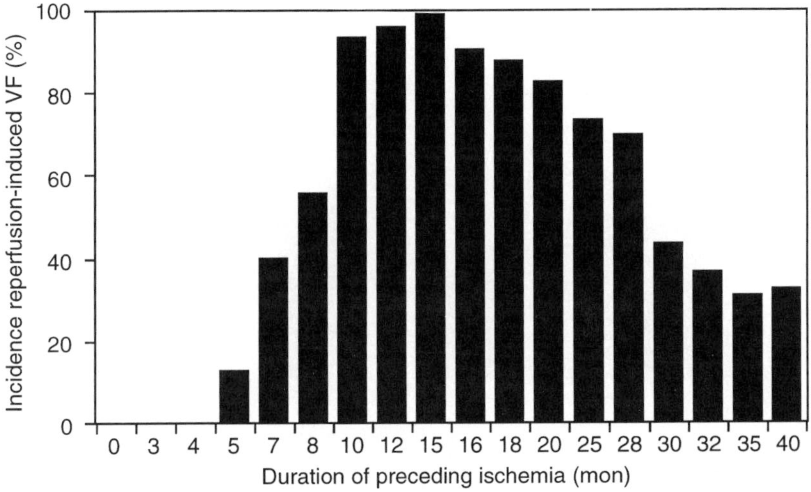

Figure 5 Duration of ischemia as a determinant of vulnerability to reperfusion-induced arrhythmias. The relationship between the incidence of reperfusion-induced ventricular fibrillation (VF) and the duration of the preceding period of regional ischemia in the isolated perfused rat heart. The profile for the rat heart in vivo is similar but displaced to the left. (From Yellon DM, Jennings RB. Myocardial Protection. The Pathophysiology of Reperfusion and Reperfusion Injury. New York: Raven Press, 1992;21.)

REPERFUSION INJURY: THERAPEUTIC CONSIDERATIONS

Clinical Background

Despite the exhaustive amount of basic science research that supports the phenomenon of reperfusion injury, the existence of myocardial reperfusion injury in human beings remains controversial. It was of great interest to early investigators after analysis of large clinical trial data to find that an "early hazard" existed in the administration of thrombolytic therapy (Fig. 6). Treated patients in ISIS-3 had a higher mortality in the first 24 hours than did untreated patients (120). A systematic overview had indicated that in patients treated late (beyond 6 to 12 hours from symptom onset), the risk of myocardial rupture appears to be increased by thrombolytic therapy (121). When one considers these findings from the early experience with thrombolytic therapy, there was some suggestion that the process of reperfusion may be deleterious in the early period. More recent data from ASSET (122) and GUSTO-1 (123) have not identified such an "early hazard" with the use of t-PA. In fact, one of the most interesting findings of the GUSTO-1 angi-

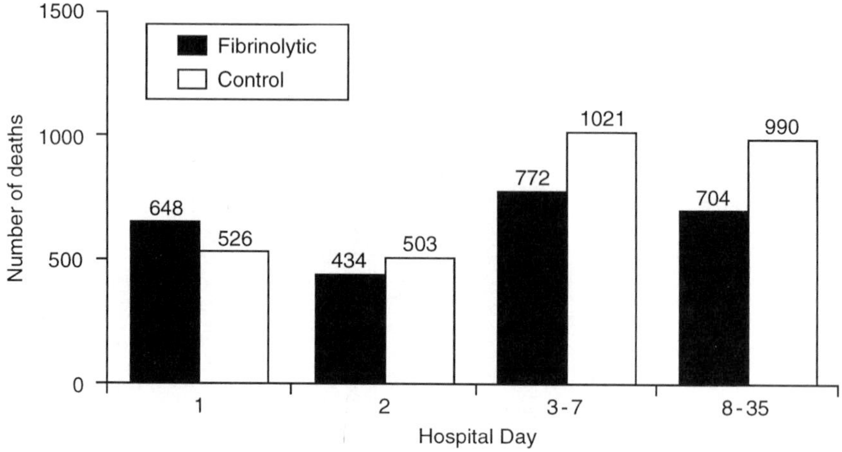

Figure 6 Data from an overview of seven major randomized, controlled thrombolytic trials, demonstrating the paradoxically increased mortality risk during the first day of hospitalization among patients treated with streptokinase or t-PA, compared to placebo therapy ("early hazard"). (From Lincoff AM, Topol EJ. Illusion of reperfusion: does anyone achieve optimal reperfusion during acute myocardial infarction? Circulation 1993;87:1792–1805.)

ographic substudy was that more rapid reperfusion associated with accelerated t-PA therapy led to better regional and global function by the time of the 90-min angiogram, with little change beyond that point (124).

Studies of Agents to Prevent Reperfusion Injury

Superoxide Dismutase

Free radical scavengers are cellular protective enzymes that efficiently and specifically scavenge the cytotoxic free radicals produced within cells. A recombinant form of superoxide dismutase (SOD) has been produced, allowing for extensive animal and human experimentation. Several experimental animal studies have demonstrated a reduction in reperfusion arrhythmias (125,126). The beneficial effects of SOD have been shown in canine models of myocardial ischemia (127). Jolly and associates demonstrated that the infusion of SOD plus catalase, initiated either before coronary occlusion or reperfusion, significantly reduced the extent of necrosis produced by 1.5 hours of coronary ligation followed by 22.5 hours of reperfusion (21).

The first moderate-size clinical trial specifically designed to assess reperfusion injury was performed using SOD (Table 1). Flaherty and colleagues (28) randomized patients undergoing coronary angioplasty within 6 hours of the onset of acute myocardial infarction to receive either placebo or SOD (10 mg/kg bolus followed by an infusion of 0.2 mg/kg/min for 1 hour). There was no difference between groups in coronary artery patency rate, mortality rate, global left ventricular function, or regional wall motion abnormalities.

Prostacyclin

Prostacyclin, a potent, naturally occurring prostaglandin, exerts a variety of cardiovascular and cellular actions of potential value in acute myocardial ischemia. These properties include the reduction of systemic blood pressure without changing heart rate, the lowering of coronary vascular and total peripheral resistance, the inhibition of platelet aggregation and the concomitant formation of thromboxane B_2, and the reduction of the release of lysosomal enzymes which may have an important role in reducing reperfusion injury. The ability to attenuate reperfusion injury was demonstrated by Simpson (128) and colleagues, whereby infarct size in dogs following ischemia reperfusion was reduced through a mechanism related to inhibition of neutrophil migration and the inhibition of superoxide anion production.

In the TAMI-4 pilot study (129), to evaluate combined therapy, rt-PA (100 mg over 3 hours) and Iloprost (2 ng/kg/min for 48 hours) were administered to 25 patients and then rt-PA alone (same dose) was given to an additional 25 patients with evolving myocardial infarction (Table 1). Despite the previous promising experimental data, the Iloprost-treated patients had a lower 90-min patency rate (44% vs. 60%) and a high rate of complications, including flushing, headache, nausea, and hypotension. Although this was a small pilot study, not even a trend toward improvement in left ventricular function was observed.

Fluosol

Considerable progress has been made in recent years toward the development of preparations of substances to be used as respiratory gas transport carriers (130,131). The best-characterized of these are the perfluorochemicals, which are cyclic or straight-chain hydrocarbons in which hydrogen atoms have been replaced with fluoride (132). Unlike hemoglobin, perfluorochemicals have an oxygen content that rises in a linear fashion with an increase in oxygen tension, and a high level of arterial oxygen is essential for perfluorochemicals to transport quantities of oxygen that are comparable to the amount carried by red blood cells (133).

The role of Fluosol, a perfluorochemical, in reducing reperfusion injury has been investigated in animal models of ischemia reperfusion. Intracoronary and intravenous infusions of Fluosol in the perireperfusion period significantly reduced infarct size and improved ventricular function in animals that were examined for up to 2 weeks after reperfusion (134). Fluosol has also been shown to preserve endothelial structure and endothelium-dependent relaxation of large and small vessels following ischemia reperfusion in a canine model (135).

In light of the very promising animal studies, Forman undertook an initial pilot study of intravenous Fluosol in the setting of direct coronary angioplasty (136). In this study, 26 patients with first anterior myocardial infarctions were randomized to either intravenous Fluosol or placebo before primary angioplasty. In these patients, both global (54% vs. 42%) and regional (−1.6 vs. −2.9 standard deviations per chord) left ventricular function were better in the Fluosol group, and thallium infarct size (3.5% vs. 18% of the left ventricle) was much smaller in Fluosol-treated patients. Following this initial pilot study, the TAMI 9 research group (30) randomized 430 patients to either r-tPA therapy with adjunctive Fluosol or r-tPA alone aimed at preventing reperfusion injury for patients with acute myocardial infarction (Table 1). When given with r-tPA, Fluosol was not associated with improvement in ventricular systolic function, reduction in thallium infarct size, or overall clinical outcome (Fig. 7). Fluosol was, however, associated with a reduction in ischemic complications and with an increase in pulmonary edema and congestive heart failure.

Inflammatory Cell Mediators

The presence of a typical inflammatory reaction associated with reperfusion of previously ischemic myocardium has been well described (137). The neu-

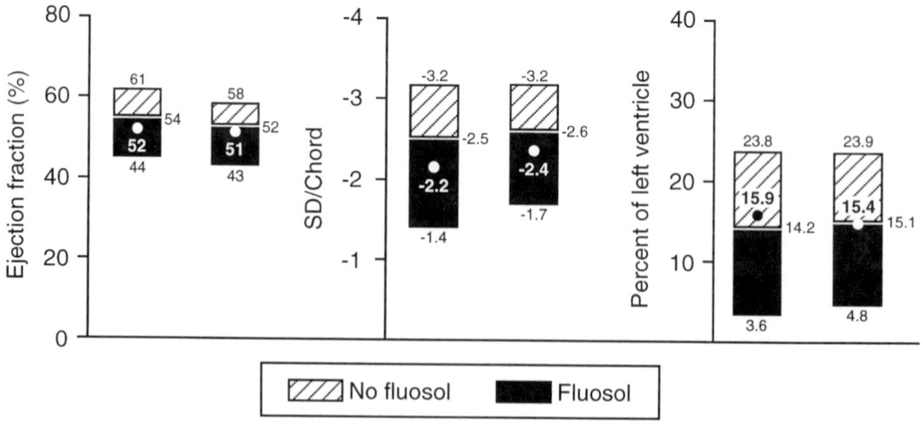

Figure 7 Median and intraquartile ranges as well as the mean values for ejection fraction, infarct zone function, and thallium estimated infarct size for patients who did and did not receive Fluosol. (From Ref. 30.)

trophil, a component of this inflammatory reaction, plays a critical role in the genesis of reperfusion injury (12,137–139). Neutrophils must adhere to endothelium before migration from circulation into tissue, where they can cause cellular damage. Agents that block the interaction of neutrophils with endothelium following ischemia reperfusion, namely, selectin blockers, have been successful in reducing infarct size in animal models of ischemia reperfusion (140,141). Given the promising experimental data, a pilot clinical trial was undertaken known as Cylexin as an Adjunct to Lytics to Prevent Super Oxide reperfusion injury (CALYPSO) which utilized primary angioplasty for the treatment of acute myocardial infarction and randomized patients to receive either the P-selectin blocker Cylexin or placebo at the time of angioplasty. Unfortunately, the trial was stopped early as there was no benefit in terms of myocardial salvage when assessed by sestamibi nuclear scanning, which was the primary endpoint of the study (Sutton, personal communication).

A novel monoclonal antibody directed against the CD11, CD18 integrin receptors has recently been studied in a clinical trial of direct coronary angioplasty for acute myocardial infarction as adjunctive therapy (142) (the HALT MI trial). A total of 374 patients with acute myocardial infarction undergoing direct PTCA within 6 hours of symptom onset were randomized to receive either 0.3 mg/kg or 1 mg/kg of Hu23F2G, or placebo by bolus injection. A total of 86 patients were excluded because of TIMI flow grade of 2 or 3 prior to angioplasty. A total of 248 patients actually received study drug. The primary endpoint was infarct size by technetium-99, Sestamibi SPECT at 5 to 9 days, with 30-day and 6-month clinical follow-up. The results of this study in regard to infarct size as a percentage of the area at risk demonstrated no significant difference between those patients receiving placebo and those receiving the CD11, CD18 receptor inhibitor (placebo 19%, low dose 16%, and high dose 17%). In addition, there was no statistically significant difference found in the peak CPK measurement or core TIMI frame count when comparing placebo to study drug. Finally, the death rate at 30 days was not different between placebo and study drug (placebo 3.3%, low dose 0.8%, and high dose 1.4%) (Table 6). Overall, there was no reduction in infarct size in those patients receiving adjunctive therapy with the CD 11/CD 18 inhibitor in this clinical trial of primary angioplasty for acute myocardial infarction. In addition, regarding the other clinical endpoints that included death and congestive heart failure, the HALT MI trial demonstrated no benefit to receiving the CD11/CD18 integrin receptor inhibitor.

Myocardial ischemia in humans is often brought about by the long-term consequences of hypercholesterolemia (i.e., endothelial function, plaque formation, fissures in arterial plaques, etc.) (143). Against this setting,

Table 6 Results from the HALT-MI Trial

	Placebo	Low dose (0.3 mg/kg)	High dose (1 mg/kg)	*P* value
Infarct size (%)	16.6	16.0	17.2	ns
Ant MI size (%)	23.3	25.3	27.7	ns
CPK (AUC)	175	175	184	ns
TIMI frame count	21.3	23.3	22.3	ns
Death rate (%)	3.3	1.4	0.8	ns

Infarct size determined by sestamibi at 7 days. The remaining variables are 30-day outcomes.

cholesterol-lowering agents have been widely used to reduce cardiovascular risk (144–146). The major action of the HMG coenzyme A reductase inhibitors (simvastatin, pravastatin), collectively known as the statins, is inhibition of cholesterol synthesis in the liver (147). Recently, however, there has been a suggestion that these statins may exert effects separate from their cholesterol lowering actions. Lefer and colleagues (148) therefore tested the hypothesis that a clinically relevant dose of a widely used statin could exert an ameliorating effect on reperfusion injury in a neutrophil-dependent model of myocardial ischemia and reperfusion. In the neutrophil-dependent isolated perfused rat heart model of ischemia (20 min) and reperfusion (45 min), the administration of simvastatin improved coronary flow and preserved left ventricular function. In addition, simvastatin significantly reduced neutrophil accumulation in the ischemic myocardium. Interestingly, simvastatin significantly attenuated P-selectin expression, CD18 upregulation in rat PMNs, and PMN adherence to rat vascular endothelium. These results by Lefer and colleagues (148) provide evidence that HMG coenzyme A reductase inhibitors are potent and effective cardioprotective agents that inhibit leukocyte endothelial cell interactions and preserve cardiac contractile function in coronary perfusion after myocardial ischemia and reperfusion. Moreover, these effects are unrelated to the cholesterol lowering action of this agent and appear to be mediated by enhanced endothelial release of nitric oxide.

Adenosine

Adenosine is recognized as an important regulator of myocardial function and coronary vascular tone in the ischemic myocardium. Stimulation of adenosine A_2 receptors coupled to G-proteins attenuates both free radical generation by activated neutrophils and platelet aggregation following myocardial ischemia reperfusion which may be beneficial in limiting reperfusion injury. Animal models have demonstrated an apparent reduction in infarct size when pretreated with adenosine (9,149). Interestingly, Norton and colleagues (150) randomly assigned rabbits undergoing ischemia reperfusion to one of three agents, each acting on different adenosine receptor sites, to determine any potential receptor specificity in blunting reperfusion injury. A significant reduction in infarct size was achieved with all three agents, notably adenosine, cyclopentyladenosine (A_1 receptor agonist), and CGS 21680C (A_2 receptor agonist). The administration of the A_1 receptor agonist may be most clinically appealing, since it would avoid the potential side effects associated with activation of A_2 receptors.

The AMISTAD trial (Acute Myocardial Infarction Study of Adenosine) was designed to determine the safety and efficacy of combining adenosine (70 mg/kg/min IV for 3 hours) with one of the thrombolytic agents, either streptokinase or tissue plasminogen activator, to further reduce the injury associated with acute myocardial infarction (151). The patients in this trial were stratified by MI location, and the primary endpoint of the study was final infarct size as determined by technetium-99 sestamibi SPECT scanning. The patients with anterior MI who were treated with adenosine plus thrombolytic therapy experienced median final infarct size of 15% (N = 39) as compared to 45.5% (N = 38) for those patients treated with thrombolytic therapy alone. Interestingly, for patients with nonanterior MI, infarct size was similar (11.5% N = 72 vs. 11.5% N = 72) regardless of the addition of adenosine. For those patients with anterior myocardial infarction, the amount of myocardium at risk was similar in the adenosine and nonadenosine groups, 49.5% versus 51%. However, the amount of heart muscles salvaged, as a percentage of myocardium at risk, was greater with the adenosine plus thrombolytic therapy (62.3%) versus thrombolytic therapy alone (15%).

Sodium/Hydrogen Exchange Inhibitors

The first clinical evaluation of cariporide involved patients undergoing primary angioplasty for anterior wall myocardial infarctions (152). This was a medium-size study with a total enrollment of 100 patients. Patients were dosed with 40 mg cariporide IV prior to opening the occluded artery. The primary endpoints were infarct size (serial CPK-MB determination) and ventricular function as determined by pre- and day 18 to 25 postangioplasty ventriculography. Patients demonstrated significant improvement in LV function parameters in the cariporide group, with no change found in the control group. Additionally, the size of the infarction, as determined by area under the CPK-MB curve, was significantly less in the active treatment arm. This study appears to demonstrate that even when administered primarily during reperfusion, cariporide reduces myocardial necrosis and reperfusion injury.

The Guard During Ischemia Against Necrosis (GUARDIAN) trial was undertaken to demonstrate that the beneficial effects seen in the preclinical models would translate into clinical benefit for patients at high risk for complications of cardiac ischemia. Patients were eligible for enrollment if they 1) had unstable angina pectoris or a non-Q-wave myocardial infarction, 2) were undergoing a high risk percutaneous coronary intervention (i.e., at least type 2 B or type C lesion characteristic), or 3) were undergoing high-risk coronary artery bypass grafting (CABG) (i.e., urgent or re-do surgery, or unstable symptoms in the last 4 weeks). Notably, patients who would have qualified for the previous study were excluded from this trial. Patients were randomized to one of three doses of cariporide (HOE 642) or placebo, with treatment lasting for 2 to 7 days at the discretion of the investigator (153,154). A total of 11,590 patients were enrolled and evaluated for events at 36 days and at 6 months.

The primary endpoint of the trial was defined as death or MI at 36 days, while secondary endpoints included events related to left ventricular dysfunction (CHF, arrhythmias, shock) at 6 months, refractory angina pectoris, infarct size determination by CPK-MB release, and death/MI at 10 days. There was no significant difference in the primary endpoint of death or MI at 36 days. Patients who were enrolled in the high-risk CABG group (n = 2918) did show a benefit in 36-day mortality at the highest dose (12.8%) versus the lower doses and placebo (18.2%, 18.1%, 16.7%).

While these results of the GUARDIAN trial are disappointing, they appear to be consistent with the findings in the animal models. As noted earlier, when animals were pretreated with cariporide, which provided adequate tissue levels of drug at the time of ischemia, outcomes were very favorable. Treatment only during the reperfusion phase, however, provided benefit to a lesser degree. Therefore, the timing of administration of cariporide to the patients in the high-risk CABG group should be closely scrutinized. Perhaps, this agent is better suited for a preventive role in patients at high risk for cardiac ischemia.

SUMMARY

Ever since Braunwald and Kloner in 1982 drew the attention of clinicians to the stunned myocardium as a manifestation of reperfusion injury (62), the debate has continued as to whether reperfusion injury is a real phenomenon or simply a laboratory artifact (6). Proponents and opponents of the concept of reperfusion injury accept that the sequence of histopathological changes following prolonged ischemia may be accelerated by reperfusion. Clearly this does not establish that these changes were caused by reperfusion per se. Theoretically, if reperfusion injury could be treated and eliminated, the outcome of patients with acute myocardial infarction might further improve. Unfortunately, there currently exists a great dissociation between clinical data and experimental results. In pilot studies, SOD does not appear to improve recovery of ventricular function in patients with acute myocardial infarction undergoing successful reperfusion by urgent angioplasty (28), whereas the perfluorochemical Fluosol may reduce myocardial infarct size after successful emergency angioplasty (136), but not following thrombolysis (30). Despite much enthusiasm and positive experimental data using the p-selectin blocker Cylexin in limiting reperfusion injury (140,141), the recently started CALYPSO trial of primary angioplasty with randomization to adjunctive Cylexin or placebo was terminated early due to a trend of larger infarcts in the Cylexin arm.

Despite the considerable gains made in reperfusion therapy for acute myocardial infarction in the past decade, there still is a remarkable gap between the large amount of experimental data and the paucity of clinical observations concerning reperfusion injury. This sobering disparity between "the bench and the bedside" will continue to challenge basic research workers and clinicians into the next century. An answer to this challenge may have considerable therapeutic implications for future patients with acute myocardial infarction.

REFERENCES

1. Jennings R, Sommers H, Smyth G, Flack H, Lynn H. Myocardial necrosis induced by temporary occlusion of a coronary artery in the dog. Arch Pathol 1960;70:68–78.
2. Sommers H, Jennings R. Experimental acute myocardial infarction: histologic and histochemical studies of early myocardial infarcts induced by temporary or permanent occlusion of a coronary artery. Lab Invest 1964;13:1491–1502.
3. Zimmerman A, Daems W, Hulsmann W. Morphological changes of heart muscle caused by successive perfusion with calcium free and calcium containing solutions (calcium paradox). Cardiovasc Res 1967;1:201–209.
4. Reimer K, Tanaka M, Murry C, Richard V, Jennings R. Evaluation of free radical injury in myocardium. Toxicol Pathol 1990;18:470–480.
5. Braunwald E, Kloner R. Myocardial reperfusion: a double-edged sword? J Clin Invest 1985;76:1713–1719.
6. Nayler W, Elz J. Reperfusion injury: laboratory artifact or clinical dilemma? Circulation 1986;74:215–221.
7. Ambrosio G, Becker L, Hutchins G, Weisman H, Weisfeldt M. Reduction in experimental infarct size by recombinant human superoxide dismutase: insights into the pathophysiology of reperfusion injury. Circulation 1986;74.
8. Olafessen B, Forman M, Ruett D. Reduction of reperfusion injury in the canine preparation by intracoronary adenosine: importance of the endothelium and the no-reflow phenomenon. Circulation 1987;80:1135–1145.

9. Babbitt DG, Virmani R, Forman MB. Intracoronary adenosine administered after reperfusion limits vascular injury after prolonged ischemia in the canine model. Circulation 1989;80:1388–1399.
10. Simpson PJ, Todd RF, Mickelson JK, et al. Sustained limitation of myocardial reperfusion injury by a monoclonal antibody that alters leukocyte function. Circulation 1990;81:226–237.
11. Simpson P, Todd R, Fantone J, Mickelson J, Griffen J, Luchessi B. Reduction of experimental canine myocardial reperfusion injury by a monoclonal antibody (anti Mo1, anti CD11) that inhibits leukocyte adhesion. J Clin Invest 1991;81:624–629.
12. Engler R, Covell J. Granulocytes cause reperfusion ventricular dysfunction after 15 minute ischemia in the dog. Circulation 1987;61:20–28.
13. Braunwald E. The stunned myocardium: newer insights into mechanisms and clinical implications [letter; comment]. J Thoracic Cardiovasc Surg 1990;100: 310–311.
14. Bolli R. Mechanism of myocardial "stunning." Circulation 1990;82:723–738.
15. Bolli R. Oxygen-derived free radicals and myocardial reperfusion injury: an overview. Cardiovasc Drugs Ther 1991;5:249–268.
16. Bolli R, Zhu W, Thornby J. Time course and determinants of recovery of function after reversible ischemia in conscious dogs. Am J Physiol 1988;254: H102–H114.
17. Kloner R, Ganote C, Jennings R. The "no-reflow" phenomenon after temporary coronary occlusion in the dog. J Clin Invest 1974;54:1496–1508.
18. Manning A, Hearse D. Reperfusion induced arrhythmias: mechanisms and prevention. J Mol Cell Cardiol 1984;16:497–518.
19. Hale S, Lange R, Alker K, Kloner R. Correlates of reperfusion ventricular fibrillation in dogs. Am J Cardiol 1984;53:1397–1400.
20. Hagar JM, Hale SL, Kloner RA. Effect of preconditioning ischemia on reperfusion arrhythmias after coronary artery occlusion and reperfusion in the rat. Circ Res 1991;68:61–68.
21. Jolly S, Kane W, Balilie M. Canine myocardial reperfusion injury: its reduction by the combined administration of superoxide dismutase and catalase. Circ Res 1984;54:277–285.
22. Myers M, Bolli R, Lekich R. Enhancement of recovery of myocardial function by oxygen free radical scavengers after reversible regional ischemia. Circulation 1985;72:915–921.
23. Przyklenk K, Kloner R. Superoxide dismutase plus catalase improve contractile function in the canine model of the "stunned myocardium." Circ Res 1986;58:148–156.
24. Meerson F, Kagan V, Kozlov Y, Belkina L, Arkhipenko Y. The role of lipid peroxidation in pathogenesis of ischemic damage and the antioxidant protection of the heart. Basic Res Cardiol 1982;77:465–485.
25. Roberts M, Young I, Trouton T. Transient release of lipid peroxides after coronary artery balloon angioplasty. Lancet 1990;336:143–145.
26. Menasche P, Grousset C, Mouas C, Piwnica A. A promising approach for improving recovery of heart transplants: prevention of free radical injury

through iron chelation by desferroxamine. J Thorac Cardiovasc Surg 1990; 100:13–21.
27. Allen B, Okamoto F, Buckberg G, et al. Studies of controlled reperfusion after ischemia. XV. Immediate functional recovery after six hours of regional ischemia by careful control of conditions or reperfusion and composition of reperfusate. J Thorac Cardiovasc Surg 1986;92:621–635.
28. Flaherty JT, Pitt B, Gruber JW, et al. Recombinant human superoxide dismutase (h-SOD) fails to improve recovery of ventricular function in patients undergoing coronary angioplasty for acute myocardial infarction. Circulation 1994;89:1982–1991.
29. Forman MB, Ingram DA, Murray JJ. Role of perfluorochemical emulsions in the treatment of myocardial reperfusion injury. Am Heart J 1992;124:1347–1357.
30. Wall T, Califf R, Blakenship J, TAMI group. Intravenous Fluosol in the treatment of acute myocardial infarction: results of the Thrombolysis and Angioplasty in Myocardial Infarction 9 Trial. Circulation 1994;90:114–120.
31. Smith E, Egan J, Bugelski P. Temporal relation between neutrophil accumulation and myocardial reperfusion injury. Am J Physiol 1988;255:H1060–H1068.
32. Dreyer W, Michael L, West M. Neutrophil accumulation in ischemic canine myocardium: insights into the time course, distribution, and mechanism of localization during early reperfusion. Circulation 1991;84:400–411.
33. Mullane K, Read N, Salmon J, Moncada S. Role of leukocytes in acute myocardial infarction in anesthetized dogs: relationship to myocardial salvage by anti-inflammatory drugs. J Pharmacol Exp Ther 1984;228:510–522.
34. Romson J, Hook B, Kunkel S. Reduction of the extent of ischemic myocardial injury by neutrophil depletion in the dog. Circulation 1983;67:1016–1023.
35. de Lorgeril M, Basmadjian A, Lavallee M, et al. Influence of leukopenia on collateral flow, reperfusion flow, reflow ventricular fibrillation, and infarct size in dogs. Am Heart J 1989;117:523–532.
36. Litt MR, Jeremy RW, Weisman HF, Winkelstein JA, Becker LC. Neutrophil depletion limited to reperfusion reduces myocardial infarct size after 90 minutes of ischemia. Evidence for neutrophil-mediated reperfusion injury. Circulation 1989;80:1816–1827.
37. Engler R, Schmid-Schonbein G, Pavelec R. Leukocyte capillary plugging in myocardial ischemia and reperfusion in the dog. Am J Pathol 1983;111:98–111.
38. Lefer A, Albertine K, Weyrich A, Ma X. Polymorphonuclear leukocytes (PMN) accumulate intravascularly but do not migrate to the myocardium following ischemia/reperfusion in the cat. FASEB J 1993;7:A344.
39. Entman M, Youker K, Shappel S. Neutrophil adherence to isolated adult canine myocytes. Evidence for a CD 18 dependent mechanism. J Clin Invest 1990;85:1497–1506.
40. Wiggers C. The interplay of coronary vascular resistance and myocardial compression in regulating coronary flow. Circ Res 1954;2:271–279.

41. Seccombe JF, Schaff HV. Coronary artery endothelial function after myocardial ischemia and reperfusion. Ann Thorac Surg 1995;60:778–788.
42. Forman MB, Puett DW, Virmani R. Endothelial and myocardial injury during ischemia and reperfusion: pathogenesis and therapeutic implications. J Am Coll Cardiol 1989;13:450–459.
43. Kloner R, Alker K, Campbell C, Figures G, Eisenhauer A, Hale S. Does tissue-type plasminogen activator have direct beneficial effects on the myocardium independent of its ability to lyse intracoronary thrombi? Circulation 1989;79:1125–1136.
44. Dauber IM, Van Benthuysen KM, McMurtry IF, et al. Functional coronary microvascular injury evident as increased permeability due to brief ischemia and reperfusion. Circ Res 1990;66:986–998.
45. Jennngs R, Scharper J, Hill M, Steenbergen C, Reimer K. Effect of reperfusion late in the phase of reversible ischemic injury: changes in cell volume, electrolytes, metabolites, and ultrastructure. Circ Res 1985;56:262–278.
46. Svendsen JH. Myocardial capillary permeability for small hydrophilic indicators during normal physiological conditions and after ischemia and reperfusion. Acta Physiol Scand Suppl 1991;603:119–123.
47. Dauber I, Lesnefsky E, Van Benthuysen K, Weil J, Horwitz L. Reactive oxygen metabolite scavengers decrease functional coronary microvascular injury due to ischemia-reperfusion. Am J Physiol 1991;260:H42–H49.
48. Hansen PR, Svendsen JH, Host NB, Hansen SH, Haunso S. Effect of 5-aminosalicylic acid on myocardial capillary permeability following ischaemia and reperfusion. Cardiovasc Res 1992;26:798–803.
49. Engler R, Dahlgren M, Morris D, Peterson M, Schmid-Schoenbein G. Role of leukocytes in the response to acute myocardial ischemia and reflow in dogs. Am J Physiol 1986;251:H314–H323.
50. Mehta J, Nichols W, Donnelly W, Lawson D, Saldeen T. Impaired canine coronary vasodilator response to acetylcholine and bradykinin after occlusion-reperfusion. Circ Res 1989;64:43–54.
51. Gassler JP, Topol EJ. Reperfusion revisited: beyond TIMI 3 flow. Clin Cardiol 1999;22:20–29.
52. Nicklas J, Gips S. Decreased coronary flow reserve after transient myocardial ischemia in dogs. J Am Coll Cardiol 1989;13:195–199.
53. Ito H, Tomooka T, Sakai N. Lack of myocardial perfusion immediately after successful thrombolysis. A predictor of poor recovery of left ventricular function in anterior myocardial infarction. Circulation 1992;85:1699–1705.
54. Schofer J, Montz R, Mathey D. Scintigraphic evidence of the "no-reflow" phenomenon in human beings after coronary thrombolysis. J Am Coll Cardiol 1985;5:593–598.
55. Kern M, Moore J, Aguirre F, et al. Determination of angiographic (TIMI grade) blood flow by intracoronary Doppler flow velocity during acute myocardial infarction. Circulation 1996;94:1545–1552.
56. GUSTO Investigators. The effects of tissue plasminogen activator, streptokinase, or both on coronary artery patency, ventricular function, and survival after acute myocardial infarction. N Engl J Med 1993;329:1615–1622.

57. Heyndrickx G, Millard R, McRitchie R, Maroko P, Vatner S. Regional myocardial functional and electrophysiological alterations after brief coronary artery occlusion in conscious dogs. J Clin Invest 1975;56:978–985.
58. Weiner J, Apstein C, Arthur J, Pirzada F, Hood W. Persistence of myocardial injury following brief periods of coronary occlusion. Cardiovasc Res 1976; 10:678–686.
59. Ellis S, Henschke C, Sandor T, Wynne J, Braunwald E, Kloner R. Time course of functional and biochemical recovery of myocardium salvaged by reperfusion. J Am Coll Cardiol 1983;1:1047–1055.
60. Bolli R. Myocardial "stunning" in man. Circulation 1992;86:1671–1691.
61. Braunwald E, Kloner R. The stunned myocardium: prolonged, postischemic ventricular dysfunction. Circulation 1982;66:1146–1149.
62. Kloner R, Ellis S, Lange R, Braunwald E. Studies of experimental coronary artery reperfusion: effects on infarct size, myocardial function, biochemistry, ultrastructure and microvascular damage. Circulation 1983;68(suppl I):8–15.
63. Taegtmeyer H, Roberts A, Raine A. Energy metabolism in reperfused heart muscle: metabolic correlates to return of function. J Am Coll Cardiol 1985; 6:864–870.
64. Ambrosio G, Jacobus W, Bergman C, Weisman H, Becker L. Preserved high energy phosphate metabolic reserve in globally "stunned" hearts despite reduction of basal ATP content and contractility. J Mol Cell Cardiol 1987;19: 953–964.
65. Arnold J, Braunwald E, Sandor T, Kloner R. Inotropic stimulation of reperfused myocardium with dopamine: effects on infarct size and myocardial function. J Am Coll Cardiol 1985;6:1026–1034.
66. Jackson C, Mickelson J, Pope T, Rao P, Lucchesi B. Oxygen free radical mediated myocardial and vascular dysfunction. Am J Physiol 1986;251: H1225–H1231.
67. Burton K, McCord J, Ghai G. Myocardial alterations due to free-radical generation. Am J Physiol 1984;246:H776–H783.
68. Bolli R, Jeroudi MO, Patel BS, et al. Marked reduction of free radical generation and contractile dysfunction by antioxidant therapy begun at the time of reperfusion. Evidence that myocardial "stunning" is a manifestation of reperfusion injury. Circ Res 1989;65:607–622.
69. Bolli R, McCay PB. Use of spin traps in intact animals undergoing myocardial ischemia/reperfusion: a new approach to assessing the role of oxygen radicals in myocardial "stunning." Free Radic Res Commun 1990;9:169–180.
70. Yasutake M, Haworth RS, King A, Avkiran M. Thrombin activates the sarcolemmal sodium/hydrogen exchanger. Evidence for a receptor mediated mechanism involving protein kinase C. Circ Res 1996;79:705–715.
71. Yokoyama H, Yasutake M, Avkiran M. Alpha-adrenergic stimulation of sarcolemmal sodium/hydrogen exchanger activity in rat ventricular myocytes: evidence for selective mediation by the alpha A-adrenoceptor subtype. Circ Res 1998;82:1078–1085.

72. Yasutake M, Ibuki C, Hearse DJ, Avkiran M. Na/H exchange and reperfusion arrhythmias: protection by intracoronary infusion of a novel inhibitor. Am J Physiol 1994;267:H2430–H2440.
73. Scholz W, Albus U, Counillon L, et al. Protective effects of HOE 642, a selective sodium-hydrogen exchange subtype I inhibitor, on cardiac ischemia and reperfusion. Cardiovasc Res 1995;29:260–268.
74. Xue YX, Aye NN, Hashimoto K. Antiarrhythmic effects of HOE 642, a novel Na/H exchange inhibitor, on ventricular arrhythmias in animal hearts. Eur J Pharmacol 1996;317:309–316.
75. Shimada Y, Hearse DJ, Avkiran M. Impact of extracellular buffer composition on cardioprotective efficacy of Na/H exchange inhibitors. Am J Physiol 1996; 270:H692–H700.
76. Sack S, Mohri M, Schwartz ER, et al. Effects of a new Na/H antiporter inhibitor on postischemic reperfusion in pig hearts. J Cardiovasc Pharmacol 1994;23:72–78.
77. Shipolini AR, Yokoyama Y, Galinanes M, et al. Na/H exchanger activity does not contribute to protection by ischemic preconditioning in the isolated rat heart. Circulation 1997;96:3617–3625.
78. Klein HH, Pich S, Bohle RM, et al. Myocardial protection by Na/H exchange inhibition in ischemic, reperfused porcine hearts. Circulation 1995;92:912–917.
79. Rohmann S, Weygandt H, Minck KO. Preischaemic as well as postischaemic application of a Na/H exchange inhibitor reduces infarct size in pigs. Cardiovasc Res 1995;30:945–951.
80. Garcia-Dorado D, Gonzalez MA, Barrabes JA, et al. Prevention of ischemic rigor contracture during coronary occlusion by inhibition of Na/H exchange. Cardiovasc Res 1997;35:80–89.
81. Miura T, Ogawa T, Suzuki K, Goto M, Shimamoto K. Infarct size limitation by a new Na/H exchange inhibitor, HOE 642: difference from preconditioning in the role of protein kinase C. J Am Coll Cardiol 1997;29:693–701.
82. Linz W, Albus U, Crause P, et al. Dose-dependent reduction of myocardial infarct mass in rabbits by the NHE-1 inhibitor cariporide (HOE 642). Clin Exp Hypertens 1998;20:733–749.
83. Gumina RJ, Mizumura T, Beier N, Schelling P, Schultz JJ, Gross GJ. A new sodium/hydrogen exchange inhibitor, EMD 851231, limits infarct size in dogs when administered before or after coronary artery occlusion. J Pharmacol Exp Ther 1998;286:175–183.
84. Klein HH, Bohle RM, Pich S, et al. Time-dependent protection by Na/H exchange inhibition in the regionally ischemic, reperfused porcine heart preparation with low residual blood flow. J Mol Cell Cardiol 1998;30:795–801.
85. Ciuffo A, Ouyang P, Becker L, Levin L, Weisfeldt M. Reduction of sympathetic inotropic response after ischemia in dogs: contributor to stunned myocardium. J Clin Invest 1985;75:1504–1509.
86. Bolli R, Triana J, Jeroudi M. Prolonged impairment of coronary vasodilation after reversible ischemia: evidence for microvascular “stunning.” Circ Res 1990;67:332–343.

87. Zhao M, Zhang H, Robinson T, Factor S, Sonnenblick E, Eng C. Profound structural alterations of the extracellular collagen matrix in postischemic dysfunctional ("stunned") but viable myocardium. J Am Coll Cardiol 1987;10: 1322–1334.
88. Fournier C, Boujon B, Hebert J, Zamani K, Grimon G, Blondeau M. Stunned myocardium following coronary spasm. Am Heart J 1991;121:593–595.
89. Touchstone D, Beller G, Nygaard T, Tedesco C, Kaul S. Effects of successful intravenous reperfusion therapy on regional myocardial function and geometry in humans: a tomographic assessment using two dimensional echocardiography. J Am Coll Cardiol 1989;13:1506–1513.
90. Pfisterer M, Zuber M, Wenzel R, Burkart F. Prolonged myocardial stunning after thrombolysis: can left ventricular function be assessed definitely at hospital discharge? Eur Heart J 1991;12:214–217.
91. Sheehan F, Doerr R, Schmidt W. Early recovery of left ventricular function after thrombolytic therapy for acute myocardial infarction: an important determinant of survival. J Am Coll Cardiol 1988;12:289–300.
92. Kloner R, Allen J, Cox T, Zheng Y, Ruiz C. Stunned left ventricular myocardium following exercise treadmill testing in coronary artery disease. Am J Cardiol 1991;68:629–634.
93. Ambrosio G, Betocchi S, Pace L. Prolonged impairment of regional left ventricular systolic function after exercise in patients with stable angina. Circulation 1991;84(suppl II):475.
94. Robertson W, Feigenbaum H, Armstrong W, Dillon J, O'Donnell J, McHenry P. Exercise echocardiography: a clinically practical addition in the evaluation of coronary artery disease. J Am Coll Cardiol 1983;2:1085–1091.
95. Roberts A, Spies M, Sanders J. Serial assessment of left ventricular performance following coronary artery bypass grafting. J Thorac Cardiovasc Surg 1981;81:69–84.
96. Wilson I, Gardner T. Stunned myocardium in cardiac surgery. In: Kloner RA, Przyklenk, K, eds. The Stunned Myocardium: Properties, Mechanisms, and Clinical Manifestations. New York: Marcel Dekker, 1993:379–399.
97. Nixon J, Brown C, Smitherman T. Identification of transient and persistent segmental wall motion abnormalities in patients with unstable angina by two dimensional echocardiography. Circulation 1982;65:1497–1503.
98. Wijns W, Serruys P, Slager C. Effect of coronary occlusion during percutaneous transluminal angioplasty in humans on left ventricular chamber stiffness and regional pressure radius relations. J Am Coll Cardiol 1986;7:455–463.
99. Sheridan D, Penkoske P, Sobel B, Corr P. Alpha adrenergic contributions to dysrhythmia during myocardial ischemia and reperfusion in cats. J Clin Invest 1980;65:161–171.
100. Corr P, Saffitz J, Sobel B. What is the contribution of altered lipid metabolism to arrhythmogenesis in the ischemic heart? In: Hearse DJ, Manning AS, Janse MJ, eds. Life Threatening Arrhythmias During Ischemia and Infarction. New York: Raven Press, 1987:91–114.
101. Opie LH. Role of calcium and other ions in reperfusion injury. Cardiovasc Drugs Ther 1991;5:237–247.

102. Hirche H, Friedrich R, Kebbel U, McDonald F, Zylka V. Early arrhythmias, myocardial extracellular potassium and pH. In: Parratt JR, ed. Early Arrhythmias Resulting from Myocardial Ischemia: Mechanisms and Prevention by Drugs. London: Macmillan, 1982:113–124.
103. Curtis MJ, Pugsley MK, Walker MJ. Endogenous chemical mediators of ventricular arrhythmias in ischaemic heart disease. Cardiovasc Res 1993;27:703–719.
104. Yamazaki S, Fujibayashi Y, Rajagopalan R, Meerbaum S. Effects of staged versus sudden reperfusion after acute coronary occlusion in the dog. J Am Coll Cardiol 1986;7:564–572.
105. Colquhoun M, Julian D. Treatable arrhythmias in cardiac arrests seen outside hospital. Lancet 1992;339:1167.
106. Burney RE, Walsh D, Kaplan LR, Fraser S, Tung B, Overmyer J. Reperfusion arrhythmia: myth or reality? Ann Emerg Med 1989;18:240–243.
107. Solimene MC, Ramires JA, Bellotti G, Tranchesi B, Jr., Pileggi F. Reperfusion arrhythmias in acute myocardial infarction—fact or coincidence? Int J Cardiol 1988;20:341–351.
108. Hackett D, McKenna W, Davies G, Maseri A. Reperfusion arrhythmias are rare during acute myocardial infarction and thrombolysis in man. Int J Cardiol 1990;29:205–213.
109. Kloner RA. Does reperfusion injury exist in humans? J Am Coll Cardiol 1993; 21:537–545.
110. Hansen PR. Myocardial reperfusion injury: experimental evidence and clinical relevance. Eur Heart J 1995;16:734–740.
111. Shiki K, Hearse D. Preconditioning of ischemic myocardium: reperfusion-induced arrhythmias. Am J Physiol 1987;253:H1470–H1476.
112. Bolli R, Myers M, Zhu W, Roberts R. Disparity of reperfusion arrhythmias after reversible myocardial ischemia in open chest and conscious dogs. J Am Coll Cardiol 1986;7:1047–1056.
113. Hagar J, Kloner R. Reperfusion arrhythmias: experimental and clinical aspects. Age Reperfusion 1990;2:1–5.
114. Murry C, Jennings R, Reimer K. Preconditioning with ischemia: a delay of lethal cell injury in ischemic myocardium. Circulation 1986;74:1124–1136.
115. Jennings R, Murry C, Reimer K. Preconditioning myocardium with ischemia. Cardiovasc Drugs Ther 1991;5:933–938.
116. Downey J. Ischemic preconditioning: nature's own cardioprotective intervention. Trends Cardiovas Med 1992;12:170–176.
117. Marber M, Latchman D, Walker J, Yellon D. Cardiac stress protein elevation 24 hours after brief ischemia or heat stress is associated with resistance to myocardial infarction. Circulation 1993;88:1264–1272.
118. Sun J, Tang X, Knowlton A, Park S, Qiu Y, Bolli R. Late preconditioning against myocardial stunning. J Clin Invest 1995;95:388–403.
119. Ottani F, Galvani M, Ferrini D, et al. Prodromal angina limits infarct size. A role for ischemic preconditioning. Circulation 1995;91:291–297.
120. ISIS-3. A randomized comparison of streptokinase vs. tissue plasminogen activator vs. anistreplase and of aspirin plus heparin vs. aspirin alone among

41,299 cases of suspected acute myocardial infarction. Lancet 1992;339:753–770.

121. Honan M, Harrell F, Reimer K. Cardiac rupture, mortality and the timing of thrombolytic therapy: a meta-analysis. J Am Coll Cardiol 1990;16:359–367.
122. Wilcox R, von der Lippe G, Olsson C. Trial of tissue plasminogen activator for mortality reduction in acute myocardial infarction: Anglo-Scandinavian Study of Early Thrombolysis (ASSET). Lancet 1988;ii:525–530.
123. Kleiman N, White H, Ohman E, GUSTO Investigators. Mortality 24 hours after thrombolysis in the GUSTO trial: corroborating evidence for the importance of early perfusion. Circulation 1993;88(suppl I):1–17.
124. GUSTO Investigators. An international randomized trial comparing four thrombolytic strategies for acute myocardial infarction. N Engl J Med 1993;329: 673–682.
125. Nejima J, Knight DR, Fallon JT, et al. Superoxide dismutase reduces reperfusion arrhythmias but fails to salvage regional function or myocardium at risk in conscious dogs. Circulation 1989;79:143–153.
126. Kusama Y, Bernier M, Hearse DJ. Exacerbation of reperfusion arrhythmias by sudden oxidant stress. Circ Res 1990;67:481–489.
127. Werns S, Shea M, Driscoll E. The independent effects of oxygen radical scavengers on canine infarct size: reduction by superoxide dismutase but not catalase. Circ Res 1985;56:895.
128. Simpson P, Mitsos S, Gallagher K, et al. Prostacyclin protects ischemic-reperfused myocardium in the dog by inhibition of neutrophil activation. Am Heart J 1987;113:129–137.
129. Topol E, Ellis S, Califf R, et al. Combined tissue type plasminogen activator and prostacyclin therapy for acute myocardial infarction. J Am Coll Cardiol 1989;14:877–884.
130. Clark L, Gollan F. Survival of mammals breathing organic liquids equilibrated with oxygen at atmospheric pressure. Science 1966;152:1755.
131. Tremper K, Friedman A, Levine E, Lapin R, Camarillo D. The preoperative treatment of severely anemic patients with a perfluorochemical oxygen transport fluid. N Engl J Med 1982;307:277–283.
132. Geyer R. Fluorocarbon-polyol artificial blood substitutes. N Engl J Med 1973; 289:1077–1082.
133. Liu JX, Tanonaka K, Ohtsuka Y, Sakai Y, Takeo S. Improvement of ischemia/reperfusion-induced contractile dysfunction of perfused hearts by class I C antiarrhythmic agents. J Pharmacol Exp Ther 1993;266:1247–1254.
134. Forman M, Pitarys C, Vildibill H, et al. Pharmacologic perturbation of neutrophils by Fluosol results in sustained reduction in infarct size in the canine model of reperfusion. J Am Coll Cardiol 1992;19:205.
135. Forman M, Puett D, Bingham S, et al. Preservation of endothelial cell structure and function by intracoronary perfluorochemical in a canine preparation of reperfusion. Circulation 1987;76:469–479.
136. Forman MB, Perry JM, Wilson BH, et al. Demonstration of myocardial reperfusion injury in humans: results of a pilot study utilizing acute coronary

angioplasty with perfluorochemical in anterior myocardial infarction. J Am Coll Cardiol 1991;18:911–918.
137. Lucchesi BR, Werns SW, Fantone JC. The role of the neutrophil and free radicals in ischemic myocardial injury. J Mol Cell Cardiol 1989;21:1241–1251.
138. Opie LH. Reperfusion injury and its pharmacologic modification. Circulation 1989;80:1049–1062.
139. Kloner RA, Przyklenk K, Whittaker P. Deleterious effects of oxygen radicals in ischemia/reperfusion: resolved and unresolved issues. Circulation 1989; 80: 1115–1127.
140. Silver M, Sutton J, Hook S, et al. Adjunctive selectin blockade successfully reduces infarct size beyond thrombolysis in the electrolytic canine coronary artery model. Circulation 1995;92:492–499.
141. Lefer AM, Weyrich AS, Buerke M. Role of selectins, a new family of adhesion molecules, in ischaemia-reperfusion injury. Cardiovasc Res 1994;28: 289–294.
142. Faxon DP, Gibbons RJ, Chronos NAF, Gurbel PA, Martin JS. The effect of a CD11/CD18 inhibitor (Hu23FG) on infarct size following direct angioplasty: the HALT MI study. Circulation 1999;100:791–792.
143. Kinlay S, Selwyn AP, Delagrange D, Creager MA, Libby P, Ganz P. Biological mechanisms for the clinical success of lipid-lowering in coronary artery disease and the use of surrogate end-points. Curr Opin Lipidol 1996;7:389–397.
144. Levine GN, Keaney JF Jr, Vita JA. Cholesterol reduction in cardiovascular disease: clinical benefits and possible mechanisms. N Engl J Med 1995;332: 512–521.
145. Treasure CB, Klein JL, Weintraub WS, Talley JD, Stillabower ME, Kosinski AS, Zhang J, Boccuzzi SJ, Cedarholm JC, Alexander RW. Beneficial effects of cholesterol-lowering therapy on the coronary endothelium in patients with coronary artery disease. N Engl J Med 1995;332:481–487.
146. Delanty N, Vaughan CJ. Vascular effects of statins in stroke. Stroke 1997;28: 2315–2320.
147. Alberts AW. Discovery, biochemistry and biology of lovastatin. Am J Cardiol 1988;62:10J–15J.
148. Lefer AM, Campbell B, Yong-Kyoo S, Scalia R, Hayward R, Lefer D. Simvastatin preserves the ischemic-reperfused myocardium in normocholesterolemic rat hearts. Circulation 1999;100:178–184.
149. Olafsson B, Forman M, Puett D. Reduction of reperfusion injury in the canine preparation by intracoronary adenosine: importance of the endothelium and the no-reflow phenomenon. Circulation 1987;76:1135–1145.
150. Norton ED, Jackson EK, Turner MB, Virmani R, Forman MB. The effects of intravenous infusions of selective adenosine A1-receptor and A2-receptor agonists on myocardial reperfusion injury. Am Heart J 1992;123:332–338.
151. Mahaffey KW. The AMISTAD study group. Does adenosine in conjunction with thrombolysis reduce infarct size? Results from AMISTAD. Circulation 1997; 96:1444.

152. Drexler H, Rupprecht HJ, Buerke M, et al. A Na/H exchange inhibitor improves recovery of ventricular function in patients undergoing coronary angioplasty for acute myocardial infarction. Circulation 1998;98:1344.
153. Erhardt LRW. Guard During Ischemia Against Necrosis (GUARDIAN) trial in acute coronary syndromes. Am J Cardiol 1999;83:23G–25G.
154. Scholz W, Jessel A, Albus U. Development of the Na/H exchange inhibitor cariporide as a cardioprotective drug: from the laboratory to the GUARDIAN trial. J Thromb Thrombol 1999;8:61–70.
155. Sakuma T, Hayashi Y, Sumii K, Imazu M, Yamakido M. Prediction of short- and intermediate-term prognoses of patients with acute myocardial infarction using myocardial contrast echocardiography one day after recanalization. J Am Coll Cardiol 1998;32:890–897.
156. Wu K, Zerhouni EA, Judd RM, Lugo-Olivieri CH, Barouch LA, Schulman SP, Blumenthal RS, Lima JA. Prognostic significance of microvascular obstruction by magnetic resonance imaging in patients with acute myocardial infarction. Circulation 1998;97:765–772.

25

Lessons from the GUSTO Trials

Vasant B. Patel and Eric J. Topol
The Cleveland Clinic Foundation
Cleveland, Ohio

INTRODUCTION

The management of acute myocardial infarction has evolved since the introduction of fibrinolytic therapy in large part propelled by unprecedented number of large-scale, multicenter, randomized trials. The Global Utilization of Streptokinase and Tissue Plasminogen Activator of Occluded Coronary Arteries (GUSTO) series of trials have been part of the pivotal collaborative work in advancing the field of cardiovascular medicine. In particular, the GUSTO trial organization incorporated substudies to provide a mechanistic understanding of the main trial's findings.

The original GUSTO trial was designed to evaluate which of the available fibrinolytic regimens was superior in restoring rapid and sustained reperfusion in the setting of acute myocardial infarction. Beyond the overall trial assessing clinical outcome, an angiographic substudy evaluated the effect of the early open artery, reocclusion, and preservation of cardiac function. The second GUSTO trial incorporated the spectrum of patients with acute coronary syndromes including patients with unstable angina and myocardial infarction with either ST-elevation, ST-depression, or T-wave inversion. The GUSTO II trial was designed to evaluate the importance of thrombin inhibition and compared hirudin, a direct thrombin inhibitor, to heparin in patients with acute coronary syndromes. An angioplasty substudy compared the efficacy of primary angioplasty with fibrinolytic therapy for acute ST-elevation myocardial infarction. The introduction of third-generation fibrinolytic agents was the foundation of the GUSTO III trial, which compared the efficacy of reteplase to alteplase in acute MI. The next significant advance in the management of acute MI led to introduction of potent platelet inhibition with glycoprotein IIb/IIIa receptor antagonist as an adjunct to fibrinolysis and hence the genesis of GUSTO IV pilot study. The GUSTO IV main trial is currently enrolling patients and is expected to resolve whether combined fibrin and platelet lysis will improve survival compared with conventional fibrinolytic therapy.

GUSTO I TRIAL

Background and Rationale

Numerous trials in the 1980s reported superior outcomes with fibrinolytic therapy for acute myocardial infarction when compared to placebo. The proposed mechanism was that fibrinolytic therapy rapidly established reperfusion to ischemic myocardium and hence myocardial preservation. Thus, the survival benefit of fibrinolysis was based on the "open-artery hypothesis" which proposed that early and durable infarct artery patency resulted in better left ventricular function and improved survival. However, this theory was challenged by the GISSI-2 (Gruppo Italiano per lo Studio della Streptochinase nell'Infarcto Miocardio) and ISIS-3 (International Study of Infarct Survival Collaborative Group) trials which reported no improvement in survival with alteplase compared to streptokinase, even though alteplase was known to yield higher patency than streptokinase (1–3). These findings were however confounded by use of conventional dosing of alteplase and lack of intravenous heparin. While GISSI-2 and ISIS-3 reported lack of survival benefit with conventional dosing of alteplase, other clinical studies using accelerated regimen of alteplase, and angiographic studies using intravenous heparin in the setting of acute MI demonstrated higher patency and lower reocclusion rates (4,5). The controversial results of these trials and clinical studies showing lower reocclusion rates with a combination of alteplase and streptokinase led to the genesis of the GUSTO I trial (6). The objective was to compare accelerated alteplase with intravenous heparin to streptokinase or combination of both agents in patients with acute ST-elevation myocardial infarction (Fig. 1). The primary endpoint was 30-day all-cause mortality. The secondary endpoints were death and nonfatal hemorrhagic or disabling strokes. The pivotal angiographic substudy enrolled a total of 2431 patients to investigate and understand the relationship between infarct artery patency, myocardial preservation, and mortality (7). Coronary artery patency and reocclusion were assessed at 90 min, 180 min, 24 hours, and 5 to 7 days after fibrinolytic administration.

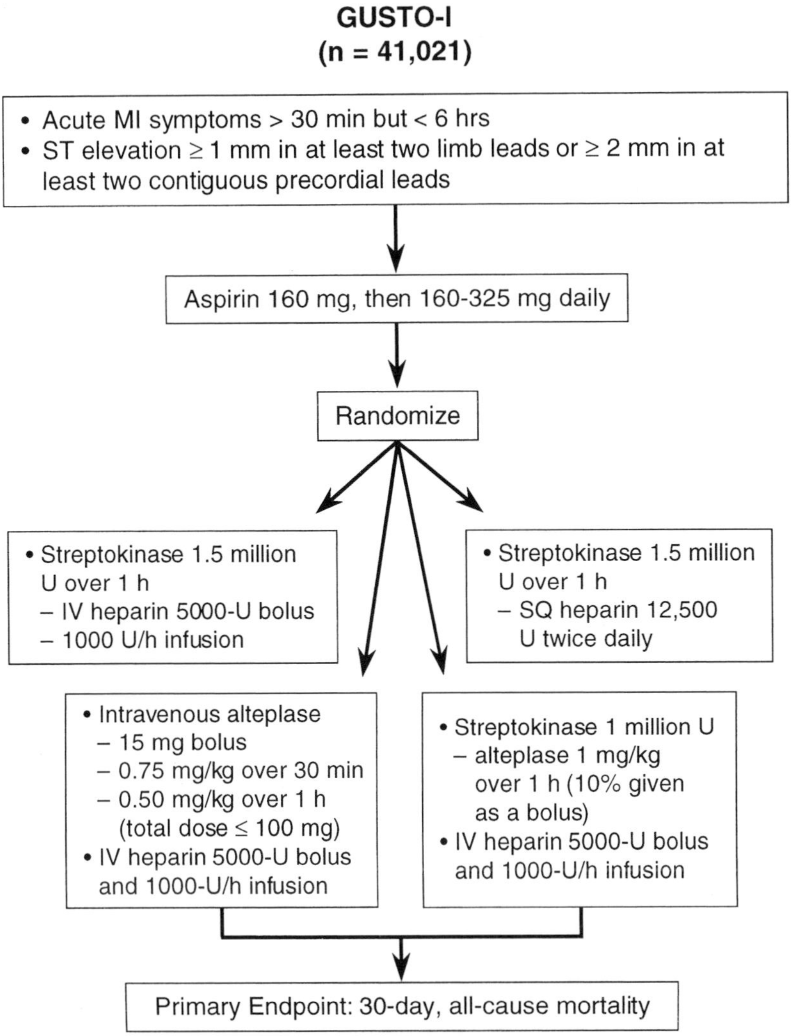
GUSTO-I
(n = 41,021)
• Acute MI symptoms > 30 min but < 6 hrs
• ST elevation ≥ 1 mm in at least two limb leads or ≥ 2 mm in at least two contiguous precordial leads
Aspirin 160 mg, then 160-325 mg daily
Randomize
• Streptokinase 1.5 million U over 1 h – IV heparin 5000-U bolus – 1000 U/h infusion
• Streptokinase 1.5 million U over 1 h – SQ heparin 12,500 U twice daily
• Intravenous alteplase – 15 mg bolus – 0.75 mg/kg over 30 min – 0.50 mg/kg over 1 h (total dose ≤ 100 mg)
• IV heparin 5000-U bolus and 1000-U/h infusion
• Streptokinase 1 million U – alteplase 1 mg/kg over 1 h (10% given as a bolus)
• IV heparin 5000-U bolus and 1000-U/h infusion
Primary Endpoint: 30-day, all-cause mortality

Figure 1 Protocol algorithm of the GUSTO I trial. MI = myocardial infarction.

Results

The principal finding of the GUSTO I trial was a 1.1% absolute and 14.6% relative reduction in 30-day mortality with accelerated alteplase (6.3%) compared with streptokinase (7.4%) (6). The mortality benefit with accelerated alteplase regimen was highly significant whether compared with streptokinase and subcutaneous or intravenous heparin ($P = .001$) or the combination of alteplase and streptokinase ($P = .04$). In streptokinase-treated patients, intravenous heparin conferred no added advantage over subcutaneous heparin. The accelerated alteplase regimen was associated with increased incidence of intracranial hemorrhage when compared with streptokinase (0.72% vs. 0.52%, $P = .03$). The survival benefit was seen as early as 24 hours after randomization and was sustained at 1-year follow-up with savings of 10 lives per 1000 patients treated with alteplase compared to streptokinase (Fig. 2) (8).

Angiographic Substudy

At 90-min angiography, the Thrombolysis in Myocardial Infarction (TIMI) grade 2 or 3 flow was 81%, 73%, 54%, and 60% for front-loaded t-PA,

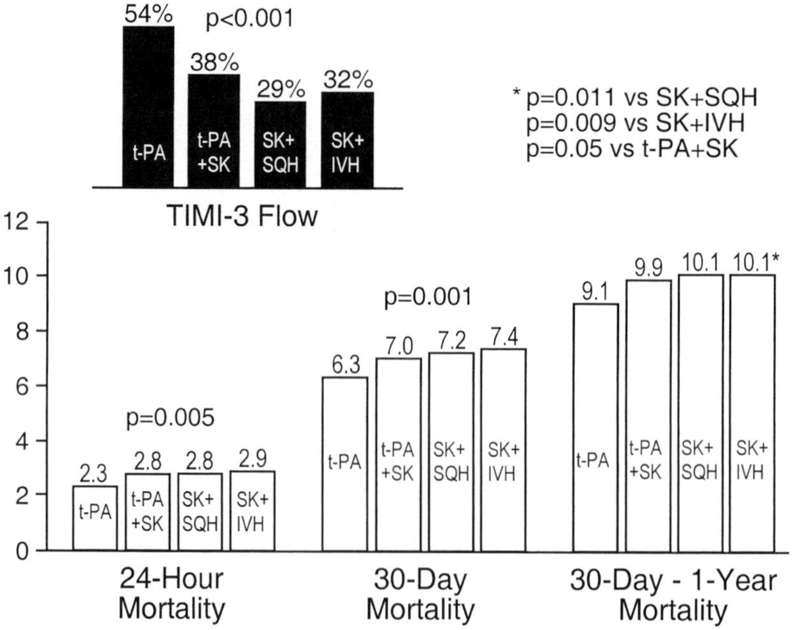

Figure 2 Mortality at 24 hours, 30 days, and 1 year in the four treatment groups of the GUSTO I trial. Complete coronary patency (TIMI grade 3 flow) was highest with accelerated alteplase regimen and correlated consistently with improved survival compared to streptokinase or combination of alteplase and streptokinase. SK = streptokinase, t-PA = alteplase, SQH = subcutaneous heparin, IVH = intravenous heparin.

combination of t-PA and streptokinase, streptokinase and subcutaneous heparin, and streptokinase and intravenous heparin, respectively. Importantly, TIMI-3 flow was present in 54%, 38%, 29%, and 32% of patients, respectively. However, at 180 min, at 24 hours, and at 5 to 7 days, the patency rates were similar irrespective of fibrinolytic regimen (7). The angiographic substudy established the linkage among infarct artery patency, preserved left ventricular function, and clinical outcome. Furthermore, it highlighted the primacy of attaining early TIMI-3 flow in acute MI. Left ventricular ejection fraction, infarct size, and 30-day mortality outcomes were favorable when TIMI-3 flow was achieved compared with TIMI 0–2 flow irrespective of fibrinolytic regimen (9). The accelerated alteplase regimen while yielding highest TIMI-3 flow, also resulted in higher left ventricular ejection fraction and lower end-systolic volume index compared to streptokinase (10). The advantage of alteplase therapy was almost entirely explained by higher coronary patency as demonstrated using simple regression model of relationship among fibrinolytic therapy, coronary patency, and survival (9). At 2-year follow-up, restoration of early TIMI-3 flow and preservation of left ventricular function resulted in 61% and 75% reduction in death beyond initial 30 days (11). Thus, early restoration of normal coronary flow was associated with reduction in ~3 lives per 100 patients in the first month and an additional 5 lives per 100 beyond initial 30 days. While early open-artery hypothesis is based on myocardial salvage, there is evidence to support restoration of coronary patency beyond the expected time for preservation of left ventricular function. In a multivariate analysis after adjusting for left ventricular ejection fraction, patients with open rather than closed infarct-related artery had significantly lower 30-day mortality ($P < .001$) (12).

GUSTO II TRIAL

Background and Rationale

The GUSTO I trial while testing the "open-artery hypothesis" established the importance of early infarct artery patency and superiority of front-loaded t-PA in achieving the highest degree of TIMI-3 flow at 90-min. However, even the best available fibrinolytic regimen yielded TIMI-3 flow in only 54% of patients. While validating the open-artery hypothesis, the GUSTO trial estimated that improving TIMI-3 flow at 90-min by 40% would yield an additional 15% reduction in mortality (13). Importantly, the GUSTO trial highlighted the major limitation of heparin as an anticoagulant. While intravenous heparin enhanced fibrinolysis with alteplase, it did not confer advantage over subcutaneous heparin with streptokinase. The challenge with heparin has been appropriate initial dosing as well as timely establishment and maintenance of therapeutic anticoagulation. Because of varying levels of antithrombin-III and plasma proteins among individuals, the degree of anticoagulation with heparin can be unpredictable. In addition, heparin is not effective against clot-bound thrombin and does not effectively suppress thrombin generation, an important limitation since fibrinolysis results in release of clot-bound thrombin (14). Recognizing these limitations of heparin, the focus shifted to a newer, more potent class of thrombin inhibitors. Direct thrombin inhibitors inactivate clot-bound thrombin and are not influenced by other mediators such as platelet factor 4. As clinical studies reported higher patency rates with hirudin compared with heparin in acute coronary syndromes, these agents became the focus of attention (15,16). The quest for strategies to enhance coronary patency led to genesis of the GUSTO II trial to test the "thrombin hypothesis": a more potent thrombin inhibition would improve clinical outcomes in acute coronary syndromes.

The GUSTO II trial incorporated a spectrum of acute coronary syndromes including unstable angina having ST-depression or T-wave inversion as well as ST-elevation myocardial infarction. The objective was to evaluate whether direct thrombin inhibitors were superior to heparin in the spectrum of acute coronary syndromes where coronary thrombus is the primary target. Patients with ST-elevation MI were eligible to receive fibrinolysis either with accelerated alteplase or streptokinase. The primary endpoint was a composite of death, nonfatal myocardial infarction, or reinfarction at 30 days.

The GUSTO IIa study initially enrolled patients to receive hirudin 0.6 mg/kg bolus followed by 0.2 mg/kg/hr infusion or heparin 5000 units bolus followed by 1000 to 3000 U/hr infusion for up to 120 hours (17). This trial, similar to TIMI 9a study, was prematurely terminated due to increased incidence of intracranial hemorrhage, especially in patients with ST-elevation MI receiving fibrinolytic therapy. Recognizing the need for a lesser degree of anticoagulation, especially during fibrinolysis, the GUSTO IIa study was resumed as GUSTO IIb with lower doses of hirudin (0.1 mg/kg bolus followed by 0.1 mg/kg/hr infusion) or heparin (5000 unit bolus followed by a standard 1000 U/hr infusion) up to 72 hours (Fig. 3) (18). Lessons from GUSTO I, which demonstrated an optimal anticoagulation between activated prothrombin time (aPTT) of 50 to 70 sec (19), and GUSTO IIa, which demonstrated high hemorrhagic stroke rates at aPTT of 60 to 90 sec (17), led to adjustment in aPTT target range of 60 to 85 sec for the GUSTO IIb study.

An important substudy evaluated the efficacy of primary angioplasty against accelerated alteplase regimen in 1138 patients with ST-elevation MI (20). While several studies had reported significant reduction in death, reinfarction, and stroke with primary angioplasty compared with fibrinolysis, these studies were largely conducted at specialized centers with small number of patients and thus its applicability to general practice remained uncer-

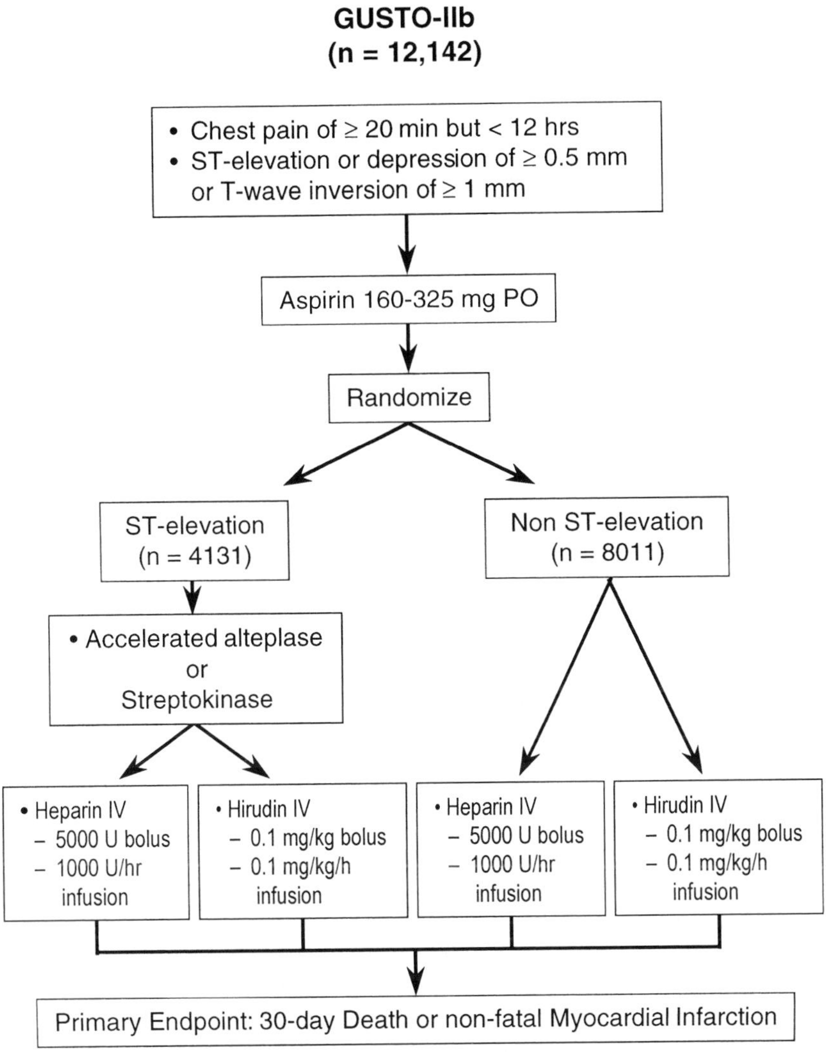

Figure 3 Protocol algorithm of the GUSTO IIb trial.

tain (21–25). The impetus for the GUSTO IIb angioplasty substudy was to provide insight into the debate about the superiority of primary angioplasty over accelerated alteplase (not previously tested) for acute ST-elevation MI. This study was unique as it incorporated many centers, various operators, large sample size, and the best available fibrinolytic regimen.

Results

GUSTO IIa

The results in this trial mainly focused on bleeding complications. Although the trial was planned to enroll 12,000 patients, it was stopped after enrolling 2564 patients due to excess of intracerebral hemorrhagic events, especially in patients receiving fibrinolysis (1.8% vs. 0.3%, $P < .001$). The 1.8% event rate was much higher than the 0.7% observed in the GUSTO I trial. The increase in incidence of intracranial hemorrhage was explained by the significantly higher aPTT in these patients compared to those who did not have intracranial hemorrhage (110 sec vs. 87 sec, $P = .03$). The overall incidence of hemorrhagic stroke was higher in patients receiving hirudin compared to heparin (1.3% vs. 0.7%, $P = .11$) (17). At higher degree of anticoagulation, the incidence of death, MI, or reinfarction was similar between hirudin and heparin (11.7% vs. 11.0%). The most important lesson from GUSTO IIa was that for both direct thrombin inhibitors and unfractionated heparin, the aPTT was useful index for predicting risk of hemorrhagic stroke in patients receiving fibrinolytic therapy.

GUSTO IIb

The results from this study represent the main trial results as 12,142 patients with a spectrum of acute coronary syndromes were enrolled according to the presence of ST elevation on presenting electrocardiogram (4131 patients) or its absence (8011 patients). The primary endpoint of death, nonfatal MI, or reinfarction at 30 days occurred in 8.9% of patients receiving hirudin and 9.8% receiving heparin ($P = .06$), an absolute 0.9% and a relative 11% reduction in events with hirudin (18). The treatment effect was similar across the spectrum of acute coronary syndromes, those with or without ST-segment elevation (Fig. 4). Though the composite endpoint did not reach statistical significance for hirudin to show superiority at 30 days, the composite endpoint was statistically significant at 24 hours (1.3% vs. 2.1%, $P = .001$), 48 hours (2.3% vs. 3.1%, $P = .001$), and at 6 months (12.3% vs. 13.6%, $P = .04$), demonstrating hirudin to be more effective than heparin (18,26). Importantly, intracranial hemorrhage occurred less frequently and it was similar among hirudin- and heparin-treated patients (0.3% vs. 0.2%, $P = .24$). The results of GUSTO IIb, therefore, are consistent with and validate the thrombin hypothesis in acute coronary syndromes.

Two crucial lessons from the main GUSTO IIb study were the interaction between hirudin and streptokinase and the influence of hirudin on thrombin activity. While clinical outcomes have been known to be better for alteplase with intravenous heparin, the GUSTO IIb results indicate superior outcomes in patients treated with streptokinase and hirudin with an absolute

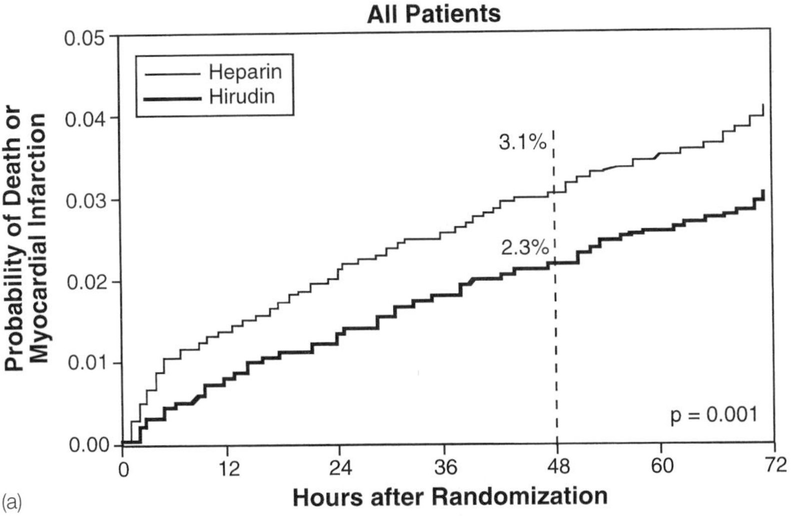

(a)

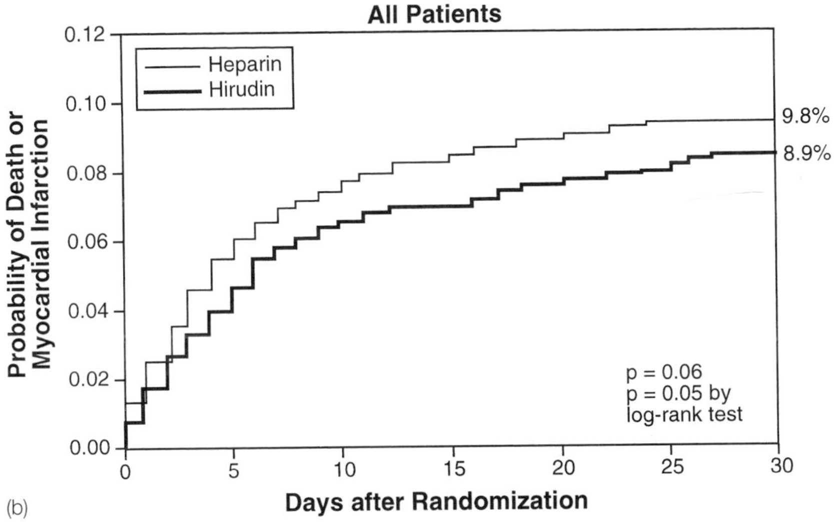

(b)

Figure 4 Kaplan-Meier estimates of the probability of death or myocardial infarction in all patients according to treatment assignment within the first 72 hours (a) and at 30 days (b). Probability of death or myocardial infarction were similar in those with ST elevation (c) and those without ST elevation (d). (From Ref. 18.)

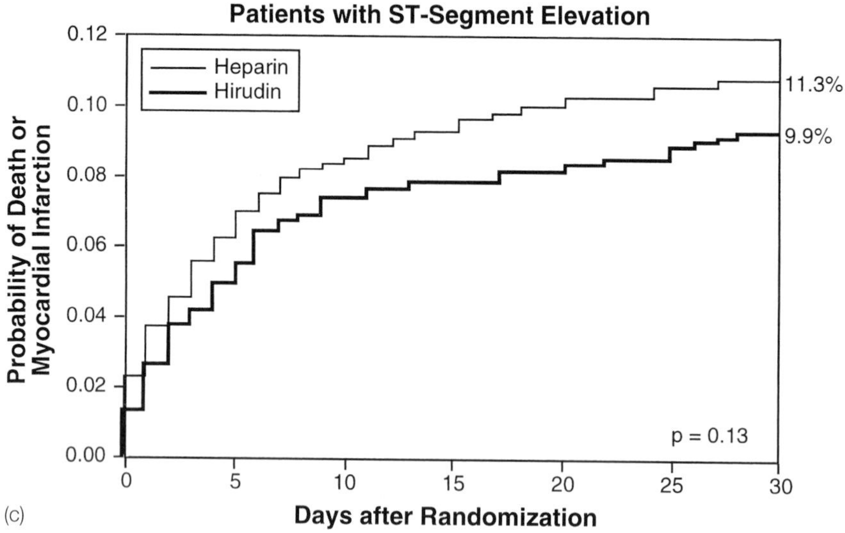

(c)

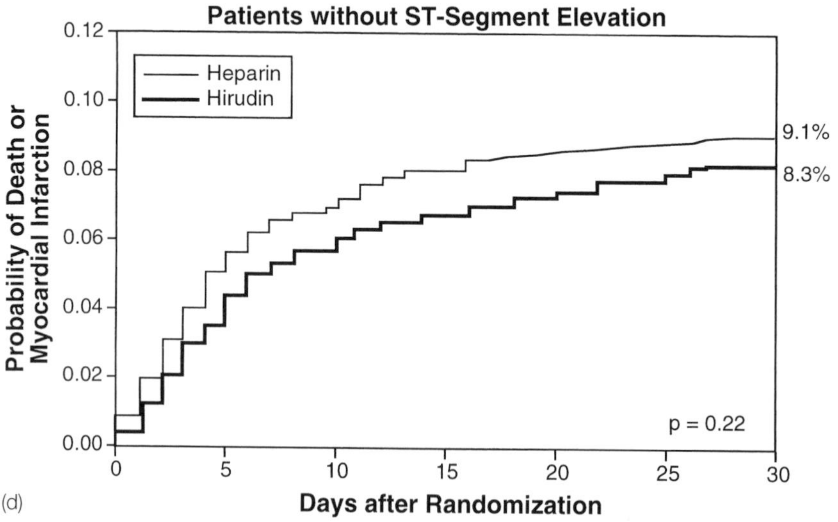

(d)

Figure 4 Continued

5.8% and a relative 40% reduction in death or reinfarction at 30 days compared with heparin (Fig. 5) (27). Similar to heparin, the efficacy of hirudin appears to largely depend on the balance between its presence in the circulation and the intrinsic coagulation state of the patient. The findings of hirudin being very effective in reducing death or myocardial infarction at

	Streptokinase + Hirudin (n=500)	Streptokinase + Heparin (n=515)	p-Value
30 Day Mortality	5.0%	7.6%	0.092
30 Day Reinfarction	4.2%	8.4%	0.007
30 Day Mortality or Reinfarction	8.6%	14.4%	0.004
	Alteplase + Hirudin (n=1151)	**Alteplase + Heparin (n=1123)**	
30 Day Mortality	6.1%	5.9%	0.84
30 Day Reinfarction	5.3%	5.9%	0.54
30 Day Mortality or Reinfarction	10.3%	10.9%	0.68

Odds Ratio and 95% CI

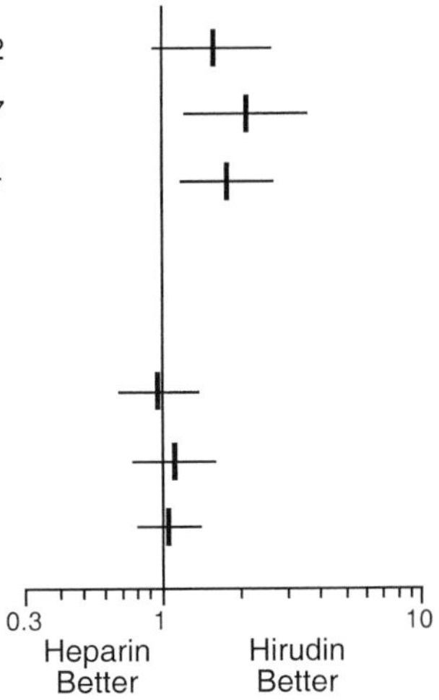

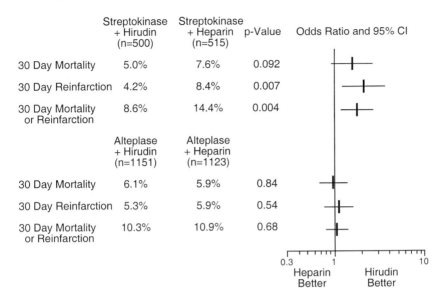

Figure 5 Unadjusted risk of death and/or reinfarction at 30 days for heparin and hirudin treatment assignments with fibrinolysis utilizing streptokinase or accelerated alteplase. (From Ref. 27.)

24 and 48 hours and not beyond the 72 hour infusion may be supported by the hemostasis substudy (unpublished data). One of many hypotheses for the lack of benefit at 30 days was rebound hypercoagulability after cessation of infusion. Though effective at suppressing thrombin activity (measured as fibrinopeptide A; FPA), hirudin did not diminish thrombin generation (measured as prothrombin fragment 1.2, F1.2). In fact, at the termination of the infusion, thrombin generation and activity returned to baseline within 24 hours for heparin and hirudin (Fig. 6). This important substudy demonstrates that hirudin is more potent than heparin at suppressing thrombin activity.

Angioplasty Substudy

The primary endpoint of death, reinfarction, and nonfatal disabling stroke at 30 days was present in 9.6% of patients randomized to primary angioplasty and 13.7% randomized to fibrinolysis, representing an absolute 4.1% and relative 30% reduction in events (20). At 6-month follow-up, the benefit from primary angioplasty was no longer significant compared with fibrinolysis (13.3% vs. 15.9%, $P = .23$).

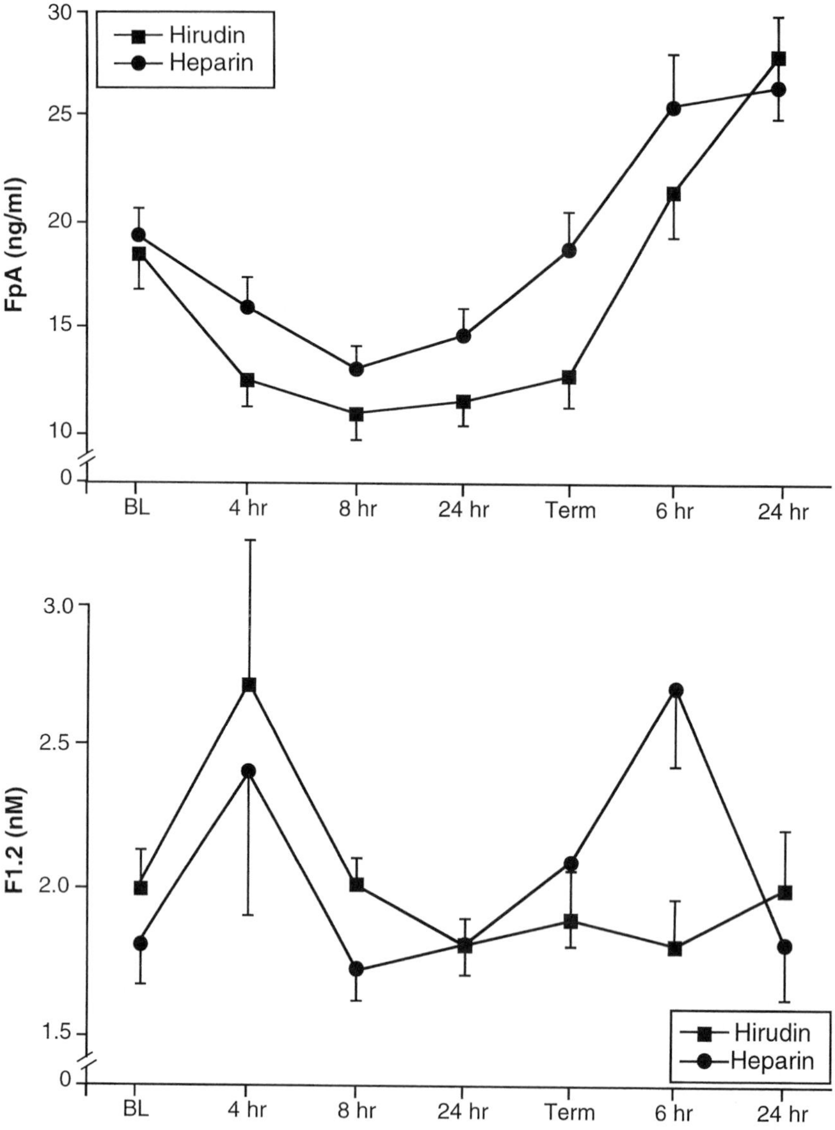

Figure 6 (Top) Thrombin activity (fibrinopeptide A) and (bottom) thrombin generation (prothrombin fragment 1.2) within the first 24 hours of treatment with heparin or hirudin.

GUSTO III TRIAL

Background and Rationale

The failure to achieve optimal reperfusion in nearly half of the treated patients with accelerated alteplase in acute myocardial infarction was an important impetus for developing new fibrinolytic agents. Agents with longer half-lives and more fibrin specificity were being introduced in an effort to achieve rapid and sustained fibrinolysis. Reteplase, a third-generation recombinant plasminogen activator, is derived by modification of the tissue-type plasminogen activator and consists of the kringle-2 and protease domains of t-PA. The deletion of kringle-1 domain yields an agent with a plasma half-life of ~15 min and lower fibrin specificity than t-PA. Reteplase is administered as double-bolus regimen of 10 units intravenously given twice 30 min apart. Reteplase was initially compared with streptokinase in a study of ~6000 patients and resulted in a statistically nonsignificant but slightly lower 35-day mortality (9.02% vs. 9.53%) (28). A subsequent angiographic study, RAPID-2, compared reteplase with accelerated alteplase. Infarct-related coronary artery patency (TIMI grade 2 or 3) and complete patency (TIMI grade 3) at 90 min after the start of fibrinolytic therapy were significantly higher in the reteplase-treated patients (83% vs. 73%, $P = .03$, and 60% vs. 45%, $P = .01$), respectively (29). Although not powered to detect differences in clinical outcome, there was a trend toward lower 35-day mortality with reteplase (4.1% vs. 8.4%, $P = .11$). The observations from INJECT and RAPID studies in part supported the open-artery hypothesis and were the foundation for the genesis of the GUSTO III trial. The GUSTO III trial was designed to test whether reteplase by achieving rapid patency of the infarct-related artery significantly reduces 30-day mortality compared with accelerated tPA regimen in a large population of patients. This trial was powered to evaluate clinical efficacy and safety of the two fibrinolytic regimens. A total of 15,059 patients with acute ST-elevation myocardial infarction were randomized to reteplase or alteplase (30). The primary endpoint of the study was 30-day mortality (Fig. 7).

Results

The primary endpoint of 30-day mortality was similar in reteplase- and alteplase-treated patients (7.47% vs. 7.24%, $P = .54$), an absolute difference of 0.23%. The combined endpoint of death or nonfatal disabling stroke were 7.89% and 7.91%, respectively (30). At 1 year, death occurred in 11.2% of patients randomized to reteplase and 11.0% to alteplase (31). Thus, the chief finding of this trial was that reteplase was not superior to alteplase; however, in terms of combined endpoints of death and stroke or bleeding complications, the results for reteplase and alteplase therapy were remarkably similar.

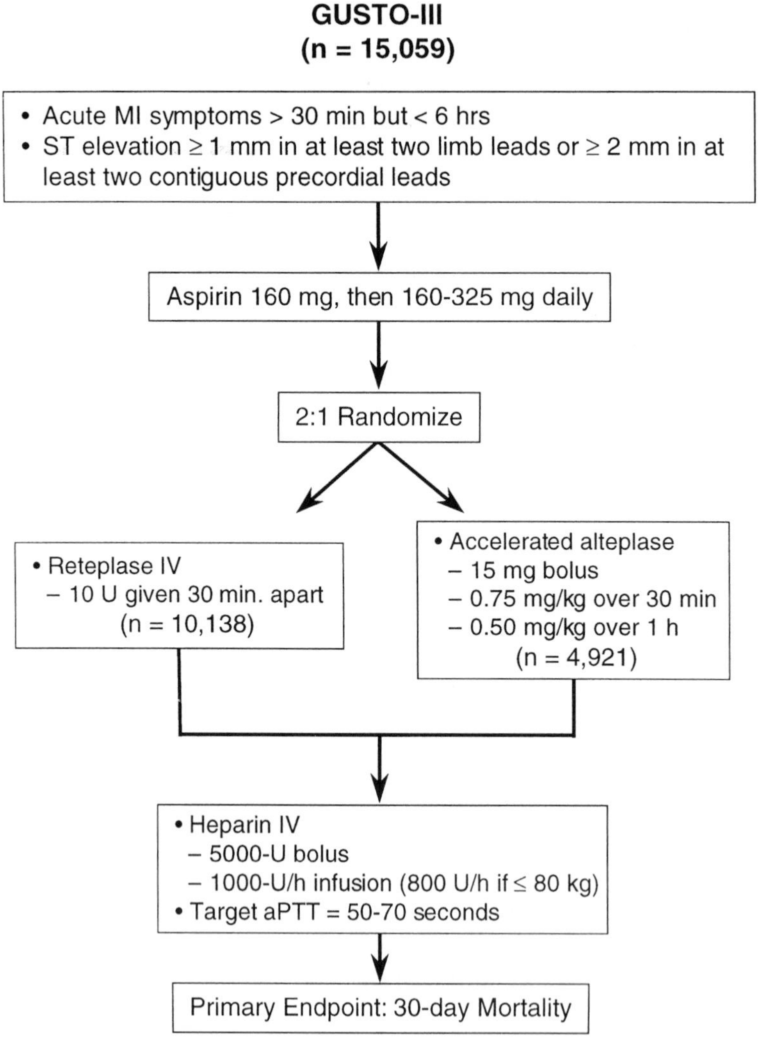
GUSTO-III
(n = 15,059)
• Acute MI symptoms > 30 min but < 6 hrs
• ST elevation ≥ 1 mm in at least two limb leads or ≥ 2 mm in at least two contiguous precordial leads
Aspirin 160 mg, then 160-325 mg daily
2:1 Randomize
• Reteplase IV
– 10 U given 30 min. apart
(n = 10,138)
• Accelerated alteplase
– 15 mg bolus
– 0.75 mg/kg over 30 min
– 0.50 mg/kg over 1 h
(n = 4,921)
• Heparin IV
– 5000-U bolus
– 1000-U/h infusion (800 U/h if ≤ 80 kg)
• Target aPTT = 50-70 seconds
Primary Endpoint: 30-day Mortality

Figure 7 Protocol algorithm of the GUSTO III trial.

The GUSTO III trial, while not designed or powered to assess equivalence between two fibrinolytic therapies, did provide important data to assess relative efficacy. Although the appropriate boundaries for definition of equivalence may be challenged, an absolute 1% difference in mortality has been the benchmark for equivalence by GUSTO I trial. The 95% confidence intervals for the 30-day mortality gap in GUSTO III range over 1.0%, so it is difficult to assert with certainty that reteplase and alteplase are equivalent or interchangeable. Nevertheless, one of the most important lessons of the GUSTO III study was that higher patency with reteplase did not translate into better survival, thus challenging the simplicity of the early open-artery hypothesis (28,29).

GUSTO IV TRIAL

Background and Rationale

In translating the results of the first three GUSTO trials, it was apparent that adjunct therapies to fibrinolysis will play an important role if clinicians were to improve upon the mortality rate of ~6% to 7%. While fibrinolytics target fibrin, heparin or hirudin targets thrombin, and aspirin thus far has been the widely used antiplatelet agent in the therapeutic armamentarium for acute MI. Release of clot-bound thrombin is a powerful activator of platelets (Fig. 8). Though aspirin has been shown to reduce mortality in the setting of evolving transmural MI, aspirin is a weak antiplatelet agent which is influenced by various agonists (32). Furthermore, chronic aspirin therapy does not fully protect against subsequent events as a substantial proportion of patients who present with acute coronary syndromes are taking aspirin (33,34). In contrast, antagonism of the glycoprotein IIb/IIIa receptor yields a more potent platelet inhibition and has been successfully utilized during percutaneous coronary interventions (35,36). Furthermore, in the setting of acute MI and stenting, IIb/IIIa inhibition with abciximab resulted in improved recovery of microvascular perfusion (potentially by inhibiting platelet interaction with leukocytes and microvasculature) and enhanced contractile function of the myocardium at risk (37). The final common pathway that leads to platelet aggregation involves externalization and functionalization of IIb/IIIa surface integrins and the binding of fibrinogen to these surface receptors on adjacent platelets (Fig. 8). Glycoprotein IIb/IIIa inhibitors bind to the fibrinogen receptor on the platelets and thereby prevent formation or progression of a platelet plug. A multifaceted approach targeting fibrin, thrombin, and platelets to achieve optimal reperfusion led to initiation of the GUSTO IV trial.

Insights from the early studies of combination strategy using low-dose fibrinolytic therapy and glycoprotein IIb/IIIa receptor antagonism were the foundation for the GUSTO IV trial. The Strategies for Patency Enhancement in the Emergency Department (SPEED) trial was a dose-finding and pilot confirmation phase of the main Phase III GUSTO IV trial which evaluated the efficacy and safety of reteplase and abciximab in treatment of acute MI. In this pilot study, 528 patients from 69 sites were treated with full-dose

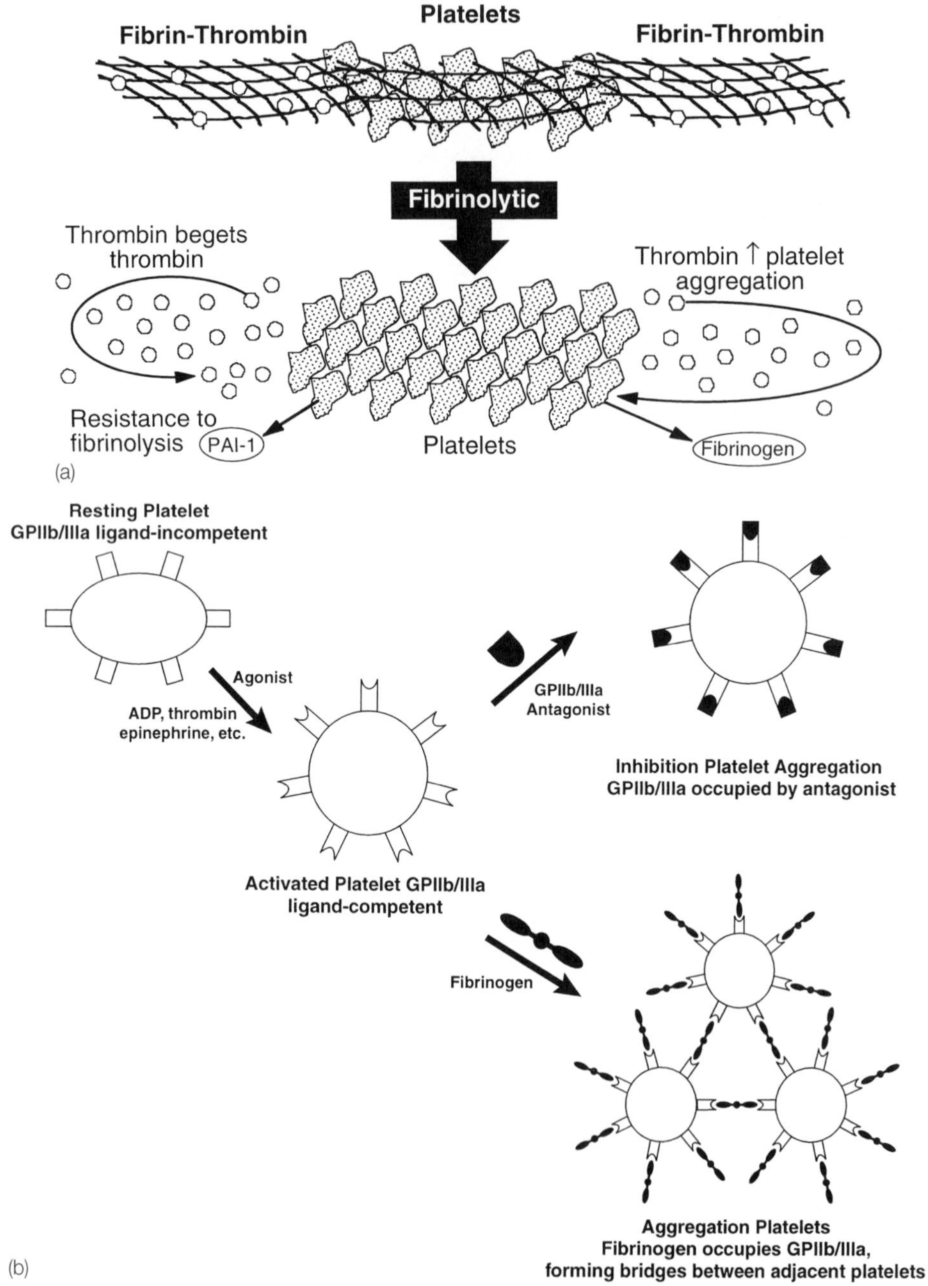

Figure 8 (a) Schematic representation of fibrinolysis leading to activation of platelets which in turn expresses thousands of glycoprotein IIb/IIIa receptors and eventually platelet aggregation. (b) Release of clot-bound thrombin further activates platelets. Glycoprotein IIb/IIIa receptor antagonism inhibits platelet aggregation.

reteplase (10 U + 10 U) alone or low-dose reteplase (5 U + 5 U) and full-dose abciximab. Patients randomized to full-dose reteplase received 70 U/kg heparin and those randomized to combination therapy either 60 U/kg or 40 U/kg. The primary endpoint was TIMI grade 3 flow at 60- to 90-min angiography. "Platelet lysis" with full-dose abciximab when given with low-dose fibrinolysis resulted in higher TIMI grade 3 flow when compared with full-dose reteplase (61% vs. 47%, $P = .05$) (38). Interestingly, abciximab alone yielded TIMI-3 flow in 27% of patients at 60- to 90-min angiography, a finding comparable to other studies (39). Furthermore, there was a trend toward reduction in mortality (3.5% vs. 5.5%), reinfarction (0.9% vs. 2.8%), and urgent revascularization (2.6% vs. 3.7%) with combination therapy compared with reteplase alone. Importantly, these ischemic endpoints were reduced without an increase in incidence of intracranial hemorrhage (0% vs. 0.9%) (38).

The cumulative effect of early infarct vessel patency, improved microvascular perfusion, and reduction in reocclusion with fibrinoplatelet lysis is being investigated in the GUSTO IV trial. The GUSTO IV AMI trial will randomize 16,600 patients with ST-elevation MI to receive either full-dose reteplase alone or half-dose reteplase plus full-dose abciximab (Fig. 9). The primary endpoint of the trial is 30-day all-cause mortality. Thus, the GUSTO IV trial is comprehensively designed to assess not only the benefit of early patency, but also the potential benefit of relieving microvascular obstruction and reducing reocclusion in evolving MI.

MORTALITY

While the linkage between coronary patency and survival was perhaps the most important message of the GUSTO I trial, it also provided considerable insights in identifying clinical variables that portend adverse outcome. In GUSTO I and IIb trials, mortality within the first 24 hours accounted for a significant proportion of death following fibrinolysis. For ST-elevation MI, in GUSTO I and GUSTO IIb trials, 39% and 36% of the total 30-day mortality occurred within the first 24 hours (40,41). In contrast, for non-ST-elevation MI, reinfarction occurred more frequently during the first 24 hours than did death. The severity of clinical presentation rather than cardiovascular risk factors appeared to predict early mortality. Hypotension and Killip class IV at presentation were the most powerful predictors of death within first 24 hours. In addition, tachycardia, anterior infarct location, diabetes mellitus, prior myocardial infarction or coronary revascularization, and female gender were also independent predictors of early mortality. Older age, tachycardia, higher Killip class, anterior infarct location, and low systolic blood pressure at presentation were strong independent predictors of 30-day mortality (42).

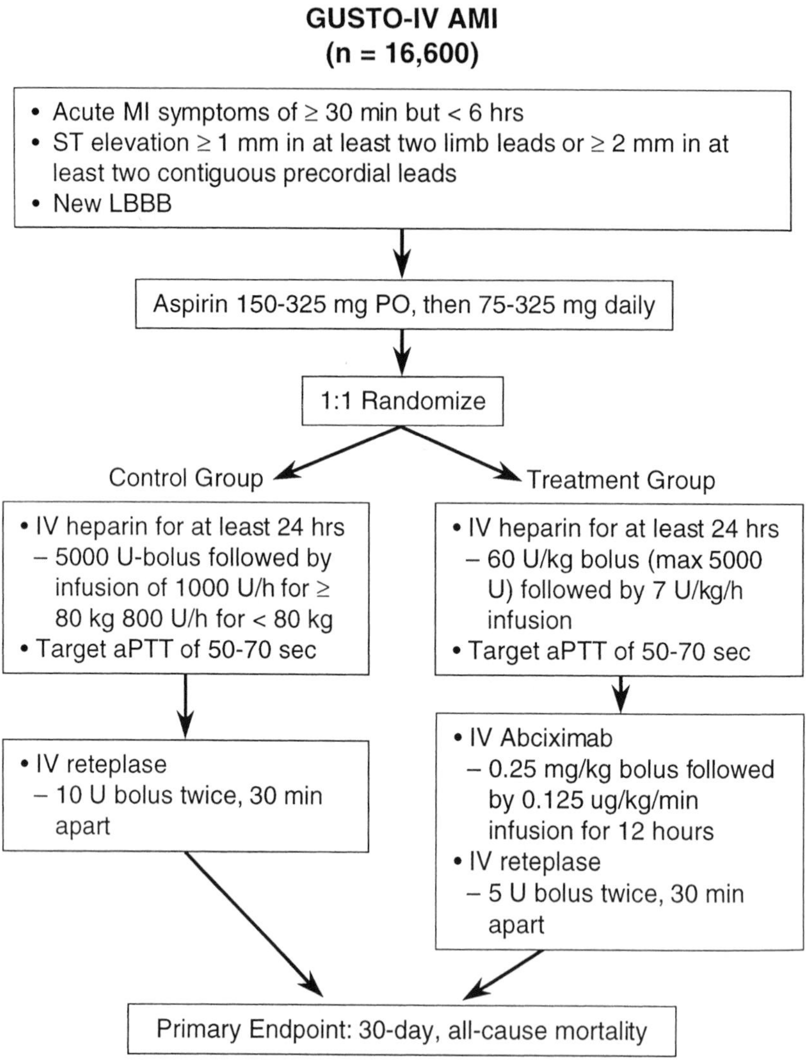

Figure 9 Protocol algorithm of the GUSTO IV AMI trial. AMI = acute myocardial infarction, IV = intravenous, LBBB = left bundle branch block.

Collectively, these variables provided 90% of the prognostic information from baseline clinical data, and the subsequent GUSTO IIb and III trials confirmed the predictive power of these baseline characteristics (18,30). Fibrinolytic agent, hypertension, time to treatment, height, weight, prior myocardial infarction, or history of cerebrovascular accident were also independent predictors of 30-day mortality. Young age, better left ventricular function, nondiabetic status, and TIMI flow grade were independent predictors of long-term survival (11).

MAJOR BLEEDING OR STROKE

In patients with ST-elevation MI receiving fibrinolysis, the incidence of moderate (requiring blood transfusion) or severe (hemodynamically significant) bleeding was 12.6% in the GUSTO I trial. The most common source of bleeding was procedure related (43). The presence of severe bleeding was associated with other undesirable outcomes such as arrhythmias, left ventricular dysfunction, or reinfarction. Advanced age, lower body weight, female gender, and African ancestry were independent predictors of moderate or severe bleeding. In GUSTO IIb and III trials, moderate or severe bleeding was present in 9.5% and 8%, respectively.

Intracranial hemorrhage (ICH) occurred in 0.65%, 0.60%, and 0.90% of patients in GUSTO I, IIb, and III trials, respectively. The willingness for clinicians to treat patients of more advanced age may explain in part the higher incidence of ICH in the latter study. In the GUSTO IIb study, moderate bleeding and intracranial hemorrhage occurred more frequently with hirudin than with heparin (8.8% vs. 7.7%, and 0.20% vs. 0.02%, respectively). In the angioplasty substudy, intracranial hemorrhage occurred in 1.4% of patients receiving fibrinolysis compared with 0% for those undergoing primary angioplasty, suggesting angioplasty to be a preferable modality for reperfusion in high-risk patients. Prior to GUSTO-I study, advanced age, low body weight, hypertension, and alteplase therapy were reported to predict risk of ICH following fibrinolysis (44). In the GUSTO I trial, 268 patients had intracranial hemorrhage (45). The median time to ICH following fibrinolysis was 10 hours. Of all strokes, 41% were fatal, 31% were disabling, and 24% were nondisabling, with no significant treatment-related differences. Intracranial hemorrhage resulted in higher mortality (60% vs. 17%) and significant disability (25% vs. 40%) compared with nonhemorrhagic stroke. Patients with moderate or severe residual deficits showed a significant decrease in quality of life. Older age, lower body weight, and prior cerebrovascular disease were strong predictors of ICH. Other, less powerful predictors were high diastolic blood pressure, accelerated alteplase or combination alteplase-streptokinase therapy, and hypertension. A systematic review of tomograhic images of patients with ICH revealed a spectrum of findings with majority of being large volumes, solitary, and supratentorial (46). In particular, higher hemorrhagic volume was present in the elderly, subdural hematomas in those with antecedent trauma or syncope, and deep intraparenchymal hemorrhage in patients with hypertension. In a multivariate analysis, independent predictors of mortality were Glasgow Coma Scale score, time from fibrinolysis to intracranial hemorrhage, volume of intracranial hemorrhage, and the various baseline clinical predictors of mortality in the overall GUSTO I trial ($P = .001$) (47). While treatment is limited for this highly lethal complication of fibrinolysis, neurosurgical evacuation should be considered in eligible patients. In GUSTO I, 46 patients underwent neurosurgical evacuation and 222 patients did not. Evacuation was associated with a significantly higher 30-day survival (65% vs. 35%) and a trend toward improved functional status (20% vs. 12%) (48).

Nonhemorrhagic stroke occurred in 0.6% of patients in the GUSTO I trial. Of the 247 patients, 17% died and another 40% were disabled at 30-day follow-up (49). In descending order of priority, advanced age, tachycardia, history of stroke or transient ischemic attack, diabetes, prior angina, and hypertension were independent predictors of ischemic stroke. A nomogram based on clinical characteristics exists to predict the risk of ischemic stroke for more aggressive diagnostic and therapeutic management (49).

CLINICAL VARIABLES AND OUTCOMES

The main results of the GUSTO trials impress upon the primacy of early coronary patency and importance of adjunct therapies to fibrinolysis. However, due to the large population of patients and use of sophisticated statistical analysis, the GUSTO trials provide substrate to study numerous clinical variables and its predictive capacity for adverse clinical outcome. Furthermore, since the inception of the original GUSTO trial, there have been noticeable changes in the patient population and clinical outcomes (Table 1).

Age

Collectively, in all the GUSTO trials, advanced age has been the most important predictor of adverse clinical outcomes. Elderly patients (age >75 years) accounted for 10.5% of the total population in GUSTO I and 13.6% in GUSTO III (30). In these trials, 30-day mortality was lower (~5%) in patients ≤75 years of age and higher (~20%) in >75 (Fig. 10) (6,30). At 1 year, mortality among the elderly was 27% in GUSTO I and 29% in GUSTO III (31). In GUSTO I, elderly patients had a higher incidence of hemorrhagic stroke with alteplase (2.1% vs. 1.2%) and lower mortality (4.4% vs. 5.5%)

Table 1 Changes in Demographics and Major Outcomes in the GUSTO Trials

Characteristic	GUSTO I	GUSTO II[a]	GUSTO III
Years of the trial	1990–1993	1993–1995	1995–1997
No. of patients	41,021	3053	15,059
Median age (yr)	62 (52, 70)[b]	62.5 (53, 71)	63 (53, 71)
Age >75 years (%)	10.5	11.8	13.6
Female sex (%)	25.2	22.4	27.4
Median systolic blood pressure (mm Hg)	130 (112, 144)	130 (115, 148)	135 (119, 150)
Median interval between onset of symptoms and treatment (hr)	2.7 (1.9, 3.9)	2.8 (1.8, 4.2)	2.7 (1.8, 3.8)
Anterior infarction (%)	39.1	40.9	47.5
Median length of hospitalization (days)	9 (7, 13)	9 (6, 13)	7 (5, 12)
30-day mortality (%)	7.0	6.2	7.4
All strokes (%)	1.4	1.2	1.7
Hemorrhagic strokes (%)	0.6	0.6	0.9

[a]Only data on patients treated with thrombolytic agents are given.
[b]Values in parentheses are the 25th and 75th percentiles.

compared with streptokinase. Furthermore, the elderly may respond differently compared with younger patients even with adequate restoration of flow in the infarct-related artery. The GUSTO I angiographic substudy demonstrated increased mortality, reduced left ventricular ejection fraction, and increased end-systolic volume index at 5- to 7-day follow-up in the elderly patients despite patency of infarct-related artery at 90-min angiography. Although the causes may be multifactorial, a more rapid progression of ischemic injury or a blunted postreperfusion recovery appears to contribute to the poorer outcomes in the elderly patients (50). The GUSTO IIb study compared outcomes in the elderly patients for primary angioplasty versus fibrinolysis. While outcomes were better with angioplasty than with alteplase, the risk of death increased with age irrespective of treatment (Fig. 11) (51). After adjusting for baseline characteristics, each incremental 10-year increase in age elevated the risk of death or myocardial infarction by 1.32% ($P = .02$).

Infarct Location

Patients with anterior myocardial infarction are a high-risk subgroup often presenting with cardiogenic shock and have a higher 24-hour and 30-day mortality (40,42). In the GUSTO I and III trials, 30-day mortality was nearly

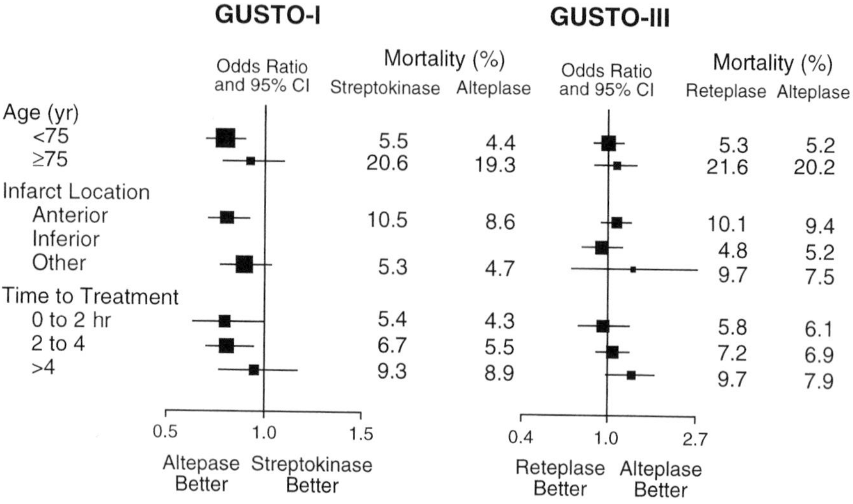

Figure 10 Hazard ratio and confidence intervals for 30-day mortality according to age, infarct location, and time to treatment. The GUSTO I compared alteplase to streptokinase. The GUSTO III trial compared alteplase to reteplase. (From Refs. 6 and 30.)

twice in patients with anterior MI compared with other MI location (Fig. 10) (6,30). While in the GUSTO I trial patients with anterior MI derived a greater benefit from accelerated alteplase therapy than streptokinase (29% relative reduction in 30-day mortality), outcomes were similar for reteplase and alteplase in GUSTO III. Aside from anterior MI, patients presenting with inferior MI but with precordial ST-segment depression (V1 to V3) appear to be at increased risk of death. In GUSTO I, patients with inferior MI and precordial ST depression on electrocardiogram had significantly higher 30-day (4.7% vs. 3.2%) and 1-year (5.0% vs. 3.4%) mortality, larger infarct size, and higher post-MI complications (congestive heart failure, cardiogenic shock, or arrhythmias) than patients without precordial ST depression (52). While the magnitude of inferior ST elevation did not correlate with the degree of precordial ST depression, the prognostic significance of precordial ST depression was superior than the magnitude of inferior ST elevation. Interestingly, the presence of ST depression in precordial leads V4 to V6 in the setting of acute inferior MI was associated with higher incidence of multivessel coronary artery disease and lower left ventricular ejection fraction compared with patients having no precordial ST depression or those with ST depression in leads V1 to V3 (53). Importantly, the presence of precordial ST depression in patients with inferior MI was associated with

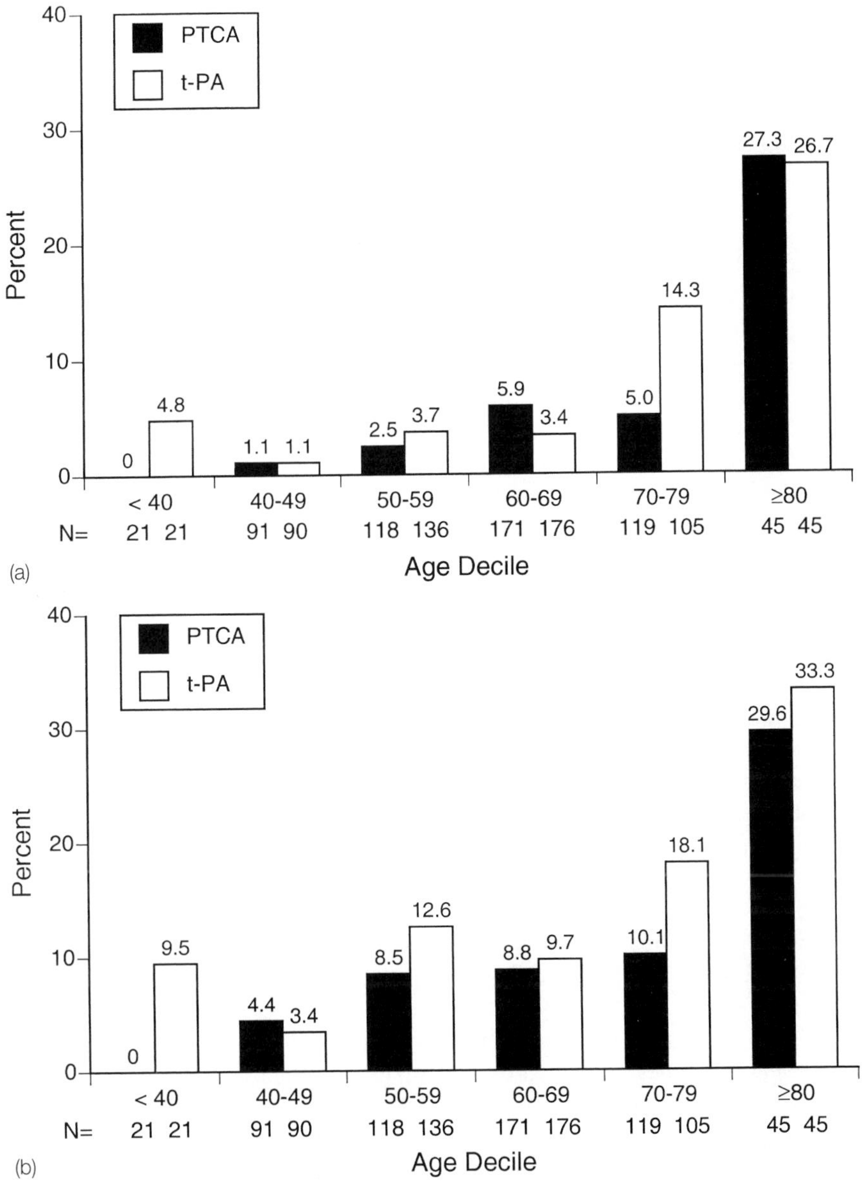

Figure 11 Histogram of 30-day mortality (a) and 30-day mortality and/or reinfarction (b) according to treatment (angioplasty vs. fibrinolysis) and age. The risk of death increased with age irrespective of treatment assignment. (From Ref. 51.)

larger infarction, reduced left ventricular function, and higher incidence of circumflex artery involvement, suggesting that this electrocardiographic pattern represents a larger inferior MI with likely extension to the posterolateral wall. Thus, patients with anterior MI or inferior MI with precordial ST depression represent a special subgroup that requires close observation and aggressive management.

Time to Treatment

Timely reperfusion remains one of the most important predictors of outcomes with early restoration of coronary patency resulting in decreased infarct size and improved left ventricular function. Initially in GUSTO I and then in GUSTO III trial, earlier fibrinolysis resulted in lower 30-day mortality (Fig. 10) (6,30). While the mortality was the lowest during the first hour of symptom onset, very few patients (<3%) received fibrinolysis during this "golden" hour in the GUSTO I trial (54). The mortality rate increased from 5.5% in the initial 2 hours from symptom onset to 9.0% when fibrinolysis was administered beyond 4 hours of symptom onset. Considerable in-hospital delays were noted in attaining electrocardiographic readings, in deciding the course of therapy, and, most of all, in the time to infuse the drug. As time to treatment increased, the incidence of recurrent ischemia or reinfarction decreased, but the rates of cardiogenic shock, heart failure, and stroke increased. Elderly, female, diabetic, and hypertensive patients tended to have longer delays in presentation and treatment. Treatment delays in GUSTO I varied according to regions. In particular, while greater proportion of patients reached hospital within 2 hours of symptom onset in Canada, administration delays were longer in Canada than in other enrolling sites in GUSTO I (55). Treatment delays in these patients resulted in higher nonfatal cardiac events such as shock, ventricular tachycardia/fibrillation, or asystole. Overall, time to treatment was a significant predictor of mortality with each additional hour of delay resulting in approximately 0.5% increase in 30-day mortality (42).

The GUSTO IIb trial contributed to our understanding of time to treatment and outcomes with regards to primary angioplasty and non ST-elevation myocardial infarction. In this study, reduction in in-hospital delays (door-to-balloon inflation time) resulted in improved survival. The 30-day mortality of patients who underwent primary angioplasty within the first 60 min from enrollment was 1% compared with 6.4% for those beyond 90 min (56). The mortality rate of patients assigned to angioplasty who never underwent the procedure was 14.1% ($P = .001$). Logistic regression analysis revealed that the time from enrollment to first balloon inflation was a significant predictor of mortality within 30 days. After adjustment for differences in baseline characteristics, the probability of death increased 1.6 times ($P = .008$) for each 15-min increase in time interval. In comparison to fibrinolysis, primary angioplasty appeared to be less advantageous in patients presenting early after symptom onset. In patients presenting within 4 hours from symptom onset (total ischemia time) and being randomized to direct angioplasty (time to treatment), 30-day mortality was similar between angioplasty and fibrinolysis (6.0% vs. 5.9%). However, patients presenting beyond 4 hours of symptom onset had marked reduction in mortality with primary angioplasty compared to fibrinolysis (5.6% vs. 11.3%) (57). The GUSTO IIb trial, by including patients with unstable angina and non-ST-elevation MI, provided the largest series to date on outcomes of patients treated aggressively early with cardiac catheterization with or without revascularization versus conservative therapy. The early aggressive strategy resulted in a significant reduction in 30-day (2.2% vs. 5.9%) and 1-year (5.0% vs. 13.3%) mortality and remained significant even after adjusting for baseline differences in clinical variables ($P < .001$) (58).

Gender

In GUSTO I, III, and IV pilot trials, women accounted for 25%, 27%, and 25% of the total population. In GUSTO IIb, women accounted for 24% of all ST-elevation MI and 33% of non-ST-elevation MI patients (18). In general, women were significantly older than men (66 vs. 59 years of age) and had longer time to treatment (1.2 vs. 1.0 hours) (59). After adjusting for age, women more often had history of diabetes, hypertension, and smoking than men. Nonfatal complications including cardiogenic shock, congestive heart failure, serious bleeding, and reinfarction were significantly higher in women than in men ($P < .001$). Unadjusted (11.3% vs. 5.5%) and age-adjusted (5.9% vs. 4.4%) 30-day mortality was higher among women than men ($P < .001$). Furthermore, women had nearly twice as many total strokes as men (2.1% vs. 1.2%) secondary to their older age at presentation; however, age-adjusted risk of hemorrhagic stroke was similar in men and women. While alteplase therapy resulted in higher incidence of stroke in women than streptokinase, this was offset by a greater relative reduction in mortality. At 1 year, age-adjusted mortality was similar in men and women (1.06, 95% CI 0.97 to 1.15) (60). Thus, it appears overall that women are a higher risk group, but the majority of the adverse events seem to occur early within the first 30 days and no significant gender difference between 30 days and 1 year. In GUSTO I, fibrinolytic therapy was associated with a need for blood transfusion in 25% of all menstruating women (12 patients) as a result of increased vaginal bleeding (61). None of these women had severe bleeding and none died. Thus, insights from this small cohort of select patients suggest that fibrinolytic therapy in menstruating women should generally not be withheld in management of acute MI.

Diabetes Mellitus

Although fibrinolysis has substantially improved mortality in acute ST-elevation MI, diabetes mellitus remains an independent predictor for increased adverse outcomes. In the GUSTO trials, diabetes was present in 15% to 20% of the total population. Diabetic patients tended to be older, more likely to be female, to present with anterior MI, to have multivessel coronary artery disease, to have delay (~15 min on average) in fibrinolysis, and to have coexisting hypertension compared with nondiabetics (62). Mortality at 30 days was higher among diabetic patients compared with nondiabetics (10.5% vs. 6.2%, $P < .001$). In particular, insulin-treated diabetics did worse than non-insulin-treated diabetics (12.5% vs. 9.7%, $P < .001$). Mortality was lowest among diabetics receiving accelerated t-PA. Congestive heart failure, cardiogenic shock, stroke, and arrhythmias were more common among diabetic patients. The proportion of patients undergoing revascularization was similar between patients with and without diabetes, although diabetic patients were more likely to undergo coronary artery bypass graft surgery (10.4% vs. 8.3%).

While mortality was similar in diabetics and nondiabetics undergoing bypass surgery, diabetics undergoing percutaneous angioplasty shortly after myocardial infarction had higher mortality than nondiabetics (13.2% vs. 4.5%). Diabetes remained an independent predictor for mortality at 1-year follow-up (14.5% vs. 8.9%, $P < .001$) (Fig. 12). In the GUSTO I angiographic substudy, congestive heart failure and mortality were higher in diabetics than nondiabetics ($P < .001$) even though coronary patency and left ventricular function were similar between diabetics and nondiabetics ($P = .70$) (63). Diabetic patients had less compensatory hyperkinesia in the noninfarct zone. Diabetes remained an independent determinant of 30-day and 1-year mortality after correction for differences in baseline clinical and angiographic variables. While bleeding remains a concern in patients with diabetic retinopathy, ocular hemorrhage occurred rarely (0.03%) in these patients (64). Thus, diabetic retinopathy should not be a contraindication in consideration for fibrinolysis.

Hypertension

Hypertension was present in 38% to 48% of patients in the GUSTO trials. In GUSTO I, patients with history of hypertension represented a higher-risk group as these patients tended to be older, more often female or diabetic, having history of prior infarction, and higher Killip class at presentation. A

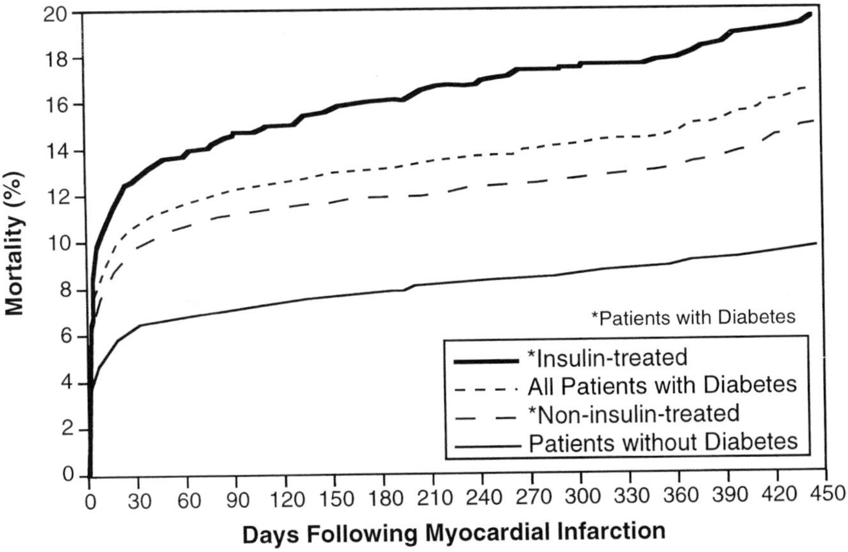

Figure 12 Kaplan-Meier estimates of mortality according to diabetic status. Diabetic patients are further categorized based on insulin treatment. (From Ref. 62.)

history of hypertension or elevated systolic blood pressure on admission (≥175 mm Hg) were associated with increased bleeding as well as stroke, including intracranial hemorrhage (65). After adjusting for baseline clinical variables, a history of hypertension, but not elevated systolic blood pressure at presentation, was an independent predictor of mortality and hemorrhagic stroke. However, elevated systolic blood pressure at entry in those receiving accelerated alteplase therapy was associated with a lower rate of death at 30 days (4.3% vs. 7.8%, $P = .04$) and a lower rate of death or disabling stroke (4.9% vs. 8.9%, $P = .03$) compared to patients receiving streptokinase. Results from the GUSTO I trial suggest that hypertensive patients with low risk for death from cardiac causes (no prior infarction or lower Killip class), the risk-to-benefit ratio with thrombolysis is about unity, with about 13 lives saved per 1000 persons treated at the risk of about 13 intracranial hemorrhages. In contrast to elevated systolic blood pressure, low systolic blood pressure (≤100 mm Hg) was associated with increased 30-day mortality. Death or nonfatal stroke occurred more frequently in patients with low systolic blood pressure compared with elevated pressure (18.7% vs. 8.8%). Whether primary angioplasty yields a marked benefit toward death or hemorrhagic stroke compared to fibrinolysis for ST-elevation MI requires further study.

Prior Myocardial Infarction

Patients with prior myocardial infarction accounted for 16%, 17%, and 18.4% of the entire cohort in the GUSTO I, IIb, and III trials. Patients with prior infarction tended to be older in age, more often males, having multivessel coronary artery disease, and overall lower left ventricular ejection fraction compared to patients with first MI. While patients with prior myocardial infarction presented to the hospital earlier than those having their first event, institution of fibrinolytic therapy was delayed (66). Prior myocardial infarction was associated with higher 30-day (11.7% vs. 5.9%) and 1-year (17.3% vs. 8.2%) mortality, and remained an independent predictor of death after adjusting for differences in baseline clinical variables (P = .001). Despite similar infarct vessel patency rates, accelerated alteplase use resulted in a significantly lower 30-day (10.4% vs. 12.2%) and 1-year (15.9% vs. 17.8%) mortality when compared with streptokinase. Thus, the lesson from GUSTO I trial is that patients with prior myocardial infarction should be educated to seek medical help early if they develop symptoms suggestive of acute myocardial infarction, and upon hospital arrival they should be promptly triaged to receive reperfusion therapy with accelerated alteplase.

Prior Coronary Revascularization

Prior coronary revascularization, while intuitively would appear to confer protective effect from subsequent events, is in reality a marker for future adverse events. Interestingly, prior percutaneous and surgical coronary revascularization patients differ in baseline clinical characteristics and clinical outcomes. Patients with prior bypass surgery tended to be older, had history of prior myocardial infarction, more often presented with pulmonary edema or cardiogenic shock, and often had delay in treatment. In contrast, patients with previous angioplasty tended to be younger, to present sooner after symptom onset, and to have lower heart rate at presentation and fewer anterior myocardial infarctions than those without prior angioplasty.

Unadjusted 30-day mortality was significantly higher in patients who had prior coronary bypass surgery compared to those who did not (10.7% vs. 6.7%, $P < .001$) (42). Angiographically, patients with prior bypass surgery had more severe coronary stenoses and higher rates of occluded vessels with graft failure, accounting for nearly half of all infarctions. Alteplase use resulted in lower mortality than streptokinase. In contrast, unadjusted 30-day mortality was significantly lower in patients with prior angioplasty compared to those without prior angioplasty (5.6% vs. 7.0%, P = .03) (67). Recurrent ischemia and reinfarction occurred more frequently in patients who had prior angioplasty, as did bypass surgery (12.2% vs. 8.5%) and repeat angioplasty (34.5% vs. 21.4%). The risk of death was similar for alteplase and streptokinase. After adjusting for differences in baseline characteristics, prior angioplasty or bypass surgery remained an independent predictor of 30-day mortality.

Smoking

In contrast to patients with history of diabetes, hypertension, or prior myocardial infarction, patients with smoking history had a lower 30-day mortality than nonsmokers (4.0% vs. 10.3%, $P < .001$) (68). One potential explanation may be that smokers tended to be younger patients, more often male, and with higher left ventricular ejection fraction following fibrinolysis compared with nonsmokers. Furthermore, smokers tended to have lower reocclusion rates than nonsmokers. After adjusting for differences in baseline clinical and angiographic variables, 30-day mortality rates were similar among smokers and nonsmokers. In GUSTO IIb angioplasty substudy, smokers who underwent primary angioplasty had higher procedural success rates ($P = .02$), lower percent stenosis of the culprit lesion before reperfusion ($P = .03$), and, less commonly, an occluded infarct-related artery ($P = .05$) compared with nonsmokers (69). Primary angioplasty was associated with a lower 30-day mortality than alteplase for current smokers, with a similar trend for former smokers and nonsmokers. Thus, primary angioplasty yielded better outcome compared to alteplase in smokers and nonsmokers.

Cardiogenic Shock

Cardiogenic shock in patients with acute myocardial infarction, whether present upon arrival to the hospital or developing during index hospitalization, presents a therapeutic challenge for clinicians. In GUSTO I, cardiogenic shock occurred in 7.2% of patients (70). Of these, 11% had shock on arrival and 89% developed this feared complication after hospital admission, which was associated with a 57% and 55% 30-day mortality. These mortality rates were significantly higher than the 3% mortality in patients without shock ($P < .001$). While shock developed less frequently in patients treated with alteplase, the 30-day mortality was lower with streptokinase than with alteplase, suggesting that alteplase may require adequate coronary perfusion to be fully effective. However, mortality was similar in patients with cardiogenic shock treated with reteplase compared with alteplase ($P = .59$) despite higher coronary patency with reteplase (71).

Interestingly, 30-day mortality was significantly lower if aggressive strategy of early angiography and if indicated revascularization was performed in patients who developed cardiogenic shock ($P < .001$) (72). In general, revascularization within 30 days for myocardial infarction complicated by shock was associated with reduced 1-year mortality ($P = .007$) (73). Adjusted 30-day and 1-year mortality was lower in patients treated in the United States than other countries ($P < .001$) (74). This difference in mortality may be due to the greater use of invasive diagnostic and therapeutic interventions in the United States. Placement of intra-aortic balloon counterpulsation (IABP) early after fibrinolysis in patients with cardiogenic shock resulted in increased risk of bleeding, but was also associated with lower 30-day and 1-year mortality (75). An algorithm has been developed using clinical and hemodynamic data to prognosticate risk for patients with cardiogenic shock (76). In this analysis, older age, prior myocardial infarction, oliguria, and altered sensorium were independent predictors of 30-day mortality.

Arrhythmias

Atrial fibrillation, though not very common in the setting of acute MI, is a predictor of adverse clinical outcome. Atrial fibrillation was present in 2.5% of patients presenting with acute myocardial infarction and in 7.9% of patients during hospitalization (77). Patients with atrial fibrillation were older and had higher peak creatine kinase levels, higher Killip class, increased heart rate, and multivessel coronary artery disease. In-hospital stroke, mainly ischemic stroke, occurred more frequently in patients with atrial fibrillation (3.1% vs. 1.3%, $P < .001$). Unadjusted 30-day (14.3% vs. 6.2%, $P < .001$) and 1-year (21.5% vs. 8.6%, $P < .001$) mortality rates were higher in patients with atrial fibrillation than in those without. After adjusting for baseline characteristics, atrial fibrillation after enrollment but not at baseline was a predictor of 30-day mortality.

Sustained ventricular tachycardia or fibrillation occurs in up to 20% of patients with acute myocardial infarction and has been associated with a poor prognosis. In GUSTO I, 10.2% of patients had sustained ventricular tachycardia, fibrillation, or both. Advanced age, hypertension, prior myocardial infarction, higher Killip class, anterior infarct location, and diminished left ventricular ejection fraction were associated with a higher risk of sustained ventricular tachycardia and fibrillation. These ventricular dysrhythmias were associated with higher in-hospital, 30-day, and 1-year mortality (78). Mortality was higher with early or late occurrence of these dysrhythmias, as well as with both sustained ventricular tachycardia and fibrillation compared to tachycardia or fibrillation alone ($P < .001$).

Prophylactic lidocaine has been used to treat ventricular arrhythmias in the setting of acute MI; however, its use remains controversial. In GUSTO I and IIb, 16% and 3.5% of patients, respectively, received prophylactic lidocaine. Though not statistically significant, prophylactic lidocaine use was associated with lower in-hospital and 30-day mortality (79). After adjusting for differences in baseline characteristics, the risk of death was similar with or without prophylactic lidocaine use.

Recurrent Ischemia or Reinfarction

Ischemic symptoms recur often following fibrinolysis due to its prothrombotic properties. In GUSTO I, 20% of patients had recurrent ischemia assessed by angina, electrocardiographic changes, or hemodynamic instability. Patients with reischemia were more often females, had more cardiovascular risk factors, and less often received intravenous heparin. Reinfarction and 30-day mortality were significantly higher in patients with recurrent ischemia ($P < .001$) (80). Importantly, mortality markedly increased when angina was associated with hemodynamic changes compared to angina alone (29.1% vs. 5.4%).

In GUSTO IIb, recurrent ischemia was more common in patients without ST elevation than with ST elevation on electrocardiogram (35% vs. 23%, $P < .001$) (81). In contrast, 30-day mortality was higher in patients with ST-elevation MI (6.1% vs. 3.8%, $P < .001$); however, at 1 year, no difference in mortality was noted in patients with or without ST elevation. Non ST-elevation MI was associated with higher incidence of reinfarction at 6-month follow-up (9.8% vs. 6.2%). In GUSTO I, reinfarction occurred in 11% of patients who developed cardiogenic shock, compared with 3% of patients without shock (70).

THE FUTURE

In the GUSTO trials performed thus far, the common theme has been early patency of infarct-related artery with stacking of adjunct medical therapies which targeted fibrin, thrombin, and platelets. While the original GUSTO trial validated the open-artery hypothesis, the third GUSTO trial challenged it with equivalence in clinical outcomes with reteplase despite higher coronary patency rates. The present, GUSTO IV, pilot study brings about the highest complete coronary patency rates achieved thus far with the use of full-dose glycoprotein IIb/IIIa receptor antagonism along with reduced-dose fibrinolytic agent. While there is optimism for reduction in hemorrhagic stroke with this strategy, whether it will significantly reduce mortality remains to be seen. The future of therapeutic armamentarium for acute myocardial infarction includes intravenous and oral glycoprotein IIb/IIIa receptor antagonists, low-molecular-weight heparins or other improved anticoagulants, and potentially anti-inflammatory agents. In addition, subsequent GUSTO trials may include intravenous and/or oral anti-inflammatory agents as adjunct therapy to reduce subsequent ischemic complications and to halt progression of atherosclerosis.

Fortunately, the international collaboration of the GUSTO trials has brought us a wealth of new insights in the management of acute coronary syndromes. The continued alliance between clinicians and industry in inventing and implementing new pharmacologic and mechanical strategies for acute reperfusion therapy has tremendous potential not only to improve long-term survival but also to enhance quality of life. The lessons learned thus far and those to come will hopefully positively impact clinical practices throughout the world.

REFERENCES

1. GISSI-2 Investigators. GISSI-2: a factorial randomised trial of alteplase versus streptokinase and heparin versus no heparin among 12,490 patients with acute myocardial infarction. Lancet 1990;336:65–71.
2. ISIS-3 Collaborative Group. ISIS-3: a randomised comparison of streptokinase vs tissue plasminogen activator vs anistreplase and of aspirin plus heparin vs aspirin alone among 41,299 cases of suspected acute myocardial infarction. Lancet 1992;339:753–770.
3. Granger CB, Califf RM, Topol EJ. Thrombolytic therapy for acute myocardial infarction. A review. Drugs 1992;44:293–325.
4. Neuhaus KL, von Essen R, Tebbe U, Vogt A, Roth M, Riess M, Niederer W, Forycki F, Wirtzfeld A, Maeurer W. Improved thrombolysis in acute myocardial infarction with front-loaded administration of alteplase: results of the rt-PA-APSAC patency study (TAPS). J Am Coll Cardiol 1992;19:885–891.
5. Bleich SD, Nichols TC, Schumacher RR, Cooke DH, Tate DA, Teichman SL. Effect of heparin on coronary arterial patency after thrombolysis with tissue plasminogen activator in acute myocardial infarction. Am J Cardiol 1990;66: 1412–1417.
6. GUSTO Investigators. An international randomized trial comparing four thrombolytic strategies for acute myocardial infarction. N Engl J Med 1993;329: 673–682.
7. GUSTO Angiographic Investigators. The effects of tissue plasminogen activator, streptokinase, or both on coronary-artery patency, ventricular function, and survival after acute myocardial infarction. N Engl J Med 1993;329:1615–1622.
8. Califf RM, White HD, Van de Werf F, Sadowski Z, Armstrong PW, Vahanian A, Simoons ML, Simes RJ, Lee KL, Topol EJ. One-year results from the Global Utilization of Streptokinase and TPA for Occluded Coronary Arteries (GUSTO-I) trial. Circulation 1996;94:1233–1238.
9. Simes RJ, Topol EJ, Holmes DR Jr, White HD, Rutsch WR, Vahanian A, Simoons ML, Morris D, Betriu A, Califf RM. Link between the angiographic substudy and mortality outcomes in a large randomized trial of myocardial

reperfusion. Importance of early and complete infarct artery reperfusion. GUSTO-I Investigators. Circulation 1995;91:1923–1928.
10. Migrino RQ, Young JB, Ellis SG, White HD, Lundergan CF, Miller DP, Granger CB, Ross AM, Califf RM, Topol EJ. End-systolic volume index at 90 to 180 minutes into reperfusion therapy for acute myocardial infarction is a strong predictor of early and late mortality. The Global Utilization of Streptokinase and t-PA for Occluded Coronary Arteries (GUSTO)-I Angiographic Investigators. Circulation 1997;96:116–121.
11. Ross AM, Coyne KS, Moreyra E, Reiner JS, Greenhouse SW, Walker PL, Simoons ML, Draoui YC, Califf RM, Topol EJ, Van de Werf F, Lundergan CF. Extended mortality benefit of early postinfarction reperfusion. GUSTO-I Angiographic Investigators. Circulation 1998;97:1549–1556.
12. Puma JA, Sketch MH Jr, Thompson TD, Simes RJ, Morris DC, White HD, Topol EJ, Califf RM. Support for the open-artery hypothesis in survivors of acute myocardial infarction: analysis of 11,228 patients treated with thrombolytic therapy. Am J Cardiol 1999;83:482–487.
13. Topol EJ. Validation of the early open infarct vessel hypothesis. Am J Cardiol 1993;72:40G–45G.
14. Granger CB, Becker R, Tracy RP, Califf RM, Topol EJ, Pieper KS, Ross AM, Roth S, Lambrew C, Bovill EG. Thrombin generation, inhibition and clinical outcomes in patients with acute myocardial infarction treated with thrombolytic therapy and heparin: results from the GUSTO-I Trial. GUSTO-I Hemostasis Substudy Group. J Am Coll Cardiol 1998;31:497–505.
15. Cannon CP, McCabe CH, Henry TD, Schweiger MJ, Gibson RS, Mueller HS, Becker RC, Kleiman NS, Haugland JM, Anderson JL. A pilot trial of recombinant desulfatohirudin compared with heparin in conjunction with tissue-type plasminogen activator and aspirin for acute myocardial infarction: results of the Thrombolysis in Myocardial Infarction (TIMI) 5 trial. J Am Coll Cardiol 1994;23:993–1003.
16. Topol EJ, Fuster V, Harrington RA, Califf RM, Kleiman NS, Kereiakes DJ, Cohen M, Chapekis A, Gold HK, Tannenbaum MA. Recombinant hirudin for unstable angina pectoris. A multicenter, randomized angiographic trial. Circulation 1994;89:1557–1566.
17. GUSTO-IIa Investigators. Randomized trial of intravenous heparin versus recombinant hirudin for acute coronary syndromes. Circulation 1994;90:1631–1637.
18. GUSTO-IIb Investigators. A comparison of recombinant hirudin with heparin for the treatment of acute coronary syndromes. N Engl J Med 1996;335:775–782.
19. Granger CB, Hirsch J, Califf RM, Col J, White HD, Betriu A, Woodlief LH, Lee KL, Bovill EG, Simes RJ, Topol EJ. Activated partial thromboplastin time and outcome after thrombolytic therapy for acute myocardial infarction: results from the GUSTO-I trial. Circulation 1996;93:870–878.
20. GUSTO-IIb Angioplasty Substudy Investigators. A clinical trial comparing primary coronary angioplasty with tissue plasminogen activator for acute myocardial infarction. N Engl J Med 1997;336:1621–1628.

21. Zijlstra F, de Boer MJ, Hoorntje JC, Reiffers S, Reiber JH, Suryapranata H. A comparison of immediate coronary angioplasty with intravenous streptokinase in acute myocardial infarction. N Engl J Med 1993;328:680–684.
22. Gibbons RJ, Holmes DR, Reeder GS, Bailey KR, Hopfenspirger MR, Gersh BJ. Immediate angioplasty compared with the administration of a thrombolytic agent followed by conservative treatment for myocardial infarction. The Mayo Coronary Care Unit and Catheterization Laboratory Groups. N Engl J Med 1993;328:685–691.
23. Grines CL, Browne KF, Marco J, Rothbaum D, Stone GW, O'Keefe J, Overlie P, Donohue B, Chelliah N, Timmis GC. A comparison of immediate angioplasty with thrombolytic therapy for acute myocardial infarction. The Primary Angioplasty in Myocardial Infarction Study Group. N Engl J Med 1993;328: 673–679.
24. Ribeiro EE, Silva LA, Carneiro R, D'Oliveira LG, Gasquez A, Amino JG, Tavares JR, Petrizzo A, Torossian S, Duprat Filho R. Randomized trial of direct coronary angioplasty versus intravenous streptokinase in acute myocardial infarction. J Am Coll Cardiol 1993;22:376–380.
25. Weaver WD, Simes RJ, Betriu A, Grines CL, Zijlstra F, Garcia E, Grinfeld L, Gibbons RJ, Ribeiro EE, DeWood MA, Ribichini F. Comparison of primary coronary angioplasty and intravenous thrombolytic therapy for acute myocardial infarction: a quantitative review. JAMA 1997;278:2093–2098.
26. Granger CB, Van de Werf F, Armstrong PW. Hirudin reduces death and myocardial (re)infarction at 6-months: follow-up results of the GUSTO-IIb trial. J Am Coll Cardiol 1998;31:79A.
27. Metz BK, White HD, Granger CB, Simes RJ, Armstrong PW, Hirsh J, Fuster V, MacAulay CM, Califf RM, Topol EJ. Randomized comparison of direct thrombin inhibition versus heparin in conjunction with fibrinolytic therapy for acute myocardial infarction: results from the GUSTO-IIb trial. J Am Coll Cardiol 1998;31:1493–1498.
28. INJECT Investigators. Randomised, double-blind comparison of reteplase double-bolus administration with streptokinase in acute myocardial infarction: trial to investigate equivalence. International Joint Efficacy Comparison of Thrombolytics. Lancet 1995;346:329–336.
29. Bode C, Smalling RW, Berg G, Burnett C, Lorch G, Kalbfleisch JM, Chernoff R, Christie LG, Feldman RL, Seals AA, Weaver WD. Randomized comparison of coronary thrombolysis achieved with double-bolus reteplase (recombinant plasminogen activator) and front-loaded, accelerated alteplase (recombinant tissue plasminogen activator) in patients with acute myocardial infarction. The RAPID II Investigators. Circulation. 1996;94:891–898.
30. GUSTO-III Investigators. A comparison of reteplase with alteplase for acute myocardial infarction. N Engl J Med 1997;337:1118–1123.
31. Ohman E. Durability of treatment effect of thrombolysis for acute myocardial infarction: The GUSTO trials. J Am Coll Cardiol 1999;33:380A.
32. Antiplatelet Trialists' Collaboration. Collaborative overview of randomised trials of antiplatelet therapy. I. Prevention of death, myocardial infarction, and

stroke by prolonged antiplatelet therapy in various categories of patients. BMJ 1994;308:81–106.
33. Alexander JH, Harrington RA, Tuttle RH, Berdan LG, Lincoff AM, Deckers JW, Simoons ML, Guerci A, Hochman JS, Wilcox RG, Kitt MM, Eisenberg PR, Califf RM, Topol EJ, Karsh K, Ruzyllo W, Stepinska J, Widimsky P, Boland JB, Armstrong PW. Prior aspirin use predicts worse outcomes in patients with non-ST-elevation acute coronary syndromes. PURSUIT Investigators. Am J Cardiol 1999;83:1147–1151.
34. Garcia-Dorado D, Theroux P, Tornos P, Sambola A, Oliveras J, Santos M, Soler J. Previous aspirin use may attenuate the severity of the manifestation of acute ischemic syndromes. Circulation 1995;92:1743–1748.
35. EPILOG Investigators. Platelet glycoprotein IIb/IIIa receptor blockade and low-dose heparin during percutaneous coronary revascularization. N Engl J Med 1997;336:1689–1696.
36. EPISTENT Investigators. Randomised placebo-controlled and balloon-angioplasty-controlled trial to assess safety of coronary stenting with use of platelet glycoprotein-IIb/IIIa blockade. Lancet 1998;352:87–92.
37. Neumann FJ, Blasini R, Schmitt C, Alt E, Dirschinger J, Gawaz M, Kastrati A, Schomig A. Effect of glycoprotein IIb/IIIa receptor blockade on recovery of coronary flow and left ventricular function after the placement of coronary-artery stents in acute myocardial infarction. Circulation 1998;98:2695–2701.
38. Ohman E, Topol E. Trial of abciximab with and without low-dose reteplase for acute myocardial infarction. Circulation 2000. In press.
39. Verheugt F, Ohman E, Antman E. Emergency room infusion of abciximab speeds up reperfusion in acute myocardial infarction eligible for primary PTCA. Eur Heart J 1999;20:616.
40. Kleiman NS, White HD, Ohman EM, Ross AM, Woodlief LH, Califf RM, Holmes DR Jr, Bates E, Pfisterer M, Vahanian A. Mortality within 24 hours of thrombolysis for myocardial infarction. The importance of early reperfusion. The GUSTO Investigators. Circulation 1994;90:2658–2665.
41. Kleiman NS, Granger CB, White HD, Armstrong P, Ardissino D, de Werf FV, Zoldeyhi P, Thompson TD, Califf RM, Topol EJ. Death and nonfatal reinfarction within the first 24 hours after presentation with an acute coronary syndrome: experience from GUSTO-IIb. Am Heart J 1999;137:12–23.
42. Lee KL, Woodlief LH, Topol EJ, Weaver WD, Betriu A, Col J, Simoons M, Aylward P, Van de Werf F, Califf RM. Predictors of 30-day mortality in the era of reperfusion for acute myocardial infarction. Results from an international trial of 41,021 patients. GUSTO-I Investigators. Circulation 1995;91:1659–1668.
43. Berkowitz SD, Granger CB, Pieper KS, Lee KL, Gore JM, Simoons M, Armstrong PW, Topol EJ, Califf RM. Incidence and predictors of bleeding after contemporary thrombolytic therapy for myocardial infarction. GUSTO I Investigators. Circulation 1997;95:2508–2516.
44. Simoons ML, Maggioni AP, Knatterud G, Leimberger JD, de Jaegere P, van Domburg R, Boersma E, Franzosi MG, Califf R, Schroder R. Individual risk

assessment for intracranial haemorrhage during thrombolytic therapy. Lancet 1993;342:1523–1528.

45. Gore JM, Granger CB, Simoons ML, Sloan MA, Weaver WD, White HD, Barbash GI, Van de Werf F, Aylward PE, Topol EJ. Stroke after thrombolysis. Mortality and functional outcomes in the GUSTO-I trial. Circulation 1995;92: 2811–2818.
46. Gebel JM, Sila CA, Sloan MA, Granger CB, Mahaffey KW, Weisenberger J, Green CL, White HD, Gore JM, Weaver WD, Califf RM, Topol EJ. Thrombolysis-related intracranial hemorrhage: a radiographic analysis of 244 cases from the GUSTO-I trial with clinical correlation. Stroke 1998;29:563–569.
47. Sloan MA, Sila CA, Mahaffey KW, Granger CB, Longstreth WT, Jr., Koudstaal P, White HD, Gore JM, Simoons ML, Weaver WD, Green CL, Topol EJ, Califf RM. Prediction of 30-day mortality among patients with thrombolysis-related intracranial hemorrhage. Circulation 1998;98:1376–1382.
48. Mahaffey KW, Granger CB, Sloan MA, Green CL, Gore JM, Weaver WD, White HD, Simoons ML, Barbash GI, Topol EJ, Califf RM. Neurosurgical evacuation of intracranial hemorrhage after thrombolytic therapy for acute myocardial infarction: experience from the GUSTO-I trial. Am Heart J 1999; 138:493–499.
49. Mahaffey KW, Granger CB, Sloan MA, Thompson TD, Gore JM, Weaver WD, White HD, Simoons ML, Barbash GI, Topol EJ, Califf RM. Risk factors for in-hospital nonhemorrhagic stroke in patients with acute myocardial infarction treated with thrombolysis: results from GUSTO-I. Circulation 1998;97:757–764.
50. Lesnefsky EJ, Lundergan CF, Hodgson JM, Nair R, Reiner JS, Greenhouse SW, Califf RM, Ross AM. Increased left ventricular dysfunction in elderly patients despite successful thrombolysis: the GUSTO-I angiographic experience. J Am Coll Cardiol 1996;28:331–337.
51. Holmes DR Jr, White HD, Pieper KS, Ellis SG, Califf RM, Topol EJ. Effect of age on outcome with primary angioplasty versus thrombolysis. J Am Coll Cardiol 1999;33:412–419.
52. Peterson ED, Hathaway WR, Zabel KM, Pieper KS, Granger CB, Wagner GS, Topol EJ, Bates ER, Simoons ML, Califf RM. Prognostic significance of precordial ST segment depression during inferior myocardial infarction in the thrombolytic era: results in 16,521 patients. J Am Coll Cardiol 1996;28:305–312.
53. Birnbaum Y, Wagner GS, Barbash GI, Gates K, Criger DA, Sclarovsky S, Siegel RJ, Granger CB, Reiner JS, Ross AM. Correlation of angiographic findings and right (V1 to V3) versus left (V4 to V6) precordial ST-segment depression in inferior wall acute myocardial infarction. Am J Cardiol 1999;83: 143–148.
54. Newby LK, Rutsch WR, Califf RM, Simoons ML, Aylward PE, Armstrong PW, Woodlief LH, Lee KL, Topol EJ, Van de Werf F. Time from symptom onset to treatment and outcomes after thrombolytic therapy. GUSTO-I Investigators. J Am Coll Cardiol 1996;27:1646–1655.
55. Cox JL, Lee E, Langer A, Armstrong PW, Naylor CD. Time to treatment with thrombolytic therapy: determinants and effect on short-term nonfatal outcomes

of acute myocardial infarction. Canadian GUSTO Investigators. CMAJ 1997; 156:497–505.
56. Berger PB, Ellis SG, Holmes DR Jr, Granger CB, Criger DA, Betriu A, Topol EJ, Califf RM. Relationship between delay in performing direct coronary angioplasty and early clinical outcome in patients with acute myocardial infarction: results from the global use of strategies to open occluded arteries in Acute Coronary Syndromes (GUSTO-IIb) trial. Circulation 1999;100:14–20.
57. Granger C, Phillips H, Betriu A, Ellis S, Weaver W, Aylward P, Stebbins A, Lee K, Califf R, Topol E. Direct angioplasty may be less advantageous in patients presenting early after symptom onset: Results from GUSTO-IIb. J Am Coll Cardiol 1997.
58. Cho L, Marso S, Bhatt D, Hsu C, Topol E. An early invasive strategy is associated with decreased mortality: GUSTO-IIb trial. Circulation 1999;100:I-359.
59. Weaver WD, White HD, Wilcox RG, Aylward PE, Morris D, Guerci A, Ohman EM, Barbash GI, Betriu A, Sadowski Z, Topol EJ, Califf RM. Comparisons of characteristics and outcomes among women and men with acute myocardial infarction treated with thrombolytic therapy. GUSTO-I Investigators. JAMA 1996;275:777–782.
60. Moen EK, Asher CR, Miller DP, Weaver WD, White HD, Califf RM, Topol EJ. Long-term follow-up of gender-specific outcomes after thrombolytic therapy for acute myocardial infarction from the GUSTO-I trial. J Womens Health 1997;6:285–293.
61. Karnash SL, Granger CB, White HD, Woodlief LH, Topol EJ, Califf RM. Treating menstruating women with thrombolytic therapy: insights from the global utilization of streptokinase and tissue plasminogen activator for occluded coronary arteries (GUSTO-I) trial. J Am Coll Cardiol 1995;26:1651–1656.
62. Mak KH, Moliterno DJ, Granger CB, Miller DP, White HD, Wilcox RG, Califf RM, Topol EJ. Influence of diabetes mellitus on clinical outcome in the thrombolytic era of acute myocardial infarction. GUSTO-I Investigators. J Am Coll Cardiol 1997;30:171–179.
63. Woodfield SL, Lundergan CF, Reiner JS, Greenhouse SW, Thompson MA, Rohrbeck SC, Deychak Y, Simoons ML, Califf RM, Topol EJ, Ross AM. Angiographic findings and outcome in diabetic patients treated with thrombolytic therapy for acute myocardial infarction: the GUSTO-I experience. J Am Coll Cardiol 1996;28:1661–1669.
64. Mahaffey KW, Granger CB, Toth CA, White HD, Stebbins AL, Barbash GI, Vahanian A, Topol EJ, Califf RM. Diabetic retinopathy should not be a contraindication to thrombolytic therapy for acute myocardial infarction: review of ocular hemorrhage incidence and location in the GUSTO-I trial. J Am Coll Cardiol 1997;30:1606–1610.
65. Aylward PE, Wilcox RG, Horgan JH, White HD, Granger CB, Califf RM, Topol EJ. Relation of increased arterial blood pressure to mortality and stroke in the context of contemporary thrombolytic therapy for acute myocardial infarction. A randomized trial. GUSTO-I Investigators. Ann Intern Med 1996;125: 891–900.

66. Brieger DB, Mak KH, White HD, Kleiman NS, Miller DP, Vahanian A, Ross AM, Califf RM, Topol EJ. Benefit of early sustained reperfusion in patients with prior myocardial infarction (the GUSTO-I trial). Am J Cardiol 1998;81: 282–287.
67. Labinaz M, Sketch MH Jr, Stebbins AL, DeFranco AC, Holmes DR Jr, Kleiman NS, Betriu A, Rutsch WR, Vahanian A, Topol EJ, Califf RM. Thrombolytic therapy for patients with prior percutaneous transluminal coronary angioplasty and subsequent acute myocardial infarction. GUSTO-I Investigators. Am J Cardiol 1996;78:1338–1344.
68. Barbash GI, Reiner J, White HD, Wilcox RG, Armstrong PW, Sadowski Z, Morris D, Aylward P, Woodlief LH, Topol EJ. Evaluation of paradoxic beneficial effects of smoking in patients receiving thrombolytic therapy for acute myocardial infarction: mechanism of the "smoker's paradox" from the GUSTO-I trial, with angiographic insights. J Am Coll Cardiol 1995;26:1222–1229.
69. Hasdai D, Lerman A, Rihal CS, Criger DA, Garratt KN, Betriu A, White HD, Topol EJ, Granger CB, Ellis SG, Califf RM, Holmes DR Jr. Smoking status and outcome after primary coronary angioplasty for acute myocardial infarction. Am Heart J 1999;137:612–620.
70. Holmes DR Jr, Bates ER, Kleiman NS, Sadowski Z, Horgan JH, Morris DC, Califf RM, Berger PB, Topol EJ. Contemporary reperfusion therapy for cardiogenic shock: the GUSTO-I trial experience. J Am Coll Cardiol 1995;26:668–674.
71. Hasdai D, Holmes DR Jr, Topol EJ, Berger PB, Criger DA, Hochman JS, Bates ER, Vahanian A, Armstrong PW, Wilcox R, Ohman EM, Califf RM. Frequency and clinical outcome of cardiogenic shock during acute myocardial infarction among patients receiving reteplase or alteplase. Results from GUSTO-III. Eur Heart J 1999;20:128–135.
72. Berger PB, Holmes DR Jr, Stebbins AL, Bates ER, Califf RM, Topol EJ. Impact of an aggressive invasive catheterization and revascularization strategy on mortality in patients with cardiogenic shock in the GUSTO-I trial. An observational study. Circulation 1997;96:122–127.
73. Berger PB, Tuttle RH, Holmes DR Jr, Topol EJ, Aylward PE, Horgan JH, Califf RM. One-year survival among patients with acute myocardial infarction complicated by cardiogenic shock, and its relation to early revascularization: results from the GUSTO-I trial. Circulation 1999;99:873–878.
74. Holmes DR Jr, Califf RM, Van de Werf F, Berger PB, Bates ER, Simoons ML, White HD, Thompson TD, Topol EJ. Difference in countries' use of resources and clinical outcome for patients with cardiogenic shock after myocardial infarction: results from the GUSTO trial. Lancet 1997;349:75–78.
75. Anderson RD, Ohman EM, Holmes DR Jr, Col I, Stebbins AL, Bates ER, Stomel RJ, Granger CB, Topol EJ, Califf RM. Use of intraaortic balloon counterpulsation in patients presenting with cardiogenic shock: observations from the GUSTO-I study. J Am Coll Cardiol 1997;30:708–715.
76. Hasdai D, Holmes DR Jr, Califf RM, Thompson TD, Hochman JS, Pfisterer M, Topol EJ. Cardiogenic shock complicating acute myocardial infarction: predictors of death. GUSTO Investigators. Am Heart J 1999;138:21–31.

77. Crenshaw BS, Ward SR, Granger CB, Stebbins AL, Topol EJ, Califf RM. Atrial fibrillation in the setting of acute myocardial infarction: the GUSTO-I experience. J Am Coll Cardiol 1997;30:406–413.
78. Newby KH, Thompson T, Stebbins A, Topol EJ, Califf RM, Natale A. Sustained ventricular arrhythmias in patients receiving thrombolytic therapy: incidence and outcomes. The GUSTO Investigators. Circulation 1998;98:2567–2573.
79. Alexander JH, Granger CB, Sadowski Z, Aylward PE, White HD, Thompson TD, Califf RM, Topol EJ. Prophylactic lidocaine use in acute myocardial infarction: incidence and outcomes from two international trials. The GUSTO-I and GUSTO-IIb Investigators. Am Heart J 1999;137:799–805.
80. Betriu A, Califf RM, Bosch X, Guerci A, Stebbins AL, Barbagelata NA, Aylward PE, Vahanian A, Van de Werf F, Topol EJ. Recurrent ischemia after thrombolysis: importance of associated clinical findings. GUSTO-I Investigators. J Am Coll Cardiol 1998;31:94–102.
81. Armstrong PW, Fu Y, Chang WC, Topol EJ, Granger CB, Betriu A, Van de Werf F, Lee KL, Califf RM. Acute coronary syndromes in the GUSTO-IIb trial: prognostic insights and impact of recurrent ischemia. The GUSTO-IIb Investigators. Circulation 1998;98:1860–1868.

26

Treatment of Acute Myocardial Infarction

International and Regional Differences

Louise Pilote
McGill University Health Centre
Montreal, Quebec, Canada

INTRODUCTION

Multiple randomized clinical trials have examined whether aggressive approaches to the treatment of acute myocardial infarction (MI)—using invasive and costly procedures such as angiography in all patients and revascularization in most patients—added a benefit compared with more conservative approaches that use cardiac procedures more selectively (1–10). The results of these studies have called into question whether there is any clinical advantage to an aggressive approach. Thus, the clinical practice guidelines of authoritative bodies such as the American Heart Association and American College of Cardiology have recommended the use of angiography only in patients who develop complications and show evidence of inducible ischemia after acute MI (11,12). Despite the results of these studies and the publication of practice guidelines for the use of angiography and revascularization after acute MI, wide international and regional variations in the treatment of acute MI persist.

Comparing the treatment of acute MI in different regions highlights differences in practice patterns. Such differences provide natural experiments that allow for the assessment of the impact of practice variations on clinical outcomes in an actual clinical setting rather than in the context of a clinical trial. In addition, evaluating these differences informs patients about the care they receive, provides health care policy makers with data for making decisions about the distribution of health care resources, and informs physicians who are interested in delivering the best possible care. However, geographic variations in care suggest that in some areas, patients receive suboptimal care while patients in other areas might receive care that is not cost-effective. Thus, given the present health care climate, finding the level of care that provides the best outcomes at minimal cost is a timely challenge.

This chapter will describe the results of several studies that examined practice patterns in the treatment of acute MI in different countries and different regions of the United States, with a particular focus on the use of angiography, revascularization procedures, and cardiac medications. In addition, this chapter will investigate the impact of these practice variations on clinical outcomes, as well as on quality-of-life measurements and cost of care. Finally, potential reasons for these differences in practice patterns and the determinants of the use of cardiac procedures in clinical practice will be identified and discussed.

VARIATIONS IN TREATMENT OF ACUTE MI

International Variations in Angiography, Revascularization, and Cardiac Medications

The initial studies to report international variations in the treatment of acute MI compared the treatment practices between the United States and Canada. Such comparisons are useful in assessing practice patterns in different health care systems; Canada has a universal single-payer health insurance system, whereas the United States has multiple insurance coverage systems. These studies were published at a time when U.S. health care policy makers were looking to Canada for a potential model for changes in the American health care system.

In one of the first study comparing the treatment of acute MI in the United States and Canada, Rouleau et al. studied patients from 19 Canadian and 93 U.S. hospitals participating in the Survival and Ventricular Enlargement (SAVE) study (13). Despite the similarity of the 1573 U.S. patients and 658 Canadian patients participating in the study, coronary angiography was more commonly performed in U.S. patients than in Canadian patients (68% vs. 35%; $P < .001$); revascularization procedures were also more common among U.S. patients (31% vs. 12%; $P < .001$) (Table 1). These differences did not result in any apparent differences in mortality (22% vs. 23%)

Table 1 Coronary Arteriography and Revascularization Procedures Performed After the Index Infarction

Procedure or procedures	Before randomization			During follow-up after randomization			Entire period after infarction		
	United States	Canada	Prevalence ratio (95% CI)	United States	Canada	Prevalence ratio (95% CI)	United States	Canada	Prevalence ratio (95% CI)
	No. (%)			No. (%)			No. (%)		
Coronary arteriography	1069 (68)	232 (35)	1.93 (1.73–2.15) $P < .001$	496 (32)	144 (22)	1.44 (1.23–1.69) $P < .001$	1227 (78)	317 (48)	1.62 (1.49–1.76) $P < .001$
PTCA	350 (22)	53 (8)	2.76 (2.10–3.63) $P < .001$	112 (7)	32 (5)	1.46 (1.00–2.15) $P = .033$	417 (27)	75 (11)	2.33 (1.85–2.92) $P = .001$
CABG	159 (10)	32 (5)	2.08 (1.44–3.01) $P < .001$	180 (11)	51 (8)	1.48 (1.10–1.99) $P = .005$	339 (22)	83 (13)	1.71 (1.37–2.13) $P < .001$
Revascularization	482 (31)	80 (12)	2.52 (2.03–3.14) $P < .001$	270 (17)	79 (12)	1.43 (1.13–1.81) $P = .001$	674 (43)	148 (22)	1.19 (1.63–2.22) $P < .001$
PTCA per coronary arteriogrpahy	(33)	(23)	1.43 (1.11–1.84) $P = .001$	(23)	(22)	1.02 (0.72–.144)	(34)	(24)	1.44 (1.16–1.78) $P < .001$
CABG per coronary arteriography	(15)	(14)	1.08 (0.76–1.53)	(36)	(35)	1.02 (0.80–1.32)	(28)	(26)	1.06 (0.86–1.30)
Revascularization per coronary arteriography	(45)	(34)	1.31 (1.08–1.58) $P = .002$	(54)	(55)	0.99 (0.84–1.17)	(55)	(47)	1.18 (1.04–1.34) $P = .009$

Source: Ref. 13.

CI, confidence interval; PTCA, percutaneous transluminal coronary angioplasty; CABG, coronary-artery bypass grafting.

Table 2 Relative Risk of Death, Recurrent Myocardial Infarction, or Activity-Limiting Angina

Event	After 1 year			After 2 years			Entire follow-up period		
	United States No. (%)	Canada No. (%)	Relative risk (95% CI)	United States No. (%)	Canada No. (%)	Relative risk (95% CI)	United States No. (%)	Canada No. (%)	Relative risk (95% CI)
Death	173 (11)	72 (11)	0.98 (0.73–1.30)	246 (16)	107 (16)	1.03 (0.81–1.31)	357 (23)	146 (22)	1.00 (0.82–1.23)
Recurrent myocardial infarction	121 (8)	57 (9)	1.22 (0.88–1.17)	159 (10)	79 (12)	1.31 (0.99–1.74)	210 (13)	93 (14)	1.19 (0.92–1.53)
Death or recurrent myocardial infarction	251 (16)	105 (16)	1.02 (0.80–1.29)	346 (22)	153 (23)	1.09 (0.89–1.33)	479 (30)	191 (29)	1.01 (0.85–1.20)
Angina	285 (18)	154 (23)	1.31 (1.06–1.61) $P = .012$	359 (23)	189 (29)	1.29 (1.07–1.56) $P = .007$	427 (27)	217 (33)	1.27 (1.06–1.51) $P = .008$
Death, recurrent myocardial infarction, or angina	490 (31)	237 (36)	1.19 (1.01–1.41) $P = .034$	628 (40)	295 (45)	1.19 (1.02–1.37) $P = .023$	774 (49)	347 (53)	1.15 (1.01–1.32) $P = .042$

Source: Ref. 13.
Relative risks represent values after adjustment for minor baseline differences among population groups.
CI, confidence interval.

or reinfarction incidences over 1 year (14% vs. 13%) (Table 2). However, the incidence of activity-limiting angina was more common in Canada than in the United States (33% vs. 27%; $P < .007$).

The more intensive use of cardiac procedures such as bypass surgery suggests a more expensive treatment strategy for acute MI in the United States than in Canada. Given the absence of significant differences in cumulative mortality and reinfarction incidences, this study raised questions as to whether the frequent use of cardiac procedures after acute MI was in fact cost-effective; the results also raised questions about potential overuse of cardiac procedures in the United States and underuse in Canada.

The next study to compare the practice patterns in the United States and Canada was a retrospective cohort study performed in two university hospitals: Stanford Medical Center (Palo Alto, CA) and the Royal Victoria Hospital at McGill University (Montreal) (14). This 1994 study extended the results of Rouleau's study, obtaining more extensive data on patient functional status. Moreover, in contrast to the above study, which used a clinical trial as a source of patients, this study examined 518 consecutive patients treated for acute MI in the coronary care unit of those two hospitals over 2 years, thus providing a closer look at actual clinical practice. This study confirmed findings of a more invasive approach in the United States than in Canada, but also found an increased use of noninvasive tests in Canada compared with the United States. Among comparable patient groups, invasive procedures were more commonly performed at Stanford (angiography 55% vs. 34%; angioplasty 30% vs. 13%; bypass surgery 10% vs. 4%; $P < .001$ for all comparisons). In contrast, noninvasive tests were more commonly performed at McGill (exercise tests 56% vs. 20%; tests of left ventricular function 86% vs. 59%; $P < .001$ for both) (Table 3). In-hospital and 1-year reinfarction and mortality cumulative incidences were similar at Stanford and McGill. In contrast, angina was reported less commonly at Stanford (33% vs. 40%; $P = .15$), and the functional status of Stanford patients was superior to that of McGill patients (Duke Activity Status Index mean: 28.8 and 22.9, respectively; $P = .006$).

Several studies have used the database provided by the first Global Utilization of Streptokinase and t-PA (tissue plasminogen activator) for Occluded Coronary Arteries (GUSTO I) study to examine practice patterns internationally and in different regions of the United States (15). This large international randomized clinical trial (>40,000 patients) compared four different thrombolytic strategies. Because the treatment of patients after thrombolysis was left to the discretion of the treating physician, this study provided an opportunity to study practice patterns in a large number of patients with acute MI.

Table 3 Patients with In-Hospital Procedures and Events

	Stanford,[a] % (n = 233)	McGill,[a] % (n = 285)
Invasive procedures		
Coronary angiogram[b]	55	34
Coronary angioplasty[b]	30	13
Coronary artery surgery[b]	10	4
Noninvasive procedures		
Exercise tests[b,c]	20	56
Left ventricular function tests[b,d]	59	86
Events		
Recurrent myocardial infarction	1	1
Death	12	11

Source: Ref. 14.
[a]Stanford indicates Stanford (Calif.) University Hospital; McGill, Royal Victoria Hospital (McGill University, Montreal, Quebec).
[b]$P < .05$.
[c]Includes the exercise treadmill test and exercise thallium scan.
[d]Includes the echocardiogram and multiple-gated radionuclide ventriculogram.

In the first study making use of the GUSTO I database, Van de Werf et al. (16) compared the treatment of acute MI between the United States (N = 23,105) and 14 other countries (N = 17,916) involved in the GUSTO I study. Patterns of use of cardiac medications were different in the United States and in these other countries: during hospitalization, antiarrhythmics were used in 46% of patients in the United States and 27% of patients elsewhere; calcium antagonists were used in 38% and 21% of patients; digitalis and other inotropes were used in 26% and 18% of patients; and angiotensin-converting enzyme (ACE) inhibitors were used in 22% and 25% of patients. Angioplasty and bypass surgery were used more commonly in the United States than elsewhere (angioplasty in 31% of U.S. patients, compared with 10% elsewhere; bypass surgery in 13% compared with 3%). Despite the more aggressive use of cardiac medications and procedures in the United States than in the other countries, enrollment in the United States was only a marginally significant predictor of improved survival (30-day mortality was not significantly different: 6.8% in the United States vs. 7.2% elsewhere; $P = .09$). Another study of the GUSTO I database compared the Canadian to the American coronary angiography practices in the detection of severe coronary artery disease (CAD) (17). Seventy-one percent of Americans underwent angiography, compared with 27% of Canadians. Yet, the prevalence of severe CAD was the same, 17%, in the two countries. This suggests that the Canadian approach does not lead to detection of the more severe cases and that patients with severe CAD might go undetected.

Finally, studies of administrative databases in Canada and in the United States which provide population-based analyses of patients with acute MI at different points in time have confirmed the findings drawn from secondary analyses of randomized trials. Tu et al. compared 224,258 elderly Medicare beneficiaries in the United States to 9444 elderly patients in Ontario, Canada, in 1991 (18). The higher use of cardiac procedures in the United States did not appear to affect prognosis. Although the 30-day mortality was slightly lower in the United States (21.3% vs. 22.3%, $P = .03$), the 1-year mortality was similar (34.3% vs. 34.4%, $P = .94$). Furthermore, Pilote et al. looked at temporal trends in technology use for the treatment of acute MI in the elderly in the United States (n = 1.7 million Medicare beneficiaries) and Quebec, Canada (n = 34,856), between 1988 and 1994 (19). Growth in technology use was greater in the United States than in Quebec. For example, use of PTCA increased from 7% to 18% in the United States compared with 2% to 6% in Quebec. Yet, downward trends in mortality were similar; 1-year mortality went from 39.1% to 32.8% in the United States and from 37.6% to 32.1% in Quebec.

Thus, the more frequent use of invasive cardiac procedures among U.S. patients with acute MI did not improve reinfarction and mortality incidences when compared with those rates resulting from a much lower use of these procedures among Canadian patients. The more frequent use of noninvasive cardiac procedures and the longer length of hospital stay in Canada compared with the United States, suggesting that the differences in cost of care might not be as large as previously thought. Viewed together, these studies raise questions about the potential benefit of an aggressive approach to the treatment of acute MI in terms of increased functional status and reduced post-MI angina.

International variations in MI management have been reported between countries other than the United States and Canada. These studies drew information from various databases. For example, Heller et al. examined the practices of doctors in Australia, Brazil, Chile, India, and Thailand and found both between- and within-country variation in the use of most cardiac interventions (20).

Regional Variations in the Use of Angiography, Revascularization, and Cardiac Medications

International variations in care are largely a result of the different health care systems. Whether variations in the treatment of acute MI existed within the United States—that is, within the same health care system is a question addressed by several investigators. Pilote et al. merged the databases of the GUSTO I trial and the American Hospital Association in order to link patient and hospital characteristics and examine the treatment of acute MI among the major census regions in the United States (21). The proportion of patients undergoing cardiac procedures varied greatly across the United States and was lowest in New England (Table 4). The percentage of patients who had coronary angiography ranged from 52% to 81%, coronary angioplasty ranged from 22% to 35%, and coronary artery bypass surgery ranged from 9% to 17%. With the exception of New England, interregional variation was closely related to on-site availability of cardiac procedures (Fig. 1). After statistical adjustment for clinical and hospital facilities characteristics, and with Mid Atlantic as a reference, patients in New England were still less likely to undergo angiography than in the other regions (Fig. 2).

Medication use during the initial hospitalization varied greatly across regions (Fig. 3). In New England, oral beta-blockers (55% to 81% of patients), nitrates (61% to 77%), and ACE inhibitors (18% to 23%) were used most often; calcium channel blockers (31% to 42%), lidocaine (14% to 43%), and digitalis (14% to 20%) were used least often. Clinical trials have shown an improved survival with the use of beta-blockers and ACE inhibitors (22,23) yet in many regions of the United States these medications are not used routinely. Compared with other regions, the practice in New England was closer to evidence-based medical practice and, in that way, followed a pattern similar to that among Canadian patients enrolled in the GUSTO I trial.

Finally, differences in the frequency of cardiac procedures were not clearly related to clinical outcomes. In-hospital, 30-day, and 1-year mortality cumulative incidences ranged from 5.4% to 7.2%, 3.3% to 4.1%, 5.8% to 7.7%, and 8.6% to 10.3%, respectively. Thus, among acute MI patients enrolled in a large clinical trial in which the postthrombolysis treatment was left to the discretion of the treating physicians, wide variation was found in the use of cardiac procedures and medications within the United States. The impact of these variations on mortality was minimal.

Regional variations in the treatment of acute MI within the United States have also been observed in other databases. Using the Medicare database, Guadagnali et al. studied U.S. patients between the ages of 65 and 79 and covered by Medicare who were admitted to 478 different hospitals in the states of Texas and New York for the treatment of acute MI (24). While coronary angiography was performed more often among patients with acute MI in Texas than in New York, the risk of death at 2 years was lower in New York. Furthermore, in contrast with the findings of other studies, the patient group that underwent the more aggressive approach (Texans) had

Table 4 Use of Cardiac Procedures in the Treatment of the Study Patients, by Region of the United States

Variable	New England (N = 2318)	Mid Atlantic (N = 3758)	South Atlantic (N = 5296)	East North Central (N = 3616)	South Central (N = 1333)	West North Central (N = 1551)	Mountain (N = 1839)	Pacific (N = 2061)
Procedure (% of patients)								
Angiography	52	67	77	79	81	72	72	66
Angioplasty	22	26	33	33	34	35	34	24
Coronary surgery	9	12	14	14	17	14	13	12
Characteristics of angioplasty								
Elective (% of patients)	73	77	87	84	88	75	81	86
Diseased coronary vessels (% of patients)								
None	12	11	13	11	11	10	12	13
One	33	34	35	36	35	34	37	35
Two	31	31	29	30	31	28	28	29
Three	21	22	22	21	21	24	20	22
Left Main	3	2	2	2	3	3	3	2
Left ventricular ejection (%)[a]	50	50	51	50	50	51	53	55
Procedure following angiography (% of patients)								
Angioplasty	43	39	43	42	42	48	47	37
Coronary artery bypass surgery	18	18	18	18	21	19	18	18

Source: Ref. 21.
[a]Values represent the median left ventricular ejection fractions.

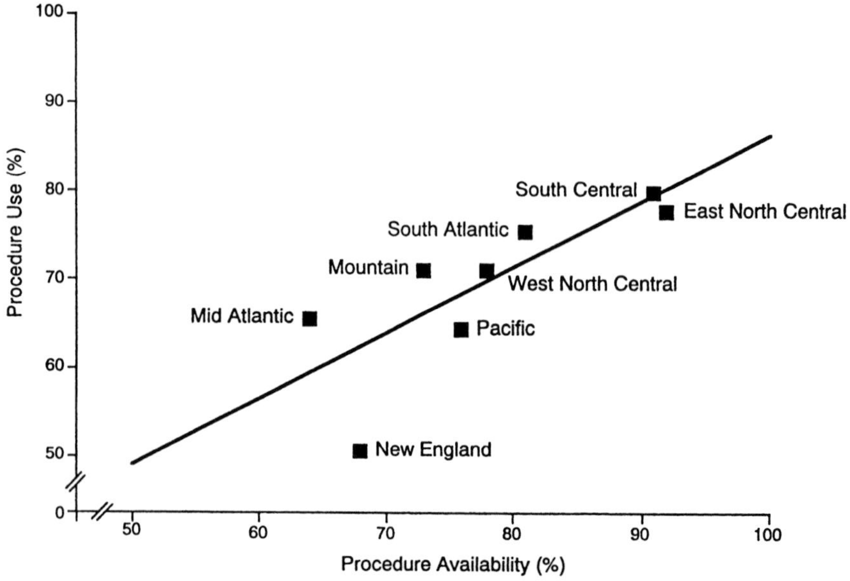

Figure 1 Depiction of a positive association between regional use and availability of coronary angiography. (From Ref. 21.)

more angina and more difficulty with performing activities requiring high energy expenditure than the New York patient group.

Even within the same region, marked variations in the use of angiography for acute MI have been reported; for example, Selby et al. found that the rates of angiography in 16 Kaiser Permanente hospitals in Northern California were inversely related to the risk of heart disease events ($P < .001$) and death ($P = .03$) (25). Use of angiography within the first 3 months after MI ranged from 30% to 77%. Unlike all studies described so far, the 1-year cumulative incidence of mortality was lower at hospitals with higher procedure rates.

In hospitals with high frequency of angiography in this study, the use of thrombolysis and of ACE inhibitors was higher than in hospitals with lower angiography rates. This may explain the lower mortality incidences in hospitals with more frequent use of angiography in this particular study.

Geographic Variations in Other Cardiac Procedures

Aside from the use of angiography and revascularization procedures, other cardiac procedures used in the coronary care unit have also been shown to vary. Data from the GUSTO I study demonstrate international and regional

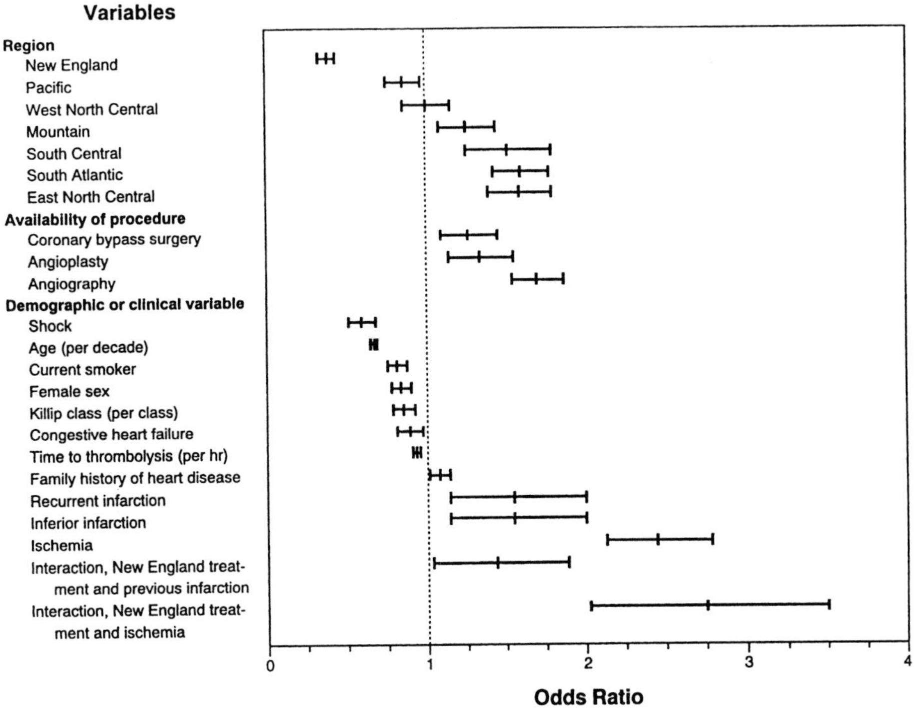

Figure 2 Odds ratios and 95% confidence intervals for various factors that influenced the use of angiography before hospital discharge in 21,772 study patients with acute myocardial infarction. (From Ref. 21.)

variations in these other cardiac procedures. For example, across U.S. regions, temporary transvenous pacemaker use ranged form 7% to 14%, pulmonary artery catheters ranged from 15% to 22%, intra-aortic balloon pumps ranged from 3% to 7%, and mechanical ventilators from 14% to 22%.

There is widespread use of many of the above-mentioned procedures; however, their benefit has not been demonstrated despite their attendant costs. The use of pulmonary artery catheterization, for example, is very controversial. This procedure is performed frequently in post-MI patients, yet its benefits have not been demonstrated in a randomized clinical trial. At this time, a widely shared clinical belief of benefits makes the performance of a clinical trial evaluating pulmonary artery catheterization difficult because physicians are reluctant to enroll patients in studies comparing use

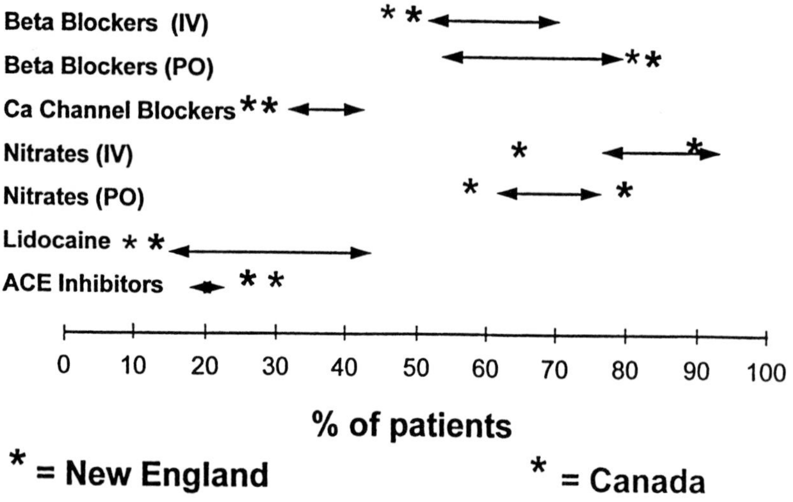

Figure 3 Comparison across regions of the United States and Canada showing the range in the percentage of patients on any given medication. (Data from Ref. 21.)

and nonuse of this procedure. A prospective cohort study concluded that pulmonary artery catheterization led to higher hospital costs and was not associated with superior outcomes (26). Selection bias is among the problems associated with observational studies of this type; high-risk patients are more likely to receive the procedure. However, the authors used subgroup analysis and multivariate modeling techniques as well as sensitivity analysis and came to similar conclusions.

Many aspects of the management of patients with acute MI have not been studied in detail. Variations in the use of such elements of care is not surprising, given the absence of evidence favoring one therapy over another. Yet variations also exist in areas of care, particularly the use of certain medications with strong supporting evidence for their use. Quality indicators have been identified to access practice in relationship with the scientific evidence. These included pharmacologic therapy, reperfusion, and smoking cessation advice (27). A striking example of underuse is the use of beta-blockers after acute MI, which has clearly been shown to improve survival. As previously mentioned, in the GUSTO I study, oral beta-blocker use ranged from 55% to 81%. Discharge prescriptions of beta-blockers were also suboptimal, ranging from 49% to 71% of patients. In the Cooperative Cardiovascular Project, a study of 186,800 Medicare beneficiaries with acute MI, discharge prescription of beta-blockers was 49.5%, and that of ACE inhibitors was 59.3% (27). Most post-MI patients are eligible for beta-blocker and ACE inhibitor use, and their use should be higher. Thus, similarly to cardiac procedures, widespread variations in medication use suggest a lack of agreement between evidence-based therapy and actual clinical practice.

In summary, several studies have demonstrated wide geographic variations in the use of cardiac procedures and medications for the treatment of acute MI. Several regions in the United States and in several other countries take an approach to the care of MI patients that is more in accordance with an evidence-based medicine; results of clinical trials and meta-analyses seem to be applied in clinical practice in these centers. In contrast, a number of patients received medical treatment that is not based on the results of recent clinical trials.

IMPACT OF PRACTICE PATTERN VARIATIONS ON CLINICAL OUTCOMES

Mortality

In all studies described thus far, marked variations in practice have not been associated with any differences in mortality and reinfarction cumulative incidences. This observation is consistent with the findings of the Thrombolysis in Myocardial Infarction II B (TIMI-II B) study, in which patients were randomized to an invasive or conservative strategy of treatment after thrombolysis for acute MI. The patients in the invasive strategy arm had more angiography than patients in the conservative strategy (93% vs. 33%), more angioplasty (57% vs. 16%), and slightly more bypass surgery (11.9% vs. 10.5%) (1). Despite the more extensive use of invasive procedures, the cumulative incidence of mortality was equivalent in the invasive-strategy and the conservative-strategy arms at both 21 days (4.9% vs. 4.1%) and 1 year (6.9% vs. 7.4%) (2).

Functional Status and Quality of Life

Mortality and reinfarction cumulative incidences are important measurements in any study of cardiovascular diseases. Yet, much of medical care after acute MI is directed at relieving symptoms and improving functional status and quality of life (14). Although differences in practice patterns may not affect mortality, they may affect the quality of life of surviving patients. A GUSTO I substudy investigated the impact of practice variations on medical outcomes including measurement of quality of life and use of medical resources during the year after acute MI (28). The investigators obtained data on a total of 2600 U.S. and 400 Canadian patients randomly selected from the GUSTO I trial. Length of hospital stay was, on average, 1 day longer in

Canada than in the United States, but the procedure rate was much lower in Canada (angiography: 25% vs. 72%; angioplasty: 11% vs. 29%; coronary bypass surgery: 3% vs. 14%; $P < .001$ for all comparisons). At 1 year after enrollment, 24% of the Canadian patients and 53% of the U.S. patients had undergone angioplasty or bypass surgery at least once. After 1 year, several measures of quality of life suggested that the quality of life of U.S. patients was superior to that of Canadian patients (Table 5). For example, the prevalence of chest pain and dyspnea at 1 year was higher among the Canadian patients (34% vs. 21%, and 45% vs. 29%; $P < .001$), and the Canadian patients also had worse functional status than U.S. patients (Fig. 4). The Canadian patients also had more visits to physicians during the follow-up year but fewer visits to specialists. These results suggest that the more frequent use of cardiac procedures and of specialty care in the United States may confer a better quality of life in post-MI patients.

A major question raised by this study is whether the differences in quality of life between Canadian and U.S. patients with MI are due to cultural differences rather than to differences in medical care. Given the subjective nature of quality-of-life questionnaires, cultural differences could theoretically affect responses (29).

The study of subjective outcomes brings an added level of uncertainty. While there are outcomes that are easy to measure—such as mortality—other outcomes, such as disability, distress, and dissatisfaction with health care, are more difficult to measure. In fact, most databases used in these types of analyses do not routinely record outcomes relating to functional status and quality of life (30). Furthermore, unlike the predictors of mortality, which are beginning to be well understood, predictors of functional status and quality of life have not been as clearly defined. This lack of knowledge about predictors makes statistical adjustment for differences between groups difficult. Consequently, uncertainty about outcomes other than mortality exists because of both poor documentation and lack of knowledge about predictors. More work is needed on outcomes that better describe the burden of illness.

Cost

Underlying the issues of appropriate care is the issue of cost. In today's society, the cost of care is a pivotal issue. Patient management must optimize outcomes at the lowest possible cost. Studies of geographic variations offer a look at styles of patient management. However, measuring the cost of care as it relates to practice styles is a difficult undertaking, requiring measurement of the whole process of care. In addition, similar to the measurement of clinical outcomes, long-term follow-up is necessary to define the eco-

Table 5 Changes in Quality of Life over the Course of 1 Year

Measure	Canadian patients (N = 311)	U.S. patients (N = 2165)	*P* value
	% of patients		
General health vs. before MI			.007
Much better	24	25	
Somewhat better	23	23	
About the same	31	36	
Somewhat worse	16	3	
Physical capacity vs. before MI			<.001
Much better	12	15	
Somewhat better	18	15	
About the same	35	48	
Somewhat worse	25	18	
Much worse	10	4	
Emotional state or mood vs. before MI			.03
Much better	17	18	
Somewhat better	15	17	
About the same	49	52	
Somewhat worse	13	10	
Much worse	6	3	
Change in functioning due to health (1-yr vs. 30-day status)[a]			<.001
Improved by ≥1 category	31	44	
Unchanged	54	43	
Worse by ≥1 category	15	13	
Working conditions vs. before MI, if employed or homemaker			
Amount of work same or more	63	69	.29
Working less or less hard	51	43	.06
Quality of work same or better	94	95	.51
Changes in work activities due to health	57	37	<.001

Source: Ref. 28.
[a]Effect of health on functioning.

nomic implications of various practice patterns. Given the constraint of resources, the most costly care must be allocated to the patients that are more likely to benefit most from the therapy. Indiscriminate use of costly procedures no longer has its place in health care systems facing shrinking budgets (31).

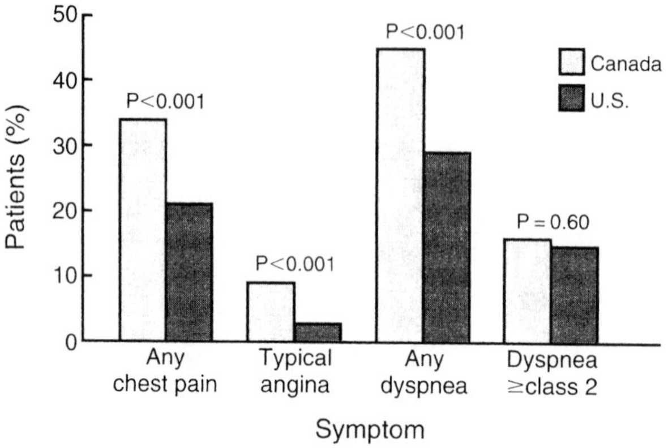

Figure 4 Status of cardiac symptoms at 1 year in a random sample of Canadian (n = 400) and U.S. (n = 2600) patients who were randomized in the GUSTO I trial. (From Ref. 28.)

Limitations of Studies of Geographic Variations

Even though the results of geographic variation studies agree with the results of randomized clinical trials, problems arise when studies use secondary analyses of large databases to study geographic variation and make inferences on the effects of practice patterns on infrequent outcomes such as mortality. The problems relate to the nonrandomized nature of the treatment allocation, the lack of statistical power afforded by the few endpoint events, and the absence of long-term follow-up; these difficulties create obstacles to making conclusive statements about the impact of variations on outcome.

Nonrandomized Nature of Treatment Allocation

In studies of geographic variations, patients are not randomized to one system of care or another. Consequently, statistical analyses cannot adjust for unknown differences in severity of disease or other clinical variables. Subgroup analyses may allow the identification of groups that are more comparable and less subject to inadequate control for differences in severity of illness. For example, a study by Holmes et al. revealed favorable outcomes as a result of an aggressive approach in a subset of GUSTO I patients who had acute MI complicated by cardiogenic shock (32). The more aggressive treatment of U.S. patients with this complication resulted in better outcome compared with the more conservative approach in non-U.S. patients; the 1-year survival cumulative incidences were 44% in the United States and 30% elsewhere. In a subgroup of patients with a similar severity of illness, an aggressive approach was beneficial. Perhaps the inability to adjust for severity of illness in a large group of patients, as seen in previous studies, explains the lack of impact of an aggressive approach to the treatment of acute MI on mortality. Subgroup analyses, such as the one by Holmes, allow the identification of groups that are more comparable. In this particular case, they allowed the identification of high-risk groups that are more likely to benefit from an aggressive approach.

Lack of Statistical Power to Make Inferences on Mortality Rate Differences

Another problem with linking outcome to differences in practice patterns is that in cardiovascular care, outcomes of major importance—such as mortality—are relatively rare. Thus, large sample sizes are necessary to improve the precision of the estimates of effect. Most studies of geographic comparisons are too small; thus, the lack of differences in mortality and reinfarction incidences may be due to a lack of statistical power. In looking more closely at the 1-year mortality incidence across regions of the United States, New England had the lowest rates of revascularization at 1 year but had one of the highest cumulative incidence of mortality. The difference between the highest and the lowest was not statistically significant, but a larger study might have confirmed a statistically significant difference in the cumulative incidence of mortality.

Unavailability of Long-Term Follow-Up

Finally, the absence of long-term follow-up in most studies is an issue that prevents definitive conclusions about the effectiveness of various intensities of care. Most studies comparing practice patterns do not have data exceeding 1 year of follow-up. Although data consistently show a lack of differences in in-hospital mortality and reinfarction 1-year cumulative incidences, trends in some studies hint at a superior survival rate in patients treated aggressively. For example, Mark et al. reported a slightly higher 1-year survival in the sample of U.S. patients compared with Canadian patients ($P = .02$); this difference was not present at 30 days (28). Perhaps, longer-term follow-up would uncover greater differences in survival according to aggressiveness of use of invasive cardiac procedures. Thus, larger numbers of patients and longer-term follow-up are the only way of verifying whether variations in intensity of care of patients with acute MI has any effect on clinical outcomes such as mortality.

Determinants of the Use of Cardiac Procedures

Wide variations in patterns of care raise questions about the reasons for differing methods of treating patients (Table 6). A number of hypotheses

Table 6 Potential Reasons for Variations in Diagnostic and Therapeutic Cardiac Procedures

Environmental factors	Physician factors	Patient factors
Medical insurance status (fee for service vs. managed care)	Medical uncertainty	Patient preference
Availability of needed procedure	Specialist vs. generalist	Demographics
Proximity of medical centers with appropriate expertise	Physician's skills	Severity of illness
	Inappropriate use	Patient attitude toward disease
	Physician's beliefs and interpretation of medical evidence	Heterogeneity of disease expression
		Illness and medical care

could explain the observed variations in management of acute myocardial infarction (33). Physicians may remain uncertain about how well clinical guidelines or the findings of a study apply to their patients. The interpretation and applications of the information may be affected by the presence of leading medical centers in a given region or by the ratio of specialists to generalists (34,35). Physician testing patterns and attitudes and patient preferences may vary across regions, thus affecting treatment selections. Inappropriate use of cardiac procedures may be responsible for some of the variation (36). Finally, nonclinical factors, including the patient's insurance status and state regulations, may influence the decision-making process (37). These wide variations question whether evidence-based medicine is widely and strictly practiced. Thus, the determinants of the use of cardiac procedures and the influences on physicians' behavior need to be identified in order to promote the practice of medicine that is evidence based.

Another study used the GUSTO I database to identify the variables that best predict angiography and revascularization use (38). Among 21,772 U.S. patients in GUSTO I, 71% underwent angiography before hospital discharge. Of these, 58% underwent revascularization and 73% underwent angioplasty. Age divided the group according to the use of angiography (Fig. 5); only 53% of patients aged at least 73 years underwent angiography, compared with 76% of patients <73 years of age. In older patients, age was again most predictive; in younger patients, the availability of angioplasty was a stronger predictor (67% of patients at sites without angioplasty received angiography, vs. 83% at sites with angioplasty). The next-most-important predictor was recurrent ischemia, a more powerful predictor at sites without angioplasty than at sites with angioplasty.

Both models of revascularization use and type identified coronary anatomy as the most predictive variable (Fig. 6). Based on this analysis in the

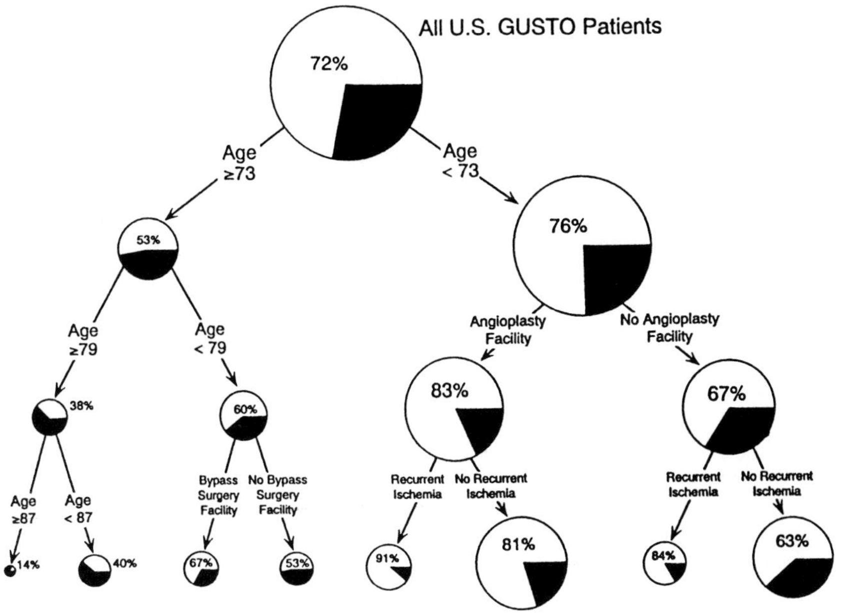

Figure 5 Classification and regression tree model showing the variables that discriminate between subgroups according to their likelihood of undergoing angiography after thrombolysis for acute myocardial infarction. The white area of the pie chart represents the percent use of angiography; the overall area indicates the sample size of the subgroup relative to the total population. (From Ref. 38.)

United States, younger age and availability of procedures appear to be the major determinants of angiography, while coronary anatomy largely drives the use and type of revascularization. In other patient populations, on-site availability of angiography facilities has been shown to be a major determinant of the use of cardiac procedures as well (39,40). This process of being more aggressive in young patients without complication after acute MI tends to select low-risk patients for a cardiac procedure rather than higher-risk patients, who would most likely benefit from a given procedure.

Finally, a survey of 332 U.S. and 200 Canadian physicians involved in the GUSTO I trial investigated the physicians' decision making regarding procedure use (41). As expected, American physicians were found to recommend coronary angiography after uncomplicated MI significantly more. Cardiac procedures were more available in the United States both in terms of access and waiting for procedures. American physicians rated more highly the importance of patient requests, malpractice, and insurance coverage as

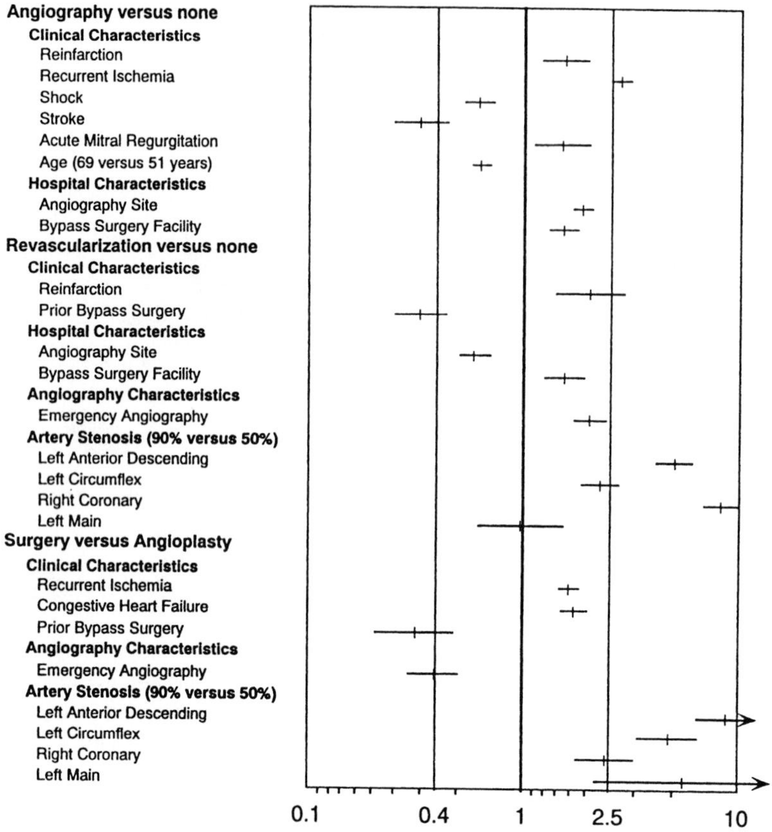

Figure 6 Odds ratios with the 95% confidence intervals for factors influencing angiography use and the use and type of revascularization before hospital discharge in the U.S. GUSTO I patients with acute MI. To the left of odds ratio, a cardiac procedure is less likely; to the right it is more likely. (From Ref. 38.)

influencing clinical decisions; Canadian physicians rated more highly availability of cardiac procedures. Thus, although the practice environment partially explains physicians' behavior, American and Canadian physicians appear to have different conceptions of what care is appropriate.

CONCLUSION

The treatment of acute MI has been the subject of many randomized clinical trials. Despite extensive data on the relative efficacies of the various therapies, extensive regional and international practice variations exist in the treatment of this condition. These geographic variations are not related to severity of illness or clinical presentation. Several studies have failed to relate a more aggressive approach to the treatment of acute MI to a reduction in mortality compared with a more conservative approach; however, the available data suggest that the quality of life of patients treated aggressively is superior to the quality of life of patients treated conservatively. Nonclinical factors, such as availability of cardiac procedures, appear to be a major determinant of the use of these procedures. Such variations in the treatment of a clinical condition suggest that certain patterns of care for MI patients are inappropriate and might lead to outcomes not commensurate to medical expenses. These variations may also suggest that limited resources may restrict access to cardiac procedures, and that might have a negative impact on the quality of life of patients with acute MI. The extent of cardiac procedures that will optimize outcomes, including mortality and quality of life, at the lowest level of resource use has yet to be identified.

REFERENCES

1. TIMI Study Group. Comparison of invasive and conservative strategies after treatment with intravenous tissue plasminogen activator in acute myocardial infarction. Results of the thrombolysis in myocardial infarction (TIMI) Phase II trial. N Engl J Med 1989;320:618–627.
2. Williams DO, Braunwald E, Knatterud G, et al. One-year results of the Thrombolysis in Myocardial Infarction Investigation (TIMI) Phase II trial. Circulation 1992;85:533–542.
3. SWIFT Trial Study Group. SWIFT trial of delayed elective intervention vs conservative treatment after thrombolysis with anistreplase in acute myocardial infarction. Br Med J 1991;302:555–560.
4. Ellis SG, Mooney MR, George BS, et al. Randomized trial of late elective angioplasty versus conservative treatment for patients with residual stenosis after thrombolytic treatment of myocardial infarction. Circulation 1992;86: 1400–1406.
5. Barbash GI, Roth A, Hod H, et al. Randomized controlled trial of late in-hospital angiography and angioplasty versus conservative treatment after treatment with recombinant tissue-type plasminogen activator in acute myocardial infarction. Am J Cardiol 1990;66:538–545.
6. Topol EJ, Holmes DR, Rogers WJ. Coronary angiography after thrombolytic therapy for acute myocardial infarction. Ann Intern Med 1991;114:877–885.
7. Rogers WJ, Baim DS, Gore JM, et al. Comparison of immediate invasive, delayed invasive, and conservative strategies after tissue-type plasminogen activator. Results of the Thrombolysis in Myocardial Infarction (TIMI) Phase II-A trial. Circulation 1990;81:1457–1476.

8. Simoons ML, Arnold AE, Betriu A, et al. Thrombolysis with tissue plasminogen activator in acute myocardial infarction: no additional benefit from immediate percutaneous coronary angioplasty. Lancet 1988;i:197–202.
9. Topol EJ, Califf RM, George BS, et al. A randomized trial of immediate versus delayed elective angioplasty after intravenous tissue plasminogen activator in acute myocardial infarction. N Engl J Med 1987;317:581–588.
10. Califf RM, Topol EJ, Stack RS, et al. Evaluation of combination thrombolytic therapy and timing of cardiac catheterization in acute myocardial infarction. Results of Thrombolysis and Angioplasty in Myocardial Infarction Phase 5 randomized trial. Circulation 1991;83:1543–1556.
11. Gunnar RM, Bourdillon PD, Dixon DW, et al. ACC/AHA guidelines for the early treatment of patients with acute myocardial infarction. Circulation 1990; 82:664–707.
12. Guidelines for coronary angiography: a report of the American College of Cardiology/American Heart Association Task Force on assessment of diagnostic and therapeutic cardiovascular procedures. Circulation 1987;76:963A–977A.
13. Rouleau JL, Moye LA, Pfeffer MA, Arnold JM, Bernstein V, Cuddy TE. A comparison of treatment patterns after acute myocardial infarction in Canada and the United States. N Engl J Med 1993;328:779–784.
14. Pilote L, Racine N, Hlatky MA. Treatment of acute myocardial infarction in the United States and Canada: a comparison of two university hospitals. Arch Intern Med 1994;154:1090–1096.
15. GUSTO Investigators. An international randomized trial comparing four thrombolytic strategies for acute myocardial infarction. N Engl J Med 1993;329: 673–682.
16. Van de Werf F, Topol EJ, Lee KL, et al. Variations in patient treatment and outcomes for acute myocardial infarction in the United States and other countries. Results from the GUSTO trial. JAMA 1995;273:1586–1591.
17. Batchelor WB, Peterson ED, Mark DB, Knight JD, Granger CB, Armstrong PW, Califf RM. A comparison of US and Canadian cardiac catheterization practices in detecting severe coronary artery disease after myocardial infarction: efficiency, yield, and long-term implications. J Am Coll Cardiol 1999;34: 12–19.
18. Tu JV, Pashos CL, Naylor CD, Chen E, Normand SL, Newhouse JP, McNeil BJ. Use of cardiac procedures and outcomes in elderly patients with myocardial infarction in the United States and Canada. N Engl J Med 1997;337:1008–1009.
19. Pilote, L, Lavoie F, Saynina O, Eisenberg M, McClellan M. Procedures and outcomes for the treatment of the elderly with acute myocardial infarction in the United States and Canada between 1988 and 1994. Circulation 1998;98:I-195. Abstract.
20. Heller RF, O'Connell RL, Lim LI, Atallah A, Lanas F, Joshi P, Tatsanavivat P. Variation in stated management of acute myocardial infarction in five countries. Int J Cardiol 1999;68:63–67.

21. Pilote L, Califf RM, Sapp S, et al. Regional variation across the United States in the treatment of acute myocardial infarction. N Engl J Med 1995;333:565–572.
22. Beta-Blocker Heart Attack Trial Research Group. A randomized trial of propranolol in patients with acute myocardial infarction. Mortality results. JAMA 1982;247:1707–1714.
23. Garg R, Yusuf S, for the Collaborative Group on ACE Inhibitor Trials. Overview of randomized trials of angiotensin-converting enzyme inhibitors on mortality and morbidity in patients with heart failure. JAMA 1995;273:1450–1456.
24. Guadagnoli E, Hauptman PJ, Ayanian JZ, Pashos CL, McNeil BJ, Cleary PD. Variation in the use of cardiac procedures after acute myocardial infarction. N Engl J Med 1995;333:573–578.
25. Selby JV, Fireman DH, Lunstrom R, et al. Variation among hospitals in coronary angiography practices and outcomes after myocardial infarction in a large health maintenance organization. N Engl J Med 1996;335:1888–1895.
26. Connors AF Jr, Speroff T, Dawson NV, et al. The effectiveness of right heart catheterization in the initial care of critically ill patients. JAMA 1996;276:889–897.
27. O'Connor GT, Quinton HB, Traven NH, Ramunno LD, Dodds TA, Marciniak TW, Wennberg JE. Geographic variation in the treatment of acute myocardial infarction: the Cooperative Cardiovascular Project. JAMA 1999;281:627–633.
28. Mark DB, Naylor CD, Hlatky MA, et al. Medical resource and quality of life outcomes following acute myocardial infarction in Canada versus the United States: the Canadian-U.S. GUSTO substudy. N Engl J Med 1994;331:1130–1135.
29. Pilote L, Bourassa MG, Bacon C, Hlatky MA. Better functional status in American than in Canadian patients after myocardial infarction: an effect of medical care? J Am Coll Cardiol 1995;26:1115–1120.
30. Naylor CD, Guyatt GH, for the Evidence-Based Medicine Working Group. User's guide to the medical literature. X. How to use an article reporting variations in the outcomes of health services. JAMA 1996;275:554–559.
31. Eisenstein EL, Newby KL, Pilote L, Peterson ED. Do regional differences in invasive cardiac procedure rates drive costs of care for the acute myocardial infarction patient? Circulation 1996;94:I-506. Abstract.
32. Holmes DR, Califf RM, Van de Werf F, et al. Differences in countries' use of resources and clinical outcome for patients with cardiogenic shock after myocardial infarction: results from the GUSTO trial. Lancet 1997;349:75–78.
33. Detsky AS. Regional variation in medical care. N Engl J Med 1995;333:589–590.
34. Ayanian JZ, Hauptman PJ, Guadagnoli E, Antman EM, Pashos CL, McNeil BJ. Knowledge and practices of generalist and specialist physicians regarding drug therapy for acute myocardial infarction. N Engl J Med 1994;331:1136–1142.
35. Jollis JG, Delong ER, Peterson ED, et al. Outcome of acute myocardial infarction according to the specialty of the admitting physician. N Engl J Med 1996;335:1880–1887.

36. Leape LL, Park RE, Solomon DH, Chassin MR, Kosecoff J, Brook RH. Does inappropriate use explain small-area variations in the use of health care services? JAMA 1990;263:669–672.
37. Wenneker MB, Weissman JS, Epstein AM. The association of payer with utilization of cardiac procedures in Massachusetts. JAMA 1990;264:1255–1260.
38. Pilote L, Miller DP, Califf RM, Rao JS, Weaver WD, Topol EJ. Determinants of use of coronary angiography and revascularization after thrombolysis for acute myocardial infarction in the United States. N Engl J Med 1996;335: 1198–1205.
39. Every NR, Larson EB, Litwin PE, et al. The association between on-site cardiac catheterization facilities and the utilization of coronary angiography after acute myocardial infarction. N Engl J Med 1993;329:546–551.
40. Blustein J. High technology cardiac procedures: the impact of service availability on service utilization in New York State. JAMA 1993;270:344–349.
41. Pilote L, Granger C, Armstrong PW, Mark DB, Hlatky MA. Differences in the treatment of acute myocardial infarction in the United States and Canada: a physician's survey. Med Care 1995;33:598–610.

27

Quality of Coronary Disease Report Cards

David E. Kandzari and James G. Jollis
Duke University Medical Center and
Duke Clinical Research Institute
Durham, North Carolina

We know how to measure quality. . . . This is not a knowledge problem. We simply haven't decided we want to expand the necessary resources and political will.

Mark Chassin, former health commissioner of New York State
Wall Street Journal, Oct. 24, 1996, p. R18

INTRODUCTION

The shift of the U.S. health care system to capitated insurance has provided only a partial solution to rising medical costs. While managed care organizations have lowered costs through limits on utilization and negotiation of lower prices, no system is in place to assure that health care quality does not suffer as a result of the lower costs. This critical need for information about quality, as well as dramatic advances in computerized data, techniques with which to make balanced comparisons among these data, and electronic media have ushered in the "report card era." Beginning with publicly reported comparisons of hospital mortality by the Health Care Financing Administration in 1986, a precedent was established whereby medical care providers are scrutinized according to their outcomes. A large number of reports have focused on cardiology, including the New York State Cardiac Surgery and Coronary Angioplasty Reporting Systems, the Pennsylvania Health Care Cost Containment Council's Focus on Heart Attack and Hospital Performance Report, the California Hospital Outcomes Project, and the Health Care Financing Administration Cooperative Cardiovascular Project (CCP) (1–6).

Most recently, physician and hospital specific ratings are becoming a prominent feature of the internet through sites such as HealthGrades.com and Healthscope.org. With the presentation of these "report cards," interest has intensified among patients, providers, payers, and the general public concerning the validity and implications of such comparisons. Differences between providers identified in current outcome reports can be attributed to at least three factors, differences in the illness severity of patients, differences in the quality and technical abilities of providers, and chance variation. The ideal outcomes system will take into account both illness severity and chance variation, such that providers identified as "outliers" represent better or worse practice. This chapter will examine how close current outcomes systems come to this ideal, and identify areas for future improvement to cardiac report cards that will enable them to reliably identify best practice.

MEASURES OF QUALITY

Outcomes comparisons can be viewed as one of at least three perspectives by which to measure quality. Other methods by which to gauge quality include structural measures (e.g., physician credentials and the availability of specialized services) and process measures (e.g., use of medications associated with better outcomes in clinical trials). The inference of systems that measure structure and process is that adherence to such standards will lead to improved outcomes for patients. Measuring quality of care according to outcomes represents the most difficult and resource-intensive approach of these alternatives.

AMI REPORT CARDS

Three of the most notable regional acute myocardial infarction (AMI) report cards are the Pennsylvania "Focus on Heart Attack" and Hospital Performance Report, the California Hospital Outcomes Project, and the Cooperative Cardiovascular Project. The Pennsylvania and California systems focus on outcomes, while the CCP measures process of care. With the public release of the Pennsylvania and California studies, they are designed to serve as a type of "consumer's report," comparing hospitals, and in the case of Pennsylvania, physicians across the states. A typical report involves a listing of hospitals or physicians by region, followed by some indication of whether the outcome measure lies outside of the predicted normal range. The Pennsylvania report provides details regarding actual, expected, and risk-adjusted rates of death with confidence intervals, and additional comparisons according to costs and length of hospital stay (Table 1). The California report rates hospitals according to two different risk models, flagging hospitals for which 30-day death rates are felt to represent outliers. The California study also published the comments of hospitals and medical staffs regarding the limitations of the study with respect to their specific institution. Both reports include descriptions targeted to the public concerning the potential uses and limitations of the outcomes comparisons. The CCP involved elderly Medicare patients treated in 1994 and 1995 in all 50 states, and the findings were presented to individual hospitals through state peer review organizations. Process "indicators" such as use of thrombolytic therapy or beta-blockers for the individual hospitals were compared to regional rates of use, and hospitals were asked to respond with a plan to address any one deficiency identified by the CCP data.

REVASCULARIZATION REPORT CARDS

A number of report cards focus on coronary revascularization, a key procedure in the treatment of acute coronary syndromes. The prototypical regional angioplasty scorecard is the New York State Coronary Angioplasty Reporting System (Fig. 1). Beginning in 1991, all hospitals performing angioplasty in the state were required to provide demographic, illness severity, complication, and outcome data concerning all procedures. Each year, the health department publishes a brochure that contains hospital specific outcome information including number of procedures and deaths, as well as expected and risk-adjusted mortality rates with confidence intervals. As comparisons according to mortality are difficult due to the low death rate associated with coronary angioplasty, future reports will also include a more frequent outcome, procedural myocardial infarction, by requiring the reporting of creatine-phosphokinase MB levels.

OUTCOMES COMPARISONS

The fundamental issue regarding outcomes reporting involves balancing comparisons, or "leveling the playing field." By using mathematical models to account for differences between patients and hospitals, report cards attempt to provide a control group by which outcomes can be compared. Issues regarding data collection as well as model derivation can have substantial influence on outcome estimates. Report cards need to be considered

Table 1 Pennsylvania Hospital Performance Report 1999

SOUTHWESTERN HOSPITALS	Heart Attack				Heart Failure and Shock				Major Vessel Operations Except Heart	
	CASES	Risk-adjusted MORTALITY	Risk-adjusted LENGTH OF STAY	Average CHARGE	CASES	Risk-adjusted MORTALITY	Risk-adjusted LENGTH OF STAY	Average CHARGE	CASES	Risk-adjusted MORTALITY
AUMC - Allegheny Valley	276	⊙	7.7	$15,370	464	●	5.8	$9,962	10	⊙
AUMC - Canonsburg	96	⊙	5.7	$10,301	177	⊙	5.1	$8,717	0	
Allegheny General	393	⊙	5.7	$16,490	463	⊙	5.8	$12,288	312	●
Armstrong County Memorial	163	⊙	6.4	$9,755	348	⊙	5.3	$6,409	11	⊙
Brownsville General	73	⊙	8.4	$9,341	187	⊙	7.0	$7,830	0	
Butler Memorial	226	⊙	5.6	$11,714	381	⊙	5.4	$8,474	26	⊙
Children's - Pittsburgh	2	**Not	Rated		8	⊙	6.7	$8,683	46	⊙
Citizens General	196	⊙	6.7	$13,116	389	⊙	5.5	$9,248	9	⊙
Forbes Regional	337	⊙	6.6	$11,314	666	⊙	5.9	$8,424	26	⊙
Frick	176	⊙	7.2	$10,650	444	⊙	6.3	$7,540	5	⊙
Greene County Memorial	51	⊙	3.8	$7,040	145	⊙	3.8	$5,572	0	
Highlands	63	⊙	5.0	$8,325	137	⊙	5.5	$8,261	0	
Jeannette District Memorial	127	⊙	6.8	$9,306	319	⊙	5.6	$7,204	6	**Not Rated
Jefferson	381	⊙	6.5	$11,000	722	⊙	5.0	$7,151	66	○
Latrobe Area	333	⊙	6.2	$13,815	647	⊙	4.9	$8,450	32	⊙
Magee-Womens	0				2	**Not	Rated		1	**Not Rated
McKeesport	202	⊙	8.0	$15,205	438	⊙	6.7	$9,928	12	⊙
Medical Center - Beaver	181	⊙	7.2	$13,425	668	⊙	6.0	$8,305	86	⊙
Mercy - Providence	34	⊙	8.5	$15,335	161	○	6.6	$9,365	3	**Not Rated
Monongahela Valley	227	⊙	8.3	$13,591	529	⊙	6.3	$10,293	33	⊙

Major Vessel Operations Except Heart: the Risk-adjusted LENGTH OF STAY and Average CHARGE columns are headed but contain no entries.

● Mortality significantly greater than Expected
⊙ Mortality not significantly different than Expected
○ Mortality significantly less than Expected
* Did not submit required data
** Had fewer than five cases evaluated

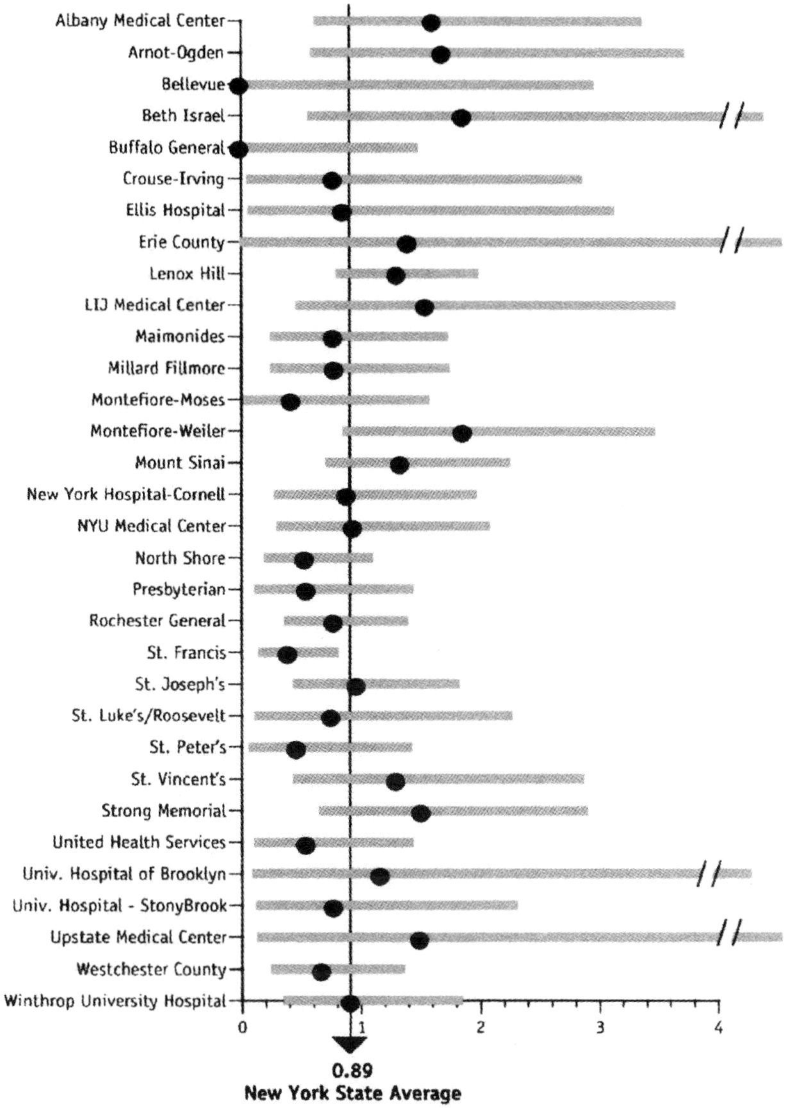

Figure 1 Risk-adjusted mortality rates and related confidence intervals by hospital for angioplasty in New York State (1995, all cases). ● = Risk-adjusted mortality rate, 1995; gray bar = potential margin of statistical error.

according to their methodology in order to understand the validity of their findings.

Insurance Claims Data

Most regional outcomes reporting systems rely on insurance claims data in some part to identify patients, adjust for illness severity, or determine outcome. The typical elements of insurance claims include patient identifiers, dates, diagnoses, procedures, charges, and discharge status. Diagnoses are coded according to the *International Classification of Diseases* (ICD) system, and procedures may be coded according to either the ICD system, or Current Procedural Terminology codes (7,8). This coding system may be used to derive Diagnosis-Related Groups (DRG), an illness classification system adopted and modified by the federal government for standard health care billing and reporting. The advantages of insurance claims include their routine collection in a computerized format, and their geographically dispersed, population-based samples. Using patient identifiers and dates, longitudinal records of patient care can be constructed. In fee-for-service health care systems, patient bills are often the only available source of information to identify patients who underwent procedures of interest or were hospitalized with conditions of interest. For the Pennsylvania Focus on Heart Attack and Hospital Performance Report, the Cooperative Cardiovascular Project, HealthGrades.com Hospital Report Cards and the California Hospital Outcomes Project, patients for study were identified by hospital claims.

Comorbidity Versus Complication

As insurance claims are generated for the purpose of determining reimbursement rather than risk adjustment, they have many limitations in outcomes comparisons. The greatest limitation involves the difficulty in distinguishing comorbid conditions from complications among claims diagnoses. For example, conditions such as congestive heart failure or cardiogenic shock may represent illnesses present on admission, or "predictors," or they may be the result of a complication that occurred during hospitalization, or "postdictors." While a number of approaches have attempted to separate complications from comorbidities, there is no reliable way to entirely distinguish between these two entities. By considering complications to represent comorbidities in outcomes comparisons, hospitals and physicians may be given "credit" for complications and assigned a lower mortality estimate. Thus, problems with quality apparent in unadjusted data may be obscured by risk adjustment. The inclusion of complications in risk adjustment models will also enhance the apparent performance characteristics of these models, as they reinforce the tautology that "patients with the most complications have the most complications."

Other Claims Data Limitations

Other significant limitations of insurance claims data in risk adjustment have been previously documented (9–11). These include the lack of definitions, undercoding of many conditions, biases in coding such that diagnoses that increase compensation are more likely to be coded and chronic conditions in acutely ill patients are less likely to be coded, and inadequate surveillance of accuracy. Potential approaches to the proper use of claims data include the recognition of these limitations and a focus on claims data elements that are most likely to be reliable such as age, gender, the performance of higher priced procedures, and mortality (12).

Two studies that use claims data to identify acute myocardial infarction patients potentially fail to include a substantial portion of complicated patients. Both the CCP and Pennsylvania Focus on Heart Attack rely on a principal diagnosis of acute myocardial infarction to identify patients. Patients who were assigned a principal diagnosis involving a complication of acute myocardial infarction such as cardiogenic shock or papillary muscle rupture were excluded from these studies. Using the Medicare database as a reference, we found that patients with complications of acute myocardial infarction listed as the principal diagnosis represented an additional 21% of patients with 28% in-hospital mortality compared to the 14% mortality for patients identified according to a principal diagnosis acute myocardial infarction alone. By excluding these complicated patients, both systems miss the opportunity to identify outcome differences among a high-risk group of patients. Studies using claims data to identify acute myocardial infarction patients should be broadened to include such patients with complications.

Other Data Sources

In an effort to overcome the limitations of insurance claims data, a number of outcomes systems obtain patient data from additional sources. For the New York State Cardiac Surgery and Coronary Angioplasty Reporting Systems, each hospital submits data to the Health Department following all coronary revascularization procedures according to a standard data collection form that includes definitions of each data element. In Pennsylvania, hospitals are required to submit data according to the MediQual System, a proprietary chart review system that measures illness severity according to the presence of a number of key clinical findings. For the Cooperative Cardiovascular Project, contracted chart abstracters extracted >200 data elements from medical charts. While additional data collection requires substantial resources, the improved data concerning illness severity allow more balanced and meaningful comparisons among patients, hospitals, and physicians that would not be possible with claims data alone.

Report card systems that collect additional data represent a substantial improvement over systems that rely on claims data alone, but they still have some limitations. The MediQual system shares the same limitation as claims data in distinguishing comorbidities from complications. While the exact methodology is not publicly available, the MediQual system assigns an Admission Severity Group among five levels of risk (0–4), and is based on 23 key clinical findings involving vital signs, physical examination, and laboratory studies identified by chart review. Reviewers are instructed to select the most abnormal value during the first 48 hours of hospitalization, and missing variables are considered to be normal by default. By assigning the most abnormal value during the 48-hour review period, complications may potentially be considered comorbidities. For example, low systolic blood pressure or mechanical ventilation that is the result of complications within the first 48 hours would be included in Admission Severity Group calculation, attributing higher risk to the patient "on admission." Other systems for risk adjustment such as All Patient Refined Diagnosis Related Groups used by many insurers and hospitals share the same difficulty in distinguishing comorbidities and complications (13). To overcome the problem of confusing complications for comorbidities as noted above, illness severity indicators in the MediQual system should be limited to those present on admission, and data elements that may represent complications should be excluded from risk adjustment models whenever possible.

Potential for Gaming

A limitation of any system that relies on self-reporting, such as the New York system, insurance claims, and catheterization laboratory databases, is the potential for "gaming." Gaming is defined as the specification of risk factors to achieve the highest estimate of expected mortality. In the case of New York, the prevalence of a number of risk factors increased substantially since the initial public release of provider-specific outcomes (14). Risk factors that are most susceptible to manipulation involve elements that are subjective, or involve broad definitions such as angina class or urgent procedure (15). To the extent that "gaming" encourages more complete specification of risk, comparisons among providers will improve. However, gaming also carries great potential to skew risk estimates for individual providers. There are a number of approaches to minimize the potential for gaming to confound comparisons.

First, whenever possible, risk adjustment models should focus on objective measures of severity. For example, "admission systolic blood pressure" may represent a more objective measure of circulatory state than "cardiogenic shock." Second, precise definitions of risk factors should be specified to the extent possible. Third, risk models should be periodically recalculated on more recent data. Risk factors that become overly reported by all providers will fall in prognostic importance. Fourth, some level of independent data auditing should be routinely applied to all outcomes systems. In addition to identifying potential discrepancies, the "Hawthorne effect" of such an audit is likely to encourage accurate risk factor specification among all providers. In the case of New York, hospitals that were felt to have inaccurately reported procedural data according to independent audit were requested to resubmit their data in a corrected format.

Missing Data

Missing data is a common occurrence among all of the current scorecard systems. Systems that use MediQual consider missing data to be within normal limits, while systems that rely on insurance claims consider missing diagnoses to signify the absence of such a diagnosis. Risk may be improperly assigned if the biases that led to missing data are also related to the outcome of interest. For example, in MediQual, ejection fraction may be missing for patients who do not survive long enough to undergo ventricular function measurement, and such patients would be expected to have lower ejection fractions on average, rather than the value of 70% assigned by the system (3,16). For claims data, conditions such as hypertension have been found to be associated with lower mortality, a finding that runs counter to clinical intuition (17). It has been postulated that chronic conditions are associated with lower mortality because they are less likely to be coded for severely ill patients.

To improve risk adjustment, missing data may be accounted for in a number of ways. Characteristics that are missing for a substantial number of patients should be excluded from risk adjustment models. From a statistical approach, missing information can sometimes be imputed from other available data. For example, estimating left ventricular ejection fraction based on other measures of the circulatory state such a Killip class, infarct location, or systolic blood pressure may result in a less biased risk estimate than assuming ejection fraction to be normal. The reliability of insurance claims in identifying a particular disease can be determined by examining a sample of claims for which more detailed clinical data are available. Previous work has shown that more severe illnesses such as acute myocardial infarction and diabetes were more likely to be identified, while other diagnoses such as tobacco use disorder were less reliable (18). Finally, routine data checks can be used to identify missing data elements at the point of collection, possibly serving to target efforts at improved collection of such missing items.

"Small-Numbers Problem": Low-Volume Providers

Report cards are limited in their ability to reliably identify quality of care in the setting of a small number of outcomes. This situation arises for conditions in which outcomes are rare such as death following angioplasty, or situations where providers are infrequently involved with the condition of interest as in the case of low-volume angioplasty operators. Due to small numbers, outcomes estimates have wide confidence intervals.

The issue of small numbers takes on particular significance in the debate about angioplasty volume guidelines. In the United States, it is estimated that approximately one-half of physicians and one-quarter of hospitals performing coronary angioplasty fail to meet the volume limits proposed by expert panels. There is also an increasing amount of data from regional and national studies to suggest that patients treated by low-volume operators have worse outcomes. Studies involving California, Medicare, New York State, and Society for Coronary Angiography and Intervention have found higher rates of bypass surgery and death for low-volume hospitals, and studies from New York State, northern New England, Medicare, and an academic registry have found worse outcomes for low-volume physicians (19–25). However, a few reports have failed to find such a relationship regarding physician volume (20,27).

These latter studies were less likely to identify a volume relationship, as they involved relatively few low-volume physicians and were conducted in relatively high-volume hospitals. While the majority of evidence indicates that low-volume physicians and hospitals are associated with worse outcomes *on average*, some of these low-volume operators have mortality and complication rates that are better than the average. The argument against volume limits is that they potentially restrict high-quality, low-volume operators from practice. Opponents of volume limits believe that individual operators should be judged on the basis of their outcomes, rather than strict volume limits. Proponents of volume limits note that the absence of proof of a difference (outlier status) is not the same as proof of no difference. As low-volume operators have worse outcomes on average, and quality low-volume operators are difficult to identify due to wide confidence intervals around individual outcome estimates, they believe that adherence to a process measure such as volume limits is the most reliable approach to assuring quality angioplasty.

In order to increase the chances of identifying quality low-volume providers, systems will need to incorporate additional outcomes that occur more frequently, can be reliably identified, and are considered to represent negative outcomes. While it is difficult to arrive at consensus as to which outcomes represent significant complications, possible endpoints include bypass surgery prior to discharge, or creatine-phosphokinase MB release as proposed for forthcoming New York angioplasty reports. Another approach to reliably identifying quality low-volume operators is to combine angioplasty experience over a number of years.

Identification of Providers

One important component of report cards involves the identification of the appropriate physician or hospital involved in a patient's care. Ideally, the physician or hospital most likely to influence a patient's outcome should be examined. In the case of a major procedure, the angioplasty operator and surgeon are compared. For acute coronary syndromes where survival may be influenced by early therapeutic decisions, the physician or hospital initially involved in patient care should be examined. Given the complex interactions among health care providers, with the potential for multiple physicians and hospitals to interact in a patient's care, the issue of identifying the responsible provider becomes confounded.

The greatest potential bias regarding provider identification involves the "Will Rogers effect," based upon the humorous comment that when people migrated from Oklahoma to California, the intelligence quotient of both states increased. In the case of report cards, certain physicians or hospitals may be more likely to be selected for complicated patients, with the potential for such providers to become associated with worse outcomes. The same bias may also overestimate the performance of providers who transfer complicated patients. Such a bias may be present in the Pennsylvania Heart Attack and Hospital Performance studies, where the patients who died after transfer to another hospital were attributed to the receiving hospital and excluded from comparisons involving the transferring hospital. Worse outcomes may have been attributed to the receiving hospital that were actually due to practice issues in the initial hospital such as failure to initiate reperfusion therapy. Thus, such a system misses the opportunity to identify hospitals in which early acute myocardial infarction treatment could be improved. In order to avoid the biases introduced by the transfer of patients, outcomes systems should include comparisons that attribute care to the earliest provider.

To identify hospitals, most systems rely on hospital identification submitted with hospital claims or mandatory hospital reports. The ideal outcomes system will link all hospitals involved in an episode of care, relying on admission and discharge dates, the admission source, and the discharge status. The identification of physicians is somewhat more difficult, partly because a given patient may receive care from a number of physicians involved in a variety of relationships including group practice, consultation, emergency department, and transfers among services. Various state systems rely on state license numbers to identify the physician associated with care. Beginning in 1992, all physicians submitting claims to Medicare were required to include their Unique Physician Identification Number (UPIN) with their bills. Given the prevalence of coronary disease in Medicare patients, most physicians treating acute coronary syndromes outside of federal and staff-model health maintenance organization hospitals participate in the UPIN system. The federal initiative to identify providers of care is being extended to physicians in training, nurse practitioners, and physician assistants according to a National Provider Identifier. For Medicare patients, there are at least two sources for physician identification. Hospital claims (Part A) identify a procedure physician and an attending physician, the latter defined as "the clinician who is primarily and largely responsible for the care of the patient from the beginning of the hospital episode" (28). All physician claims (Part B), including claims for initial hospital evaluation, consults, and procedures, identify the physician submitting the claim. When we compared admitting physician according to hospital or physician bills, we found that the two sources agreed approximately 80% of the time. When the two sources disagreed, it is likely that the physician associated with the majority of care was other than the admitting physician. As noted above, to attribute care to the provider most able to influence outcome, as well as to avoid biases involved in transfer, the earliest hospital and physician involved in an episode of care should be identified in outcomes comparisons. This may be accomplished through definitions which include the earliest provider, as well as through the use of physician and hospital bills to identify the earliest provider.

Risk Adjustment Models

There are a number of statistical approaches to making balanced comparisons. Most current report cards examine dichotomous endpoints such as the occurrence of death or a complication, and use logistic regression models to balance comparisons. Estimated outcomes are subject to wide variation, depending on a number of factors including patient and provider identification, data quality, risk factor and outcome selection, and model development. Regardless of the statistical approach, the most important element of any outcomes comparison involves the concurrent publication of the methodology involved in making the comparison. Such information allows readers to understand whether differences in outcome were due to methodological factors, differences between patients, or differences in the quality of care. Risk adjustment systems that restrict the publication of the underlying methodology represent "black boxes." Given the potential for differences in outcome to be attributable to methodology rather than quality of care, such systems cannot be used to reliably identify "best practice" in a peer-reviewed fashion. If the methodology behind comparisons cannot be released due to proprietary considerations, we believe that resources should be directed to a system that can be fully scrutinized as part of scorecard reporting.

The methodological reports accompanying the Pennsylvania Focus on Heart Attack and the California Hospital Outcomes Project represent excellent examples of the information that should be provided in order to understand scorecard comparisons. These reports included clear descriptions of inclusion and exclusion criteria, prevalence of risk factors across hospitals, unadjusted outcomes, and model derivation and performance. While there is no consensus as to the optimal measure of model performance, standard measures include discrimination, reliability, and validation.

"Discrimination" can be described according to the shape and area of the Receiver Operator Characteristic (ROC) curve, with 1 indicating perfect discrimination among all possible pairs of patients, and 0.5 indicating no discrimination. Most models yield ROC areas in the 0.70 to 0.85 range. "Reliability" refers to the ability of a model to predict outcomes that closely follow observed outcomes. This can be illustrated by dividing patients into same-size groups based on their level of estimated risk, and then comparing estimated to observed outcomes within each group. A model with excellent reliability will yield estimated outcomes that are similar to the observed outcomes. "Validation" refers to the ability of a model derived in one population to perform in a different population. Well-derived models should show similar performance among populations, while models that contain statistically spurious associations will show a decline in performance in other populations. Common approaches to validating include a split-sample approach, where the model may be derived on one-half of the population, and tested on the other half. Other approaches include "bootstrapping," a technique whereby the model is repeatedly derived on randomly selected subgroups of the original sample, and performance characteristics are estimated among these smaller samples. Finally, models may be "externally" validated by applying the model to an entirely separate population, such as patients treated in another state or at different times.

STRUCTURE AND PROCESS MEASURES: PHYSICIAN SPECIALTY AND VOLUME

A common strategy to reduce costs by managed care organizations involves limiting access to specialty care. This shift in medical care represents a fundamental alteration in structure (specialty certification) and process (specialty care). Quality of care is likely to improve to the extent that primary care physicians provide better care to an individual patient across a broad range of illnesses. Costs have fallen as primary care physicians use fewer resources (29). If specialists continue to be associated with higher costs in the era of managed care, specialty certification may no longer suffice as a measure of quality, unless such care can be shown to favorably influence outcome.

Better outcomes for specialty care are most likely to be seen with severe illnesses, such as acute coronary syndromes. The potential impact of specialty care on acute coronary syndromes has been examined in a number of studies. In a survey of 1211 physicians in Texas and New York, Ayanian and colleagues reported that family practitioners and internists were less aware of or less certain about effective and life-saving drugs in the treatment of acute myocardial infarction than cardiologists (30). As part of the Pennsylvania Focus on Heart Attack, Nash and colleagues reported that in-hospital mortality was lower for acute myocardial infarction patients cared for by cardiologists (31). After adjusting for illness severity for all 40,684 hospital admissions for acute myocardial infarction in Pennsylvania in 1993, cardiology patients had lower adjusted mortality than internal medicine patients (risk ratio 1.26, 95% confidence interval 1.17 to 1.35) or family practitioners (risk ratio 1.29, 95% confidence interval 1.18 to 1.40). The study also found improved survival for physicians who treated 12 or more myocardial infarction patients per year, regardless of specialty (32). Specialty and volume were related, as 80% of the higher-volume physicians were cardiologists.

Our study also found that Medicare patients admitted by a cardiologist were 12% more likely to survive to 1 year than those admitted by a primary care physician, after adjusting for patient and hospital characteristics ($P < .001$) (Fig. 2) (33). Patients who were admitted by a primary care physician and underwent cardiology consultation had an intermediate survival. We also identified two potential mechanisms for the better survival. Cardiology patients were more likely to be treated with medications associated with improved survival including thrombolytic therapy, beta-blockers, and aspirin. With the increased use of coronary angiography, a greater proportion of cardiology patients were identified to have left main or three-vessel coronary artery disease, and more cardiology patients went on to revascularization.

There are three possible explanations for the relationship between specialty and outcome. First, as suggested by the Ayanian and Medicare studies, specialists are more familiar with the management of acute myocardial infarction, and their treatment decisions lead to improved survival. A second

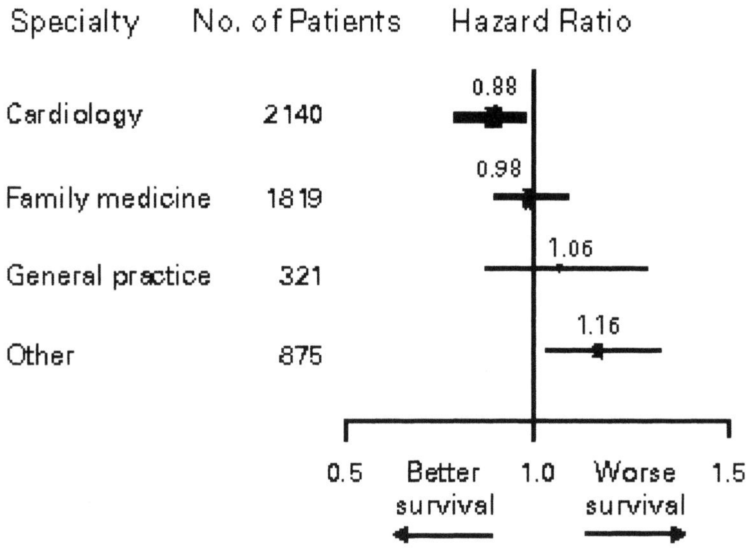

Figure 2 Hazard ratios for adjusted 1-year mortality among patients with acute myocardial infarction in the Cooperative Cardiovascular Project cohort, according to the specialty of the admitting physician. The bars indicate the 95% confidence intervals. The hazard ratios have been adjusted for indicators of severity of illness; availability of facilities for coronary angiography, angioplasty, or bypass surgery at the hospital; and urban or rural location. Patients admitted by physicians specializing in internal medicine served as the reference category. (From Ref. 31.)

explanation may be that patients cared for by specialists have better survival due to lower illness severity. While both the Pennsylvania and Medicare studies adjusted for illness severity in their mortality comparisons, it is possible that factors related to illness severity that were not measured by these observational studies led to the improved survival. A third explanation is that other factors associated with specialty care lead to better survival, such as hospitals that care for larger numbers of acute myocardial infarction patients, have emergency room physicians who are more likely to recognize acute myocardial infarctions and initiate early treatment, and have on-site resources available for the management of complications, such as coronary angioplasty or bypass surgery. For Medicare patients with acute coronary syndromes, Thiemann and colleagues showed that hospitals with more experience treating myocardial infarction, reflected by their case volume, had lower mortality than low-volume hospitals (Fig. 3). These findings persisted after consideration of physician specialty, availability of invasive procedures, clinical factors, and geographic location (34).

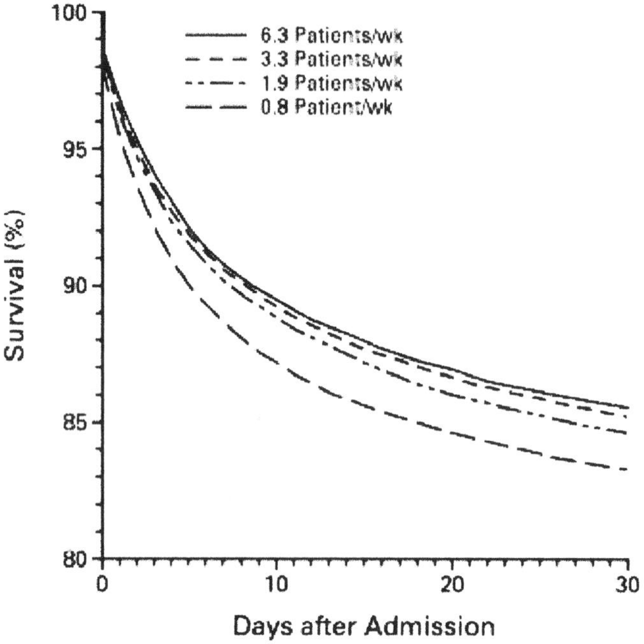

Figure 3 Kaplan-Meier 30-day survival curves according to hospital volume of Medicare patients with acute myocardial infarction. Each quartile represents the median hospital volume of Medicare patients with myocardial infarction per week. (From Ref. 34.)

INTERNET-BASED REPORT CARDS

Increased consumer interest and Internet access have sparked the emergence of web-based report cards using both structural and outcomes measures. Healthscope.org, supported by a consortium of California employers, compares hospitals, physician groups, and health plans according to consumer surveys, health maintenance organization ratings (the Health Plan Employer Data and Information Set—HEDIS), and California government reports. Viewers are presented with simple menus that provide ready access to a broad array of comparative information including patient satisfaction, waiting time to see a specialist, treatment of hyperlipidemia and hypertension, angioplasty volume, and myocardial infarction mortality comparisons (derived from the California Hospital Outcomes Project noted above).

Another Internet site that rates hospitals and physicians on a national basis is HealthGrades.com. Hospital mortality is rated on a five-star scale from "poor" to "best" according to a number of discharge diagnoses and procedures including myocardial infarction and coronary angioplasty. The methodology is similar to the initial HCFA hospital comparisons of the 1980s, using Medicare ICD-9 discharge data to identify patients and adjust for illness severity. Physicians are rated according to simple structural criteria. Physicians who have practiced for more than 2 years and have specialty board certification, the absence of Medicare or medical board sanctions, and affiliation with a hospital whose performance is rated equal to or better than predicted models are listed as "leading physicians." While the site provides a stunning array of hospital- and physician-specific data, the underlying methodology shares all of the limitations of rudimentary, insurance claims-based outcomes comparisons. As the Internet evolves and sites continue to compete for viewers of health-related "portals," the content of Internet report cards is likely to substantially improve.

DO REPORT CARDS IMPROVE OUTCOMES?

The first regional report cards involving bypass surgery were published in 1990, and a number of studies have attempted to gauge their impact according to trends in mortality following this publication. Bypass surgery mortality declined following the reporting of outcomes in New York State and northern New England, and O'Connor and Hannan have suggested that scorecarding efforts in these regions have been responsible for the improved outcomes. Peterson and colleagues also showed improved bypass surgery outcomes within New York despite an increased preoperative risk profile with elderly patients more likely to undergo revascularization since the program's initiation (35). Increased procedural access for New York Medicare patients suggested that declining early postoperative mortality rates were due to improved quality of care rather than changes in patient selection (35–37). A study by Ghali and colleagues, however, found that surgical mortality declined during the same period in Massachusetts, a state that lacked a regional scorecard. These findings suggested that the improved outcomes in New York and northern New England may have been due to factors other than outcomes reporting (38).

While the findings of declining surgical mortality in states with and without scorecard systems are intriguing, the impact of outcomes systems cannot be fully understood based on current literature. Comparisons of the relative decline in surgical mortality between regions are hampered by differences in patient population that cannot be resolved with the available data. It is likely that national trends of improved mortality are due to technical enhancements, advancement along the "learning curve," and local quality improvement efforts. Regional report cards may have also played a role in the improved outcomes. Based on their observations, Ghali suggested that outcomes systems be evaluated according to a randomized comparison, taking into account the cost of information systems relative to the measured improvement in outcome. Such randomized trials are unlikely to be conducted, and the potential benefits of measuring outcomes would be difficult to measure. Regardless of the results of such trials, scorecard systems are likely to expand for the reasons outlined above.

RATING REPORT CARDS

While this chapter highlights opportunities to improve current scorecard systems, it should be noted that all of the current outcomes systems are far superior to systems in which health care is administered without any attempt at measurement or comparison. An appropriate analogy for the latter situation is driving at night without the use of headlights; it is difficult to know where the vehicle is heading, and there is little potential to avoid hazardous situations. Keeping in mind the tenet that any outcome system is better than no outcome system, Table 2 compares representative scorecarding efforts in coronary disease. Among the current scorecard initiatives, systems that rely on risk adjustment data beyond insurance claims go a long way toward providing meaningful comparisons. Given the potential limitations of all current scorecarding efforts, their findings should only serve to direct additional study and review in identifying best practice.

FUTURE OF REPORT CARDS

With the growing demand for information about quality of care, governmental and commercial entities are likely to continue to expand efforts to compare providers. The techniques by which to make comparisons among observational data are fairly well established. As outlined above, we understand how to attribute differences in outcomes to differences in illness severity, differences in care, and chance variation. However, there are a number of obstacles to scorecarding which must be overcome before such efforts can realize their full potential in identifying best practice. The greatest impediment involves the allocation of adequate resources to properly compare outcomes. Current efforts would be greatly enhanced if additional resources were directed toward data collection and validation. Such resources are essential to obtain reliable information about patient identification, risk adjustment, and outcomes.

A second obstacle to better report cards involves the issue of patient confidentiality. As computer databases expand, there is great concern that confidential health information may be publicly released. Due to this concern, efforts such as the federal "Standards for Privacy of Individually Iden-

Table 2 Report Card of Report Cards

Scorecard	Disease or procedure	Patient identification	Risk adjustment	Outcome	Potential to consider complications as comorbidities	Grade	Comments
New York CARS CSRS	Angioplasty Bypass surgery	Hospitals	Hospital-reported data	Death, complications	—	B	Self-reported data with some potential for gaming
Cooperative Cardiovascular Project	Acute MI	Medicare hospital claims	Chart review Hospital claims	Medication use	—	B	Chart review; missing data elements not recorded in charts
Pennsylvania Focus on Heart Attack Consumers Guide to CABG and Hospital Performance Report	Acute MI Bypass surgery Heart failure	State hospital claims	MediQual Systems, Inc. Hospital claims	Death Charges Length of stay	++	B	Both hospital claims and MediQual may consider complications to represent comorbidities
California Hospital Outcomes Project	Acute MI	State hospital claims	Hospital claims	Death	+	C+	Based on hospital claims Methodology incorporates thorough consideration of strengths and weaknesses of claims data; new coding guidelines identify comorbidities with an additional digit
HealthGrades.com Hospital Report Cards and Leading Physicians	Acute MI Angioplasty Heart failure	MEDPAR Medicare hospital claims State hospital claims	Hospital claims	Death	+	D	Promotes flawed claims data adjustment abandoned by HFCA one decade earlier
Healthscope.org	Acute MI Angioplasty Evidence-based treatment patterns	State hospital claims HEDIS data	Hospital claims	Death Evidence-based treatment patterns	+	A−	Combines best available data in user-friendly format
No outcomes system	—	—	—	—	—	F	

tifiable Health Information" are under way to exclude patient identifiers from medical databases. Without patient identifiers, outcomes comparisons are severely restricted. Such identifiers are required to link episodes of care, combine data sources, and track long-term outcomes. Adequate safeguards exist, such as encryption, access barriers, and peer oversight, whereby privacy can be maintained. We believe that the potential benefit of patient identifiers in improving care far outweighs the potential risk of lost privacy.

A third obstacle involves maintaining active participation among providers to properly execute outcomes comparisons. With any comparison, a number of providers are likely to fall toward the lower end of quality measures, and the potential to be identified as such may motivate some to hinder outcomes comparisons. Over the long term, comparisons among providers will continue to expand, regardless of the willing participation of providers. Private-sector initiatives, including Internet-based services that are not subject to the political process or public scrutiny, are more likely to expand in the absence of public or physician-supported systems. We believe that the best approach to ensuring the long-term success of physicians and hospitals, as well as the best approach to improving patient care, is for physicians to collaborate fully with outcomes comparisons. The active involvement of health care providers will assure that comparisons are properly derived, permit physicians and hospitals to demonstrate their abilities to patients and health care purchasers, and allow physicians to determine best practice.

REFERENCES

1. Chassin MR, Hannan EL, DeBuono BA. Benefits and hazards of reporting medical outcomes publicly. N Engl J Med 1996;334:394–398.
2. State of New York, Department of Health Cardiac Advisory Committee, Angioplasty in New York state 1995, June 1997.
3. Focus on heart attack in Pennsylvania, the technical report. Pennsylvania Health Care Cost Containment Council, June 1996.
4. Pennsylvania Health Care Cost Containment Council. A hospital performance report: 15 common medical procedures and treatments, June 1999.
5. State of California, Office of Statewide Planning and Development, Annual report of the California hospital outcomes project. December 1993.
6. Ellerbeck EF, Jencks SF, Radford MJ, Kresowick TF, Craig AS, Gold JA, Krumholz HM, Vogel RA. Quality of care for Medicare patients with acute myocardial infarction. A four-state pilot study from the Cooperative Cardiovascular Project. JAMA 1995;273:1509–1514.
7. International Classification of Diseases, 9th Revision, Clinical Modification. Los Angeles: Practice Management Information Corp., 1991.
8. Physicians' Current Procedural Terminology 1994. Chicago: American Medical Association, 1994.

9. Jenks SF, Williams DK, Kay TL. Assessing hospital-associated deaths from discharge data. JAMA 1988;260:2240–2246.
10. Iezzoni LI, Foley SM, Daley J, Hughes J, Fisher ES, Heeren T. Comorbidities, complications, and coding bias. JAMA 1992;267:2197–2203.
11. Jollis JG, Ancukiewicz M, DeLong ER, Pryor DB, Muhlbaier LH, Mark DB. Discordance of databases designed for claims payment versus clinical information systems. Implications for outcomes research. Ann Intern Med 1993; 119:844–850.
12. Hannan EL, Kilburn H Jr, Lindsey ML, Lewis R. Clinical versus administrative databases for CABG surgery. Does it matter? Med Care 1992;30:892–907.
13. Iezzoni LI, Ash AS, Shwartz M, Daley J, Hughes JS, Mackiernan YD. Predicting who dies depends on how severity is measured: implications for evaluating patient outcomes. Ann Intern Med 1995;123:763–770.
14. Green J, Wintfeld N. Report cards on cardiac surgeons. Assessing New York State's approach. N Engl J Med 1995;332:1229–1232.
15. Ellis SG, Omoigui N, Bittl JA, Lincoff M, Wolfe MW, Howell G, Topol EJ. Analysis and comparison of operator-specific outcomes in interventional cardiology. From a multicenter database of 4860 quality-controlled procedures. Circulation 1996;93:431–439.
16. Focus on heart attack in Pennsylvania, research methods and results. Pennsylvania Health Care Cost Containment Council, April 1996.
17. Jenks, Iezzoni LI, Foley SM, Daley J, Hughes J, Fisher ES, Heeren T. Comorbidities, complications, and coding bias. JAMA 1992;267:2197–2203.
18. Jollis JG, Ancukiewicz M, DeLong ER, Pryor DB, Muhlbaier LH, Mark DB. Discordance of databases designed for claims payment versus clinical information systems. Implications for outcomes research. Ann Intern Med 1993; 119:844–850.
19. Ritchie JL, Phillips KA, Luft HS. Coronary angioplasty. Statewide experience in California. Circulation 1993;88:2735–2743.
20. Jollis JG, Peterson ED, DeLong ER, Mark DB, Collins SR, Muhlbaier LH, Pryor DB. The relationship between hospital volume of coronary angioplasty and short term mortality in patients over age 65 in the United States. N Engl J Med 1994;331:1625–1629.
21. Kimmel SE, Berlin JA, Laskey WK. The relationship between coronary angioplasty procedure volume and major complications. JAMA 1995;274:1137–1142.
22. Hannan EL, Racz M, Ryan TJ, McCallister BD, Johnson LW, Arani DT, Guerci AD, Sosa J, Topol EJ. Coronary angioplasty volume-outcome relationships for hospitals and cardiologists JAMA 1997;277:892–898.
23. McGrath PD, Wennberg DE, Malenka DJ, Kellett MA Jr, Ryan TJ Jr, O'Meara JR, Bradley WA, Hearne MJ, Hettleman B, Robb JF, Shubrooks S, VerLee P, Watkins MW, Lucas FL, O'Connor GT. Operator volume and outcomes in 12,998 percutaneous coronary interventions. Northern New England Cardiovascular Disease Study Group. J Am Coll Cardiol 1998;31:570–576.
24. Jollis JG, Peterson ED, Nelson CL, Stafford JA, DeLong ER, Muhlbaier LH, Mark DB. Relationship between physician and hospital coronary angioplasty volume and outcome in elderly patients. Circulation 1997;95:2485–2491.

25. Ellis SG, Weintraub W, Holmes D, Shaw R, Block PC, King SB 3d. Relation of operator volume and experience to procedural outcome of percutaneous coronary revascularization at hospitals with high interventional volumes. Circulation 1997;95:2479–2484.
26. Malenka DJ, McGrath PD, Wennberg DE, Ryan TJ, Kellett MA, Shubrooks SJ, Bradley WA, Hettlemen BD, Robb JF, Hearne MJ, Silver TM, Watkins MW, O'Meara JR, VerLee PN, O'Rourke DJ. The relationship between operator volume and outcomes after percutaneous coronary interventions in high volume hospitals in 1994–1996. The northern New England experience. J Am Coll Cardiol 1999;34:1471–1480.
27. Grines CI. Thrombolysis or primary angioplasty for acute myocardial infarction. N Engl J Med 1997;336:1102–1103.
28. Iezzoni LI. Data sources and implications: administrative databases. In: Iezzoni LI, ed. Risk Adjustment for Measuring Health Care Outcomes. Ann Arbor, MI: Health Administration Press, 1994:122.
29. Greenfield S, Nelson EC, Zubkoff M, et al. Variations in resource utilization among medical specialties and systems of care. JAMA 1992;267:1624–1630.
30. Ayanian JZ, Hauptman PJ, Guadagnoli E, Antman EM, Pashos CL, McNeil BJ. Knowledge and practices of generalist and specialist physicians regarding drug therapy for acute myocardial infarction. N Engl J Med 1994;331:1136–1142.
31. Nash IS, Nasy DB, Fuster V. Do cardiologists do it better? J Am Coll Cardiol 1997;29(3):475–478.
32. Casale PN, Jones JL, Wolf FE, Pei Y, Eby LM. Patients treated by cardiologists have a lower in-hospital mortality for acute myocardial infarction. J Am Coll Cardiol 1997;29(suppl A):392A.
33. Jollis JG, DeLong ER, Peterson ED, Muhlbaier LH, Fortin DF, Califf RM, Mark DB. Outcome of acute myocardial infarction according to the specialty of the admitting physician. N Engl J Med 1996;335:1880–1887.
34. Thiemann DR, Coresh J, Oetgen WJ, Powe NR. The association between hospital volume and survival after acute myocardial infarction in elderly patients. N Engl J Med 1999;340:1640–1648.
35. Peterson ED, DeLong ER, Jollis JG, Muhlbaier LH, Mark DB. The effects of New York's bypass surgery provider profiling on access to care and patient outcomes in the elderly. J Am Coll Cardiol 1998;32:993–999.
36. Hannan EL, Kilburn H, Racz M, Shields E, Chassin MR. Improving the outcomes of coronary artery bypass surgery in New York State. JAMA 1994;271:761–766.
37. O'Connor GT, Plume SK, Olmstead EM, Morton JR, Maloney CT, Nugent WC, Hernandez F, Clough R, Leavitt BJ, Coffin LH, Marrin CA, Wennberg D, Birkmeyer JD, Charlesworth DC, Malenka DJ, Quinton HB, Kasper JF. A regional intervention to improve the hospital mortality associated with coronary artery bypass graft surgery. JAMA 1996;275:841–846.
38. Ghali WA, Ash AS, Hall RE, Moskowitz MA. Statewide quality improvement initiatives and mortality after cardiac surgery. JAMA 1997;277:379–382.

28

Cost-Effectiveness of New Diagnostic Tools and Therapies for Acute Coronary Syndromes

Eric L. Eisenstein and Daniel B. Mark
Duke Clinical Research Institute
and Duke University Medical Center
Durham, North Carolina

INTRODUCTION

Three 20th-century trends have converged to create today's technology-driven health care system (1). First, increasing life expectancy (49.2 years in 1900 vs. 76.5 years in 1997 for U.S.) means that people live long enough to develop chronic diseases (2). Second, greater societal wealth permits a larger portion of society's resources to be spent on health care (3% of U.S. gross domestic product in 1900 vs. 13.6% in 1997) (1–3). And, finally, the development of medical insurance provides a large pool of funds for medical expenses (paying 0% of U.S. medical expenses in 1900 vs. 83% in 1990) (1). These trends are particularly important for ACS patients, who are typically older and whose 30-day medical costs ($17,251 in 1995) (4) are 4.7 times annual per-capita health expenditures in the United States (5).

In the past, the incremental value of new ACS therapies was not questioned. The introduction of intensive care units, external defibrillators, and CPR in the late 1950s and early 1960s reduced short-term acute MI mortality by 20% (32% to 12%) (6–9). The addition of thrombolytic and aspirin therapy in the 1980s resulted in a further 5% reduction (12% to 7%). However, reperfusion innovations (i.e., tissue plasminogen activator and direct angioplasty) of the 1990s have reduced short-term acute MI mortality by

2% at best (from 7% to 5%) (10,11). This progression illustrates the diminishing returns that accrue when new medical therapies are layered upon a mature technological infrastructure. Thus, because of past successes, the ability of new technologies to reduce short-term mortality in ACS patients will be limited and cardiologists will need to develop alternative, more sophisticated means for placing a value on the care they provide.

In this chapter, we will introduce a framework for evaluating the economic attractiveness of new medical therapies, define its elements (medical costs and health benefits) and compare different methods for their measurement. We will then use this framework to evaluate the economics of new diagnostic tools and therapies for ACS patients.

CLINICAL ECONOMICS CONCEPTS

Appraisers use one of three approaches to determine the value of financial and real assets (12,13). *Asset-based methods* estimate the costs of individual components and then sum them to arrive at a cost for the whole. *Market methods* begin with the prices of similar products then adjust for differences between the current product and its competitors. Lastly, *income methods* estimate the present value of future benefits that will be derived from investing in the product. Health economists combine elements from each approach into the cost-effectiveness ratio, used to evaluate the economic attractiveness of medical goods and services. The cost-effectiveness ratio essentially measures the costs for each additional unit of health benefit offered to patients by a new medical therapy. While most would agree that this is a fair way to evaluate medical goods and services, differences frequently arise regarding which costs and health benefits to include in the analysis as well as how to measure them.

Economic Evaluation Framework

The cost-effectiveness ratio, as shown below, compares the incremental cost per incremental unit of health benefit gained by the new therapy versus the standard of care.

$$\frac{C_{\text{New}} - C_{\text{Old}}}{E_{\text{New}} - E_{\text{Old}}}$$

where C = cost and E = effectiveness. While the theoretical time frame for assessing costs and health benefits is the patient's lifetime, this approach leads to obvious practical limitations in data collection. Thus, most economic studies measure costs and health benefits to a point at which the differences in strategies become negligible. For ACS patients, the acute period typically lasts 30 to 60 days with sequelae continuing from 6 to 12 months after which they return to a chronic CAD state (14,15). Thus, economic studies of ACS therapies typically do not measure costs beyond 1 year and assume no difference in costs between treatment strategies after that point. However, the health benefits of ACS therapies may extend well beyond 1 year and should be accounted for in the analysis.

Types of Economic Analysis

There are several possible relationships between incremental costs and incremental health benefits (Fig. 1). When a new strategy reduces health benefits in comparison to usual care, no economic analysis is performed. When there is no difference in health benefits between patient management strategies, the analysis reduces to a comparison of the difference in costs ($C_{New} - C_{Old}$). This is called a *cost minimization analysis*. When the new therapy has greater health benefits and costs more than the standard of care, a trade-off is involved between the new strategy's greater health benefits and its greater costs, and a *cost-effectiveness analysis* is required. Finally, when the new strategy has greater health benefits and costs less, it is known as a *dominant strategy* (better in both cost and health benefit) and no further analysis is required. Although the term cost-effectiveness has been used colloquially to denote something perceived to be a good economic value, this usage is incorrect (16). To avoid confusion, we will use the term "econom-

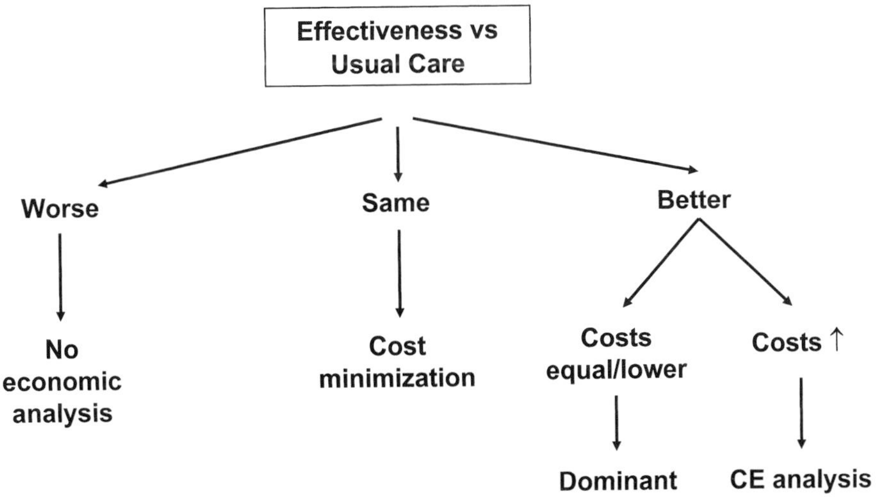

Figure 1 Types of economic analysis.

ically attractive" when a therapy is a dominant strategy or when an economic analysis (cost minimization or cost-effectiveness) has a favorable result.

Economic Attractiveness Criteria

Various criteria have been proposed for assessing the relative economic attractiveness of new medical therapies that improve outcomes but also increase costs. Cost-effectiveness analyses produce a ratio of cost per unit of health benefit, and therefore need to be assessed versus an external standard to determine if the new therapy is comparable with other accepted medical therapies.

Tengs and colleagues, in an analysis of 587 lifesaving interventions, found that the median cost per year of life saved (YOLS) varied by type of intervention ($19,000 per YOLS for medical interventions, $48,000 for injury reduction interventions, and $2,800,000 for toxin control interventions) (17). These researchers concluded that the range for acceptable cost per YOLS for a lifesaving intervention was attributable to the amount of legislation and litigation in an area. Thus, the economic attractiveness criterion is lower for medical interventions where there has been less direct government involvement and fewer class action lawsuits. Within medicine, various methods have been proposed for establishing a cost-effectiveness threshold above which new technologies would not be economically attractive (18–20). The most straightforward method is one proposed by Goldman that uses the cost of dialysis for treating end stage renal disease (now covered by the federal government regardless of patient age) as a benchmark for economic attractiveness (19). In 1995, annual Medicare costs per renal dialysis patient were $52,000 (21). In general, most experts consider therapies that cost <$50,000 per YOLS to be economically attractive, those in the $50,000 to $100,000 per YOLS range borderline, and those costing >$100,000 per YOLS economically unattractive (22).

League tables, which rank health care alternatives by ascending cost-effectiveness ratios, are frequently used to compare the economic attractiveness of therapeutic options (Table 1). It is important to note that the economic attractiveness of a new therapy is not fixed, but a function of the alternative against which it is being compared as well as the patient population in which it is administered. For example, a therapy will generally be more economically attractive in a higher-risk than in a lower-risk population (e.g., secondary versus primary prevention) and when it is compared against placebo versus an active therapy. Health care policy makers find league tables attractive guides in resource allocation decisions because of their simplicity (23–25). However, they actually oversimplify a complex problem and can mislead decisionmakers (26). For example, they virtually never in-

Table 1 Acute Coronary Syndromes League

New technology	Existing technology	Patient population	Cost[a] ($)/YOLS	Reference
Beta-blockers	No therapy	Myocardial infarction survivors	1,000	Wilhelmsson (1981)
CABG	Medical therapy	Left main coronary artery disease	6,700	Weinstein (1982)
PTCA	Medical therapy	Men age 55 with severe angina	8,900	Wong (1990)
Hypertension screening	No screening	Asymptomatic men age 60	13,200	Littenberg (1990)
Exercise stress test	No testing	Age 60 with mild pain and no left ventricular dysfunction	15,600	Lee (1988)
Beta-blockers	No therapy	Hypertensive age 35–64 no heart disease and ≥95 mm Hg	16,800	Edelson (1990)
Lovastatin	No therapy	Men age 55–64 with heart disease and <250 mg/dL	24,000	Goldman (1991)
t-PA	Streptokinase	Anterior myocardial infarction, age 61–75	24,800	Mark (1995)
Lovastatin	No therapy	Men age 45–54 with no heart disease and ≥300 mg/dL	40,900	Goldman (1991)
t-PA	Streptokinase	Anterior myocardial infarction, age 41–60	60,000	Mark (1995)
CABG	Medical therapy	Two-vessel coronary artery disease	90,200	Weinstein (1982)
Hypertension screening	No screening	Asymptomatic women age 20	104,600	Littenberg (1990)
PTCA	Medical therapy	Men age 55 with mild angina	132,200	Wong (1990)

[a]Costs adjusted to 1998 dollars using the consumer price index.

clude any measure of the uncertainty around a cost-effectiveness estimate (e.g., confidence intervals). And they do not alert the user when substantially different methods have been used to estimate costs and outcomes. Because of these limitations, league tables should only be used for illustrative purposes and not to guide decision making (26,27).

Perspective

The perspective is the viewpoint from which an economic analysis is conducted. Although economic analyses have been performed from the patient, employer, payer, and provider perspectives, they most often use a societal perspective because it is the most comprehensive (28). All other perspectives omit certain costs or health benefits from their analyses or count transfer payments between societal members as cash inflows or outflows. The societal perspective accounts for all economic elements including costs associated with the current episode of care (index costs) as well as all downstream medical costs (follow-up costs).

Although insurance and income transfers (e.g., welfare or disability payments) are frequently the most important cash flows for patients, payers, employers, and providers, they are not included in analyses performed from the societal perspective because they are not costs of care. However, they should be included when analyses are performed from any other perspective (28).

Medical Costs

As shown above, the perspective of an analysis also determines the economic elements it will include. The remainder of this section will discuss the measurement of those elements and will be limited to analyses from the societal perspective.

Medical Cost Terminology

Cost accountants use different classification systems for different types of analyses. *Product costing systems* seek to identify all costs involved with providing specific medical goods and services (e.g., primary PTCA) to patients. *Marginal analysis systems* are concerned with the relationship between changes in patient volume and changes in costs (e.g., how costs in chest pain units increase as the number of patients increases) (29).

Product costing systems have their origin in the mechanized integrated textile mills of the early 19th century, when managers wanted to determine all of the costs involved with converting raw materials into finished yarn and fabric (30). Then, as now, the problem was how to allocate costs that were shared by multiple end products. It is a relatively easy task to identify *direct costs* associated with specific patients (e.g., technician time or volume of heparin used during a diagnostic catheterization). However, it is more difficult to allocate *indirect costs* (e.g., catheterization laboratory administrator or clerical time used in scheduling procedures) to specific patients. The problem is further complicated because some indirect costs occur in the same cost centers as the direct costs (e.g., in the catheterization laboratory) but others occur in different cost centers (e.g., patient accounting, medical records, human resources, or the hospital laundry). Because of these difficulties, accountants develop formulas for allocating portions of the indirect costs to individual patients so that a total cost per patient can be calculated.

When product costing was initially developed, direct costs (labor and materials) accounted for 80% or more of a textile mill's total costs; therefore, accuracy in indirect cost allocation was not essential. However, in modern hospitals direct costs are typically <70% of total patient costs and in patients undergoing PCI or CABG procedures, they may be as little as 50% of direct costs (31) (E. Eisenstein, unpublished). Thus, the importance of accurate indirect cost allocation is increasing in health care.

Traditionally, hospitals have used simple metrics (e.g., revenue dollars) to allocate indirect costs. However, these methods frequently lead to overallocations of indirect costs to high-revenue-generating departments (e.g., cardiovascular services) and underallocations of indirect costs to lower-revenue hospital departments. The result is that higher-revenue-generating departments appear to be less profitable than they actually are. Activity-based costing (ABC), which assigns costs to activities (e.g., 1 hour of stepdown unit care) instead of resources, appears to overcome many of the problems with traditional indirect cost allocation algorithms (32–35).

Marginal analysis is a cost classification system in which costs varying in direct proportion with the number of patients seen are called *variable costs* (e.g., contrast medium and catheters in a catheterization laboratory) whereas costs that remain stable regardless of changes in patient volume are called *fixed costs* (e.g., equipment and facilities in a catheterization laboratory). Since fixed costs are always defined for a specific capacity (e.g., number of beds in a chest pain unit), all costs will necessarily become variable in the long run with extreme variation in patient volume. Some costs are hybrids and exhibit characteristics of both variable and fixed costs. *Semivariable costs* have both fixed and variable components (e.g., utilities in which there is a fixed connection fee and a variable fee based upon volume used). *Semifixed costs*, the other type of hybrid cost, vary in a semifixed (stepwise) way with changes in patient volume (e.g., nursing middle-management staffing, which varies with the number of nurses).

Medical Cost Calculation

The results of an economic analysis will be sensitive to the costing method used. For example, when it is anticipated that the difference in costs between two patient management strategies will be driven by differences in the rates of rehospitalization, a general costing method that does not require the collection of detailed costing data may be satisfactory. However, when it is anticipated that cost differences in the analysis will be driven by the utilization of specific resources (e.g., balloons or stents within the catheterization laboratory), a more detailed costing method will be required.

Three methods are used for estimating medical costs: *bottom-up*, *top-down*, and *imputation models*. Bottom-up methods estimate the costs of individual components and then sum them to arrive at a cost for the whole episode; top-down methods estimate aggregate costs from aggregate charges; and imputation models use patient characteristics and resource utilization as inputs for models which estimate costs.

Three bottom-up methods have been used in economic analyses. Microcosting (the gold standard) uses industrial engineering techniques to estimate the unit cost of each resource used and sums them to yield departmental and total case costs. The advantage of microcosting is its precision; the disadvantage is the cost of collecting and maintaining this level of data. Modern hospital cost accounting systems typically combine industrial engineering techniques with expert opinion to estimate average costs for resources used. Although not as precise as microcosting, hospital cost accounting systems yield results which are close approximations with lower data collection costs. The third bottom-up method, "big ticket" costing, assigns fixed costs to major health care products (e.g., CABG, PTCA , ICU room-day) and uses them to estimate case costs in the economic analysis. The advantage is the low cost of data collection; its disadvantage is its lack of detail. For example, if a standard cost is used for all PCI procedures, the analysis would not be able to differentiate among PTCA, stent, and rotablator procedures.

Two top-down methods have been used in U.S. economic analyses: ratio of cost to charge (RCC) and Medicare standard costs. The RCC method estimates costs from the line item charges on the patient's bill using conversion factors (typically aggregate ratios for institutional departments). The advantage of this method is its ease of use because all U.S. hospitals treating Medicare patients file annual cost reports that contain department level cost conversion factors. The disadvantage of RCC is that it sacrifices some of the accuracy of microcosting. Several studies have used Medicare DRG and/or Physician Fee Schedule reimbursements as surrogates for costs. Again, the advantage in these methods is the ease of data collection. The disadvantage of the DRG approach is its lack of detail (e.g., all CABG surgeries without catheterization are assigned the same costs) and the fact that Medicare doesn't include all costs in its reimbursements. Since Medicare reimburses physicians at the CPT code level, they are a reasonable estimate of physician costs.

Two studies have compared bottom-up and top-down costing methods. In a single institution study of CABG and PTCA costs, Lipscomb and colleagues found that average case costs were approximately the same when using results from a hospital cost accounting system and the RCC method, however, costs at the department level varied (36). In a study of 14 hospitals with automated bottom-up cost accounting systems, Ashby found that the average case costs across 40 DRGs were 4.4% higher using the top-down methods than they were using a bottom-up method (37). However, the differences in average costs between methods varied by DRG. Because the reported differences between hospital cost accounting and RCC methods are relatively small, most experts consider the results comparable.

Various imputation models have also been used to estimate costs in economic analyses. The two principal approaches are the use of case mix-adjusted cost functions (38) and the use of resource-based regression equations (39). The obvious advantage to these methods is that they don't require the collection of detailed cost data. The disadvantages relate to imprecisions of the estimates due to differences between the patient population under study and that represented in the database used in the model.

Lost-Productivity Costs

The value of lost productivity is the cost associated with lost or impaired ability to work or engage in leisure activities due to morbidity or mortality (28). Typically, these costs are measured as lost wages (patient and caregiver). Although measuring lost wages is conceptually simple, it is fraught with many practical difficulties and researchers are frequently forced to make assumptions which significantly affect their results. In many illnesses, the patient gradually rather than suddenly loses his ability to work. This presents a problem for the economic researcher who must determine whether to evaluate the lost productivity as the patient's wage rate (if any) before symptom onset, the wage rate before the patient became totally disabled, the potential wages had the patient not become disabled, or the wage rate had the patient been working. Because of these issues, many researchers evaluate all lost productivity at a common rate (e.g., average national income) which may inflate the value of lost productivity in patients with chronic illnesses. An additional problem with this approach is that patients past retirement age have no wage-earning capacity, and their lost productivity is just the value of their housekeeping services (40,41). In general, cost-effectiveness analyses ignore these costs.

Health Benefits

Measuring health benefits is even more difficult than measuring costs (42). This is because there is no universal health care outcome that can be used in all economic analyses. An additional difficulty is the inherent variability in many outcome measurements (42,43). While survival is an easily identifiable clinical outcome, many commonly used medical therapies have no effect on patient life expectancy. Even when therapies do increase patient life expectancy, the gains are typically modest (44–46). Table 2 shows differences in incremental life expectancy associated with prevention of and treatment for CAD.

Although exercising and quitting smoking both produce modest gains in life expectancy for 35-year-old patients at average-risk, life expectancy gains in higher-risk patients are much greater. This is because these therapies are targeted at patients who will benefit whereas the benefits of therapies in lower-risk patients are averaged across those who will and will not benefit. Interestingly, life expectancy gains in patients with CAD are modest at best and decline significantly when the comparison is between therapies (e.g., t-PA vs. streptokinase) rather than therapy and placebo (e.g., thrombolysis with t-PA). Because of this, quality-adjusted life years (QALYs) have been adopted as a standard measure of effectiveness. QALYs assign a weight to a patient's life expectancy representing their health-related quality of life (with 1 denoting perfect health and 0 denoting death). This adjustment allows all life expectancy estimate comparisons to be made from the same base (i.e., deviations from life years in perfect health). The rationale behind using QALYs is that therapies may improve the patient's overall quality of life without affecting longevity.

Adjusting for Differences in Timing

Patient management strategies often require different resources and produce different health benefits over time. For example, in a comparison of CABG surgery versus PCI for patients with multivessel CAD, CABG patients typically will incur higher index costs and greater short-term mortality whereas PCI patients will incur greater follow-up costs and long-term mortality. Discounting (the reverse of compound interest) is used to adjust for cost and health benefits that occur at different times and treats all costs and health benefits as if they occurred at baseline. Although various discount rates have been used, a 3% rate has become the standard when making comparisons using a societal perspective (28).

Table 2 Gains in Life Expectancy

Treatment/prevention strategy	Patient population	Gains in life expectancy (years added) Men	Women
	Average-risk patients		
Exercise consuming 2000 kcal/wk for 30 yrs	35-year-old men	0.517	—
Quitting cigarette smoking	35-year-olds	0.833	0.667
	High-risk patients		
Reduction of diastolic BP to 88 mm Hg	35-year-olds with		
	Diastolic BP of 90–94 mm Hg	1.083	0.917
	Diastolic BP >150 mm Hg	5.333	5.667
Reduction of cholesterol to 200 mg/dL	35-year-olds with		
	Cholesterol level of 200–239 mg/dL	0.500	0.417
	Cholesterol level of >300 mg/dL	4.167	6.333
Reduction of weight to ideal level	35-year-olds		
	<30% over their ideal weight	0.667	0.500
	>30% over their ideal weight	1.667	1.083
	Patients with established disease		
Revascularization with CABG or PTCA	Men with 2 VD	0.333	—
	Men with 3 VD	0.750	—
Routine beta-blocker therapy	55-year-old male AMI survivor with:		
	Low risk of recurrence	0.100	—
	Medium risk of recurrence	0.342	—
	High risk of recurrence	0.467	—
Thrombolysis with t-PA	Men or women with suspected AMI	1.250	1.250
t-PA versus streptokinase	Men or women with suspected AMI		
	Inferior	0.163	0.163
	Anterior	0.196	0.196
Heart transplant	Men or women with end-stage heart failure	5.417	5.417

Source: Data from Refs. 45,74,135–139.

Cost-Effectiveness Calculations

Table 3 shows the cost-effectiveness ratio calculations for comparing two patient management strategies. The new therapy has higher index costs but lower follow-up costs than the usual care strategy, but their cumulative costs at two years are identical. (For the purpose of this analysis, we will assume that there is no difference in follow-up costs after 2 years.) After discounting, the new therapy has $777 higher cumulative costs since the timing of its cash flows were earlier than those for usual care. Although the two strategies yield identical life expectancies (10 years undiscounted and 8.53 years discounted), the new therapy produces a slightly higher QALY for its patients (7.7 vs. 7.3). Thus, there is a 0.4 QALY benefit for the new therapy versus usual care. Although usual care costs $777 less, the new therapy is favored because it produces greater quality of life at an acceptable cost of $1822 per QALY, well below the accepted threshold for "economic attractiveness."

ECONOMIC STUDIES OF ACUTE CORONARY SYNDROMES

General Considerations

Acute coronary syndromes typically resolve within 30 to 60 days (14,15). Nonetheless, treatment decisions made by healthcare professionals during

Table 3 Cost-Effectiveness Computations

	New therapy	Usual care
Index costs	$45,000	$30,000
Follow-up costs		
Year 1	$0	$3000
Year 2	$0	$12,000
Cumulative costs	$45,000	$45,000
Discounted costs		
Year 1	$0	$2913
Year 2	$0	$11,310
Present value	$45,000	$44,223
Cost difference	$777	
Life expectancy	10 years	10 years
Discounted life expectancy	8.530 LY	8.530 LY
Quality of life	0.92	0.85
Discounted quality-adjusted life expectancy	7.7 QALY	7.3 QALY
QALY difference	0.4 QALY	
Cost per QALY (cost-effectiveness ratio)	$1822	

this period will account for 35% to 40% of the total medical costs these patients will incur over the next 12 years (39). Conceptually, ACS medical costs can be divided into five major resource utilization components (Fig. 2).

Prehospitalization

Preadmission Evaluation

Annually, 5 million to 6 million acute chest pain patients are evaluated in U.S. emergency departments at a total cost of >$6 billion (47,48). Most will be admitted to a hospital, where they will stay for an average of 1.9 days and incur $4,135 in charges (49). Ultimately, 15% will be identified as having acute myocardial infarction, 45% unstable angina or nonacute CAD, and 40% chest pain without an underlying coronary etiology (50). The annual cost for those found to be free of acute disease is $600 million (50). At the same time, 5% of chest pain patients will have an undiagnosed MI and be inappropriately discharged (51,52), one of the leading causes of malpractice suits against physicians (53,54).

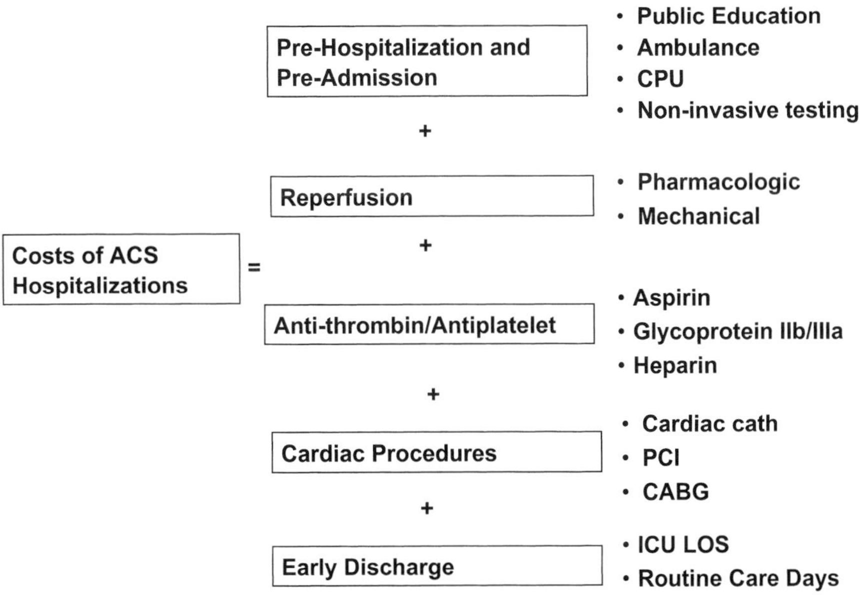

Figure 2 Economic components of ACS hospitalization.

Chest Pain Units

For the ED physician, one of the benefits of chest pain units is that they delay the hospital admission decision and provide an alternative to either discharging patients prematurely or admitting the patient and committing expensive cardiac care unit resources. Several studies have demonstrated the safety and economic viability of chest pain units (Table 4) (55–59). In the Duke program, Newby found that the use of a chest pain unit diagnostic strategy compared with conventional admission and rule-out resulted in a 2.3-day reduction in mean length of stay and a 47% reduction in hospital costs (59). Mikhael and colleagues (57) investigated the incremental value of routine stress testing in chest pain unit patients already ruled out for MI and found that the cost per year of life saved was less than $2000. Thus, the combination of chest pain unit evaluation with early exercise stress testing is both a clinically and economically attractive strategy.

The success of chest pain units has created interest in extending them to include patients at intermediate risk. In a study that applied the Agency for Health Care Policy and Research's Unstable Angina Guidelines to 457 consecutive patients receiving an emergency department physician's diagnosis of unstable angina or rule out unstable angina, Katz and colleagues found that only 6% met guideline criteria for low risk and were suitable for direct home discharge (60,61). Fifty-four percent met intermediate-risk cri-

Table 4 Chest Pain Unit Reductions in Length of Stay (LOS) and Costs

		Reduction	
Study	Publication year	LOS	Average costs ($)
Gaspoz et al.	1994		
CCU		4.0	7274
Step-down		2.0	2104
Wards		3.0	2785
Gomez et al.	1996	0.5	981
Newby	1996	2.3	1765
Mikhail	1997	ND	1470
Roberts	1997	0.5	567

ND = No data recorded.
Reduction in LOS and costs are for initial hospitalization except for Gaspoz, which includes follow-up through 6 months.
Source: Adapted from Newby, 1996.

teria and 40% met high-risk criteria, requiring intensive care unit admission. Thus, there remains great potential to expand the use of chest pain units to include the majority of chest pain patients, those at intermediate risk, who were excluded by earlier protocols.

Farkouh and colleagues randomized 424 intermediate-risk Mayo Clinic patients to chest pain unit or standard hospital admission (52). After 6 hours, 60 of the 212 patients randomized to the chest pain unit were admitted because of positive CK-MB assays or symptoms of recurrent chest pain. The remaining patients underwent stress testing (either exercise treadmill or pharmacologic) after which 55 were admitted. Ninety-seven patients had a negative stress test and were discharged to their homes with outpatient follow-up within 72 hours. The use of selected cardiac tests and procedures and cardiac rehospitalizations was greater in patients randomized to initial hospital admission through 6 months follow-up ($P = .003$). During the 6-month study duration, patients randomized to initial hospital admission incurred 61% more costs (measured with cumulative cost weights) than patients randomized to the chest pain unit. This study's 38% reduction in cost from use of a chest pain unit versus standard care diagnostic strategy is similar to results from previous studies reported in Table 4.

Previous studies have shown that cardiac troponins can provide additional prognostic information in chest pain patients over that available from creatine kinase assays (CK) alone (62–64). However, the incremental value of these biochemical markers has not been assessed in a randomized study. Polznczyk and colleagues developed a decision-analytic model to evaluate seven triage strategies employing CK-MB and Troponin I assays and early exercise testing in chest pain patients admitted to the emergency department (65). They found that the use of CK-MB mass with early exercise testing was the most competitive strategy ($43,000 per YOLS) for younger patients (55 to 64 years of age) and for all patients with a low to moderate probability of acute MI. Troponin I was an economically attractive second test ($47,400 per YOLS) in patients 65 to 74 years of age and in high risk patients where exercise testing could not be performed, CK-MB values were normal, or ischemic changes were seen on electrocardiograms.

Reperfusion Therapies

Pharmacologic Reperfusion

Several studies have assessed the relative economic attractiveness of streptokinase versus conventional therapy for acute myocardial infarction patients (66–71). Assuming that 10 years of life would be gained for each death prevented, Naylor and colleagues estimated the incremental cost-effectiveness of streptokinase versus no reperfusion therapy at $2000 to $4000 per

YOLS (70). In an analysis that looked at the cost-effectiveness of streptokinase according to MI location, the cost per additional life saved was $9900 for anterior infarctions, $56,600 for inferior infarctions, and $28,400 for infarctions in other locations (71).

Krumholz and colleagues used the GISSI and ISIS-2 clinical results to estimate the cost-effectiveness of streptokinase in the very elderly, a group at higher risk of complications, particularly hemorrhage, with thrombolytic therapy (69). They observed that streptokinase had a smaller relative reduction in mortality for elderly than younger patients although their absolute mortality risk remained much higher. Assuming a mean life expectancy of 5.5 years for 70-year-olds and 2.7 years for 80-year-olds, Krumholz estimated the cost-effectiveness of streptokinase versus no thrombolytic therapy at $21,600 per YOLS in 70-year-olds and $21,200 per YOLS in 80-year-olds.

Although previous studies attempted to estimate the incremental economic attractiveness of t-PA versus streptokinase (72,73), GUSTO I was the first clinical trial to prospectively collect detailed resource utilization information (baseline to 1 year) (74). Resource utilization (length of stay [ICU and regular], procedure use, [coronary angiography, PTCA, and CABG]) and cumulative 1-year inpatient costs exclusive of thrombolysis were similar for patients treated with streptokinase and t-PA (average $24,575 streptokinase and $24,990 t-PA). However, because of the disparity in thrombolytic agent costs (AWP of streptokinase $320; t-PA $2,750) (75), the incremental 1-year cost of the t-PA treatment strategy was $2845 greater than streptokinase. Using 1-year survival from GUSTO I and the experience of similar patients treated at Duke University, these investigators estimated a mean survival for t-PA patients of 15.41 years and for streptokinase patients 15.27 years. After discounting at 5% per annum, there was a 0.09-year estimated survival advantage for t-PA-treated patients with a resulting cost-effectiveness ratio of $32,678 per YOLS. Sensitivity analyses indicated that t-PA was generally more economically attractive for older patients and for those with anterior versus inferior infarctions.

The next generation in pharmacologic reperfusion is the combination of thrombolytic agents with glycoprotein IIb/IIIa platelet inhibitors (76–78). Although early clinical results are promising, none of these has included formal economic analysis. Because this combination therapy will significantly increase baseline hospital costs of AMI patients, such data will undoubtedly be an important factor in the acceptance of these therapies.

Mechanical Reperfusion

Meta-analyses of pharmacologic versus mechanical reperfusion in AMI patients have reported that primary angioplasty yields significant reduction of inhospital and 30-day rates of death and reinfarction when compared with thrombolysis (10,79). However, it is unclear if these results could be replicated in community settings and whether the incremental health benefits of mechanical reperfusion justify their incremental costs.

Initial studies concluded that primary angioplasty was economically neutral (80–84). In the Zwolle trial of 301 patients, cumulative hospital and pharmaceutical costs at one year were almost identical for patients treated with primary angioplasty and thrombolytic therapy (\$17,316 vs. \$16,668, respectively, $P = .22$) (81). However, in a community-based observational analysis of 1050 primary angioplasty and 2095 thrombolytic therapy patients, Every and colleagues observed that patients receiving thrombolysis had 1.1 days longer index length of stay (7.9 vs. 6.8 days) but lower baseline hospital costs (median \$12,600 vs. \$16,300, $P < .001$) (85). These patients also had lower cardiac procedure use and costs at discharge and after 3 years (30% fewer coronary angiographies, 15% fewer percutaneous interventions, and 13% lower costs). Cumulative inpatient costs at 3 years were also lower for patients initially receiving thrombolysis (median \$16,500 vs. \$19,600, $P < .001$).

In the GUSTO IIb Direct Angioplasty Substudy, the 30-day primary endpoint (death, nonfatal MI, or disabling stroke) was significantly lower for primary angioplasty patients (9.6% vs. 13.6%, $P = .033$), but by six months this benefit had attenuated and was no longer significant (13.3% vs. 15.7%, P = ns). A prospective economic substudy conducted in U.S. GUSTO IIb patients observed that patients receiving primary angioplasty had lower lengths of stay during their index hospitalizations (7.2 vs. 7.6 days, $P = .001$) and lower hospital costs (\$13,765 vs. \$14,404, $P = .009$) but higher physician fees (\$3,989 vs. \$3,355, $P = .0008$) resulting in similar baseline costs (\$17,753 vs. \$17,398, $P = .25$) (86). During 6 months follow-up, primary angioplasty patients had slightly higher, although not statistically significant, rates of cardiac procedures; nonetheless, follow-up costs were similar (\$2,886 vs. \$2,381, $P = .50$). At 6 months, hospital costs were lower for primary angioplasty patients (\$15,399 vs. \$16,101, $P = .022$) while physician fees were higher (\$4,339 vs. \$3,693, $P = .007$), yielding similar cumulative inpatient costs (\$19,738 vs. \$19,795, $P = .232$). Thus, contrary to earlier smaller clinical trials, GUSTO IIb demonstrated no significant long-term clinical or economic difference between mechanical and pharmacologic reperfusion (86).

Differences between the GUSTO IIb results and those for the PAMI, Zwolle, and Mayo Clinic studies have led some to conclude that the site's overall experience level is an important determinant of whether primary angioplasty will be a superior reperfusion strategy (81,83,87,88). These conclusions were verified in a recent decision analysis which found that primary angioplasty would be cost saving versus thrombolytic therapy in a hospital with an existing catheterization laboratory, night/weekend staffing coverage, and admitting more than 200 MI patients annually. However, primary angioplasty would not be economically attractive in a lower volume institution (89).

Recent clinical trials have demonstrated significant clinical benefits for primary stenting versus primary angioplasty (90–92). In a randomized study of 227 patients, Suryapranata and colleagues found a significant reduction in six-month event-free survival (95% vs. 80%, $P = .012$ for death, re-MI, subsequent CABG, or TVR) (91). In this trial's economic substudy, Van't Hof and colleagues compared resource utilization and costs through 12 months of follow-up and observed that in-hospital costs were lower for patients treated with primary angioplasty ($15,322 vs. $17,508). However, at 1 year costs were similar between patient groups (primary angioplasty $22,107 vs. primary stenting $21,418) due to higher follow-up rates of re-MI, re-PTCA, and CABG for primary angioplasty patients (93).

Antithrombin and Antiplatelet Therapies

Unfortunately, neither the most commonly used antithrombin (unfractionated heparin) or antiplatelet (aspirin) therapies has been the subject of a formal economic analysis. Thus, while there is strong belief among practitioners that aspirin is cost saving (if not dominant) and that heparin may be cost-effective in certain populations, there is no evidence to substantiate these beliefs (94). In this section, we will review the results from economic studies of newer direct antithrombin low-molecular-weight heparin, and glycoprotein IIb/IIIa platelet inhibitor therapies in non-ST elevation ACS patients as well as the use of glycoprotein IIb/IIIa platelet inhibitors as adjunctive therapies in percutaneous coronary interventions.

Antithrombin Therapy

Recent research in antithrombins has focused on novel anticoagulants (e.g., direct antithrombins and low-molecular-weight heparins) in non-ST elevation ACS patients. Although the early benefits of the direct thrombin hirudin were shown to diminish over time, the low-molecular-weight heparin enoxaparin has demonstrated a durable treatment effect versus unfractionated heparin (95–100).

The ESSENCE clinical trial reported an initial 16% relative reduction (16.6% vs. 19.8%, $P = .019$) in the composite endpoint of death, myocardial infarction, or recurrent angina at 14 days which was sustained at 30 days (19.8% vs. 23.3%, $P = .016$) for patients receiving low-molecular-weight heparin versus those receiving unfractionated heparin (98). A prospective economic analysis using U.S. patients enrolled in ESSENCE examined whether the increased cost of enoxaparin versus unfractionated heparin ($155 vs. $80 per patient) would be offset by cost savings in the initial 30 days after treatment (99). During the index hospitalization, patients receiving enoxaparin consumed fewer medical resources than patients receiving heparin (e.g., PTCA 15% vs. 20%, $P = .04$) and had lower inpatient (hospital and physician) costs ($11,857 vs. $12,620, $P = .18$). Through 30 days follow-up the trend toward less medical resource consumption with enoxaparin persisted (e.g., diagnostic catheterization 57% vs. 63%, $P = .04$, and ICU days 2.4 vs. 2.8, $P = .05$), resulting in significantly lower cumulative inpatient costs for enoxaparin-treated patients ($13,155 vs. $14,357, $P = .04$). Since the enoxaparin treatment strategy demonstrated both a clinical and an economic ($1,202 cost saving) benefit versus unfractionated heparin, it was considered a dominant strategy (99).

Antiplatelet Therapy

Although the economic attractiveness of glycoprotein IIb/IIIa platelet inhibitors has been demonstrated in decision-analytic and other economic models, PURSUIT is the only clinical trial to include a prospective economic analysis in its design (4,101,103).

The PURSUIT clinical trial randomized ACS patients (unstable angina or non-Q-wave myocardial infarction) to eptifibatide therapy or placebo and observed a 1.5% absolute reduction (15.7% vs. 14.2%, $P = .042$) in the composite endpoint of death or MI at 30 days for patients treated with eptifibatide (104). In the U.S. PURSUIT economic analysis, no significant difference in average inpatient costs (hospital plus physician) was found between eptifibatide-treated and placebo patients exclusive of the cost of eptifibatide (index hospitalization $14,729 vs. $14,957, $P > .10$; cumulative 6-month costs $18,456 vs. $18,828, $P > .10$). Thus, the only cost difference between treatment strategies was that of the drug itself ($1217) (103). Using the 6-month PURSUIT follow-up data, the PURSUIT investigators estimated that the life expectancy for patients receiving eptifibatide would be 15.96 years (vs. 15.85 years for patients receiving placebo), resulting in a cost-effectiveness ratio of $16,491 per YOLS. Since ACS survivors rated their health at 0.84 on a 0 (death) to 1 (excellent health) utility scale, the corresponding cost utility ratio was $23,449 per QALY.

The economic attractiveness of glycoprotein IIb/IIIa platelet inhibition as an adjunctive therapy for percutaneous coronary intervention has been assessed in five clinical trials with prospective economic studies (Table 5) (105–109). EPIC investigated the use of abciximab in PTCA patients who were at high risk for abrupt vessel closure (110). The cost for abciximab therapy ($1407) and an increased risk of bleeding contributed to a $1550

Table 5 Economic Analysis of Glycoprotein IIb/IIIa Platelet Inhibition in Percutaneous Coronary Intervention

	Study name and treatment				
				EPISTENT	
	EPIC abciximab	EPILOG abciximab	RESTORE tirofiban	Stent + abciximab PTCA + abciximab	Stent + abciximab Stent + placebo
Clinical endpoint	Composite	Composite	Composite	Death	Death
Significance	Yes	Yes	No	No	Yes
Therapy costs ($)					
Active	1,407	1,489	700	3,598	$3,598
Control				1,997	$2,219
Increment				1,601	$1,279
Baseline costs ($)					
Active	14,984	10,247	12,230	13,229	13,229
Control	13,474	9,632	12,145	11,357	11,924
Increment	1,550	615	85	1,872	1,305
Total costs ($)					
Follow-up	6 months	6 months	30 days	1 year	1 year
Active	18,269	14,477	12,446	17,952	17,952
Control	17,976	13,200	12,402	17,370	17,020
Increment	293	1,277	44	582	932
Incremental LE				0.11 years	0.15 years
Cost-effectiveness				$5291/YOLS	$6,213/YOLS

cost increment for abciximab-treated versus placebo patients at baseline. During the 6-month follow-up period, patients receiving abciximab were less likely than placebo patients to be rehospitalized (24.1% vs. 31.2%, $P = .004$) or undergo additional revascularization procedures (15.6% vs. 19.9%, $P = .04$). These resource utilization differences led to \$1270 ($P = .018$) higher follow-up medical costs for placebo patients and similar cumulative costs for both treatment regimens at 6 months (105).

The EPILOG clinical trial was designed to test the hypothesis that weight-adjusted heparin would reduce the increased rate of bleeding observed in EPIC. The EPILOG economic analysis reported a significant reduction in baseline hospital costs for abciximab patients treated with low-dose heparin versus placebo patients ($P = .005$). After including the cost of abciximab, there was only a \$615 difference between the active and control arms. However, EPILOG patients treated with abciximab and weight-adjusted heparin did not have the same reduction in follow-up hospitalizations and revascularization procedures that was observed in EPIC and the cost increment actually increased during follow-up (106). The RESTORE trial, which looked at the agent tirofiban, had results similar to EPILOG: baseline costs for patients receiving tirofiban and placebo were similar, but the treatment effect for tirofiban attenuated at 30 days so there was no economic difference (108).

EPISTENT compared three treatment strategies: stent plus abciximab, stent plus placebo, and PTCA plus abciximab (109,111). One-year mortality was 1.0% for stent plus abciximab; 2.4% for stent plus placebo ($P = .037$); and 2.1% for PTCA plus abciximab patients. In a prospective U.S. economic analysis, the baseline costs for the stent plus abciximab treatment strategy were largely driven by the incremental cost of these therapies (\$1305 vs. stent alone and \$1871 vs. PTCA plus abciximab). At the end of 1-year follow-up, cost differences among the three treatment strategies had diminished due to lower 30-day rates of cardiac events (death, MI, urgent revascularization) in patients receiving abciximab and lower long-term follow-up rehospitalization and repeat PCI rates in patients receiving stents. Thus, at 1 year the incremental cost for the stent plus abciximab strategy was \$582 versus PTCA plus abciximab and \$932 versus stent plus placebo. Projecting the 1-year differences in mortality, these investigators estimated that the incremental life expectancy benefit for the stent plus abciximab strategy was 0.11 years versus the PTCA plus abciximab and 0.15 years versus the stent plus placebo strategy (both discounted at 3% per annum). The resulting cost-effectiveness ratios for the stent plus abciximab strategy were \$5291 per YOLS versus the PTCA plus abciximab and \$6213 versus the stent plus placebo strategy. Thus, in this study the stent plus abciximab strategy was a highly economically attractive therapy.

Cardiac Procedures and Lengths of Stay

Cardiac procedures and hospital lengths of stay are the two most expensive decisions that clinicians make and thus have been the focus of several important cost management studies. Calvin and colleagues used four variables from the Braunwald unstable angina classification system along with patient age and history of diabetes to predict the occurrence of major in-hospital cardiac complications in unstable angina patients (112,113). Although these clinical variables accurately predicted major complications, collectively they explained only 4.7% of the variance in these patients' total hospital costs. In contrast, the use of cardiac procedures alone explained an additional 32.9% of the variance (114). When these researchers compared resource utilization across four risk groups defined by their probability of major complication (i.e., 2.0%, 2.1–5.0%, 5.1–15.0%, and ≥15.1%), they found that more than half of the patients in each group were admitted to the CCU, but there were no differences in the use of coronary angiography and percutaneous coronary interventions among risk groups. The principal risk-based resource use difference was that higher-risk patients were more likely to undergo CABG surgery than lower-risk patients. These results confirm that treatment-related factors (i.e., cardiac procedures and lengths of stay) rather than patient-related factors are the primary determinants of ACS patient costs (39,115,116).

Cardiac Procedures

Coronary angiography has received a great deal of attention from those seeking to control ACS patient costs because it functions as a gatekeeper for the more expensive cardiac revascularization procedures (117). Although large variances in the use of coronary angiography have been well documented, higher usage rates have not been associated with better patient outcomes (118–121), but appear to be a direct relationship between the availability of coronary angiography and its use (122–125).

The TIMI IIIB clinical trial investigated the relative effectiveness of an early invasive versus an early conservative patient management strategy in patients with unstable angina and non-Q-wave myocardial infarction and found no difference in cardiac event rates (i.e., death and nonfatal MI) between patient management strategies (126). Despite a 0.7-day longer length of stay and 6.3% greater 6-week rehospitalization rate, back-of-the-envelope estimates have suggested that there may be a significant cost reduction through use of the initial conservative patient management strategy (127). Unfortunately, neither TIMI IIIB nor the more recent VANQWISH trial contained a prospective economic analysis which would have assessed the relative economic attractiveness of a conservative patient management strategy for ACS patients (128).

Kuntz and colleagues used decision-analytic modeling techniques to investigate the cost-effectiveness of routine coronary angiography after acute myocardial infarction (129). Their model compared two diagnostic strategies: coronary angiography and treatment guided by its results, versus initial medical therapy without coronary angiography. The resulting cost-effectiveness ratios varied from $17,000 to >$1 million per QALY depending on the patient population. The routine coronary angiography diagnostic strategy was found to be economically attractive versus the initial medical strategy for patients with mild postinfarction angina, a strongly positive ETT result, and a prior AMI (except those with a LVEF 0.20 to 0.49 aged >74 years). However, the routine coronary angiography diagnostic strategy was only economically unattractive for patients with mild postinfarction angina, a negative ETT result, and LVEF $\geq$ 0.50 when they had a prior MI and were older (>45 for men and >65 for women). Generally, in patients with severe postinfarction angina or a strongly positive ETT and patients with a prior MI (even if their ETT was negative), the routine coronary angiography diagnostic strategy had cost-effectiveness ratios <$50,000 per QALY (i.e., was "economically attractive").

Length of Stay

Reductions in length of stay (ICU and regular room) have been a primary focus of many ACS patient management strategies (130). For example, lengths of stay at Duke University Medical Center for acute MI patients were reduced from 10.6 days in 1986 to 7.8 days in 1997, and those for unstable angina patients were reduced from 11.7 to 4.7 days during that period (E. Eisenstein, unpublished data).

Newby and colleagues used clinical data from GUSTO I to investigate the potential for early discharge in acute MI patients who were uncomplicated at 96 hours (59). Early discharge criteria included the absence of death, reinfarction, ischemia, stroke, shock, heart failure (Killip class > 1), CABG surgery, balloon pumping, emergency catheterization, or cardioversion/defibrillation in the first 4 days. Patients meeting these criteria had 1.0% mortality at 30 days and 3.6% mortality at 1 year. Using these risk stratification criteria, 57.3% of GUSTO I patients were "uncomplicated" and eligible for discharge on day 4; their actual mean length of stay was 8.9 days (131). Eisenstein and colleagues (131) used information from the GUSTO I economic substudy to simulate the cost effects of Newby's early discharge criteria. Average costs for U.S. uncomplicated patients were $15,825 versus $24,582 for complicated patients before implementing Newby's early discharge criteria. Assuming uncomplicated AMI patients were discharged on day 4, their average index hospitalization costs could be reduced by 26.5% to $11,624.

In a subsequent analysis, Newby et al. (132) estimated the cost-effectiveness of hospital day 4 for the uncomplicated acute MI patients. This analysis was based on GUSTO I data and assumed that only preventable in-hospital deaths were patients who had VT/VF on day 4. The incremental cost of a regular room with telemetry and physician care was $624 and the life expectancy benefit of hospital day 4 was 0.006 years, yielding a cost-effectiveness ratio of $105,629 per YOLS for hospital day 4 in uncomplicated acute MI patients. However, this analysis assumed that all required testing and patient education can be completed by 72 hours, and most hospitals in the United States would be unable to achieve this level of efficiency at present.

CONCLUSION

In 1992, George Lundberg, then the editor of JAMA, predicted that without major change U.S. heath expenditures would reach $1.4 trillion by 1996 and cause a meltdown in the U.S. health care system (133). However, due to the advent of the "managed care era," the annual percentage increase in health expenditures declined, reaching a low of 4.4% in 1995–96, and total U.S. health expenditures were only $1.039 billion in 1996 (134). It is now clear that this short-term effect of managed care expansion is ending, and current projections are that health expenditures will be 15.5% of the U.S. gross domestic product in 2007 (134). Thus, questions of value in health expenditures will likely become more acute in the next decade.

ACKNOWLEDGMENT

The authors acknowledge the editorial assistance of Tracey Simons, M.A.

REFERENCES

1. Getzen TE: Health Economics: Fundamentals and Flow of Funds. New York: John Wiley, 1997.
2. CDC Fastats A to Z. Centers for Disease Control National Center for Health Statistics. Available at http://www.cdc.gov/nchs/fastats/hexpense.htm. Accessed March 6, 2000.
3. Jacobs E, Shipp S: How family spending has changed in the US. Monthly Labor Review 1990;March:20–27.
4. Eisenstein EL, Peterson ED, Jollis JG, Tardiff BE, Califf RM, Mark DB. Evaluating the potential economic attractiveness of newer therapies in non-ST elevation acute coronary syndrome patients. PharmacoEconomics 2000; 17(3):263–272.

5. Health Care Financing Administration. Health, United States, 1998 with socioeconomic status and health chartbook. Available at: www.cdc.gov/nchs/fastats/pdf/hu98t119.pdf. Accessed March 6, 2000.
6. Day HW. An intensive coronary care area. Dis Chest 1963;44:423–427.
7. Koch EB, Reiser SJ. Critical care: historical development and ethical considerations. In: Fein IA, Strosbers MA, eds. Managing the Clinical Care Unit. Rockville, MD: Aspen, 1987:3–20.
8. Hilberman M. The evolution of intensive care units. Crit Care Med 1975;3:159–165.
9. Reiser SJ. The intensive care unit. Int J Tech Assess Health Care 1992;8:382–394.
10. Weaver WD, Simes RJ, Betriu A, Grines CL, Zijlstra F, Garcia E, Grinfeld L, Gibbons RJ, Ribeiro EE, DeWood MA. Comparison of primary coronary angioplasty and intravenous thrombolytic therapy for acute myocardial infarction: a quantitative review. JAMA 1998;278:2093–2098.
11. ASSENT-2 Investigators. Single-bolus tenecteplase compared with front-loaded alteplase in acute myocardial infarction: the ASSENT-2 double-blind randomised trial. Lancet 1999;354:716–722.
12. American Medical Association: Assessing the Value of Medical Practice: The Physician's Handbook for Measuring and Maximizing Practice Value. Norcross, GA: Coker Publishing, 1996.
13. Unland JJ. The valuation of hospitals and medical centers: analyzing and measuring hospital assets and market value. Chicago: Probus Publishing, 1993.
14. Mark DB, Topol EJ. Chronic coronary artery disease. In: Talley JD, Mauldin PD, Becker ER (eds). Cost Effective Diagnosis and Treatment of Coronary Artery Disease. Baltimore: Williams & Wilkins, 1997:168–177.
15. Califf RM, Eisenstein EL. Cost-effectiveness of therapy for acute ischemic heart disease. In: Talley JD, ed. Cost-Effective Diagnosis and Treatment of Coronary Artery Disease. New York: Igaku-Shoin, 1997:139–167.
16. Doubilet P, Weinstein MC, McNeil BJ. Use and misuse of the term "cost effective" in medicine. N Engl J Med 1986;314:253–256.
17. Tengs TO, Adams ME, Pliskin JS, Safran DG, Siegel JE, Weinstein MC, Graham JD. Five hundred life-saving interventions and their cost-effectiveness. Risk Anal 1995;15:369–390.
18. Kaplan RM, Bush JW. Health-related quality of life measurement for evaluation research and policy analysis. Health Psychol 1981;1:61–80.
19. Goldman L, Weinstein MC, Goldman PA, Williams L. Cost effectiveness of HMG-CoA reductase inhibition for primary and secondary prevention of coronary heart disease. JAMA 1991;265:1145–1151.
20. Laupacis A, Feeny D, Detsky AS, Tugwell PX. How attractive does a new technology have to be to warrant adoption and utilization?: tentative guidelines for using clinical and economic evaluations. Can Med Assoc J 1992;146:473–481.
21. US Renal Data System. USRDS 1999 Annual Data Report. Bethesda, National Institutes of Health, 1999.

22. Mark DB. Medical economics in cardiovascular medicine. In: Topol EJ, ed. Textbook of Cardiovascular Medicine. New York, Lippincott-Raven, 1997: 1033–1062.
23. Hadorn DC. Setting health care priorities in Oregon: cost-effectiveness meets the rule of rescue. JAMA 1991;265:2218–2225.
24. Eddy DM: Oregon's methods: did cost effectiveness analysis fail? JAMA 1991;266:2135–2141.
25. Leichter HM. Oregon's bold experiment: whatever happened to rationing? J Health Politics Policy Law 1999;24:147–160.
26. Mason J, Drummond M, Torrance G. Some guidelines on the use of cost effectiveness league tables. Br Med J 1993;306:570–572.
27. Glassman PA, Model KE, Kahan JP, Jacobson PD, Peabody JW. The role of medical necessity and cost-effectiveness in making medical decisions. Ann Intern Med 1997;126:152–156.
28. Gold MR, Siegel JE, Russell LB, Weinstein MC. Cost-effectiveness in health and medicine. New York: Oxford University Press, 1996.
29. Finkler SA. Cost Accounting for Health Care Organizations. Gaithersburg, MD: Aspen Publishers, 1994.
30. Johnson HT, Kaplan RS. Relevance lost: the rise and fall of management accounting. Boston: Harvard Business School Press, 1987.
31. Roberts RR, Frutos PW, Ciavearella GG, Gussow LM, Mensah EK, Kampe LM, Strauss HE, Joseph G, Rydman RJ. Distribution of variable versus fixed costs of hospital care. JAMA 1999;281:644–649.
32. Baker JJ, Boyd GF. Activity-based costing in the operation room at Valley View Hospital. J Health Care Finance 1997;24:1–9.
33. Asadi MJ, Baltz WA. Activity-based costing for clinical paths. An example to improve clinical cost and efficiency. J Soc Health Sys 1996;5:1–7.
34. Alanen J, Keski-Nisula L, Laurila J, Suramo I, Standerskjold-Nordenstam CG, Brommels M. Costs of plain-film radiography in a partially digitized radiology department. An activity-based cost analysis. Acta Radiol 1998;39:200–207.
35. Zeller TL, Senagore AJ, Siegel G. Manage indirect practice expense the way you practice medicine: with information. Dis Colon Rectum 1999;42:579–589.
36. Lipscomb J, Mark DB, Cowper PA. Comparison of hospital costs derived from cost-to-charge ratios and from a detailed cost accounting system for patients undergoing cardiac procedures. Assoc Health Svc Res 1994.
37. Ashby JL. The accuracy of cost measures derived from Medicare cost report data. Hospital 1992;3:1–8.
38. Barnett PG. Research without billing data: econometric estimation of patient-specific costs. Med Care 1997;35:553–563.
39. Eisenstein EL, Shaw LK, Nelson CL, Hakim Z, Hasselblad V, Mark DB. Assessing the clinical and economic burden of coronary artery disease. 1986–1998. Submitted 2000.
40. Rice DP. Cost-of-illness: fact or fiction? Lancet 1994;344:1519–1520.
41. Rice DP. Estimating the cost of illness. Am J Pub Health 1967;57:424–440.

42. Detsky AS. Using cost-effectiveness analysis for formulary decision making: from theory to practice. PharmacoEconomics 1994;6:281–288.
43. Hornberger JC, Redelmeier DA, Petersen J. Variability among methods to assess patients' well-being and consequent effect on a cost-effectiveness analysis. J Clin Epidemiol 1992;45:505–512.
44. Naimark D, Naglie G, Detsky AS. The meaning of life expectancy: what is a clinically significant gain? J Gen Intern Med 1994;9:702–707.
45. Tsevat J, Weinstein MC, Williams LW, Tosteson ANA, Goldman L. Expected gains in life expectancy from various coronary heart disease risk factor modifications. Circulation 1991;83:1194–1201.
46. Wright JC, Weinstein MC. Gains in life expectancy from medical interventions—standardizing data on outcomes. N Engl J Med 1998;339:380–386.
47. Barish RA, Doherty RJ, Browne BJ. Reeingineering the emergency evaluation of chest pain. J HealthCare Quality 1997;19:6–12.
48. National Center for Health Statistics, Stussman BJ. National Hospital Ambulatory Medical Care Survey: 1995 Emergency Department Survey. Advance Data from Vital Health Statistics. Hyattsville, MD: Public Health Service, 1997.
49. DRG Handbook. Comparative Clinical and Financial Standards. Baltimore: HCIA, 1997.
50. Newby LK, Gibler WB, Christenson RH, Ohman EM. Serum markers for diagnosis and risk stratification in acute coronary syndromes. In: Cannon CP, ed. Contemporary Cardiology: Management of Acute Coronary Syndromes. Totowa, NJ: Humana Press, 1998:147–17.
51. Jesse RL, Kontos MC. Evaluation of chest pain in the emergency department. Curr Prob Cardiol 1997;22:149–236.
52. Farkouh ME, Smars PA, Reeder GS, Zinsmeister AR, Evans RW, Meloy TD, Kopecky SL, Allen M, Allison TG, Gibbons RJ, Gabriel SE, for the CHEER Investigators. A clinical trial of a chest pain unit observation for patients with unstable angina. N Engl J Med 1998;339:1882–1888.
53. McCarthy BD, Beshansky JR, D'Agostino RB, et al. Missed diagnoses of acute myocardial infarction in the emergency department: results from a multicenter study. Ann Emerg Med 1993;22:579–582.
54. Rusnak RA, Stair TO, Hansen K, Fastow JS. Litigation against the emergency physician: common features in cases of missed myocardial infarction. Ann Emerg Med 1989;18:1029–1034.
55. Gomez MA, Anderson JL, Karagounis LA, Muhlestein JB, Mooers FB, for the ROMIO Study Group. An emergency department-based protocol for rapidly ruling out myocardial ischemia reduces hospital time and expense: results of a randomized study (ROMIO). J Am Coll Cardiol 1996;28:25–33.
56. Gaspoz JM, Lee TH, Weinstein MC, Cook EF, Goldman P, Komaroff AL, Goldman L. Cost-effectiveness of a new short-stay unit to "rule out" acute myocardial infarction in low risk patients. J Am Coll Cardiol 1994;24:1249–1259.
57. Mikhail MG, Smith FA, Gray M, Britton C, Frederiksen SM. Cost-effective-

ness of mandatory stress testing in chest pain center patients. Ann Emerg Med 1997;29:88–98.
58. Roberts RR, Zalenski RJ, Mensah EK, Rydman RJ, Ciavarella G, Gussow L, Das K, Kampe LM, Dickover B, McDermott MF, Hart A, Straus HE, Murphy DG, Rao R. Costs of an emergency department-based accelerated diagnostic protocol vs. hospitalization in patients with chest pain. JAMA 1997;278: 1670–1676.
59. Newby LK, Califf RM. Identifying patient risk: the basis for rational discharge planning after acute myocardial infarction. J Thromb Thrombol 1996; 3:107–115.
60. Braunwald E, Mark DB, Jones RH, Cheitlin MD, Fuster V, McCauley K, Edwards C, Green LA, Mushlin AI, Swain JA, Smith EE III, Cowan M, Rose GC, Concannon CA, Grines CL, Brown L, Lytle BW, Goldman L, Topol EJ, Willerson JT, Brown J, Archibald N. Unstable angina: diagnosis and management. AHCPR 1994;94–0682.
61. Katz DA, Griffith JL, Beshansky JR, Selker HP. The use of empiric clinical data in the evaluation of practice guidelines for unstable angina. JAMA 1996; 276:1568–1574.
62. Green BG, Beaudreau RW, Chan DW, DeLong DM, Kelley CA, Kelen GD. Use of troponin T and creatine kinase-MB subunit levels for risk stratification of emergency department patients with possible myocardial ischemia. Ann Emerg Med 1998;31:19–29.
63. Tucker JF, Collins RA, Anderson AJ, Hauser J, Kalas J, Apple FS. Early diagnostic efficiency of cardiac troponin I and troponin T for acute myocardial infarction. Acad Emerg Med 1997;4:3–5.
64. Hamm CW, Goldmann BU, Heeschen C, Kreymann G, Berger J, Meinertz T. Emergency room triage of patients with acute chest pain by means of rapid testing for cardiac troponin T or troponin I. N Engl J Med 1998;337:1687–1689.
65. Polanczyk CA, Kuntz KM, Sacks DB, Johnson PA, Lee TH. Emergency department triage strategies for acute chest pain using creatine kinase-MB and troponin I assays: a cost-effectiveness analysis. Ann Intern Med 1999;131: 909–918.
66. Vermeer F, Simoons ML, de Zwaan C, van Es GA, Verheught FWA, van der Laarse A, van Hoogenhuyze DCA, Azar AJ, van Dalen FJ, Lubsen J, Hugenholtz PG. Cost benefit analysis of early thrombolytic treatment with intracoronary streptokinase: twelve month follow-up report of the randomised multicentre trial conducted by the Interuniversity Cardiology Institute of the Netherlands. Br Heart J 1988;59:527–534.
67. Herve C, Castiel D, Gaillard M, Boisvert R, Leroux V. Cost-benefit analysis of thrombolytic therapy. Eur Heart J 1990;11:1006–1010.
68. Simoons ML, Vos J, Martens LL. Cost-utility analysis of thrombolytic therapy. Eur Heart J 1991;12:694–699.
69. Krumholz HM, Pasternak RC, Weinstein MC, Friesinger GC, Ridker PM, Tosteson ANA, Goldman L. Cost effectiveness of thrombolytic therapy with

streptokinase in elderly patients with suspected acute myocardial infarction. N Engl J Med 1992;327:7–13.
70. Naylor CD, Bronskill S, Goel V. Cost-effectiveness of intravenous thrombolytic drugs for acute myocardial infarction. Can J Cardiol 1993;9(6):553–558.
71. Midgette AS, Wong JB, Beshansky JR, Porath A, Fleming C, Pauker SG. Cost-effectiveness of streptokinase for acute myocardial infarction: a combined meta-analysis and decision analysis of the effects of infarct location and of likelihood of infarction. Med Decis Making 1994;14:108–117.
72. Laffel GL, Fineberg HV, Braunwald E. A cost-effectiveness model for coronary thrombolysis/reperfusion therapy. J Am Coll Cardiol 1987;10:79B–90B.
73. Steinberg EP, Topol EJ, Sakin JW, Kahane SN, Appel LJ, Powe NR, Anderson GF, Erickson JE, Guerci AD. Cost and procedure implications of thrombolytic therapy for acute myocardial infarction. J Am Coll Cardiol 1988;12:58A–68A.
74. Mark DB, Hlatky MA, Califf RM, Naylor CD, Lee KL, Armstrong PW, Barbash G, White H, Simoons ML, Nelson CL, Clapp-Channing NE, Knight JD, Harrell FE Jr, Simes J, Topol EJ. Cost effectiveness of thrombolytic therapy with tissue plasminogen activator as compared with streptokinase for acute myocardial infarction. N Engl J Med 1995;332:1418–1424.
75. 1994 Drug Topics Red Book. Montvale, NJ: Medical Economics Data, 1994.
76. Antman EM, Guigliano RP, Gibson CM, McCabe CH, Coussement P, Kleiman NS, Vahanian A, Adgey AA, Menown I, Rupprecht HJ, van der Wieken LR, Ducas J, Schereer J, Anderson K, Van de Werf F, Braunwald E, for the TIMI I4 Investigators. Abciximab facilitates the rate and extent of thrombolysis: results of the thrombolysis in myocardial infarction (TIMI) 14 trial. Circulation 1999;99:2720–2732.
77. Ohman EM, Kleiman NS, Gacioch G, Worley SJ, Navetta FI, Talley JD, Anderson HV, Ellis SG, Cohen MD, Spriggs D, Miller M, Kereiakes D, Yakubov S, Kitt M, Sigmon KN, Califf RM, Krucoff MW, Topol EJ, for the IMPACT II AMI Investigators. Combined accelerated tissue-plasminogen activator and platelet glycoprotein IIb/IIIa integrin receptor blockade with Integrilin in acute myocardial infarction. Results of a randomized, placebo-controlled, dose-ranging trial. Circulation 1997;95:846–854.
78. SPEED Group. Trial of abciximab with and without low-dose reteplase for acute myocardial infarction. Circulation 2000. In press.
79. Michels KB, Yusuf S. Does PTCA in acute myocardial infarction affect mortality and reinfarction rates? A quantitative overview (meta-analysis) of the randomized clinical trials. Circulation 1995;91:476–485.
80. Reeder GS, Bailey KR, Gersh BJ, Holmes DR, Christianson J, Gibbons RJ, for the Mayo Coronary Care Unit and Catheterization Laboratory Groups. Cost comparison of immediate angioplasty versus thrombolysis followed by conservative therapy for acute myocardial infarction: a randomized prospective trial. Mayo Clin Proc 1994;69:5–12.
81. de Boer MJ, van Hout BA, Liem AL, Suryapranata H, Hoorntje JCA, Zijlstra F. A cost-effective analysis of primary coronary angioplasty versus thrombolysis for acute myocardial infarction. Am J Cardiol 1995;76:830–833.

82. Zijlstra F, de Boer M, Hoorntje JCA, Reiffers S, Reiber JHC, Suryapranata H. A comparison of immediate coronary angioplasty with intravenous streptokinase in acute myocardial infarction. N Engl J Med 1993;328:680–684.
83. Stone GW, Grines CL, Rothbaum D, Browne KF, O'Keefe J, Overlie PA, Donohue BC, Chelliah N, Vlietstra R, Catlin T, O'Neill WW, for the PAMI Investigators. Analysis of the relative costs and effectiveness of primary angioplasty versus tissue-type plasminogen activator: the Primary Angioplasty in Myocardial Infarction (PAMI) trial. J Am Coll Cardiol 1997;29:901–907.
84. Beatt KJ, Fath-Ordoubadi F. Angioplasty for the treatment of acute myocardial infarction. Heart 1997;78:12–15.
85. Every NR, Parsons LS, Hlatky MA, Martin JS, Weaver WD, for the Myocardial Infarction Triage and Intervention Investigators. A comparison of thrombolytic therapy with primary coronary angioplasty for acute myocardial infarction. N Engl J Med 1996;335:1253–1260.
86. Mark DB, Granger CB, Ellis SG, Phillips HR, Knight JD, Davidson-Ray L, Topol EJ. Costs of direct angioplasty versus thrombolysis for acute myocardial infarction: results from the GUSTO II randomized trial. Circulation 1996; 94:168A.
87. Grines CL, Browne KF, Marco J, Rothbaum D, Stone GW, O'Keefe J, Overlie P, Donohue B, Chelliah N, Timmis GC, Vlietstra RE, Strzelecki M, Puchrowicz-Ochocki S, O'Neill WW. A comparison of immediate angioplasty with thrombolytic therapy for acute myocardial infarction. N Engl J Med 1993; 328:673–679.
88. Gibbons RJ, Holmes DR, Reeder GS, Bailey KR, Hopfenspirger MR, Gersh BJ. Immediate angioplasty compared with the administration of a thrombolytic agent followed by conservative treatment for myocardial infarction. N Engl J Med 1993;328:685–691.
89. Lieu TA, Gurley J, Lundstrom RJ, Ray GT, Fireman BH, Weinstein MC, Parmley WW. Projected cost-effectiveness of primary angioplasty for acute myocardial infarction. J Am Coll Cardiol 1997;30:1741–1750.
90. Steinhubl SR, Topol EJ. Stenting for acute myocardial infarction. Lancet 1997;350:532–533.
91. Suryapranata H, van't Hof AW, Hoorntje JC, de Boer MJ, Zijlstra F. Randomized comparison of coronary stenting with balloon angioplasty in selected patients with acute myocardial infarction. Circulation 1998;97:2482–2485.
92. Grines CL, Cox DA, Stone GW, Garcia E, Mattos LA, Giambartolomei A, Brodie BR, Madonna O, Eijgelshoven M, Lansky AJ, O'Neill WW, Morice MC, for the Stent Primary Angioplasty in Myocardial Infarction Study. N Engl J Med 1999;341:1949–1956.
93. van't Hof AW, Suryapranata H, de Boer MJ, Hoorntje JC, Zijlstra F. Costs of stenting for acute myocardial infarction. Lancet 1998;351:1817–1822.
94. Krumholz HM. Cost-effectiveness analysis and the treatment of acute coronary syndromes. In: Cannon CP, ed. Contemporary Cardiology: Management of Acute Coronary Syndromes. Totowa, NJ: Human Press, 1998:601–610.

95. Antman EM. Hirudin in acute myocardial infarction. Thrombolysis and Thrombin Inhibition in Myocardial Infarction (TIMI) 9B trial. Circulation 1996;94:911–921.
96. Antman EM. Low-molecular-weight heparins: an intriguing new twist with profound implications. Circulation 1998;98:287–289.
97. GUSTO IIb Investigators. A comparison of recombinant hirudin with heparin for the treatment of acute coronary syndromes. N Engl J Med 1996;335:775–782.
98. Cohen M, Demers C, Gurfinkel EP, Turpie AGG, Fromell G, Goodman S, Langer A, Califf RM, Fox KAA, Premmereur J, Bigonzi F, for the ESSENCE Study Group. Enoxaparin (low molecular weight heparin) versus unfractionated heparin for unstable angina and non-q-wave myocardial infarction: primary endpoint results from the ESSENCE trial. N Engl J Med 1997;337:447–452.
99. Mark DB, Cowper PA, Berkowitz S, Davidson-Ray L, DeLong ER, Turpie AGG, Califf RM, Weatherly B, Lee KL, Cohen M. Economic assessment of low molecular weight heparin (enoxaparin) versus unfractionated heparin in acute coronary syndrome patients: results from the ESSENCE randomized trial. Circulation 1998;97:1702–1707.
100. Fox KAA. Implication of the Organization to Assess Strategies for Ischemic Syndromes-2 (OASIS-2) study and the results in the context of other studies. Am J Cardiol 1999;84:26M–31M.
101. McElwee N, Johnson ER. Potential economic impact of glycoprotein IIb-IIIa inhibitors in improving outcomes of patients with acute ischemic coronary syndromes. Am J Cardiol 1997;80:39B–43B.
102. Szucs TD, Meyer BJ, Kiowski W. Economic assessment of tirofiban in the management of acute coronary syndromes: an analysis based on the PRISM PLUS trial. Eur Heart J 1999;20:1217–1219.
103. Mark DB, Harrington RA, Lincoff AM, Califf RM, Nelson CL, Tsiatis AA, Buell HE, Mahaffey KW, Davidson-Ray L, Topol EJ. Cost effectiveness of platelet glycoprotein IIb/IIIa inhibition with eptifibatide in patients with non-ST elevation acute coronary syndromes. Circulation 2000;101:366–371.
104. PURSUIT Investigators. Inhibition of platelet glycoprotein IIb/IIIa with eptifibatide in patients with acute coronary syndromes without persistent ST-segment elevation. N Engl J Med 1998;339:436–443.
105. Mark DB, Talley JD, Topol EJ, Bowman L, Lam LC, Jollis JG, Cleman MW, Lee KL, Aversano T, Untereker WJ, Davidson-Ray L, Califf RM, for the EPIC Investigators. Economic assessment of platelet glycoprotein IIb/IIIa inhibition for prevention of ischemic complications of high risk coronary angioplasty. Circulation 1996;94:629–635.
106. Lincoff AM, Mark DB, Califf RM, Tcheng JE, Ellis SG, Davidson-Ray L, Anderson K, Stoner GL, Topol EJ. Economic assessment of platelet glycoprotein IIb/IIIa receptor blockade during coronary intervention in the EPILOG trial. J Am Coll Cardiol 1997;29:240A.
107. IMPACT II Investigators. Effects of competitive platelet glycoprotein IIb/IIIa inhibition with integrilin in reducing complications of percutaneous coronary intervention. Lancet 1997;349:1422–1428.

108. Weintraub WS, Culler S, Boccuzzi SJ, Cook JR, Kosinski AS, Cohen DJ, Burnette J. Economic impact of glycoprotein IIb/IIIa blockade after high-risk angioplasty: results from the RESTORE trial. J Am Coll Cardiol 1999;34:1061–1066.
109. EPISTENT Investigators. Randomised placebo-controlled and balloon-angioplasty-controlled trial to assess safety of coronary stenting with use of platelet glycoprotein IIb/IIIa blockade. Lancet 1998;352:87–92.
110. Topol EJ, Califf RM, Weisman HF, Ellis SG, Tcheng JE, Worley S, Ivanhoe R, George BS, Fintel D, Weston M, Sigmon K, Anderson KM, Lee KL, Willerson JT, on behalf of the EPIC Investigators. Randomised trial of coronary intervention with antibody against platelet IIb/IIIa integrin for reduction of clinical restenosis: results at six months. Lancet 1994;343:881–886.
111. Topol EJ, Mark DB, Lincoff AM, Cohen E, Burton J, Kleiman N, Talley JD, Sapp S, Booth JE, Cabot CF, Anderson K, Califf RM, for the EPISTENT Investigators. Outcomes at 1 year and economic implications of platelet glycoprotein IIb/IIIa blockade in patients undergoing coronary stenting: results from a multicentre randomized trial. Lancet 1999;354:2019–2024.
112. Calvin JE, Klein LW, Vandenberg BJ, Meyer P, Condon JV, Snell RJ, Rameriz-Morgen LM, Parillo JE. Risk stratification in unstable angina: prospective validation of the Braunwald classification. JAMA 1995;273:136–141.
113. Braunwald E. Unstable angina. A classification. Circulation 1989;80(2):410–414.
114. Calvin JE, Klein LW, Vandenberg BJ, Meyer P, Rameriz-Morgen LM, Parillo JE. Clinical predictors easily obtained at presentation predict resource utilization in unstable angina. Am Heart J 1998;136:373–381.
115. Spertus JA, Weiss NS, Every NR, Weaver WD. The influence of clinical risk factors on the use of angiography and revascularization after acute myocardial infarction. Arch Intern Med 1995;155:2309–2316.
116. Mark DB. Implications of cost in treatment selection for patients with coronary heart disease. Ann Thorac Surg 1996;61:S12–S15.
117. Wennberg DE, Kellett MA, Dickens JD, Malenka DJ, Keilson LM, Keller RB. The association between local diagnostic testing intensity and invasive cardiac procedures. JAMA 1996;275:1161–1164.
118. Guadagnoli E, Hauptman PJ, Ayanian JZ, Pashos CL, McNeil BJ, Cleary PD. Variation in the use of cardiac procedures after acute myocardial infarction. N Engl J Med 1995;333:573–578.
119. Pilote L, Califf RM, Sapp S, Miller DP, Mark DB, Weaver WD, Gore JM, Armstrong PW, Ohman EM, Topol EJ, for the GUSTO I Investigators. Regional variation across the United States in the management of acute myocardial infarction. N Engl J Med 1995;333:565–578.
120. McClellan M, McNeil BJ, Newhouse JP. Does more intensive treatment of acute myocardial infarction in the elderly reduce mortality? Analysis using instrumental variables. JAMA 1994;272:859–866.
121. Marrugat J, Sanz G, Masia R, Valle V, Molina L, Cardona M, Sala J, Seres L, Szescielinski L, Albert X, Lupon J, Alonso J. Six-month outcome inpatients

with myocardial infarction initially admitted to tertiary and nontertiary hospitals. J Am Coll Cardiol 1997;30:1187–1192.

122. Gatsonis CA, Epstein AM, Newhouse JP, Normand SL, McNeil BJ. Variation in the utilization of coronary angiography for elderly patients with an acute myocardial infarction. An analysis using hierarchical logistic regression. Med Care 1995;33:625–642.

123. Every NR, Fihn SD, Maynard C, Martin JS, Weaver WD. Resource utilization in the treatment of acute myocardial infarction: staff-model health maintenance organization vs. fee-for-service hospitals. J Am Coll Cardiol 1995;26: 401–406.

124. Pilote L, Miller DP, Califf RM, Rao JS, Weaver WD, Topol EJ. Determinants of the use of coronary angiography and revascularization after thrombolysis for acute myocardial infarction. N Engl J Med 1996;335:1198–1205.

125. van Miltenburg AJ, Simoons ML, Bossuyt PM, Taylor TR, Veerhoek MJ. Variation in the use of coronary angiography in patients with unstable angina is related to differences in patient population and availability of angiography facilities, without affecting prognosis. Eur Heart J 1996;17:1828–1835.

126. TIMI IIIB Investigators. Effects of tissue plasminogen activator and a comparison of early invasive and conservative strategies in unstable angina and non-Q-wave myocardial infarction. Results of the TIMI IIIB trial. Circulation 1994;89(4):1545–1556.

127. McFalls EO, Braunwald E. Cost effectiveness of TIMI IIb strategies. Circulation 1994;90:2569.

128. Boden WE, O'Rourke RA, Crawford MH, Blaustein AS, Deedwania PC, Zoble RG, Wexler LF, Kleiger RE, Pepine CJ, Ferry DR, Chow BK, Lavori PW. Outcomes in patients with acute non-Q-wave myocardial infarction randomly assigned to an invasive as compared with a conservative management strategy. Veterans Affairs Non-Q-Wave Infarction Strategies in Hospital (VANQWISH). N Engl J Med 1998;338:1785–1792.

129. Kuntz KM, Tsevat J, Goldman L, Weinstein MC. Cost-effectiveness of routine coronary angiography after acute myocardial infarction. Circulation 1996;94: 957–965.

130. Newby LK, Califf RM, Guerci AD, Weaver WD, Col J, Horgan JH, Mark DB, Stebbins A, Van de Werf F, Gore JM, Topol EJ. Early discharge in the thrombolytic era: an analysis of criteria for uncomplicated infarction from the Global Utilization of streptokinase and t-PA for Occluded Arteries (GUSTO) Trial. J Am Coll Cardiol 1996;27:623–632.

131. Eisenstein EL, Newby LK, Knight JD, Shaw LJ, Califf RM, Topol EJ, Mark DB. Cost avoidance through early discharge of the uncomplicated acute myocardial infarction patient. J Am Coll Cardiol 1996;27:330A.

132. Newby LK, Eisenstein EL, Califf RM, Thompson TD, Nelson CL, Peterson ED, Armstrong PW, Van de Werf F, White HD, Topol EJ, Mark DB. Cost effectiveness of early discharge after acute myocardial infarction in patients with no complications. N Engl J Med 2000;342(11):749–755.

133. Lundberg GA. National health care reform: the aura of inevitability intensifies. JAMA 1992;267:2521–2524.

134. Health Care Financing Administration. National Health Expenditures 1960–1998. Available at: www.hcfa.gov/stats/NHE-OAct./tables/t1.htm. Accessed: March 7, 2000.
135. Hatziandreu EI, Koplan JP, Weinstein MC, Caspersen CJ, Warner KE. A cost-effectiveness analysis of exercise as a health promotion activity. Am J Public Health 1988;78:1417–1421.
136. Wong JB, Sonnenberg FA, Salem DN, Pauker SG. Myocardial revascularization for chronic stable angina: an analysis of the role of percutaneous transluminal coronary angioplasty based on data available in 1989. Ann Intern Med 1990;113:852–871.
137. Goldman L, Sia STB, Cook EF, Rutherford JD, Weinstein MC. Costs and effectiveness of routine therapy with long-term beta-adrenergic antagonists after acute myocardial infarction. N Engl J Med 1988;319:152–157.
138. Levin LA, Jonsson B. Cost-effectiveness of thrombolysis—a randomized study of intravenous rt-PA in suspected myocardial infarction. Eur Heart J 1992;13:2–8.
139. O'Brien BJ, Buxton MJ, Ferguson BA. Measuring the effectiveness of heart transplant programmes: quality of life data and their relationship to survival analysis. J Chron Dis 1987;40:137S–158S.

Index